OCULAR PHARMACOLOGY

OCULAR PHARMACOLOGY

WILLIAM H. HAVENER
B.A., M.D., M.S. (Ophth.)

Professor and Chairman, Department of Ophthalmology,
Ohio State University; Member, Attending Staff,
University Hospital; Member, Consulting Staff,
Children's Hospital and Mt. Carmel Hospital,
Columbus, Ohio

FOURTH EDITION

with 377 illustrations

THE C. V. MOSBY COMPANY

Saint Louis   1978

FOURTH EDITION

Previous editions copyrighted 1966, 1970, 1974

Printed in the United States of America

The C. V. Mosby Company
11830 Westline Industrial Drive, St. Louis, Missouri 63141

Library of Congress Cataloging in Publication Data

Havener, William H.
    Ocular pharmacology.

    Includes bibliographical references and index.
    1.   Materia medica, Ophthalmological.
2. Ocular pharmacology. I. Title. [DNLM:
1. Eye diseases—Drug therapy.   WW166 H386o]
RE994.H35 1978   617.7'061   78-7208
ISBN 0-8016-2105-4

GW/CB/B 9 8 7 6 5 4 3 2 1

TO
Phyllis Ann

PREFACE *to fourth edition*

This fourth edition of *Ocular Pharmacology* contains reasonably comprehensive references to the ophthalmic literature of the past 20 years with respect to the use of ophthalmic medications and the responses of eye diseases to such treatments. This information has been reviewed, classified, and presented as fairly as possible, although the prejudices that accrue from one's own clinical experiences cannot help but bias the presentation.

The pharmacology of drugs is reasonably straightforward, allowing for some idiosyncrasies and sensitivities of response. Unfortunately, diseases and the host response are almost infinitely variable. Medical education has attempted to cope with this problem by a prolonged period of clinical experience under supervision—the residency system of education. Demonstration and practical application of the skills of examination, diagnosis, properly balanced medical and surgical therapy, and reassurance are best accomplished in a context of personal guidance, such as is found in a good residency.

My goal as an author has been to provide a readily accessible reference that will be useful in these circumstances of continuous clinical learning and patient care.

This edition contains a half million words and 2573 references, a truly monumental task of typing and arranging. Mrs. Ruth Davis accomplished this enormous feat within a year, in addition to helping me care for our patients during this time. I am most appreciative of her cheerful, enthusiastic, and accurate support.

William H. Havener, M.D.

PREFACE *to first edition*

Only twelve years have passed since I completed my own residency training; yet during my brief span in ophthalmology a remarkable number of new drugs have become available for general clinical use. These include the secretory inhibitors, the osmotic hypotensive drugs, most of the antibiotics, antifungal and antiviral agents, the ever-more-potent corticosteroids, and new synthetic autonomic drugs, as well as better vehicles for these medications. Simultaneously, a number of the old faithful drugs have been discredited, for example, dionin, vasodilators, iodides, and indiscriminately used vitamins. The effects of these various medications upon the eye and the general body, both favorable and adverse, have been studied in great detail, thereby permitting more precise and rational clinical use.

Improved diagnostic methods have led to better understanding of disease processes and consequently more effective treatment. For instance, spontaneous vitreous hemorrhage in the absence of recognizable bilateral retinopathy due to systemic disease is now recognized commonly to be caused by vessel rupture by a retinal tear. Recognition of such tears permits prophylactic treatment with photocoagulation rather than by blood-in-the-vitreous placebos.

The purpose of this book is to compile for ready reference the pharmacologic information which has appeared in the eye literature during the past several decades. Such knowledge is quite essential for the intelligent medical therapy of eye problems and should supersede the "cookbook" approach to treatment. Residents, particularly, but also some practicing ophthalmologists may be heard to advise a given medication because a quoted authority "always uses it for this disease." Surprisingly often, the authoritative "cookbook" advice is either misquoted or inappropriately applied.

I hope this book will help to develop sound pharmacologic judgment, which will permit scientifically rational use of preferred medications for the treatment of accurately diagnosed ocular problems. Nothing less is good enough for our patients.

Recognition of assistance in preparing this volume must first be given to the innumerable physicians and scientists who have discovered and organized our knowledge of the response of the eye to medications. The enormous amount of secretarial work was expertly performed by Miss Marjorie Hendricks. The illustrations were prepared by Miss Sallie Gloeckner, whose ability has contributed greatly to our teaching program. Dr. Arthur Culler contributed his entire collection of journals for use in the preparation of the files of material upon which this text is based.

William H. Havener, M.D.

CONTENTS

PART ONE

DRUGS IN
OPHTHALMIC PRACTICE

1

EVALUATION OF THERAPEUTIC RESPONSE*

Somewhere long ago I read of an early American physician who prescribed cabbage for the relief of certain symptoms suffered by a blacksmith. The blacksmith recovered. In due time a preacher became ill with similar symptoms. Cabbages were prescribed but, alas, the preacher died. The physician thereupon concluded that for these symptoms cabbages would cure blacksmiths but would kill preachers. I hope that this book will help somewhat to put ophthalmic medication on a more rational basis than cabbages for symptoms.

CONTROLLED OBSERVATION

Do clinical coincidences unjustifiably influence our treatment of patients today? Of course, they will always do so. The emotional impact of a single dramatic clinical occurrence often creates lasting but unwarranted impressions as to the effect of a given medication or procedure. As an example of the fallacy of such *post hoc, ergo propter hoc* (after this, therefore because of this) thinking, the following actual case is cited.

An 84-year-old woman underwent an uncomplicated cataract extraction. The surgeon had planned to use alpha-chymotrypsin for zonulysis but decided against it at the last minute because he had never previously

*Reprinted in part from New Orleans Academy of Ophthalmology: Symposium on ocular pharmacology and therapeutics, St. Louis, 1970, The C. V. Mosby Co.

used it. Although there had been no bleeding and the eye looked perfect at the close of surgery, at the first dressing on the following day the anterior chamber was almost filled with fresh red blood. No history of trauma could be obtained. (One is reminded that postoperative hemorrhages usually originate from new vessels growing across the incision and therefore appear 5 to 7 days postoperatively. Postcataract hyphema is rarely massive.) The hemorrhage grew progressively worse, filling the anterior chamber. On the seventh postoperative day, bright red blood still completely filled the anterior chamber, and no trace of iris detail was visible. Miraculously, on the eighth day the blood had entirely disappeared, and the eye was in perfect condition without even the tiniest hyphema. No medication was responsible for this amazing improvement.

Clearly evident is the unpredictability of an individual case. Had the surgeon used alpha-chymotrypsin he would have been sure that it caused the hemorrhage. Any medication (carbonic anhydrase inhibitor, trypsin, blood transfusion, miotic, and the like) used on the seventh day would have received credit for the cure. Similarly, surgical evacuation of the blood would have been interpreted as the cause of improvement. Obviously a carefully controlled and adequately extensive series of cases are necessary to draw any valid clinical conclusions.

3

Controlled and *random* are concepts that appear to be most unclear to a large number of medical writers and readers. The basic question is, With what patient should the treated patients be compared? Ideally, the control group should be virtually identical to the treated patients in all respects. "Controls" cannot be an equal number of patients accumulated 5 years ago or the patients who did not get better with treatment. Because of observer bias, *controlled* does not mean strictly alternated groups of patients. Rather, a random selection (designed in an orderly fashion to invoke the laws of chance and not synonymous with haphazard) is important to eliminate the observer and patient factors that are not related to the treatment response being evaluated.[1]

INACCURATE OBSERVATION

Even when the known distortions of prejudice and bias are excluded, our own ability to perceive details is far more limited and less reliable than we think it is. One needs only to discuss a series of previously observed patients with a group of competent ophthalmologists to realize the amazing differences of opinion as to the physical findings in a given eye. Our own record when compared with objective documentation such as a photograph is little better. I am quite certain that *at least a 50% change*, for better or worse, must occur before I myself can reliably say the eye has improved or worsened since yesterday's observation. Repeatedly we have been convinced that a fundus lesion was substantially better or worse; yet when the photograph was returned, the lesion was found to be entirely unchanged. Many studies have documented these considerable variations in clinical and laboratory observations.

The accuracy of competent clinical and laboratory work is high, and the following comments should not be construed as adverse criticism of medical skills. Indeed, recognition of the possibility of faulty determination and observations is part of the skill of an astute physician.

It is instructive and sobering to specify the magnitude of potential clinical error. The interpretation of x-ray films lends itself well to such critical evaluation, for the same films remain available for repeated study. In a study of the effectiveness of x-ray methods for mass survey detection of chest disease, experienced physicians were found to miss 25% of the cases of x-ray–visible pulmonary disease. Reading the same films 3 months later, individual physicians missed 20% of the positive findings they had themselves previously diagnosed.

Still more thought-provoking were the results of comparison of full-sized serial chest x-ray films to determine whether pulmonary disease had improved, had worsened, or was unchanged. In such comparisons, experienced radiologists disagreed with each other in 30% of the cases, and a single physician disagreed with his own previous interpretation 20% of the time.

Similar study of the histopathologic diagnosis of cancer suggests that an expert pathologist is about 85% reliable in his diagnoses. Clinical diagnoses suffer equal variability. Five pediatricians classified 221 children as to nutritional status. Malnutrition was diagnosed in 90 children by one or another physician, but all five physicians agreed on the diagnosis of malnutrition in only 7 children.

Laboratory reports, often accepted at face value, are found to be even more variable than medical observations. In one study of 59 hospital laboratories a standardized sample of hemoglobin, accurately prepared to contain 9.8 g/100 ml, was reported to measure from 8.0 to 15.5. Of these reports, 67% were considered to be beyond the reasonable range of error, and 22% were in gross error.[2]

Many other examples of variations in clinical and laboratory observations were cited in the same article. Although no reference was made to ophthalmology, the significance of these facts to ophthalmic therapy is clear. In our search for the scientific truths on which our medical or surgical treatments should be based, we must distinguish between the truly reliable and well-written paper and the potboiler that purports to reach a conclusion through "clinical impressions." We must admit, at least to ourselves, the possibility that our case of unilateral chronic simple glaucoma might turn out to be a carotid-cavernous fistula, that pyrimethamine may do more harm than good in a given case of uveitis, or that convergence exercises in a particular case of exophoria may simply be of psychologic value. It is uncomfortable but stimulating to have residents perpetually ask, "Why do you do this?" In short, this is a plea for continuing self-evaluation of our diagnostic and therapeutic habits.

DOUBLE-BLIND CONTROLLED OBSERVATION

The ultimate in scientific objectivity and indisputable accuracy is supposedly represented by the double-blind tests. Obviously (supposedly) such a format will eliminate errors of judgment, control, and prejudice. To quote Spaeth, "Since the design of this study was of the double-blind, placebo-controlled type, the coded medication and placebo were identical in appearance and their identity was not known to the investigator, the nursing staff, or the patient until the termination of the study, at which time the code was broken and the findings recorded."[3] When the code was broken, the author reports that of the total 111 patients, 52 had received placebo medication and 59 active medication. Most pertinent to the present evaluation of double-blind studies is the fact that all 52 placebo patients were male and all 59 active medication patients were female! The possibility that this distribution occurred by chance is about 1 in 10^{33}—not very likely. This means that despite all the care and work lavished on this experiment, someone, probably the nurse assigned to give medications, misunderstood the instructions and introduced a methodical error by giving the medications on the basis of sex. This methodical error apparently was undetected by the author until he broke the code and discovered the impossible male-female distribution. A reasonable inference from this accident would be that one is justified

in regarding with caution even the most careful scientific study if its results conflict with other sources of information or if it is not subsequently confirmed by other studies.

In this study there were two large wards segregated for men and women. The placebo box was placed on the male ward and the active medication box on the female ward. As Murphy's law states, if anything can go wrong, it will do so.

STATISTICAL SIGNIFICANCE

Statistical significance is another misunderstood term. Often it is accepted as sort of a seal of approval that verifies the conclusion of the author. Actually, all that is established by a "statistically significant difference" is that the control and experimental groups do indeed differ in some respect. This difference is not necessarily the use or nonuse of the given treatment but often will be another factor in selection of the two groups. These factors may be obvious to the reader or may be quite subtle, perhaps even concealed completely by inadequate reporting of selection methods. To cite a well-known example, there is a statistically significant correlation between the number of marriages performed by the Church of England and the new cases of venereal disease that occur during the same year. However, this does not mean that the marriage ceremony causes disease—rather, both marriage and disease rates are related to the number of individuals existing in the marriageable age group in a given year.

A statistical dilemma particularly relevant to ophthalmology disputes whether we should count eyes or subjects. The answer depends on the experiment. Since the eyes of an individual usually react very similarly, any analysis of the *sum* or *average* of measurements should be based on the number of subjects. Calculating this type of study on the basis of two eyes rather than one individual does not result in twice as much information. On the other hand, comparison of *differences* in response to a given treatment is ideally carried out by observing the differences in response of the paired eyes of a series of individuals.[4]

Statistical significance and gambling are both governed by the laws of chance. Just as the most enthusiastic gambler would hesitate to take on odds of a thousand to one, so the statistician says a finding is "significant" if it occurs by chance only once in a thousand times. For practical purposes we may rely on statistical significance—if the experiment is properly designed. However, let us consider what one in a thousand chances means.

If any of us had only one patient in the hospital, his last initial could be any of the 26 letters and would occasion no statistical speculation. Admission of a second patient with the same last initial might arouse comment, for this could happen only once in 26 times (assuming all letters in the alphabet were equally common, which is not true). Chance admission of only three patients, each with the same initial, could occur only once in 26^2 (676) times. Actually, this has happened to me on three occasions during the past 14 years of practice. On one of these occasions a fourth patient of mine with the same initial was admitted to the hospital. Unfortunately the admitting office changed his status from private to clinical and he entered the hospital on the ward service. Except for this happenstance, I would have had four hospital patients with the same last initial, an event expected once in 26^3 (17,576) times.

PATIENT (UN)RELIABILITY

A delightful and ostensibly true anecdote describes an elderly lady, something of a hypochondriac, who regularly and frequently, with multiple complaints, visited her favorite physician. Upon her death, her will specified that a very large, securely locked trunk in her attic was to be given to the faithful physician. With great anticipation and considerable difficulty, he forced open the heavy lid. Lo, within he found, unused, every single bottle of medication he had dispensed to her over the years.

This lady is representative of 30% to 40% of our patients. Multiple independent investigations document the astonishing fact that one third of our patients fail to use the medications we prescribe. This failure to cooperate cannot be detected by inquiry because the patients lie. Failure to cooperate cannot reliably be correlated with environment, education, socioeconomic status, or patient characteristics such as age or sex. Reliability of clinic attendance and of obtaining drugs does not correlate with cooperation in actually taking the medication. About the only consistent factor is duration of therapy. Patients become progressively less cooperative in using medication during a long course of treatment. (Glaucoma is a classic example of a long-term treatment disease.) Also, multiple medications are less likely to be taken properly.

Antituberculous medications are suitable for accurate scientific determination of patient cooperation, since the drugs are easily detectable in the urine. Absence of a drug in the urine sample means the patient has failed to take the preceding two doses of medication. In a study of 75 outpatients on isoniazid and/or aminosalicylic acid, 30% of the isoniazid patients and 42% of the aminosalicylic acid patients had negative urine tests for the presence of the drug at least 40% of the times tested.[5]

A case report illustrates the problem. After 1 month of hospital treatment for culture-proved tuberculous pericarditis, a 41-year-old woman was discharged to outpatient treatment with isoniazid and aminosalicylic acid. She never missed an appointment, gained weight, remained afebrile, and showed nonprogressive chest x-ray films. The outpatient pharmacy dispensed 1170 isoniazid tablets and 5005 aminosalicylic acid tablets to her. In her 7-month summary was written "TB pericarditis, healing, on ℞, asymptomatic." In all respects this patient seemed quite cooperative and a therapeutic triumph.

During this period, however, 15 separate urine specimens showed *no trace* of medications. At the close of the study she was given a dose of isoniazid and aminosalicylic acid under observation. She objected strenuously to taking these medications, exclaiming these were "the pills that made me sick." Three hours later her urine was strongly positive for both drugs. (No false negative tests were ever encountered in hospital patients known to be taking medication.)

The author of this report cites other studies confirming this high incidence of patient unreliability in the use of a variety of medications (penicillin, antacids, prednisone, chlorpromazine, meprobamate, and placebos). Patients also deny taking medications when they have taken them. Of 38 patients found to have blood serum evidence of meprobamate, a barbiturate, or phenothiazine, 29 denied taking such medications!

Hence in the evaluation of therapeutic response (either favorable or unfavorable) we must not fail to consider the possibility (nay, the great probability) that the patient is not using his medication properly. Physicians who say to themselves, "My patients follow my instructions," are gullible individuals with unwarranted faith in human nature and with egotistical notions of their own omnipotence. (I confess to believing that my patients do as I tell them, but it is a shock to hear the nurses report to me what the patients describe as my instructions—despite repetition and mimeographed instructions!)

In spite of such evidence, you are probably skeptical—you think your glaucoma patients use pilocarpine faithfully. Let us cite yet another study of inpatient peptic ulcer patients instructed to take their own antacid medication 10 times daily.[6] As determined by actual consumption of medicine, the median patient took *only 46%* of the prescribed antacid. The reliability of these patients was assessed by 27 physicians. Of the 27 physicians, 22 greatly overestimated patient reliability. Of greatest importance, the physicians were totally unable to distinguish the reliable patient from the unreliable one—these judgments were no better than if blind chance alone had been used to rank the patients. (Are you still an unbeliever? If so, find out how often your own wife gives your child the antibiotic for his sore ear—or some comparable medication.)

A practical suggestion: Check your own appointment schedule at the end of each day to see how many broken or cancelled appointments have occurred. One form of patient noncompliance is disappearance. In one group of 89 patients with ocular hypertension and glaucoma, 37% failed to return within a period of 12 to 21 months following diagnosis.[7] Obviously, loss to follow-up of more than one third of patients with such a potentially serious eye problem cannot be dismissed lightly. I, personally, have been reluctant to send missed appointment notices, thinking that it was the patient's privilege not to return to me. However, the implications of neglected glaucoma are so great that perhaps the matter should be reconsidered. Should we institute selective reminder and recall systems in our own office practice, as many dentists do? It might not be a bad idea, especially for glaucoma patients.

GENERIC INEQUIVALENCE

Discrepancies between reports of the effects of a given drug occur both in experimental situations and in clinical therapy. Such discrepancies may sometimes be explained by differences in preparation of the drug by different manufacturers. Many factors may influence the therapeutic usefulness of a drug even though the preparation contains the stated amount of the active ingredient. Such factors include solubility of the dosage form, effect of other ingredients, pH, particle size, stability, age, compression of the tablet, binders, thickness and type of enteric coating, taste, comfort of use (for eye drops), appearance, uniformity of suspension, and type of liquid vehicle.

As an example of the great effect of differences in formulation, two lots of tolbutamide (Orinase) tablets were prepared, each containing 0.5 g of drug and both meeting *United States Pharmacopeia* (USP) specifications. All composition and manufacturing details of these two preparations were identical except that one lot contained only half the amount of disintegrant gum. This single and seemingly minor pharmacy change more than

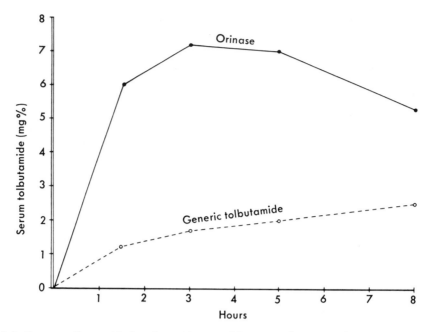

Fig. 1-1. Serum tolbutamide levels in 10 normal human volunteers after ingestion of commercial tolbutamide (Orinase) and USP equivalent experimental drug without disintegrant. (Modified from Varley, A. B.: J.A.M.A. **206:**1745, 1968.)

tripled the tablet disintegration time from 2 to 7.6 minutes. An even more important but less conspicuous change occurred in dissolution time—from 3.8 to 103 minutes.[8]

As would be expected, this solubility difference was reflected in greatly reduced serum levels after administration of the less soluble drug. As shown in Fig. 1-1, the serum levels of commercial tolbutamide rose much more rapidly and reached much higher levels. During the 8-hour period after tablet administration the cumulative drug content in the serum was three and one-half times greater for the commercial preparation than for the experimental preparation with half the amount of disintegrant gum. Serum glucose levels were measured in these normal subjects. The cumulative 8-hour glucose drop was more than twice as great for the commercial preparation as for the experimental preparation.

The generic inequivalence of different brands of chloramphenicol has been the subject of much comment in the medical literature and presumably is well known to all physicians. Another significant generic in-

equivalence exists in penicillin preparations. The *United States Pharmacopeia* requires penicillin G preparations to contain at least 85% penicillin G. In fact, commercially available penicillin G from reputable manufacturers contains 98% or more of penicillin G. The less pure generic equivalent preparations offered inexpensively from other sources may contain many contaminating allergens. These contaminants are believed to be responsible for some of the allergic reactions attributed to penicillin, inasmuch as the pure drug may not cause a comparable allergic response.[9]

DRUG STABILITY

To cite an example of variation in drug effect relevant to ophthalmology, isoflurophate is dispensed in anhydrous peanut oil because water rapidly destroys the molecule. If the pharmaceutical dispenser dilutes the preparation with water or if the patient contaminates the dropper with tears, the isoflurophate will hydrolyze and no therapeutic effect will result. Absence of miosis is a readily observed sign that will alert the ophthalmologist to faulty medication or method of use.

The early reports on idoxuridine stated that the drug effect on herpes simplex was so reliable that failure of a dendritic ulcer to respond should arouse suspicion of the use of outdated medication. Resistant virus strains have since been demonstrated, but the clinician should still suspect an inactive bottle of drug when therapy fails.

The deterioration of epinephrine is well known to all of us and can be recognized by obvious discoloration of the solution. But how many ophthalmologists alert the patient to this easily observed sign of loss of potency?

Even well-known incompatibilities are commonly disregarded. Preoperative surgical cleaning may include consecutive scrubbing of the skin with pHisoHex and Zephiran. These are, of course, anionic and cationic detergents, respectively. Their combined effect is to neutralize each other.

MEDICATION ERRORS

Despite mimeographed reference sheets, repeated instructions, and personal attention to the proper bedside medications to be continued in home use, I find errors of frequency of use and even of the medication to be used not uncommon. Confusion is especially likely in the case of multiple medications.

Unlabeled drugs are a particularly dangerous source of error. As a consultant, I often see a patient who brings a purseful of bottles, some old, some new, labeled only with the frequency for use. Invariably such patients do not know which medications they should use. Accurate identification of something so important as a medical prescription should be legally required.

Tribute to the accuracy and conscientiousness of our nurses and pharmacists is certainly appropriate. Nevertheless, allowance must be made for occasional human errors. Do not exclude the possibility of error in medication if the response of a given eye is greatly different than expected.

The problem of counterfeit drugs is of unknown magnitude, but it is known to exist in our nation. Penalties for drug counterfeiting are only token and potential profits are great. Detection of a spurious antibiotic or corticosteroid preparation would be beyond my capability, except insofar as the expected therapeutic response is absent.

PHARMACOGENETICS

Even if we are certain the proper medication has been administered as directed, constitutionally determined individual variations in response occur. Allergy, idiosyncrasy, and hypersensitivity are common examples of pharmacogenetic differences.[10]

The hyperreactivity of a person with Down's syndrome (mongolism) to atropine is an example of a pharmacogenetic response of ophthalmologic interest. Topical atropine will produce abnormally great mydriasis in a mongoloid. This finding has been attributed to a structural anomaly of the iris. However, the cardioacceleratory effects of atropine are twice the normal magnitude in mongoloids indicating that a difference in drug response is present throughout the body and not just within the iris.[11] Such pharmacogenetic differences are an often unappreciated cause of response variation.

Succinylcholine, the muscle relaxant routinely used before intubation of patients during general anesthesia, is inactivated within minutes by cholinesterase. However, individuals who have a genetic deficiency of cholinesterase may be paralyzed and apneic for many hours following succinylcholine administration.

THE PLACEBO EFFECT

Lest we forget the importance of our interpersonal relationship with patients and assume that medical care is accomplished only with drugs or surgery, I quote from Dr. Charles Dunlap, "Among the tools used by a doctor, words both heard and spoken are as necessary and as powerful as drugs or instruments. Used carelessly, they can produce deep wounds that fester and never heal. But when skillfully and gently used, they can ease pain, inspire hope, bring joy, allay despair, and even put a fretful child to sleep."[12]

The words as well as the attitudes and the actions of a physician cause a measurable patient response that may be termed the placebo effect. A placebo is defined as a medication given to please the patient. The physician knows the mechanism of action of the placebo is psychologic. Actually, of course, the placebo effect will also account for part of the response of a patient to a potent drug. Even if the potent drug is ineffectual against the given disease, measurable subjective improvement can be expected in a significant number of cases. Here exists a trap for the unwary physician, who may readily confuse the placebo response with specific therapeutic benefit. This explains many of the enthusiastic but subsequently unconfirmed reports in the literature. In general, the greater a physician's interest in a treatment, particularly if it is his own discovery or if the physician has recently been converted to its use, the more effective that treatment will appear to be.[13]

About 35% of patients will show a significant response to placebo therapy.[14] Stated in another way, almost any drug (provided that it is not harmful) will cause subjective improvement in one of every three patients suffering from almost anything. Objective improvements will also occur in the parameters ordinarily recognized as psychosomatic (for example, pulse, respiration, gastric acid secretion, and fatigue). Interestingly, toxic side effects such as drowsiness, dry mouth, and nausea can be elicited in substantial numbers (10% to 50%) of patients receiving a placebo, depending on the amount of suggestion present. Even skin rashes (dermatitis medicamentosa and angioneurotic edema) may be precipitated by placebo therapy of predisposed individuals. The placebo effect is greatest in situations where the stress and psychologic reaction of the patient are greatest. It does not matter in the least of what the placebo is made or how large the dose so long as it is not detected as a placebo by the patient.

Use of the placebo effect in ophthalmology is obviously not to be condemned, since it does benefit a considerable number of patients. In the management of vitreous hemorrhage, for instance, prescription of some harmless medication may be comforting. However, I do not believe it fair to the patients to select an inordinately expensive placebo, since cheap ones work just as well (if supported by the physician's attitude). Furthermore, placebos are no substitute for accurate diagnostic recognition of a retinal tear, which requires sealing and not a blood-in-the-vitreous placebo. In practice, I almost never use a placebo for major eye problems but reserve such treatment for the annoying, vague, minor, common symptoms that have no obvious basis yet cause persistent complaint, particularly in nervous and worried persons. Whether the placebo is a cold compress or a harmless eye drop does not seem to matter. This approach is certainly easier than trying to convince some people they do not need "something for my tired eyes."

The recent widespread acceptance of the value of acupuncture, by layman and physician alike, was undreamed of only a few short years ago and will probably be incomprehensible and unbelievable to the reader a few short years hence. Acupuncture will at least temporarily benefit and may even permanently cure as many as 35% of patients suffering from almost any ophthalmic disorder. Do not be skeptical, for I am about to prove this to you.

Some 7000 years ago a chronically ill oriental warrior recovered miraculously from his primary disease following an arrow wound. Fortunately the arrow struck him at the acupuncture site specific for the cure of his disease. Subsequent empirical clinical trials led to the discovery of the multiple acupuncture sites that are recorded on the charts of the traditional practitioners of Chinese medicine. The almost unbelievable capability of acupuncture to counteract virtually any type of disease or disorder is attested to by veteran reporters and by experienced physicians, including ex-President Nixon's own personal doctor.[15-17]

But why does acupuncture work? Is it a mysterious technique, the details of which are unknown to science? Or is it but a variant of well-established principles of medical management? Without further ado, let us define acupuncture for what it is and then proceed with a well-documented scientific explanation of the process. Acupuncture is simply the Chinese version of placebo therapy. The clever Orientals have skillfully perfected a format within which the placebo effect is maximized.

A placebo effect may be defined as the result of a therapy (or a component of a therapy) that has a demonstrable effect but that objectively is without specific activity for the condition being treated.

Do not minimize the value of the placebo effect. For centuries physicians have held an honored place in society despite the worthlessness of their remedies. No treatment of any specific value is found in the writings of Hippocrates. Witness the bloodletting and the purges that were advocated in comparatively modern times. As recently as 1952, a full third of 17,000 prescriptions in England were considered to have only placebo value.[18] The skill of the physician was (and still is) to treat illness by encouragement and ineffective medications. Many therapeutic successes can be attributed to the enthusiasm and support of the physician and the faith of the patient. Indeed, we are still faith healers.

Lest we fail to comprehend the potency of emotional attitudes and believe that only psychosomatic illnesses respond to placebo therapy, let us refer to the control of pain from severe wounds. At the Anzio beachhead during World War II only 25% of the severely injured battle casualties required morphine.[19] In contrast, of the civilians studied, 80% required analgesic medication postoperatively. The difference was attributed to the fact that pain caused civilians to become apprehensive about their operations, whereas the wounded soldier knew his injury represented a ticket to the shelter of a hospital and then to home.

The therapeutic effect of the placebo is by no means limited to the management of disorders commonly accepted as being psychosomatic. A significant placebo therapeutic effect was demonstrated in 35% of 1082 patients suffering from such diverse afflictions as wound pain, angina pectoris, headache, nausea, cough, seasickness, the common cold, and anxiety.[14] This placebo effect was demonstrable in 26% to 58% of the patients suffering from these various conditions. Please note that this percentage variability was not related to the responsiveness of the given medical condition. Placebo responsiveness is a property of the patient and the environment and not a characteristic of the disease (except insofar as the cure of a self-limited condition may be attributed to an unrelated factor, such as a placebo).

What makes a placebo work? Is it always effective in about one third of patients? What circumstances make it more or less effective?

The importance of psychic influences on gastric function is well known, even to the layman. Yet, in a careful study of 18 volunteers, placebo medication with lactose, glucose, or barium sulfate capsules did not alter the volume of gastric secretion, pepsin secretion, or the amount of free hydrochloric acid.[20] In other words, the placebo had no effect whatsoever. The reason for the lack of response was that these volunteers were not told to expect any result from taking the capsule. In the absence of any psychic suggestion, no placebo effect occurred.

Angina pectoris also responds to placebo therapy—38% of 90 patients experienced pain relief. In view of the emotional aspects of the disorder, such a placebo response is not surprising. The technique of selective coronary arteriography is now available and permits separation of patients with the anginal syndrome into two distinct groups— one with coronary atherosclerosis and the other with no detectable coronary abnormalities. Placebo therapy of 95 patients with angina and coronary vessel disease helped only 4%, whereas 25% of 27 patients with the anginal syndrome and normal coronary arteries responded to placebo therapy.[21] Perhaps the relatively low rate of placebo response was due to the fact that the amount of psychic suggestion was deliberately minimized. However, the primary reason for commenting on this study is to emphasize that diagnostic inaccuracies may greatly alter the therapeutic (and placebo) response obtained in a given report.

In four separate studies of psychiatric outpatients, placebo response rates were 24%, 35%, 74%, and 76%.[22] In these studies the placebo effect was at least comparable to the results obtained with active drugs. For example, in one study the placebo rate of response was 76%, the Stelazine response was 67%, the Librium response was 87%, and the Equanil response was 44%. Note that variability in response is characteristic of clinical studies.

The difference in response in these various studies was a result of the management of the patients. The lowest rate of placebo reactivity, 24%, was obtained in a study that included no testing of the patients. The highest rate of placebo reactivity, 76%, was achieved in a study that included detailed psychologic testing (eight separate tests, including such impressive examinations as the Minnesota Multiphasic Personality Inventory and the Wechsler Adult Intelligence Scale) at the time of each clinic visit. These multiple tests and contacts with the research personnel caused the emotional impact that resulted in relief of the symptoms.

Not only the placebo response but also the effect of the active tranquilizer medication is affected by the circumstances of patient care. Specifically, the effectiveness of the tranquilizing medications also varied from 30% to 87%, depending on the amount of attention given the patient. Obviously a very large proportion of the measured drug response in these patients was a placebo response entirely unrelated to specific drug activity. As an example, in one series of patients the placebo response was 76% and the Librium response 87%. This means that the true Librium response was only 11%, as 76% of the responses were attributable to the placebo effect. (This difference is statistically significant providing it is reproducible.)

Clearly, the clinical setting in which a new drug is evaluated is of great importance. Comparison of drug evaluations performed under different circumstances may be quite misleading.

Sir William Osler advised that new remedies be used quickly, while they are still efficacious.[23] This astute, tongue-in-cheek statement illustrates this great clinician's understanding of the placebo effect, which is related to the enthusiasm and confidence of the physician.

So much for documentation of the placebo principle; now, what good is this knowledge to the ophthalmologist?

Wise physicians realize that they, themselves, cause the placebo effect. They do not really need sugar pills or to twirl acupuncture needles. All they must do is present themselves to the patient as trustworthy, knowledgeable, genuinely interested persons who are offering specific recommendations for the patient. Reasonably detailed, rational explanations and discussions of the patient's problem are appropriate but probably benefit the patient via a placebo mechanism and not because of their intellectual value. Acquiring identical knowledge by reading a book from the library is not an adequate substitute for the physician-placebo.

Let me give specific examples. Permit me to select a patient who is truly psychologically ready for cataract extraction—a patient who fully realizes that he is no longer willing or able to tolerate the visual handicap. The placebo ritual appropriate to this patient is a reasonably thorough, confidence-inspiring examination. Bear in mind that the patient does not know what the lights we use actually do. We might just as well expose him to a battery of multicolored nonsense lights and lenses connected to an impressive oscilloscope face. Subsequent to the examination ritual, we discuss the management of the cataract in terms of what will be experienced. Perhaps this could be compared to the discussions entailed in the comparable technique of "natural" childbirth. The net effect is a patient who will often spontaneously verbalize, "I'm not afraid at all. I have complete confidence in you. I know everything will turn out all right."

With a minimum of sedation and local anesthesia, patients prepared in this manner will go through surgery as easily as if they were being treated with acupuncture.

Another example of the physician-placebo involves the patient who following surgery is depressed, apprehensive, withdrawn, and complains of eye pain. His low morale is transmitted to his wife and magnified by her concern. The gloom is so tangible you could almost cut it with a knife. You know the rest of the scenario. Physician walks in, changes bandage, reassures that all will be well, bids patient to rise from bed of pain and walk, patient does. Something genuine has occurred—a psychologic response achieved without the placebo pill.

The placebo does not have to be the physician or a pill. The physician can invest patients or their relatives and attendants with the placebo mantle. One does this via specific instructions such as the application of warm compresses for 15 minutes four times a day, daily walks, etc. What patients do is irrelevant so long as they believe it will help them. If you advise sensible, moderate physical exercise and intellectual contact with friends, so much the better, for this actually is beneficial.

A particularly excellent and comprehensive review of the placebo effect[24] presents an overwhelmingly convincing outline of the power of the placebo, which deserves conscious use in the therapy of conditions that do not respond to specific treatment. A remarkable list of severe toxic side effects associated with placebo use is also presented. The physician should be aware that such side effects will be encountered. There is even the apocryphal tale of the psychologist who committed suicide by taking an overdose of a placebo.

In summary, intelligent and understanding use of the placebo effect can greatly benefit and comfort even those patients with genuine and serious eye problems. To avoid misunderstanding, I am not suggesting that psychologic hocus pocus is any substitute for accurate diagnosis and specific therapy of eye disease. As we have already established, specific therapy automatically has placebo value but, by definition, placebo therapy has no specific pharmacologic value.

REASSURANCE THERAPY

I have devoted so much time to the placebo because it is indeed a vital part of our therapy and of our evaluation of therapy. A knowledgeable internist has described the nature and the usefulness of the reassurance approach more elegantly.[25] He says that to be effective, reassurance therapy requires the following six steps. Omission of any of these steps detracts from or nullifies the value of the reassurance.

1. Obtain a sufficiently detailed history of the symptoms. Never try to reassure the patient during the initial history. Premature attempts at reassurance inhibit the patient from continuing with the history, usually reflect anxiety or impatience on the part of the physician, and are not effectively reassuring to the patient.

2. Determine the affective meaning of the symptoms. Although this step can be done almost simultaneously with step one, it is commonly overlooked or poorly performed. One reason for this is that the physician is concentrating on the verbal description and not on the affect. A second reason is that affect is communicated nonverbally—by tone of voice and mannerisms (body language). You must be aware that no patients come to you unless they are concerned or frightened by something. Therefore it is necessary to *evaluate consciously* the amount of patient concern in every history. The amount of patient concern will, of course, determine the amount of reassurance therapy required.

3. Examine the symptomatic portion of the body. Appropriate steps in physical diagnosis are necessary to establish the presence or absence of disease. Furthermore, touching the patient (laying on of hands) is in itself therapeutic and will dramatically enhance the effectiveness of the subsequent verbal reassurance.

4. Make a diagnosis. You should identify the presence or absence of disease in the

traditional medical manner. Obviously you are unable to give reassurance or explanation until you are reasonably sure of the nature of the problem.

5. Explain the pathophysiology of the symptom to the patient. Paradoxically, patients do not really need to understand all of the details, but they must receive three attitudes from the physician. First, they must believe that the physician understands the symptoms. Second, they must believe that the physician is concerned about them as individuals but is not anxious, frightened, or uncertain as to the management of the symptoms. Third, patients must believe that the physician is sympathetic about the symptom. We tend to be annoyed by patients whose symptoms persist—they frustrate us and we convey an attitude of displeasure. Physicians must accept the fact that they cannot eradicate all physical and emotional symptoms and not be affronted by the audacity of the persistent symptom.

6. Only after this preamble of history, examination, diagnosis, and explanation is reassurance appropriate. Reassurance may be defined as a credible and acceptable prognosis. Essentially, reassurance is a prediction of the future, an outline of the reasonable expectations of the patient. For benign conditions, reassurance may be categorical and absolute. For proposed surgery, reassurance must be qualified, perhaps with regard to the percentage of successful outcome or some comparable conditional prediction. In some conditions the prognosis is hopeless—the eye is irreparably damaged. Even (and especially) under such circumstances reassurance is appropriate and consists of a reasonable outline of the anticipated care and convalescence and of the type of lifetime activity subsequently possible. Reassurance cannot deny the facts of life and no attempt should be made to evade genuine problems. Reassurance does stress the positive aspects of the situation and banishes the fears that are without foundation.

Do not neglect reassurance, for it is one of the most important contributions you make to the welfare of every patient. Do not over-look the component of reassurance in the evaluation of therapy or otherwise you will grossly overestimate the value of your medications.

EVALUATION OF VITAMIN A TREATMENT OF RETINITIS PIGMENTOSA

The difficulty of making a true evaluation of therapeutic response is well illustrated by the history of a 10-year research project concerning the effect of 11-*cis* vitamin A in the treatment of retinitis pigmentosa.[26] As background for this project, recall that we ordinarily ingest vitamin A in the all-*trans* form, which is then isomerized in the eye to the 11-*cis* form. Only the 11-*cis* form can be utilized to manufacture retinene, the visual pigment. One theory of the causation of retinitis pigmentosa has postulated an inherited biochemical defect of the isomerization of vitamin A, with consequent degeneration of the retinal rods.

Animal experimentation demonstrated that retinal degeneration in vitamin A–deficient rats could be prevented by extremely small doses of 11-*cis* vitamin A but not by comparable doses of all-*trans* vitamin A.

An exploratory clinical experiment was performed by treating seven patients with retinitis pigmentosa with oral 11-*cis* vitamin A, 100,000 units daily for 1 month and then 50,000 units daily during a 2-year period. Of these seven patients, three showed significant improvement in visual acuity, three showed significant improvement in visual field, and one showed significant improvement in the dark adaptation curve.

Another group of eight patients with retinitis pigmentosa received intramuscular injections of 11-*cis* vitamin A, 100,000 units twice weekly for 1 year. Two of these patients showed significant improvement in visual fields, and two showed significant improvement in dark adaptation.

Understandably encouraged by these results, the authors undertook a 2-year study of 20 patients, administering 100,000 units of 11-*cis* vitamin A intramuscularly twice weekly. Vision improved significantly in six patients, visual fields improved in eight patients, and dark adaptation improved in two patients. Three patients interrupted treatment, suffered relapses, and improved when treatment was resumed.

From these data is it safe to conclude that 11-*cis* vitamin A treatment will at least arrest the progress of retinitis pigmentosa over a 2-year period, if not actually improve the condition, in approximately one third of patients? Certainly this would seem to be a conservative conclusion and would apparently justify such treatment of this previously hopeless disease.

Fortunately these authors were critical scientists and formulated a rigidly controlled study of 88 retinitis pigmentosa patients matched in pairs according to history, progress, and status of the disease. The treatment group received 11-*cis* vitamin A, 100,000 units intramuscularly twice weekly, for 3 years. The control group received an identical dosage of all-*trans* vitamin A. The final results, shown in Table 1-1, indicate absolutely no benefit from treatment with 11-*cis* vitamin A.

This 10-year study illustrates an all too common sequence of events. An attractive basic hypothesis receives initial confirmation from animal experimentation. Preliminary clinical studies show encouraging results. Additional clinical studies, still uncontrolled, independently verify the encouraging results. At this stage, unfortunately, the given therapy usually is released from the laboratory and becomes generally used in medical practice. Established in the medical literature and in drug handbooks, the treatment acquires the respectability of usage and inevitably receives credit for an encouraging number of satisfied patients. But, alas, as years go by some skeptical clinician finally arranges a controlled clinical study. (Can you imagine the effort required to evaluate 88 patients with retinitis pigmentosa, match them in severity, and inject them twice weekly for 3 years!) Of such experiences is skepticism of new treatments born.

You may think that this example of 11-*cis* vitamin A treatment of retinitis pigmentosa is not representative—and, after all, it has not been recommended. Preliminary reports from a committee on therapeutic evaluation suggest that two thirds of the older drugs available today are of unproved value and probably worthless. Presumably the lipotropic and iodide preparations widely advertised for management of ocular degenerative diseases will fall into this category. These useless drugs entered our armamentarium via the path outlined in the 11-*cis* vitamin A example. Perhaps we are not as far from the bad old days of purging and bloodletting as we would like to imagine.

TOXIC EFFECTS

Finally, the evaluation of therapeutic response must also take into account the possibility of adverse side effects. Recognize that pilocarpine toxicity may cause nausea and vomiting wrongly attributed to acute glaucoma. Glaucoma secondary to corticosteroid therapy is well publicized but not always recognized. The somewhat confused mental state of the unreliable old lady with glaucoma could be caused by acetazolamide toxicity.

Table 1-1. Final results of 11-*cis* vitamin A treatment of patients with retinitis pigmentosa

	3 years		*2½ years or less*	
	11-cis	*All-trans*	*11-cis*	*All-trans*
Improved	1	1	2	1
Same	4	9	0	1
Regressed	21	17	7	3
Not qualified	1	3	0	0
Total	27	30	9	5

Continuing superficial punctate keratitis may be due to irritation from the medication long after the primary disease etiology has vanished. Do not permit your glaucoma patient with cholinesterase deficiency to undergo exploratory abdominal surgery seeking the cause of stomach pains.

A compact review of toxic drug effects is presented in the apocryphal story of a physician who treated himself.

About ten years ago this busy physician developed acute pharyngitis and, seeking quick relief, self-medicated himself with penicillin. The pharyngitis improved rapidly; but to his great distress, forty-eight hours later he developed a severe urticarial reaction to the penicillin and was confined to his bed for one week. After several days of misery, hydrocortisone was administered and in due course the urticaria subsided. Not long thereafter he experienced abdominal pain and gastrointestinal bleeding, and radiographic studies demonstrated a duodenal ulcer, a well-known complication of steroid therapy. Because of headaches resulting from the loss of blood, he was given acetophenetidin and to his utter chagrin developed a fixed drug eruption on the genitalia, which consisted of a painful ulceration persisting for several weeks. But the worst was yet to come. The duodenal ulcer was treated with Sippy powders containing calcium carbonate and calcium phosphate to control gastric acidity; shortly thereafter he experienced painful urethral calculi, which fortunately subsided when these powders were discontinued. In addition, probanthine was administered to control gastric secretion. The patient then noted some visual disturbances; after several months, it was discovered that he had glaucoma. The intraocular pressure was controlled with physostigmine salicylate solution; however, the use of these drops created a severe conjunctival congestion, resulting in great embarrassment and damage to the psyche.

One wonders if he might not have been better off had the original pharyngitis been treated with simple aspirin gargles and rest.*

THE RANDOMIZED CONTROLLED CLINICAL TRIAL

Knowing about all these pitfalls, how do we avoid them? Anyone planning a clinical

*From Dunphy, E. B.: Trans. Am. Acad. Ophthalmol. Otolaryngol. **70:**9, 1966.

study really should prepare for the ordeal by reading a symposium devoted to the subject, such as one published by the National Eye Institute.[27] It is sobering to realize that we do not really know whether radical or simple mastectomy is better, whether coronary artery surgery is beneficial, or whether emergency surgery is good for bleeding peptic ulcers. In our own field, we do not even know whether we should use photocoagulation for retinal holes (I do not think that asymptomatic holes discovered on routine examination should be treated, unless the other eye is already detached—and even then I am not sure), let alone whether we should photocoagulate venous occlusions, chorioretinitis, senile macular degeneration, or diabetic retinopathy. I realize that the Cooperative Diabetic Retinopathy Study (cost—1 million dollars per year) came to the widely publicized conclusion that disc vascularization was improved by extensive photocoagulation, and yet in the National Eye Institute Symposium a physician reported seeing 3 patients who were dropouts from the Diabetic Retinopathy Study because their treated eye had not done well. These patients refused to return to the study. Obviously, greater attrition of patients who did not do well will unavoidably bias a study toward a more favorable result than actually exists. Unfortunately, all clinicians know of the tendency of patients who do poorly to look elsewhere for their salvation. Since you need to know my prejudices in order to assess my credibility, let me state that I am unconvinced that the net effect of photocoagulation of diabetic retinopathy is beneficial.

Paradoxically, for 20 years I have tried to teach rational ophthalmic therapy and yet am daily unable to define what is rational. I know that osmotherapy will reduce intraocular pressure, but I am not convinced that intravenous mannitol is desirable before cataract extraction. So how should this be dealt with? The only answer that I can offer is that a medical or surgical treatment should not be used unless the physician is reasonably sure that it will be of benefit. That the treatment "might not hurt" is not enough indication for its use. Unfortunately, it is very difficult to prove that antibiotics do or do not favorably alter the normal surface bacterial flora preoperatively, that corticosteroids are or are not good for toxoplasmosis, and that pilocarpine is or is not good for hyphema.

Ultimately I must admit that I will never know whether a given retinal hole should be treated, even though I have personally operated on more than 10,000 retinal detachments. There are so many clinical variations, limitations of follow-up and of technique, problems of informed consent, and malpractice hazards that there is just no way to answer the question except with vague generalizations. I do not mean to condemn scientific attempts to seek knowledge but rather to place them in a proper perspective. Do not worship randomized controlled trials but recognize that they are better than clinical impressions, which are truly misleading. Most importantly and most practically, make clear to the bureaucrats and lawyers who believe that a Professional Standards Review Organization will identify the one perfect treatment that medicine is an imperfect science and that the perfect treatment is not known.

SUMMARY

We have an unfortunate tendency to permit our diagnostic and therapeutic responses to become stereotyped to such a degree that these intellectual exercises degenerate into conditioned reflexes. When vitreous hemorrhage automatically means placebo pills and a waiting period of 2 weeks, our patients are in trouble. The scientific method is applicable to each patient. Gather all available facts (history and physical examination). Formulate a tentative hypothesis (preliminary diagnosis). On the basis of the hypothesis, seek additional corroborative or conflicting facts (look at the patient again to confirm the findings pertinent to the diagnosis). From this information, assemble a theory (presume the diagnosis is correct). Finally, check the theory against other known facts (prescribe the appropriate medi-

cation and observe whether the expected therapeutic response occurs).

Most faults in patient management originate from insufficient fact-gathering. The step most overlooked is the second check of the patient, intended to elicit subtle corroborative or conflicting facts. These inconspicuous details usually determine whether a macular lesion is a melanoma or a disciform degeneration. Such details require intellectually guided seeking (for example, are sinusoids present?) rather than hopeful looking. This intellectually guided seeking is mandatory in evaluation of therapeutic response. Otherwise, if the patient finally recovers at the end of the self-limited disease, the unwary physician will attribute the "cure" to the final medication prescribed—but it will not work the next time (just as the cabbages at the beginning of this chapter failed to cure the preacher).

REFERENCES

1. Shimkin, M. B.: Numerical method in therapeutic medicine, J.A.M.A. **188**:100, 1964; Trans. Stud. Coll. Physicians Phila. **31**:204, 1964.
2. Garland, L. H.: Clinical and laboratory observer variations, J. New Drugs **1**:65, 1961.
3. Spaeth, G. L.: The effects of bromelains on the inflammatory response caused by cataract extraction: a double-blind study, Eye Ear Nose Throat Mon. **47**:634, 1968.
4. Ederer, F.: Shall we count numbers of eyes or numbers of subjects? Arch. Ophthalmol. **89**:1, 1973.
5. Maddock, R. K., Jr.: Patient cooperation in taking medicines—a study involving isoniazid and aminosalicylic acid, J.A.M.A. **199**:169, 1967.
6. Caron, H. S., and Roth, H. P.: Patient's cooperation with a medical regimen, J.A.M.A. **203**:120, 1968.
7. Bigger, J. F.: A comparison of patient compliance in treated vs untreated ocular hypertension, Trans. Am. Acad. Ophthalmol. Otolaryngol. **81**:OP-277, March-April, 1976.
8. Varley, A. B.: The generic inequivalence of drugs, J.A.M.A. **206**:1745, 1968.
9. Friend, D. G.: Generic drugs and therapeutic equivalence, J.A.M.A. **206**:1785, 1968.
10. Wessler, S., and Avioli, L. V.: Pharmacogenetics, J.A.M.A. **205**:679, 1968.

11. Harris, W. S., and Goodman, R. M.: Hyperreactivity to atropine in Down's syndrome, N. Engl. J. Med. **279:**407, 1968.
12. Dunlap, C.: Med. World News, July 3, 1964.
13. Shapiro, A. K.: Etiologic factors in placebo effect, J.A.M.A. **187:**712, 1964.
14. Beecher, H. K.: The powerful placebo, J.A.M.A. **159:**1602, 1955.
15. Thach, W.: I have seen acupuncture work, Today's Health **50:**50, 1972.
16. Dimond, E. G.: Medical education and care in People's Republic of China, J.A.M.A. **218:**1552, 1971.
17. Dimond, E. G.: Acupuncture anesthesia, J.A.M.A. **218:**1558, 1971.
18. Dunlop, D.: Survey of 17,301 prescriptions, Br. Med. J. **1:**292, 1952.
19. Beecher, H.: Control of suffering in severe trauma, J.A.M.A. **173:**534, 1960.
20. Rider, J. A.: Placebo gastric analysis, Am. J. Gastroenterol. **56:**364, 1971.
21. Amsterdam, E.: New aspects of the placebo response in angina pectoris, Am. J. Cardiol. **24:**305, 1969.
22. Lowinger, P., and Dobie, S.: What makes a placebo work? Arch. Gen. Psychiatry **20:**84, 1969.
23. Editorial: Br. Med. J. **2:**437, 1970.
24. Honigfeld, G.: Nonspecific factors in treatment, Dis. Nerv. Syst. **25:**145, 1964.
25. Sapira, J. D.: Reassurance therapy, Ann. Intern. Med. **77:**603, 1972.
26. Chatzinoff, A., Nelson, E., Stahl, N., and Clahane, A.: Eleven CIS vitamin A in the treatment of retinitis pigmentosa, Arch. Ophthalmol. **80:**417, 1968.
27. National Eye Institute: The randomized controlled clinical trial, Am. J. Ophthalmol. **79:**752, May, 1975.

2
ROUTES OF ADMINISTRATION

PERMEABILITY OF OCULAR STRUCTURES

Administration of drugs intended to affect different portions of the eye must be guided by knowledge of the permeability of the various ocular structures. For example, the penetration of medications through the intact cornea is not a matter of simple diffusion but is best explained by a differential solubility concept. The cornea may be thought of as a fat-water-fat sandwich. Chemical analysis shows the lipid content of the epithelium and endothelium to be 100 times greater than that of the corneal stroma. As a result, the epithelium and endothelium are relatively impermeable to electrolytes but are readily penetrated by fat-soluble substances. The stroma is readily penetrated by electrolytes but not by fat-soluble substances. The differential solubility theory of penetration of the cornea by an alkaloid (for example, homatropine) is illustrated in Fig. 2-1, in which R_3N represents the nonionized, fat-soluble, water-insoluble form of the alkaloid.[1] This exists in equilibrium with the ionized, water-soluble, fat-insoluble form, R_3NH^+. The relative proportion of ionized and nonionized substance is determined by the pH.

Although both ionized and nonionized alkaloids exist in the tears, only the nonionized form penetrates into the epithelium. The stroma resists entry by the nonionized form, until it again ionizes. Traversing the stroma freely, the ionized alkaloid is again blocked by endothelium until it changes to the fat-soluble, nonionized form.

All medications that readily enter the eye after topical application have this ability to exist in equilibrium in solution as ionized or nonionized forms. Substances that are exclusively electrolytes or nonelectrolytes will not penetrate the intact cornea. Fluorescein, a negatively charged ion that can easily be seen clinically, nicely demonstrates the resistance of the intact cornea to penetration by electrolytes. Biomicroscopy shows no staining of the cornea or aqueous after fluorescein instillation on the normal cornea. If the epithelium is damaged, fluorescein enters the stroma. Should damage be sufficient to disturb the endothelium, fluorescein will be recognized within the aqueous also.

The structural and physiologic similarity of the conjunctival epithelium to that of the cornea is well known. That this similarity includes permeability characteristics is demonstrated clinically with every application of fluorescein. The normal, intact conjunctiva and the underlying subconjunctival, episcleral, and scleral tissues do not color with fluorescein; hence the surface must be resistant to the penetration of this electrolyte.

A more sophisticated demonstration of the resistance of the intact conjunctiva to the passage of electrolytes evaluated the movement of radioactive hydrocortisone from a subconjunctival depot to the tear fluid.[2] The subconjunctival injection was given by two approaches: by the usual transconjunctival penetration of the hypodermic needle and by introduction of the needle through the lid skin to the subconjunctival space, taking

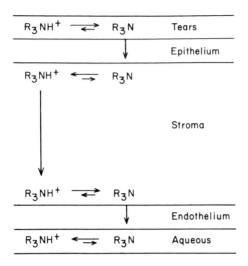

Fig. 2-1. Penetration of an alkaloid through the cornea, illustrating differential solubility characteristics.

Table 2-1. Accumulation of ^{14}C hydrocortisone in teardrops after subconjunctival injection*

Time interval after injection (min)	Hydrocortisone (conjunctiva punctured) (μg)	Hydrocortisone (conjunctiva intact) (μg)
30	122.6	0
45	287.7	0
60	339.0	0

*From Wine, N. A., Gornall, A. G., and Basu, P. K.: Am. J. Ophthalmol. **58**:362, 1964.

care not to puncture the conjunctiva. Equal doses were positioned in similar locations by these two approaches. The teardrops were collected by applying filter paper to the conjunctiva immediately after the drug injection. No hydrocortisone entered the tear fluid across the intact conjunctiva, in contrast to the leakage of 5.5% of the total dose into the tears within 1 hour after transconjunctival injection (Table 2-1).

Barriers with a differential solubility resistance comparable to that of the cornea also surround the entire eye. The existence of these barriers may be visualized by the intravenous injection of fluorescein. Fluorescein fundus angiography shows this dye flowing through but confined within the normal retinal vessels. The retinal vessel walls constitute a blood-eye barrier posteriorly. In contrast, the choroidal circulation appears to leak fluorescein, which cannot, however, pass through the retinal pigment layer, representing another part of the blood-eye barrier.

The sclera, although a tough structural component of the eye, does *not* act as a differential solubility barrier. Experimental injection of human serum albumin labeled with radioactive iodine and Evans blue dye into the suprachoroidal space of rabbits resulted

in rapid escape of the albumin across the sclera into the orbital tissues. Within 1 hour, only 10% of the radioactive albumin remained within the eye.[3] At 1 hour, 25% of the radioactivity was recoverable from the orbital tissues, 50% was within the sclera, and 10% had already entered the body beyond the orbit (Fig. 2-2). As judged by the visible location of the dye, the albumin moved directly across the sclera toward the exterior of the eye, apparently propelled by the intraocular pressure. Study of the curves in Fig. 2-2 confirms this impression that suprachoroidal injections leave the eye via the sclera rather than through the choroidal circulation. Similar suprachoroidal injections of dextran (mol. wt. 40,000) also resulted in rapid transscleral escape. Hence we may conclude that the sclera is quite a porous barrier, permitting free passage of even very large molecules. However, do not overlook the effect of the strong unidirectional flow generated by the relatively high intraocular pressure. Even from the suprachoroidal position, the labeled molecules did *not* penetrate readily inward. Note the rapid drop of the intraocular curve (Fig. 2-2), indicating only 30% of radioactivity at 5 minutes, 10% at 1 hour, and almost 0% at 8 hours. Clearly, intraocular penetration of medications injected into Tenon's space will be minimal because of this rapid transscleral outflow.

The thick-walled iris vessels constitute another part of the blood-eye barrier. Biomicroscopy after intravenous fluorescein injection shows that no fluorescein enters the

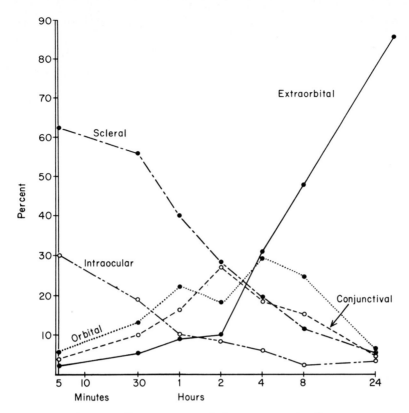

Fig. 2-2. Location of serum albumin at specified time intervals after injection into supra-choroidal space. (Modified from Bill, A.: Arch. Ophthalmol. **74**:248, 1965.)

aqueous from the normal iris surface. In contrast, the inflamed iris conspicuously leaks fluorescein into the aqueous chamber.

The ciliary epithelium occupies a unique position in the blood-eye barrier; it actively secretes some ions and permits free passage of others in accordance with the secretion-diffusion theory of aqueous formation. Fluorescein readily enters the posterior chamber from the ciliary processes and can be seen to flow forward through the pupil in a normal eye. Nevertheless, the ciliary epithelium still blocks entry of most molecules (for example, protein and most antibiotics) into the aqueous humor.

Consideration of these facts about permeability of the various eye structures will permit accurate deductions as to the penetration into the eye of a given medication, depending on its differential solubility characteristics. However, the penetration of medica-

tions into the normal eye may differ greatly from penetration into a diseased eye. Damage to the blood-eye barrier results from injury or inflammation, is manifested clinically by aqueous flare (caused by protein leakage into the aqueous), and may result in greatly increased entry of normally excluded molecules (for example, antibiotics) into the eye. With electron microscopy, the anatomic basis of blood-eye barrier breakdown can be demonstrated. The capillary endothelial cells as well as the epithelial layers of the ciliary processes separate from each other, leaving enlarged intercellular spaces that permit leakage of protein and of fine particulate material.[4]

Not only the ease of drug penetration but also the rate of its removal will determine intraocular concentrations of a medication. The two main sources of drug loss are diffusion into the circulating blood and escape via the aqueous into the canal of Schlemm. Diffusion into the blood takes place at all vessels—conjunctival and episcleral as well as intraocular. Because of these blood and aqueous losses of drug, topically applied medications do not penetrate in useful concentrations to the back of the eye. The dilated vessels of an inflamed eye carry away medication more rapidly than normal and are responsible for such practical clinical problems as the difficulty of maintaining local anesthesia of a red eye.

Drugs are not uniformly distributed within the eye but may selectively concentrate in certain parts (for example, phenothiazine concentration in pigmented cells and silver in Descemet's membrane). Presumably this selective binding of drugs is responsible for such well-known clinical effects as the prolonged cycloplegia of atropine, which persists long after the alkaloid has disappeared from the aqueous. Quantitative pharmacologic studies should take into consideration this uneven intraocular distribution. Specifically, studies of aqueous concentration of a given drug are not necessarily representative of its intraocular penetration or persistence.

TOPICAL APPLICATION

The act of placing a drop of medication directly on the eye incorrectly suggests that this drug is indeed delivered to the eye and remains there to carry out its function. A manifestation of this misconception is the commonly heard admonition that after atropine instillation on a child's eye the mother should press on the tear sac "to prevent systemic absorption."

Radioactive labeling of medications documents the very rapid spread of topical drops to all parts of the body. For example, 30 minutes after instillation of radioactive corticosteroid on rabbit eyes, only 1.6% was present within eye tissues. This medication was applied by pooling 0.25 ml of solution between the lids, held open by sutures; yet only 29% of drug remained in the conjunctival sac after 30 minutes. Nasal washings recovered only 0.5%, indicating that systemic absorption did *not* occur by nasal flow and gastrointestinal absorption. Liver, kidneys, adrenals, and the gallbladder contained 21% of the radioactivity. The remaining 47% was not specified but was presumably distributed throughout the other body tissues.[5] As shown in Fig. 5-1, absorption of tetracaine across a mucous membrane is more rapid than that following subcutaneous hypodermic injection and is comparable to a moderate rate of intravenous injection.

Despite the astonishingly rapid escape of a topically applied drug from the eye, therapeutic levels persist for clinically effective durations of time. Fig. 2-3 documents the persistence of dexamethasone after ocular instillations of 2 drops of 0.1% solution.[6] Note that iris and aqueous levels in the range of 0.5 to 1.0 μg/g of tissue were maintained for several hours. For comparison of surface and intraocular concentrations, a 0.1% solution contains 1000 μg/g.

Vehicle

The vehicle in which a drug is applied affects its penetration. More viscous vehicles prolong ocular contact and thereby increase drug absorption. Oily vehicles compete with the corneal epithelium for fat-soluble medications and may retard absorption somewhat. This competition is not of great clinical importance, since it may be offset by increasing drug concentration.

Many other factors such as pH, tonicity, electrolyte composition, wetting effect, and stability enter into the design of a vehicle.[7] Preservatives and antioxidants may be added. Drug incompatibilities must be avoided. Optimal drug concentrations and useful drug combinations are selected. Accuracy is vital. Sterility in the original container is expected. Because of these many requirements, drug compounding for ophthalmic use has become the responsibility of the large commercial manufacturers rather than of the local pharmacist, who usually has neither the equipment nor background to prepare competitive eye solutions.

As an example of the importance of pH, the penetration of radioactive labeled pilo-

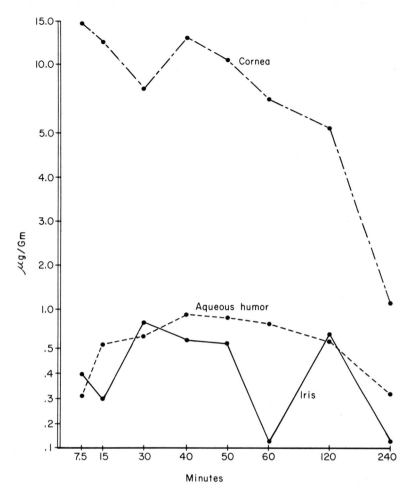

Fig. 2-3. Dexamethasone levels after single topical application of 0.1% solution. (Modified from Short, C., and associates: Arch. Ophthalmol. **75:**689, 1966.)

carpine into rabbit aqueous was compared for eye drops of pH 4 and 7.5.[8] Aqueous pilocarpine concentrations were approximately twice as high with use of the more alkaline solution. The explanation of this is not entirely clear. A weak acid, such as pilocarpine, is less ionized at the lower pH than at the physiologic 7.5. Hence, passage across the epithelium and endothelium should be enhanced at pH 4 and passage across the stroma should be hindered. Perhaps the greater thickness of the stroma is a greater barrier to nonelectrolyte passage than the thinner epithelium-endothelium barriers are to electrolyte passage. The reader should be aware of other constraints on pH adjust-

ment, such as the instability and deterioration of alkaline pilocarpine solutions.

The experimental method used to study corneal drug penetration will greatly modify the results obtained. For example, 90 minutes after topical application of 0.1% fluorometholone to the rabbit cornea, aqueous drug levels were 0.1 μg/ml in anesthetized upright animals and 1.0 μg/ml in anesthetized recumbent animals. The tenfold difference was a result of more rapid medication loss from the conjunctival sac in the upright position.[9] In another experiment,[10] topical application of 0.1% dexamethasone resulted in 1-hour postapplication aqueous levels of 0.4 μg/ml when the tested solution contained a radioactivity of 200 μC/mg. In contrast, a tested solution with radioactivity of less than 10 μC/mg resulted in aqueous radioactivity no different from the background, leading to a false assumption that the drug had not penetrated the cornea. These reports illustrate how conflicting reports in biologic experiments are easily explained by differences in methodology.

Ointment

Clinically significant enhancement of drug penetration results from the prolonged contact time achievable with the use of an ointment vehicle. For example, a 2% tetracycline suspension in ointment produced bacteriostatic drug levels within the anterior chamber lasting for several hours when applied to the intact rabbit eye. In contrast, solutions of tetracycline produced only trace levels of the drug, insufficient for effective antibacterial action.[11,12] Photofluorometric measurements of the normal human eye showed attainment of aqueous fluorescein levels twice as high with an ointment vehicle as with an aqueous vehicle for fluorescein topical application.[13]

However, the enhanced penetration resulting from the prolonged contact of an ointment vehicle may be counteracted by failure of the ointment to release the drug. Higher corneal and aqueous concentrations of dexamethasone sodium phosphate[14] and of dexamethasone alcohol[15] result from use of an aqueous vehicle than from an ointment vehicle. This is apparently because of inability of the ointment to release the dexamethasone, whether it exists as a water-soluble form (dexamethasone sodium phosphate) or a lipid-soluble form (dexamethasone alcohol).

The waxy grades of petrolatum and the unwashed lanolin used in ophthalmic ointments prepared many decades ago demonstrably slowed the healing of corneal epithelial wounds. However, currently used ophthalmic ointment vehicles do not slow the rate of reepithelialization of experimental corneal injuries or the healing of experimental keratectomies.[16] Concern has also been expressed that ointment particles may be entrapped beneath healing epithelium or under conjunctival wounds. Experimentally, ointment entrapment could not be produced as a consequence of epithelial abrasions or corneal incisions.[17] The ointment was rejected by the wound surfaces, which would not engulf ointment particles. Actual injection of the ointment was required before it would be retained within the corneal stroma or beneath the conjunctiva. Even here, the only consequence was transient neovascularization.

The commonly used ophthalmic ointment bases and liquid oily vehicles (petrolatum, lanolin, and peanut oil) are toxic to the interior of the eye, causing endothelial damage, corneal edema, vascularization, and scarring. For this reason, ophthalmic medications in ointment or oily liquid vehicles should not be instilled into the interior of the eye or used in such a way during surgery that they may accidentally enter the eye. Experimental studies showed that introduction of 0.1 ml of any of these substances into rabbit eyes caused a severe reaction with secondary glaucoma and eventual loss of the eye (Fig. 2-4). Smaller amounts were less destructive.[18]

It is my practice to instill antibiotic ointment at the close of every eye operation. Such usage provides a prolonged antibiotic presence and softens or eliminates crusts of bloody discharge. I have witnessed no adverse effects from the ointment on wound healing. A comparably strong endorsement of the postoperative use of ointment has been made by a surgeon with personal experience in the care of 20,000 patients.[19]

Continuous irrigation

Constantly high concentrations of medications on the surface of the eye may be maintained by a technique of continuous irrigation[20] in which No. 190 polyethylene tubing is passed diagonally through the lower lid with the aid of a long, curved surgical needle. The end of the tubing enters the conjunctival sac 2 mm below and temporal to the lower punctum and lies against the bulbar conjunctiva at this point. The tubing is anchored

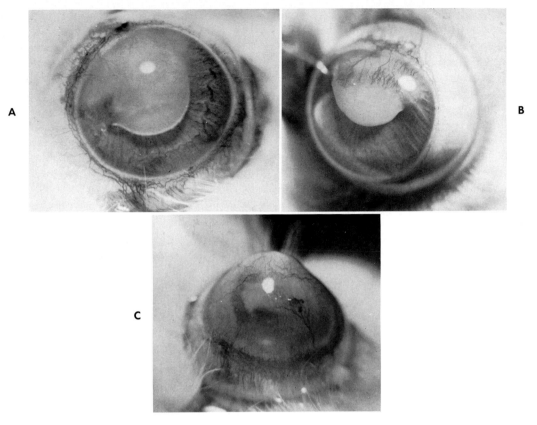

Fig. 2-4. Effect of lanolin in rabbit anterior chamber. **A,** After 1 week. **B,** After 8 weeks. **C,** After 12 weeks. (From Scheie, H. G., Rubenstein, A., and Katowitz, J. A.: Arch. Ophthalmol. **73:**36, 1965.)

to the lid skin by a 4-0 suture. The desired antibiotic solution runs from a bottle suspended as for intravenous drip at a rate of 4 or 5 drops/minute. The outflow is absorbed in a towel held near the eye. This constant irrigation technique is said also to benefit the eye by washing away contaminated debris.

What is the effect of irrigation on the healing of the corneal defects? Should conjunctival secretions and discharge be considered undesirable and frequently washed from the surface of a wound? We associate "pus" with the undesirable effects of an infection and ordinarily take steps to clean it from the eye. The accumulations of dried crusts of dead leukocytes and protein on the lid margins serve no useful purpose, are uncomfortable, and may harbor bacteria; hence they should be removed. However, it is apparent that leukocytes in the precorneal tear film are part of the ocular defense against infection. Excessive and prolonged irrigation or use of toxic chemicals may interfere with this defense mechanism.

Observation of the movement of polymorphonuclear leukocytes into corneal wounds suggest that the leukocytes originate in conjunctival vessels, pass into the tear fluid, and enter the stromal wound from the precorneal tear film.[21] Their migration is then through corneal lamellae from wound to limbus, not in the reverse direction. In large central corneal wounds, leukocytes also migrate inward from the limbus but reach the wound hours later than leukocytes from the tear film. If the precorneal tear film is continuously washed away by a saline drip, leukocytes do not reach a corneal wound, although they are present in increased numbers in the conjunctiva and the washings from the eye, as in nonirrigated wounded eyes. Many types of antibodies have been demonstrated to exist in normal tears.[22] The lysozyme enzymatic defenses of tear fluid are well known. I am reluctant to advise the constant washing away of all these normal defense mechanisms.

The same concern may be expressed about the use of a constant perfusion pump delivering 3 to 8 ml of fluid per day, although such a device has been used for as long as 2 years in the treatment of a patient with severe tear deficiency.[23] Although still experimental, this method may be superior to parotid duct transplant and is certainly more effective than repeated topical instillations of artificial tears.

Iontophoresis

Application of electromotive force will enhance corneal penetration of antibiotics that ionize in solution. This technique has never achieved clinical popularity. For more detail, the interested reader is referred to previous editions of this book.

Massage

Apparently *vigorous* massage of the eye through the closed lids may cause sufficient corneal epithelial damage to permit better penetration of poorly soluble substances. Without massage, a 1.5% solution of carbachol (with benzalkonium chloride) is required to produce complete miosis.[24] With massage, miosis is produced by a 0.09% solution. However, self-massage by the average patient was found to be ineffective and undependable. Ocular massage after instillation of the common ophthalmic drugs is unnecessary, since these preparations have solubility characteristics that permit adequate corneal penetration.

Surgical manipulation similarly increases drug penetration.

HYDROPHILIC CONTACT LENS DRUG APPLICATION

"Soft" contact lenses have the capability to absorb and slowly release chemicals in solution. This does not occur with "hard"

lenses. This capability of prolonging contact of medication with the cornea was first noted as an adverse effect since the corneal epithelium was damaged by the preservatives normally used in eye drops. Please note that preservatives, which are metabolic poisons, should not be present in medications to be applied by the contact lens vehicle.

Fluorescein, because its presence and concentration are visible and easily measured by fluorometric techniques and because it is representative of the lipid-insoluble, poorly penetrating class of drugs, was used to evaluate the effectiveness of drug application via the soft lens.[25] After repeated topical application, the corneal concentration of fluorescein was less than 0.0001 of the concentration of the applied solution. However, when the fluorescein was applied by instillation on a soft lens worn on the eye or by presoaking the lens before fitting it to the cornea, drug concentrations observed in the cornea and aqueous were up to 10 times greater than those seen after simple topical instillation. Furthermore, such concentrations could be maintained for as long as 24 hours. This preliminary experiment confirmed the expectation that soft lenses could act as a vehicle to increase the amount of drug delivered to the eye and might also eliminate the need for frequent topical application.

Soft lenses of different chemical composition have different vehicle properties. For example, the Soflens took up twice as much fluorescein on a weight basis as did the Griffin lens. (The uptake of either type of dry soft lens is almost the same as that of a fully hydrated lens.) The rate of release also differs. Within 1 hour, the Griffin lens released 70% of its fluorescein, while the Soflens had released only 25%. Presumably related to its more rapid release, anterior segment fluorescein concentrations were three to four times greater with this Griffin lens than with the Soflens. Please be aware that contamination of a soft lens with fluorescein, as may occur during clinical examination, may cause permanent staining of the lens, rendering it useless.

The Griffin lens as a vehicle in the administration of pilocarpine has been studied in detail.[26] A lens soaked in 0.5% pilocarpine solution for 10 minutes will absorb about 1 mg of pilocarpine. More prolonged soaking in more concentrated solutions results in more absorption; for example, 10 minutes in 4% pilocarpine solution results in an absorption of 3 mg per lens (mean value).

When the pilocarpine-impregnated lens is placed in water or in the eye, the time required to release 50% of the pilocarpine is about 30 minutes. Within 4 hours, over 90% of the pilocarpine has been eluted from the lens. Hence a soft lens is a relatively short-term pilocarpine repository.

The capability of a soft lens to take up and release drugs depends on the size of the openings within the soft lens substance and the molecular size of the drug.[27] These openings will permit entry of molecules about 4 Å in size, such as fluorescein (molecular weight 376). Smaller molecules (pilocarpine —molecular weight, 244; chloramphenicol— molecular weight, 323) also enter well, whereas larger molecules (colistin—molecular weight, 1431) cannot enter the lens matrix and do not exhibit prolonged contact when used with a soft lens. Prednisone (molecular weight, 360) delivery can also be enhanced by application of a soft lens presoaked in the medication.[28] Presoaking of the lens for at least 2 minutes is preferable to instillation of the medication on the lens already present on the cornea, which results in drug binding within the lens and a lesser concentration within the eye.

The use of a presoaked soft lens to deliver medication to the eye does prolong delivery time and results in longer presence (up to 4 hours) of small molecular weight drugs within the eye. This is of doubtful clinical value, since the same goal can be achieved much more easily by more frequent application of topical medication. However, the use of soft lenses is becoming widespread, and these drug interactions with the lens deserve comment.

Membrane-controlled diffusional systems

Unlike the presoaked soft contact lens, which has a drug delivery half-life of only 20 minutes, the concept of a drug reservoir will permit preparation of a device that will release the drug at a constant rate for up to a week.[29] The rate of release is dependent on the permeability of the membrane to the drug and the area of the membrane and will remain constant until the drug reservoir is exhausted, providing the osmotic and permeability relationships do not draw water into the delivery system. Devices can be fabricated that will deliver 20 μg of pilocarpine per hour within a 10% tolerance, continuing for as long as a week (Fig. 2-5).

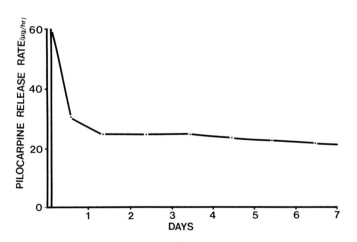

Fig. 2-5. The rate of release of pilocarpine (μg/hr) from Ocusert. (Modified from Shell, J. W., and Baker, R. W.: Ann. Ophthalmol. **6:**1037, October 1974.)

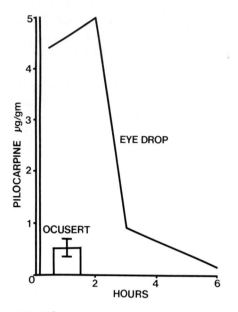

Fig. 2-6. Pilocarpine concentration in aqueous humor attained with 2% eye drop (line), compared with 8-day average value with 20 μg/hr Ocusert (bar). (Modified from Sendelbeck, L., Moore, D., and Urquhart, J.: Am. J. Ophthalmol. **80:**274, August 1975.)

Fig. 2-6[30] shows the aqueous humor concentrations of pilocarpine when administered as a 2% solution, 1 drop every 6 hours (the line), or as a 20 μg/hr Ocusert (the bar). The bar represents the mean value over a period of 8 days. The difference between intermittent drop administration and the controlled diffusion device is evident. The traditional drop method of delivery results in dramatic high peaks of medication alternating with valleys. Controlled, constant diffusion results in constant medication at a very much lower level, except for the peak delivery (Fig. 2-5) occurring during the first 12 hours of use of an Ocusert. This initial peak is caused by the rapid escape of pilocarpine already within the membrane. Actually, this initial peak delivers an amount of drug less than that contained within 1 drop of 2% solution.

Clinically, this constant low level presence of pilocarpine appears to be equivalent to the traditional eye drop in its ability to control the pressure of human glaucoma.[31,32] The effect of the 20 μg/hr or the 40 μg/hr devices cannot be exactly correlated with the previous use of 1% to 4% pilocarpine but must be evaluated empirically. Most cases controlled with 1% pilocarpine drops will be controlled with the 20 μg/hr Ocusert, but some require the 40 μg/hr unit. Most cases requiring 2% or stronger eye drops will require the 40 μg/hr Ocusert. Try the 20 μg/hr strength first and see if it works, as determined by pressure measurement at 1 week.

If pressure control is not achieved with the 40 μg/hr Ocusert, supplemental epinephrine or acetazolamide may be used, just as with the traditional eye drop. Concomitant use of the Ocusert and of any other type of eye drop does not result in incompatibility problems.

When the Ocusert is first prescribed, patients must receive detailed instruction in its insertion and removal, and their ability to do this must be confirmed. They must change the units regularly every 7 days, since their drug content becomes unreliable after about 8 days. Patients must check for the continuing presence of the Ocusert both morning and evening, since as high as 20% of patients will lose their Ocuserts from time to time. A position in the upper cul-de-sac will retain the device more securely than in the lower conjunctival sac. Insertion of a new Ocusert at bedtime will eliminate the transitory myopic blur resulting from the initial medication peak.

The advantages of this prolonged release system include better patient compliance with therapy, since the bother of repeated instillation of drops is not required. The incapacitating myopia from accommodative spasm, as occurs in younger patients, is minimized.

The disadvantages include the possibility of unrecognized loss of the device from the conjunctival sac, with resultant escape from therapy for some days. A practical problem is the cost, which is much greater than eye drops.

Patients with heavily pigmented irides are resistant to pilocarpine Ocusert therapy, just as they respond poorly to eye drops.[33]

The amount of induced accommodation

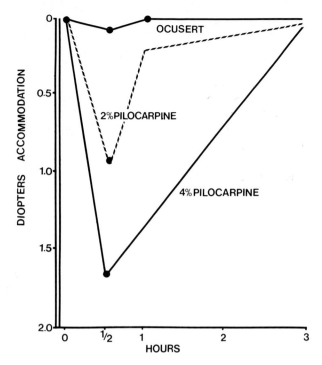

Fig. 2-7. Accommodative spasm resulting from 1 drop of 4% pilocarpine, 1 drop of 1% pilocarpine, or Ocusert. (Modified from Brown, H. S., and associates: Arch. Ophthalmol. **94:** 1716, October 1976. Copyright 1976, American Medical Association.)

associated with pilocarpine medication was evaluated in 18 patients with visual complaints related to therapy of their glaucoma. As would be expected, two thirds of these patients were under 50 years of age. Fig. 2-7[34] shows the refractive errors induced by 20 μg/hr and 40 μg/hr Ocuserts and 1% and 4% pilocarpine drops. As indicated, at 30 minutes the average accommodative response to 1% pilocarpine was 1.00 D, resulting in drop of vision to less than 20/40. The 30-minute accommodative response to 4% pilocarpine was 1.80 D, dropping vision to less than 20/50. No appreciable change in refraction resulted from the Ocuserts.[34]

Since continuous presence of the antimetabolite idoxuridine is necessary for control of herpes simplex keratitis, an Ocusert vehicle is particularly well suited to this clinical need. A delivery rate of 30 μg/hr has been empirically determined to be optimal.[35] As with previous regimens of drops or ointment, therapy must be continued for at least 2 weeks, or else relapses will occur.

SUBCONJUNCTIVAL, SUB-TENON'S, AND RETROBULBAR INJECTION

Evaluation of the relative effect of topical application versus subconjunctival injection of drugs is difficult because of the variable amounts of medication used, the uncontrollable factor of injury to ocular barriers during injection, the arbitrary selection of frequency of topical application, and the like. I have the impression that a single subconjunctival injection will achieve higher intraocular drug levels than will a few topical applications. However, repeated topical applications of most ophthalmic drugs will achieve intraocular levels that compare respectably with those of subconjunctival injection. Obviously subconjunctival injection would be considered only in the case of drugs (such as antibiotics) that penetrate poorly. Injection of a mydriatic, for instance, would be ridiculous, since such medications readily penetrate transcorneally.

In contrast, subconjunctival injection of 20 mg of gentamicin in 0.5 ml of solution will give corneal concentrations of 15 μg/g of tissue lasting for 6 hours after injection, compared with 1 μg/g 1 hour after topical instillation of a drop of 0.3% solution.[36]

The disadvantages of subconjunctival injection (patient apprehension, subsequent inflammation and pain, inconvenience, expense and possible intraocular perforation) are great enough to nullify almost all advantages that might be expected from this route of administration. Probably its greatest clinical value is realized in the emergency management of acute infection of the anterior segment.

Subconjunctival injection may be a misnomer. An early author recommended that such an injection should be given beneath Tenon's capsule, since in this position the drug is effectively closer to the eye, is absorbed more rapidly, suffers less loss into the conjunctival circulation, and reaches greater intraocular concentrations.[37] The technique of anterior subcapsular injection utilizes topical anesthesia. Both the conjunctiva and Tenon's capsule are elevated using forceps. The needle enters Tenon's capsule 3 or 5 mm behind the limbus, bevel down, to avoid pricking episcleral vessels. Comparison of the penetration of subconjunctival or sub-Tenon's capsule injection of epinephrine can be made by observing pupil response. Mydriasis began 5 to 6 minutes after sub-Tenon's capsule injection but only 10 to 16 minutes after injection between the conjunctiva and Tenon's capsule.[37]

How does a subconjunctivally injected drug penetrate into the eye? One would suppose diffusion across the sclera would be the main route, with possibly a small amount entering via systemic absorption and arterial return to the eye. No doubt drugs of differing solubility or other characteristics may be absorbed differently. Surprisingly, subconjunctival hydrocortisone enters the eye almost entirely by leaking through the conjunctival puncture into the tear fluid, from which it apparently enters the eye transcorneally.[2] This was determined by subconjunctival injection in rabbits of 0.25 ml of 2.5% hydrocortisone identified by radioactive ^{14}C labeling. In one group of rabbits the subconjunctival depot was delivered by transconjunctival injection; in the other group the needle was introduced through the skin and beneath the conjunctiva, taking care not to perforate the conjunctiva. In both groups the hydrocortisone depot was positioned in the upper temporal quadrant 2 mm from the limbus. At specified intervals the eyes were enucleated, thoroughly washed, homogenized, and measured for radioactivity by scintillation counting. Unfortunately this method does not evaluate drug distribution in the various parts of the eye. As seen in Table 2-2, enormously higher ocular drug concentrations were attained in the rabbits with punctured conjunctivas.

So many variables affect the intraocular penetration of drugs that different experiments lead to diametrically opposite conclusions. For example, when given by subconjunctival injection, radioactive chloramphenicol penetrates the rabbit aqueous in amounts twice as great as those achieved by a sub-Tenon's injection.[38] Unfortunately the exact details of the injection technique were not specified. This report suggested that the route of drug entry was either via the limbal conjunctival overlap or transcorneally via the tears. Affecting the outcome of this experiment were the facts that chloramphenicol is highly lipid soluble and penetrates the intact cornea well and that the rabbit has a

Table 2-2. Ocular penetration of ^{14}C hydrocortisone after subconjunctival injection*

Time (hr)	Hydrocortisone (conjunctiva punctured) (μg)	Hydrocortisone (conjunctiva intact) (μg)
½	176.7	3.9
1	68.0	0.7
2	41.1	0.7
24	33.8	2.8
48	14.5	2.9
72	1.8	0.8
120	1.7	0.8

*From Wine, N. A., Gornall, A. G., and Basu, P. K.: Am. J. Ophthalmol. **58:**362, 1964.

substantial orbital venous plexus capable of rapidly carrying away any medication behind the eye. The values given in this experiment are stated as radioactivity counts per 10 minutes per gram. The sub-Tenon's injection yielded counts averaging 1400 as compared to an average of 3000 obtained by subconjunctival injection. Topical instillation of the chloramphenicol yielded a count of 5700— far greater than that resulting from either route of injection. Once again, this emphasizes that no advantage accrues from injection of drugs whose solubility characteristics readily permit transcorneal passage.

Using comparable techniques with radioactive benzyl penicillin, one of the same authors again demonstrated greater aqueous concentrations in rabbits receiving medication by the subconjunctival rather than by the sub-Tenon's route.[39] Almost 50% more penicillin entered the anterior chamber from the subconjunctival site.

Another study evaluated the effectiveness of different injection sites with the use of radiopaque contrast media (diatrizoate meglumine) and radioactive cortisone.[40] The radiologic studies revealed that contrast material injected anterior to the equator (0.2 ml volume) tended to stay in that position, whereas the retrobulbar injection diffused throughout the entire orbit and contacted the entire posterior sclera. These authors do not report a distinction between the sub-Tenon's and subconjunctival routes of injection but advocate a scleral sieve concept, postulating direct transfer of the corticosteroid across the sclera.

In this study, retrobulbar injections of radioactive cortisone revealed a very rapid drug movement within the tissues. A maximum intraocular concentration was reached within 5 minutes and amounted to 1.2% of the total dose in noninflamed eyes but only 0.45% of the total dose in eyes badly inflamed by experimental uveitis. We usually think of the inflamed eye as offering less resistance to drug entry, but the authors postulated rapid loss into the systemic circulation via the inflamed orbital vessels. Within the eye, the noninflamed uvea-retina

contained 92% of the steroid and the vitreous 8%. The inflamed uvea-retina contained 80% and the inflamed vitreous 20%. The intraocular steroid level dropped rapidly, the 6-hour value being less than 2% of the 5-minute value. Intravenous injection of corticosteroid was ineffective, achieving intraocular levels only one fortieth of those attained by retrobulbar injection (intravenous dosage, 50 μC; retrobulbar injections, 2 μC).

Injection of equal amounts of radioactive zinc by retrobulbar and anterior chamber routes resulted in 10 times greater radioactivity of the retina and choroid via the latter.[41] This indicates the presence of a considerable anteroposterior exchange within the eye itself. As might be expected, the anterior chamber route maintained iris and ciliary body levels several hundred times greater than could be achieved by retrobulbar injection.

Another autoradiographic study indicates that subconjunctivally injected hydrocortisone can penetrate directly through the sclera from the injection depot. Tritium-labeled hydrocortisone was injected subconjunctivally in rabbits, and frozen sections of the eyes were positioned against photographic plates to identify the tissue location of the radioisotope. The penetration of hydrocortisone in normal and inflamed eyes is diagrammatically presented in Fig. 2-8. Demonstrable radioactivity penetrated to the retina within 30 minutes in the inflamed eye (inflammation induced by intravitreal injection of 0.2 ml of 30% bovine albumin 8 days before) but only after 4 hours in the normal eye. Only a very small proportion of the drug penetrates the eye—probably in the range of 1% to 2%. Because the drug penetration seems maximal at the site of injection, a subconjunctival depot should be positioned as closely as possible to the area of inflammation to be treated rather than in the superior temporal quadrant that is usually chosen arbitrarily.[42]

On the other hand, repeated injections of antibiotics cannot readily be given at the same site because of the inflammatory reaction. To determine the drop in intracorneal

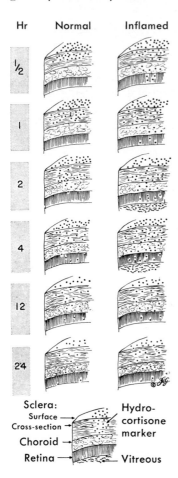

Fig. 2-8. Autoradiographic demonstration of hydrocortisone penetration from subconjunctival depot. (From McCartney, H. J., and associates: Invest. Ophthalmol. 4:297, 1965.)

antibiotic concentration with distance from the injection site, 2 mm corneal buttons were trephined from the cornea 30 minutes after limbal antibiotic injection. After injection of 30 mg of gentamicin, levels of 100 μg/g were achieved 2 mm from the injection site, dropping to 30 μg/g 8 mm away. Injection of 50 mg of penicillin G gave 500 μg/g 2 mm from the injection, dropping to 100 μg/g at 8 mm. Injection of 50 mg of chloramphenicol gave 150 μg/g at 2 mm and 50 μg/g at 8 mm. These are all enormous concentrations of antibiotic and indicate that adequate intracorneal antibiotic levels can be attained throughout the cornea regardless of the meridian of limbal subconjunctival injection.[43]

A sub-Tenon's injection of 0.25 ml of a repository suspension of methylprednisolone (Depo-Medrol) produced drug concentrations in the general range of 20 μg/g of tissue in the anterior uvea, posterior uvea-retina, cornea, and sclera 2 days after injection (radioactive measurements in monkeys).[44] Nine days after injection, corticosteroid levels of 2 to 9 μg/g persisted in these tissues. No detectable increase of radioactivity occurred in the fellow eye, indicating that corticosteroid intraocular penetration after the sub-Tenon's injection is by direct extension into the adjacent eye tissues and not by systemic absorption and hematogenous entry. This suggests that for the greatest therapeutic concentrations the repository corticosteroid should be injected at a sub-Tenon's site directly external to the position of the intraocular inflammation. Since sub-Tenon's injections can be given very far posteriorly, the author recommended this route rather than retrobulbar injection, except in cases of optic nerve or macular inflammation.

Anatomically, I see little difference between a retrobulbar injection and a posterior sub-Tenon's injection insofar as proximity to the macula is concerned. These tissue spaces freely intercommunicate, as can easily be demonstrated by the retrobulbar injection of 5 ml of anesthetic solution prior to cataract extraction. Because of the curvature of the eye, the tip of a retrobulbar needle is unlikely to be any closer to the macula than is a needletip in the posterior sub-Tenon's space. A sub-Tenon's injection can be given painlessly after instillation of topical anesthetic drops and is therefore more comfortable than a retrobulbar injection. A sub-Tenon's injection is safer than is the retrobulbar injection.

During 1973, six cases of needle scleral perforation were seen by our retina service, three of which were associated with depot corticosteroid injection for uveitis. The intravitreal depot vehicle remains visible for at least many months but seems nontoxic. The mechanical trauma to the retina and vitreous caused retinal detachment in these cases. Severe vitreoretinal traction irreparably damaged macular function despite anatomic reposition of the retina. These cases are cited to suggest caution when plunging a sharp needle toward the retrobulbar space, whether this act is performed before cataract extraction or in treatment of posterior uveitis. Incidentally, the retina surgeon finds that either a subconjunctival or sub-Tenon's injection of lidocaine (Xylocaine) in the equatorial location of a retinal tear will permit pain-free transcleral cryotherapy within several minutes.

The clinical value of retrobulbar corticosteroid injection is not clearly established. Individual case reports suggest improved control of posterior segment inflammation[45] without the systemic complications of oral corticosteroid therapy. Adequately controlled studies would be difficult to perform and are as yet unreported. Provocation of open angle glaucoma that is difficult to control may result from depot corticosteroid injection. Surgical excision is the only way to remove this material, but is a bloody and destructive undertaking.

INTRAOCULAR INJECTION

The dangers inherent in intraocular injections far outweigh possible benefits in almost all circumstances. Probably the only clear indication for this route is the administration of antibiotics during surgery required for correction of an infected laceration or a ruptured surgical wound. Only minute amounts of antibiotic are tolerated within the eye (Table 6-2). For example, the maximum safe dose of polymyxin B is 0.1 mg. Even penicillin G is toxic within the eye, which will tolerate only 4000 units (24 mg).

I have destroyed an eye by anterior chamber injection of 4000 units of what was labeled penicillin G used for prophylactic irrigation of an eye with a cilium lying quietly on the iris. A perfectly dreadful toxic reaction ensued.

Twelve cases of fungal endophthalmitis (*Paecilomyces lilacinus*) have followed implantation of intraocular lenses rinsed in a contaminated neutralizing solution.[46]

Treatment of disease of the posterior eye requires systemic administration of either oral or parenteral medication. The principles of such treatment are the same regardless of the organ to be treated and need not be repeated here.

INTRAMUSCULAR INJECTION

The penetration of systemically administered medications into the eye is qualitatively and quantitatively retarded by the blood-aqueous and blood-vitreous barriers. These barriers particularly resist penetration by electrolytes. The various intraocular endothelial and epithelial membranes and the specialized blood vessel walls constitute these barriers. The ocular hypotony after systemic administration of osmotic agents is a good example of a clinically useful effect attributable to the blood-aqueous and blood-vitreous barriers. Resistance to penetration of antibiotics is a well-known undesirable problem caused by these barriers. Fortunately the barrier is at least partially broken by the inflammation resulting from infections.

Attention should be called to the possibility of permanent injury to the sciatic nerve from intragluteal injections in infants. Evidently this tragic accident occurs easily, since two separate reports published in the same year cited a total of 22 cases.[47,48] The sciatic nerve lies near the surface in infants and is readily damaged by the traditional upper outer quadrant injection. Such injury is usually mistakenly diagnosed as a congenital lesion or the result of unrecognized poliomyelitis; however, surgical exploration has disclosed the site of needle injury in several cases. If intramuscular injections are necessary in infants, they should be given in the midportion of the quadriceps, anteriorly. This muscle mass is free of major vessels and motor nerves.

INTRAVENOUS INJECTION

We have tended to assume that the continuous intravenous administration of an antibiotic is an effective way of maintaining intraocular levels. At any rate it is certainly a dramatic and conspicuous route to the pa-

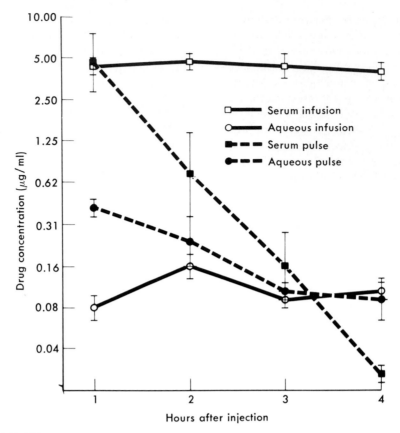

Fig. 2-9. Ampicillin concentrations in serum and aqueous following continuous intravenous infusion of 21 mg/kg in rabbits (solid lines) or following administration of the same total amount of ampicillin as 1-minute intravenous injection (dashed lines). (From Goldman, J., and associates: Ann. Ophthalmol. **5:**147, 1973.)

tient, who can see and feel continuing evidence of this constant treatment. Because of the barrier and reservoir effects of the eye, however, antibiotics such as ampicillin, chloramphenicol, and erythromycin penetrate into the eye at higher initial levels and maintain at least comparable intraocular levels for 4 hours when given as a single intravenous "pulse" rather than by continuous infusion. Rabbits were given 21 mg/kg of ampicillin either by continuous infusion over 4 hours in 150 ml of solution or by an intravenous injection completed during a 1-minute period.[49] The various antibiotic levels measured in serum and aqueous during the subsequent 4 hours are recorded in Fig. 2-9. Note that the 1-hour aqueous levels were four times as high (the chart scale is logarith-

mic) by pulsed administration as by continuous infusion. Earlier values were not measured, but the peak aqueous levels should have occurred about 15 to 30 minutes after injection and were probably much higher, as judged by the slope of the curve.

Comparable slopes, indicating better aqueous entry and a 4-hour persistence of aqueous levels with pulsed dosage, were obtained for erythromycin and chloramphenicol. The chloramphenicol levels shown in Fig. 2-10 reflect the values obtained after administration of 500 mg/kg of antibiotic. While this is 25 times the dosage of ampicillin previously discussed, the peak aqueous levels are 100 times greater. Presumably this indicates better intraocular penetration of chloramphenicol.

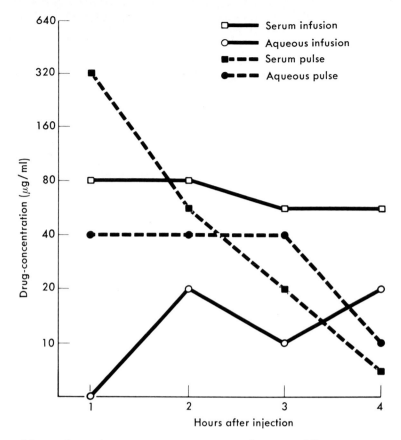

Fig. 2-10. Chloramphenicol concentrations in serum and aqueous following continuous intravenous infusion of 500 mg/kg in rabbits (solid lines) or following administration of the same total amount of chloramphenicol as 1-minute intravenous injection (dashed lines). (From Goldman, J., and associates: Ann. Ophthalmol. **5:**147, 1973.)

At any rate these findings strongly suggest the superiority of a single intravenous injection as compared to continuous intravenous infusion for the purpose of achieving high initial intraocular drug levels that will be maintained for at least 4 hours.

DELAYED-RELEASE ORAL PREPARATIONS

The practical value of sustained-release preparations should be noted. For example, a single dose of acetazolamide will reduce intraocular pressure for up to 10 hours, whereas a single dose of sustained-release acetazolamide will produce a comparable effect lasting 20 hours (Fig. 25-8). Currently available sustained-release dosage forms make the medication available at a reliable rate, equivalent to more frequent fractional dosage. Delivery of the sustained-release medication is more even than the peaks and valleys of uncoated medication.[50] Since it is less inconvenient for the patient to take a single pill than multiple pills at frequent intervals, hopefully, patient cooperation will be improved.

RETROGRADE ARTERIAL PERFUSION

Retrograde perfusion via the infraorbital artery (Fig. 2-11) attains high intraocular drug concentration of the medication (Fig. 2-12). Whether this experimental approach is clinically practicable remains to be seen. However, regional infusion might be a useful method for treatment of acute intraocular

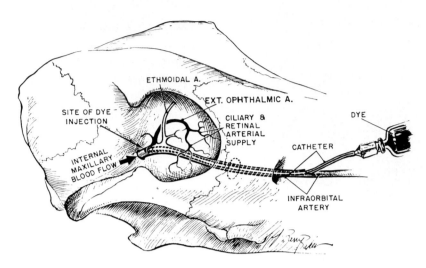

Fig. 2-11. Method of retrograde arterial perfusion of the dog eye by catheterization of infraorbital artery. (From Pilkerton, R., and associates: Am. J. Ophthalmol. **55**:338, 1963.)

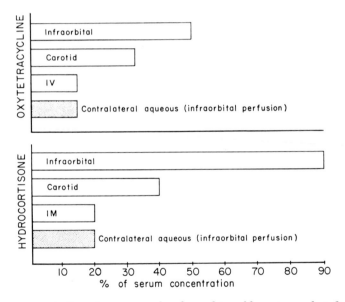

Fig. 2-12. Drug concentrations in aqueous chamber achieved by retrograde infraorbital artery perfusion, carotid perfusion, intravenous infusion, and intramuscular injection. (Expressed as percent of serum concentration.) (Modified from Pilkerton, R., and associates: Am. J. Ophthalmol. **55**:388, 1963.)

infection or in the chemotherapy of intraocular malignancy.[52]

REFERENCES

1. Moses, R. A.: Adler's physiology of the eye, ed. 6, St. Louis, 1975, The C. V. Mosby Co.
2. Wine, N. A., Gornall, A. G., and Basu, P. K.: The ocular uptake of subconjunctivally injected C^{14} hydrocortisone, Am. J. Ophthalmol. **58**:362, 1964.
3. Bill, A.: Movement of albumin and dextran through the sclera, Arch. Ophthalmol. **74**:248, 1965.
4. Smelser, G. K., and Pei, Y. F.: Cytological

basis of protein leakage into the eye following paracentesis, Invest. Ophthalmol. **4:**249, 1965.

5. Janes, R. G., and Stiles, J. F.: The penetration of cortisol into normal and pathologic rabbit eyes, Am. J. Ophthalmol. **56:**84, 1963.

6. Short, C., Keates, R. H., Donovan, E. F., Wyman, M., and Murdick, P. W.: Ocular penetration studies, Arch. Ophthalmol. **75:**689, 1966.

7. Morrison, W. H.: Stability of aqueous solutions commonly employed in the treatment of primary glaucoma, Am. J. Ophthalmol. **37:**557, 1954.

8. Ramer, R. M., and Gasset, A. R.: Ocular penetration of pilocarpine: the effect of pH on the ocular penetration of pilocarpine, Ann. Ophthalmol. **7:**293, February 1975.

9. Sieg, J. W., and Robinson, J. R.: Corneal absorption of fluorometholone in rabbits, Arch. Ophthalmol. **92:**240, September 1974.

10. Krupin, T., Waltman, S. R., and Becker, B.: Ocular penetration in rabbits of topically applied dexamethasone, Arch. Ophthalmol. **92:**312, October 1974.

11. Hardberger, R. E., Hanna, C., and Goodart, R.: Effects of drug vehicles on ocular uptake of tetracycline, Am. J. Ophthalmol. **80:**133, July 1975.

12. Massey, J. Y., Hanna, C., Goodart, R., and Wallace, T.: Effect of drug vehicle on human ocular retention of topically applied tetracycline, Am. J. Ophthalmol. **81:**151, February 1976.

13. Waltman, S. R., Buerk, K., and Foster, C. S.: Effects of ophthalmic ointments on intraocular penetration of topical fluorescein in rabbits and man, Am. J. Ophthalmol. **78:**262, August 1974.

14. Cox, W. V., Kupferman, A., and Leibowitz, H. M.: Topically applied steroids in corneal disease II. The role of drug vehicle in stromal absorption of dexamethasone, Arch. Ophthalmol. **88:**549, November 1972.

15. Kupferman, A., and Leibowitz, H. M.: Topically applied steroids in corneal disease. V. Dexamethasone alcohol, Arch. Ophthalmol. **92:**329, October 1974.

16. Hanna, C., Fraunfelder, F. T., Cable, M., and Hardberger, R. E.: The effect of ophthalmic ointments on corneal wound healing, Am. J. Ophthalmol. **76:**193, August 1973.

17. Fraunfelder, F. T., Hanna, C., Cable, M., and Hardberger, R. E.: Entrapment of ophthalmic ointment in the cornea, Am. J. Ophthalmol. **76:**475, October 1973.

18. Scheie, H. G., Rubenstein, A., and Katowitz, J. A.: Ophthalmic ointment bases in the anterior chamber, Arch. Ophthalmol. **73:**36, 1965.

19. Castroviejo, R.: Ointment bases in the anterior chamber, Arch. Ophthalmol. **74:**143, 1965.

20. Lippas, J.: Continuous irrigation in the treatment of external ocular diseases, Am. J. Ophthalmol. **57:**298, 1964.

21. Robb, R. M., and Kuwabara, T.: Corneal wound healing. Arch. Ophthalmol. **68:**636, 1962.

22. Sapse, A. T., Ivanyi, J., Stone, W., Jr., Bonavida, B., and Sercarz, R. E.: Tears as carriers of antibodies, Arch. Ophthalmol. **77:**526, 1967.

23. Ralph, R. A., Doane, M. G., and Dohlman, C. H.: Clinical experience with a mobile ocular perfusion pump, Arch. Ophthalmol. **93:**1039, October 1975.

24. O'Brien, C. S., and Swan, K. C.: Carbaminoyl choline chloride in the treatment of glaucoma simplex, Arch. Ophthalmol. **27:**253, 1942.

25. Waltman, S. R., and Kaufman, H. E.: Use of hydrophilic contact lenses to increase ocular penetration of topical drugs, Invest. Ophthalmol. **9:**250, 1970.

26. Podos, S. M., Becker, B., Asseff, G., and Hartstein, J.: Pilocarpine therapy with soft contact lenses, Am. J. Ophthalmol. **73:**336, 1972.

27. Mizutani, Y., and Miwa, Y.: On the uptake and release of drugs by soft contact lenses, Contact Intraocular Lens Med. J. **1:**177, January 1975.

28. Hull, D. S., Edelhauser, H. F., and Hyndiuk, R. A.: Ocular penetration of prednisolone and the hydrophilic contact lens, Arch. Ophthalmol. **92:**413, November 1974.

29. Shell, J. W., and Baker, R. W.: Diffusional systems for controlled release of drugs to the eye, Ann Ophthalmol. **6:**1037, October 1974.

30. Sendelbeck, L., Moore, D., and Urquhart, J.: Comparative distribution of pilocarpine in ocular tissues of the rabbit during administration by eyedrop or by membrane-controlled delivery systems, Am. J. Ophthalmol. **80:**274, August 1975.

31. Macoul, K. L., and Pavan-Langston, D.: Pilocarpine Ocusert system for sustained con-

trol of ocular hypertension, Arch. Ophthalmol. **93:**587, August 1975.

32. Quigley, H. A., Pollack, I. P., and Harbin, T. S., Jr.: Pilocarpine Ocuserts, Arch. Ophthalmol. **93:**771, September 1975.

33. Place, V. A., Fisher, M., Herbst, S., Gordon, L., and Merrill, R. C.: Comparative pharmacologic effects of pilocarpine administered to normal subjects by eyedrops or by ocular therapeutic systems, Am. J. Ophthalmol. **80:** 706, October 1975.

34. Brown, H. S., Meltzer, G., Merrill, R. C., Fisher, M., Ferre, C., and Place, V. A.: Visual effects of pilocarpine in glaucoma, Arch. Ophthalmol. **94:**1716, October 1976.

35. Pavan-Langston, D., Langston, R. H., and Geary, P. A.: Idoxuridine ocular insert therapy: use in treatment of experimental herpes simplex keratitis, Arch. Ophthalmol. **93:**1349, December 1975.

36. Baum, J. L., Barza, M., Shushan, D., and Weinstein, L.: Concentration of gentamicin in experimental corneal ulcers, Arch. Ophthalmol. **92:**315, October 1974.

37. Swan, K. C., Chrisman, H. R., and Bailey, P. F., Jr.: Subepithelial versus subcapsular injections of drugs, Arch. Ophthalmol. **56:** 26, 1956.

38. Hardy, R. G., Jr., and Paterson, C. A.: Ocular penetration of ^{14}C-labeled chloramphenicol following subconjunctival or sub-Tenon's injection, Am. J. Ophthalmol. **71:**1307, 1971.

39. Paterson, C. A.: Intraocular penetration of ^{14}C-labeled penicillin after sub-Tenon's or subconjunctival injection, Ann. Ophthalmol. **5:**171, 1973.

40. Levine, N. D., and Aronson, S. B.: Orbital infusion of steroids in the rabbit, Arch. Ophthalmol. **83:**599, 1970.

41. O'Rourke, J., Durrani, J., Benson, C., Bronzino, J., and Miller, C.: Studies in uveal physiology, Arch. Ophthalmol. **88:**185, 1972.

42. McCartney, H. J., Drysdale, I. O., Gornall, A. G., and Basu, P. K.: An autoradiographic study of the penetration of subconjunctivally injected hydrocortisone into the normal and inflamed rabbit eye, Invest. Ophthalmol. **4:** 297, 1965.

43. Oakley, D. E., Weeks, R. D., and Ellis, P. P.: Corneal distribution of subconjunctival antibiotics, Am. J. Ophthalmol. **81:**307, March 1976.

44. Hyndiuk, R. A.: Radioactive depot-corticosteroid penetration into monkey ocular tissue, Arch. Ophthalmol. **82:**259, 1969.

45. Deutsch, A. R.: Evaluation of retrobulbar repository steroid injections, Eye Ear Nose Throat Mon. **48:**219, 1969.

46. Pettit, T. H., and Martin, W. J.: Alert issued on fundus in intraocular lens solution, Clin. Trends, January 1976, p. 6.

47. Combes, M. A., Clark, W. K., Gregory, C. F., and James, J. A.: Sciatic nerve injury in infants, J.A.M.A. **173:**1336, 1960.

48. Curtiss, P. H., Jr., and Tucker, H. J.: Sciatic palsy in premature infants, J.A.M.A. **174:** 1586, 1960.

49. Goldman, J. N., Broughton, W., Javed, H., and Lauderdale, V.: Ampicillin, erythromycin and chloramphenicol penetration into rabbit aqueous humor, Ann. Ophthalmol. **5:**147, 1973.

50. Rosen, E., Tannenbaum, P., Ellison, T., Free, S. M., and Crosley, A. P., Jr.: Absorption and excretion of radioactively tagged dextroamphetamine sulfate from a sustained-release preparation, J.A.M.A. **194:**1203, 1965.

51. Pilkerton, R., Bulle, P. H., Jones, J. H., and O'Rourke, J.: Intraocular drug levels, Am. J. Ophthalmol. **55:**338, 1963.

52. O'Rourke, J., Pilkerton, R., Simmons, R., and Kraus, A.: Anatomic features relating to cannulation-infusion of the orbital arteries, Am. J. Ophthalmol. **60:**592, 1965.

3
ADHESIVES

Synthetic surgical glues have a variety of promising applications in ophthalmology. However, at the present time most of the uses of surgical adhesives in ophthalmology are experimental. The acceptability of gluing techniques is determined not only by the virtues and faults of the adhesive but also by the technologic advances in the alternate method of wound closure (sutures) and by improvements in the general techniques of ophthalmology (for example, smaller, beveled cataract incisions and the replacement of epikeratoprostheses by soft lenses).

OCULAR TOLERANCE

Various cyanoacrylate derivatives have been evaluated for surgical use on the eye. Methyl-2-cyanoacrylate, an early discovery, produces a rather marked tissue reaction and is definitely more toxic than are the longer chain derivatives. Butyl-2-cyanoacrylate is currently the most readily available derivative and is quite well tolerated. Hexyl, octyl, and decyl derivatives are even less irritating.

Although reasonably well tolerated on the corneal surface, the various cyanoacrylates may cause considerable irritation when injected within the stroma or into the anterior chamber.[1] Variable degrees of vascularization, ulceration, edema, and inflammation result.

Small amounts of cyanoacrylate adhesives are quite well tolerated by the eye. Relatively large amounts, covering a quarter or more of the corneal area, cause intense in-flammatory reaction with vascularization and erosion of adjacent tissues. Topical corticosteroid therapy adequately controlled the inflammation induced by reasonably small amounts of adhesive. The methyl derivative is considerably more toxic than the butyl and heptyl cyanoacrylates and should not be used in corneal surgery.[2]

When small amounts of isobutyl, hexyl, octyl, and decyl cyanoacrylates were injected into the corneal midstroma of rabbits by means of a 27-gauge needle, no more tissue reaction resulted than was caused by silk or catgut sutures.[3] As might be expected, epithelial downgrowth entered the intracorneal tract of the adhesive (Fig. 3-1). Introduction of 0.1 ml of cyanoacrylate into the rabbit anterior chamber usually caused a moderate inflammatory reaction. Localized corneal edema and neovascularization developed, associated histologically with loss of the corneal endothelium. In one eye, permanent and total corneal opacity and vascularization resulted.

To exclude the effects of infection, germ-free guinea pigs were selected for cyanoacrylate toxicity studies.[4] Intracorneal injection of 0.01 ml or surface application (corneal epithelium removed) of 0.015 ml were the adhesive techniques used. The characteristic result was a diffuse polymorphonuclear cellular response accompanied by heavy corneal neovascularization. This severe corneal scarring occurred with all three polymers—isobutyl, octyl, and decyl.

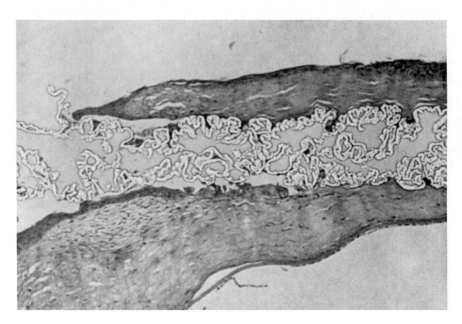

Fig. 3-1. Intracorneal needle tract filled with decyl cyanoacrylate adhesive 2 months postoperatively. (From Gasset, A., and associates: Invest. Ophthalmol. **9:**3, 1970.)

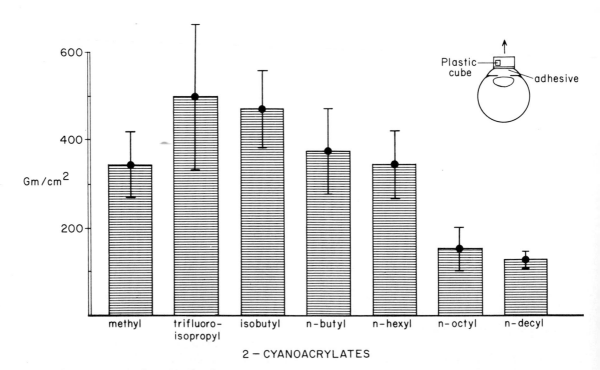

Fig. 3-2. Tensile strength of various cyanoacrylate adhesive joints between corneal stroma and polymethylmethacrylate. (Modified from Refojo, M. F., and Dohlman, C. H.: Am. J. Ophthalmol. **68:**248, 1969.)

When used to seal experimental choroidal perforations in rabbits, small amounts of isobutyl cyanoacrylate entered the eye.[5] Localized choroidal disorganization and retinal degeneration resulted, and vitreous inflammation with subsequent band formation caused focal crumpling of the retina.

Ocular tolerance of plastic substances is dependent not only on their chemical reactivity but also their shape. A smooth-surfaced implant may be well tolerated, whereas the same implant with irregular, sharp edges may produce severe inflammation.[6] The cyanoacrylate adhesives are unable to penetrate the intact cornea or sclera, and the tissue toxicity they cause is ordinarily limited to the immediate vicinity of the adhesive. These authors implanted radioactive cyanoacrylate intrastromally in rabbit corneas and demonstrated that no radioactivity had entered the intraocular tissues after 9 weeks.

ADHESIVE STRENGTH

The tensile strength of these various adhesives has been evaluated by gluing a polymethylmethacrylate cube to dried corneal stroma. As shown in Fig. 3-2, the trifluoroisopropyl and the isobutyl derivatives were much stronger than the octyl and decyl derivatives.[7]

A considerably stronger bond may be achieved by permitting the cornea to dry for several minutes before applying the adhesive. In Fig. 3-3, zero time refers to immediate application on the corneal stroma (epithelium removed) after wetting with Neosporin antibiotic solution. Note that drying

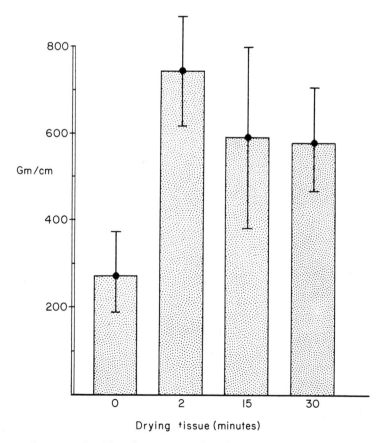

Fig. 3-3. Tensile strength of butyl-2-cyanoacrylate bonds between polymethylmethacrylate and corneal stroma after varying periods of drying. (Modified from Refojo, M. F., and Dohlman, C. H.: Am. J. Ophthalmol. **68:**248, 1969.)

for 2 minutes more than doubled the strength of the bond. Further drying, for as long as 30 minutes, did not confer additional strength but actually weakened the bond. Since the test rupture of these bonds commonly tore within the superficial stroma, one might conclude that excessive drying damages and weakens the stromal surface.

Octyl cyanoacrylate monomer (Ethicon) is a well-tolerated tissue adhesive that is non-irritating to the cornea. This adhesive remains liquid so long as it is in a pool on a plastic surface. Polymerization occurs instantly when it is squeezed into a thin film or when it is exposed to water. However, water causes the adhesive to become whitish and powdery; hence the surfaces to be bonded should be kept absolutely dry until several minutes after application of the adhesive. Since polymerization is immediate, no adjustments are possible after the initial contact.

This octyl cyanoacrylate monomer has been used to glue a plastic keratoprosthesis to Bowman's membrane.[8] Such prostheses have remained adherent for as long as 5 months. The duration of the bond depends, of course, not only on the persistence of the adhesive but also on the survival of the tissue to which the adhesive is bonded. Corneal epithelium, for instance, is such transient tissue that it will not sustain a bond for any length of time. Bowman's membrane, in contrast, is a very inert and long-lasting tissue and will maintain a prolonged bond. The octyl monomer loses its ability to polymerize firmly when the original container has been opened for some time; hence a new tube of adhesive should be used for each day's work.

TECHNIQUES OF USE

Experience in application of the cyanoacrylate adhesives is important to their successful use. Improper technique will result in failures. The following general principles[9] are helpful in use of adhesives:

1. Loose tissue and cellular layers must be removed from the ocular surface to be glued. An adhesive bond can be no more durable than its recipient surface.

2. The field must be dry. Moisture causes polymerization of the cyanoacrylate before it can contact and adhere reliably to the surface.

3. *Minimal* amounts of adhesive must be used. Toxicity is directly related to the amount of glue present. The thinnest possible film of polymer will be effective and must be sought in order to achieve an acceptable level of tissue response. The spread of excess adhesive to surrounding areas must be avoided.

4. Since the polymer will adhere immediately to tissue and to metal, contact with surrounding tissues and instruments must be avoided.

5. Appropriate instrumentation is necessary.

6. Precise and skillful surgical technique is necessary and must be performed with great speed. These adhesives set within seconds.

Cyanoacrylate application to a corneal wound is aided by use of a small, disposable polyethylene disc of whatever size needed to cover the lesion.[10] The disc is used as a carrier for the glue, permits pressure to be applied during the 15 seconds of polymerization, and readily separates from the glue surface. The disc is manipulated by an ordinary applicator stick, made to adhere loosely to the outside of the disc with a small amount of any ophthalmic ointment (Fig. 3-4).

It is possible to smooth the rough edges that may exist after application of adhesive to the ocular surface by wiping the adhesive surface with a cotton swab moistened with acetone.[11] Acetone is a good solvent for polymerized cyanoacrylate and will rapidly dissolve surface irregularities. Acetone will rapidly damage the corneal epithelium and causes temporary stromal haziness that disappears within 4 to 6 days. Introduced into the anterior chamber, acetone causes immediate corneal opacity, followed by severe iritis, glaucoma, and corneal necrosis. Clearly, acetone should not be used in the presence of a perforating wound. Also, acetone application to experimental corneal perfora-

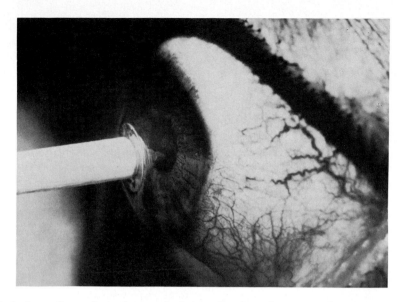

Fig. 3-4. Sealing of a perforated corneal ulcer with n-heptyl-cyanoacrylate, applied with the aid of a polyethylene disc. (From Boruchoff, S. A.: Trans. Am. Acad. Ophthalmol. Otolaryngol. **73:**499, 1969.)

tions sealed with adhesive patches results in reopening of the wound leak.

Acetone swabbing may also be used as a substitute for mechanical excision of adhesive from a tissue surface. Two to five minutes of gentle swabbing is necessary.

OCULAR USES
Corneal surgery

Closure of small corneal perforating wounds has been achieved clinically with thin films of cyanoacrylate adhesive. In one reported case a 1 × 2 mm perforation in a necrotic chronic herpetic ulcer was closed with cyanoacrylate.[12] Although the adhesive patch fell off on the second postoperative day, the aqueous leak had stopped. Successful keratoplasty was performed 7 months later, at a time when the recipient cornea had become less necrotic and friable.

In treating corneal wounds one must choose between adhesive repair, 10-0 nylon suturing, and watchful waiting. A small, slanting, spontaneously closed wound requires no surgery. A large laceration requires sutures. Perhaps the best indication for adhesive closure is a small, ragged, stellate perforation of the type difficult to make watertight with sutures.

For a brief time one of the most promising uses of adhesives was in the placement of epikeratoprostheses. The entire cornea, denuded of epithelium, can be covered by a hard contact lens cemented to Bowman's membrane about its periphery. Such a prosthesis may remain in place for months as a substitute for irreparably damaged epithelium (as in Fuchs' dystrophy). Minor problems of epithelial and vascular undergrowth occur, but in general epikeratoprostheses are surprisingly well tolerated and optically beneficial.[13-15] With the advent of the soft contact lens, comparable protection of the corneal surface has been achieved more easily by applying a soft lens, aptly termed a "bandage" lens.

Cataract incision closure

An incision of the length required in cataract surgery requires apposition by several sutures before an adhesive can be applied. In an experiment with dogs a thin line of isobutyl cyanoacrylate was applied to the cataract incision and then closed with two sutures.[16] Technical difficulty was encountered as the adhesive spreads uncontrollably and runs onto the surface of the eye. Proportionately to the amount of adhesive used, initial inflammatory and subsequent granulomatous response occurred. With the use of minimal amounts of adhesive, the inflammation subsided within 3 weeks, leaving a well-healed wound. The cyanoacrylate did not penetrate into a well-approximated wound but did bridge the corneoscleral junction.

The tensile strength of the wound was measured with an air injection bursting technique. The bursting pressure was between 200 and 300 mm Hg immediately after surgery and remained at this level for at least 10 days, at which time the experiment was ended. In contrast, the bursting strength of the incision closed with two sutures was only 10 to 50 mm Hg for as long as 4 days following surgery. Only after 10 days did the strength of the sutured incision approach that of the glued incision.

In comparison to current 10-0 nylon suturing techniques, the inflammation resulting from adhesive application is unacceptable. Nevertheless, the principle of adhesive closure has been demonstrated as practicable in the case of corneoscleral incisions.

Muscle surgery

Because of the thin sclera not uncommonly found beneath muscles and because of the ever-present hazard of scleral perforation, sutureless muscle surgery is an attractive concept. The bond strength achieved with isobutyl or decyl cyanoacrylate was studied in 63 rabbit eyes.[17] An end-on gluing technique was used rather than side-to-side gluing. Measurement of the tensile strength of the adhesion produced disappointing findings. Half of the adhesions separated with less than 12 g of pull; almost none resisted 60 g. In contrast, standard suture approximations withstood 100 to 200 g of pull before rupturing. Five days elapsed before the glued muscles adhered to the sclera with as much as 100 g of strength.

Since the normal movements of a human eye generate 40 to 65 g of pull and a wide sweep of the eye may generate as much as 100 g of pull, it is apparent that these glue bonds are not strong enough to be reliable in surgery on humans.

While not useful for the adherence of muscles to sclera, a thin cyanoacrylate film may be valuable in preventing adhesions.[18] In this technique a thin film of adhesive is painted on the bare sclera underneath the muscle. The adhesive must be allowed to polymerize before the muscle or conjunctiva contact it. During experimental periods of up to 7 months no adhesions developed between the treated sclera and the overlying muscles. The authors believed that this technique would be feasible in selected human cases with restricted motility caused by extensive fibrovascular scarring.

Retinal detachment surgery

The scleral surface is suitable for the type of adhesive application useful in a variety of scleral buckling techniques.[5,19,20] Various shapes of silicone or scleral donor material can be glued on the recipient sclera for patching, reinforcing, or indenting purposes. Accidental scleral perforations can be closed with thin cyanoacrylate films. Circling elements can be anchored to the sclera or fastened together with adhesive. The sclera is quite inert, and I would expect the use of adhesives in this area to be limited only by the ingenuity of the surgeon.

Extraction of nonmagnetic foreign bodies

A glass tube with a 0.9 mm external diameter that is connected to a microsyringe has been devised for the extraction of nonmagnetic foreign bodies.[21] The instrument is filled with silicone oil, a small amount of butyl cyanoacrylate is aspirated into the tip, and finally a tiny air bubble is aspirated (this prevents premature contact with moisture and setting of the adhesive). Under indirect ophthalmoscopic observation the tip of the glass tube is approximated to the intravitreal foreign body or dislocated lens. Extrusion of the tiniest droplet of adhesive to contact the foreign body spontaneously initiates polymerization because of the intraocular moisture. Within a few seconds, the adhesive develops a frosted appearance, indicating that it has set. The glass tube and adherent particle may then be withdrawn from the pars plana incision. The vitreous does not adhere to the cyanoacrylate. The strength of the adhesion between the glass tube and a dislocated lens was 5.7 g, approximately that achieved by a capsule forceps grip.

Update

No significant new uses of tissue adhesives have developed since the last edition, and these glues have not been approved by the Food and Drug Administration, except for experimental use. High-quality sutures and bandage soft lenses have virtually eliminated any useful place for these adhesives in ophthalmology.

REFERENCES

1. Girard, L. J., Cobb, S., Reed, T., Williams, B., and Minaya, J.: Surgical adhesives and bonded contact lenses: an experimental study, Ann. Ophthalmol. **1:**65, 1969.
2. Refojo, M. F., Dohlman, C. H., Ahmad, B., Carroll, J. M., and Allen, J. C.: Evaluation of adhesives for corneal surgery, Arch. Ophthalmol. **80:**645, 1968.
3. Gasset, A., Hood, C. I., Ellison, E. D., and Kaufman, H. E.: Ocular tolerance to cyanoacrylate monomer tissue adhesive analogues, Invest. Ophthalmol. **9:**3, 1970.
4. Aronson, S. B., McMaster, P. R. B., Moore, T. E., Jr., and Coon, M. A.: Toxicity of the cyanoacrylates, Arch. Ophthalmol. **84:**342, 1970.
5. Seelenfreund, M. H., Refojo, M. F., and Schepens, C. L.: Sealing choroidal perforations with cyanoacrylate adhesives, Arch. Ophthalmol. **83:**619, 1970.
6. Sani, B. P., and Refojo, M. F.: B[14] C-isobutyl 2-cyanoacrylate adhesive, Arch. Ophthalmol. **87:**216, 1972.
7. Refojo, M. F., and Dohlman, C. H.: The tensile strength of adhesive joints between eye tissues and alloplastic materials, Am. J. Ophthalmol. **68:**248, 1969.
8. Kaufman, H. E., and Gasset, A. R.: Clinical experience with the epikeratoprosthesis, Am. J. Ophthalmol. **67:**38, 1969.
9. Refojo, M. F., Dohlman, C. H., and Koliopoulos, J.: Adhesives in ophthalmology: a review, Surv. Ophthalmol. **15:**217, 1971.
10. Boruchoff, S. A., and Refojo, M.: Clinical applications of adhesives in corneal surgery, Trans. Am. Acad. Ophthalmol. Otolaryngol. **73:**499, 1969.
11. Turss, U., Turss, R., and Refojo, M. F.: Removal of isobutyl cyanoacrylate adhesive from the cornea with acetone, Am. J. Ophthalmol. **70:**725, 1970.
12. Ferry, A. P., and Barnert, A. H.: Granulomatous keratitis resulting from use of cyanoacrylate adhesive for closure of perforated corneal ulcer, Am. J. Ophthalmol. **72:**538, 1971.
13. Kaufman, H. E., and Gasset, A. R.: Clinical experience with the epikeratoprosthesis, Trans. Am. Acad. Ophthalmol. Otolaryngol. **73:**1133, 1969.
14. Dohlman, C. H., Carroll, J. M., Richards, J., and Refojo, M. F.: Further experience with glued-on contact lens (artificial epithelium), Arch. Ophthalmol. **83:**10, 1970.
15. Bloome, M. A., and Piepergerdes, L. G.: Epikeratoprosthesis in rhesus monkeys, Am. J. Ophthalmol. **70:**997, 1970.
16. Price, J. A., Jr., and Wadsworth, J. A. C.: Evaluation of an adhesive in cataract wound closure, Am. J. Ophthalmol. **68:**663, 1969.
17. Dunlap, E. A., Dunn, M., and Rossomondo, R.: Adhesives for sutureless muscle surgery, Arch. Ophthalmol. **82:**751, 1969.
18. Dunlap, E. A., Dunn, M., and Rossomondo, R.: New uses for ocular adhesives, Arch. Ophthalmol. **82:**756, 1969.
19. Calabria, G. A., Pruett, R. C., Refojo, M. F., and Schepens, C. L.: Sutureless scleral buckling, Arch. Ophthalmol. **83:**613, 1970.
20. Spitznas, M.: Cyanoacrylate in retinal surgery, Trans. Am. Acad. Ophthalmol. Otolaryngol. **77:**114, 1973.
21. DeGuillebon, H., Zauberman, H., and Refojo, M. F.: Cyanoacrylate adhesive: use in the removal of lens and foreign particles from the vitreous cavity, Arch. Ophthalmol. **87:**407, 1972.

4
ALPHA-CHYMOTRYPSIN

Alpha-chymotrypsin is a proteolytic enzyme useful in ophthalmology because of its relatively selective lytic action on zonular fibers.

PHARMACOLOGY
Enzymatic action

The main proteolytic effect of alpha-chymotrypsin is to split peptide bonds only at the location of certain amino acids. The most susceptible bonds are those of L-tyrosine, L-phenylalanine, and L-tryptophan; L-methionine and L-leucine may also be affected. Alpha-chymotrypsin may also hydrolyze some other types of chemical linkage. These amino acids occur widely throughout ocular tissues and not only in the zonular fibers; therefore it would be expected that alpha-chymotrypsin would damage other protein structures within the eye besides the zonular fibers.

Potency

The potency of commercial preparations of alpha-chymotrypsin is measured in Armour proteolytic activity (APA) units. One unit releases 1 μg of tyrosine from a hemoglobin substrate. Assay of alpha-chymotrypsin powders shows their potency to vary between 750 and 1300 APA units/mg. Because of this variability, concentrations are expressed as units rather than by weight. For instance, crystalline Alpha-Chymar assays at 1150 APA units/mg, whereas Quimotrase assays at 750 APA units/mg. Optimum zonulysis is obtained with 150 APA units/ml, which is the strength of a 1:5000 dilution of Quimotrase. The so-called comparable to 1:5000 concentrations of the other brands also contain 150 APA units/ml, but the actual weight of drug dispensed in the commercial vial varies, depending on its potency. Hence the 150 APA units/ml or 1:5000 dilution of the various preparations will by definition provide equal proteolytic activity for all, regardless of the potency per milligram of drug.[1]

Stability

Solutions of alpha-chymotrypsin are relatively unstable. After 9 days at room temperature, solutions have lost half of their enzymatic activity.[2] Refrigeration at 2° C maintains full activity of the solution for at least a month. The rate of loss in enzyme activity occurring at 2° and 25° C is depicted in Fig. 4-1. From the practical standpoint these findings indicate that the surgeon need not fear decomposition of alpha-chymotrypsin during the course of an operation, even if a solution is not prepared immediately before use. Since alpha-chymotrypsin is relatively inexpensive, it is usually no more practical to save it from one operation to another than it is to save other solutions. However, if the surgeon wishes, such solutions may be used after as long as a week of storage at room temperature without loss of clinical effectiveness. The commercial preparations are sterilized by filtration, do not contain preservative

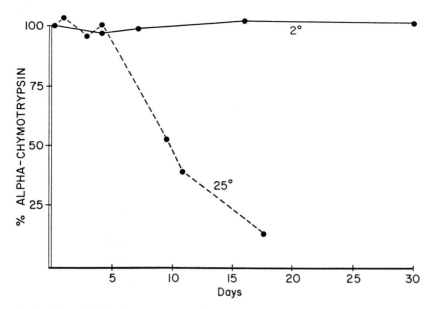

Fig. 4-1. Stability of alpha-chymotrypsin. Lines represent percent of enzyme activity remaining after storage at room temperature (25° C) and under refrigeration (2° C). (Data from Watts, L. F., Jr., and Martin, C. J.: Arch. Ophthalmol. **65**:24, 1961.)

chemicals, and therefore may easily become contaminated if saved for multiple use. To ensure sterility, solutions should be prepared immediately before use.

Preparation

The enzymatic effect of alpha-chymotrypsin is readily inactivated by many chemicals present in operating rooms, and inactivation has been reported to cause instances of complete failure of zonulysis. Inactivating chemicals include soaps, detergents, alkalies, acids, and antiseptics (such as alcohol). If a detergent is used to cleanse containers and syringes, it should be rinsed off before sterilization. If chemical sterilization is employed, naturally the equipment used in preparation of the enzyme must be thoroughly rinsed before use.

Inexperienced operating room personnel not infrequently will give the surgeon the diluent solution and discard unused the "empty" bottle containing the alpha-chymotrypsin powder! Mistakes also occur in identification of the various solutions on the operating table, which may include local anesthetic, special irrigating saline solutions, and epi-

nephrine in addition to the alpha-chymotrypsin. Confusion may arise between the two enzymes hyaluronidase and alpha-chymotrypsin; hence the surgeon should not ask for "the enzyme."

Autoclaving of powdered alpha-chymotrypsin or of the reconstituted solution destroys enzymatic activity.

The reconstituted solution should not be used if it is cloudy or contains a precipitate.

Inactivators

The activity of alpha-chymotrypsin is inhibited by a number of chemicals, including isoflurophate (also known as diisopropyl fluorophosphate, DFP) and chloramphenicol. These inhibitors could be used, if desired, to inactivate the enzyme after zonulysis. The reaction of isoflurophate and alpha-chymotrypsin is on a mol/mol basis. Since the molecular weight of alpha-chymotrypsin is 25,000 and that of isoflurophate is 250, a neutralizing amount of isoflurophate would weigh only as much as 1/100 of the amount of enzyme being inactivated. Specifically, a 1:5000 solution of alpha-chymotrypsin (1 mg/ 5 ml) would be inactivated by an equal volume of a 1:500,000 concentration of isofluro-phate.[3] In clinical usage, chemical neutral-ization of the enzyme is not necessary, since simple irrigation with saline solution is suf-ficient to remove excess enzyme. In fact, the normal structure of the eye rapidly inac-tivates alpha-chymotrypsin. Fluid aspirated from the anterior chamber immediately after cataract extraction has no proteolytic activ-ity.[4]

The other medications commonly used during cataract surgery do not inhibit alpha-chymotrypsin. These medications include pilocarpine, tetracaine, acetylcholine, and a 1:1000 concentration of epinephrine. Al-pha-chymotrypsin is inactivated by a 1:100 concentration of epinephrine. Although the rate of inactivation is not stated, experimen-tally[5] no proteolytic activity remains after 1 hour. Serum and blood rapidly inactivate alpha-chymotrypsin, and if they are present within the eye at the time of surgery, they may interfere with zonulysis.

Systemic toxicity

Alpha-chymotrypsin is quite nontoxic, requiring intravenous injection of 24,000 units/kg as a median lethal dose for rabbits. Death results from hemorrhage, presumably caused by fibrinogen depletion.

Although allergic reaction to chymotrypsin is extremely rare, classic cases have been reported. One such patient had received 17 intramuscular injections of chymotrypsin for treatment of acute epididymitis.[6] Five min-utes after the last injection he became dys-pneic, developed a generalized rash, and progressed to pulmonary edema with cyano-sis and unconsciousness. Intravenous hydro-cortisone and epinephrine were given and proved lifesaving. The patient had no other history of allergy. Other reports confirm the presence of anaphylactic reaction to alpha-chymotrypsin.[7] A similar case occurred after 11 injections.[8,9]

No allergic reactions have been known to follow intraocular use of alpha-chymotrypsin during cataract extraction. Guinea pigs have been hypersensitized to alpha-chymotrypsin and then challenged by enzyme injection

into the vitreous and anterior chamber. No noticeable allergic response resulted.[10] This finding suggests that a clinically serious al-lergic response to alpha-chymotrypsin zonu-lysis is unlikely to happen.

EFFECTS ON EYE

While the clinical use of alpha-chymotryp-sin with appropriate precautions is surpri-ingly free of undesirable side effects, it must not be assumed that the enzyme is nontoxic. Extensive experimental studies of the ocular response to alpha-chymotrypsin indicate that it is a highly potent and destructive drug that must be used with caution and respect.

Cornea

Fortunately the corneal epithelium and endothelium are resistant to the effect of 1:5000 concentrations of alpha-chymotryp-sin, and when they are intact, they protect the corneal stroma against the enzymatic ef-fect. When the epithelium and endothelium have been damaged, or if the enzyme is in-jected directly into the corneal stroma, con-siderable destruction and swelling of the cor-nea ensues. The marked thickening pro-duced by an intralamellar alpha-chymotryp-sin injection of a rabbit cornea is shown in Fig. 4-2.[11]

Irrigation of rabbit anterior chambers with 1:5000 solutions of alpha-chymotrypsin for 3 minutes, followed by rinsing with a 0.9% solution of sodium chloride, caused extensive corneal edema that persisted for weeks in 5 of 17 eyes, while similar edema occurred in 4 of the opposite control eyes irrigated with saline solution alone.[10] The eyes with corneal edema were shown histologically to have gaps in the endothelial lining. There was no demonstrable difference between histologic sections of the enzyme-irrigated eyes and of the saline-irrigated eyes. Whole flat corneal endothelial mounts show disarrangement of the endothelial mosaic and considerable increase in cellular mitosis after alpha-chy-motrypsin irrigation and less frequently after saline irrigation.[10]

Irrigation of a human eye with 1:500 al-pha-chymotrypsin resulted in full dilation of

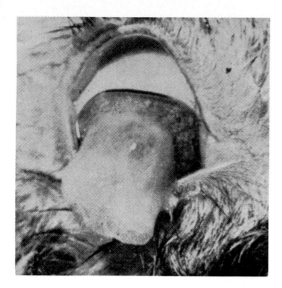

Fig. 4-2. Injection of a 1:5000 concentration of alpha-chymotrypsin into rabbit cornea caused this pronounced edema. (From Radnot, M., and Pajor, R.: Am. J. Ophthalmol. **51:**598, 1961.)

the pupil within a few minutes. Subsequently, the iris atrophied, leaving the appearance of aniridia. The cornea and vitreous were undamaged.[12]

Since most cataracts are removed through limbal incisions, evaluation of limbal rather than of corneal wound strength would seem most logical in a study of the effect of alpha-chymotrypsin on wound healing. This was done in a series of 10 white rabbits.[13] An 8 mm limbal incision was irrigated with 0.2 ml of a 1:25,000 solution of alpha-chymotrypsin at 2-minute intervals for four doses. The control incisions in the fellow eyes were irrigated with the saline-heparin diluent. Wound disruption was induced 6 days after suture removal by means of oxygen introduced intraocularly under gradually increasing pressure. Pounds per square inch required to burst the alpha-chymotrypsin incisions averaged 10.9 as compared to 11.1 for the controls—an insignificant difference.

Similarly, healing of experimental corneal incisions is not impaired by enzyme treatment. Experimental bathing of rabbit corneal wounds in a 1:5000 solution of alpha-chymotrypsin for 30 minutes caused no decrease in wound strength at 14 days, as compared to saline controls.[14] Wound strength was measured as the weight required to break a 5 mm strip excised perpendicularly across the suture line. Control strips ruptured at an average of 240 g and chymotrypsin strips at 245 g (10 eyes each).

Alpha-chymotrypsin has been evaluated experimentally to determine whether its use would clean bacterial corneal ulcers and promote their healing.[15] In this study a concentration of 10,000 units/ml of enzyme was used to bathe the cornea for 2 minutes three times a day. *Pseudomonas aeruginosa* ulcers were created by surface abrasions of the upper limbus of albino rabbits. Both enzyme-treated and control eyes were also treated with polymyxin B and neomycin. The enzyme did not hasten destruction of the bacteria and had no beneficial effects on the course of these bacterial ulcers. The enzyme treatment resulted in stromal corneal destruction and subsequently more extensive corneal ectasia and scarring than occurred in the control eyes.

A daily 5-minute corneal bath with a 1:10,000 solution of alpha-chymotrypsin was evaluated in 21 rabbits with herpetic keratitis.[16] The opposite, similarly infected eye was treated with idoxuridine (IDU) or with saline solution or was left untreated as a control. In all 21 cases the alpha-chymotrypsin-treated eye became rapidly worse than the fellow eye. Severe bullous keratopathy, stromal dissolution, and descemetocele were seen in the eyes treated with alpha-chymotrypsin, and six of them perforated. There were no perforations in the fellow eyes.

Perforation in metaherpetic keratitis after 5 days of treatment with topical alpha-chymotrypsin has been described in a human eye.[17]

Iris

The iris is relatively resistant to alpha-chymotrypsin injected into the anterior chamber. Iritis frequently accompanies the posterior ocular inflammation caused by intravitreal enzyme injection.

Zonular membrane

Zonulysis with alpha-chymotrypsin is a diffusely occurring fragmentation of the entire length of the zonular fiber.[18] These fibers are broken into relatively uniform fragments approximately 1000 Å in length. This uniformity suggests the presence of a regularly located amino acid linkage that is selectively destroyed by the enzyme.

The fragmentation does not become visible until 10 to 15 minutes after enzyme application, in contrast to destruction of the equatorial pericapsular membrane of the lens within 5 minutes. Up to 30 minutes is required for complete lysis of the entire zonular membrane. Such complete destruction of the zonular membrane is neither necessary nor desirable in clinical cataract extraction.

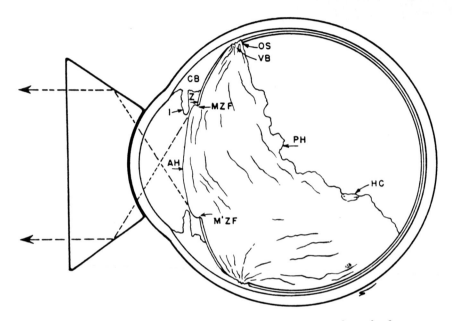

Fig. 4-3. Gonioscopic view of aphakic eye. *MZF* and *M'ZF*, Margin of zonular foramen remaining after cataract extraction; *AH*, anterior hyaloid face; *Z*, zonules; *PH*, posterior hyaloid; *HC*, hyaloid canal; *CB*, ciliary body; *I*, iris; *OS*, ora serrata; *VB*, vitreous base. (From Thorpe, H.: Am. J. Ophthalmol. **49:**531, 1960.)

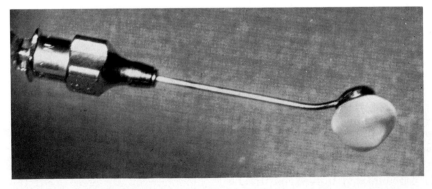

Fig. 4-4. Rabbit lens after 3-hour incubation in 1:5000 alpha-chymotrypsin solution. Note separation of zonules and vitreous from lens. (From Bedrossian, R. H.: Arch. Ophthalmol. **62:**216, 1959.)

Although one might conclude that clinical use of alpha-chymotrypsin would dissolve the entire zonular membrane, such is not the case. Gonioscopic observation of the aphakic eye permits visualization of the circular edge of the zonular membrane, which remains in its normal position even after the lens has been removed (Fig. 4-3). In all of 52 eyes examined after cataract extraction using zonulysis, this circular edge of the zonular membrane was still present. The surface of the zonular membrane was somewhat grayish and etched, and the thickness of the membrane seemed slightly less than usual after zonulysis. Also, its free margin appeared irregular. The anterior hyaloid face was intact in these cases. Examination of 42 cataracts extracted by zonulysis showed them to be entirely free of zonular remnants or to have no more than 15 zonular fibers still attached to the peripheral lens capsule.

These findings indicate that the effective site of the action of alpha-chymotrypsin in cataract surgery is the zonular attachment to the lens. In these patients only 0.3 ml of a 1:5000 solution of alpha-chymotrypsin was used, and it was thoroughly irrigated out after 2 to 4 minutes of action.

Histologic sections of rabbit eyes incubated in a 1:5000 solution of alpha-chymotrypsin for 3 hours after removal of the cornea and iris still show the zonular fibers to be microscopically unchanged in appearance. The effectiveness of the zonulysis in these eyes was proved by the fact that the lenses would fall out spontaneously if the eyes were turned to their side (Fig. 4-4).

Ciliary body

Electron microscopy of the nonpigmented ciliary epithelium of monkey eyes after zonulysis by a 1:5000 solution of alpha-chymotrypsin shows no change in this membrane.[18] When the centripetal pull of the zonules is destroyed, the ring of ciliary processes increases in diameter.

Lens

Electron microscopy of the lens capsule shows that there is a pericapsular membrane near the equator identical in structure to the zonular fibers. This membrane is not demonstrable in the central portions of the capsule. After zonulysis with alpha-chymotrypsin, the equatorial pericapsular membrane fragments and disappears, but the lens capsule proper shows no recognizable changes.[18]

Lens-vitreous attachments

The lens-vitreous attachments of the young monkey and also of young humans after autopsy are very resistant to alpha-chymotrypsin. These attachments are not lysed even when the enzyme exposure time is prolonged far beyond the time required to disintegrate the zonules completely.[18]

The result of lens extraction in young rabbits without enzymatic aid is shown in Fig. 4-5; almost always the vitreous body is firmly adherent to the lens, and both lens and vitreous are simultaneously extracted from the eye. Four injections of 0.4 ml of a 1:10,000 solution of alpha-chymotrypsin at 5-minute intervals (20 minutes of enzyme action) permitted intracapsular lens removal without vitreous loss in 20 rabbit eyes.[13] In all of 20 control eyes irrigated with saline solution, it was impossible to remove the lens without withdrawing the adherent entire vitreous body. In separating lens and vitreous, the best method of increasing enzyme effectiveness was the giving of multiple injections spaced several minutes apart. Two injections of a 1:5000 enzyme solution permitted clean extraction of 8 of 10 lenses as compared to 2 of 10 when only one injection was given. Enough alpha-chymotrypsin solution to flood the posterior chamber (0.2 ml on each side) was as effective as larger volumes. Enzymatic activity apparently is lost within 2 minutes—waiting 10 minutes did not produce more lysis than had been attained in 2 minutes. A concentration of 1:5000 was twice as effective as a 1:10,000 concentration. Isotonic saline and balanced salt solutions were equally effective diluents.

The clinician should bear in mind that the most effective method of intraocular proteolysis is not necessarily the safest method

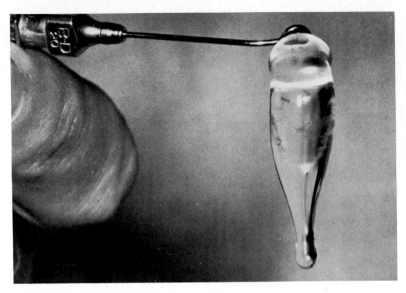

Fig. 4-5. Massive vitreous loss caused by vitreolenticular adhesions in young rabbit eye. (From Bedrossian, R. H., and Lalli, R. A.: Arch. Ophthalmol. **67:**616, 1962.)

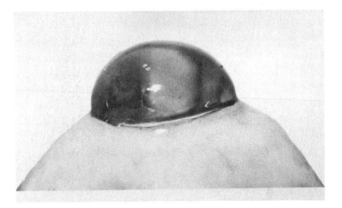

Fig. 4-6. Experimental vitreous protrusion from human eye. No rupture or weakness of the anterior hyaloid membrane is demonstrable after continuous application of a 1:1000 solution of alpha-chymotrypsin for 40 minutes. (From Geeraets, W. J.: South. Med. J. **53:**82, 1960.)

and that entry of the enzyme into the vitreous body will result in serious intraocular damage.

Vitreous face

The effect of alpha-chymotrypsin on the anterior hyaloid face has been studied in human eyes enucleated within 2 hours postmortem.[19] The cornea, iris, and lens were removed, and the vitreous was caused to protrude by equatorial pressure on the eye (Fig. 4-6). Alpha-chymotrypsin in the higher concentration of 1:1000 was then continuously applied to the exposed vitreous face for 40 minutes. Even 1 hour later there was still no noticeable decrease in the strength of the vitreous face nor any increased tendency to protrusion of the vitreous. Such findings suggest that use of alpha-chymotrypsin could not predispose the eye to vitreous loss resulting from rupture of its face.

The resistance of the vitreous structure to

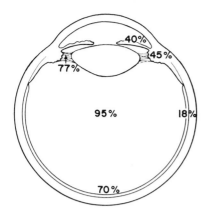

Fig. 4-7. Diagrammatic representation of data given in Table 4-1. Incidence of lesions after intravitreal injection of 0.4 ml of a 1:5000 solution of alpha-chymotrypsin into rabbit vitreous. (Modified from O'Malley, C., Moskovitz, M., and Straatsma, B.: Arch. Ophthalmol. **66:**539, 1961.)

dissolution by alpha-chymotrypsin is caused by its collagen content (collagen is not readily susceptible to the action of alpha-chymotrypsin).[20]

Retina

Although relatively innocuous in the anterior chamber, alpha-chymotrypsin in even small quantities is quite toxic when injected intravitreally. As little as 0.002 mg in the rabbit vitreous causes infiltration of inflammatory cells into the retina and irregular partial destruction of the ganglion cell layer.[21] Increased dosage causes greater damage, until at the level of 2 mg the entire retina is destroyed, leaving only Müller's fibers, and the optic nerve itself is necrotic. Intermediate doses cause varying amounts of retinal hemorrhage, inflammation, and permanent destruction. By contrast, 0.2 mg injected into the rabbit anterior chamber causes no recognizable retinal damage. Presumably this results because the outflow of aqueous carries the enzyme anteriorly, and it does not readily diffuse into the intact vitreous body.

Comparing these milligram values with clinically used concentrations, somewhat less than 1 mg of alpha-chymotrypsin is contained in 5 ml of the comparable to 1:5000

Table 4-1. Incidence of intraocular changes after intravitreal injection of normal saline solution and of alpha-chymotrypsin in saline solution*

	Control (%)	Alpha-chymotrypsin (%)
Iritis	15	40
Cyclitis	15	45
Zonulysis	0	77
Hyalitis	61	95
Retinal holes	7	18
Retinolysis	0	70

*Modified from O'Malley, C., Moskovitz, M., and Straatsma, B.: Arch. Ophthalmol. **66:**539, 1961.

solution used clinically. Only 0.01 ml of this clinically used concentration is required to contain 0.002 mg of enzyme—the amount that causes recognizable damage to the rabbit retina when injected intravitreally.

The intraocular damage resulting from injection of 0.4 ml of a 1:5000 solution of alpha-chymotrypsin into the anterior axial rabbit vitreous is outlined in Table 4-1 and Fig. 4-7. The most serious of the enzyme-induced changes was retinal degeneration. During the 14 days of this experiment, 70% of the alpha-chymotrypsin–treated eyes developed definite retinal damage.[22]

Injection of 0.1 ml of a 1:5000 solution of alpha-chymotrypsin into the vitreous of 20 rabbit eyes resulted in marked retinal damage in about three fourths of the eyes, with spontaneous retinal detachment in one eye.[23] In some eyes the retina became almost completely atrophic.

Intravitreal injection of 0.5 ml of 1:5000 alpha-chymotrypsin was found to abolish the monkey electroretinogram.[24] Apparently this enzyme diffuses through the monkey retina, for the photoreceptor layer was more severely damaged than were the inner retinal layers. This damage was permanent, extensive, and consistently reproducible with this dosage of enzyme. The selective affinity of alpha-chymotrypsin for the outer segments of the rods and cones is another example of the enzymatic specificity that permits zonulysis but not dissolution of the equally delicate vitreous structure.

The clinical implications of the pharmacologically predicted and experimentally demonstrated intraocular damage caused by alpha-chymotrypsin are clear. Enzymatic zonulysis should not be employed in the delivery of cataracts that can readily be extracted without its aid, for example, in the senile cataract of a very old patient. When it is used—and surely its use is indicated in difficult extractions, particularly in younger patients—care must be taken to irrigate the anterior chamber thoroughly to remove all of the partially digested fragments of the zonular fibers that have been shown to be responsible for enzyme-induced glaucoma through the mechanism of trabecular obstruction. This enzyme solution must *not* be injected into the human vitreous! A disputed clinical point concerns the need to irrigate the anterior chamber to remove alpha-chymotrypsin after it has been allowed 2 minutes of action.[25] Such irrigation has been advocated to reduce potential toxic effects to the interior of the eye. However, it seems likely that spontaneous enzyme inactivation occurs, providing that only small amounts have been introduced into the eye.

Table 4-2. Comparison of tensile strength of suture materials incubated in alpha-chymotrypsin solution and saline solution with nonincubated suture materials*

Mean tensile strength (g)	*Plain 6-0 gut*	*Chronic 6-0 gut*	*6-0 silk*
Nonincubated	209	255	238
Saline incubated (96 hr)	176	229	238
Alpha-chymotrypsin incubated			
1 hr	210		
10 hr	191	228	
32 hr	144	206	247
96 hr	93	197	236

*Modified from Drance, S. M., Murray, R. G., and Smith, T. R.: Am. J. Ophthalmol. **49:**64, 1960.

The enzyme-inhibiting property of human aqueous humor was evaluated after a 15-minute incubation period of equal volumes of 1:5000 alpha-chymotrypsin and of human secondary aqueous. The resulting inhibitory activity destroyed from 5% to 67% of the alpha-chymotrypsin potency in the aqueous samples studied from 10 eyes. No enzyme activity could be detected in secondary aqueous obtained from five eyes in which alpha-chymotrypsin had been used for cataract extraction (0.4 ml of a 1:5000 solution, allowed to stand for 2 minutes). On the basis of these findings, the authors question the need to irrigate or neutralize the enzyme when it is used for cataract extraction.[4]

Primary human aqueous has also been shown to inactivate alpha-chymotrypsin.[26]

EFFECT ON SUTURES

Since alpha-chymotrypsin is a proteolytic enzyme, weakening of surgical gut sutures by its action might be expected. Weakening might contraindicate use of gut sutures when the enzyme is used in cataract surgery. Numerous reports evaluating the effect of alpha-chymotrypsin on catgut sutures may be summarized as indicating that the short exposures expected in clinical usage do not significantly alter tensile strength or microscopic appearance of the sutures.[14,27]

Enzymatic damage to catgut suture can easily be demonstrated after prolonged incubation in a 1:5000 solution of alpha-chymotrypsin at 37° C (Table 4-2).[28] Plain catgut is more susceptible to this proteolytic destruction than is chromic catgut. The strength of silk sutures is unaffected by alpha-chymotrypsin. The clinical significance of these results is doubtful, since under normal conditions of usage the sutures are exposed to enzyme action for only a very few minutes. The increased incidence of wound rupture attributed to use of alpha-chymotrypsin cannot be attributed to suture weakening by enzymatic action.

CLINICAL USE

Relatively specific dissolution of the zonular attachments to the lens may be achieved without causing the intraocular toxic effects resulting from experimental use.[29]

Method

The preliminary steps of incision, suture placement, iridectomy, etc. are performed according to the surgeon's preference. Either a 1:5000 or 1:10,000 concentration of enzyme may be used. Different authors advocate amounts ranging from 0.3 to 4.0 ml of solution. The good results reported with such different amounts indicate that the enzymatic action results from a relatively small amount of solution, and that large excesses of fluid run harmlessly out of the incision.

Since the site of zonulysis is at the equatorial insertion of the fibers, the solution is introduced by various types of irrigating tips that are inserted behind the iris and are manipulated so as to direct the solution about the anterior lens equator. This distribution of the enzyme behind the iris is important; it should not simply be placed into the anterior chamber.

The irrigating cannula should not be inserted too deeply. The ora serrata is only 5 or 6 mm farther back than the proper site for enzyme placement in the peripheral posterior chamber. Remember the experimental demonstration of formation of retinal holes by enzyme action. I have observed one experienced surgeon insert the cannula so far that he must have accidentally separated the zonular fibers mechanically. Traversing the peripheral iridectomy with the alpha-chymotrypsin irrigator has two advantages—it achieves good access to the superior zonules and also guarantees patency of the iridectomy.

Immediately after enzyme injection the conjunctiva and the incision edges may be irrigated with saline solution. Despite the previously noted animal experiments indicating that alpha-chymotrypsin does not interfere with corneoscleral wound healing, there is a clinical suspicion that wound complications are more frequent after zonulysis. For this reason, multiple sutures and a limbus-based conjunctival flap are advised.

Zonulysis is usually achieved within 1 to 2 minutes and is recognized either by anterior displacement of the lens, by a more rounded lens contour, or by the ease with which it may be removed. At the end of 2 minutes, or sooner if zonulysis is recognized, gentle saline irrigation may be used to remove excess enzyme from the anterior chamber. If the zonule is unusually resistant, a second application of enzyme may be helpful.

Whether erysiphake, forceps, or cryoextraction is used for extraction depends on the surgeon's preference. No instrument should be permitted to touch the endothelium, which may be rendered more susceptible to mechanical injury by the enzymatic action.

When alpha-chymotrypsin is used in cataract extraction, serious consideration should be given to changing the usual technique of lens delivery. Whereas the tumbling method is probably safest when the zonules are to be mechanically ruptured, the sliding method permits better visualization and less corneal trauma when the lens is partially or completely dislocated by zonulysis.[30] Tumbling a lens when the upper zonules are lysed risks vitreous loss superiorly, damages the endothelium since the lens is displaced forward near the cornea, makes instrument introduction difficult, and increases the possibility of displacing the dislocated lens back into the vitreous cavity.

Results

In a double-blind statistical evaluation by the technique of sequential analysis, it was established that there is a 99% probability that alpha-chymotrypsin does, indeed, facilitate cataract extraction (Fig. 4-8).[31] (Sequential analysis is a technique in which experimental results are plotted as data are obtained. When the plotted line leaves the neutral band, this confirms or denies the supposition that the medication is effective.) Furthermore, the time required for lens delivery was recorded in the 68 patients used in this study. The mean time of delivery during control operations was 3.2 minutes, as compared with 1.6 minutes with the aid of zonulysis.

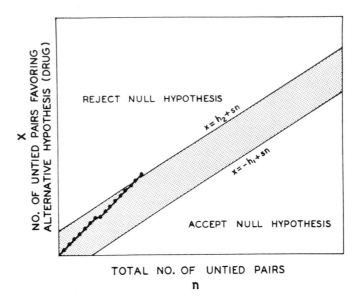

Fig. 4-8. Sequential analysis graph confirming effect of alpha-chymotrypsin on facility of cataract extraction. (From Schwartz, B., Corwin, M., and Israel, R.: Trans. Am. Acad. Ophthalmol. **64**:46, 1960.)

In 1960 the effect of alpha-chymotrypsin in cataract surgery was evaluated in a coordinated study of 1581 cataract extractions performed by more than 200 ophthalmologists throughout the United States.[32] In this series only 7% of the extractions were extracapsular, as contrasted with 19% in a previously reported large series without zonulysis.[33] The percentage of intracapsular extraction was the same whether a 1:5000 or 1:10,000 concentration of alpha-chymotrypsin was used. Use of the 1:10,000 dilution is therefore recommended, since it is equally effective and presumably less likely to cause toxic side effects. The incidence of postoperative complications was not significantly greater in this enzyme series than in a previous series of 2000 cases, with the exception that wound disruption was more common if fewer than three sutures were used for closure.[33]

A very large number of cataracts extracted using zonulysis by one group of ophthalmologists probably provides statistics as reliable as any others available. This group reported two series of 432 and 491 eyes.[34,35] Their data are presented in Table 4-3.

After extracting these 923 cataracts, the authors definitely endorse zonulysis as a routine procedure. They consider use of the enzyme to be the greatest advance in cataract surgery since the advent of intracapsular extraction and the generous use of sutures in closing the corneoscleral incision. In documenting the higher percentage of intracapsular extractions obtained with alpha-chymotrypsin, they analyzed 186 of the patients who had previous cataract surgery in the other eye without zonulysis. Only 78% of these unaided extractions were intracapsular.

To avoid giving the impression that cataract extraction is now an easy procedure, the authors add, "Although alpha-chymotrypsin is a valuable aid in obtaining an intracapsular extraction, its use does not minimize the knowledge, skill, and manual dexterity which are still necessary for good surgery and which can only be obtained through study, training, and experience."[35]

Indications

Since any additional step prolongs the operation and introduces slight hazards, the decision as to which steps should be included in a given cataract extraction should be made by weighing risks against benefits. Depend-

Table 4-3. Results of cataract extraction with aid of zonulysis*

Clinical data	First series (432 eyes)	Second series (491 eyes)
Intracapsular	93.3%	97.4%
Visual acuity 20/50 or better	360 eyes	386 eyes
Wound rupture	2 cases	4 cases
Uveitis	18 cases	6 cases
Striate keratopathy	28 cases	25 cases
Retinal detachments	4 cases (3 more during ensuing year)	3 cases
Posterior dislocation of lens requiring looping	8 cases	4 cases
Vitreous loss	3 cases	7 cases

*Data from Kennedy, P. J., and associates: Arch. Ophthal. **64:**342, 1960; and Kennedy, P. J., and associates: Arch. Ophthalmol. **65:**801, 1961.

ing on the surgeon's viewpoint, alpha-chymotrypsin may be used routinely or may be reserved for cases in which the surgeon anticipates difficulty in doing an intracapsular procedure. After the age of 60 years, the zonule is usually sufficiently fragile so that intracapsular extraction is quite easy and there is no need to resort to zonulysis.

In the past, traumatic cataracts in young adults have been treated by extracapsular extraction or by needling. With the aid of alpha-chymotrypsin, these cataracts may successfully be removed in toto with no more difficulty than is encountered in the usual intracapsular extraction. Even if the cataract is a result of a penetrating injury, in many cases an iris-lens adhesion may be separated with a spatula or may be eliminated by a local iridectomy, with subsequent complete removal of the lens. Posterior synechiae, scar tissue, and secondary membranes are *not* dissolved by alpha-chymotrypsin.

The problem of removing retained lens material at the time of an unplanned extracapsular cataract extraction is simplified by enzymatic zonulysis. Irrigation with 5 ml of a 1:5000 solution of alpha-chymotrypsin will often permit almost complete removal of such residual cortex and capsule.[36] However, many younger surgeons are unaware of the good visual results that may follow extracapsular extraction. If the anterior capsule is removed within the pupillary area, and if the nucleus and all the visible cortex have been removed, further manipulation is definitely unwise. When it is time to proceed with permanent refraction, the posterior lens capsule will be invisible except to slit-lamp examination, the vitreous face will be held back securely, and the visual result will be quite as good as without the posterior capsule. Zonulysis is advocated only if a considerable amount of ruptured anterior capsule and adherent cortex remains within the pupil. Under these circumstances, establishing the presence of a secondary membrane that will interfere with vision warrants taking the very real risk of serious complications resulting from further manipulation.

The possibility of "intracapsular" removal of an extensive secondary cataract with the aid of zonulysis should be considered. Good results were reported in 16 eyes so treated.[37] I have personally found the results of this technique to be most encouraging.

Contraindications

Zonulysis is inadvisable in patients with fluid vitreous, since posterior loss of the lens could easily occur. Should fluid vitreous be anticipated, the surgeon should certainly secure a firm grip on the cataract before applying the alpha-chymotrypsin. The possibility of posterior diffusion of the enzyme, with resultant retinal damage, should also be considered. Irrigation of only the lower zonules with a very small amount of alpha-chymotrypsin has been suggested as an effective and safe method of facilitating cataract removal in a younger patient with resistant zonules who is known to have fluid vitreous caused by myopic degeneration or inflammation.[38]

The commonest contraindication to zonulysis is the youth of the patient. Because of their dense lens-vitreous adhesions, patients younger than 20 years are not good candidates for intracapsular cataract extraction.[39] Better alternatives are an extracapsular type of procedure or postponement of surgery until the patient is older.

When used in lens extraction in 16 eyes of children removed at autopsy, 2 ml of a 1:500 concentration of alpha-chymotrypsin injected beneath the iris, followed by a 5-minute wait, satisfactorily lysed the zonular fibers, but did not free the vitreous-lens adhesions.[40] The children ranged in age from newborn to 10 years. In all 16 eyes the vitreous was firmly adherent to the posterior lens surface, causing vitreous loss in seven of the extractions. The clinical counterpart of these statistics was provided by a listing of 88 congenital cataracts removed with alpha-chymotrypsin as reported by four other surgeons. In these 88 cases, vitreous was lost 30 times! Vitreous loss occurs as commonly among patients 10 to 20 years of age as in the patients less than 10 years of age. Hence the conclusion is reached that intracapsular extraction with enzymatic zonulysis is not advisable in patients younger than 20 years. While intracapsular extraction in the young is certainly possible, the complications of vitreous loss make the procedure extremely hazardous. Cited in the report is a 14-year-old patient who suffered irreparable retinal detachment 5 months after intracapsular extraction with vitreous loss.

Although the surgeon is tempted to display technical skill by intracapsular removal of these youthful cataracts, the damage sustained by the intraocular structures is so great as to make this attempt foolhardy. This is true even when the best reduction of intraocular pressure, excellent anesthesia, the greatest surgical dexterity, and complete zonulysis are assumed. Extracapsular techniques of extraction are definitely safer for congenital cataracts. As an example, a cataract was successfully removed with zonulysis in a 16-year-old patient; however, alarming vitreous loss immediately followed lens delivery and the final vision achieved was only perception of hand movements.[41]

COMPLICATIONS OF ZONULYSIS

After cataract surgery with or without zonulysis, the surgeon expects to encounter complications. Whether these problems are caused by faulty technique, are simply the ordained percent of incidence, or are promoted by alpha-chymotrypsin toxicity is often difficult to prove.

Glaucoma

Use of alpha-chymotrypsin predisposes the eye to develop transient glaucoma during the postoperative period. In a series of 343 cataract extractions (178 with alpha-chymotrypsin and 165 without), this glaucoma (defined as a pressure of at least 24.4 mm Hg Schiøtz and detected by daily tonometry) was found in 72.5% of enzyme-treated eyes, in contrast to 23.6% of control eyes.[42] Carefully controlled analysis excluded the possibility that other factors might have caused the increased pressure (including type of iridectomy, instruments used, preexisting glaucoma, age of patient, number of sutures, technique of extraction, and so forth). That the diluent vehicle or the irrigating cannula did not cause the glaucoma was proved by irrigation with diluent alone in 17 eyes, only 17.6% of which developed glaucoma. Apparently postenzyme glaucoma is a specific complication of the use of excessively large amounts of enzyme, since routine use of 0.25 to 0.5 ml of 1:5000 alpha-chymotrypsin has not been reported to cause significant postoperative glaucoma.[43]

Alpha-chymotrypsin–induced glaucoma is dose related in that its frequency and severity increase with use of a larger volume of enzyme solution. Fig. 4-9 charts the highest (not average) pressure encountered in groups of 20 cataract extractions performed with a given volume of 1:5000 alpha-chymotrypsin. Obviously the use of greater volumes causes very substantial pressure increases. Even the smallest volume used (0.25 ml) caused postoperative pressures of 24 mm Hg or higher in 55% of cases. Use of 1.5 ml increased this to 70%. The cataract surgeon is advised to use the smallest dose of alpha-chymotrypsin necessary to produce satisfac-

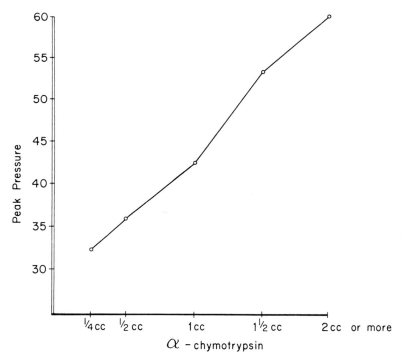

Fig. 4-9. Highest intraocular pressure occurring in each dosage group of alpha-chymotrypsin–treated patients undergoing cataract extraction. (Modified from Kirsch, R. E.: Arch. Ophthalmol. **75:**774, 1966.)

tory zonulysis. The reader is reminded that 2 to 4 ml of 1:5000 alpha-chymotrypsin was routinely used when Kirsch[44] discovered this form of postoperative glaucoma.

The mechanism whereby alpha-chymotrypsin produces glaucoma has remained unexplained for several years. Experimental injections of the enzyme into various portions (anterior chamber, posterior chamber, anterior vitreous, and posterior vitreous) of the owl monkey eye resulted in glaucoma most often after posterior chamber injections. (Second in frequency were the anterior vitreous injections.) Enzyme injections into the anterior chamber of miotic eyes did not cause glaucoma. These findings appear to exclude trabecular damage by the enzyme as the cause of glaucoma (at least in the monkey). The concentration of enzyme appeared significant, since 750 APA units of enzyme in 0.2 ml of solution caused much more severe pressure elevations than did 750 APA units in a 5 ml volume.[45] A logical explanation of

the known facts concerning enzyme-induced glaucoma would be that posterior chamber introduction of sufficient enzyme causes tissue breakdown. This tissue debris then flows forward and becomes trapped in the trabecular structure. Glaucoma ensues and lasts until this debris is absorbed. Pilocarpine benefits the glaucoma because it opens the trabecular spaces. Corticosteroids are not beneficial because the mechanism is noninflammatory.

Confirmation of this hypothesis was achieved through scanning electron microscopy. Both in monkeys[46] and in human eyes,[47] scanning electron microscopy shows that the zonular fibers, especially those near the lens, swell up into a very loose, spongelike mass (Fig. 4-10). Fragments of these partially digested zonular fibers become trapped in the trabecular meshwork (Fig. 4-11).

Further evidence supporting the hypothesis of trabecular blockage by zonular

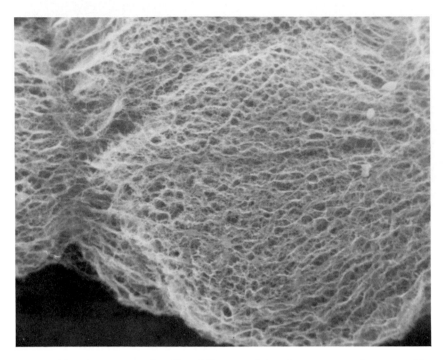

Fig. 4-10. Swollen human zonular fiber following alpha-chymotrypsin digestion. (Scanning electron microphotograph, ×2000.) (From Worthen, D. M.: Am. J. Ophthalmol. **73:**637, 1972.)

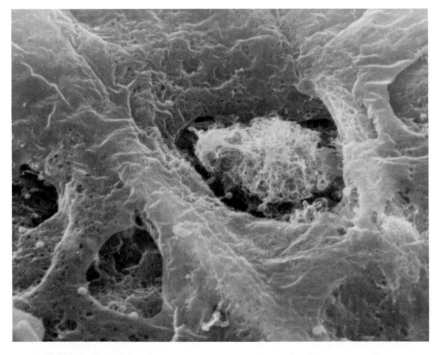

Fig. 4-11. Fluffy mass of alpha-chymotrypsin digested zonular fiber trapped in interstices of trabecular meshwork. (Scanning electron microphotograph, ×2000.) (From Worthen, D. M.: Am. J. Ophthalmol. **73:**637, 1972.)

debris was obtained by injections of the enzyme into the anterior chamber of monkey eyes.[48] Dissected specimens of the lens, zonular membrane, and ciliary body were placed in alpha-chymotrypsin solution until the lens dislocated. The lens and ciliary body were discarded. Injection of the residual solution into the anterior chamber of a monkey eye resulted in typical enzyme-induced glaucoma. When this solution was cleared of particulate debris by microfiltration (Millipore filter), it did not cause glaucoma when injected.

If a monkey eye is already aphakic (zonular membrane already digested and removed), injection of alpha-chymotrypsin will not cause any pressure elevation. Aqueous from a monkey with enzyme-induced glaucoma will not cause pressure elevation when injected into another eye.

A practical implication derived from the hypothesis of trabecular blockage by zonular debris is that irrigation of the anterior chamber following cataract extraction should remove this debris and lessen the severity of postoperative enzyme-induced glaucoma. In practice, a particulate suspension of pigmented debris is readily observed in the anterior chamber after lens delivery. I have always considered this material to be unphysiologic and have routinely removed it by irrigation with approximately 1 ml of saline solution.

Enzyme-induced glaucoma is accompanied by a decrease in facility of outflow (Fig. 4-12).[49] A deep anterior chamber and an open angle differentiate enzyme glaucoma from pupil-block glaucoma. Enzyme-induced glaucoma may or may not respond to 4% pilocarpine therapy, which should be initiated if high pressures are encountered. Although trabecular inflammation has been suggested as a possible cause, corticosteroid therapy is not of benefit.

Enzyme-induced glaucoma is usually asymptomatic. The patients with very high pressures may have ocular pain and headache and may show epithelial edema. The anterior chamber is normally deep, and the chamber angle is gonioscopically open. The peak pressures are ordinarily attained from 2 to 5 days postoperatively and in 28% of cases are as high as 40 to 60 mm Hg. The average duration of glaucoma is about 1 week. The longest case lasted 19 days. Acetazolamide, 10% phenylephrine, and cortico-

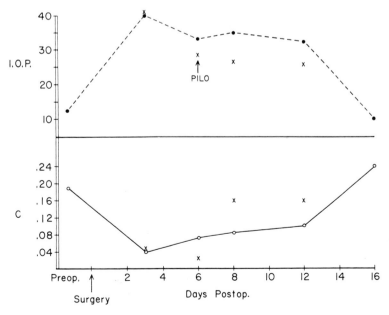

Fig. 4-12. Representative case of enzyme glaucoma. (Modified from Kirsch, R. E.: Trans. Am. Acad. Ophthalmol. Otolaryngol. **69:**1011, 1965.)

steroid therapy do not prevent pressure elevation.[50] The condition appears to be a self-limited disease that requires no treatment other than the usual postoperative care. A tonographic survey of 25 eyes 1 year postoperatively showed no significant permanent changes in outflow facility.

No correlation exists between preoperative intraocular pressure and susceptibility to enzyme-induced glaucoma.[51] Hence, if indicated, the use of alpha-chymotrypsin need not be avoided during cataract extraction in patients with glaucoma. In a series of 15 patients with bilateral cataracts and intraocular pressures ranging from 21 to 29 mm Hg in each eye, enzymatic zonulysis was used in the right eye but not in the left. In only two of the eyes treated with zonulysis was there a transient 6 mm elevation above the pressure of the control eye.[52] In a series of 200 cataract extractions performed without the use of alpha-chymotrypsin, postoperative glaucoma (undetected prior to surgery) was found in six patients within 8 weeks after surgery. Three such cases of glaucoma occurred in the control series of 200 operations performed with 0.75 to 1 ml of a 1:5000 solution of Chymar.[53] Such a late onset of glaucoma is not characteristic of enzyme-induced glaucoma and obviously does not represent a delayed type of enzyme damage, since it occurred in even greater frequency in patients not receiving the enzyme.

The clinical importance of enzyme-induced glaucoma relates to differential diagnosis and wound problems. It must be differentiated from the postoperative pupil-block and angle-closure acute glaucomas that require immediate care. It is apparently responsible for the higher incidence of wound closure problems that are clinically well recognized to follow enzymatic zonulysis. These problems include postoperative hyphema, flat anterior chamber, iris prolapse, wound rupture, and subsequent late aphakic glaucoma. Such wound complications were present in 11% of cataract extractions performed with alpha-chymotrypsin and in 4% of cases without enzyme. These complications occurred only in cases

with glaucoma, indicating that wound disruption resulted from pressure and not from an effect of the enzyme on the wound edges. From the practical standpoint, such findings support the empirical conclusion that multiple sutures help to prevent the more frequent wound problems that follow use of alpha-chymotrypsin.

A somewhat different form of alpha-chymotrypsin glaucoma in rabbits is apparently due to some type of inflammatory reaction dependent on prostaglandin synthetase. This reaction could be avoided by pretreatment with indomethacin (25 mg twice daily for 2 days) with the intent of stabilizing the blood-aqueous barrier.[54] This particular rabbit phenomenon with alpha-chymotrypsin does not appear to have a human counterpart of clinical significance, but I wonder if there is a place for indomethacin pretreatment of inflamed or injured human eyes before surgery?

Wound rupture

Delayed rupture of the cataract incision has been attributed to enzymatic impairment of wound healing. Use of multiple corneal sutures is advised to prevent this complication. In one series of 42 cases there were four extensive iris prolapses that occurred as late as 1 month postoperatively.[55] (Only one iris prolapse had occurred in 200 cases previously performed by the same authors without zonulysis.) These incisions were closed with six to nine sutures of 6-0 *plain* catgut. This suture material dissolved "much more quickly than it had in the past." Greater than usual corneal edema and reaction to surgery were present in the enzyme-treated patient. Possibly this inflammatory reaction hastened suture absorption. In two cases of postoperative wound infection I have observed the disappearance within several weeks of the 6-0 chromic sutures, which usually last well over a month.

A very high incidence of serious complications was encountered in a series of 67 cataract extractions done with the aid of 0.3 ml of a 1:5000 solution of alpha-chymotrypsin, which was left in the anterior chamber for 3 minutes before irrigation.[56] Four iris prolapses and an additional four wound disruptions occurred. Three patients had striate keratitis sufficiently severe to cause permanent corneal scarring. No complications of this sort were encountered in the 67 cataract operations immediately preceding the series in which alpha-chymotrypsin was used. The technique used in most of these cases was corneal incision closed by two sutures. The author concluded that the enzyme retards corneal healing and that a limbal incision closed by at least five sutures is necessary when alpha-chymotrypsin is used.

Gonioscopic examination of the cataract incision 2 months after surgery showed that a small cleft persisted between the posterior wound edges in 28.8% of 71 eyes in which alpha-chymotrypsin was used.[1] In a previous series of 316 cases in which the enzyme was not used, 21% of the patients had such a cleft still persisting at 2 months. These figures may indicate a slight delay in wound healing or may represent chance variations.

Although these problems in wound healing were originally attributed to some type of enzymatic effect on the incision, they are now believed to result from disruption of the wound by a transient enzyme-induced glaucoma. In a consecutive series of 100 cataract extractions performed without zonulysis, 4% of the eyes had complications attributable to wound healing.[49] In 100 comparable cases of surgery with zonulysis (using 2 to 4 ml of 1:5000 alpha-chymotrypsin), 11% had wound-healing complications. Furthermore, all 11 of these wound complications occurred in cases in which enzyme glaucoma had been demonstrated. Other authors have reported this threefold increase of incisional complications after enzyme use.[51] There is general agreement that use of multiple corneoscleral sutures is an effective method of preventing wound disruption, whether resulting from enzyme-induced glaucoma or other causes.

Vitreous loss

Vitreous loss attributable to alpha-chymotrypsin occurs when it is used for intracapsular cataract extraction in patients so young that the hyaloid attachments to the lens have not yet separated. Such vitreolenticular adhesions may persist up to the age of 20 years. Although the enzyme effectively lyses the zonular attachments to the lens, removal of the cataract withdraws a considerable portion of the anterior vitreous body.

Varying percentages of vitreous loss are reported with zonulysis in older patients, sometimes considerably in excess of control experience. Five instances of loss of formed vitreous complicated zonulytic extraction of 42 cataracts.[55] Two additional eyes in this series suffered vitreous loss during repair of iris prolapse. This 17% incidence of vitreous loss is compared with a 5% incidence in the 200 eyes operated on by the same method before enzyme use.

In another series of 32 cases, vitreous was lost only once, and it was considered related to faulty surgical technique.[57]

In small series of cases the incidence of vitreous loss varies sufficiently with chance to make comparisons of doubtful significance. Variations in preoperative preparation, surgical technique, and the weight of the surgeon's heavy hand also contribute to the uncertainty of statistics. I think that if the surgical methods used make allowance for the fact that the lens is dislocated by zonulysis, the frequency of vitreous loss should not be dangerously increased by alpha-chymotrypsin.

Keratopathy

Corneal damage followed the use of Quimotrase in 8 of 56 cataract extractions but did not occur in 76 cases with use of Alpha-Chymar or Zolyse.[58] In these patients, haziness of the upper third of the cornea was evident on the first postoperative day, progressed to the severity of bullous keratopathy by the first month (Fig. 4-13), and usually subsided by the third month, leaving faint nebular scars of the upper cornea. During the active period these patients had photophobia and tearing. The author states that this complication was unrelated to surgical technique; however, both erysiphake and capsule forceps were used in these cases,

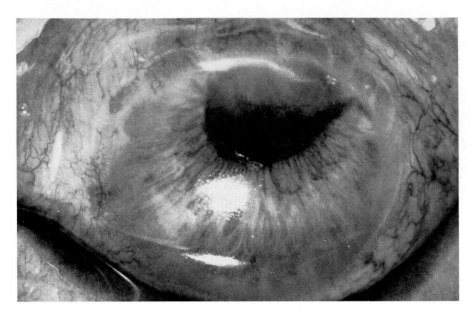

Fig. 4-13. Keratopathy 3 weeks after cataract extraction with a 1:5000 solution of Quimotrase. (From Kara, G. B.: Arch. Ophthalmol. **63:**122, 1960.)

which were published before Thorpe's report, which is summarized in the following paragraph. (Incidentally, Kara used 4 to 5 ml of enzyme and Thorpe, 0.25 to 0.3 ml.)

Thorpe noted striate keratopathy in 60% of 40 extractions with zonulysis and erysiphake.[1] Although all but one of these corneas cleared within several weeks, this incidence of keratopathy was considerably higher than had previously been experienced. Subsequently, the author changed to use of the capsule forceps, and the incidence of striate keratopathy dropped to only 3 of 37 eyes. (His technique of cataract extraction included folding the cornea behind the emerging lens.) Apparently the use of alpha-chymotrypsin increases the susceptibility of the cornea to mechanical trauma.

Corneal dystrophy

Theoretical objections to the use of alpha-chymotrypsin in patients with endothelial dystrophy do not seem to be confirmed by clinical experience. In a series of 224 cataract extractions with enzymatic zonulysis, no patient developed corneal dystrophy within a year postoperatively.[59] Included in this series were 8 eyes with large numbers of Hassall-Henle bodies and 11 eyes with a moderate number. The authors believe that alpha-chymotrypsin facilitates lens removal with a minimum of mechanical endothelial trauma and therefore is to be recommended in eyes predisposed to Fuchs' dystrophy.

Further evidence that enzymatic zonulysis does not damage the endothelium is its frequent use in cataract extraction after successful keratoplasty for Fuchs' dystrophy.[60]

Iris fragmentation

Fragmentation of the posterior pigment layer of the iris occurred in 14 of 50 cataract extractions performed with Quimotrase.[58] Since similar pigment fragmentation occurred in only 2 of 76 cases using Alpha-Chymar or Zolyse, this complication was ascribed to some impurity in the first preparation. When this occurs, large clumps of pigment float forward from the posterior chamber soon after irrigation is begun. This pigment dissolution may occur even though utmost care is taken to avoid mechanical trauma to the iris. Apparently the pigment loss is of no clinical significance.

Endophthalmitis

It has been hinted that postoperative endophthalmitis might have been caused by introduction of contaminated enzyme, and indeed faults in technique may occur when it is used, just as with any other solution introduced into the eye. A report of only one infection developing in three patients in whom the same solution of alpha-chymotrypsin was used seems to exonerate the drug solution. The infected patient was 80 years old, was a chronic alcoholic in poor general health, and probably was the source of her own infection.[41]

Retinal detachment

In a series of 425 cataract extractions, 286 were performed with the aid of alpha-chymotrypsin and 139 without. Five cases of retinal detachment developed following these 425 cataract operations—all five patients had received alpha-chymotrypsin.[61] Three detachments occurred in 39 patients who suffered vitreous loss, while two occurred in the 244 without vitreous loss. The number of cases of vitreous loss without alpha-chymotrypsin is not stated.

Since the method of selection of these patients for enzyme use is not stated, the higher incidence of detachment may be due to selection of complicated cases for use of alpha-chymotrypsin. Unless the decision to use alpha-chymotrypsin is made by a prearranged and rigidly followed system of alternate enzyme and control cases, conclusions as to the incidence of subsequent complications, such as retinal detachment, will be invalid. At the present time our information is only speculative; however, I would not anticipate an increased incidence of retinal detachment after use of alpha-chymotrypsin in cataract extraction, provided that the enzyme is not introduced into the vitreous space. Indeed, by decreasing operative traction on the zonular fibers and distortion of the eye from external pressure, zonulysis should reduce the number of detachments caused by surgical trauma to the peripheral retina. However, I believe the majority of aphakic detachments are caused by preexist-

ing retinal and vitreous faults and not by operative complications either with or without zonulysis, excluding cases resulting from excessive pull on the zonules and problems related to vitreous loss.

In a series of 5541 cases of cataract extraction performed with the routine use of alpha-chymotrypsin,[62] the frequency of postoperative retinal detachment was 2.2%. This frequency compares favorably with that generally reported in the literature (0.4% to 3.5%), indicating that use of alpha-chymotrypsin most likely neither increases nor decreases the probability of subsequent development of retinal detachment.

Allergy

No allergic response was noted when alpha-chymotrypsin was used to extract the second cataract in a series of 71 patients previously exposed to the drug at the time of zonulysis for the first cataract.[35]

Despite widespread clinical use of alpha-chymotrypsin, no cases of allergic response have been reported. Experimental efforts to sensitize rabbits and guinea pigs to this enzyme have failed. Intraocular, intraperitoneal, and intravenous routes of injection did not produce local or general allergic responses, nor could precipitating antibodies be detected.[63] No known contraindication exists, therefore, to the use of alpha-chymotrypsin as an aid to cataract extraction in allergic persons, nor should the surgeon fear to use it again during operation on the second eye.

Delayed complications

Apparently there are no significant late complications after the use of alpha-chymotrypsin (for instance, a greatly increased incidence of chronic simple glaucoma resulting from trabecular damage). In this respect, recent experience has confirmed the findings of the first physician to use enzymatic zonulysis in August 1955.[64]

CLINICAL IMPLICATIONS

Extracapsular extraction that results in retention of a massive amount of cortex and capsule is just as bad as any complication attributed to alpha-chymotrypsin. Although enzymatic damage to other structures within the eye definitely occurs, under the carefully specified conditions of clinical use, significant complications are most infrequent. Experience has modified surgical techniques so that zonulysis is utilized most effectively and safely. The usefulness of alpha-chymotrypsin in cataract surgery has been firmly established.

REFERENCES

1. Thorpe, H. E.: Enzymatic zonulolysis, Am. J. Ophthalmol. **49:**531, 1960.
2. Watts, L. F., Jr., and Martin, C. J.: Stability of alpha-chymotrypsin, Arch. Ophthalmol. **65:**24, 1961.
3. Schwartz, B., and Schwartz, J. B.: A review of the biochemistry and pharmacology of alpha-chymotrypsin, Trans. Am. Acad. Ophthalmol. **64:**17, 1960.
4. Bedrossian, R. H., and Weimar, V.: Inhibitory effect of aqueous humor on alpha-chymotrypsin, Trans. Am. Acad. Ophthalmol. **67:** 822, 1963.
5. Damaskus, C. W.: Various laboratory aspects of alpha-chymotrypsin, Am. J. Ophthalmol. **49:**1117, 1960.
6. Liebowitz, D., and Ritter, H., Jr.: Anaphylactic reaction to chymotrypsin, J.A.M.A. **172:**159, 1960.
7. Raiford, M. B.: The use of alpha-chymotrypsin in cataract surgery, J. Med. Assoc. Ga. **48:**163, 1959.
8. Rose, K.: Anaphylactic reaction to aqueous chymotrypsin injection, J.A.M.A. **173:**796, 1960.
9. Howell, I. L.: Anaphylactic reaction to chymotrypsin, J.A.M.A. **175:**322, 1961.
10. von Sallmann, L.: Experimental studies of some ocular effects of alpha-chymotrypsin, Trans. Am. Acad. Ophthalmol. **64:**25, 1960.
11. Radnot, M., and Pajor, R.: Effect of alpha-chymotrypsin on the cornea, Am. J. Ophthalmol. **51:**598, 1961.
12. Barraquer, J., Troutman, R. C., and Rutllan, J.: Surgery of the anterior segment of the eye, vol. 1, McGraw-Hill Book Co., 1964.
13. Bedrossian, R. H., and Lalli, R. A.: Clinical application of new laboratory data on alpha-chymotrypsin, Arch. Ophthalmol. **67:**616, 1962.
14. Bedrossian, R. H.: Alpha-chymotrypsin, Arch. Ophthalmol. **62:**216, 1959.
15. Binion, W. W., and Fleming, T. C.: Enzyme treatment of corneal ulcers, Am. J. Ophthalmol. **55:**795, 1963.
16. Ing, M. R., Deiter, P., and Wong, A. S.: Chymotrypsin for experimental herpes simplex keratitis, Arch Ophthalmol. **71:**554, 1964.
17. Havener, W. H., Stambaugh, N. F., and Beil, H.: Corneal perforation in metaherpetic keratitis with virus inclusions treated with alpha-chymotrypsin, Am. J. Ophthalmol. **54:** 756, 1962.
18. Ley, A. P., Holmberg, A. S., and Yamashita, T.: Histology of zonulolysis with alpha-chymotrypsin employing light and electron microscopy Am. J. Ophthalmol. **49:**67, 1960.
19. Geeraets, W. J., Chan, G., and Guerry, D.: The effect of alpha-chymotrypsin on zonular fibers and anterior hyaloid membrane, Guildcraft, September 1960, p. 35.
20. Hogan, M. J., and Zimmerman, L. E.: Ophthalmic pathology, ed. 2, Philadelphia, 1962, W. B. Saunders Co.
21. Sekiguchi, J.: Histological studies on the ocular toxicity of alpha-chymotrypsin, Jap. J. Ophthalmol. **4:**104, 1960.
22. O'Malley, C., Moskovitz, M., and Straatsma, B.: Experimentally induced adverse effects of alpha-chymotrypsin, Arch. Ophthalmol. **66:** 539, 1961.
23. Maumenee, A. E.: Effect of alpha-chymotrypsin on the retina, Trans. Am. Acad. Ophthalmol. **64:**33, 1960.
24. Hamasaki, D. I., and Ellerman, N.: Abolition of the electroretinogram, Arch. Ophthalmol. **73:**843, 1965.
25. Bedrossian, R. H.: Irrigation after chymotrypsin? Arch. Ophthalmol. **74:**882, 1965.
26. Scheie, H. G., Yanoff, M., and Tsou, K. C.: Inhibition of alpha-chymotrypsin by aqueous humor, Arch. Ophthalmol. **73:**399, 1965.
27. Fleming, T. C.: Effect of alpha-chymotrypsin on catgut sutures, Am. J. Ophthalmol. **47:** 898, 1959.
28. Drance, S. M., Murray, R. G., and Smith, T. R.: The effect of alpha-chymotrypsin on suture materials, Am. J. Ophthalmol. **49:**64, 1960.
29. Barraquer, J.: Enzymatic zonulolysis in lens extraction, Arch. Ophthalmol. **66:**32, 1961.
30. Taylor, D. M.: Principles of lens delivery, Am. J. Ophthalmol. **50:**649, 1960.
31. Schwartz, B., Corwin, M., and Israel, R.: A double-blind therapeutic trial of the effect of

alpha-chymotrypsin on the facility of cataract extraction, Trans. Am. Acad. Ophthalmol. **64**:46, 1960.

32. Troutman, R. C.: National survey on the facility of cataract extraction, operation, and immediate postoperative complications, Trans. Am. Acad. Ophthalmol. **64**:37, 1960.

33. Hughes, W. F., Jr., and Owens, W. C.: The extraction of senile cataract: a statistical comparison of various techniques and the importance of preoperative survey, Am. J. Ophthalmol. **28**:40, 1945.

34. Kennedy, P. J., Jordan, J. S., Morrison, J. F., Mulberger, R. D., and Boland, S. W.: Enzymatic zonulolysis as an aid in cataract surgery, Arch. Ophthalmol. **64**:342, 1960.

35. Kennedy, P. J., Jordan, J. S., Morrison, J.F., Mulberger, R. D., and Boland, S. W.: Enzymatic zonulolysis as an aid in cataract surgery, Arch Ophthalmol. **65**:801, 1961.

36. Byron, H. M.: Management of retained lenticular material by enzymatic zonulolysis, Arch. Ophthalmol. **66**:509, 1961.

37. Mendelblatt, F. I.: Enzymatic zonulolysis, Am. J. Ophthalmol. **59**:1106, 1965.

38. Hill, H. F.: Cataract extraction with limited enzymatic zonulolysis, Arch. Ophthalmol. **75**:89, 1966.

39. Girard, L. J., Neeley, W., and Sampson, W. G.: The use of alpha-chymotrypsin in infants and children, Am. J. Ophthalmol. **54**:95, 1962.

40. Cassady, J.: Alpha-chymotrypsin for lens extraction in infants and children, Arch. Ophthalmol. **68**:730, 1962.

41. Cogan, J. E. H., Symons, H. M., and Gibbs, D. C.: Intracapsular cataract extraction using alpha-chymotrypsin, Br. J. Ophthalmol. **43**:193, 1959.

42. Kirsch, R. E.: Glaucoma following cataract extraction associated with use of alpha-chymotrypsin, Arch. Ophthalmol. **72**:612, 1964.

43. Barraquer, J., and Rutllan, J.: Enzymatic zonulolysis and postoperative ocular hypertension, Am. J. Ophthalmol. **63**:159, 1967.

44. Kirsch, R. E.: Dose relationship of alpha-chymotrypsin in production of glaucoma after cataract extraction, Arch. Ophthalmol. **75**:774, 1966.

45. Kalvin, N. H., Hamasaki, D. I., and Gass, J. D. M.: Experimental glaucoma in monkeys, Arch. Ophthalmol. **76**:82, 1966.

46. Anderson, D. R.: Scanning electron microscopy of zonulolysis by alpha-chymotrypsin, Am. J. Ophthalmol. **71**:619, 1971.

47. Worthen, D. M.: Scanning electron micros-copy after alpha-chymotrypsin perfusion in man, Am. J. Ophthalmol. **73**:637, 1972.

48. Chee, P., and Hamasaki, D. I.: The basis for chymotrypsin-induced glaucoma, Arch. Ophthalmol. **85**:103, 1971.

49. Kirsch, R. E.: Further studies on glaucoma following cataract extraction associated with the use of alpha-chymotrypsin, Trans. Am. Acad. Ophthalmol. **69**:1011, 1965.

50. Bloomfield, S.: Failure to prevent enzyme glaucoma, Am. J. Ophthalmol. **65**:405, 1968.

51. Galin, M.: Enzymatic zonulolysis and intraocular pressure, Am. J. Ophthalmol. **61**:690, 1966.

52. Gombos, G. M., and Oliver, M.: Cataract extraction with enzymatic zonulolysis in glaucomatous eyes, Am. J. Ophthalmol. **64**:68, 1967.

53. Koke, M. P.: Alpha-chymotrypsin combined with penicillin in cataract extraction, Am. J. Ophthalmol. **63**:1706, 1967.

54. Sears, D., and Sears, M.: Blood-aqueous barrier and alpha-chymotrypsin glaucoma in rabbits, Am. J. Ophthalmol. **77**:378, March 1974.

55. Murray, R. G., and Drance, S. M.: The use of alpha-chymotrypsin in cataract surgery, Arch. Ophthalmol. **63**:910, 1960.

56. Townes, C. D.: Unfavorable effects of alpha-chymotrypsin on cataract surgery, Arch. Ophthalmol. **64**:109, 1960.

57. Rizzuti, A. B.: Alpha-chymotrypsin (Quimotrase) in cataract surgery, Arch. Ophthalmol. **61**:135, 1959.

58. Kara, G. B.: Alpha-chymotrypsin in cataract surgery, Arch. Ophthalmol. **63**:122, 1960.

59. Stocker, F. W., Matton-Van Leuven, M. T., and Georgiade, H.: Influence of alpha-chymotrypsin on endothelial corneal dystrophy, Am. J. Ophthalmol. **55**:547, 1963.

60. Fine, M.: Therapeutic keratoplasty in Fuchs' dystrophy, Am. J. Ophthalmol. **57**:371, 1964.

61. Tjanidis, T., Konstas, K., and Papageorgio, T.: On retinal detachments after operation for cataract, Arch Ophthalmol. Soc. Northern Greece **10**:200, 1961.

62. Scheie, H. G., Morse, P. H., and Aminlar, A.: Incidence of retinal detachment following cataract extraction, Arch. Ophthalmol. **89**:293, 1973.

63. Fleming, T. C., and Riddel, G. H.: Studies on the antigenic properties of alpha-chymotrypsin, Am. J. Ophthalmol. **51**:1104, 1961.

64. Jenkins, B. H.: The use of alpha-chymotrypsin in cataract surgery, South. Med. J. **53**:44, 1960.

5
ANESTHESIA

LOCAL ANESTHESIA

The great majority of ocular diagnostic and surgical procedures may be performed under local anesthesia. Superficial manipulations (for example, suture removal, tonometry, spudding of superficial corneal foreign bodies, and irrigation of the lacrimal canaliculi) require only topical instillation of a surface-active anesthetic. When more extensive procedures are to be undertaken, injection anesthesia is necessary. This may consist of nerve block (facial nerve akinesia and retrobulbar injection) or of local tissue infiltration (as for pterygium transplant and chalazion surgery). The surgeon should be aware that an inflamed eye is more difficult to anesthetize with local agents, as they are rapidly carried away by the increased circulation of blood and may be inactivated by pH changes.

Topical anesthetics

A considerable variety of surface-active anesthetics are available and they have many characteristics in common. All act quite readily on mucosal surfaces and are relatively ineffective when applied on the less permeable skin surfaces. The surface-active anesthetics are relatively toxic and should *not* be injected. Furthermore, the application of excessive amounts of topical anesthetics to mucosal surfaces may result in the absorption of enough drug to cause severe systemic reactions. (Such problems are not encountered with the few drops of anesthetic used for ocular procedures but result when large mucosal surfaces are anesthetized as, for example, during examination and treatment of the throat.)

Mechanism of action

The drugs suitable for use as local anesthetics cause a reversible block of conduction through nerve fibers. The potency of a local anesthetic parallels its affinity for the nerve receptor protein when both are isolated in solution.[1]

Tetracaine and related local anesthetics are quite similar in structure to acetylcholine. (Procaine differs from acetylcholine only in the substitution of an aniline ring for a methyl group.) The acetylcholine system is ordinarily thought of as mediating neural impulses at synapses only. Actually it also controls the ion movements within nerve fibers and is therefore important within axons and nerve fibers as well as at synapses and junctions. One theory suggests that local anesthetics block nerve conduction by successfully competing with acetylcholine for the receptor protein.

Another suggested mechanism of action is that local anesthetics compete with calcium ions for a receptor site that controls the permeability of the cell membrane. The fundamental process in the transmission of a nerve impulse is a propagated decrease in permeability of the surface membrane of the nerve axon to sodium ions. This propagated permeability decrease is prevented by the action of a local anesthetic.[2]

The long-recognized fact that nerve fibers of small size (and greater surface area) are more readily anesthetized than are larger fibers is in accordance with a chemical combination or competition concept of local anesthetic action.

Duration of action

The duration of the anesthetic effect is determined by the length of time the drug remains bound to the nerve protein. This varies with the chemical structure of the drug, its concentration and amount, and the rate of removal by diffusion and circulation.

The rapidity of onset and the duration of anesthesia increase in proportion to the concentration of a given drug until a maximal concentration is reached.[3] No further increase in duration results when this maximal effective concentration is exceeded. Hence using more than the maximal effective concentration achieves nothing but greater systemic toxicity. The maximal effective concentration of tetracaine is 1%; of cocaine, 20%; and of proparacaine, 0.5%. In the interest of safety and practical efficiency of anesthesia, the optimal concentration of a drug may be less than the maximal effective concentration. Less than maximal concentrations (for example, 0.5% tetracaine) may be less irritating to the eye, for instance, and therefore better suited to clinical practice. Repeated instillation of anesthetic drops will enhance and prolong anesthesia.

Combination of two or more local anesthetic drugs does not enhance activity beyond that which would be obtained by an equivalent concentration of the stronger drug. Since the toxic systemic effect of multiple drugs is additive, the therapeutic index is not improved by using mixtures of anesthetic agents.

Although vasoconstrictors retard the absorption of injected anesthetic solutions, they do not influence the systemic absorption of anesthetics applied topically to normal mucous membranes, nor do they materially prolong the duration of anesthesia. For instance, the duration of anesthesia of the tip of the tongue was 53 minutes after application of 1% tetracaine solution and 49 minutes (insignificant difference) after application of 1% tetracaine solution with a 1:10,000 concentration of epinephrine.[3]

When tested on the tongue, a methylcellulose vehicle was found not to prolong the anesthetic action of tetracaine. However, this testing surface is not really comparable to the conjunctival sac with respect to the effect of a viscous solution.

Toxicity

Fortunately in ophthalmology it is not necessary to use large quantities of topical anesthetics. Indeed, excessive amounts are not retained in the cul-de-sac but run harmlessly down the check. One should be aware, nevertheless, that these drugs are extremely toxic. For instance, 100 mg of tetracaine is regarded as a potentially lethal dose. This is only 5 ml of a 2% solution! Fatal reactions are rarely a result of idiosyncrasy or allergy but rather occur from ignorant use of excessive quantities of anesthetic (as during an endoscopic examination). Since generalized reactions to the topical application of anesthetic solutions are due to systemic absorption of excessive quantities of drug, such reactions are virtually nonexistent after topical ocular anesthesia. However, syncope may be mistaken for drug reaction—I have seen a patient faint in anticipation of tonometry.

The rate of drug absorption across mucous membranes is almost unbelievably rapid and is comparable to intravenous administration. Fig. 5-1 shows the blood levels in dogs after 30 mg of tetracaine was administered by rapid (30 seconds) intravenous injection, slow (20 minutes) intravenous injection, pharyngeal and tracheal instillation, and subcutaneous injection.[4] Obviously absorption across mucous membranes is far more rapid than that following subcutaneous injection! The blood level attained is a function of total dosage and not of the concentration applied. Addition of epinephrine

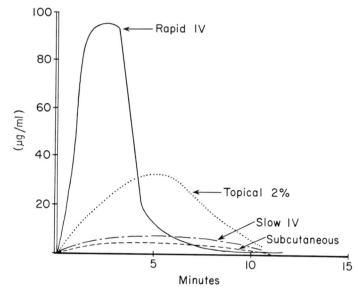

Fig. 5-1. Blood levels attained with 30 mg of tetracaine by different routes of administration (in dogs). (Modified from Adriani, J., and Campbell, D.: J.A.M.A. **162:**1527, 1956.)

(concentration 1:7500) to tetracaine solution does not materially retard its absorption across mucosal surfaces.

Since a minimal lethal dose of a local anesthetic is destroyed by the liver within 20 to 60 minutes,[5] recovery from local anesthetic poisoning is rapid if the patient can be kept alive by emergency measures.

Tetracaine reactions are characterized by a sudden onset of cardiac and respiratory collapse and may quickly prove fatal. Convulsions usually do not occur, and in this respect tetracaine toxicity differs from that of cocaine and most other topical anesthetics. Cocaine reactions usually begin with excitement, apprehension, and convulsions.

Treatment. Artificial respiration is the most important emergency measure; it must be instituted immediately and must be continued throughout the period of apnea. Intravenous administration of barbiturates is of value in controlling convulsions only and should *not* be given to the collapsed patient, since depression of vital functions is only made worse. Intravenous administration of vasopressors (for example, ephedrine, 15 mg intravenously) may help hypotension, but respiratory stimulants are considered ineffec-

tual. Further details concerning the management of anesthetic reactions will be found in the discussion of local anesthesia by injection.

Tetracaine (Pontocaine)

Tetracaine is one of the most popular topical anesthetics used in ophthalmology. Solutions of 0.5% to 2% may be instilled directly into the conjunctival sac. The majority of patients will complain of a burning sensation that lasts about 30 seconds, but this is not of clinical significance except in some children or apprehensive patients who may become frightened and uncooperative. The initial discomfort is less severe if the eyes are closed after instillation. A peculiar numb sensation persists for 10 to 20 minutes, depending on the number of drops used, and the patient may rub the eyes in annoyance. Since the corneal epithelium can be injured in this manner, the patient should be instructed to pat away tears from the closed lids with a tissue but not to rub the open eye.

Within a minute after instillation of a single drop of 0.5% tetracaine solution, anesthesia is ordinarily adequate for tonometry. Generally the patient first squeezes shut the eyes and then opens them comfortably as soon as anesthesia occurs. At this point the pressure may be measured.

Since additional manipulation is required for removal of embedded corneal foreign bodies, 2 drops or more of tetracaine at 30-second intervals should be used. When probing the nasolacrimal duct of an adult, the initial topical anesthesia should be supplemented by irrigation of the lacrimal sac with 0.25 ml of tetracaine, 0.5% solution. Care must be taken not to force tetracaine into the tissues by rough manipulations of the lacrimal needle.

Tetracaine instillations on the conjunctival surface may fail to achieve effective scleral anesthesia. For example, surface cautery of symptomatic intrascleral nerve loops was said to be painful when only topical tetracaine anesthesia was employed.[6]

Tetracaine should not be injected hypodermically for ophthalmologic procedures. One physician who did this had two patients die after injection of tetracaine for minor surgery in his office.

Corneal toxicity. As every biomicroscopist knows, the transitory presence of tiny superficial corneal epithelial lesions is commonly seen after tetracaine anesthesia. Repeated and prolonged anesthesia will intensify this epithelial damage. For this reason, it is unwise to prescribe topical anesthetics for the patient's home use to relieve pain from a corneal abrasion. Healing is significantly retarded by such medication, and normal epithelium may be damaged—both by chemical toxicity and by the patient's rubbing of the anesthetized eye. I have seen severe cases of corneal damage with accompanying iritis presumably caused by such unwise home use of topical anesthetics. Subsequent healing may be delayed for many days.

Experimental proof of the deleterious effects of topical anesthesia on epithelial regeneration is readily obtained. Both mitosis and cellular migration are inhibited.[7] Regeneration of the anesthetized rat corneal epithelium after minute puncture wounds has been studied.[8] One drop of each anesthetic solution was instilled every 15 minutes for 3 hours, at which time the rat was killed and the eyes fixed and studied microscopically. No healing occurred during this 3-hour period with solutions of 2% butacaine (Butyn), 4% cocaine, 0.4% benoxinate (Dorsacaine), 1% phenacaine (Holocaine), 0.1% dibucaine (Nupercaine), and 0.5% proparacaine (Ophthaine).[8] Partial healing was noted in patients treated with a 0.5% solution of tetracaine. Almost complete healing, with only slight distortion of the restored epithelium, occurred within 3 hours in the controls and with use of solutions of 2% piperocaine (Metycaine) and 2% lidocaine (Xylocaine).

Tetracaine seriously impairs the ability of the corneal epithelium to oxidize glucose and pyruvate. In the presence of a 0.0003M concentration of tetracaine, corneal epithelial oxidation of these vital carbohydrates was reduced by more than 80%.[9] During tetracaine anesthesia the oxygen uptake of the cornea is inhibited (17% inhibition with 0.0001M tetracaine, 62% with 0.002M tetracaine, and 75% with 0.004M tetracaine) and lactic acid accumulates within the tissue.[10]

Clinical evidence of this anesthetic-induced failure of epithelial healing was provided by a series of six patients who had sought relief of pain through the home use of tetracaine.[11] The sequence of events was remarkably similar in all patients. Initially the tetracaine was instilled every 2 hours for relief of pain. Gradually the discomfort became more annoying, and tetracaine was required after shorter intervals. Within several days the pain was extremely severe and could not be relieved by tetracaine—which several patients used as often as every 10 minutes in a vain effort to find comfort. Duration of the tetracaine treatment varied from several days to 2 weeks. The corneas of these patients showed extensive erosions of the epithelium and grayish stromal infiltration, were completely insensitive to touch, but were most painful. Healing was slow in all patients and required several months in the patients who had used tetracaine for 2 weeks. Epithelial growth from the borders was delayed and in every case was further retarded by faulty adherence to Bowman's membrane. Loose flaps of epithelium about the borders were subject to recurrent erosion, and these repeated breakdowns greatly prolonged the time of healing.

In rabbit experiments the same gradually diminishing effect of topical anesthesia was duplicated (with tetracaine, cocaine, and dibucaine), accompanied by epithelial erosion and stromal infiltration, prolonged insensitivity, and delayed healing.[12]

It seems evident that topical anesthetics should not be prescribed for prolonged home use! Ultraviolet corneal burns are the only conditions for which I have prescribed topical anesthetics. These injuries may be excruciatingly painful and can often be made much more comfortable by using tetracaine *sparingly.* Cold compresses, aspirin and codeine, and sedatives should be used during the 12 to 24 hours of severe discomfort.

Allergy. Although local allergy to tetracaine may develop because of repeated use, as in patients with glaucoma, these reactions are extremely uncommon. The ophthalmologist should suspect tetracaine allergy when the glaucoma patient complains of reddened, swollen, irritated, and itching lids that persist for some days after the office visit and tonometry. Often this will happen several times before the patient remembers to mention it. If the history is sufficiently typical, the simplest management is to note on the record the reason for changing to another anesthetic and avoid future tetracaine instillation.

Effect on microorganisms. Whenever possible, material to be cultured should be obtained without the prior instillation of an anesthetic. Not only are all commercial topical anesthetic preparations compounded with added preservatives but also the anesthetic drugs themselves are often toxic to microorganisms. Tetracaine, 0.5%, without added preservatives, completely inhibited all subsequent growth of *Staphylococcus albus,* *Pseudomonas,* and *Candida albicans* when the drug and organisms were incubated together for 24 hours. In contrast, 0.5% proparacaine did not significantly inhibit growth of any of these organisms. In commercial preparations, proparacaine contains 0.2%

chlorobutanol, which partially inhibits these organisms in a 24-hour culture. (Chlorobutanol, 0.4%, is a much more effective preservative, completely inhibiting all three organisms mentioned above for 24 hours.) Benoxinate, 0.4%, inhibited *Staphylococcus* and *Candida* but not *Pseudomonas.* Cocaine hydrochloride, 2.5%, inhibited all organisms.[13] In this study the practical effect of instillation of anesthetic drops for a brief period was not evaluated; certainly less than a 24-hour incubation is required for a corneal scraping. No doubt considerably less inhibition would occur in a shorter period of time; regardless, corneal scraping is impossible without an anesthetic.

Another study was designed to simulate the clinical conditions of anesthetic use. The amount of growth inhibition resulting from a 2-minute exposure and a subsequent 10 times dilution of the anesthetic was determined.[14] Under these circumstances the growth of *Staphylococcus albus* was inhibited by both tetracaine and proparacaine. Proparacaine also inhibited the growth of *Candida albicans.* Cocaine and benoxinate did not inhibit the growth of bacteria or fungi.

Proparacaine (Ophthaine)

Proparacaine is a synthetic topical anesthetic with characteristics essentially similar to those of tetracaine. It is supplied in a 0.5% solution, the sterility of which is maintained by addition of 0.2% chlorobutanol and 1:10,000 benzalkonium chloride.

Topical instillation of proparacaine and of tetracaine (each a 0.5% solution) produced similar anesthetic effects.[15] The time until onset of anesthesia after tetracaine instillation ranged from 9 to 26 seconds (average 14.7); that of proparacaine ranged from 6 to 20 seconds (average 12.9). The duration of action of tetracaine ranged from 9 to 24 minutes (average 15.2).

Instillation of proparacaine is considerably more comfortable than the use of tetracaine. Rated on a 4+ pain scale, discomfort with tetracaine averaged 1.5+ as compared with 0.5+ for proparacaine used in the fellow

eye.[15] Proparacaine causes much less stinging and squeezing of the lids than tetracaine
and is often completely painless. In a series
of 40 patients anesthetized with tetracaine
in one eye and proparacaine in the other,
30 reported tetracaine burned more, 4 said
proparacaine burned more, and 6 could tell
no difference. Ten of the 40 patients reported
no discomfort at all with proparacaine, a
statement made by only 2 patients with regard to tetracaine. The quality of anesthesia
was good with either drug.*

In Fig. 5-2 the anesthetic action of proparacaine is compared with that of tetracaine
and benoxinate, as measured with nylon
threads of graded rigidity. Obviously there is
no clinically significant difference in potency
between these three anesthetics.[16]

Patients allergic to tetracaine are not necessarily allergic to proparacaine, and vice
versa. Proparacaine has not been found to
cause a significant incidence of allergy. The
first patient I recognized to be sensitive to
proparacaine had undergone repeated tonometry for chronic simple glaucoma. After

several years she developed marked sensitivity to proparacaine. This manifested itself
as marked epithelial stippling and slight stromal edema, appearing within 5 to 10 minutes
after instillation. Considerable conjunctival
hyperemia and slight swelling were also
present. The lids were slightly puffy but
showed absolutely no redness or irritation,
such as typically occurs with atropine allergy.
Pain and profuse tearing were so severe as to
incapacitate the patient for many hours—
even walking was difficult. These symptoms
usually were quite severe for about half a
day and did not completely abate in less than
24 hours. Topical application of corticosteroid helped only slightly. This typical reaction developed at least four times before I
realized that it was unquestionably a result
of the use of proparacaine. The patient is
also allergic to pilocarpine. She is not allergic to tetracaine, carbachol, epinephrine, or
any other medication that she has taken.

Subsequent patients with proparacaine
allergy have exhibited comparable symptoms. Invariably the patient will have several
such episodes before I realize the existence
of the problem, which is finally revealed

*Unpublished personal observation, 1960.

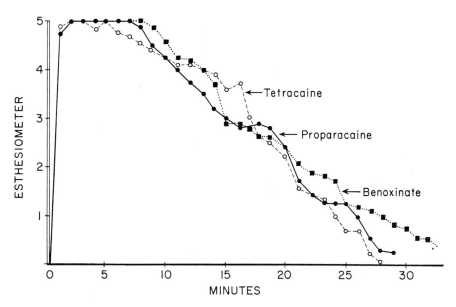

Fig. 5-2. Comparison of duration and intensity of anesthesia obtained with solutions of 0.5%
tetracaine, 0.5% proparacaine, and 0.4% benoxinate. (Modified from Linn, J. G., and Vey, E.
K.: Am. J. Ophthalmol. **40:**697, 1955.)

when the patient complains of the symptoms that followed past office visits. In two patients these repeated allergic responses over a 6-month period resulted in permanent stenotic occlusion of all four lacrimal puncta associated with epiphora.

Because it causes relatively little burning and discomfort on instillation, proparacaine is currently the anesthetic of choice in many ophthalmology offices.

Benoxinate (Dorsacaine)

Benoxinate has clinical characteristics that are essentially similar to those of proparacaine. Both drugs are less irritating than tetracaine and definitely cause less punctate epithelial damage. Since punctate staining may be confusing during applanation tonometry, this procedure is more accurately performed with benoxinate or proparacaine than with tetracaine.

A concentration of 0.4% benoxinate is most satisfactory for clinical use, giving corneal anesthesia essentially identical in intensity, time of onset, and duration to that of a 0.5% proparacaine solution. In a series of 85 patients receiving benoxinate in one eye and tetracaine in the other, no irritation was reported by 22 persons receiving benoxinate and 13 receiving tetracaine.[17] In patients reporting discomfort the duration of benoxinate burning or stinging averaged 9.8 seconds, as compared to 23 seconds for tetracaine.

In a series of 25 patients, solutions of 0.5% proparacaine were instilled in one eye and 0.4% benoxinate in the other. Thirteen patients reported more stinging with benoxinate, four experienced more stinging with proparacaine, and eight recognized no difference.*

If the ophthalmologist's objective is to reduce discomfort after ocular instillation of drops, patients should be instructed to close the eye after instillation. Thirty patients closed one eye and kept the other open after instillation of the same solution.[16] All 30 patients reported less stinging in the closed eye.

---

*Unpublished personal observation, 1960.

Table 5-1. Anesthetic concentrations 10 minutes after subconjunctival injection of 0.3 ml of 0.5% solution*

	Cornea	Iris	Aqueous
Benoxinate (mg/100 ml)	19	6	1.6
Procaine (mg/100 ml)	18	4	1.6

*Data from Schlegel, H. E., and Swan, K. C.: Arch. Ophthalmol. **51**:663, 1954.

In a series of more than 1000 patients anesthetized with benoxinate, no toxic effects were encountered, either locally or systemically.[18] Six of these patients who were allergic to other topical anesthetics (tetracaine, butacaine, and cocaine) had no reaction to benoxinate. Chemical analyses demonstrated ready penetration of benoxinate into the eye. Within 3 minutes of the application of a 1% solution to the intact rabbit cornea, concentrations of 70 mg/100 ml existed in the corneal epithelium and 7.5 mg/100 ml in the stroma. Rapid diffusion occurred, and within 15 minutes the corneal concentrations dropped to one third of their initial value. For this reason, effective anesthesia lasts not more than 10 to 15 minutes. The tissue distribution of benoxinate and procaine in rabbits 10 minutes after subconjunctival injection of 0.3 ml of a 0.5% concentration is shown in Table 5-1. Obviously both drugs penetrate well. Attention is directed to the low aqueous concentration, which indicates the inadequacy of the time-honored method of evaluating intraocular drug penetration through aqueous assay.

Cocaine

Cocaine, a naturally occurring alkaloid, was the first drug to be used successfully as a local anesthetic.[19-21] Excellent surface anesthesia is obtained by use of the 1% to 4% solutions that are employed in ophthalmology. This anesthesia is sufficiently complete to permit painless grasping of the eye with a forceps for about 10 minutes. Incomplete anesthesia persists for another 5 to 10 minutes. The indications and procedure for use of cocaine are essentially the same as those

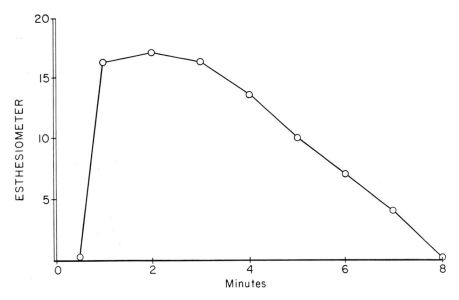

Fig. 5-3. Onset and duration of corneal anesthesia obtained from 1 drop of a 2% solution of cocaine, as measured by Frey's hairs. (Modified from Bellows, J. G.: Arch. Ophthalmol. **12:** 824, 1934.)

described previously for tetracaine. For ophthalmologic use, the newer synthetic anesthetics have replaced cocaine because of its deleterious effect on the cornea, its sympathomimetic properties, and its addicting potential.

The rate of onset and duration of cocaine anesthesia have been studied with Frey's hairs, which are calibrated as to strength. A No. 2 hair causes perceptible pain when touched to any part of the normal cornea. Tonometry is completely painless when the cornea is insensitive to a No. 2 hair. The average effect of 1 drop of a 2% solution of cocaine is illustrated in Fig. 5-3.[22] Within 30 seconds the No. 2 hair is no longer felt. The depth of anesthesia rapidly increases during the first minute, reaches a maximum at 2 minutes, and begins to decline by 3 minutes. After 8 minutes, the No. 2 hair again causes perceptible pain.

Use of 2 drops or more or use of a higher drug concentration substantially increased the duration of anesthesia. In general, this curve showing a brief latent period, a rapid onset of peak anesthesia, and a gradual decline is characteristic of all local anesthetics, with minor variations in duration. For practical purposes, within a minute the average cornea is rendered quite insensitive by an effective anesthetic.

Epithelial damage. The epithelial damage resulting from corneal anesthesia appears in its most exaggerated form when cocaine is used. Grossly visible grayish corneal pits and irregularities are readily produced by cocaine. Loosening of the epithelium may result in large erosions. In fact, this characteristic of cocaine proves useful in the treatment of dendritic ulcers, where it is used to remove the epithelium. Repeated instillation of cocaine over a period of several minutes will produce excellent anesthesia. It is then possible to dislodge the infected epithelium with an iodine-impregnated swab. Inasmuch as cocaine iodide is an insoluble precipitate, the previous cocainization protects against stromal damage by the iodine. (This protection is by no means complete, and excessive use of iodine may leave a stromal scar. Particular care should be taken in cauterizing the thin cornea of a child or dense and permanent scars may result.)

Sympathomimetic effect. About 15 to 20 minutes after instillation of cocaine, the pupil begins to dilate, reaching a maximum size within the first hour and returning to normal size within several hours. The pupil is never maximally dilated and responds to light and convergence at all times. Widening of the interpalpebral fissure is also produced in some patients by ocular instillation of cocaine.

This sympathomimetic action is said to be indirect because it occurs only in the presence of actively functioning sympathetic innervation. Cocaine, itself, has no sympathomimetic effect on denervated structures[23]; it acts by blocking the nerve terminal uptake of norepinephrine. Consequently, a greater than normal concentration of norepinephrine will accumulate at the sites of its normal production and will cause the sympathomimetic responses characteristic of this drug.

When strips of ciliary muscle are suspended in a water bath, muscle tension is not affected by cocaine in a concentration of 10 μg/ml.[24] However, such cocainization may sensitize the muscle to epinephrine. Response to a subthreshold concentration of epinephrine is obtained only after 30 minutes of cocainization. This delay in response is compatible with the possibility that cocaine may act indirectly by altering cellular permeability rather than by preventing the uptake of epinephrine.

Cocaine is clinically useful in the differential diagnosis of a miotic pupil. If the miosis is caused by sympathetic denervation affecting the second or third neuron (for example, Horner's syndrome and Raeder's paratrigeminal syndrome), there is no spontaneous liberation of norepinephrine at the

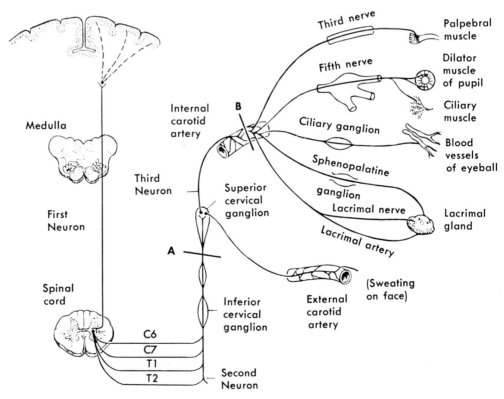

Fig. 5-4. Sympathetic pathway, indicating first, second, and third neurons for ocular sympathetic innervation. Lesions before the superior cervical ganglion, *A*, will produce Horner's syndrome with homolateral loss of facial sweating. Lesions distal to this ganglion, *B*, will not affect facial sweating. (From Boniuk, M., and Schlezinger, N. S.: Am. J. Ophthalmol. **54:** 1074, 1962.)

nerve terminals; hence its action cannot be enhanced by cocaine and the pupil does not dilate. The failure of the pupil to respond to 2% cocaine is best observed by comparison with the response of the patient's normal pupil, which will begin to dilate within 20 minutes and continue to increase in size for about an hour.

The effect of cocaine and epinephrine on the sympathetically denervated pupil is best explained by reference to Fig. 5-4, which outlines the cervical sympathetic pathway.[25] The first neuron extends from the hypothalamus to the spinal cord; the second neuron extends from the spinal cord to the superior cervical ganglion; and the third neuron is peripheral to this ganglion. Although Horner's syndrome of miosis and ptosis results from damage to any of the three neurons, testing with cocaine and epinephrine will differentiate first neuron damage from lesions of the second and third neurons. Presence or absence of facial sweating is also helpful in differentiation, since this function separates from the ocular pathway at the superior cervical ganglion. (Facial sweating may be detected by dusting starch-iodine powder on the face—the typical color change will appear when perspiration moistens the powder.)

Raeder's syndrome is caused by a lesion of the third sympathetic neuron adjacent to the trigeminal nerve (Fig. 5-4, *B*). This syndrome, of course, gives the typical cocaine and epinephrine responses expected with third neuron sympathetic denervation (Fig. 5-5).

If miosis is caused by a unilateral Argyll Robertson syndrome, the anisocoria is not eliminated by cocaine. Rather, cocainization causes dilation of both pupils (although anisocoria persists), which indicates that sympathetic innervation is unimpaired (Fig. 5-6).[26]

A 2% solution of cocaine should be used in testing the miotic pupil for evidence of sympathetic denervation. Large amounts of cocaine (several drops of 4% or 5% solution) will dilate the sympathectomized pupil by paralyzing the sphincter muscle. This dila-

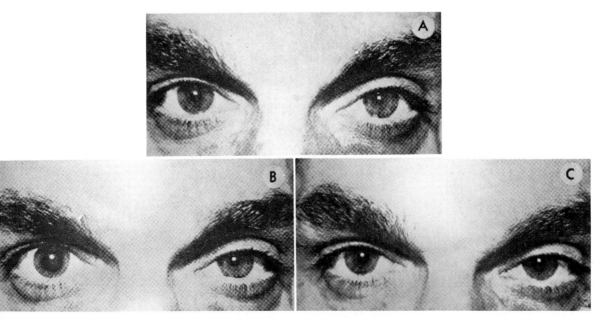

Fig. 5-5. A, Raeder's syndrome, with left ptosis and miosis. **B,** Solution of 4% cocaine dilates right eye but not left eye. **C,** Solution of 1:1000 epinephrine dilates left eye but not right eye. (From Boniuk, M., and Schlezinger, N. S.: Am. J. Ophthalmol. **54:**1074, 1962.)

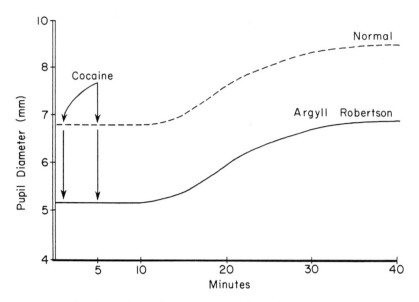

Fig. 5-6. Response of unilateral Argyll Robertson pupil to solution of 2% cocaine in each eye. Solid line: miotic, abnormal pupil. Broken line: normal pupil. (Modified from Lowenstein, O.: Am. J. Ophthalmol. **42:**105, 1965.)

tion represents a false negative test and misleads the clinician into believing that the sympathetic pathway is intact.[27]

Cocaine should not be used in ocular surgery if the surgeon does not wish the pupil to dilate or if good visualization of the fundus is necessary (as in retinal detachment procedures).

As is true with many other drugs, cocaine has less effect on a darkly pigmented iris than on one with less melanin. It is thought that the pigmented iris resists dilation by cocaine by inactivating the drug through its selective binding to the melanin granules.[28] In studies with radioactive cocaine the pigmented guinea pig iris will bind up to 18 times as much cocaine as will an albino iris. Furthermore, this cocaine binding in the pigmented iris is of long duration, whereas the albino iris permits a rapid washout of cocaine (half-life of 10 minutes). That cocaine binds to the melanin granules was established by incubating the drug with a suspension of bovine melanin granules (7 mg melanin/ml). Within 15 minutes, 61% of the cocaine was bound to the melanin and could be separated by centrifugation.

An enhanced nerve terminal site for co-

caine binding in the pigmented iris was excluded by blocking the sympathetic terminal with phenoxybenzamine or by destroying it with 6-OH-dopamine. Neither procedure reduced the cocaine binding by the pigmented iris.

Binding of radioactive ephedrine by the pigmented iris has been demonstrated previously. When the binding capacity of the pigmented iris has been saturated with ephedrine, its capacity to bind cocaine is reduced by 41%. (Cocaine binding occurs with melanin derived from the rat, guinea pig, and steer.)

This demonstration of drug binding by melanin is the most likely explanation for the well-known resistance of the pigmented iris to cycloplegics and miotics. A large proportion of the medication is simply inactivated by combination with the melanin and becomes unavailable for pharmacologic purposes.

Central nervous system effect. Considerable central nervous system stimulation results from systemic absorption of cocaine. This effect is sought by the cocaine addict. Apparently, withdrawal symptoms do not occur as in the case of morphine addiction, and the cocaine addict does not need to be tapered off of the drug. Cocaine distribution is subject to federal narcotic regulations.

Central nervous system stimulation with excitement, anxiety, convulsions, and circulatory and respiratory collapse characterizes cocaine toxicity. Severe reactions have followed doses as low as 20 mg (1 ml of a 2% solution) of cocaine. Doses in excess of 1 g are said to be fatal. One minimal lethal dose may be detoxified by the liver in an hour.[5]

Other local anesthetics

A number of other local anesthetics are no longer popular because of various faults: causing excessive irritation, having a high incidence of allergy, toxicity, etc. These medications include solutions of 2% butacaine sulfate, 2% piperocaine, 1% phenacaine, and 0.1% dibucaine.

Injection agents

The majority of ophthalmic operations can easily be performed with the patient under local anesthesia, which is clearly the method of choice. Obviously uncooperative patients (children, the mentally incompetent, and deaf persons) must have general anesthesia. A strong argument in favor of local anesthesia is the fact that each year in the United States at least 45 deaths from general anesthesia occur during eye operations performed by certified ophthalmologists.[29] Other less severe complications are far more frequent and add to the hazard of surgery performed with the patient under general anesthesia. Nausea, vomiting, and severe discomfort commonly distress patients during the day after general anesthesia. The metabolism of diabetic patients is particularly upset by fasting and general anesthesia.

Furthermore, cost to the patient and scheduling difficulties are substantially reduced if the services of the anesthesiologist and the recovery room nurses are not needed.

The ease and apparent safety with which local anesthesia may be achieved with injection techniques can lead to a false sense of security. Without appropriate safeguards, ophthalmologists performing minor surgery

in the office may find themselves in serious trouble. Local anesthetic injections should not be used unless the physician has immediately available an effective method for performing artificial respiration, a short-acting injectable barbiturate, and a vasopressor medication.[30] Appropriate premedication (for example, pentobarbital, 100 mg, and meperidine, 75 mg, for the average adult) will reduce apprehension and may increase the patient's resistance to the toxic central nervous system effects of local anesthetics. (Chloral hydrate does *not* antagonize this central nervous system toxicity.)

Under the stress of dealing with the emergency problems of acute glaucoma the ophthalmologist may forget that effective relief from severe acute ocular pain can be obtained by retrobulbar anesthesia. Such relief is free of the systemic depression caused by narcotics and is even more effective in blocking the pain. CAUTION! Do not relieve patients of their pain until they have agreed to emergency hospitalization and iridectomy, lest they refuse care because they are comfortable. Delay resulting from such a refusal could cause serious optic nerve damage. Retrobulbar anesthesia alone will probably not significantly reduce intraocular pressure and in no way substitutes for definitive therapy of glaucoma.

Procaine (Novocain)

This potent and relatively nontoxic anesthetic achieved wide popularity in injection anesthesia. Procaine penetrates poorly and is unsatisfactory for simple topical application to mucous membranes. When injected, procaine is only one fourth as toxic as cocaine[5] and furthermore is detoxified more rapidly by the body. If caution is exercised to avoid intravenous injection, 0.5 g of procaine is considered an entirely safe dose. This is the equivalent of 50 ml of a 1% solution—far more than is necessary in ophthalmic surgery. A further margin of safety is gained by simultaneous injection of epinephrine, thus retarding absorption.

Procaine may be used in concentrations varying from 0.5% to 4%. There is rarely a need to use a solution stronger than 1% for ophthalmologic anesthesia. Obviously stronger concentrations introduce a greater amount of potentially toxic drug. Toxic reactions are somewhat similar to those described for the other anesthetics. Cardiovascular collapse may occur shortly after the injection of procaine.

Lidocaine (Xylocaine)

Lidocaine is an increasingly popular drug for local injection anesthesia. Although similar to procaine in its anesthetic effect, lidocaine diffuses more readily through tissue and therefore produces a wider area of anesthesia. Its duration is longer than that of procaine. As would be expected from its greater potency, lidocaine is about 50% more toxic than is procaine.

One percent lidocaine solutions are adequate for all ophthalmic uses. For practical purposes, use of a 2% solution does not further increase the anesthetic effect; yet it doubles the dosage and the potential toxic effect. For some irrational reason, many ophthalmologists persist in the use of 2% lidocaine. Not more than 0.5 g of lidocaine should be given to a patient during an operation. This is 50 ml of a 1% solution. Obviously a large margin of safety exists for the usual ophthalmic procedures, which rarely require more than 10 to 15 ml. Accidental intravenous injection or unusual patient sensitivity may greatly reduce the tolerated dose. Systemic absorption after lidocaine injection regularly produces general drowsiness due to its effect on the central nervous system. Overdosage may cause a variety of toxic effects, including drop in blood pressure, nausea and vomiting, and convulsions.

Ophthalmologists generally express concern that accidental intravenous injection of lidocaine may occur. Relevant to this concern is the fact that lidocaine is an important antiarrhythmic agent in the management of acute myocardial infarction. For this purpose, a bolus of 100 mg (10 ml of a 1% solution) is rapidly injected intravenously. This is actually more than is used in most cataract surgery. Within 20 minutes, plasma levels have often dropped below that required to treat the arrhythmia, and a second bolus of 100 mg is advised.[31] Obviously, we have a wide margin of safety in using lidocaine for ophthalmic surgery.

Mepivacaine (Carbocaine)

Mepivacaine is a synthetic anesthetic administered by injection. [32] Its toxicity and tissue tolerance are comparable to those of procaine or lidocaine. Although adequate, its anesthetic potency (in a dosage of 1.5 ml of a 2% solution) seems slightly less than other commonly used anesthetics when evaluated in terms of akinesia of extraocular muscles or reduction of intraocular pressure.[33] The average duration of sensory anesthesia after retrobulbar injection of 1.5 ml of a 2% solution was 2 hours. This was measured by grasping with forceps the conjunctiva of human subjects every 10 minutes until sensation returned. An indication for the use of mepivacaine would be allergy to other local anesthetic agents.

Bupivacaine (Marcaine)

The advantage of bupivacaine is very prolonged duration of anesthesia. The disadvantage is slowness and incompleteness of anesthetic onset.

Less than 2 ml of 0.75% bupivacaine failed to give a consistent and reasonably prompt anesthetic. This amount produced anesthesia lasting for 8 to 12 hours, with a sufficient residual at 24 hours to permit routine Schiøtz tonometry without any topical anesthetic. Partial paralysis of the extraocular muscles might also last for 24 to 48 hours. The greatest advantage of bupivacaine was the complete freedom from postoperative pain during the first day after surgery.

Use of 0.5% bupivacaine resulted in incomplete akinesia, sometimes requiring 30 minutes or more for onset, and was unsatisfactory. Combinations of 0.5% bupivacaine (1.25 ml) with mepivacaine 0.5% (1.25 ml) or lidocaine 0.5% resulted in acceptably rapid onset of anesthesia together with long duration. Addition of hyaluronidase potentiated the effect of bupivacaine.

The prolonged effect of bupivacaine is due to the duration of its binding to nerve tissue. No local complications were observed during the use of bupivacaine in the performance of 500 cataract extractions.[34]

Because of its long duration of action, bupivacaine was used as the anesthetic in 10 patients undergoing cyclocryotherapy for glaucoma and did prevent postoperative pain for up to 7 hours. However, the postoperative pain associated with this procedure lasted for an unusually long time (average 28 days) in these patients. The average duration of postoperative pain in comparable patients treated under lidocaine anesthesia was only 4 days. The authors could not explain this unusual reaction but speculated on some alteration in the nerve fibers caused by the combination of freezing and bupivacaine.[35]

Associated medications

Epinephrine and hyaluronidase are commonly added to anesthetic solutions injected for ophthalmic surgery.

Epinephrine

The desired effects of local anesthetics such as procaine and lidocaine may be enhanced by the concomitant use of epinephrine. Such mixtures are commercially available, or the surgeon may add epinephrine to the anesthetic solution just prior to injection, in a concentration of 1:50,000 or 1:100,000. Mixing 1 ml of a 1:1000 concentration of epinephrine with 50 ml of lidocaine produces a 1:50,000 dilution. Use of epinephrine is particularly desirable in highly vascular areas such as exist about the eye. The resulting vasospasm slows drug absorption from the injected area, thereby prolonging anesthesia. This decreased rate of systemic absorption permits time for the drug to be detoxified or excreted and thereby reduces the chance of toxic reaction to the anesthetic.

If an infiltration type of injection is used directly at the operative site, a great deal of bloody oozing is prevented by epinephrine injection. This is particularly true in lid surgery. Although dacryocystorhinostomy is ordinarily carried out with the patient under general anesthesia, the operative site should be infiltrated with a local anesthetic containing epinephrine. (An epinephrine pack should also be placed high in the nose, adjacent to the lacrimal fossa.) With such a preparation, it may be possible to perform an almost bloodless dacryocystorhinostomy, in contrast to the usual bloody confusion. Similarly, postenucleation bleeding is reduced by a retrobulbar injection containing epinephrine. I believe that the increased duration of anesthesia obtained with the use of epinephrine clearly justifies its use in retrobulbar anesthesia for cataract surgery.

The patient with coronary artery disease or thyrotoxicosis should have local anesthesia without epinephrine. If a patient is under general anesthesia, it is important to inform the anesthesiologist of your intent to inject epinephrine, since it elevates blood pressure and may cause cardiac fibrillation when agents such as cyclopropane and halothane are being used. Some surgeons warn the patient that after local injection of epinephrine they may experience tachycardia, palpitation, nervousness, and apprehension. Such symptoms are transient and do not interfere with subsequent surgery. It is wise to wait for any undue restlessness to subside before beginning surgery—the patient will be more quiet, a toxic anesthetic reaction is ruled out, and it is less likely that the patient will begin to vomit during surgery or have some other undesirable reaction resulting from apprehension.

The side effects of epinephrine may mistakenly be diagnosed as the early stages of a toxic reaction to the anesthetic drug. Epinephrine does cause tremor, apprehension, pallor, and tachycardia but does not result in convulsions, twitching, or disorientation. Epinephrine reactions produce marked elevation of blood pressure in contrast to the cardiovascular collapse of procaine toxicity.

Hyaluronidase

Hyaluronic acid is a polysaccharide found in the interstitial spaces of tissue as well as in the vitreous body. Hyaluronidase is an enzyme that depolymerizes this polysaccharide. Removal of hyaluronic acid from tissues greatly increases their permeability to injected fluids. The permeability returns to normal within 24 to 48 hours because of formation of new hyaluronic acid. Hyaluronidase is nontoxic and does not damage or inflame tissues in any way. Since there is no hyaluronic acid in capillary walls, hyaluronidase does not affect capillary permeability.

Mechanical pressure (as from the volume of injected solution or from massage) is needed to spread hyaluronidase through tissue. Without pressure, it does not diffuse any great distance. The extent of fluid spread is more closely proportional to the amount of injected fluid than to the dosage of hyaluronidase. Hyaluronidase will not promote passage of fluids across fascial barriers (such as Tenon's capsule) or through fibrin clots.

Hyaluronidase is measured in turbidity reducing units (TRU). Within 30 minutes, 1 TRU will reduce the turbidity of a 0.2 mg hyaluronic acid suspension in serum to that of a 0.1 mg suspension. The enzyme is marketed in 150 TRU vials. This amount is sufficient to aid in the administration of the usual hypodermoclysis, or it may be added to a 20 ml bottle of lidocaine before ocular injection. As little as 7 TRU/ml will effectively dissolve hyaluronic acid barriers. More than 2 million TRU/kg can be tolerated intravenously by mice.[36]

Intraocular tolerance. The eye reacts minimally to intraocular injection of hyaluronidase. Anterior chamber injection of 5 TRU, repeated daily for 7 days, caused only slight iris hyperemia in rabbits.[37]

Intravitreal injection of 100 TRU of hyaluronidase partially liquefied rabbit vitreous in 4 hours.[38] Moderate uveitis ensued, and veil-like condensations of the vitreous framework were noted subsequent to these injections. Relatively impure preparations of hyaluronidase were used in earlier experiments and caused more inflammation than did the currently available enzyme.

Ophthalmic uses. In ophthalmology, hyaluronidase is useful in enhancing the effect of local injection anesthesia and in increasing the hypotony resulting from retrobulbar anesthesia. Hyaluronidase may increase the effective area of an injected anesthetic by as much as 40%.[39] Additionally, the time of onset of anesthesia may be considerably shortened—not uncommonly orbicularis paralysis will be almost complete within as little as 1 minute after injection by the van Lint or Atkinson techniques. Distortion of tissues by the injected fluid rapidly disappears, especially if external pressure is briefly applied.

Effect on duration of anesthesia. The duration of local anesthesia may be reduced by hyaluronidase alone, but the simultaneous use of epinephrine and hyaluronidase maintains the usual duration of anesthesia. The duration of motor paralysis produced by retrobulbar injection of 0.75 ml of various anesthetics was studied by observation of opticokinetic nystagmus in monkeys.[40] This technique permitted accurate evaluation of the duration of anesthesia under circumstances comparable to clinical usage. As seen in Fig. 5-7, a 2% solution of procaine produces anesthesia that lasts somewhat longer than anesthesia obtained with 1%, but 4% produces no additional effect. Solutions of 2% lidocaine have a duration comparable to 2% solutions of procaine. Although the anesthetic effect of tetracaine, 0.1% solution, lasted considerably longer, this drug is toxic and caused tissue irritation. The authors were favorably impressed with mepivacaine, a new chemical relative of lidocaine. The data given in Fig. 5-8 indicate that combination of hyaluronidase with procaine greatly reduces the duration of anesthesia but that addition of epinephrine in a 1:100,000 concentration prolongs activity. Epinephrine vasoconstriction slows the removal of anesthetic from the orbit despite breakdown of the hyaluronic acid tissue barriers. Lidocaine and mepivacaine, however, react differently in combination with these additives; the duration of anesthesia is actually shortened (Fig. 5-9). These graphs do not indicate the percentage of satisfactory blocks attained by retrobulbar injections because unsuccessful injections were discarded from the statistics. Hyal-

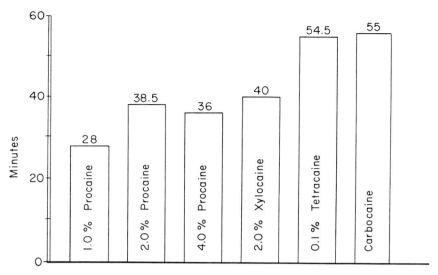

Fig. 5-7. Duration of akinesia after retrobulbar anesthesia in monkey. (Modified from Everett, W. G., Vey, E., and Finlay, J.: Trans. Am. Acad. Ophthalmol. **65**:308, 1961.)

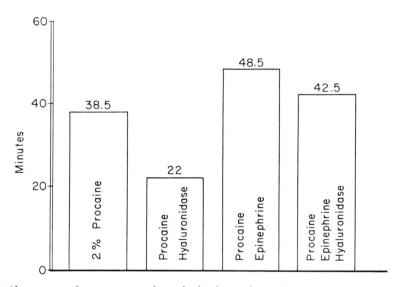

Fig. 5-8. Shortening of procaine anesthesia by hyaluronidase and prolongation by epinephrine. (Modified from Everett, W. G., Vey, E., and Finlay, J.: Trans. Am. Acad. Ophthalmol. **65**: 308, 1961.)

uronidase did enhance the effect of procaine injection but was reported not to augment the effect of lidocaine or mepivacaine. Lidocaine and mepivacaine penetrate tissue more readily than procaine and are said not to require the aid of hyaluronidase. However, regardless of which anesthetic is chosen, hy-aluronidase is still of value in retrobulbar injection because it reduces orbital tension.

Effect on intraocular penetration of medications. Hyaluronidase will not increase the intraocular penetration of subconjunctivally injected procaine.[41] Qualitative chemical analyses were made at intervals of 5,

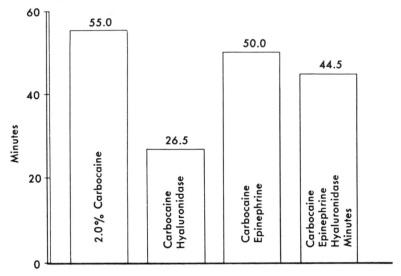

Fig. 5-9. Effect of hyaluronidase and epinephrine on mepivacaine anesthesia. (Modified from Everett, W. G., Vey, E., and Finlay, J.: Trans. Am. Acad. Ophthalmol. **65:**308, 1961.)

10, and 20 minutes after subconjunctival injections of 1% solutions of procaine alone, with a 1:5000 concentration of epinephrine, and with hyaluronidase (Table 5-2). Hyaluronidase did not alter iris concentrations of procaine at 5 or 10 minutes but caused appreciably lower concentrations at 20 minutes, presumably because of drug loss through diffusion into the bloodstream. The limbal circulation in the living animal rapidly carried away the procaine, whereas in dead animals significantly higher iris concentrations were readily attained. Use of epinephrine markedly increased the iris concentra-

Table 5-2. Qualitative analyses 10 minutes after subconjunctival injection of a 1% solution of procaine (mg/100 ml)*

	Cornea	Iris	Aqueous
Living rabbits	32	5.5	2
Dead rabbits	17	17	3
Living rabbits with epinephrine	35	12.5	2.5
Living rabbits with hyaluronidase	21	6	1

*Data from Swan, K. C.: Arch. Ophthalmol. **52:**774, 1954.

tion of procaine. The highest iris concentrations of procaine (17 mg/100 ml) were lower than the level required for anesthesia of small sensory nerves (35 mg/100 ml). This explains why subconjunctival injection alone is not a consistently satisfactory method of anesthesia for intraocular surgery. Note that aqueous studies do not accurately indicate the concentrations of medications in the iris or cornea.

Antibiotic penetration into the eye following subconjunctival injection is not enhanced by use of hyaluronidase. This fact was established by microbiologic assay of the rabbit aqueous following subconjunctival injection of lincomycin.[42] It was also determined that intraocular penetration of radioactive mannitol was not increased when hyaluronidase was added to the solution.

Hypotony. In addition to ensuring better sensory and motor nerve blocks, addition of hyaluronidase to the anesthetic solution will produce a softer eye than will a similar retrobulbar injection without hyaluronidase. Since retrobulbar injection of hyaluronidase alone has no effect on intraocular pressure, the hypotony must be due to enhancement of the anesthetic effect.[43] The very soft eye obtainable by addition of hyaluronidase to the retrobulbar anesthetic, followed by massage, is an extremely valuable safeguard against vitreous loss during cataract surgery.

Effect on eyelid skin. Loosening of the tissue bonds between the eyelid skin and the orbicularis muscle may be achieved by injection of about 1 ml of hyaluronidase-containing anesthetic solution about 30 minutes before surgery is to begin. This is a critical point in the "pinch" technique of cosmetic removal of excess lid skin.[44] This technique simply involves use of a toothed forceps to pinch the redundant skin into a ridge parallel to the lid margin. Loosened by the hyaluronidase injection, the skin will remain in a standing ridge, which can be adjusted to contain exactly the amount of skin available for excision.

Response of glaucoma. A hyaluronidase-sensitive substance may exist in the normal chamber angle and has been demonstrated to be present in abnormally large amounts in eyes enucleated for choroidal melanoma. In a series of 70 glaucomatous eyes, 10 TRU of hyaluronidase was injected subconjunctivally.[45] In almost every case, tonographic measurement showed a reduced resistance to outflow. The pressure-reducing effect persisted for about 30 hours and disappeared 2 to 3 days after injection.

A similar pressure drop was observed in 20 glaucomatous eyes after administration of hyaluronidase by iontophoresis.[46]

Because of the difficulty of administration and the short duration of response, hyaluronidase has no clinical value in the management of glaucoma.

Effect on chemosis. Hyaluronidase may be used to reduce conjunctival edema and chemosis after ocular surgery. Injection of 150 TRU subconjunctivally has been reported to cause prompt clearing of such edema.[47]

Effect on vitreous hemorrhage. In rabbits, hyaluronidase injection does not aid in the absorption of intravitreal hemorrhage.[48]

Techniques of local injection

Local injection anesthesia for ophthalmic surgery may involve the general technique of regional infiltration or the specialized techniques of orbicularis block and retrobulbar injection. Regional infiltration is simply injection of the area to be operated on, for example, the lid for chalazion surgery. This technique is too obvious to require further description.

Preceding intraocular surgery, orbicularis block and retrobulbar injection are necessary to prevent the serious complications that may result from squeezing or eye movement. Such injections should precede intraocular surgery, even if the patient is also under general anesthesia, to help prevent problems should the patient become "light" and move at a critical stage of the operation.

Orbicularis block

Orbicularis paralysis can be achieved by blocking the facial nerve anywhere along its course. Most commonly a vertical injection is made about a centimeter lateral to the orbital rim (Fig. 5-10).[49] Four to ten milliliters of anesthetic solution may be injected as the needle advances deep into skin and muscle. Injection in this area gives excellent orbicularis paralysis and does not cause lid edema, which could interfere with surgical exposure.

An alternate method, blocking the facial nerve below the ear (O'Brien technique), is less convenient, causes annoying weakness of the entire face, and is more likely to cause prolonged nerve damage.

When orbicularis paralysis is achieved by injection about the facial nerve near its exit from the stylomastoid foramen, prolonged facial paralysis may ensue. In 4 of 150 patients receiving such injections the paralysis lasted up to 3 months and tarsorrhaphy was necessary to protect the cornea. This prolonged facial paralysis is not due to the toxic effect of the anesthetic but to needle injury of the nerve, which is fixed in unyielding surrounding tissue at this site and therefore cannot roll away from the needle.[50]

Retrobulbar injection

The technique of injection will, of course, determine the portion of the orbit that is

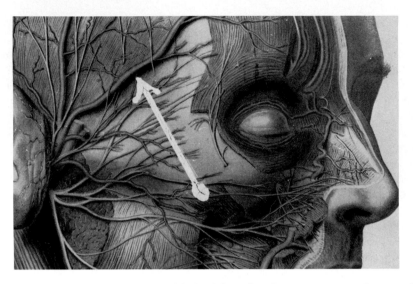

Fig. 5-10. Site of injection for effective block of the orbicularis innervation. (From Atkinson, W. S.: Trans. Am. Acad. Ophthalmol. **60:**376, 1956.)

anesthetized. A retrobulbar injection may be intended to produce sensory anesthesia alone or a combination of sensory and motor anesthesia. Two positions into which the retrobulbar needle may be introduced are shown in Fig. 5-11.[51] An anterior retrobulbar injection is placed in the relatively avascular region just behind the globe. A small quantity of solution (for example, 1 ml) in this anterior retrobulbar position will cause only sensory anesthesia. In contrast, posterior (or apical) retrobulbar injection will produce both sensory and motor anesthesia. Since the vessels of the apex of the orbit are larger and more fixed in position and cannot be so readily displaced by a needle, they are much more readily pierced than the anterior vessels. This is the reason retrobulbar hemorrhage is more frequent after deep injections, although it may also result from injury to a vortex vein.

Slicing movements of the needle within the orbit may result in retrobulbar hemorrhage, as the sharp tip and edge of the needle are dragged across tissue. Such faulty injection technique is commonly reported by observers as being the cause of retrobulbar hemorrhage, although the operator usually vigorously denies any such error.

Since no tissue barriers exist between the anterior and posterior portions of the retrobulbar space, it is obvious that the motor anesthesia of a posterior block may be achieved simply by injecting a larger volume of solution anteriorly. Indeed, there is no valid reason to risk a posterior retrobulbar injection. Four to six milliliters of 1% solution of lidocaine with hyaluronidase may safely be injected into the anterior retrobulbar space. After 3 to 5 minutes of massage, such an injection will produce almost total muscular akinesia and ocular anesthesia. The slight proptosis that results actually facilitates cataract surgery, especially if the patient has deeply sunken eyes. If massage is continued until hypotony is present, this volume of injection definitely does not increase the hazard of vitreous loss.

The distinction between anterior and posterior retrobulbar injection is particularly important when alcohol injections (see discussion of ethanol, Chapter 16) are given for relief of pain. Such an injection *must* be given anteriorly to produce a sensory block without causing disfiguring paralysis. I know of cases in which deep alcohol injections have caused ptosis and extraocular muscle paralysis. The alcohol must be confined within the retrobulbar space, for if it leaks anteriorly, severe chemosis and pain result.

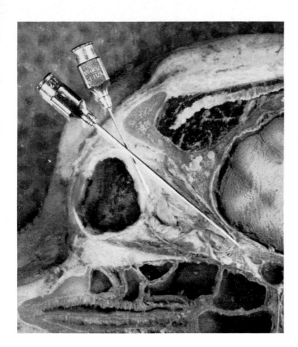

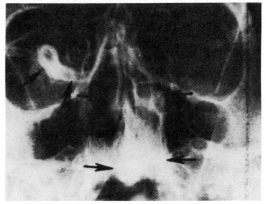

Fig. 5-12. Outline of right optic nerve after accidental intrasheath injection of contrast material that has extended intracranially. (From Reed, J. W., MacMillan, A. S., Jr., and Lazenby, G. W.: Arch. Ophthalmol. **81**:508, 1969.)

Fig. 5-11. Coronal section of orbit showing needles in position for anterior and posterior retrobulbar injections. (From Swan, K. C.: Trans. Am. Acad. Ophthalmol. **60**:368, 1956.)

The possibility of damaging the optic nerve by retrobulbar injection must always be remembered. Such an injury may be avoided by introducing the needle no more deeply than necessary to penetrate the intermuscular septum (recognizable by suddenly decreased resistance). Accidental injection into the sheaths of the optic nerve with intracranial extension during contrast orbitography has been documented by subsequent x-ray studies (Fig. 5-12).[52] Transitory lidocaine anesthesia of the right optic nerve (loss of vision), the right parasympathetic innervation (mydriasis), and innervation of both sixth nerves (loss of abduction) resulted.

Posterior subcapsular injection[51] refers to placement of the needle between sclera and Tenon's capsule. This is done by lifting the equatorial conjunctiva and Tenon's capsule with forceps and introducing the needle between forceps and eye. Injection in this space will cause sensory anesthesia without motor block but will diffuse forward to cause swelling anteriorly beneath Tenon's cap-

sule. This is a particularly good approach for blocking a given rectus muscle, since the needle may easily be introduced further back and beneath the given muscle. Attempts to inject directly into a muscle have been advocated but are more likely to injure the muscle or cause hemorrhage and therefore should be avoided. Supplementary injections of this type are unnecessary after retrobulbar injection of a large volume (4 to 6 ml) of anesthetic.

Sensory block of the optic nerve is well known to accompany retrobulbar anesthesia.[53] This is the reason that the bright operating lights are so easily tolerated by a patient during cataract extraction. Photocoagulation usually requires retrobulbar injection. I customarily inject 4 ml of 1% lidocaine solution. This almost completely eliminates light perception and permits treatment without the exasperation of continuous movements. The proptosis induced by retrobulbar injection facilitates aiming the photocoagulator into the far periphery, unhampered by the facial contours.[54]

An objective method of studying the effect of retrobulbar anesthesia consists of measuring optic nerve potentials in the cat.[55] This technique was used to evaluate the effect of various concentrations of procaine or

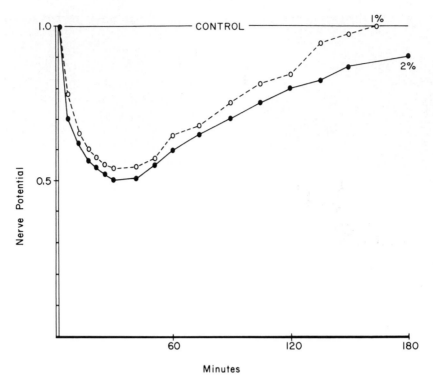

Fig. 5-13. Intensity and duration of anesthetic effect on optic nerve. (Modified from Pruett, R. C.: Arch. Ophthalmol. **77:**119, 1967.)

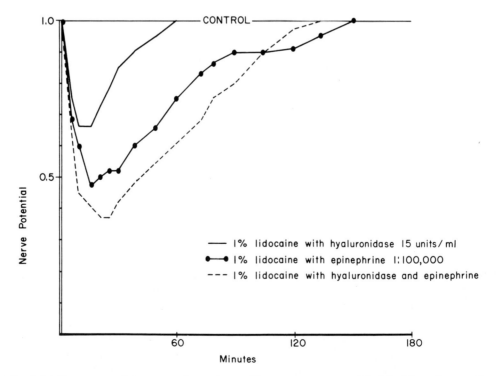

Fig. 5-14. Intensity and duration of anesthetic effect on optic nerve. (Modified from Pruett, R. C.: Arch. Ophthalmol. **77:**119, 1967.)

lidocaine, with or without hyaluronidase and epinephrine. The reader is reminded that the optic nerve is very much larger than the other sensory and motor nerves in the orbit and is therefore more resistant to complete conduction block. The maximum anesthetic effect of lidocaine on the optic nerve was attained in 20 to 30 minutes and a progressively decreasing anesthetic effect was demonstrable for as long as 3 hours (Fig. 5-13). Increasing the lidocaine concentration from 1% to 2% did not materially increase the anesthetic effect. Addition of hyaluronidase greatly shortens the lidocaine effect, but this loss may be neutralized by addition of 1:100,000 epinephrine to the anesthetic mixture (Fig. 5-14). Epinephrine alone does *not* increase the duration of lidocaine anesthesia, but it does increase the duration of procaine anesthesia.

Volume. The importance of properly injecting an adequate volume of anesthetic solution before cataract extraction is so great as to warrant some repetition. The volume of solution injected for retrobulbar anesthesia need not be limited to 1 or 1.5 ml. As much as 4 or 5 ml may be safely introduced into the muscle cone and massaged into the tissues if hyaluronidase is added to the anesthetic preparation.[56] These larger injections produce better anesthesia, akinesia, and hypotony. After injection, massage should be continued until the eye and orbit are soft rather than for a given number of minutes. Pressure should frequently be interrupted to avoid prolonged interference with retinal circulation. Injection of large volumes without the aid of hyaluronidase creates a proptosed orbit, which is quite undesirable and dangerous in intraocular surgery.

In over 200 cataract extractions performed with 4 ml or more of retrobulbar anesthetic injection, there was no instance of vitreous loss.[57] If the eye is sunken into an atrophic orbit, as much as 6 ml may be injected to raise the eye to a position more surgically accessible. As much as 8 ml may be injected into the orbit without operative complications, provided that hyaluronidase is used.[58] I have personally used retrobulbar injections of 4 to 6 ml preceding cataract

surgery for some years and am very pleased with the results. CAUTION! Be certain to use hyaluronidase; otherwise the orbit will become undesirably tense.

Hypotony. One of the truly important milestones in the development of cataract surgery was recognition of the importance of the soft eye, which can be achieved with a combination of retrobulbar anesthetic, hyaluronidase, and external pressure.[59] The factors responsible for this hypotony are multiple.

Immediately after retrobulbar anesthetic injection, intraocular pressure drops rapidly and spontaneously, generally reaching a minimum level within 5 minutes (Fig. 5-15).[60] A pressure drop comparable to that following retrobulbar anesthesia accompanies thiopental sodium–induced general anesthesia (Fig. 5-16).[60] Retrobulbar anesthesia given during thiopental general anesthesia caused only an insignificant additional drop in pressure (averaging 1.4 mm Hg in 10 patients).

Because of the similar magnitude of the pressure drop with general and local anesthesia and because there is no significant additive effect, it is reasonable to assume their mechanism of action is identical. Since relaxation of the extraocular muscles results from both types of anesthesia and because the degree of hypotony is related to the completeness of paralysis of the extraocular muscles, relaxation of the normal tonus of the extraocular muscles may reasonably be specified as the cause of the initial hypotony after anesthesia. Conversely, every ophthalmologist will agree that increased tonus of these muscles may readily increase intraocular pressure.

In a series of 100 glaucomatous eyes, intraocular pressure was measured before and after retrobulbar injection of various percentages of procaine with or without hyaluronidase.[43] In many, but not in all, cases there was some drop of intraocular pressure after the retrobulbar block. Of particular interest is the fact that injection of hyaluronidase alone did *not* alter the intraocular pressure. In general, higher concentrations of procaine or the combination of procaine with

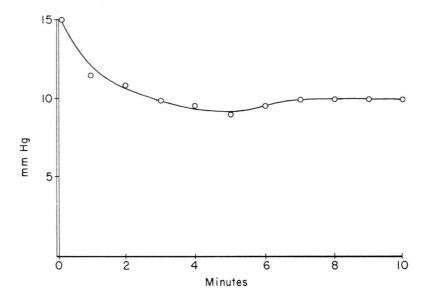

Fig. 5-15. Spontaneous fall of intraocular pressure after retrobulbar anesthesia. (Modified from Everett, W. G., Vey, E. K., and Veenis, C. Y.: Trans. Am. Acad. Ophthalmol. **63**:286, 1959.)

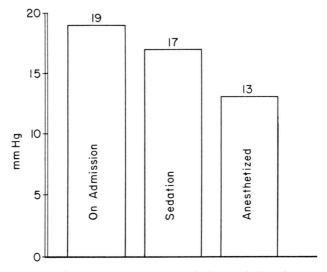

Fig. 5-16. Average intraocular tension in 46 patients before and after thiopental sodium anesthesia. (Modified from Everett, W. G., Vey, E. K., and Veenis, C. Y.: Trans. Am. Acad. Ophthalmol. **63**:286, 1959.)

hyaluronidase (15 TRU/ml) produced the greatest drop in pressure. This indicates that the well-recognized softening of the globe after hyaluronidase and procaine retrobulbar injections is due to spreading of the procaine anesthetic effect rather than to hyaluronidase per se. Facility of aqueous outflow,

tonographically measured, was not affected by these injections in glaucomatous patients.

Tonography before and after retrobulbar injection of procaine and hyaluronidase in 20 nonglaucomatous eyes failed to confirm any increased facility of outflow. Indeed, 15 of the 20 eyes had a lower facility of outflow

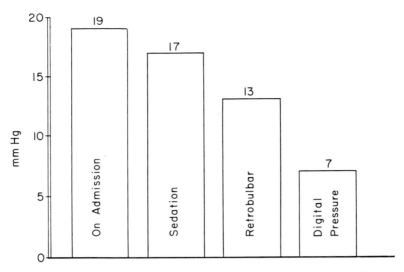

Fig. 5-17. Average intraocular pressure in 100 eyes after injection of 1.5 ml of a 15% solution of butethamine (Monocaine) with hyaluronidase and epinephrine for cataract extraction. (Modified from Everett, W. G., Vey, E. K., and Veenis, C. Y.: Trans. Am. Acad. Ophthalmol. **63:**286, 1959.)

after injection. However, in all but one eye the rate of aqueous flow decreased after retrobulbar injection.[43] Hence decreased aqueous secretion is a second mechanism whereby hypotony may be produced. If epinephrine is used in the solution, this may also inhibit aqueous secretion.

External pressure will cause a marked additional decrease of intraocular pressure even after retrobulbar anesthesia has attained its full effect. As shown in Fig. 5-17, the average postinjection pressure of 13 mm Hg was further reduced to 7 mm Hg by external pressure. The rate of fall in intraocular pressure in response to external compression is initially quite rapid. The surgeon can actually feel this softening occur during the first minute of pressure. As illustrated in Fig. 5-18, within 5 minutes after retrobulbar injection (of 2% lidocaine, epinephrine, and hyaluronidase; volume not reported) and external pressure, the intraocular pressure of the average eye drops to only a few millimeters of mercury.[61] Further gradual decrease in pressure may be obtained by prolonging the external pressure. Although 5 minutes is the average optimal time for external pressure, the time varies depending

on the eye and the amount of pressure exerted. Ideally, the surgeon should continue pressure until the eye is mushy soft. Presumably, external pressure accelerates aqueous outflow. Vitreous volume is also reduced.

The surgeon should release external pressure at frequent intervals (perhaps every 30 seconds) to guard against possible retinal damage from prolonged collapse of the central retinal circulation. Actually, the pressure required to produce hypotony need not be sufficient to collapse the circulation; nevertheless, this precaution seems worthwhile.

The duration of pressure-induced hypotony is rather short. In a series of 20 normal human eyes subjected to 5 minutes of digital pressure (released for 2 seconds every 30 seconds), the intraocular pressures had returned to base-line levels approximately 15 minutes after the pressure was released.[62] No rebound increase in pressure occurred. Comparable pressure was applied to the eyes of 30 rabbits. Initial pressures in these rabbit eyes ranged in the mid-20's. After 5 minutes the pressure had dropped to below 10 mm Hg and the vitreous weight had decreased by an average of 2.3%. However, 10 minutes following massage the pressures

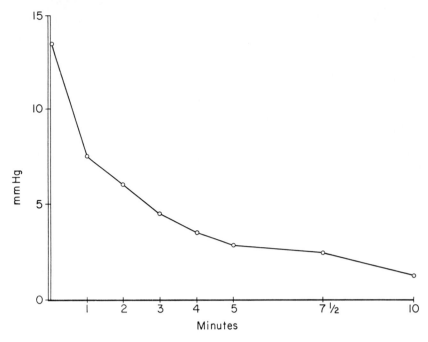

Fig. 5-18. Average intraocular pressures after retrobulbar anesthesia and digital pressure. (Modified from Kirsch, R. E.: Arch. Ophthalmol. **58:**641, 1957.)

ranged in the mid-30's and the vitreous weight had increased by an average of 4.4%. The authors calculated that aqueous outflow alone would have been adequate to reduce the pressures by the measured amount. They questioned the value of massage except as a means to achieve good akinesia of the extraocular muscles. (Neither the patients nor the rabbits received a retrobulbar anesthetic in this study.)

Culture of meibomian secretions expressed during digital pressure prior to cataract surgery in 25 patients revealed no pathogenic microorganisms.[63] The fear of possible endophthalmitis from this source seems unfounded.

Use of carbonic anhydrase inhibitors has been advocated further to reduce intraocular pressure before cataract extraction. By decreasing aqueous flow, such drugs might prolong hypotony for some hours after cataract surgery. Whether this is of any practical value in promoting initial wound healing will depend on the individual surgeon's philosophy and perhaps on the number of sutures used to close the cataract incision.

PREANESTHETIC PREPARATION

Although hypnosis is too time-consuming and unreliable to be endorsed as an anesthetic routine, it does demonstrate dramatically that psychologic methods can reduce or eliminate even severe pain and apprehension. Proper preoperative explanation and discussion will reassure patients and establish their confidence in the surgeon. Periodic reassurance during the operation is encouraging to patients. Occasional nervous individuals do much better if their attention is diverted by discussing their grandchildren, hobbies, and the like during the procedure.

The history and physical examination should be directed toward uncovering factors that might interfere with surgery or the postoperative period. Examples of such factors include previous reactions to local anesthetics, intolerance of sedatives or antibiotics, conditions that might produce coughing or vomiting, cardiac or skeletal difficulties that preclude lying flat, deafness, undue fear of and resistance to manipulations about the eyes, blood dyscrasias with

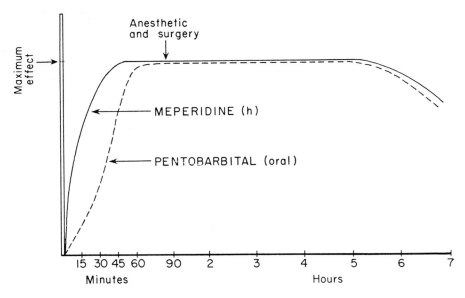

Fig. 5-19. Onset and duration of effect of preoperative medication indicating desirability of giving it 1 to 1½ hours before surgery. (Modified from Atkinson, W. S.: Arch. Ophthalmol. 49:481, 1953.)

hemorrhagic tendencies, mental disorders, and so forth.

Attention to details in the operating room is important when local anesthesia is being used. Banging of pans, gossip, criticism of the quality of instruments and help, quarreling, mention of errors in technique, and the like do not contribute to the patient's peace of mind. "Oops" is occasionally heard in our operating room, and one surgeon characteristically delivers a heartfelt and vigorous "Damn!" at critical moments. The conscious patients' responses to these expletives have not been tabulated. Although such comments may seem irrelevant in a book on medical therapy, inadvertent remarks and disturbances prior to surgery can certainly undo the benefits expected from preoperative sedation.

Premedications

Preoperative medications are given to decrease pain, to relieve anxiety, to counteract possible toxic effects of injection anesthesia, to reduce secretions (in the case of general anesthesia), and to minimize postoperative nausea and vomiting. The commonly used drugs include narcotics, barbiturates, para-

sympatholytics, and tranquilizers. Representatives of each group will be discussed.[64,65]

Meperidine (Demerol)

Because morphine not infrequently causes nausea and vomiting, meperidine has become a more popular analgesic for use in ocular surgery. Probably the most common error in the use of meperidine is giving it too late. Usually this injection is given just before the orderly arrives to take the patient to surgery. The patient is therefore fully awake and unsedated during this journey, which is dreaded by many patients.

After intramuscular administration of meperidine, its analgesic effect appears within 15 minutes, but the maximum effect may not be reached for as long as an hour. Therefore meperidine should be given 45 to 90 minutes before the start of surgery. Actually, the time of greatest need for analgesia is at the beginning of surgery, when the various local or intravenous injections are being given. Since the duration of the narcotic effect is 2 to 6 hours depending on the size of the dose, the surgeon need not fear loss of the meperidine effect if the start of surgery is delayed (Fig. 5-19).[66] Furthermore, if meperidine is given at least an hour before the operation, any untoward effect such as vomiting or confusion will become evident before the surgical incision is started.

Because the sedative effect of meperidine is relatively slight, it is usually accompanied by a barbiturate for preanesthetic medication. Solutions of meperidine hydrochloride and sodium phenobarbital cannot be mixed in the same syringe, since the phenobarbital will precipitate, making the mixture unsuitable for administration. Hence it is necessary that each drug be given separately.

Meperidine may be administered intravenously preceding or during intraocular surgery in amounts from 25 to 100 mg. Prompt drowsiness and relaxation occur. This procedure is of value in the management of a patient who is unduly apprehensive or restless before or during cataract surgery under local anesthesia.[67] The injection should be given slowly, over a period of 1 to 2 minutes. Complete relaxation is achieved within 2 or 3 minutes. Such intravenous use is not superior to adequate premedication with meperidine but has the advantage of quickly relaxing a patient who has received insufficient premedication. Nausea and vomiting may follow intravenous administration of meperidine, especially if injection has been rapid, and this may cause problems if the eye is surgically open.

When given orally, meperidine acts within 20 to 60 minutes.

The dose of meperidine is 1 mg/pound for children. The usual adult dose is 75 to 100 mg, depending on the size of the individual and the degree of apprehension. Very elderly patients tend to require proportionately less drug, particularly if they are frail and underweight. Conversely, higher dosage is tolerated and desirable for young, muscular or heavy, apprehensive persons.

Pentobarbital (Nembutal)

For the purposes of preoperative medication, the effects of barbiturates almost perfectly complement those of meperidine. Barbiturates are effective sedatives but have no significant analgesic power. Hence the combination of meperidine and pentobarbital induces both sedation and analgesia.

Pentobarbital is rapidly absorbed from the gastrointestinal tract or from the site of the hypodermic injection. It is destroyed by the liver and therefore has an unduly prolonged effect in patients with hepatic disease. A hypnotic dose will induce sleep in 20 to 60 minutes if the patient is undisturbed. Because the effect of pentobarbital will last 5 hours or more, the drug can be (and should be) given an hour or more preoperatively without fear of loss of effect. Considerable individual variations in response exist; however, 100 mg is the usual adult dose (approximately 1 mg/pound in children). Infrequently barbiturates will cause delirium and confusion rather than sedation, particularly in elderly patients. Such a response may be detected if a test dose is given on the evening preceding surgery.

Premedication with barbiturates is said to increase the threshold of toxic reaction to injected local anesthetics. I find this difficult to document precisely. Most authorities say the usual 100 mg dose is inadequate and that 300 to 500 mg is required to counteract such toxicity. Actually, only the convulsive component of an anesthetic reaction is alleviated by barbiturates. Barbiturate overdosage will actually worsen respiratory and cardiac depression; therefore, not more than 300 to 500 mg of pentobarbital should be given intravenously to control such convulsions, and no barbiturate should be given if convulsions are not present. Regardless of whether premedication with meperidine and pentobarbital increases resistance to toxic local anesthetic responses, I am absolutely convinced that such premedication strikingly reduces the incidence of apprehension, fainting, and shocklike responses that commonly are encountered during local anesthetic procedures done without such premedication. Such emotional responses may be mistaken for toxic drug responses. Although unpleasant, these reactions are not dangerous (unless the patient is injured by falling during a fainting episode).

The degree of sedation and tranquility

desired varies with the surgeon. I personally become apprehensive when patients fall asleep during cataract surgery. All too often they will awaken and move suddenly in surprise—perhaps at a critical part of the operation. I would prefer my patients to be sufficiently awake and concerned so that they are consciously trying to cooperate by lying quietly.

The physician should be aware that barbiturates are popular for suicidal purposes. Because of variable gastrointestinal absorption, the fatal dose is inconstant, but as little as 1.5 g of pentobarbital would be most dangerous. If given very rapidly intravenously, only 200 to 300 mg may cause respiratory arrest.

Atropine

To prevent respiratory problems caused by mucus secretion during general anesthesia, an adequate dosage of a parasympatholytic drug such as atropine is essential. The preoperative dosage of atropine is 0.1 mg/10 pounds, with a usual maximum of 0.6 mg. (Scopolamine dosage is roughly half that of atropine—0.1 mg/20 pounds.)

Systemic atropine premedication is not contraindicated in patients with glaucoma, since the usual dose is insufficient to counteract the effect of topical miotics.

Since the patient can swallow effectively and because secretions are not stimulated, atropine is unnecessary preceding local anesthesia.

Chlorpromazine (Thorazine)

As reported in 1961, tranquilizers were the major ingredient in 13% of all prescriptions in the United States and in frequency of use were second only to antibiotics.[68] Chlorpromazine was the first of the large number of phenothiazine derivatives to be recognized for its tension-relieving, antiemetic, and anesthetic-potentiating effects. Knowledge of the phenothiazines is important to the ophthalmologist because their therapeutic effects may be valuable in treatment of eye patients and because their toxic complications may involve the eyes.

Ocular hypotensive effect. When given to rabbits, intramuscularly (but not topically) in a dosage of 0.3 to 0.5 mg/kg, chlorpromazine reduces aqueous flow by an average of 72%.[69] In a series of 19 rabbits the average pretreatment intraocular pressure of 18 mm Hg decreased to 13 mm Hg within an hour after chlorpromazine administration and remained at this reduced level for at least 3 hours. A compensatory decrease in the facility of outflow (pretreatment facility of outflow was 0.30; posttreatment, 0.18) occurred, thereby excluding increased facility as the mechanism of pressure decrease. Possibly chlorpromazine blocks aqueous secretion through a sympatholytic action.

Bicarbonate concentration in the posterior chamber of the rabbit is not decreased during the hypotensive effect of chlorpromazine.[70] The ocular hypotensive effect of chlorpromazine lasts for 5 to 7 hours.[71] The magnitude of pressure drop is increased by a larger dosage, being as great as a 9 mm Hg average drop per rabbit (weight not reported) with 15 mg of drug.

Because this intraocular pressure drop is not sustained, tranquilizers are not used in the management of glaucoma.

Antiemetic effect. The incidence of postoperative nausea, vomiting, and retching was studied in 554 patients receiving chlorpromazine, 50 mg; placebo; pentobarbital, 100 or 150 mg; or dimenhydrinate (Dramamine).[72] These medications were administered as unknown units in a random sequence and were given intramuscularly 10 to 30 minutes before conclusion of nitrous oxide and ether anesthesia. The occurrence of symptoms was verified by constant observation by special technicians. The problem of placebo reaction was eliminated, since all patients were completely unaware of the medication or the study. Interestingly, most patients were subsequently unaware of nausea or vomiting that occurred during the first 4 hours postoperatively, a fact that may account for the lower incidence of vomiting in series of cases studied by questioning the patient rather than by continuous observation.

As seen in Table 5-3, 50 mg of chlorpro-

Table 5-3. Incidence of nausea, vomiting, and retching; incidence of hypotension; and awakening time after administration of specific medications*

Medication	Incidence of nausea, vomiting, and retching (%)		Hypotension (%)	Awakening time (min)
	Within 4 hours	Within 24 hours		
Placebo	58	82	7	87
Chlorpromazine, 50 mg	34	59	30	144
Dimenhydrinate, 100 mg	61	75	16	112
Pentobarbital, 100 mg	52	75	9	112
Pentobarbital, 150 mg	43	67	20	132

*Modified from Knapp, M. R., and Beecher, H. K.: J.A.M.A. **160:**376, 1956.

mazine effectively and significantly reduced the frequency of postanesthetic nausea, vomiting, and retching. However, this drug also prolonged recovery time from anesthesia by an average of almost 1 hour and caused a 30% incidence of disturbing hypotension. The authors considered the potential dangers of aspiration and vascular occlusion sufficiently great that routine prophylactic use of chlorpromazine was not advised. Pressor amines, including levarterenol, are not effective against chlorpromazine-induced arterial hypotension, which usually improves spontaneously in 2 to 4 hours (duration 15 hours in one patient). (However, none of this series of patients suffered any hypotensive complication.)

Comparable conclusions were reached in another study of 725 patients. Particular caution was advised in patients with labile blood pressure, especially if systolic pressure was above 160 or below 100 mm Hg.[73]

Some anesthesiologists consider the intensified and prolonged sedation and the hypotensive effects of the phenothiazine tranquilizers so disturbing that they advocate discontinuing such medications for 10 days before surgery.[74] Since one person in seven uses these tranquilizers, inquiry as to routinely used drugs is in order before preanesthetic medications are prescribed.

Since phenothiazine antiemetics are effective even after severe vomiting has started, the routine prophylactic use of such drugs is not ordinarily justified and subjects many patients to the hazards of a drug they do not

need. In a series of 2230 patients, 23% had retching and temporary vomiting after general anesthesia without use of tranquilizers. However, only 3.5% had persistent and severe vomiting.[75] In ordinary anesthetic practice the antiemetics are limited to treatment of nausea and vomiting as it occurs postoperatively.[76]

Control of nausea and vomiting is achieved equally well with any of the phenothiazine drugs.[77] Hypotension is less likely with promethazine (Phenergan), 12.5 or 25 mg, than with chlorpromazine.

Value in cataract surgery. Use of chlorpromazine prior to cataract surgery with local anesthesia has been advocated because it relieves anxiety, reduces nausea and vomiting, and causes a soft eye.[78] Two consecutive series of 100 cataract extractions were performed with and without chlorpromazine (25 mg orally before surgery, intramuscularly immediately after surgery, and every 3 hours thereafter as required for nausea and vomiting).[79] The optimum tranquilizing effect was reached from 30 minutes to 2 hours after medication and lasted for 4 to 8 hours. In addition, both series of patients received pentobarbital, 100 mg, the night before surgery and again 4 hours and 1 hour preceding surgery. Meperidine, 50 to 100 mg, was given 30 minutes preoperatively.

The study showed that chlorpromazine reduced postoperative nausea from 27% to 19%, postoperative vomiting from 18% to 8%, and apprehension from 20% to 9%. A significant disadvantage of chlorpromazine

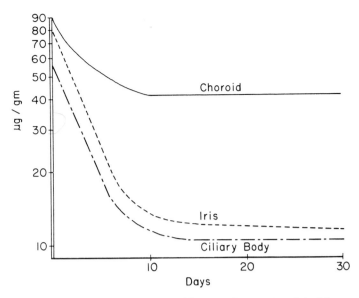

Fig. 5-20. Persistence of chlorpromazine in rabbit uveal tract. (Modified from Potts, A. M.: Invest. Ophthalmol. **1:**522, 1962.)

premedication for cataract extraction is the tendency to excessive sedation, during which the patient may make unpredictable and dangerous movements. This potentiating effect on sedation is particularly troublesome in older patients.

The surgeon must be aware that hypodermic administration of phenothiazines, as in the treatment of postoperative nausea, may cause postural hypotension. Specifically, such medication may cause postoperative cataract patients to faint and fall on their face while attempting to go to the bathroom.

Toxic effects. A great number of uncommon, troublesome, and potentially serious complications have been described after chlorpromazine therapy. These include urticaria, contact dermatitis, photosensitivity, agranulocytosis, convulsive seizures, catalepsy, restlessness and agitation, fatigue, drowsiness, mental depression, parkinsonism, assorted bizarre muscle spasms and tics particularly common about the face but also involving trunk muscles, jaundice, and liver disease. However, in view of the fact that chlorpromazine has been given to more than 50 million patients during its first 10 years of use, the frequency of these complications is

small (for instance, agranulocytosis occurs in 1 of 250,000 cases).[80]

Histologic study of liver tissue obtained at autopsy or by biopsy suggests that chlorpromazine-induced jaundice is characterized by intrahepatic canalicular obstruction of bile flow.[81] Apparently, chlorpromazine hepatitis is an acute process, which may subside without residual effects (although it may rarely be fatal), and may not recur with subsequent use of the drug.

Ocular complications of phenothiazine therapy vary from transient blurred vision (due to transient myopia) that disappears promptly when treatment is stopped[82,83] to permanent chorioretinal atrophy.[84] Two of the phenothiazine tranquilizers, NP-207 (never released for commercial use) and thioridazine, will in high dosage cause decreased visual acuity and impaired dark adaptation. These symptoms become progressively more severe during the course of prolonged medication. With the initial symptoms, ophthalmoscopic examination is essentially normal, although some hyperemia and edema of the retina and optic nerve may be present. Subsequently, pigment granularity develops, ultimately coalescing into peculiar, large, irregularly circular areas. At this stage the visual loss is irreversible.

Phenothiazine retinopathy has not been reported except after high doses of drug. Thioridazine requires a dosage of 2000 mg/day; NP-207, 200 mg/day.[85] Even at high-dosage levels, a month or more of treatment may be required before visual symptoms appear.[86] Such toxic changes have never been reported to follow use of the common phenothiazine tranquilizers (promethazine, chlorpromazine, prochlorperazine, and trifluoperazine).

The following study of the intraocular distribution of phenothiazine derivatives is significant because it helps to explain this remarkably localized toxicity and because it illustrates the extraordinary affinity of drugs for certain tissues. The data given in Fig. 5-20 indicate that the concentration of chlorpromazine in pigmented rabbit choroid may attain 84 μg/g of tissue 48 hours after administration of 5 mg/kg.[87] By comparison, the blood concentration at this time was 0.17 μg/g, and the retinal concentration was 0.79 μg/g. Not only was the initial choroidal concentration of drug enormously higher than that in other tissues but it also lasted for a much greater time. After 30 days, choroidal concentration of chlorpromazine was still 45 μg/g, although blood values had dropped to 0.006 μg/g. Obviously selective concentration and retention of phenothiazine derivatives occur in pigmented uveal tissue.[87]

Diazepam (Valium)

Various combinations of tranquilizers, narcotics, and sedatives have been advocated for use during eye surgery. As an example, diazepam (Valium) is a tranquilizer that was used in combination with meperidine and local injection anesthesia in 160 eye operations.[88] These medications were given intravenously in variable dosages titrated to meet the patient's needs. Most patients received less than 10 mg of diazepam and 15 mg of meperidine. In addition, premedication up to 100 mg of pentobarbital or 1 g of chloral hydrate was given.

Good patient cooperation was achieved in 91% of these 160 patients. Four patients were restless and uncooperative and could not be controlled by this medication. Half of the patients had complete amnesia for the operation, and one fourth had only slight recall of the procedure.

Let me stress that an anesthesiologist was monitoring these patients and was responsible for determining individualized intravenous dosages, control of hypotension, oxygen administration, and similar highly important details. While the attention and hands of the ophthalmologist are fully occupied by the surgery, the ophthalmologist is not able to control safely a patient brought to the verge of general anesthesia. Resist the temptation to sedate and tranquilize your patient into immobility, for the next step is into eternity.

Hypotension is not only an immediate hazard to life but may initiate future cerebral or cardiac problems. To quote Sadove, "I caution you that, if on the night of surgery the patient is given heavy sedation, it is possible that 3 months later the patient may die of a coronary attack which was begun that night silently, only to kill many weeks or months later."[89]

Summary

Probably the best preoperative sedative and tranquilizer is the surgeon, who reassures the patient by careful explanation and attention.[90] Preoperative medications only supplement the confidence of the patient in the physician.

However, adequate sedation (for example, 100 mg of pentobarbital), analgesia (for example, 75 mg of meperidine), and antiemetic (for example, promethazine, 25 mg hourly as needed for nausea) can make eye surgery much more pleasant.

GENERAL ANESTHESIA

The decision to use general anesthesia should be tempered with the knowledge that primary anesthetic death occurs in 1 of 3000 patients.[91] Lesser complications (for example, pneumonia, thrombophlebitis, pressure damage to peripheral nerves, exposure keratopathy, and prolonged nausea and vomiting) are not rare. Without exception, all anesthesiologists in my acquaintance have stated emphatically their preference for local anesthesia, if possible, for any procedure to be performed on themselves.

On the other hand, the development of more complex techniques of cataract surgery (for example, phacoemulsification and anterior chamber lens implants) has resulted in a definite trend toward the use of more general anesthesia, or at least standby anesthesia. I am honestly not quite sure why this is, but I think it represents a preoccupation with the machinery and technology we use, to the extent that the surgeon cannot devote attention to the existence of the patient. I do not mean this to sound critical—after all, there are only so many things that can be done at the same time. As a consequence, in busy centers the anesthesiologists have learned the needs of an ophthalmic surgeon and deliver a properly quiet patient, reliably and safely.[92-94] Under these circumstances the risks of general or of local anesthesia are essentially the same (although there is the occasional patient whose lungs are so bad that an anesthesiologist refuses to administer a general anesthetic and the ophthalmologist proceeds with an uneventful operation using a local anesthetic).

The prolonged convalescence that occurs after general anesthesia is often unnoticed or disregarded but is nevertheless real. For as long as 1 month following anesthesia, many patients do not feel well, have no endurance, and generally feel as if they are recovering from a severe case of the flu. In the case of elderly patients, this period of debility may be prolonged, lasting many months. I am acutely aware of this, since the detachment surgeon usually follows the patients during these months. In contrast, the anesthesiologist never sees the patient again after discharge from the hospital and may be entirely unaware of the existence of this recovery period. These late aftereffects of general anesthesia cannot be lightly disregarded in the decision as to the type of anesthetic the ophthalmologist honestly recommends as best for the patient.

Combination of local with light general anesthesia is, of course, another option. If a normal depth of general anesthesia is contraindicated by the health of the patient, sometimes relief of pain with a local anesthetic will permit carrying the patient with a relatively light general anesthetic. This decision will require consultation with the anesthesiologist.

Clearly, the techniques of general anesthesia are the province of the trained anesthesiologist and are not properly considered in an ophthalmology text. Description of the ocular side effects of general anesthetic agents and indications for general anesthesia in ophthalmology are pertinent, however.

Most ophthalmologists prefer local anesthesia alone whenever it is possible to secure good patient cooperation. This is because a local anesthetic can easily be given by the ophthalmologist (a particularly important consideration if the facilities of a medical center are not available), is less expensive, is safer (particularly in poor-risk patients), and has fewer aftereffects (such as nausea, vomiting, and sickness). General anesthesia is necessary whenever one is dealing with a potentially uncooperative patient such as a child[95,96] or a deaf person, emotionally unstable and apprehensive patients, or psychotic persons. Especially with intraocular surgery, it is not permissible to risk the patient's moving at a critical time. Long and uncomfortable procedures (such as performed for retinal detachment) or emotionally unpleasant operations (enucleation) are better done with the patient asleep.

Even if the surgery is done with the patient under general anesthesia, supplemental injection of local anesthesia is often desirable for the following reasons:

1. A lighter plane of anesthesia is possible without the hazard of the patient's moving in response to occasional painful stimuli.
2. Postoperative pain will be less during the first few hours, which are the most likely to be uncomfortable.
3. Squeezing of the lids during the immediate postoperative period is prevented by local akinesia.
4. Oculocardiac reflexes may be decreased.

5. If epinephrine is contained in the local injection, bleeding is decreased.

Effects on intraocular pressure

Anesthesia produced by intravenous administration of thiopental sodium (Pentothal) causes a significant drop of intraocular pressure in both normal and untreated glaucomatous eyes. Apparently the mechanism of this pressure decrease is improved facility of outflow. The aqueous humor dynamics in 20 patients with chronic simple glaucoma (not operated on for glaucoma and not given miotics within 48 hours before anesthesia) were studied before and after thiopental anesthesia.[97] Preanesthetic pressures in these patients varied from a low of 29 mm Hg to a high of 66 mm Hg. Within 20 minutes after the start of anesthesia, a marked drop of pressure (average, 19 mm Hg) occurred in all patients. This decrease in intraocular pressure was accompanied in all but one patient by an increased facility of outflow. Cardiovascular changes could not have been responsible for the intraocular pressure drop, since the systolic blood pressure dropped an average of only 9 mm Hg in contrast to the 19 mm Hg intraocular drop. Evaluation of the effect of preanesthetic medication in these glaucoma patients indicated that premedication with atropine and scopolamine did *not* alter the intraocular pressure (atropine or scopolamine in a 0.5 mg dose was used in each of these 20 patients). Obviously the common fear of increased intraocular pressure resulting from parasympatholytic preanesthetic medication is completely unfounded, even if additional miotics are not used. Premedication with meperidine, morphine, or secobarbital did cause a decrease in the intraocular pressure of these glaucomatous patients. Interestingly, 0.1 or 0.2 g of secobarbital did not alter pressure or outflow facility in 11 normal eyes. The authors concluded that these findings indicated the action of a neurovascular factor in chronic simple glaucoma.

General anesthesia with any of the commonly used agents also causes a marked drop of intraocular pressure in normal eyes. This drop increases as deeper levels of anesthesia are attained (Fig. 5-21).[98] After anesthesia, the intraocular pressure rapidly returns to normal. Table 5-4 shows that this drop in pressure averages 5 to 7 mm Hg and essentially is produced equally by cyclopropane, diethyl ether, thiopental sodium, and vinyl ether.[99] Tonography suggested that the mechanism of this pressure drop was an increase in the facility of outflow. Intraocular pressure correlated closely with the depth of anesthesia, being lowest in deep anesthesia and rising when the anesthesia lightened. These authors speculate that anesthesia may depress a hypothalamic region that controls aqueous outflow. Respiratory disturbances such as coughing or straining resulted in increased intraocular pressure that persisted for some minutes.

The implications of these findings in respect to the diagnosis of congenital glaucoma (a disease in which tonometry is often done with the patient under anesthesia) deserve comment. Elevated readings during the early stages of anesthesia, even several minutes after struggling and breath-holding, may be artifactual and cannot be relied on as indicative of glaucoma. Elevated readings taken during deep anesthesia, several minutes after any muscular activity has ceased, represent a genuine elevation of intraocular pressure. Any reading taken during deep general anesthesia is probably lower than the patient's normal intraocular pressure;

Table 5-4. Drop in intraocular pressure during deep anesthesia with different anesthetic agents*

Anesthetic agent	Number of eyes	Average pressure (mm Hg)
Preanesthetic state	140	17.7
Cyclopropane	20	11.4
Diethyl ether	32	12.0
Thiopental sodium	78	10.7
Vinyl ether	10	11.6

*Data from Kornblueth, W., and associates: Arch. Ophthalmol. **61:**84, 1959.

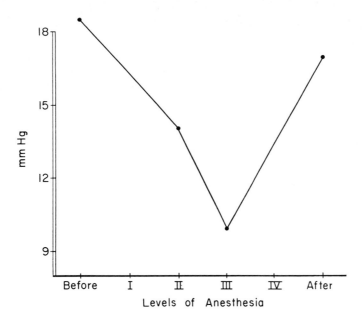

Fig. 5-21. Progressive drop of intraocular pressure at descending levels of general anesthesia with halothane (Fluothane). (Modified from Magora, F., and Collins, V.: Arch. Ophthalmol. **66:**806, 1961.)

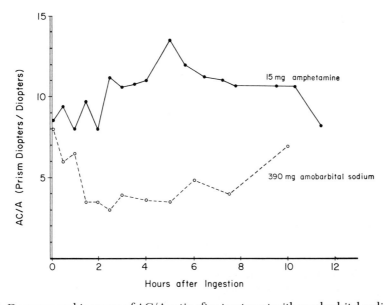

Fig. 5-22. Decrease and increase of AC/A ratio after treatment with amobarbital sodium (Amytal) and amphetamine, respectively. With these drugs, a normal AC/A ratio of 8 was reduced as low as 3 or increased as high as 13 in this subject. (Modified from Westheimer, G.: Arch. Ophthalmol. **70:**830, 1963.)

therefore, a borderline pressure under these conditions probably represents an abnormal elevation. The average pressure of 140 eyes under deep anesthesia was only 10 to 12 mm Hg.

Autonomic effects

The parasympathetic stimulation resulting from general anesthesia is well known to manifest itself as pupillary miosis. In a study of 36 patients, general anesthesia was found to cause varying degrees of accommodation, reaching values as high as 5 diopters.[100] Children were particularly likely to accommodate strongly during anesthesia. The practical implication of this finding is that adequate cycloplegia is essential in obtaining an accurate refraction with the patient under anesthesia. This fact should be remembered if a pediatric examination under anesthesia is to include refraction.

The accommodative convergence/accommodation (AC/A) ratio may also be altered by drugs that act on the central nervous system (presumably, the convergence center). Barbiturates decrease convergence and amphetamines enhance convergence (Fig. 5-22).[101] This effect explains why a convergent strabismus may disappear completely when the patient is anesthetized prior to surgery. I anticipate that convergence stimulating and depressing drugs will be developed that will be clinically useful in controlling strabismus.

Effect on intraocular gases

The laws of diffusion and partial pressure of gases require that equilibration of concentration will occur whenever a new gas is introduced into a biologic system. Specifically, if 60% nitrous oxide is used as an anesthetic, nitrous oxide will enter every gas-filled space in the body until it equilibrates with a content of 60% nitrous oxide. If the eye contains a bubble of air or sulfur hexafluoride, the gas within the eye cannot escape and to it is added 60% more nitrous oxide. The only possible consequence is a precipitous rise of pressure, actually measured at 101 mm Hg in a detachment operation entailing intravitreal injection of a large

air bubble during nitrous oxide anesthesia.[102,103] The practical consequence is that a gaseous anesthetic must not be given to a patient with a large volume (certainly less than 1 ml, or serious pressure problems will result) of intraocular air or other gas, or else the intraocular pressure will rise, probably to dangerous levels.[104]

Muscle relaxants for supplementary use
Curare

Curare blocks myoneural transmission (via acetylcholine) to skeletal muscle. Transmission of impulses may also be blocked in the autonomic ganglia. Therapeutic doses of curare depress consecutively the muscles supplied by the cranial nerves, the general musculature, and finally the diaphragm. Hence it is possible to obtain simultaneous and almost complete paralysis of lids and extraocular muscles with relatively little respiratory handicap.

Reliable response requires intravenous administration. The maximal effect is reached in 3 to 5 minutes and will persist for 20 to 30 minutes. Because of individual variations in susceptibility, a test dose is given, with a 5-minute wait before the next increment. A representative test dose is 3 mg (20 rabbit head-drop units) of purified tubocurarine chloride. The same dose may be repeated at 5-minute intervals until the desired relaxation is obtained. Curare produces muscle relaxation without the preliminary spasmodic the synthetic depolarizing drugs such as succinylcholine.

Facilities for adequate artificial respiration *must* be immediately available whenever muscle-relaxing drugs such as curare are used. These drugs are dangerous! Oxygen and positive pressure respiration (via endotracheal intubation) will effectively prevent death from apnea. Because of the rapid renal elimination of curare, antidotes such as physostigmine or neostigmine are unnecessary and undesirable in treatment of respiratory collapse. Furthermore, such antidotes also have undesirable parasympathomimetic actions, are inadequate in treatment of a great overdosage of curare, and under some circumstances (notably in myasthenia) may increase the curarizing effect.

Circulatory collapse may complicate curare overdosage, does not always readily respond to vasoconstrictor drugs, and may be responsible for the slight increase in operative mortality reported to follow use of muscle relaxants in general anesthesia.[105]

Myasthenia gravis may increase susceptibility to curarization by as much as 20-fold. Renal and hepatic disease slow its excretion and detoxification.

When cataract surgery is performed with the patient under general anesthesia, the supplementary relaxing effect of cuarare, relatively specific for the extraocular muscles, may give added protection against vitreous loss. In a series of 586 cataract extractions with the patients under general anesthesia, the amount of curare required to give complete ocular relaxation varied from 6 to 21 mg.[106] It should be given in small increments, with maximum relaxation being achieved before the time of cataract delivery.

Although curare and general anesthesia may effectively control the patient during surgery, they do not prevent postoperative pain and squeezing of the eyes. I personally believe that local injection anesthesia and massage should be used in addition to general anesthesia for intraocular surgery. The cataract surgeon should seek a very soft and completely motionless eye, which will safely permit whatever delicate intraocular maneuvers may be required.

In the past, curare was advocated as a supplement to local anesthesia for cataract extraction.[107,108] Without intubation, the use of curare requires careful titration of the individual patient by an anesthesiologist experienced in this technique and familiar with the pace of the surgeon. Overdosage may cause the terrifying sensation of respiratory paralysis during full consciousness. Pharyngeal relaxation may result in pooling of excess saliva induced by curarization. Prevention of salivation requires preoperative atropinization, as would be used for general anesthesia. Apparently, experience minimizes such complications, since these authors considered curare to be worthy of routine use. However, five instances of vitreous loss occurred in 85 cataract extractions done with curare and local anesthesia. Such results hardly seem worth the very great hazard, expense, and bother. (Since the advent of hyaluronidase, large-volume retrobulbar anesthetic injections with massage achieve total relaxation quite consistently.)

The effect of curare (6 to 9 mg intravenously) on intraocular pressure was studied in five patients by tonography.[99] No other medications or anesthetic agents were used in these patients. Curare decreased the intraocular pressure by 1 to 5 mm Hg (average 2.8 mm Hg). Since the coefficient of facility of outflow decreased by 18% and the rate of flow dropped by 30%, the pressure-lowering effect was attributed to relaxation of extraocular muscles and not to improved outflow.

Succinylcholine chloride

Succinylcholine, an acetylcholine competitor, blocks the myoneural junction through depolarization, thereby causing temporary paralysis of skeletal musculature. It is widely used to attain muscular relaxation during general anesthesia. Initially the extraocular muscles react to succinylcholine with increased activity. Intravenous injection of succinylcholine produces a steep rise of intraocular pressure resulting from this demonstrable contraction of the extraocular muscles.[109,110] Proof that this is the mechanism of succinylcholine-induced ocular hypertension is derived from the experimental sectioning of the extraocular muscle tendons, which virtually eliminates the hypertensive response.[111]

Shown in Fig. 5-23 is the tonographic record of a human eye in which a marked increase in intraocular pressure occurred after intravenous injection of 5 mg of succinylcholine.[112] The duration of elevated intraocular pressure is sufficiently short (only a few minutes) that use of succinylcholine for intubation will not cause difficulty during subsequent surgery.

When the patient is deeply anesthetized, succinylcholine has no pressure-elevating

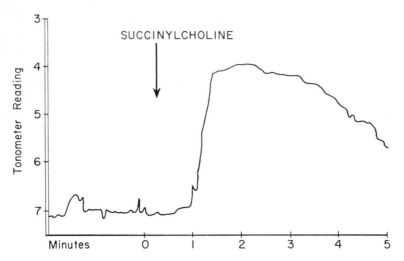

Fig. 5-23. Tonographic record of unanesthetized patient showing marked increase of intraocular pressure following 5 mg of succinylcholine intravenously. (Modified from Kornblueth, W., and associates: Am. J. Ophthalmol. 49:1381, 1960.)

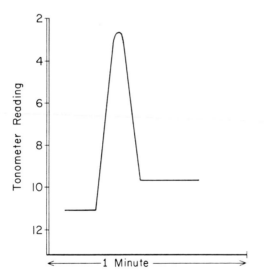

Fig. 5-24. Increase in intraocular pressure of normal eye in response to Valsalva stress during tonography.

effect on the eye. This has been confirmed in a series of 82 patients.[113] This difference in response of anesthetized and nonanesthetized extraocular muscles apparently accounts at least partially for the conflicting reports as to the safety of succinylcholine in ocular surgery. Apparently, general anesthesia paralyzes the extraocular muscles sufficiently to prevent their contraction.

After the initial stage of contraction, the extraocular muscles are paralyzed by succinylcholine and may be maintained in this relaxed condition by continuous administration of the drug. It is therefore safe to use succinylcholine during intraocular surgery if it is started well in advance of opening the eye and if effective levels are maintained throughout the operation. Succinylcholine should not be started after the eye has been opened because of the hazard of losing intraocular contents. Its administration is *particularly contraindicated* if the anesthesia becomes light during the operation and the patient begins to move, for in this lightly anesthetized state the extraocular muscles will contract strongly in initial response to the drug.

If the eye is already open at the start of anesthesia (because of laceration, iris prolapse, incision disruption, and the like), use of succinylcholine may be extremely dangerous. Before intubation of such a patient, the level of anesthesia should be sufficiently deep to achieve complete relaxation. Bucking of the patient during intubation is similar to the Valsalva effect, which may induce venous back pressure sufficient to raise intraocular pressure as high as 50 mm Hg (Fig. 5-24).

That danger to the eye from succinylcholine is not only theoretical was proved in the case of a 70-year-old patient who coughed on the intratracheal tube after cataract extraction had been uneventfully concluded.[114] Fifty milligrams of succinylcholine was given intravenously to stop the coughing and was immediately followed by an expulsive hemorrhage and ultimate evisceration.

Certainly there is no contraindication to the use of succinylcholine during general anesthesia for extraocular surgical procedures. (This drug is never used as a supplement to local anesthesia, since it paralyzes respiration.)

Unlike curare, succinylcholine is not antagonized by anticholinesterase drugs. Cholinesterase inhibitors such as neostigmine or physostigmine *prolong* the action of succinylcholine and are therefore contraindicated in the treatment of succinylcholine overdosage.

Succinylcholine is rapidly destroyed in 3 to 4 minutes by pseudocholinesterase; hence the paralysis it induces is only of a short duration. Chronic systemic intoxication with the long-acting anticholinesterase drugs such as may be used in the treatment of glaucoma or strabismus can greatly prolong the effect of succinylcholine. The ophthalmologist should make the anesthesiologist aware of such prior drug usage. A genetic deficiency of pseudocholinesterase also exists. Such patients may remain apneic for 4 to 8 hours after a single dose of succinylcholine.[115,116]

As would be expected, succinylcholine initiates a relaxation of accommodation, beginning within 20 seconds after intravenous administration, reaching a maximal level from 45 to 210 seconds, and disappearing after 300 seconds. This was determined by ultrasonic measurement of lens thickness and anterior chamber depth.[117]

CARDIAC ARREST

A colleague once told me of the most difficult walk of his life. It was only down two flights of steps, but at the bottom waited the parents who did not yet know of the death of their child during surgery for strabismus.

Many of our friends have taken this difficult walk, and some day you and I may have our turn. Are *you* prepared to avert tragedy?

When the heart stops pumping blood, the brain has only 3 or 4 minutes to live. Unless someone in the room knows what to do, the patient will surely die. Regardless of whether the heart is in asystole or fibrillation, two problems face the physician:

1. Restoration of blood flow (including oxygenation)
2. Restoration of the normal heartbeat

The first of these is an emergency and must be met by immediate cardiac massage. The second is not urgent, since effective blood pressure may be maintained for hours, if necessary, by cardiac massage.

Steps toward cardiac massage must be started immediately whenever the pulse and blood pressure are lost. There is *no time* to take an electrocardiogram. *Do not* give artificial respiration and wait! Medication *cannot* be given by any route, including intravenously, because the circulation has stopped. There is *no time* to experiment or to look up directions; therefore you must know the technique of closed chest cardiac massage.

Closed chest defibrillation

Closed chest techniques have made open chest methods obsolete.

Brief application of an alternating current longitudinally through the heart from the external skin surfaces will effectively depolarize the myocardium and arrest fibrillation.[118] A commercial closed chest defibrillator generates a 60-cycle AC current of 5 amperes for one-fourth second (440 volts for adults and 220 volts for children). The two electrodes are positioned roughly at the top and bottom of the heart, at the suprasternal notch and about 3 cm below the left nipple.

Although use of the closed chest defibrillator eliminates the need for thoracotomy, the electric shock must be given within 3 minutes of circulatory arrest; otherwise the heart is too anoxic to resume its normal beat. Since in most instances this time interval is too short to permit transportation and use of the defibrillator, closed chest cardiac massage and artificial respiration must be started immediately on diagnosis of cardiac arrest and must be continued until an effective and spontaneous heartbeat has been restored.

Closed chest cardiac massage

The human heart, fixed in the mediastinum, almost completely fills the space between the sternum and thoracic spine. The chest of the unconscious adult is sufficiently flexible to permit effective cardiac compression when firm pressure is applied to the lower third of the sternum. Such external cardiac massage has maintained effective circulation for as long as 2 hours in human patients.[119]

To apply closed chest cardiac massage, the patient is placed supine on a firm surface such as an operating table or a floor. The physician stands or kneels beside the patient, being high enough above the patient so that the weight of the physician's body can be used for pressure. The heel of one hand is placed on the lower third of the sternum, and the second hand is placed on the first (Fig. 5-25). The vertical pressure applied

should be sufficient to move the sternum from 1 to 2 inches toward the vertebral column. Despite application of considerable pressure, there is little danger of rib fracture when only the heel of the hand is applied to the sternum; however, *no* pressure should be applied to the ribs by the fingers. At the end of each compression, pressure is completely removed from the chest, allowing it to reexpand fully and permitting both ventricles to fill with blood. This cycle is repeated about 60 times per minute, which is the approximate rate of a slowly beating heart. Each adequate cardiac compression should produce a palpable pulse and maintain a measurable blood pressure.

The possibility of causing damage by excessively vigorous external cardiac massage must not be forgotten. One autopsy report describes fracture of ribs 2 through 8 (inclusive and on both sides) fracture of the sternum, and a 500 ml hemopericardium due to rupture of a pulmonary vein.[120] Rib fractures were found in 40% of 348 autopsies performed after unsuccesful closed chest cardiac massage.[121] The second most com-

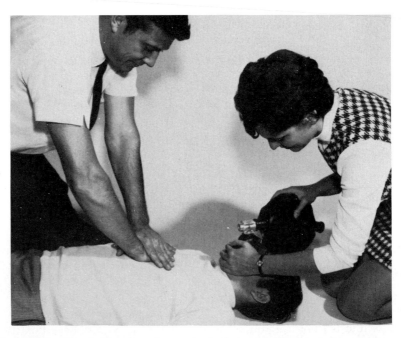

Fig. 5-25. Position of heel of hands on lower third of sternum for closed chest cardiac massage. Note the necessity for adequate artificial respiration.

mon complication (10% of cases) was gastric and esophageal laceration.

Much less force is required in resuscitation of infants. Only moderate fingertip pressure is applied to the middle third of the sternum. Excessive force may cause crushing injury, to which the liver is particularly vulnerable. The pressure of one hand alone is adequate for most children up to 10 years of age.

If the cardiac arrest is caused by asystole rather than by fibrillation, intraventricular injection of 1 ml of a 1:10,000 concentration of epinephrine may help to restore spontaneous heartbeat.

External cardiac massage* is a technique that should be familiar to all surgeons, since it is effective and simple and eliminates the problems of infection, hemorrhage, and injury that commonly accompany emergency thoracotomy. At the Johns Hopkins Hospitals, external massage has been used on more than 100 patients and has been successful in approximately two thirds of these cases.

Artificial respiration

Open chest or closed chest cardiac massage will not revive patients unless they are adequately oxygenated during the procedure. Four minutes of anoxia will cause permanent brain damage.

If the patient is already intubated, as during general anesthesia, pulmonary ventilation requires simply the rhythmic pressure of the anesthesiologist's hand on the breathing bag. In the absence of intubation, an open airway must be established. This may be done by extending the neck and pulling up the lower jaw or by inserting a plastic airway over the tongue and into the pharynx. Ventilation of the lungs can then be achieved by mouth-to-mouth breathing. Entry of the air should be free and should result in recognizable chest expansion.

A variety of respirator bags and masks, with or without oxygen, are available. It is a wise precaution to have such a bag and

mask on hand wherever local anesthetics are used. The apparatus selected *must* permit application of positive pressure. (Some masks simply provide a flow of oxygen but do not permit pressure application. Such devices will not help a patient in respiratory arrest.) The AMBU* apparatus is a sturdy, self-inflating respirator bag specifically designed for emergency treatment of respiratory arrest. A foot-operated suction pump is included and is of value in removing pharyngeal secretions. When used, such a respirator mask should snugly cover both nose and mouth. The bag is squeezed 10 to 15 times per minute, permitting intervening periods of expiration.

Should respiratory stimulants such as caffeine, nikethamide (Coramine), and pentylenetetrazol (Metrazol) be used? Anesthesiologists do not advocate the use of drugs to stimulate respiration but prefer oxygen and a clear airway.

Death from anesthesia is due to respiratory or cardiac failure. Faulty management of the airway is said to be responsible for 90% of these deaths.[122] When the oxygen need is maintained by adequate artificial respiration, animals will tolerate as much as 10 times the amount of local anesthetic that would otherwise be fatal. Bear in mind that artificial respiration corrects respiratory arrest alone, not cardiac arrest. Conversely, cardiac massage (open or closed) restores circulation alone and does not oxygenate the blood.

Oculocardiac reflex

With respect to the numbers of patients involved, prevention of cardiac arrest is more important than its treatment. Anesthesiologists are primarily responsible for establishing and maintaining the good airway that will prevent anoxia and accumulation of carbon dioxide, precursors to cardiac arrest. Furthermore, they are responsible for avoiding dangerously deep levels of anesthesia. It has been suggested that the ophthalmologist may help to prevent cardiac arrest by blocking the oculocardiac reflex.

*A 16 mm sound and color film, *External Cardiac Massage,* is available from the film library of The American Medical Association, Chicago, Ill.

*Air-Shield Inc., Hatboro, Pa.

The oculocardiac reflex is a trigeminovagal reflex that causes cardiac slowing or standstill.[123] This reflex may be elicited by pressure on the globe, traction on extraocular muscles or optic nerve, and direct pressure on the orbital contents that remain after enucleation. These cardiac responses may occur during either light or deep general anesthesia. In a series of 50 eye operations, muscle traction produced significant bradycardia in 15 patients (30%).[124] Retrobulbar injection of lidocaine or procaine was given to 12 of these patients and in each instance abolished the oculocardiac reflex.

The authors of different clinical studies do not agree as to whether intravenous administration of atropine or retrobulbar injection of lidocaine is the most effective agent in preventing cardiac irregularities resulting from the oculocardiac reflex. In a series of 50 consecutive eye operations performed with the patients under local anesthesia, attempts were made to induce cardiac slowing by pressure or traction.[125] Reproducible cardiac changes occurred in 5 of the first 25 patients and in 4 of the next 25. The first 5 were treated with a retrobulbar injection of 2 ml of a 2% solution of lidocaine, which abolished the oculocardiac reflex in all 5 patients. Atropine, 0.5 mg intravenously, was used in the group of 4 patients and prevented recurrence of the abnormalities in only 2 of these. Subsequent lidocaine retrobulbar block abolished the oculocardiac reflex in one instance of atropine failure. In the fourth patient, atropine injection was followed by tachycardia to 240 beats/minute, attributed to "atropine sensitivity" (?). The authors recommended routine retrobulbar anesthesia in all cases of eye surgery (whether a local or general anesthetic is used) to prevent cardiac disturbances resulting from the oculocardiac reflex.

Another study (in which I personally participated) suggested that atropine was considerably more effective than retrobulbar anesthesia in preventing the oculocardiac reflex.[126] In a group of 28 patients, cardiac slowing of 10% to 50% occurred in 82% of the patients during surgery on the extra-ocular muscles. This bradycardia occurred despite premedication with 0.1 to 0.4 mg of atropine or scopolamine. However, intravenous administration of atropine (0.1 to 0.2 mg) during surgery did prevent bradycardia for as long as 30 minutes in all but 1 of 17 patients. (To produce complete vagal block in an adult, 2 to 3 mg of atropine is required.) In 17 other patients, retrobulbar block with a 1% solution of lidocaine, 1 to 2 ml injected into the anterior portion of the retrobulbar space, did not significantly decrease bradycardia; 12 of 17 patients (70%) experienced bradycardia.

In a series of 14 patients with a marked oculocardiac reflex during strabismus surgery, intravenous administration of atropine, 0.003 mg/pound, abolished the cardiac slowing within 1 minute.[127]

Knowledge that the oculocardiac reflex requires a combination of eye stimulation and apnea (oculorespiratory reflex) (Fig. 5-26) leads to another effective treatment.[128] Nothing more than artificial respiration will often promptly relieve the bradycardia resulting from ocular stimulation. To be effective, the respiratory exchange must inflate the lungs widely. Immediately on detection of dangerous cardiac slowing during eye surgery, the ophthalmologist should discontinue surgical manipulation and the patient should be made to breathe deeply by pressure on the anesthesia bag. The oculocardiac reflex may occur without anoxia or hypercapnia.

A study of 810 patients receiving various types of anesthesia supported the conclusion that assisted or controlled respiration during reflex stimulation was the simplest and most useful method for routine control of oculocardiac reflex. Such respiratory control does not eliminate reflex activity but does terminate reflexly induced cardiac and respiratory arrest.[129]

Should retrobulbar anesthesia be used routinely to supplement general anesthesia for the purpose of preventing the oculocardiac reflex? Actually, the bradycardia and marked cardiac arrhythmias that commonly occur (47% of cases)[130] during the process of intubation exceed the cardiac response

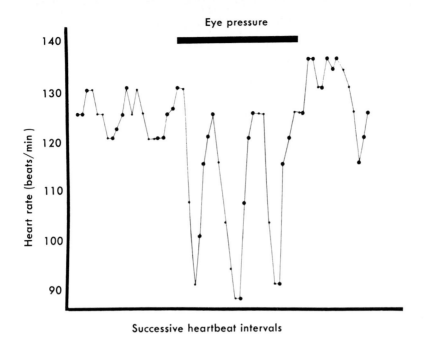

Fig. 5-26. Line represents heart rate, computed from intervals between successive beats. Occurrence of spontaneous respirations is indicated by large dots superimposed on line. When heart rate is slowed by eye pressure, it tends to return to normal with each breath. (From Aserinsky, E., and DeBias, A.: Arch. Ophthalmol. **69:**484, 1963.)

usually resulting from ocular surgery and arouse no concern. The hazard of such minor arrhythmias is slight, possibly less than the dangers of retrobulbar injection.[131] Indeed, of three cardiac arrests during eye surgery over a 20-year period at one hospital, two occurred within 5 minutes after retrobulbar injection for cataract extraction under local anesthesia. Furthermore, the incidence of cardiac arrest is approximately 1 in 3500 cases of eye surgery—despite demonstrable oculocardiac reflexes in 30% to 80% (depending on whose statistics you choose) of such patients.

I have seen several dozen retrobulbar hemorrhages, a number of optic nerve inflammations, one case of transfixion of a thin myopic sclera with resulting severe intraocular hemorrhage, and at least 12 cases of retinal detachment following ocular perforation by a retrobulbar needle. I very much doubt that routine retrobulbar injection can be justified by the supposition that it might prevent cardiac arrest.

For interest, consider that a pediatric

ophthalmologist deliberately tried with traction 623 times to induce the oculocardiac reflex in patients during routine strabismus surgery. Success was achieved 48.6% of the time.[132] Obviously, this ophthalmologist must not have feared the consequences of doing this; nor should we, so long as the patient is adequately oxygenated.

REFERENCES

1. Nachmansohn, D.: Basic aspects of nerve activity explained by biochemical analysis, J.A.M.A. **179:**145, 1962.
2. Goodman, L. S., and Gilman, A.: The pharmacologic basis of therapeutics, ed. 4, New York, 1970, Macmillan Publishing Co., Inc.
3. Adriani, J., and Zepernick, R.: Clinical effectiveness of drugs used for topical anesthesia, J.A.M.A. **188:**711, 1964.
4. Adriani, J., and Campbell, D.: Fatalities following topical application of local anesthetics to mucous membranes, J.A.M.A. **162:**1527, 1956.
5. Goodman, L. S., and Gilman, A.: The pharmacological basis of therapeutics, ed. 4,

New York, 1970, Macmillan Publishing Co., Inc.

6. Stevenson, T. C.: Intrascleral nerve loops, Am. J. Ophthalmol. **55**:935, 1963.

7. Gundersen, T., and Liebman, S. D.: Effect of local anesthetics on regeneration of corneal epithelium, Arch. Ophthalmol. **31**:29, 1944.

8. Marr, W. G., Wood, R., Senterfit, L., and Singelman, S.: Effect of topical anesthetics, Am. J. Ophthalmol. **43**:606, 1957.

9. Kinoshita, J. H.: Some aspects of the carbohydrate metabolism of the cornea, Invest. Ophthalmol. **1**:178, 1962.

10. Herrmann, H., Moses, S., and Friedenwald, J. S.: Influence of Pontocaine hydrochloride and chlorbutanol on respiration and glycolysis of cornea, Arch. Ophthalmol. **28**:652, 1942.

11. Behrendt, T.: Experimental study of corneal lesions, Am. J. Ophthalmol. **41**:99, 1956.

12. Behrendt, T.: Experimental secondary effects of topical anesthesia of the cornea, Am. J. Ophthalmol. **44**:74, 1957.

13. Kleinfeld, J., and Ellis, P. P.: Effects of topical anesthetics on growth of microorganisms, Arch. Ophthalmol. **76**:712, 1966.

14. White, J. H., and Cinotti, A. A.: The inhibition of growth of microorganisms by topical anesthetics, Eye Ear Nose Throat Dig. **49**:22, 1970.

15. Boozan, C. W., and Cohen, I. J.: Ophthaine, Am. J. Ophthalmol. **36**:1619, 1953.

16. Linn, J. G., and Vey, E. K.: Topical anesthesia in ophthalmology, Am. J. Ophthalmol. **40**:697, 1955.

17. Emmerich, R., Carter, G. Z., and Berens, C.: An experimental clinical evaluation of Dorsacaine hydrochloride (benoxinate, novesine), Am. J. Ophthalmol. **40**:841, 1955.

18. Schlegel, H. E., and Swan, K. C.: Benoxinate (Dorsacaine) for rapid corneal anesthesia, Arch. Ophthalmol. **51**:663, 1954.

19. Koller, C.: Preliminary report on local anesthesia of the eye, Arch. Ophthalmol. **12**:473, 1934.

20. Bloom, S.: Carl Koller, M.D., Arch. Ophthalmol. **31**:344, 1944.

21. Koller, K.: On the use of cocaine to anaesthetize the eye, Arch. Ophthalmol. **13**:404, 1884. (Translated by H. Knapp in On cocaine and its use in ophthalmic and general surgery, Arch. Ophthalmol. **68**:31, 1962.)

22. Bellows, J. G.: Surface anesthesia in ophthalmology, Arch. Ophthalmol. **12**:824, 1934.

23. Philpot, F. J.: The inhibition of adrenalin oxidation by local anesthetics, J. Physiol. **97**:301, 1940.

24. Van Alphen, G. W. H. M., Robinette, S. L., and Macri, F. J.: Drug effects on ciliary muscle and choroid preparations in vitro, Arch. Ophthalmol. **68**:81, 1962.

25. Boniuk, M., and Schlezinger, N. S.: Raeder's paratrigeminal syndrome, Am. J. Ophthalmol. **54**:1074, 1962.

26. Lowenstein, O.: The Argyll Robertson pupillary syndrome, Am. J. Ophthalmol. **42**:105, 1956.

27. Lowenstein, O.: Miosis in Argyll Robertson syndrome and related pupillary disorders, Arch. Ophthalmol. **55**:356, 1956.

28. Patil, P. N.: Cocaine-binding by the pigmented and the nonpigmented iris and its relevance to the mydriatic effect, Invest. Ophthalmol. **11**:739, 1972.

29. Gartner, S., and Billet, E.: A study on mortality rates, Am. J. Ophthalmol. **45**:847, 1958.

30. Adriani, J.: Seminar: local anesthetics, Seminar Report, Fall, 1956.

31. Greenblatt, D. J., Bolognini, V., Koch-Weser, J., and Harmatz, J. S.: Pharmacokinetic approach to the clinical use of lidocaine intravenously, J.A.M.A. **236**:273, July 19, 1976.

32. Council on Drugs: New drugs and developments in therapeutics, J.A.M.A. **183**:178, 1963.

33. Vey, E. K., Finlay, J., and Everett, W. G.: A clinical evaluation of mepivacaine, Am. J. Ophthalmol. **53**:827, 1962.

34. Gills, J. P., and Rudisill, J. E.: Bupivacaine in cataract surgery, Ophthalmic Surg. **5**:67, Winter 1974.

35. Abel, R., Jr., and Kaufman, H. E.: Prolonged pain after cyclocryotherapy performed with retrobulbar bupivacaine hydrochloride anesthesia, Ann. Ophthalmol. **7**:301, February 1975.

36. Seifter, J., Baeder, D. H., and Begany, A. J.: Influence of hyaluronidase and steroids on permeability of synovial membrane, J. Proc. Soc. Exp. Biol. Med. **72**:277, 1949.

37. Alfano, J. E., and Clampit, J.: Injection of hyaluronidase into the anterior chamber of the rabbit eye, Am. J. Ophthalmol. **39**:198, 1955.

38. Von Sallmann, L.: Experimental study on the vitreous, Arch. Ophthalmol. **43**:638, 1950.

39. Moore, D. C.: An evaluation of hyaluroni-

dase in local and nerve block analgesia: a review of 519 cases, Anesthesiology **11**:470, 1950.

40. Everett, W. G., Vey, E., and Finlay, J.: Duration of oculomotor akinesia of injectable anesthetics, Trans. Am. Acad. Ophthalmol. **65**:308, 1961.

41. Swan, K. C.: Ocular penetration of procaine following subconjunctival injection, Arch. Ophthalmol. **52**:774, 1954.

42. Melikian, H. E., Nowakowski, J., Boyle, G. L., and Leopold, I. H.: Use of subconjunctival hyaluronidase, Am. J. Ophthalmol. **71**: 1313, 1971.

43. De Roetth, A., and Carroll, F. D.: Effect of retrobulbar procaine injection on aqueous humor dynamics, Arch. Ophthalmol. **53**:399, 1955.

44. Parkes, M., and Fein, W.: Further experience with the pinch technique for repair of eyelid deformities, Arch. Ophthalmol. **94**: 1534, September 1976.

45. Ruiz Barranco, F., and Montero Marchena, J.: The effect of hyaluronidase on tension of glaucomatous eyes, Am. J. Ophthalmol. **47**:921, 1959 (abst.).

46. Landesberg, J.: Primary glaucoma: open-angle type, Am. J. Ophthalmol. **48**:81, 1959.

47. Tassmann, I. S.: The use of hyaluronidase in ophthalmology, Am. J. Ophthalmol. **35**: 683, 1952.

48. Planten, J. T., and Hoppenbrouwers, R.: Intraocular hyaluronidase, Am. J. Ophthalmol. **39**:135, 1955 (abst.).

49. Atkinson, W. S.: Observations on anesthesia for ocular surgery, Trans. Am. Acad. Ophthalmol. **60**:376, 1956.

50. Atkinson, W. S.: Facial nerve block, Am. J. Ophthalmol. **57**:144, 1964.

51. Swan, K. C.: New drugs and techniques for ocular anesthesia, Trans. Am. Acad. Ophthalmol. **60**:368, 1956.

52. Reed, J. W., MacMillan, A. S., Jr., and Lazenby, G. W.: Transient neurologic complication of positive contrast orbitography, Arch. Ophthalmol. **81**:508, 1969.

53. Carroll, F., and de Roetth, A. J.: The effect of retrobulbar injections of procaine on the optic nerve, Trans. Am. Acad. Ophthalmol. **59**:356, 1955.

54. Havener, W. H., and Makley, T. A.: The photocoagulator—a new clinical instrument, Guildcraft **35**:19, 1961.

55. Pruett, R. C.: The effects of local anesthetics upon the optic nerve conduction in the cat, Arch. Ophthalmol. **77**:119, 1967.

56. Atkinson, W. S.: The development of ophthalmic anesthesia, Am. J. Ophthalmol. **51**:1, 1961.

57. Van Bergen, T. M., and Swets, E. J.: Retrobulbar anesthesia, Am. J. Ophthalmol. **56**:825, 1963.

58. Atkinson, W. S.: Larger retrobulbar injections, Am. J. Ophthalmol. **57**:328, 1964.

59. Gartner, S.: Methods of inducing anesthesia and hypotony for cataract surgery, Arch. Ophthalmol. **61**:50, 1959.

60. Everett, W. G., Vey, E. K., and Veenis, C. Y.: Factors in reducing ocular tension prior to intraocular surgery, Trans. Am. Acad. Ophthalmol. **63**:286, 1959.

61. Kirsch, R. E.: Further studies on the use of digital pressure in cataract surgery, Arch. Ophthalmol. **58**:641, 1957.

62. Obstbaum, S. A., Robbins, R., Best, M., and Galin, M. A.: Recovery of intraocular pressure and vitreous weight after ocular compression, Am. J. Ophthalmol. **71**:1059, 1971.

63. Hermann, J. S.: Digital pressure prior to cataract surgery, Am. J. Ophthalmol. **55**: 1060, 1963.

64. Atkinson, W. S.: Anesthesia in ophthalmology, Springfield, Ill., 1955, Charles C Thomas, Publisher.

65. Adriani, J.: Premedication—an old idea and new drugs, J.A.M.A. **171**:1086, 1959.

66. Atkinson, W. S.: Preanesthetic sedation and analgesia for intraocular operations done with local anesthesia, Arch. Ophthalmol. **49**:481, 1953.

67. Fishof, F.: Meperidine in cataract surgery, Am. J. Ophthalmol. **53**:672, 1962.

68. Council on Drugs: New drugs and developments in therapeutics, J.A.M.A. **177**:245, 1961.

69. Constant, M. A., and Becker, B.: Experimental tonography, Arch. Ophthalmol. **56**: 19, 1956.

70. Paul, S. D., and Leopold, I. H.: The effect of tranquilizing and ganglion-blocking agents, Am. J. Ophthalmol. **42**:752, 1956.

71. Paul, S. D., and Leopold, I. H.: The effect of chlorpromazine (thorazine) on intraocular pressure in experimental animals, Am. J. Ophthalmol. **42**:107, 1956.

72. Knapp, M. R., and Beecher, H. K.: Postanesthetic nausea, vomiting, and retching, J.A.M.A. **160**:376, 1956.

73. Weiss, W. A., McGee, J. P., Jr., Branford, J., and Hanks, E. C.: Value of chlorproma-

zine in preoperative medication, J.A.M.A. **161**:812, 1956.

74. Papper, E. M.: The proper use of tranquilizers in surgical patients, Trans. Am. Acad. Ophthalmol. **64**:689, 1960.

75. Adriani, J., Arens, J., and Anthony, S. O.: Postanesthetic vomiting, J.A.M.A. **175**:666, 1961.

76. Conger, C. W., Claassen, L. G., and Hamelberg, W.: Control of postoperative nausea and vomiting, Ohio State Med. J. **57**:897, 1961.

77. Bellville, J. W., Howland, W. S., and Bross, I. D. J.: Postoperative nausea and vomiting, J.A.M.A. **172**:1488, 1960.

78. Harley, R. D., and Mishler, J. E.: The use of chlorpromazine in cataract surgery, Am. J. Ophthalmol. **43**:744, 1957.

79. Harley, R. D., and Mishler, J. E.: Ataractic and antiemetic drugs in cataract surgery, Am. J. Ophthalmol. **47**:177, 1959.

80. Ayd, F. J., Jr.: Chlorpromazine: ten years' experience, J.A.M.A. **184**:51, 1963.

81. Stein, A. A., and Wright, A. W.: Hepatic pathology in jaundice due to chlorpromazine, J.A.M.A. **161**:508, 1956.

82. Yasuna, E.: Acute myopia associated with prochlorperazine (Compazine) therapy, Am. J. Ophthalmol. **54**:793, 1962.

83. Bard, L. A.: Transient myopia, Am. J. Ophthalmol. **58**:682, 1964.

84. Apt, L.: Complications of phenothiazine tranquilizers—ocular side effects, Survey Ophthalmol. **5**:550, 1960.

85. Weekley, R. D., Potts, A. M., Reboton, J., and May, R. H.: Pigmentary retinopathy in patients receiving high doses of a new phenothiazine, Arch. Ophthalmol. **64**:65, 1960.

86. May, R. H., Selymes, P., Weekley, R. D., and Potts, A. M.: Thioridazine therapy: results and complications, J. Nerv. Ment. Dis. **130**:230, 1960.

87. Potts, A. M.: The concentration of phenothiazines in the eye of experimental animals, Invest. Ophthalmol. **1**:522, 1962.

88. McTigue, J. W., and Urweider, H. A.: The use of diazepam (Valium) in ophthalmic surgery, Trans. Am. Acad. Ophthalmol. Otolaryngol. **73**:78, 1969.

89. Sadove, M. S.: Discussion of paper, Trans. Am. Acad. Ophthalmol. Otolaryngol. **73**:84, 1969.

90. Cosgriff, S.: Society proceedings, Am. J. Ophthalmol. **49**:361, 1960.

91. Memery, H. N.: Anesthesia mortality in private practice, J.A.M.A. **194**:1185, 1965.

92. Lynch, S.: The case for general anesthesia, Trans. Am. Acad. Ophthalmol. Otolaryngol. **79**:OP-559, July-August 1975.

93. Wolf, G. L., Lynch, S., and Berlin, I.: Intraocular surgery with general anesthesia, Arch. Ophthalmol. **93**:323, May 1975.

94. Newell, F. W.: Current trends in ophthalmic anesthesia, Ophthalmic Surg. **6**:15, Summer 1975.

95. Reese, A. B.: Problems encountered in an eye clinic for children, Am. J. Ophthalmol. **43**:24, 1957.

96. Stringham, J. D.: Pediatric anesthesia, Arch. Ophthalmol. **57**:24, 1957.

97. De Roetth, A., and Schwartz, H.: Aqueous humor dynamics in glaucoma, Arch. Ophthalmol. **55**:755, 1956.

98. Magora, F., and Collins, V.: The influence of general anesthetic agents on intraocular pressure in man, Arch. Ophthalmol. **66**:806, 1961.

99. Kornblueth, W., Aladjemoff, L., Magora, F., and Gabbay, A.: Influence of general anesthesia on intraocular pressure in man, Arch. Ophthalmol. **61**:84, 1959.

100. Burch, P. G.: Accommodation during general anesthesia, Arch. Ophthalmol. **81**:202, 1969.

101. Westheimer, G.: Amphetamine, barbiturates, and accommodation-convergence, Arch. Ophthalmol. **70**:830, 1963.

102. Smith, R. B.: Nitrous oxide anesthesia with gas in the vitreous cavity, Am. J. Ophthalmol. **80**:779, October 1975.

103. Smith, R. B., Carl, B., Linn, J. G., Jr., and Nemoto, E.: Effect of nitrous oxide on air in vitreous, Am. J. Ophthalmol. **78**:314, August 1974.

104. Aronowitz, J. D., and Brubaker, R. F.: Effect of intraocular gas on intraocular pressure, Arch. Ophthalmol. **94**:1191, July 1976.

105. American Medical Association: New and nonofficial drugs, Philadelphia, 1962, J. B. Lippincott Co.

106. Mietus, C. A., Haugue, E. B., and Carbone, D. J.: Use of general anesthesia and muscle relaxants in cataract surgery, Am. J. Ophthalmol. **47**:487, 1959.

107. Cordes, F. C., and Mullen, R. S.: The use of curare in cataract surgery, Am. J. Ophthalmol. **34**:557, 1951.

108. Farquharson, H.: Curare with local anesthesia in cataract surgery, Am. J. Ophthalmol. **34**:554, 1951.

109. Lincoff, H. A., Ellis, C. H., Devoe, A. G., De Beer, E. J., Impastato, D. J., Berg, S.,

Orkin, L., and Magda, H.: The effect of succinylcholine on intraocular pressure, Am. J. Ophthalmol. **40:**501, 1955.

110. Lincoff, H. A., Breinin, G. M., and DeVoe, A. G.: The effect of succinylcholine on the extraocular muscles, Am. J. Ophthalmol. **43:** 440, 1957.

111. Macri, F. J., and Grimes, P. A.: The effects of succinylcholine on the extraocular striate muscles and on the intraocular pressure, Am. J. Ophthalmol. **44:**221, 1957.

112. Kornblueth, W., Jampolsky, A., Tamler, E., and Marg, E.: Contraction of the oculorotary muscles and intraocular pressure, Am. J. Ophthalmol. **49:**1381, 1960.

113. Lewallen, W. M., and Hicks, B. L.: The use of succinylcholine in ocular surgery, Am. J. Ophthalmol. **61:**985, 1966.

114. Norskov, K.: Expulsive haemorrhage caused by succinylcholine, Acta Ophthalmol. **38:** 285, 1960.

115. Alfano, J. E.: Pseudocholinesterase, cholinesterase and congenital glaucoma, Am. J. Ophthalmol. **61:**985, 1966.

116. Lessell, S., Kuwabara, T., and Feldman, R. G.: Myopathy and succinylcholine sensitivity, Am. J. Ophthalmol. **68:**789, 1969.

117. Abramson, D. H.: Anterior chamber and lens thickness changes induced by succinylcholine, Arch. Ophthalmol. **86:**643, 1971.

118. Kouwenhoven, W. B., Milnor, W. R., Knickerbocker, G. G., and Chestnut, W. R.: Closed chest defibrillation of the heart, Surgery **42:**550, 1957.

119. Kouwenhoven, W. B., Jude, J. R., and Knickerbocker, G. G.: Closed-chest cardiac massage, J.A.M.A. **173:**1064, 1960.

120. Herman, R., and Banks, C. N.: Massive hemopericardium due to external cardiac massage, J.A.M.A. **193:**1064, 1965.

121. Lundberg, G. D., Mattei, I. R., Davis, C. J., and Nelson, D. E.: Hemorrhage from gastroesophageal lacerations following closed-chest cardiac massage, J.A.M.A. **202:**195, 1967.

122. Atkinson, W. S.: Management of respiratory and cardiac failure, Arch. Ophthalmol. **70:** 813, 1963.

123. Gay, A. J., Joffe, W. S., and Barnet, R.: The afferent course of the oculorespiratory reflex of the third, fourth, and sixth cranial nerves, Invest. Ophthalmol. **3:**451, 1964.

124. Kirsch, R. E., Samet, P., Kugel, V., and Axelrod, S.: Electrocardiographic changes during ocular surgery and their prevention by retrobar injection, Arch. Ophthalmol. **58:** 348, 1957.

125. Mendelblatt, F., Kirsch, R., and Lemberg, L.: A study of comparing methods of preventing the oculocardiac reflex, Am. J. Ophthalmol. **53:**506, 1962.

126. Bosomworth, P. P., Ziegler, C. H., and Jacoby, J.: The oculo-cardiac reflex in eye muscle surgery, Anesthesiology **19:**1, 1958.

127. Welhaf, W. R., and Johnson, D. C.: The oculocardiac reflex during extraocular muscle surgery, Arch. Ophthalmol. **73:**43, 1965.

128. Aserinsky, E., and DeBias, A.: Suppression of oculocardiac reflex by artificial respiration, Arch. Ophthalmol. **69:**484, 1963.

129. Pontinen, P. J.: The importance of the oculocardiac reflex during ocular surgery, Acta Ophthalmol. **86**(suppl.)**:**1, 1966.

130. Landers, P. H., and Moyer, J. K.: Electrocardiographic observations, Am. J. Ophthalmol. **60:**71, 1965.

131. Beler, D. K.: The oculocardiac reflex, Am. J. Ophthalmol. **56:**954, 1963.

132. Apt, L., Isenberg, S., and Gaffney, W. L.: The oculocardiac reflex in strabismus surgery, Am. J. Ophthalmol. **76:**533, October 1973.

6
ANTIBIOTICS

Almost incredibly serious charges have been advanced against the habitual use of antibiotic prescriptions. A pharmacist who reviewed recorded antibiotic use for all (1035) patients admitted to a 500-bed private hospital during 1 month[1] found that systemic antimicrobial agents were prescribed for 340 patients, the reasons being classified as treatment of infection (36%), prophylactic (54%), or symptomatic (10%). Judgment as to the validity of the treatment classified the usage as being rational (13%), irrational (66%), or questionable (21%). The cost of the drugs used was $18,224.55. Of this, only $1677.38 (9.2%) was considered expended for rational therapy. Adverse drug reactions occurred in 48 patients (14% of those treated), and 91.7% of these reactions occurred in patients receiving therapy on an irrational or questionable basis. This information was presented to the Senate Health Subcommittee headed by Senator Edward Kennedy on February 25, 1974, thereby ensuring its consideration in the political process that governs us.

A survey article originating from the Department of Health, Education and Welfare[2] presents a variety of reasons for believing that antibiotics are being overused to our detriment. The production of medical antibiotics increased from 3,000,000 pounds in 1960 to 9,600,000 pounds in 1970. Of all prescriptions, 20% are for antibiotics. In 1972 27% of the 33,000,000 hospitalized patients received antibiotics at a cost of $218,000,000.

The mortality from bacteremia (35%) is the same now as in the era before penicillin, although the etiology is now more heavily gram-negative than in the past. Projected from a 0.3% annual death rate caused by gram-negative bacteremia in a large teaching hospital, more than 100,000 such deaths occur annually in the United States. Half of the persons with common colds who are treated by physicians receive antibiotics. The incidence of aplastic anemia following chloramphenicol administration is 1 in 80,000 "doses" (article misstatement—this is the incidence in treated patients, not doses). This study has found that, "Hundreds of thousands of patients may be unnecessarily exposed to the hazards of antibiotics because of their inappropriate use."

An attempt at rational evaluation of adverse drug reaction problems[3] criticized statistics indicating that hospitalization for adverse drug reactions costs $4.5 billion annually for room cost alone and that 140,000 patients annually suffer fatal drug reactions. Such numbers are arrived at by extrapolating from the worst statistic available to the entire population of the United States. (For example, in my operating suite, half of the surgery is for retinal detachment. Therefore, if x operations are performed annually in the United States, $0.5x$ of these are for retinal detachment.) Aside from the invalidity of such statistical approaches, the original data base is usually incomplete, arbitrary, unrepresentative, and uncontrolled.

114

How should the question of proper antibiotic use in ophthalmic practice be dealt with? My purpose in these introductory paragraphs is to ask you to consider your own indications for antibiotic usage. Should antibiotics be used for prophylactic purposes? For presumed virus infections? Are you choosing proper antibiotics? I do not think that our usage of drugs is as bad as our critics represent, but in honesty, we could do better. Please do not disregard this introduction, but reconsider your own prescribing habits.

Accurate diagnosis of the infectious nature of an ocular disorder is, of course, the first step in successful antibiotic therapy. Obviously the red eye of phacolytic glaucoma or the irritation of a burdock bur embedded in the upper lid will not respond to antibiotics.

The second step is the selection of a drug effective against the responsible microorganism. Usually this requires identification of the organism by staining and culture techniques and laboratory measurement of its antibiotic sensitivity. General knowledge of the typical appearance of some infections (for example, the hyperacute, purulent conjunctivitis of the newborn that is characteristic of gonococcal infection) and of the spectrum of various antibiotics (for example, colistin is effective against gram-negative bacilli) may be helpful while awaiting laboratory reports.

The third essential is a knowledge of the toxic effects of antibiotics. A variety of serious problems (for example, deafness) may cause the "treatment to be worse than the disease."

CHOICE OF AGENT

The decision as to which antibiotic to use for a given infection will be guided by general knowledge (for example, almost all gonococci are sensitive to penicillin). However, each case requires individual assessment (for example, the patient may be allergic to penicillin). Except for initial emergency treatment, arbitrary choice of an antibiotic for a serious infection is unwise, since such a decision is based only on statistical generalizations, and individual strains of microorganisms vary widely in their sensitivity. If the infection is at all serious, laboratory sensitivity studies are essential for selection of the best antibiotic.

For topical use in the treatment of minor ocular infections, the antibiotics commonly administered systemically should be avoided. The widespread prescription of these antibiotics has created many resistant strains of microorganisms. The possible sensitization of patients to these drugs is an unwarranted risk when equally good results can otherwise be obtained. Finally, the unnecessary use of these valuable drugs will hasten development of new strains of resistant organisms that may later menace community health.

Laboratory studies of the antibiotic sensitivity of organisms isolated from the eye clearly indicate the superiority of the antibacterial drugs whose use is limited to topical application.[4] Such medications include bacitracin, gramicidin, the nitrofurans, neomycin, sulfacetimide, and polymyxin B.

Properly chosen combinations of these exclusively topical antibiotics will be effective against the great majority of commonly encountered bacteria. Such combinations can be prescribed with reasonable confidence for minor infections or for prophylactic purposes. A popular combination includes bacitracin (effective against gram-positive organisms), polymyxin B (effective against gram-negative organisms), and neomycin (effective against both gram-positive and gram-negative organisms, particularly *Proteus vulgaris*, which is very resistant to most other antibiotics).[5] This combination was used to treat 214 patients with surface ocular infections. Within 1 to 2 weeks virtually all infections caused by gram-positive or gram-negative organisms were successfully cleared. Only 1 of these 214 patients had a local allergic reaction to the drug combination.

Our clinical wisdom has been seriously challenged by a study of 143 patients with blepharoconjunctivitis or conjunctivitis.[6] Not only are we unable to diagnose the etiology of blepharoconjunctivitis, but we are unable to establish that there is any difference between treatment with corticosteroids, antibiotics, or both used in combination. On the basis of a detailed protocol including all of the historical and clinical data generally accepted as being of value in etiologic diagnosis, 84 cases were diagnosed as bacterial, 21 as viral, 32 as allergic, and 6 as irritative. Unfortunately, however, the laboratory studies (bacterial culture, gram and Giemsa stains) showed no correlation with the clinical diagnoses. Positive cultures for pathogenic bacteria were found in only 31% of cases diagnosed as being of bacterial etiology but in 52% of cases believed to be viral. Positive gram stain findings occurred in equal frequency in all 4 groups of patients and did not even correlate with the culture findings. Giemsa identification of leukocytes, lymphocytes, or eosinophils was of no value, since these cell types were distributed throughout all 4 diagnostic categories. One might dismiss this report as an indictment of the researchers, but they are well-known and respected academicians and have documented their work in detail.

Even more devastating is their report on therapeutic response.[7] These cases of blepharoconjunctivitis and conjunctivitis responded equally well to weak corticosteroids (0.2% hydrocortisone), potent corticosteroids (0.1% dexamethasone), corticosteroid-antibiotic combinations (Maxitrol, which is composed of dexamethasone, neomycin, and polymyxin B), or antibiotics alone (Statrol, composed of neomycin and polymyxin B). Evaluation of only patients with *Staphylococcus aureus* infection showed the confounding results that corticosteroid treatment was superior to antibiotic treatment (perhaps resistant organisms?). Control treatment with hydroxypropylmethylcellulose was not nearly as effective as treatment with any of the drugs, indicating that spontaneous cure despite any drug was not the explanation of these unexpected findings. How should rational therapy of conjunctivitis be delivered?

PROPHYLACTIC USE

Clinical wisdom indicates that antibiotic prophylaxis is of no value in routine clean general surgery performed on healthy patients with normal resistance. Should topical antibiotics be used prophylactically before intraocular surgery? To answer this question intelligently, the surgeon must know the sources of intraocular infection, the characteristics of extraocular infection, and the antibacterial spectrum of the antibiotic being used.

Certainly it is possible to introduce organisms from the environment into the eye, and for this reason, meticulous aseptic surgical techniques must be rigidly enforced. I know of a small epidemic in which three eyes were lost because *Pseudomonas* infection developed after cataract surgery. The same strain of bacteria, as judged by sensitivity characteristics, was isolated from each of the three eyes and from the interior of a rubber irrigating bulb that had been used in each of the three operations. The bulb had not been autoclaved but had been ineffectively soaked in sterilizing solution before being used in the next patient. Many other instances are known in which infection originated from an external source.

Fortunately, environmental contamination can be reduced to almost nothing in a well-run operating room. This leaves the patient as the main source of infection. This source was confirmed by a series of 11 cases of endophthalmitis that occurred in 2508 cataract extractions.[8] All 11 infections were caused by *Staphylococcus aureus*, and exactly the same organisms had been found in preoperative cultures. As a result of this confirmation of the patient as the source of infection, a policy of using topical antibiotic ointment five times preoperatively at 3-hour intervals was instituted. Only six cases of postoperative endophthalmitis occurred during performance of the next 7662 cataract extractions.

These 7662 operations were subdivided into several groups. Patients in whom preoperative cultures showed no bacteria numbered 2263, and after these operations not one case of endophthalmitis occurred. On recovery of *Staphylococcus aureus* in preoperative culture in 567 cases, prophylactic antibiotics were used until ocular cultures became negative preoperatively; no infections occurred in this series. Despite known preoperative cultures of *Staphylococcus aureus* in 978 cases, cataract extraction was done after five routine applications of prophylactic ointment; in this group only one case of postoperative infection occurred, and it was caused by *Pseudomonas aeruginosa* organisms that had *not* been cultured preoperatively. No preoperative cultures were done in 3854 cases, from which five cases of endophthalmitis resulted.

The fact that no infections occurred after the 2830 operations on eyes known to be free of virulent bacteria preoperatively warrants serious consideration. Are the cost and inconvenience of preoperative cultures too great a price to pay for this freedom from infection? Could the six infections that occurred in the cases of unknown sterility or known infection—despite prophylactic antibiotics (although the type of antibiotic used varied with different surgeons and was not specified)—have been prevented by more intensive preoperative treatment? Obviously these theoretical questions are impossible to answer.

Do other investigators likewise find a decrease in postoperative endophthalmitis when prophylactic measures are taken? Yes. Twenty-one infections in 2086 operations without prophylaxis were followed by two infections in 1200 cataract extractions with prophylaxis.[9]

How long does it take to eliminate bacteria by treatment? In a series of 507 patients with infections caused by *Staphylococcus aureus*, complete elimination of bacteria occurred in 1 day in 73 patients, in 2 days in 219 patients, in 3 days in 137 patients, in 4 days in 64 patients, and in 5 days in 14 patients. Similarly, infections resulting from *Escherichia coli* and *Proteus vulgaris* required 3 to 7 days of treatment before clearing (Table 6-1).[8]

How long does antibiotic therapy maintain ocular sterility? Of 41 patients disinfected by antibiotics, 29 were reinfected within 24 hours after treatment was stopped! In the remaining 12 patients, infection recurred within 2 to 7 days.

What is the source of reinfection? The same strains of bacteria are commonly found on all surfaces of the body. In the 507 patients with ocular *Staphylococcus* infection, the same organism was also isolated elsewhere as follows: nose, 431 isolations from 505 cultures; throat, 131 isolations from 426 cultures; and eyelids, 131 isolations from 426 cultures.

Which antibiotic should be used for prophylaxis? The development of antibiotic resistance by staphylococci is illustrated in Fig. 6-1. From the initial 86% sensitivity to penicillin, these organisms dropped to only 22% sensitivity. Similar resistance has developed in response to the other commonly used antibiotics. Existence of resistant strains of staphylococci and the possibility of infection with different types of bacteria clearly indicate that the prophylactic medication of choice should be an antibiotic combination, which can attain a broader spectrum of effectiveness than can any single antibiotic.

Antibiotic treatment of donor eyes for corneal transplantation is a special kind of prophylaxis. Despite sterile technique in removal and handling, in one study 50% of 1859 donor eyes were culture-positive.[10] One

Table 6-1. Number of days required for elimination of ocular bacteria by topical antibiotic therapy*

	Days required to sterilize eye						
Organism	*1*	*2*	*3*	*4*	*5*	*6*	*7*
Staphylococcus aureus	73†	219†	137†	64†	14†		
Escherichia coli			6†	11†	5†		
Proteus vulgaris			7†	6†	19†	4†	2†

*Modified from Locatcher-Khorazo, D., and Guiterrez, E.: Am. J. Ophthalmol. **41**:981, 1956.
†Number of eyes becoming sterile on given day.

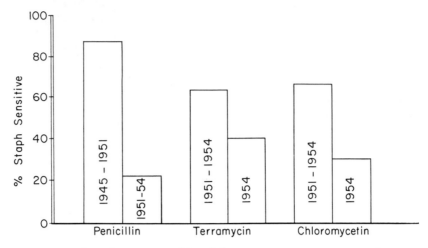

Fig. 6-1. In vitro studies of sensitivity of *Staphylococcus aureus* to various antibiotics, as measured in the years designated. Note the rapid and significant increase in resistant strains. (Modified from Locatcher-Khorazo, D., and Guiterrez, E.: Am. J. Ophthalmol. **41**:981, 1956.)

hour after washing with chloramphenicol solution, only 30% of the eyes remained culture-positive. Some of the eyes were washed with Neosporin; of these only 20% remained culture-positive after 1 hour. Reducing by one half the number of culture-positive donor eyes seems like a worthwhile result of prophylaxis.

Another circumstance would be the continuous wearing of a hydrophilic contact lens on a normal eye. What happens if a drop of Neosporin is instilled four times daily for 3 months? Apparently nothing happens, except the development of bacterial resistance.[11] In this study 17 volunteers were fitted with a continuous wear soft lens in only 1 eye. The Neosporin drops were randomly assigned to the eye with or without the contact lens. At the end of the 12-week period, the normal flora had not been displaced from any eye, nor had secondary invaders appeared. Using *Staphylococcus* epidermidis as an indicator, resistance appeared in 2 weeks in the treated eyes and in 4 weeks in the opposite, untreated eyes. Quite clearly, prophylactic antibiotics are not indicated in the routine of continuous wear cosmetic contact lenses.

Should prophylactic antibiotics be used in fractures that cause communications between the paranasal sinuses and the orbit or the intracranial cavity? Case reports[12] suggest this, but adequate controls do not exist.

How about management of intraocular foreign bodies? Again, we do not have controlled series of cases and must rely on clinical prejudices. My personal prejudice is to treat vigorously and immediately every patient with an intraocular foreign body. Why? We know that intraocular infections do develop in some such cases, that the sight of the eye is almost invariably lost if an overt infection develops, and that antibiotic treatment will sterilize most such severely infected eyes (not fungus infections) even though sight is lost. I interpret these facts to indicate that early and vigorous systemic and topical antibiotic treatment of an eye destined to be lost (if untreated) to a susceptible microorganism will prevent development of the infection and will save the eye. Not all injured eyes develop infection, and routine prophylaxis will certainly treat many patients who would have healed just as well without treatment. Unfortunately, there is no way to differentiate these patients before infection develops, hence I treat them all.

INTRACAMERAL INJECTION

The usual treatment of intraocular infection consists of intensive use of systemic and

Table 6-2. Amount of antibiotic tolerated on injection into anterior chamber*

Agent	Dosage
Bacitracin	500-1000 units
Chloramphenicol	1-2 mg
Colistin	0.1 mg
Erythromycin	1-2 mg
Neomycin	2.5 mg
Penicillin G	1000-4000 units
Methicillin	1 mg
Polymyxin B	0.1 mg
Streptomycin	0.5-5 mg
Tetracycline	2.5-5 mg

*From Leopold, I. H.: Invest. Ophthalmol. 3:504, 1964.

topical routes of antibiotic administration. Intracameral injection of antibiotics may lead to operative complications and drug irritation but has the advantage of rapidly achieving a very high intraocular antibiotic concentration. The risks and benefits of such injection must be weighed in each case. Presumably, intracameral antibiotic injection would be particularly suitable to the treatment of infected conditions that necessitate surgery (for example, closure of a ruptured operative wound or repair of a dirty laceration). Antibiotic dosages tolerated by the anterior chamber are listed in Table 6-2.[13]

Irrigation of the anterior chamber with excessive amounts of antibiotic, even penicillin, can destroy the endothelium, result in dense corneal opacity, produce destructive iritis with neovascularization, and induce cataract. Be reasonably certain that the alternative is worse than taking the risk of injecting any type of antibiotic into the anterior chamber. Most of the eyes that exhibit alarming redness and flare during the first few days after cataract surgery will do very well without any additional surgical ventures and certainly do not warrant prophylactic intracameral injections.

EFFECT ON EPITHELIAL REGENERATION

The effect of topical antibiotics on the healing of corneal epithelial wounds is of obvious practical importance, since these drugs are commonly used in the treatment of eyes with epithelial defects. Fortunately, in clinically used concentrations, antibiotics usually do not delay healing of experimental epithelial wounds.[14,15]

TOXIC CONJUNCTIVITIS

Not uncommonly chronic keratoconjunctivitis will develop after topical antibiotic treatment of a surface ocular infection. Although it is caused by the antibiotic, this inflammation is often misinterpreted as being a continuing infection. Such toxic keratoconjunctivitis may gradually become more severe during prolonged treatment. When this diagnosis is suspected, all medications should be discontinued and treatment should be limited to cold compresses. Often it will be difficult to convince these patients that treatment should be stopped, particularly because a latent period of some days may precede improvement. Conjunctival scrapings of toxic keratoconjunctivitis characteristically show mononuclear cells with typical basophilic granules.[16]

ALTERATION OF MICROFLORA

Proof of the inhibitory effect of one microorganism on another was provided by a study of 24,389 strains isolated from eye patients.[17] Forty-seven percent of these organisms produced antibiotics effective against the test organism (*Corynebacterium pseudodiphtheriticum*). The frequency of this inhibitory ability indicates that elimination of one microorganism with antibiotic treatment may permit an overgrowth of other microorganisms.

Oral administration of the broad-spectrum antibiotics (notably the tetracyclines) significantly alters the normal intestinal microflora. A most common consequence is the uninhibited multiplication of the remaining resistant species, notably the yeasts such as *Candida albicans*. Such infection usually remains confined to the intestinal tract but may rarely disseminate systemically.

Direct potentiation of fungi by antibiotics has been suspected but cannot be regarded as established. The concept of antibiotic potentiation of fungus growth is based on suggestive, but as yet incomplete, experimental work. In one such experiment, both corneas of 11 young rabbits were infected by intrastromal injection of *Candida albicans*.[18] Oxytetracycline (Terramycin), 1% solution, was added to the inoculum of the right eyes, while the left eyes remained untreated as controls. Corneal perforation occurred in eight treated eyes and in one control eye. Although on first glance this 8:1 ratio appears to indicate fungus potentiation by antibiotics and has frequently been referred to as providing such proof, this is not necessarily the case. Intralamellar injection of tetracyclines is irritating, and this nonclinical method of application may have caused enough damage to the thin corneas of these young rabbits to account for the higher incidence of perforation. Furthermore, this experimental result was obtained only in infection with *Candida albicans* and after treatment with oxytetracycline by intralamellar injection. Infection of adult rabbits with other types of fungi (including *Aspergillus*) treated with chlortetracycline (Aureomycin) showed no increased growth resulting from the presence of the antibiotic. These experiments, characterized by the author as "exploratory," certainly cannot be interpreted as a rational contraindication to the clinical use of antibiotics in ocular therapy.

The effect of chlortetracycline on fungus infections has been evaluated in mice infected with *Candida albicans*.[19] Intraperitoneal injection of 2 mg of chlortetracycline in 17 mice and of 320 million *Candida* cells in 17 other mice resulted in no deaths. However, when these doses of chlortetracycline and *Candida* were combined and injected simultaneously, 16 of 17 mice died of *Candida* infection. In a variation of this experiment, incubation of *Candida* with chlortetracycline and subsequent washing away of the antibiotic did not enhance virulence. Inactivation of chlortetracycline solutions by boiling or by being allowed to stand at room temperature destroyed its fungus-enhancing properties. Chlortetracycline did not alter *Candida* growth in vivo. Intraperitoneal injections of chlortetracycline and *Candida* at separate times gave the results shown in Table 6-3.

This experiment indicates that chlortetracycline interferes for at least a day with the normal defense mechanisms. However, chlortetracycline given 8 to 24 hours after infection does not enhance *Candida* growth. Whether these experiments indicate that chlortetracycline is a biologic activator of fungus infections or simply damages resistance as a nonspecific irritant cannot be determined from the facts available.

A claim for possible neomycin potentiation of *Candida* keratitis was based on a study of seven rabbits, four of which were made somewhat worse with neomycin treatment, whereas three were not.[20] Such a finding is statistically insignificant and it remains to be confirmed that antibiotics potentiate the ocular growth of the fungi commonly encountered in mycotic keratitis.[21] Furthermore, a very high proportion of corneal infections are caused by bacteria and a very small proportion by fungi. To withhold antibiotic therapy in a patient with a corneal infection of unknown etiology appears to be extremely poor clinical judgment.

From the practical standpoint, the fear of fungus potentiation should not deter the ophthalmologist from topical use of antibiotics.

Table 6-3. Survival of mice infected with *Candida* organisms and receiving chlortetracycline at various intervals*

	Mice	
Time receiving chlortetracycline	*Living*	*Dead*
24 hr before infection	5	4
8 hr before infection	4	5
2 hr before infection	1	9
Simultaneously with infection	1	9
4 hr after infection	3	7
8 hr after infection	9	1
24 hr after infection	10	0

*From Seligmann, E.: Proc. Soc. Exp. Biol. Med. **79:**481, 1952.

Bacterial ocular infection is far more common than fungus infection, cannot be excluded with certainty in clinical eye infections, and usually responds well to properly selected antibiotics. The unproved concept of fungus potentiation is a *poor* excuse for permitting bacterial corneal destruction.

Is fungus growth potentiated by topical antibiotic therapy in clinical practice? Fungus cultures were taken twice, at intervals of 3 to 6 weeks, from the eyes of 245 Indian children.[22] Of these children, 102 had trachoma and were treated with topical erythromycin or tetracycline ointments or with parenteral triple sulfonamides. Negative fungus cultures were obtained both before and after treatment in 70% of the antibiotic-treated patients, and in 61% of the nontrachomatous, untreated controls. In 30% of the treated patients, the initial tests were fungus negative but became fungus positive after antibiotic treatment. However, an even higher proportion of untreated patients, 39%, developed ocular fungus contamination during the same period of time. Hence this study fails to show any potentiation of ocular fungus infection by antibiotic therapy.

Although many of these Indian children had fungi on their lids and/or conjunctiva, in only 7 of the 245 children was the same type of fungus found at both sites. This indicates that fungal contamination of the extraocular tissues is transient and presumably of environmental origin, in contrast to the true carrier state of infection characteristic of bacteria.

INFANT SUSCEPTIBILITY TO ANTIBIOTIC TOXICITY

The relative safety with which antibiotics can be prescribed for adults apparently does not extend to treatment of the infant or unborn fetus. As examples, colistimethate sodium causes abnormalities of infantile renal tubular cells, the eighth nerve of the newborn is particularly sensitive to streptomycin, tetracycline may cause pseudotumor cerebri and dental defects, pyrimethamine damages cerebral development, novobiocin increases the chance of developing kernicterus,

and chloramphenicol may kill a newborn child. Obviously this means that the ophthalmologist should use systemic antibiotics in the treatment of pregnant women or of infants only when clearly and definitely required.[23]

AMPHOTERICIN B (FUNGIZONE)

Amphotericin B is an antibiotic substance derived from strains of *Streptomyces nodosus*. It has a wider spectrum of activity against the yeastlike fungi than any other presently available antifungal agent. Amphotericin B is the drug of choice in therapy of infections resulting from *Coccidioides immitis*, *Histoplasma capsulatum*, *Cryptococcus neoformans*, *Blastomyces dermatitidis*, *Candida* species, and many other less common fungi. Growth of these organisms in vitro is inhibited by amphotericin B concentrations of 0.02 to 0.5 μg/ml. Isolated cases of sporotrichosis, mucormycosis, chromoblastomycosis, and aspergillosis have responded favorably to amphotericin B.[24] Viruses, protozoa, and bacteria are not affected by amphotericin B,[25] nor do actinomycosis and nocardiosis respond to this drug.

Mechanism of action

Amphotericin B causes increased permeability of cytoplasmic membranes, thereby permitting leakage of essential intracellular constituents. The antibiotic binds rapidly to susceptible cellular membranes such as those of vulnerable yeasts. The extent to which permeability is damaged is dose related. However, a more rapid death of the yeasts cannot be achieved clinically by increasing drug dosage because the same cytoplasmic membrane damage also affects human cells (the mechanism of toxicity). Synthetic derivatives with reduced toxicity also have a reduced chemotherapeutic effect, further indicating the similar mechanisms of the toxic and therapeutic effects.[26]

Administration

Being relatively insoluble in water, amphotericin B is poorly absorbed from the gastrointestinal tract and therefore should be administered intravenously. For intravenous infusion, a solution of 0.1 mg/ml in a 5% solution of dextrose is used. Saline solution cannot be used since it causes the amphotericin B to precipitate. (Unused solutions should be discarded after 24 hours. Amphotericin B is both heat labile and light sensitive, and the dry powder should therefore be refrigerated and protected from light.) The rate of intravenous administration should be so adjusted that the total dose is received over a period of 3 to 6 hours.

Since the tolerance to amphotericin B varies greatly among patients, dosage must be individually adjusted. The routine recommendation is 0.25 mg/kg, to be increased by increments of 5 to 10 mg/day as tolerated. The objective is to reach a daily dosage of 1 mg/kg, which will result in blood levels of 1 to 2 μg/ml. Dosage of less than 1 mg/kg may be relatively ineffective. Failure of the disease to respond necessitates a gradual increase to 1.5 mg/kg/day. This dose should not be exceeded—indeed, many patients can never achieve it. Since renal excretion is slow and demonstrable blood levels persist for 18 hours or more after a single dose, treatment need be given only once a day or perhaps every other day. The latter schedule of alternate-day therapy is suggested when clinical improvement is noted. Relapse may occur if amphotericin B is discontinued too soon. Alternate-day therapy is advised for at least 2 months, with administration of a total dose of at least 3 g of amphotericin B.

Amphotericin B is fungistatic rather than fungicidal, and therefore quick cures are not to be expected. Therapy will be prolonged for weeks or months. The clinician should not increase dosage to the highest possible level in the hope of obtaining more prompt remission. Rather, dosage should be adjusted to avoid renal damage and permit a prolonged fungistatic effect.

For topical administration, a 0.15% solution of amphotericin B may be freshly prepared with sterile water. (Do not use saline—it precipitates.) The preparation must be refrigerated in a dark bottle to slow its disintegration. Drops are instilled every 30 minutes for the first 3 days of treatment of a fungus keratitis. When improvement is evident, the frequency of administration may be reduced, but a level of four times daily instillation is necessary for at least a month.[27] In passing, note that of the 12 persons with keratomycosis who were successfully treated with this regimen, none had responded to previous antibiotic or corticosteroid therapy. Gentamicin is the currently popular wonder drug for eye infections, but it is not effective against fungus infections.

Toxicity

Unpleasant and potentially dangerous side effects are almost inevitable when the drug is given at therapeutic levels; therefore amphotericin B should be used only under close clinical supervision. Headaches, chills and fever, and anorexia are common and may be minimized by the use of antipyretics and antihistaminics. Acetylsalicylic acid, 0.64 g, and promethazine (Phenergan), 25 mg, may be given orally 30 minutes before the infusion is started. Severe symptoms during the course of intravenous infusion may necessitate temporary interruption of the flow or a decrease in the dose given.

Most patients on a high dosage of amphotericin B for prolonged periods show renal damage as manifested by rising blood urea nitrogen levels and other indicators; kidney function tests should be done periodically during such therapy. Blood urea nitrogen levels up to 30 mg/100 ml occur in the majority of patients during the second or third week of treatment. Values higher than this require interruption of treatment until the blood urea nitrogen has dropped below 30, lest serious renal failure result. Blood urea nitrogen estimations should be obtained every 2 to 3 days.

Moderate anemia is frequently encountered during amphotericin B therapy (75% of 30 patients).[28] The mechanism of this appears to be bone marrow depression and decreased red cell production. Fortunately this anemia is usually self-limited, does not progress to dangerous levels, and disappears after therapy is stopped. Sometimes a transfusion of whole blood is necessary. Complete blood counts should be a weekly routine—more often if values drop to borderline levels.

Gastrointestinal cramps, nausea, vomiting, and diarrhea may force reduced treatment. Alternate-day dosage will often permit the patient to recover from these symptoms and to eat relatively normally on the intervening days.

Hypokalemia may cause weakness or electrocardiographic changes. Supplemental potassium is curative.

Local chemical thrombophlebitis may result from the irritating nature of amphotericin B solutions. The phlebitis may be minimized by decreasing the drug concentration, by reducing the rate of infusion, and by avoiding reuse of the same vein.

Because of its toxicity, amphotericin B should be given in treatment of reasonably well-substantiated cases of susceptible mycotic infection. Diagnosis is preferably made by culture of the organism. Vague, undiagnosed diseases (such as uveitis) associated with a positive skin test for one of the fungi do not usually justify the use of such a poisonous drug.

Ocular penetration

The blood-eye barrier is highly resistant to the passage of amphotericin B. After intravenous administration in 1 mg/kg of amphotericin B, no antibiotic entered the normal rabbit aqueous nor was any demonstrable in eyes with severe hydrochloric acid keratitis. However, in animals with an intense uveitis induced by intravitreal albumin injection, aqueous levels of 0.16 μg/ml were attained and levels of 0.13 μg/ml persisted for 24 hours.[29]

In one study, trace amounts of amphotericin B, too small for reliable measurement, were found in the aqueous of normal and inflamed eyes after subconjunctival injection of 150 μg. Transcorneal penetration after topical application was not evaluated in this paper.[29]

Ocular tolerance

The effect of intraocular (anterior chamber) amphotericin B injections in rabbits has been studied.[30] A single injection of 25 μg in 0.05 ml of distilled water caused transitory and reversible iritis and slight clouding of the lens but no permanent sequelae. Increasing the injection to 50 μg considerably increased the severity of reaction, but it subsided after 4 days. Further increase to 125 μg of amphotericin B caused irreversible opacification of the cornea and interior of the eye. Anterior chamber injections of 25 μg may be repeated after 3 days, since the effect of the preceding dose will have subsided by that time.

Treatment of a human postcataract *Volutella* fungus infection with intraocular injection of 40 μg of amphotericin B was successful in sterilizing the eye.[30] Unfortunately there developed a corneal pannus, an updrawn pupil, a vitreous retraction, and a total funnel-shaped retinal detachment. Whether these complications were caused by the infection or by the treatment is hard to determine.

Conjunctival application of ointments containing amphotericin B, 5 mg/g (0.5%), is safely tolerated with only slight irritation. Topical application of such an ointment is obviously much safer than systemic or intraocular injection and is the route of choice in treatment or corneal infection. Topical application of amphotericin B ointment in as great a concentration as 50 mg/g (5%) causes corneal edema and iritis that may persist for a week.[30]

Intravitreal injection of amphotericin B can be highly destructive. Injection of 250 μg caused immediate clouding of the vitreous and retinal detachment. The vitreous remained clear with injections of 25 to 100 μg, but retinal detachments occurred within 5 days. The mechanism of retinal detachment is necrosis of the retina, which can be observed as a white patch appearing almost immediately after positioning of even a small dose near the retina. Of clinical importance is the absolute necessity that an intravitreal injection of amphotericin B *must* be placed exactly in the center of the vitreous (as far as possible from the retina) and should be injected slowly to avoid spurting toward the retina. Doses as small as 5 to 10 μg, placed in the center of the vitreous, were well tolerated by the rabbit eye, resulting in no detectable clinical, microscopic, or electroretinogram (ERG) changes. Sodium deoxycholate is used as a solubilizing agent in the commercial preparation of amphotericin B. The intraocular damage described occurred with pure crystalline amphotericin B alone and did not result from sodium deoxycholate injections, indicating that the damage is caused by the antibiotic and not by the vehicle.[31]

The practical reason for intravitreal injections is that a single injection of 5 μg of amphotericin B into the center of the vitreous will cure experimental *Candida albicans* endophthalmitis with retention of vision if treatment is given within 5 days of the infecting inoculation.[32] Even if the vitreous is slightly cloudy before treatment, the infection was reversible. After the retina has been destroyed by infection, it is too late for successful treatment. From the standpoint of the clinician, this allows very little time to decide whether or not a fungus infection is present, to diagnose it by aspiration, and to institute effective treatment.

Clinical use

Clinical reports[33-35] describe the use of amphotericin B in the sterilization of corneal ulcers caused by a wide variety of fungi. Apparently topical use is quite effective. Because of the devitalized condition of the cornea after the usual prolonged course of a fungus infection, healing is markedly delayed. Secondary bacterial infection must be prevented by routine antibacterial therapy during the period of epithelial defect. Sometimes the weakened cornea will require the structural reinforcement of a lamellar graft. The availability of an antifungal agent as effective as amphotericin B makes apparent the importance of cultures and smears (including techniques for fungus identifica-

tion) in serious ocular infection. A search for fungi should be instituted early in the management of every case of resistant corneal infection, especially in the presence of hypopyon. Persistent, slowly developing intraocular infection after trauma or surgery should arouse suspicion of fungus etiology, and, if sufficiently severe, it may warrant diagnostic surgical aspiration of material for culture.

Combined therapy with nystatin (25,000 units/ml) and amphotericin B (0.1 mg/ml) cured hypopyon keratitis caused by the mold *Allescheria boydii*.[34] Because the case history is very characteristic of fungus keratitis and since it is well documented, the following abstract is presented.

The patient was first seen 3 weeks after injury from a fish scale; a deeply infiltrating central corneal ulcer and severe iritis were present.[34] Systemic administration of penicillin, streptomycin, and chloramphenicol as well as topical administration of chloramphenicol, sulfisoxazole (Gantrisin), and atropine were started. On the second day hypopyon was present and topical hydrocortisone and neomycin were added to the treatment. Central corneal necrosis was present the third day, and by the sixth day perforation seemed imminent. At this time examination of corneal scrapings in a potassium hydroxide mount revealed fungus hyphae and spores. Thereafter all drugs except atropine were discontinued, and nystatin and amphotericin B were used in a frequency varying from every 15 minutes to every 3 hours. Improvement began on the ninth hospital day, was definite by the fifteenth day, and was sufficient to permit discharge on the twenty-first day. A dense central leukoma about half the thickness of normal cornea and 20/200 vision were the end results.

Obviously the assumption that hypopyon ulcers are a result of bacterial infection is invalid. Examination for fungi by culture and potassium hydroxide examination of the corneal scrapings should be part of the early management of every severe corneal ulcer. This is particularly true if pathogenic bacteria cannot readily be demonstrated on initial microscopic examination and becomes urgent if the ulcer progresses despite antibiotic therapy; under these circumstances, eyes may be unnecessarily lost by shotgun therapy with antibiotic-corticosteroid combinations.[36]

Hourly instillation of amphotericin B solution (1 mg/ml, 0.1%) resulted in the clinical cure of five patients with mycotic keratitis caused by *Curvalaria lunata, Penicillium spinulosum, Gibberella fujkuroi, Fusidium terricola,* and *Aspergillus versicolor.*[33] This conclusion is supported by the facts that previous antibiotic therapy did not cure these ulcers, that pathogenic bacteria could not be cultured, that the fungi were identified by culture prior to amphotericin B therapy, that the fungi disappeared with treatment, and that improvement of the ulcers coincided with eradication of the fungi. Some weeks are required for final healing of fungus corneal ulcers. This delay is because of toxic substances that are quite damaging to the cornea even when applied as an extract of killed fungi. The extensive tissue destruction resulting from fungus infection of the cornea may be partially due to a proteolytic toxin that may be isolated in extracts of fungus (for example, *Cephalosporium*).[37] Corneal perforation may occur if the keratitis has been severe—such eyes can sometimes be saved by lamellar keratoplasty.

Subacute nodular granulomatous conjunctivitis may be a complication of systemic coccidioidomycosis. The diagnosis must be made by biopsy and a microscopic examination of the tissue, supplemented by culture on Sabouraud's medium or by animal inoculation.[38] Since the infection described in this study was a generalized infection, therapy was by intravenous administration of amphotericin B, 1 mg/kg, given daily or several times weekly as tolerated by the patient. After 1 month of therapy, this conjunctival lesion almost completely disappeared; however, treatment was continued for 7 months to ensure cure of systemic lesions. Although the diagnosis in this patient was established beyond question by repeated examinations over a 7-year period, the coccidioidin skin

tests were always *negative* until a test done 6 months after completion of amphotericin B therapy was positive.

Chorioretinitis. Use of amphotericin B in the treatment of uveitis is difficult to evaluate because of the usual problems of clinical diagnosis. Nine cases of chorioretinitis were thought to be of histoplasmic etiology because skin tests and complement fixation tests were positive and the chest x-ray findings were compatible with histoplasmosis.[39] Amphotericin B therapy did not seem to alter significantly the clinical course of the chorioretinitis. The amphotericin B was administered intravenously in doses of 50 mg/day (in 500 ml of a 5% concentration of glucose) up to a total dosage of not more than 1 g. Because of the rather marked toxicity of this drug, it would seem best to limit its use to the treatment of patients with a most convincing diagnosis of histoplasmosis, preferably those with systemic manifestations in whom the organism can be recovered from the other tissues. Chills, fever, vomiting, abdominal and head pain, azotemia, hemorrhagic gastroenteritis, and hematologic disturbances result from amphotericin B therapy, which should not be lightly undertaken.

The effectiveness of amphotericin B in the treatment of intraocular histoplasmosis has been proved by its successful use in the therapy of rabbits infected by anterior chamber inoculation with *Histoplasma capsulatum.* Amphotericin B (0.5 mg/kg) was given intravenously once daily for 15 days. This treatment was started 2 weeks after inoculation. In eight treated rabbits, various organ cultures were negative for *Histoplasma* organisms, and six of eight inoculated eyes were sterile. In contrast, viable organisms were recovered from all untreated inoculated eyes and from the lung, liver, spleen, kidney, and heart blood of the untreated animals. Marked clinical improvement was grossly evident in the treated eyes, in contrast to the extensive necrosis of the untreated eyes. The authors of this report emphasize, however, that *Histoplasma capsulatum* had never been isolated from a human eye and that amphotericin B therapy of experimentally induced mycotic ophthalmitis is not the same as treatment of supposedly histoplasmic immunogenic eye involvement.[40]

Orbital infection. A patient with proved histoplasmosis of the lacrimal gland and adjacent orbital tissues was successfully treated with 1 mg/kg amphotericin B intravenously, for a total of 35 doses over a period of 12 weeks.[41]

Lid infection. When the fungus infection to be treated is small and well localized, amphotericin B may be applied by local injection. In this way effective concentrations are achieved locally, yet systemic toxicity is avoided. For example, in treatment of an *Aspergillus* granuloma of the lid, 1 cm in size, 1 mg of amphotericin B diluted in distilled water was injected directly into the granuloma and surrounding tissue.[42] Repeated at weekly intervals, this dosage completely cured the *Aspergillus* granuloma within 2 months. Of practical interest was the initial failure to diagnose the fungal nature of this infection, which was recognized only with special fungus stains of the second biopsy specimen.

Summary

Amphotericin B is a moderately effective drug for combating yeastlike fungi. Superficial keratomycoses may respond well to this drug. Because its intraocular penetration is poor and its intraocular injection highly toxic, use of amphotericin B for fungus endophthalmitis is of limited value. Theoretically, fungus uveitis (for example, that caused by *Histoplasma* and *Candida*) should respond to systemic administration of amphotericin B. Unfortunately the medication is very poisonous and troublesome to administer systemically.

In the treatment of most superficial ocular fungus infections, pimaricin is more effective than amphotericin B.

BACITRACIN

Bacitracin is a bactericidal antibiotic with a range of activity that closely parallels that of penicillin. It is active chiefly against gram-positive organisms but also destroys spirochetes, gonococci, *Entamoeba histolytica*, and *Actinomyces*. Bacitracin is ineffective against gram-negative bacilli. Most gram-positive organisms are inhibited by 0.001 to 0.5 unit/ml of the drug.

Resistant strains of bacteria are much less frequently encountered with the use of bacitracin than with penicillin. Of 36 strains of organisms with different resistances to penicillin and to bacitracin, 30 were more resistant to penicillin and 6 to bacitracin.[43] Bacitracin is not inactivated by blood, pus, necrotic tissue, or bacterial enzymes such as penicillinase.

Clinical use

Concentrations of 500 to 1000 units/g are nonirritating to the eye and other tissues and cause no undesirable systemic effects. Bacitracin does not penetrate the cornea in therapeutic amounts. It is not absorbed from the gastrointestinal tract but may be given orally in treatment of intestinal infections such as *Entamoeba histolytica*. Parenteral administration may achieve effective systemic antibacterial concentrations but can damage renal tubules in doses greater than 200 to 400 units/kg. Because of this systemic toxicity, use of bacitracin is ordinarily confined to topical application. Topical bacitracin is quite effective in treatment of surface ocular infections[44] and is commonly used for this purpose.

Although bacitracin solutions are unstable, reasonable potency may be maintained for 3 weeks if the solution is refrigerated. The dry powder and ointment preparations are stable for over a year at room temperature.

Summary

Although the antibacterial spectrum of bacitracin is comparable to that of penicillin, for topical ocular use, bacitracin is preferable to penicillin because fewer strains of organisms are resistant, allergy is less frequent, and sensitization that prevents future use of penicillin is avoided.

CEPHALOSPORIN DERIVATIVES

Cephaloridine and cephalothin are semisynthetic wide-spectrum antibiotics chemically similar to penicillin. Both penicillin

Table 6-4. Minimal inhibitory concentrations (MIC) of cephaloridine in vitro for various microorganisms*

Sensitive (MIC = 0.005 to 1.0 µg/ml)	Moderately sensitive (MIC = 1.0 to 8.0 µg/ml)	Resistant (MIC > 8.0 µg/ml)
Streptococcus pyogenes A	*Salmonella* spp.	*Pseudomonas* spp.
Streptococcus viridans (some)	*Shigella* spp.	*Proteus* spp.
Streptococcus faecalis (some)	*Escherichia coli* (≅70%)	*Aerobacter* spp.
Diplococcus pneumoniae	*Proteus mirabilis* (some)	*Klebsiella* spp. (some)
Clostridium spp.	*Haemophilus influenzae* (most)	*Escherichia coli* (some)
Neisseria gonorrhoeae	*Streptococcus viridans* (some)	*Haemophilus influenzae* (some)
Neisseria meningitidis	*Streptococcus faecalis* (few)	*Staphylococcus aureus* (some R)
Actinomyces spp.	*Bacillus subtilis*	
Corynebacterium spp.	*Klebsiella* spp. (most)	
Staphylococcus albus	*Staphylococcus aureus* (some R)	
Staphylococcus aureus (S and some R)†		

*From Riley, F. C., Goyle, G. L., and Leopold, I.: Am. J. Ophthalmol. **66:**1042, 1968.
†S = penicillin-sensitive; R = penicillin-resistant.

and the cephalosporins interfere with cell wall synthesis and are therefore bactericidal. These derivatives have a broader antibacterial action than most penicillins, since they are effective against a large variety of gram-positive and gram-negative microorganisms. The sensitivity of various representative microorganisms to cephaloridine is shown in Table 6-4.[45] Obviously sensitivity studies are required to determine the susceptibility of any given strain of microorganism encountered in clinical practice. Note that *Proteus* and *Pseudomonas* are resistant. However, the cephalothin derivatives will inhibit *Staphylococcus aureus* strains that are resistant to penicillin and methicillin.

Dosage

Cephaloridine and caphalothin are water soluble but poorly absorbed from the gastrointestinal tract. Hence they are administered by injection, either intramuscularly or intravenously, for emergency treatment of severe infections. The cephalosporins are incompatible with other antibiotics; therefore an antibiotic mixture should not be prepared for intravenous administration or for injection. The recommended adult human dose is 1 g every 8 hours.

Cephalexin (Keflex) is well absorbed following oral administration. However, it is less effective than is penicillin against sensitive microorganisms, and no oral drug is recommended for treatment of serious infections with resistant staphylococci.

Aqueous penetration of cephaloridine

The plasma and secondary aqueous levels attained in rabbits after a single intravenous injection of 25 mg/kg of cephaloridine are shown in Fig. 6-2.[46] Primary aqueous levels in these rabbits averaged less than 2 µg/ml throughout the 4-hour period.

Cephaloridine concentrations in human secondary aqueous were studied in patients undergoing cataract surgery. High concentrations were present within 15 minutes and useful concentrations persisted for 8 hours (Fig. 6-3). These data indicate that the recommended human dose of cephaloridine, 1 g intravenously every 8 hours, should result in effective intraocular antibiotic levels in inflamed human eyes.

Much lower aqueous levels, averaging 2 µg/ml at 4 hours after injection, were reported to follow intramuscular injection of 1 g of cephaloridine in an adult (Fig. 6-4).[45]

Cephaloridine, 50 mg in 0.25 ml distilled

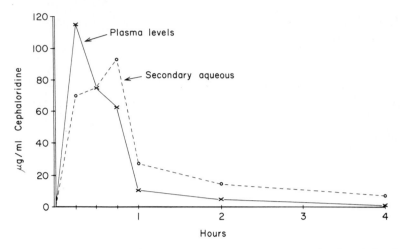

Fig. 6-2. Rabbit plasma and secondary aqueous concentrations (μg/ml) of cephaloridine after single intravenous dose of 25 mg/kg. (Data from Records, R. E.: Arch. Ophthalmol. **81**:331, 1969.)

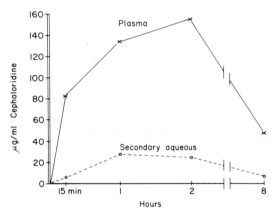

Fig. 6-3. Human plasma and secondary aqueous concentrations (μg/ml) of cephaloridine after single intravenous dose of 1 g. (Data from Records, R. E.: Arch. Ophthalmol. **81**:331, 1969.)

water, was injected subconjunctivally prior to surgery in 30 cataract patients and in 10 patients with retinal detachment.[47] Within 10 minutes after injection, all samples of aqueous humor or subretinal fluid contained sufficient antibiotic to inhibit coagulase-positive *Staphylococcus aureus,* as measured by a filter paper disc or blood agar technique.

Aqueous penetration of cephalothin

Intravenous injection of 15 mg/kg of sodium cephalothin produced no measurable primary aqueous drug concentration in rabbits.[48] In secondary aqueous, such an intravenous dosage caused a 15-minute concentration of 2 μg/ml, dropping to 0.8 μg/ml 30 minutes after injection and to 0 μg/ml at 45 minutes. Subconjunctival injection of 50 mg sodium cephalothin produced a primary aqueous concentration of 54 μg/ml at 1 hour, which persisted at a level of 35 μg/ml 4 hours after injection.

Cephalothin penetration into human aqueous was studied by aspiration of secondary aqueous at the time of cataract sur-

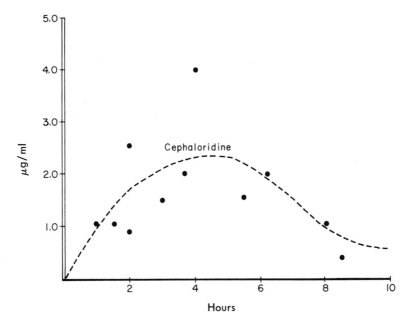

Fig. 6-4. Aqueous humor levels of cephaloridine (μg/ml) after intramuscular injection of 1 g in adult humans. (Modified from Riley, F. C., Goyle, G. L., and Leopold, I.: Am. J. Ophthalmol. **66:**1042, 1968.)

gery. Fifteen minutes after an intravenous injection of 1 g of sodium cephalothin, the mean secondary aqueous concentration in 18 patients was 0.55 μg/ml, with a range from 0 to 2.50 μg/ml. After 30 minutes the mean in 18 patients was 0.48 μg/ml, with a range from 0 to 1.00 μg/ml.[49]

Subconjunctival injection of 50 mg of cephalothin (Keflin) in humans was given at varying intervals before cataract extraction.[50] This resulted in aqueous levels of 10 to 30 μg/ml attained within 20 minutes and lasting for 2 hours after injection. The aqueous concentrations then dropped rather rapidly, maintaining bacteriostatic levels for perhaps 6 hours. Most susceptible microorganisms are inhibited by cephalothin levels of 1 to 5 μg/ml. Despite tetracaine anesthesia, these subconjunctival injections caused immediate pain lasting as long as a half hour. One third of the 22 patients complained of extremely severe ocular pain. Chemosis lasted for several hours, followed by conjunctival hyperemia and edema lasting for 4 days. Somewhat less reaction occurred following injection of 25 mg,

but this lower dosage produced some severe responses also.

Intramuscular injection in rabbits of 150 mg/kg of cephalothin results in primary aqueous levels ranging from 0.2 to 1.0 μg/ml after 45 minutes.[51]

Toxicity

Renal damage may result from dosages of cephaloridine greater than 4 g/day. Cross allergy between penicillin and cephaloridine has been suggested because of anaphylactic reactions in a few patients. However, most patients with a history of penicillin allergy will tolerate cephaloridine. Conversely, cephaloridine allergy may occur in patients not sensitive to penicillin.

Aqueous penetration of cephalexin

Cephalexin is an orally absorbed derivative of cephalosporin. Given in an oral dose of 2.0 g to patients prior to cataract surgery, cephalexin produced primary aqueous levels of 1 to 2 μg/ml 2 to 4 hours after administration. Demonstrable aqueous levels persisted for as long as 12 hours.[52]

Cost-effectiveness

At a cost of $1.00 to $3.00 per gram, cephalosporins are expensive antibiotics. During the 1973-1974 fiscal year, 12% of The Ohio State University Hospital drug budget was expended on purchase of cephalosporins. Critical examination of antibiotic usage showed that cephalosporins were frequently used for prophylaxis and treatment of conditions that either required no antibiotic at all or could have been treated equally well or even better with a less expensive antibiotic.[53]

Summary

Cephaloridine and cephalothin have a wider antibacterial spectrum than penicillin but are somewhat more toxic. Their use is advised when culture and sensitivity studies have shown the microorganism causing a serious infection to be susceptible to them. The cephalosporins are resistant to inactivation by penicillinase, hence they are effective against penicillin-resistant staphylococci. These drugs penetrate fairly well into secondary aqueous humor.

CHLORAMPHENICOL (CHLOROMYCETIN)

Because of its differential solubility characteristics, this antibiotic is one of the most effective drugs for the treatment of intraocular infections.

Antimicrobial spectrum

Chloramphenicol has a broad antimicrobial spectrum, being effective against a wide variety of gram-positive and gram-negative organisms, rickettsia, and spirochetes.[54] For example, the great majority of strains of the following organisms were sensitive to less than 16 μg/ml of chloramphenicol: *Aerobacter aerogenes, Bacillus anthracis, Bacillus subtilis, Brucella, Clostridium, Corynebacterium* (diphtheria), *Escherichia coli, Haemophilus, Klebsiella, Staphylococcus* (*aureus* as well as *albus*), *Neisseria, Pasteurella, Shigella*, and *Streptococcus*. An organism of considerable ocular significance, *Pseudomonas aeruginosa*, was quite resistant, 139 of 212 strains not being destroyed by 75 μg/ml. Since great variations occur in the sensitivity of various strains of organisms, general summaries cannot be relied on. Rather, the sensitivity of the organisms responsible for a given infection must be determined, if possible.

Intraocular penetration

The ether/water partition coefficient indicates the relative solubility of a drug in lipids or water. The ether/water coefficient of penicillin is 0.0004, whereas that of chloramphenicol is 4.25. In other words, chloramphenicol is 10,000 times more fat soluble than penicillin. Its high differential solubility results in the superior intraocular penetration of chloramphenicol.[55]

The aqueous penetration of intravenously administered chloramphenicol has been studied in rabbits.[56] One hour after intravenous injection of 50 mg/kg of chloramphenicol the serum concentration was 12 μg/ml and the aqueous concentration was 6 μg/ml. At this time no measurable concentration was detected in the vitreous. This finding suggests that aqueous penetration may be quite comparable to cerebrospinal fluid penetration (values approximately half of those found in the serum).

After systemic administration, chloramphenicol penetrates the eye more readily than do penicillin, streptomycin, chlortetracycline (Aureomycin), and oxytetracycline (Terramycin).[57-59] Such drugs enter the eye in much higher than normal concentrations when the barriers are destroyed by surgery or paracentesis. Ideally, therefore, antibiotics should be given promptly following injury, so as to attain an adequate plasma concentration at the time of surgical repair or foreign body removal.

Primary aqueous levels of 5 to 10 μg/ml were achieved in rabbits following subconjunctival injection of 10 mg/kg of chloramphenicol succinate.[60] These levels persisted from 1 to 4 hours after injection. Intraperitoneal injection of probenecid 30 minutes prior to the subconjunctival chloramphenicol injection increased the chloramphenicol aqueous levels to 20 μg/ml. (Probenecid may block the active transport of antibiotics out of the eye, just as it blocks the kidney and the cerebrospinal transport system. Its mechanism of action is inhibition of organic acid transport, which is accomplished by competition for carrier systems.) Although these aqueous concentrations of antibiotic are very high, metabolically rabbits have a great capacity to destroy chloramphenicol. Consequently, for a rabbit study to be analogous to the human situation, a rabbit must be given 20 times the human dosage of chloramphenicol. Thus it can be inferred that a much greater intraocular penetration than reported in this experiment would be seen in the human.

Aqueous chloramphenicol levels of 3 to 6 μg/ml are present 2 hours after topical administration of 0.5% drops every 5 minutes for six doses. Demonstrable antibiotic persisted for 5 hours after drug administration. This study was performed in 18 patients undergoing cataract surgery.[61]

Dosage

Blood levels of chloramphenicol in excess of 15 μg/ml are easily attained in man. The usual dosage for adults is 3 to 5 g/day, administered in divided doses every 4 hours. Chloramphenicol is readily absorbed from the gastrointestinal tract, producing a peak blood level at 2 hours and declining to insignificant levels by 8 hours. Rapid renal excretion occurs.

If an immediate, high blood level is desirable, an initial dose of 3 g may be given. Oral dosage produces concentrations comparable to the intravenous route; hence parenteral administration (intravenous or intramuscular) is indicated only if the patient cannot or should not (as preceding general anesthesia) take the drug by mouth. For parenteral administration, the highly water-soluble sodium succinate derivative is recommended.

Stability and solubility

Chloramphenicol is a fairly stable compound and will actually resist destruction by boiling for as long as 5 hours. In water at room temperature its solubility is only 0.25%; however, it is readily ether soluble.

Toxicity

The LD_{50} dose for mice is 245 mg/kg. Hence, although recommended doses are well tolerated without acute side effects, the clinician must be aware that, unlike penicillin, enormous doses cannot be given with impunity.

In high dosage, chloramphenicol causes a typical toxic reaction in infants. This is characterized by abdominal distention, cyanosis, and vasomotor collapse. If high dosage of chloramphenicol is continued, the child may die. This peculiar reaction may be related to the inadequate amount of glycuronyl transferase produced by the immature liver. This transferase is one of the enzymes involved in the detoxification of chloramphenicol. (A genetic enzyme deficiency may be a factor in chloramphenicol-induced aplastic anemia. The only test of predictive value in selecting individuals likely to develop aplastic anemia is the determination of impaired chloramphenicol clearance 4 to 6 hours after an intravenous test dose.[62]) This reaction has not been observed in any infant given divided doses of chloramphenicol not in excess of 50 mg/kg/24 hours. Half this dose is advised for premature infants.

Considerable publicity has been given to the possibility of agranulocytosis resulting from use of chloramphenicol. While the danger of this complication is not to be underestimated, the benefits of chloramphenicol in treating eye infections (because of its excellent penetration of the blood-aqueous barrier) should not be lost.

Early recognition and proper care of drug-induced agranulocytosis demands careful observation of patients receiving drugs known to cause this condition. Of the 830 cases of drug-induced agranulocytosis reported to the Council of Drugs,[63] 56 were attributed to chloramphenicol. For proper perspective, one should know that 92 cases were attributed to sulfonamides and 370 to phenothiazine tranquilizers.

The mechanism of agranulocytosis may be the formation of antibodies that agglutinate leukocytes in the presence of the drug. Hence the earliest sign is leukopenia. Hematologic recovery begins when the drug is eliminated from the body, usually within 5 to 10 days after it is discontinued. The mortality rate is very low if agranulocytosis is discovered by routine white cell count before the development of an infection. The sudden onset of a severe prostrating infection (usually a sore throat) during treatment with chloramphenicol requires immediate evaluation of the possibility of agranulocytosis.

Aplastic anemia of delayed onset, not necessarily dose related, is the most serious complication of chloramphenicol therapy. In a survey of the *Registry of Blood Dyscrasias* (a series of 284 patients), the median time of onset of blood dyscrasia was found to be 38 days after discontinuation of treatment.[64] Hence monitoring blood counts *during* chloramphenicol therapy is of little or no value in preventing mortality. The author recognizes that unavoidable bias is present in a collection of cases assembled with the expectation that a given factor is responsible, thus complicating a calculation of true incidence.

Statistical studies concerning such rare problems as chloramphenicol-induced aplastic anemia are difficult to undertake and even more difficult to evaluate. For example, all aplastic anemia deaths in California during an 18-month period were studied, with the conclusion that patients receiving 4 g of chloramphenicol had a 13 times greater chance of dying from aplastic anemia than did the population as a whole.[65] Actually, only 60 patients died of aplastic anemia during this period, and only 10 had received chloramphenicol. Three of these had received the drug 8, 9, and 24 months before the onset of anemia (related?). Perusal of the vast amount of data in this article suggests that numerous extrapolations of doubtful validity were made from uncertain data (for example, physician questionnaires, which are notoriously inaccurate, as any physician who has filled one out will testify). The frequency of fatal aplastic anemia subsequent to chloramphenicol treatment seems to be in the range of 1 in 50,000 patients.

While I would never wish a patient to be the 1 in 50,000 who dies of aplastic anemia months after chloramphenicol therapy, I believe the evil associated with the drug has been exaggerated out of context. For the sake of argument, would it be preferable to use a hypothetical antibiotic effective against fewer microorganisms (only gram positive rather than broad spectrum), capable of causing instant anaphylactic death (rather than delayed for months), and fatal in the same frequency (1 in 50,000)?[66] Obviously chloramphenicol would be a more sensible choice than this hypothetical drug, since it is more likely to be effective and no more likely to be fatal. Of course, the hypothetical drug is penicillin. Chronologically, the active condemnation of chloramphenicol coincides with its exploding the cherished generic equivalence myth, and the possibility of retribution bears consideration. Without doubt, the relative toxicity of chloramphenicol, as compared to the toxicity of alternative antibiotics, has been grossly exaggerated. A detailed review of the true facts leaves one feeling outraged.[67]

Prolonged use of chloramphenicol has been suspected to cause optic atrophy in children. More than 100 g of chloramphenicol (250 mg three times a day) was given prophylactically to two children with cystic fibrosis of the pancreas. Disabling visual loss was recognized after about 4 months of treatment. Histologic study of the optic nerves obtained at autopsy showed marked demyelination of the papillomacular bundle (Fig. 6-5).[68] Such eye changes are infrequent; recognizable bilateral optic neuritis has been reported in only 6 of 200 chloramphenicol-treated patients with cystic fibrosis. Since papilledema may occur in cases of cystic fibrosis with severe pulmonary disease (presumably these patients are antibiotic treated), it is uncertain whether the optic atrophy in these cases was part of the disease or was a manifestation of chloramphenicol toxicity.[69]

In a study of 98 cystic fibrosis patients receiving long-term chloramphenicol therapy (from approximately 1964 to 1969), 13 developed visual disturbances. Characteristically, the visual loss was sudden, bilateral,

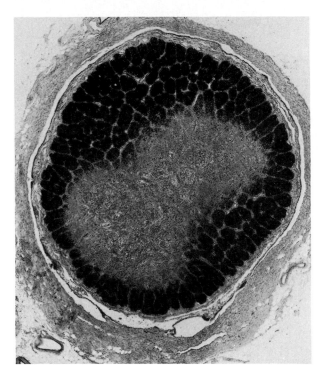

Fig. 6-5. Cross section of optic nerve 1 cm behind eye; from child with cystic fibrosis who received prolonged chloramphenicol therapy. (From Wong, V. G., and Collins, E.: Am. J. Ophthalmol. **59:**763, 1965.)

and associated with an ophthalmoscopic picture of optic neuritis. The condition was dose related, depending on the amount and duration of chloramphenicol therapy. Discontinuance of treatment resulted in a prompt improvement in vision in 11 of the 13 patients. Autopsy findings in three patients who had suffered visual disturbances included bilateral optic atrophy with primary involvement of the papillomacular bundle, loss of the retinal ganglion cells, and gliosis of the nerve fiber layer.[70]

Clinical use

Because of the potential toxicity of chloramphenicol, it should not be used systemically for trivial infections, nor should it be used for serious infections in which less toxic antibacterial drugs are equally effective. With the exception of infections of the intraocular fluids, which are not readily accessible to other antibiotics and the culture of which is ordinarily impracticable, chloramphenicol should usually be employed only after the causative organism has been isolated and determined to be sensitive to the drug. It should not be used without the precaution of frequent blood counts and evaluation of the patient for acute infections, which may herald agranulocytosis.[71]

The systemic use of chloramphenicol in ophthalmology is usually limited to the treatment of intraocular infections, which ordinarily follow penetrating trauma or surgery. Unfortunately, externally obtained cultures in such cases are usually negative or isolate surface organisms unrelated to the endophthalmitis. For this reason, in most cases of potential or existing intraocular infection, the physician must choose an antibiotic arbitrarily. The antibiotic chosen is selected on the basis of its ability to penetrate the blood-aqueous barrier and its reasonably broad antibacterial spectrum. Chloramphenicol meets both these criteria as well as any other available drug and hence is one of the best medications for treatment or prophylaxis of endophthalmitis. An oral dose of 3 g is advised initially, followed by 0.5 g every 4 hours.[72]

Topical application of chloramphenicol ointment (1%) or solution (0.2%) was well tolerated by the human eye in over 200 cases with virtually no evidence of irritation or discomfort.[73] The drug was very effective against the majority of surface bacterial infections but did not alter the course of herpes simplex keratitis or epidemic keratoconjunctivitis. No instance of toxic or allergic local reaction was encountered. Comparable results were obtained with use of 0.5% chloramphenicol solution (Chloroptic) in 46 cases of superficial ocular infection.[74]

Chloramphenicol is reported to be an effective drug against trachoma. All of a series of 19 Navajo Indians were cured by 1 g/day. An average of nine daily doses were required for cure. No topical medication was used.[75] Treatment of trachoma may be stopped when the cornea is cleared. Disappearance of the conjunctival follicular changes requires more time than does corneal clearing but will spontaneously improve without further antibiotic therapy.[76]

It is likely that antibiotics eliminate only the secondary bacterial agents that complicate trachoma. Chloramphenicol topical drops (0.25% concentration, three times a day), ointment (1% concentration, nightly), and oral capsules (1 g, every day) used concurrently resulted in complete clearance of secondary infection in 2 to 3 days and considerably relieved all symptoms. However, in only 19 of these 60 patients did the inclusion bodies disappear and the pannus regress. Similar results were obtained after therapy with oxytetracycline, chlortetracycline, and erythromycin. Sulfacetimide, 30% solution applied four times a day, was more effective, clearing inclusion bodies in 51 of 70 cases, but in this series, treatment was continued for 6 weeks.[77]

Silicone rubber is permeable to chloramphenicol. An experimental silicone implant for retinal detachment surgery was expanded by injection within it of 25% chloramphenicol sodium succinate. Upon sacrifice of the animals, as long as 2½ months later, inhibitory concentrations of chloramphenicol were found within the tissue specimens just external to the implant.[78]

Summary

Because of its differential solubility characteristics, chloramphenicol penetrates into the intraocular fluids far more readily than do most other antibiotics. Furthermore, it has a broad antibacterial spectrum. For these reasons, it is a drug of choice for treatment of intraocular infections.

CLINDAMYCIN

Clindamycin (7-chlorolincomycin) is effective against toxoplasmosis in rabbits. Following suprachoroidal injection, the rabbits developed active retinochoroiditis in about 4 days. Retrobulbar injection of 150 mg clindamycin was given on the first day of recognizable activity, followed by 100 mg/kg/day intramuscularly for 8 days. Three fourths of the treated animals rapidly improved, clearing being evident by the sixth day, and retained normal retinal architecture and function. In contrast, complete disruption of the retina occurred in two thirds of the untreated eyes. No organisms could be recovered from any of the treated eyes, but *Toxoplasma* organisms were demonstrated by fluorescein antibody methods in 80% of the untreated eyes.[79]

Although clindamycin is considered to be a penicillin-equivalent antibiotic, strains of group A streptococci may be clindamycin resistant. This emphasizes the need for bacterial sensitivity studies in cases of serious infection.[80]

COLISTIN (COLY-MYCIN)

Colistin is an antibiotic that effectively inhibits gram-negative organisms such as *Pseudomonas aeruginosa, Escherichia coli, Aerobacter aerogenes, Klebsiella pneumoniae, Shigella,* and *Salmonella.* Colistin has little effect against gram-positive organisms or *Proteus bacilli. Pseudomonas* strains are sensi-

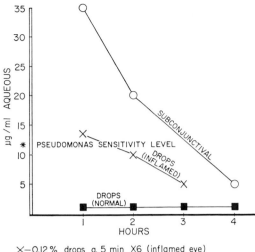

X—0.12% drops q. 5 min X6 (inflamed eye)
O—15 mg subconjunctival (normal eye)
—0.12% drops q. 5 min X6 (normal eye)
—10 mg/kg IM (normal or inflamed eye)

Fig. 6-6. Aqueous levels of colistin attained by various routes of administration in rabbits. (Modified from Pryor, J. G., Apt, L., and Leopold, I. H.: Arch. Ophthalmol. **67:**612, 1962.)

tive to colistin in concentrations of 8 to 11 μg/ml. The intraocular penetration of colistin is shown in Fig. 6-6. Therapeutically effective aqueous levels of colistin are attained by subconjunctival injection and by topical application of 0.12% drops (if the eye is inflamed). Intramuscular injection of tolerated amounts (10 mg/kg) and topical application to the normal eye did not produce effective aqueous levels. Vitreous levels were not detectable following any of these methods of administration.

Clinical use

No corneal or conjunctival irritation follows instillation of concentrations of 0.12% drops. Subconjunctival injection of 10 mg of sodium colistin methansulfonate caused no irritation after 24 hours. In contrast, subconjunctival injections of 10 mg of polymyxin B in the opposite eye of the same rabbits caused marked chemosis lasting 4 days.[81]

A series of 165 patients with ocular infections were treated with 0.12% colistin sulfate drops.[82] The average dose was 1 or 2 drops every 30 minutes to 1 hour for approximately 2 weeks. Particularly significant were the 89 patients who had *Pseudomonas* ocular infections. Of these, about 90% were cured of their infection. Only one patient was reported to develop an adverse reaction, a local allergy.

Effective systemic therapy with colistin methansulfonate (colistimethate) requires intramuscular injection of 4 to 5 mg/kg/day. In this dosage, 30% to 50% of patients show renal or central nervous system toxicity.[83] Respiratory arrest resulting from the central nervous system effect of colistin has been described.[84]

Colistin and polymyxin B are quite similar in many respects. The fatal intravenous dose (LD_{50}) for rats is 5 mg/kg for both drugs.* Their antibacterial spectrum is essentially identical. Although colistin methansulfonate is recognizably less irritating than polymyxin B sulfate, it has been suggested that polymyxin methansulfate is also less irritating and that the basic drugs (colistin and polymyxin B) are practically identical substances.[83] Both drugs are derived from species of aerobacilli.

At the present time, colistin is preferable to polymyxin B for parenteral therapy of infections caused by susceptible gram-negative organisms.

Combined treatment with both colistin and gentamicin did not result in more rapid healing of *Pseudomonas* corneal ulcers in rabbits than was achieved with use of either drug alone.[85]

ERYTHROMYCIN

Erythromycin is quite similar to penicillin in its effect against gram-positive microorganisms. Staphylococcal resistance to erythromycin develops quite as readily as it does to penicillin and is related to the frequency of use (Fig. 6-7).[86] Susceptible organisms are inhibited by minimal concentrations of erythromycin ranging from 0.1 to 3 μg/ml.[87]

Erythromycin is well tolerated in oral dosage of 200 to 600 mg every 6 hours. The 0.5% ophthalmic ointment is nonirritating. Jaun-

---

*Unpublished data from Warner-Chilcott Laboratories.

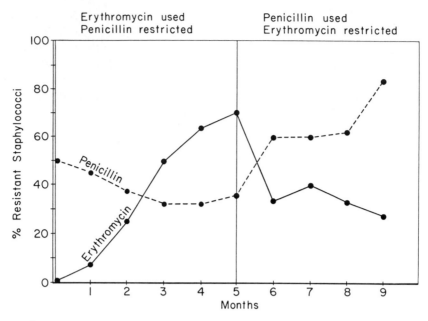

Fig. 6-7. Change in percentage of resistant staphylococci among hospital staff during period of general use of erythromycin and nonuse of penicillin, followed by period of use of penicillin and nonuse of erythromycin. (Based on data from Jackson, G. G., Lepper, M. H., and Dowling, H. E.: J. Lab. Clin. Med. **44:**41, 1954.)

dice and abnormal liver function may occasionally occur during or after erythromycin therapy. Gastrointestinal irritation with nausea and vomiting may be caused by large doses.[88]

Ocular penetration and tolerance

After intravenous injection of 100 mg, erythromycin penetrates poorly into the intact rabbit eye, achieving transient aqueous concentrations of 0.7 μg/ml and vitreous concentrations of 0.1 μg/ml.

Solutions of 2% or lesser concentrations are well tolerated as corneal baths. One hour after a 5-minute bath of the intact rabbit cornea with a 2.5% solution, erythromycin concentrations were: cornea, 9 μg/ml; aqueous, 9 μg/ml; and vitreous, 0.9 μg/ml.

Subconjunctival injection of 20 mg of erythromycin causes chemosis and corneal haze lasting at least a week. Subconjunctival injection of 5 mg causes some conjunctival congestion lasting for 2 days but gives remarkably high drug levels: at 1 hour, cornea, 95 μg/ml; aqueous, 59 μg/ml; and vitreous,

5 μg/ml; and at 4 hours, cornea, 7 μg/ml; aqueous, 9 μg/ml; and vitreous, 0.3 μg/ml.

Intracameral injections of 2.5 mg or more of erythromycin are quite destructive, resulting in prolonged keratitis and iritis. An intracameral injection of 1 mg (in 0.1 ml volumes) caused only transient mild iritis.[89]

Clinical use

Erythromycin alone has a much more limited antibacterial spectrum than the mixtures of exclusively topical antibiotics now in common use for eye infections. It is certainly not the drug of choice for treatment of an ocular infection of unknown etiology.

Twenty-one Arizona Indian children with early trachoma (stages 1, 2, and 3) were treated with oral dosages of erythromycin, 2 to 3 mg/pound, every 4 to 6 hours. No local medication was used. At least 12 days of therapy were recommended, since recurrences were noted with shorter courses. Usually within 5 days the mononuclear cells and inclusion bodies characteristic of trachomatous exudate cleared, and the clinically evident conjunctivitis subsided. Follicles and pannus persisted for some time after the cytologic findings had become normal and the conjunctivitis had disappeared. There was no relapse among the 21 patients during an 8-month follow-up period.

Summary

Erythromycin has a limited antibacterial spectrum somewhat comparable to that of penicillin. Staphylococcal resistance readily develops. The main indication for ophthalmic use is a sensitivity study that reveals it to be effective against the infecting organisms.

Erythromycin is well tolerated and relatively nontoxic.

GENTAMICIN

Another antibiotic effective against gram-negative organisms and staphylococci is gentamicin. At least three fourths of the strains of *Pseudomonas, Klebsiella, Aerobacter,* and *Escherichia coli* and all but 1 of 38 staphylococcal strains were sensitive to 4 μg/ml of gentamicin. Sixty percent of *Proteus* strains were inhibited by 9 μg/ml.[90]

Ocular penetration

Whether instilled topically as drops or ointment or given intramuscularly, gentamicin penetrates very poorly into normal rabbit eyes. Aqueous levels as high as 0.8 μg/ml may be achieved by subconjunctival injection of 0.5 ml of 0.3% gentamicin solution or by intravenous dosages of 0.5 mg/pound. Aqueous levels as high as 1.6 μg/ml may be achieved in mechanically abraded or chemically burned rabbit eyes by topical instillation of a 0.3% solution or ointment.[91] No measurable vitreous levels of gentamicin were achieved in any of the eyes. Of 53 strains of *Pseudomonas* studied by this author, 45 were inhibited by 1.6 μg/ml of gentamicin. This concentration will also inhibit growth of many penicillin-resistant staphylococci. Gentamicin should therefore be a useful drug for treatment of anterior segment infections caused by *Pseudomonas* or *Staphylococcus.*

The diffusion of a compound from the serum into the aqueous humor is inversely proportional to its insolubility in lipid, its degree of protein binding, and its molecular weight. Gentamicin is relatively insoluble in lipids, is 25% to 30% protein bound, and has an intermediate molecular weight of 425; hence it would be expected to meet considerable resistance at the blood-eye barriers. In rabbits, subconjunctival injection of 4 mg of gentamicin produced average primary aqueous levels of 3 μg/ml lasting for several hours. Increasing the subconjunctival dose to 10 mg (in 0.5 ml volumes) raised the aqueous level to 4 μg/ml. In secondary aqueous, gentamicin levels were about twice as high as in the primary aqueous and approximated 1/2000 of the concentration in the subconjunctival space. The aqueous levels achieved by subconjunctival injection were sufficient to inhibit sensitive gram-negative microorganisms.[92]

Diffusion into other ocular tissues has also been evaluated. One hour after a subconjunctival injection of 20 mg of gentamicin in the rabbit eye the following levels (in μg/ml) were achieved: aqueous, 12; vitreous, 1.3; cornea, 11.5; iris, 6.5; lens, 0.5; retina, 12; sclera, 74; and conjunctiva, 185. Levels of 0.2 to 0.6 μg/ml persisted at 24 hours. Much greater levels were achieved in an inflamed eye, for example, 20 μg/ml in the retina at 1 hour.[93]

In rabbit eyes inflamed by experimentally induced *Pseudomonas* corneal ulcers, very high aqueous levels of gentamicin can be achieved simply by topical instillation. Use of 4 drops of 2% gentamicin solution every 15 minutes gave aqueous levels averaging 9.5 μg/ml at 30 minutes and 32 μg/ml at 1 hour.[94] (Four drops of a 2% solution contain 5 mg of drug. If given every 15 minutes, 80 mg is administered in 4 hours. The allowable daily dose of gentamicin is 1 mg/kg. Obviously toxic systemic levels could be approached by generous topical instillations of gentamicin.)

Prior to cataract surgery, 15 patients received subconjunctival injection of 10 mg of gentamicin in 0.25 ml volumes. Aqueous drug levels were determined at varying time intervals and ranged from 2 to 7 μg/ml at 1 hour and from 1 to 9 μg/ml at 2½ hours.[95]

Toxicity

Gentamicin is so toxic that its recommended systemic dose is only 1 mg/kg/day. Even in life-threatening circumstances, the highest allowable dose is 5 mg/kg/day. In a study of 59 cats, nephrotoxicity appeared in most animals at a dose level of 20 mg/kg and vestibular damage at 40 mg/kg, therapy being of 14 days' duration. Thirty percent of the cats were ataxic at a dose level of 20 mg/kg, and one animal suffered a 50% hearing loss, histologic examination showing destruction of cochlear hair cells.[96]

After gentamicin therapy, 3 of 25 patients suffered disabling, permanent, bilateral, and complete labyrinthine damage. This was not accompanied by deafness.[90]

Intravitreal injection of gentamicin in the rabbit eye is highly destructive.[97] At a dose of 4.0 mg, the ERG is extinguished within 1 week. A dose of 1.0 mg extinguishes the ERG within 2 weeks. Half of the eyes receiving 0.3 mg lost their ERG within 2 weeks. With only 0.1 mg, 3 of 10 eyes showed no ERG or ophthalmoscopic changes, the other 7 being moderately damaged. The 4 eyes receiving 0.05 mg gentamicin showed no ERG or ophthalmoscopic changes. Care must be taken to inject the drug slowly into the center of the vitreous, because a forceful squirt will spread the gentamicin to the retina, causing severe local damage.

Clinical use

The clinical effectiveness of topical gentamicin in the management of common external eye infections was evaluated in a series of 101 patients. After 1 to 2 weeks of treatment, all but one of the patients were clinically cured. Bacteriologic studies showed persistence of microorganisms in 30% of the patients despite total symptomatic cure. This finding indicates that complete bacterial eradication is not clinically realistic.[98]

Comparable results were obtained in another clinical series of 89 patients. In this study, gentamicin and Neosporin were compared and found to be equally effective in the management of external ocular infections.[99]

Gentamicin is chemically incompatible with many other antibiotics, mutual destruction occurring if they are mixed in solution before administration.[100] If administered separately, antibiotic incompatibility or antagonism is probably of very little, if any, clinical significance.

Gentamicin is not absorbed from the gastrointestinal tract.

Development of bacterial resistance to gentamicin is a matter of natural selection and readily occurs with overusage in a hospital environment. Resistant strains will retain resistance for as many as 80 in vitro transfers.

Summary

Gentamicin is highly effective against gram-negative organisms and resistant staphylococci. Unfortunately, it is so toxic that its systemic use is justified only in life-threatening circumstances. Because of the development of resistant organisms, which is a very real problem in *your* hospital, just as in mine, the thoughtless use of powerful antibiotics such as gentamicin is unwise. Use of gentamicin to treat a minor blepharoconjunctivitis or as prophylaxis following a clean cataract extraction will create the resistant strain that may kill tomorrow's patient. Please do not succumb to the current trend of prescribing the newest high-powered antibiotic in such a thoughtless manner.

ISONIAZID

Isoniazid (isonicotinic acid hydrazide) has proved to be an effective antituberculous agent without significant toxicity. Oral dosage is 4 to 5 mg/kg/day (100 mg every 6 hours for an average adult). Peak plasma levels appear within 1½ hours after oral administration of isoniazid. Excretion is mainly renal and is fairly complete within 24 hours. Topical ocular application of a 10% solution or ointment is well tolerated, as is subconjunctival injection of 10 to 20 mg.

Isoniazid is completely ineffective against the common bacteria and viruses, but concentrations as low as 0.02 μg/ml are bacteriostatic for *Mycobacterium tuberculosis*. Corneal penetration of isoniazid is good, and aqueous concentrations are adequate for bacteriostasis by any route of administration.[101] Concentrations of 5 μg/ml are attained by oral and intramuscular administration, and by hourly topical application of 10% drops. Topical application of 10% ointment and subconjunctival injection will give aqueous levels as high as 30 μg/ml. All ocular tissues, including sclera, are penetrated rapidly by isoniazid. Posterior segment concentrations obtained by systemic routes are higher than those achieved by topical administration.

Clinical use

Isoniazid has been shown to inhibit the progress of experimental tuberculous (human and bovine) infection of rabbit eyes.[101] Massive inoculations led to loss of the eye despite treatment, but 2½ months of isoniazid therapy cured rabbits infected with lesser doses of bacilli. It should be emphasized that in these known tuberculous infections, clinical improvement was not noted until after 3 weeks of therapy, and 2 to 3 months elapsed before clinical cure. Combination therapy with isoniazid, streptomycin, and *p*-aminosalicylic acid seemed more effective than use of any one of the drugs alone. Other research has confirmed the beneficial effect of isoniazid in cases of ocular tuberculosis.[101]

Clinical evaluation of the antituberculous drugs is severely handicapped by the difficulty of obtaining a definite etiologic diagnosis. The problem is compounded by the fact that spontaneous subsidence of uveitis may occur within the 1 to 3 months known to be required for an isoniazid cure of tuberculosis.

Excellent response, with less residual scarring and atrophy, is reported in the treatment of supposedly tuberculous uveitis by a combination of cortisone and isoniazid.[102] Improvement was often noted in 1 week as compared to 3 weeks without cortisone. This may be explained by steroid inhibition of inflammation, permitting the antituberculous medications to act more effectively. An alternative explanation is that in these cases, tuberculous infection of the eye is not actually the cause. If corticosteroids are used in the treatment of uveitis (or for other purposes), the physician should order chest x-ray examinations to rule out active pulmonary disease.

Unfortunately resistance of tubercle bacilli to isoniazid develops rapidly. Before isoniazid therapy, 97% of the strains of tubercle bacilli were found to be susceptible to this drug. After 12 to 14 weeks of therapy, 70% to 80% had become resistant. This resistance persisted long after the cessation of treatment.[103] The development of resistant strains is significantly delayed by the use of combinations of antituberculous drugs; hence such combined use is strongly recommended (for example, streptomycin, 1 g twice weekly; *p*-aminosalicylic acid, 12 to 15 g/day; and isoniazid, 4 mg/kg/day).

LINCOMYCIN

Lincomycin is bactericidal against a wide range of gram-positive organisms but is ineffective against most gram-negative microorganisms. It may be given orally or parenterally in a dosage of 500 mg, which will result in effective serum levels lasting for as long as 6 hours (oral) or 20 hours (intramuscular).[104] Except for diarrhea that occurs in 10% of patients, few significant side effects are reported.

Aqueous penetration

Intramuscular injection of 600 mg of lincomycin several hours before cataract surgery results in primary aqueous levels of 1 to 2 μg/ml. These levels in uninflamed human eyes indicate that therapeutic amounts of lincomycin do enter the eye (1 μg/ml will inhibit most pneumocci and streptococci, and 2 μg/ml will inhibit 90% of staphylococci).[105,106] Comparable levels were achieved in rabbit studies.[107]

During a cataract extraction a syringe containing alpha-chymotrypsin and another containing 300 mg of lincomycin in 1 ml of solution were inadvertently transposed. The lincomycin was injected into the posterior chamber, the customary site for use of alphachymotrypsin. When the error was discovered, the eye was irrigated with 2.5 ml of balanced saline solution and then with alphachymotrypsin. On the first postoperative day there was eyelid swelling, conjunctival chemosis, and 2 + aqueous flare and cells. After 2 weeks of corticosteroid therapy the ocular reaction subsided. The final corrected vision was 20/25.[108]

NALIDIXIC ACID

Nalidixic acid is a new antibacterial agent effective against a variety of gram-negative microorganisms. Concentrations as high as 4% are tolerated reasonably well by the rabbit eye, causing only transient mild conjunctival congestion. Hourly instillation of 4% nalidixic acid effectively controlled well-established *Proteus mirabilis* infections in rabbit corneas, sterilizing the corneal ulcers within 6 hours. In comparison, one third of similar ulcers treated with 4% ampicillin drops showed positive cultures 24 hours after therapy was started. Nalidixic acid therapy of *Pseudomonas* ulcers was ineffective.[109]

NEOMYCIN

Neomycin is a broad-spectrum antibiotic effective against a variety of gram-positive and gram-negative microorganisms. Its antibacterial spectrum is broader than that of bacitracin, penicillin, or streptomycin. Neomycin is more likely to be effective against *Proteus vulgaris* than is polymyxin B. It is not fungistatic. Staphylococcal resistance does not develop to neomycin. The drug is very stable at room temperature and is not inactivated by body fluids.

Nephrotoxicity[110] and ototoxicity are sufficiently severe to contraindicate parenteral use. Neomycin-induced deafness is comparable to that resulting from dihydrostreptomycin, and the two drugs appear to have additive ototoxic effects. Absorption via topical or oral administration is not sufficient to cause any toxic systemic effects.

Topical use of neomycin has been reported to cause improvement in one patient with conjunctival tuberculosis.[111]

NITROFURANS

The nitrofurans are synthetic antimicrobial drugs effective against a variety of gram-positive and gram-negative microorganisms. Staphylococci are ordinarily susceptible to nitrofurans (average inhibitory concentration, 1 mg/100 ml or 0.001%) and do not readily develop resistance. *Pseudomonas* strains are usually resistant. Depending on concentration, nitrofurans may be either bacteriostatic or bactericidal. They are effective despite the presence of blood, pus, and serum. These drugs are quite stable and will withstand autoclaving. Unfortunately the nitrofurans are quite toxic and are not well suited for systemic use.

Typical drugs

Nitrofurazone (Furacin) is available in ophthalmic preparations that include a 1% ointment and a 0.02% solution. Both are well tolerated after topical ocular application. This drug may be used for the control or prophylaxis of surface infections of or about the eye. A considerable number of the commonly encountered surface bacteria will be controlled by nitrofurazone, and the frequency of its application should be in proportion to the severity of the infection. Fungi and viruses are not susceptible to nitrofurazone.

In a clinical study of 596 patients, surface bacterial infections were treated with topical nitrofurazone.[112] The frequency of application varied from four times daily to every 30 minutes, depending on the severity of the disease. Good response was obtained in 85% of these patients. Virus infections were not alleviated. Only 5 of these 596 patients developed local drug allergy. All five had used the ointment form. No allergy was encountered after the use of drops alone. No toxic effects (such as retarded corneal epithelial healing) were clinically recognizable. The ophthalmic preparations are subjectively nonirritating. Nitrofurazone was considered to be comparable to the antibiotics commonly used for the treatment of surface ocular infections.

Nitrofurazone-impregnated gauze dressings (Furacin soluble dressing) were applied to half the area of 50 skin donor sites, while the other half of each wound was covered with ordinary petrolatum gauze.[113] At the end of 2 weeks an average of 90% of the area covered with nitrofurazone was epithelialized, as compared to an average of 80% of the petrolatum-covered area. Presumably the greater healing occurred as a result of the prevention of secondary infection. Staphylococci were completely absent from the cultures of these wounds. In two instances, extensive infection with *Pseudomonas aeruginosa* occurred despite nitrofurazone dressing. None of the 50 patients developed allergy. Use of nitrofurazone dressings could be considered in the treatment of injuries such as burns or abrasions of the skin surfaces about the eye.

Furaltadone (Altafur), a nitrofuran derivative, can be given orally for treatment of staphylococcal infections and is one of the medications used in the management of resistant strains. Blood levels after oral administration are too unreliable to classify furaltadone as a first-choice medication for serious infections. On the other hand, its side effects are too serious to warrant its use for trivial infections.

Intraocular penetration of furaltadone was studied in rabbits after oral, intravenous, subconjunctival, and topical administration.[114] In no instance were detectable vitreous or aqueous levels of the drug achieved by safe doses. Aqueous levels of 6 μg/ml were measured in one animal an hour after intravenous dosage of 125 mg/kg; however, this dose killed the animal within 1½ hours. Subconjunctival injection of 0.5 ml of a 10% solution of furaltadone hydrochloride gave aqueous levels of 90 μg/ml at 1 hour but resulted in necrosis of the cornea and sclera and in rupture of the eye.

Thirteen patients received furaltadone (250 mg, four times a day) for treatment or prophylaxis of ocular infection.[114] No blood levels of the drug could be detected with a minimal sensitivity test of 4 μg/ml.

Of interest to ophthalmologists is the development of paresis of the sixth cranial nerve during furaltadone treatment. In the reported cases, paresis cleared after the drug was stopped.[115,116]

Summary

The nitrofuran derivatives may be useful for treatment of surface ocular infections, particularly those caused by antibiotic-resistant staphylococci. *Pseudomonas* strains are usually resistant to nitrofuran treatment.

Intraocular penetration is insignificant in safe dosage; hence these drugs are of no value in the treatment of intraocular infection.

NOVOBIOCIN (ALBAMYCIN)

Novobiocin is effective against a variety of gram-positive and gram-negative organisms. It is tolerated topically in concentrations up to 1.2%. Corneal vascularization has followed experimental use of 10% solutions. As much as 12.5 mg of novobiocin may be given subconjunctivally; this dose causes transitory corneal staining for 1 day. Subconjunctival injection of 25 mg will cause severe damage to the anterior segment of the eye. As much as 0.2 mg of novobiocin is tolerated intracamerally and 0.1 mg intravitreally. Intraocular injection of 25 mg will cause blindness.[117]

Topical application of novobiocin in a concentration tolerable to the normal eye causes no measurable aqueous penetration. Subconjunctival injection of 12.5 mg results in aqueous concentrations of 30 to 90 μg/ml. Systemic dosage results in poor intraocular penetration; only very large doses (0.5 g intravenously in rabbits) achieve useful levels.

NYSTATIN (MYCOSTATIN)

Nystatin is a *Streptomyces*-derived antibiotic highly active in inhibiting the growth of a wide variety of fungi, molds, and yeasts. It has little or no effect on other types of microorganisms. Nystatin is fungistatic, not fungicidal.[118]

Despite the broad antifungal spectrum of nystatin, its therapeutic effect in systemic mycoses has been disappointing because toxicity prevents administration of adequate quantities of the drug. Oral preparations are poorly absorbed, intravenous injections cause chills and fever, and intramuscular injections cause local reactions. Therefore, for ophthalmic use, nystatin is administered topically in the treatment of surface fungus infections.

The solubility and stability of nystatin are of clinical importance. As much as 200,000 units may be dissolved in 1 ml of a special commercial diluent (N-methyl glucamine, Tween 20, and dimethyl acetamide),* while only 300 to 600 units will dissolve in 1 ml of water. If the nystatin solution in the diluent is placed into isotonic saline solution or water, a fine suspension results. (This type of suspension was used in the rabbit tolerance experiments to be presented next.) Refrigerated aqueous suspensions retain 90% of their original activity after storage for 2 weeks.

Experimental therapy

Intraocular infections. The use of nystatin for experimental therapy of intraocular *Aspergillus fumigatus* infections in the albino rabbit has established the therapeutic effectiveness of the drug as well as the eye's tolerance of it.[119] Nystatin is reasonably well tolerated as a topical ointment containing 100,000 units/g and as a single subconjunctival dose of 5000 units in a 0.5 ml saline solution. Two hundred units of nystatin in a 0.1 ml solution were injected into the vitreous or aqueous chamber without causing excessive reaction. Histopathologically demonstrable hyperemia and leukocytic infiltration persisted for 48 hours after injection of the anterior chamber and for a week after intravitreal injection. Vitreous assays suggested that nystatin levels sufficient to inhibit *Aspergillus* growth persisted for only 24 hours after

*E. R. Squibb & Sons.

injection. A second intravitreal injection of 200 units of nystatin, 36 hours after the first, caused vitreous degeneration. Single intravitreal injection of 400 units of nystatin caused cloudiness of the vitreous that persisted for at least a week.

Aspergillus growth is inhibited by a nystatin concentration of 6 to 12 units/ml. Intravitreal injection of 1000 *Aspergillus* spores will destroy all untreated rabbit eyes, with clinical evidence of severe infection recognizable within 3 days (Fig. 6-8, *A*). Eyes infected in this manner were injected intravitreally with 200 units of nystatin at 30 minutes or 24, 48, or 72 hours after infection. Seven of the eight eyes treated 24 hours after infection (Fig. 6-8, *B*) showed no evidence of fungus growth during observation periods for as long as 7 weeks. Treatment 2 days or more after infection temporarily reduced the severity of infection but did not protect the eyes from destruction. Therapy 30 minutes after infection delayed, but did not prevent, endophthalmitis. Possibly this can be explained by the resistance of *Aspergillus* spores to nystatin before they have germinated; after germination, when the organisms are finally susceptible, the antibiotic is no longer present.

The greater the number of *Aspergillus* spores injected, the more rapid is the inflammatory response. Proximity to vascular structures such as the iris or ciliary body resulted in more rapid growth than did inoculations into the central vitreous. The variable incubation period of human ocular fungus infections may be explained by differences in the size and location of the inoculum as well as by variations in resistance and virulence.

Corneal infections. The effectiveness of nystatin against corneal infections has been evaluated in rabbits infected with *Candida albicans*.[35] This study reports no toxicity after topical instillation of 100,000 units of nystatin/ml, but states that subconjunctival injection of 2000 units or more may cause localized necrosis. Subconjunctival injection of 800 units caused only transitory conjunctivitis. Bioassay failed to detect nystatin in aspirated aqueous after treatment by either

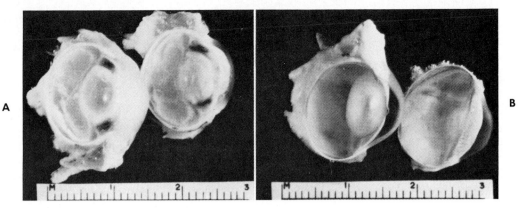

Fig. 6-8. A, Experimental *Aspergillus* endophthalmitis in untreated rabbit eye 6 days after standard intravitreal inoculation. Vitreous abscesses and retinal exudate are prominent. **B,** Nystatin-treated rabbit eye 6 days after standard intravitreal inoculation with *Aspergillus* spores. Intravitreal injection of 200 units was given 24 hours after fungus inoculation. Intraocular inflammation is absent. (From Fine, B., and Zimmerman, L.: Arch. Ophthalmol. **64:** 849, 1960.)

Table 6-5. Results of treatment with nystatin of rabbit corneas infected with *Candida* organisms*

Time between inoculation and start of treatment (hr)	Eyes treated (No.)	Treated eyes developing infection (No.)	Degree of infection
0	8	0	—
4	6	1	Mild
24	10	6	Mild
48	5	5	Severe
72 (or longer)	6	6	Severe

*From Montana, J. A., and Sery, T. W.: Arch. Ophthalmol. **60:**1, 1958.

topical or subconjunctival injection. (The assay method was sensitive to 80 units/ml and would therefore have failed to detect smaller amounts. *Candida albicans* is inhibited by 8 units nystatin/ml.)

Treatment with nystatin ointment, 100,000 units/ml applied three times a day, was begun either immediately after corneal inoculation with *Candida* or after delays of 4, 24, 48, or 72 hours. As seen in Table 6-5, no infection developed in those eyes treated immediately.[35] Mild infections, which were controlled by treatment, occurred in 1 of 6 eyes treated 4 hours after inoculation and in 6 of 10 eyes treated after 24 hours. Severe infection destroyed all eyes untreated during

the first 48 hours, regardless of subsequent therapy. Microscopic sections of untreated eyes showed Descemet's membrane to be intact at 24 hours, but at 48 hours mycelial penetration into the anterior chamber was evident.

The ineffectiveness of topical nystatin therapy after 48 hours is compatible with the belief that the cornea blocks drug penetration. When *Candida* organisms enter the anterior chamber, they are beyond the reach of topical nystatin.

The method of inoculation was intracorneal injection of 100,000 *Candida* organisms. This invariably caused infection of prednisolone-treated corneas, with an hypopyon ulcer appearing by the fourth day and perforation usually by the seventh day. *Candida* infection of the rabbit cornea could *not* be produced in this way without the aid of steroids. Prednisolone, 30 to 60 μg, was injected intracorneally just before fungus inoculation. The facilitation of corneal infection produced by a single prednisolone injection was found to last for at least 2 weeks.

Clinical use

A patient with *Aspergillus fumigatus* keratitis was cured after a month of treatment with nystatin.[120] Since no ophthalmic preparation of this antifungal drug is commercially available, a concentration of 50,000 units/ml was prepared by suspending sterile nystatin powder in an aqueous solution of 1.2% sodium chloride and 0.5% chlorobutanol. This nystatin suspension was instilled every 2 hours. (Would use of an ointment vehicle have prolonged effective therapeutic contact with the cornea? We have applied to the human eye a commercial ointment of 100,000 units/g intended for skin use.) Nystatin was also administered orally, 500,000 units every 8 hours. The effectiveness of nystatin was indicated by the facts that smears and cultures were negative by the fifth day of treatment (both smears and cultures were initially positive for *Aspergillus*) and that the hypopyon and corneal infiltrate cleared, recurred, and again cleared as nystatin was used, discontinued, and again administered. Atropine, hot compresses, and narcotics (for severe pain) were also used. Corticosteroid therapy was not used.

Summary

Nystatin inhibits the growth of a variety of molds, yeasts, and fungi. Unfortunately it is poorly absorbed orally and quite toxic when administered parenterally. Topical application of nystatin ointment, 100,000 units/g is of value in the treatment of corneal mycoses.

PENICILLINS

Penicillin is a generic term often used without the realization that a number of natural and synthetic derivatives of 6-aminopen-

icillanic acid exist. All of the clinically useful penicillins effectively inhibit certain bacteria, resist inactivation by human tissues, and are remarkably nontoxic. Considerable variations exist in solubility, stability, and resistance to destruction by penicillinase.[121]

Types

Potassium penicillin G is very water soluble and is ideal for attaining high plasma concentrations rapidly. This form of penicillin is absorbed and excreted rapidly; therefore it must be administered intramuscularly at least every 6 hours to maintain satisfactory blood levels. As much as 100 million units/day may be given intravenously for overwhelming or resistant infections. Intramuscular doses greater than 500,000 units may be very painful.

Although potassium penicillin G may be given orally, its absorption is limited because of its instability in gastric acid. Only about 15% of the orally administered drug can be recovered in the urine. To avoid destruction of the drug, oral doses should always be given at least 1 hour before or 2 hours after meals. For treatment of infections caused by sensitive bacteria, the minimal recommended oral dose is 400,000 units four times a day.

Procaine penicillin G (Crysticillin, Depopenicillin, Diurnal, Lentopen) is less soluble in water and is therefore absorbed more slowly than potassium penicillin G. Intramuscular doses of 600,000 units every 24 hours will maintain demonstrable plasma concentrations, comparable to those attained by oral administration of 250 mg four times a day of phenoxymethyl penicillin or potassium phenethicillin. If higher blood levels are desired, large injections of potassium penicillin G should be used. Giving doses of procaine penicillin G larger than 600,000 units and more often than every 12 hours is an inefficient method of achieving high plasma concentrations.

A 2% solution of aluminum monostearate, a water repellant, may be added to procaine penicillin G. This form of penicillin is absorbed slowly over a period of several days and therefore produces lower plasma levels.

Benzathine penicillin G (Bicillin) is only slightly water soluble and produces very low blood levels, which may last for several weeks. A single injection of 2,400,000 units will cure early syphilis in most cases. The longer acting forms of penicillin are more likely to produce hypersensitivity reactions.

Phenoxymethyl penicillin (penicillin V; Pen-Vee, V-Cillin) is much more acid stable than is penicillin G; hence it is well suited for oral use. As much as 75% of an oral dose may be recovered in the urine, indicating absorption two to five times that of oral penicillin G. Phenoxymethyl penicillin may be given without regard to the time of meals. An oral dose of 250 mg four times a day is adequate for most infections. The oral route may be considerably more economical than the parenteral route (and more comfortable!).

Phenoxyethyl penicillin (potassium phenethicillin; Alpen, Chemipen, Darcil, Dramcillin-S, Maxipen, Semopen, Syncillin) is pharmacologically comparable to phenoxymethyl penicillin.

The types of penicillin described to this point differ in solubility and stability. Their antibacterial effect, however, is essentially the same, as all are effective against most gram-positive cocci (with the noteworthy exception of penicillinase-producing and therefore resistant staphylococci), gonococci, enterococci, *Haemophilus*, *Clostridium*, and spirochetes. Most gram-negative bacteria (specifically, *Pseudomonas*) are resistant to these forms of penicillin.

Sodium methicillin (Dimocillin, Staphcillin) is resistant to destruction by penicillinase and is a first-choice agent against resistant staphylococci (unless the patient is allergic to penicillin). Minimal dosage is 1 g intramuscularly every 6 hours. Serious infections may require 2 g every 4 hours, given by continuous intravenous drip. The renal excretion of methicillin is rapid, half being excreted within 2 hours after intramuscular injection and 1 hour after intravenous administration.

Methicillin is extremely unstable in even slightly acid solutions and therefore should be dissolved just before use. When added to infusion fluids, it may be inactivated within several hours.

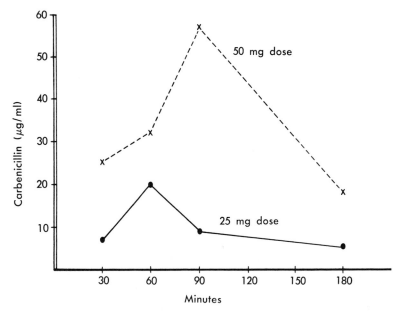

Fig. 6-9. Primary aqueous levels (rabbit) obtained after subconjunctival injection of carbenicillin in 25 and 50 mg dosages. (Modified from Rich, A. M., Dunlap, W. A., and Partridge, J. R.: Am. J. Ophthalmol. **75:**490, 1973.)

Sodium oxacillin (Prostaphlin, Resistopen) is pharmacologically comparable to methicillin, except that it is more acid stable and may therefore be given orally (500 mg every 2 hours). Frequent dosage is necessary because of the rapid excretion of the drug.[122]

Oxacillin is not excreted in sweat and therefore is not effective against skin-surface infections.

Ampicillin (Penbritin) is an acid-stable, orally absorbed synthetic penicillin with broad-spectrum antibacterial activity. It is effective against a variety of gram-negative bacteria, particularly *Escherichia coli* and *Proteus*.[123] The drug is administered orally, 0.75 g every 6 hours. It is chiefly indicated for the treatment of infections caused by tetracycline-resistant, gram-negative bacteria.

Minimal inhibitory concentrations of ampicillin for the common gram-positive organisms range from 0.01 to 0.05 μg/ml.[124] The majority of gram-negative organisms are considerably more resistant, requiring from 0.5 to 5 μg/ml.

Carbenicillin is a semisynthetic penicillin that acts against gram-negative pathogens. Inhibition of most strains of *Pseudomonas* requires doses of up to 50 μg/ml. *Proteus* and *Escherichia coli* may respond to carbenicillin therapy. Penicillinase-producing staphylococci are resistant. Gentamicin and carbenicillin are incompatible in solution.

The drug has low toxicity and may be used in doses of 20 to 40 g/day. Because of acid instability, carbenicillin must be given parenterally. The intravenous route is ordinarily used. Fig. 6-9 shows the aqueous levels achieved following subconjunctival injection.[125]

Ocular penetration

The blood-aqueous and blood-vitreous barriers severely limit passage of nonlipoid-soluble drugs such as penicillin into the vitreous, aqueous, and lens. A comparable barrier separates the healthy vitreous from the aqueous.[55] A common error is to think of the entire eye as being within the blood-aqueous barrier; this is not true. The uveal tract is freely accessible to blood-borne medications.

The semisynthetic penicillin derivatives vary considerably in their intraocular penetration. Methicillin, carbenicillin, cloxacillin, and amoxicillin do not penetrate nearly as well as does ampicillin.[126-128]

When an ointment containing 100,000 units/ml of penicillin is applied to the surface of the healthy rabbit eye, aqueous drug levels will reach only about 4 units/ml and will have dropped to 1 unit/ml in 2½ hours (Fig. 6-10).[129] Similar low levels are obtained in the intact sclera, cornea, and uveal tract. Fortunately the common infections of the corneal surface either are outside the blood-aqueous barrier or destroy it and are therefore more than normally accessible to penicillin therapy. Purified crystalline penicillin is virtually nontoxic to the exterior of the eye and can be used in very high concentrations without ocular irritation. Topical application achieves much higher concentrations on the corneal surface than the systemic routes of

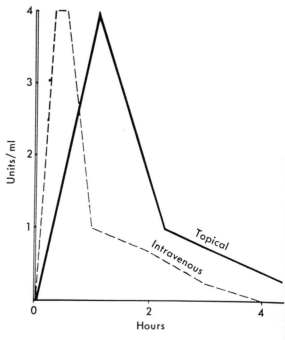

Fig. 6-10. Penicillin in rabbit aqueous (units/ml) after topical application of ointment, 100,000 units/ml, and intravenous administration of 50,000 units. (Modified from Sorsby, A., and Ungar, J.: Br. Med. J. **114**:4480, 1946.)

administration. For these reasons, topical penicillin therapy is effective against keratitis but is ineffective against endophthalmitis.

Subconjunctival injection of 1,000,000 units of crystalline penicillin G in 1 ml of a 1:1000 concentration of epinephrine produces effective intraocular levels of penicillin.[130] These levels persist for as long as 48 hours. Smaller amounts of penicillin without epinephrine produce substantially lower intraocular levels. As noted in Figs. 6-11 and 6-12, an intramuscular injection of penicillin results in much lower intraocular concentrations than those obtained by subconjunctival injection of an equal amount of drug. Intraocular concentrations of penicillin obtained by retrobulbar injection were higher than those achieved by intramuscular injection but lower than those following subconjunctival injection. As a specific example, 24 hours after treatment, 16 units/ml of drug persisted in the aqueous after the subconjunctival injection, compared to less than 0.1 unit/ml after intramuscular injection. One should realize that these figures were obtained in normal rabbits and that a comparable intramuscular dose for humans would require many millions of units. The penetration of the subconjunctival dose should be less directly related to the size of the body. These penicillin levels were obtained in healthy eyes, and higher values should result in inflamed eyes with damaged blood-aqueous barriers.

Twenty-four hours after subconjunctival injection of 1,000,000 units of penicillin in an epinephrine solution, the corneal concentration was more than 500 units of tissue and the posterior uveal concentration more than 300 units/g. The lens had the lowest level of all eye tissues, only 4 units after 24 hours.

Vitreous levels are lower than those of the aqueous, for instance, 8 units/ml after 24 hours (Fig. 6-12). It is noteworthy that by the second day quite similar vitreous levels are produced by subconjunctival injection of 1,000,000 units in epinephrine and by 5000 units injected intravitreally. This is a most practical point, for subconjunctival injection is far simpler, more convenient, and safer than intravitreal injection. In view of the effective levels of penicillin obtained by the two routes, intravitreal injections can be justified only when the vitreous cavity is already opened, as by trauma. Even under these circumstances, manipulation of the remaining vitreous may have undesirable effects. Although intravitreal injection of 5000 units of crystalline penicillin produces good levels within the vitreous cavity for up to 48 hours, it diffuses poorly to the anterior segment of the eye.[130] At 24 hours the vitreous penicillin concentration is more than 32 units/ml, at 48 hours it is 16 units/ml, and at 64 hours it remains as only a trace. At 24 hours only 4 units/ml are in the aqueous.

After systemic administration, penicillin levels are far higher in the vascular tissues of the eye than in the internal fluids. Two hours after intramuscular injection of penethamate (a synthetic penicillin ester) in rabbits the following concentrations in units/g of wet tissue

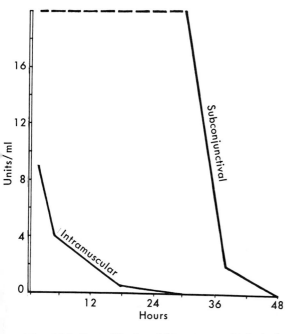

Fig. 6-11. Penicillin in rabbit aqueous (units/ml) after injection of 1 million units in a 1:1000 solution of epinephrine by subconjunctival and intramuscular routes. (Modified from Sorsby, A., and Ungar, J.: Br. J. Ophthalmol. **32:**864, 1948.)

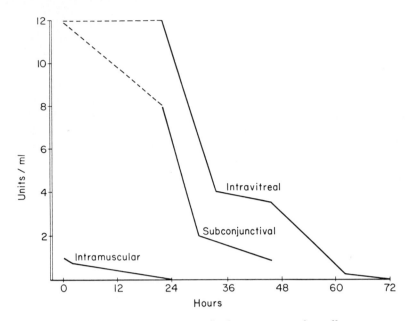

Fig. 6-12. Penicillin in rabbit vitreous (units/ml) after injection of 1 million units in a 1:1000 solution of epinephrine by subconjunctival and intramuscular routes. Intravitreal injection was 5000 units. (Modified from Sorsby, A., and Ungar, J.: Br. J. Ophthalmol. **32:**864, 1948.)

were measured: blood, 0.38; cornea, 0.12; aqueous, 0.04; anterior uvea, 3.8; lens, less than 0.01; vitreous, 0.09; posterior uvea, 1.82; and sclera, 0.39. Note that aqueous levels are not representative of concentrations in the surrounding tissues and that this particular compound was selectively concentrated in the uveal tract in concentrations higher than in the blood.[55]

Selective concentration also occurs on the surface of susceptible microorganisms. Although radioisotope studies show ion exchange within living tissues to proceed with almost unbelievable rapidity, this does not necessarily mean that particles of medication diffuse freely away from their target tissues. By the use of radioisotope-labeled penicillin, it has been shown that within 60 seconds of treatment time the penicillin may become firmly absorbed to the surface of the cell wall of *Bacillus subtilis.*[131]

The application of penicillin by iontophoresis (2 milliamperes for 5 minutes) increased the aqueous concentrations to levels eight times higher than those attained by simply

bathing the cornea in the same concentration of penicillin.[132]

Plasma levels of penicillin may be increased by blocking renal excretion. Each hour, approximately 60% of the circulating penicillin is excreted. Probenecid and carinamide will increase penicillin plasma levels from 2 to 10 times.[133] Dosage of probenecid is 500 mg four times a day and of carinamide, 2 g every 3 hours. In practice, these tubule-blocking drugs are rarely used, since the same effect can be achieved just as economically by giving more penicillin. Furthermore, these drugs may cause allergy or renal stones, and their action is inconstant.

The differences in antibiotic concentrations in various parts of the eye were evaluated using both radioactive and bioassay techniques.[134] The inadequacy of aqueous levels as a measure of the antibiotic concentration within the eye was emphasized. For example, following systemic administration of penicillin, the iris concentrations averaged 2.5 times those of the aqueous, whereas the vitreous levels were less than 0.1 of the aque-

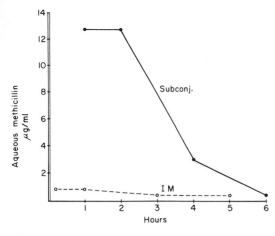

Fig. 6-13. Aqueous concentrations (μg/ml) of methicillin after subconjunctival injection of 20 mg and intramuscular injection of 40 mg/kg. (Modified from Green, W. R., and Leopold, I. H.: Am. J. Ophthalmol. 60:800, 1965.)

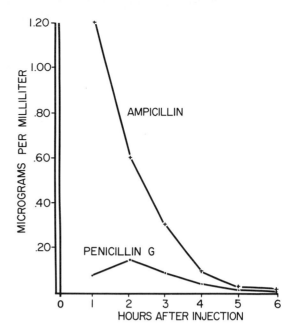

Fig. 6-14. Aqueous drug concentrations (rabbit) following intramuscular injection of 21 mg/kg of antibiotic. (Modified from Goldman, J. N., and Klein, J. O.: Ann. Ophthalmol. 2:35, April 1970.)

ous levels. Choroid and retina levels approximated aqueous levels.

Methicillin

A therapeutic concentration of methicillin (sodium dimethoxyphenyl penicillin) will penetrate into the normal rabbit aqueous after subconjunctival injection of 20 mg (Fig. 6-13).[135] Intraocular penetration is less effective when the route of administration is intramuscular.

The intraocular penetration of methicillin in the human was studied by bioassay of aqueous obtained at cataract surgery.[136] Continuous intravenous infusion over a 24-hour period of 8 g of methicillin (with oral probenecid) achieved an average serum concentration of 45 μg/ml but an aqueous level of only 0.46 μg/ml. A concentration of 4 μg/ml inhibits growth of most gram-positive organisms. In an eye with iridocyclitis the aqueous concentration was 6 μg/ml. Two diabetic eyes with cataract, but otherwise clinically normal, demonstrated aqueous concentrations of 6.5 μg/ml, presumably indicating abnormal vascular permeability in the diabetic eye. These data indicate that therapeutic concentrations of methicillin do not enter the

normal human eyes but may be achieved when the blood-aqueous barriers are broken down by inflammation.

Oxacillin

No measurable levels of oxacillin could be detected in aqueous humor obtained from 40 patients during cataract extraction. The drug had been administered by intramuscular injection before surgery, resulting in serum levels as high as 5.7 μg/ml at the time of surgery. In man, approximately 93% of the oxacillin in the blood is bound to plasma protein. The protein-bound oxacillin is completely blocked from entry into the aqueous. Clearly, oxacillin is not likely to be an effective drug in the treatment of intraocular infection. Indeed, oxacillin does not penetrate even into the inflamed animal eye.[137]

Ampicillin

Ampicillin is reported to produce aqueous humor levels approximately twice as high as

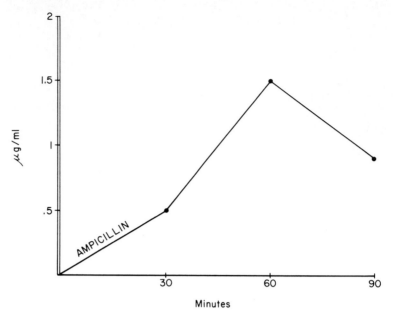

Fig. 6-15. Aqueous humor (rabbit) concentrations of ampicillin given intramuscularly in a dosage of 50 mg/kg. (Modified from Goldman, E. E., McLain, J. H., and Smith, J. L.: Am. J. Ophthalmol. **65:**717, 1968.)

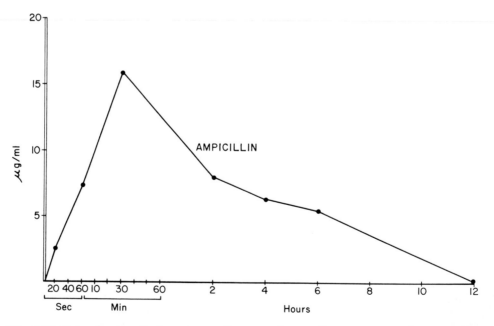

Fig. 6-16. Rate of entry of subconjunctivally injected ampicillin into aqueous humor (rabbit). (Modified from McPherson, S. D., Jr., Presley, G. D., and Crawford, J. R.: Am. J. Ophthalmol. **66:**430, 1968.)

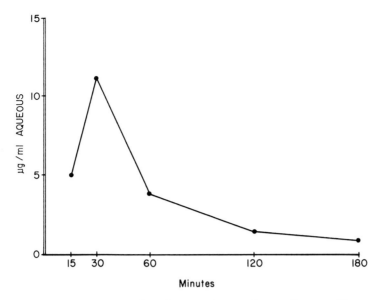

Fig. 6-17. Aqueous levels after topical application of 2 mg of ampicillin on rabbit cornea. (Data from Kurose, Y., and Leopold, I. H.: Arch. Ophthalmol. **73:**361, 1965.)

those achieved with comparable doses of aqueous penicillin G.[138] Blockage of renal tubular excretion by oral probenecid (35 mg/kg given 30 minutes before ampicillin injection) resulted in aqueous humor levels two to five times greater than those achieved without probenecid. There is considerable variation in the format and the results of experimental determinations. Fig. 6-14[139] shows an even greater ampicillin penetration as compared to penicillin G.

The aqueous levels shown in Fig. 6-15 resulted from a single, intramuscular ampicillin dosage of 50 mg/kg, which would be 3500 mg for a 70 kg man.[138] A titer of 2 μg/ml will inhibit most gram-positive cocci.

Subconjunctivally injected ampicillin penetrates the anterior chamber with remarkable rapidity. After a subconjunctival injection of 100,000 units (62.5 mg) of ampicillin in a 0.25 ml solution, bacteriostatic concentrations of antibiotic are demonstrable in the rabbit aqueous within 30 seconds. Peak levels are reached in 30 minutes, declining to zero in about 12 hours (Fig. 6-16).[140]

Incidentally, it was noted in this study that

if antibiotic levels are of value during and after cataract surgery, it is more rational to give a subconjunctival injection before rather than after the operation.

Topical application of 2 mg of ampicillin on the rabbit cornea resulted in the concentrations shown in Fig. 6-17.[124]

Human aqueous concentrations of ampicillin were measured by securing aqueous samples at the time of cataract extraction.[124] The aqueous levels achieved by different oral doses are shown in Fig. 6-18. These data suggest that an oral dosage of 1 g of ampicillin every 4 hours should maintain antibiotic concentrations in the anterior segment of the eye sufficient to inhibit the common gram-positive organisms. Consistent aqueous levels effective against relatively resistant gram-negative organisms cannot be maintained with reasonable dosage schedules.

Plasma protein binding of antibiotics renders them biologically inactive and also excludes the bound portion from entry into the primary aqueous. The proportion of ampicillin bound to protein is 17%; of methicillin, 30%; of penicillin G, 55%; and of oxacillin, 92%. Similarly, a decrease in intraocular

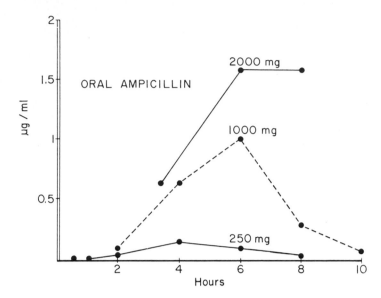

Fig. 6-18. Aqueous levels after single oral dose of ampicillin. (Data from Kurose, Y., and Leopold, I. H.: Arch. Ophthalmol. **73:**361, 1965.)

penetration follows systemic administration of the drugs.[141] There is a critical free plasma level, approximately 21 μg/ml, below which ampicillin does not cross the blood-aqueous barrier. These authors also measured the primary aqueous levels of the rabbit following subconjunctival injection of antibiotic and found the following levels of antibiotics 1 hour after injection: ampicillin, 1000 μg/ml; methicillin, 166 μg/ml; and oxacillin, 145 μg/ ml. Four hours after subconjunctival injection, no detectable levels of ampicillin or methicillin were present in the aqueous.

Dicloxacillin

Dicloxacillin, which is highly effective against penicillinase-producing *Staphylococcus aureus*, will not penetrate into primary aqueous when given intravenously or orally but will enter secondary aqueous in concentrations as high as 12 μg/ml 2 hours after administration.[142] Subconjunctival injection of 50 mg will give aqueous concentrations as high as 181 μg/ml at 1 hour and 50 μg/ml at 4 hours. A concentration of 0.5 μg/ml will inhibit most gram-positive cocci, including penicillinase-producing *Staphylococcus aureus*.

Carbenicillin

Intraocular penetration of carbenicillin following intravenous administration is poor, in the same range as that of penicillin G. One hour after intravenous administration of 30 mg/kg, primary aqueous levels were 2 to 3 μg/kg. Probenecid, 200 mg, did not increase levels significantly. In the inflamed eye, aqueous levels reached 33 μg/ml, but vitreous levels were less than 3 μg/ml. Subconjunctival injection of 100 mg gave aqueous levels averaging 172 μg/ml in normal primary aqueous and 196 μg/ml in the inflamed eye. Vitreous levels were poor, less than 4 μg/ml even in the inflamed eye. The half-life of carbenicillin in the aqueous was found to be 40 minutes.[143] Since most strains of *Pseudomonas* require more than 50 μg/ml of carbenicillin for inhibition, it is evident that vitreous concentrations of antibiotic adequate to control this microorganism were not achieved.

Twenty cataract patients received subconjunctival injections of carbenicillin varying from 50 to 500 mg. Immediate, severe, burning pain resulted, followed by a marked local chemosis that persisted for 2 to 11 days. Aqueous levels were quite variable, but in most cases the 100 mg dosage level resulted in primary aqueous levels of about 150 μg/ml from 30 minutes to 2 hours after injection.[144]

Therapy of intraocular infections

The use of penicillin in the treatment of eye infections is limited by several factors. Most important is the susceptibility of the offending microorganism, for, of course, there will be no therapeutic response to penicillin if the organism is resistant (or if the disease is misdiagnosed and not of infectious etiology). A very practical limitation is the 5% incidence of allergy after topical ocular use of penicillin. Because of this, other antibiotics and antibacterials have completely replaced penicillin in the local treatment of minor surface ocular infections. The most complex limiting factor is the resistance of the blood-aqueous barrier to the passage of penicillin. That this barrier can be bypassed is experimentally demonstrable, as shown in the following discussion.

Experimental use

Experimental intraocular infections produced by injection of 50,000 *Staphylococcus aureus* organisms into the aqueous or vitreous were treated by subconjunctival injection of 1,000,000 units of penicillin.[145] As would be expected from knowledge of the attainable intraocular concentrations, the infection was arrested with preservation of normal eyes when the penicillin was administered 4 hours after infection. If treatment was delayed for 24 hours, the anterior chamber infections cleared but left varying degrees of synechiae and corneal scarring. The 24-hour treatment of vitreous infections resulted in opaque, organized vitreous. Untreated control eyes were all destroyed by panophthalmitis. These findings are compatible with those of other studies.[146]

It is evident that the time at which treatment is initiated is a determining factor in the outcome of an intraocular infection. Antibiotics should be given prophylactically as soon as possible after a penetrating injury, preferably by the general physician who first sees the patient. The physician will, of course, have to use the intramuscular or oral routes rather than subconjunctival injection, which will be given later by the ophthalmologist.

An instructive quantitative experiment was carried out by inoculating the anterior chambers of rabbits with gonococci and then determining the least amount of penicillin required to sterilize the eye when given by various routes. Intramuscular injection required 150,000 units of penicillin; subconjunctival injection required 100,000 units; and direct inoculation into the anterior chamber required *only* 2.5 units. It is obvious that very effective barriers to aqueous penetration by penicillin exist, even in an infected eye.

Clinical use

Clinical use of penicillin in the treatment of corneal and anterior segment infections indicated that the human eye tolerates well the subconjunctival injection of 500,000 units of crystalline penicillin in 0.5 ml of 1:1000 concentration of epinephrine at intervals of 24 hours.[147] Topical anesthesia with cocaine was used. (The modern synthetic anesthetics should be equally effective.) Injection of 0.5 ml of a 1:1000 concentration of epinephrine is apparently safe, although some patients (cardiac and thyrotoxic) may be more sensitive to its effects than others. Although it is not specified in these articles, a sub-Tenon's capsule injection should result in more effective intraocular penetration than an injection just beneath the conjunctiva.

A practical point is that concentrated solutions of penicillin should be made up in water rather than in normal saline solution; otherwise they will be quite hypertonic and therefore more irritating.

Currently accepted doses of penicillin for the treatment or prophylaxis of eye infections are very high.[148] One million units of crystalline penicillin administered intramuscularly or intravenously every 8 hours is recommended. Concomitant oral use of probenecid, 2 g initially and 0.5 g every 6 hours, blocks elimination of penicillin and thereby helps to maintain high concentrations within the body. After a penetrating eye injury, penicillin should be given as just described for the first 48 hours. Should no signs of infection be present at that time, penicillin may be discontinued or reduced in dosage, depending on the circumstances. Simultaneously with penicillin, an initial dose of 2 g of streptomycin followed by 1 g every 8 hours was recommended to give a wider antibacterial spectrum. However, the toxicity of streptomycin in this dosage is unacceptable.

Differences of opinion exist as to whether prophylactic antibiotics should be utilized after routine cataract surgery. Statistics indicate that there is a 0.5% incidence of intraocular infection after cataract surgery even when performed with the best of technique. In view of this known possibility, a series of 1202 patients were injected subconjunctivally immediately after cataract extraction with 100,000 units of penicillin G in a 0.25 ml volume, which contained 1 drop of a 1:1000 concentration of epinephrine.[149] Four of these eyes (0.24%) developed intraocular infection, and three of the four infections

were caused by penicillin-resistant organisms. Subsequently, streptomycin, 10 mg, was added to the injection. Combined penicillin and streptomycin injections were then given to 3226 patients over a 3-year period, and not one case of intraocular infection developed! A control series of 1773 patients who were operated on in the same institution received no antibiotics and had a 0.51% incidence of infection (9 eyes). The injection caused slight postoperative conjunctival congestion, but no instance of damaging allergic or toxic reaction occurred in this large series.

Eight cases of postoperative staphylococcal endophthalmitis were reported to follow prophylactic subconjunctival injection of penicillin (100,000 units) and streptomycin (10 mg) solution.[150] In four of these cases there was a latent period of 21 to 40 days between surgery and infection. The long period of latency caused some clinical confusion, since the time interval was more characteristic of fungus than of bacterial infection. The incidence of infection was 3% of the operated eyes, which indicates that anti-

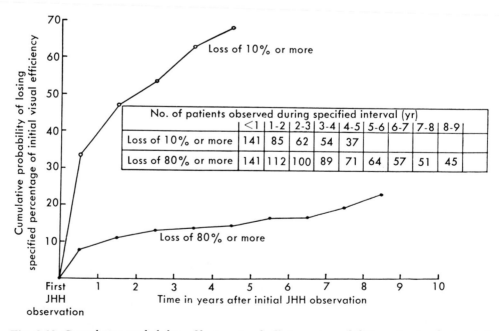

Fig. 6-19. Cumulative probability of losing visual efficiency in syphilitic optic atrophy treated with penicillin. *JHH* refers to Johns Hopkins Hospital. (From Hahn, R. D., and associates: J. Chronic Dis. **1:**601, 1955.)

biotic prophylaxis will not reliably protect against faults in sterile operative technique.

Penicillin is effective in slowing the progress of syphilitic optic atrophy. After 8 years, only 25% of penicillin-treated patients with syphilitic optic atrophy will have lost 80% of their initial vision (Fig. 6-19), whereas in this same period of time, 65% of untreated patients will likely become blind.[151] Combining malaria fever therapy with the penicillin treatment of syphilitic optic atrophy[151] does not alter the results obtained (Fig. 6-20) and is not warranted because of the risks inherent in malaria therapy.[152] Early stages of optic atrophy respond to treatment much better than do advanced stages (Fig. 6-21).[153]

Benzathine penicillin (900,000 units intramuscularly every 2 weeks for 4 months) has been used for the treatment of trachoma.[154] Of 18 patients so treated, 12 were completely cured, and 2 showed great improvement at the end of 4 months. Two years later, all but 1 of the 18 were cured. Whether penicillin acts directly on the virus or merely arrests secondary bacterial infection is not clear.

Toxic effects

For practical purposes, external application of penicillin in any concentration is nontoxic to the eye.

Definite toxic effects were noted in the majority of rabbit eyes receiving intravitreal injections of 2000 to 5000 units of the various

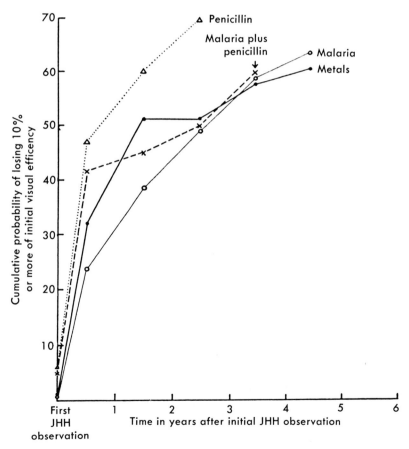

Fig. 6-20. Effect of various types of treatment of syphilitic optic atrophy. Differences are *not* significant. *JHH* refers to Johns Hopkins Hospital. (Modified from Hahn, R. D., and associates: J. Chronic Dis. **1**:601, 1955.)

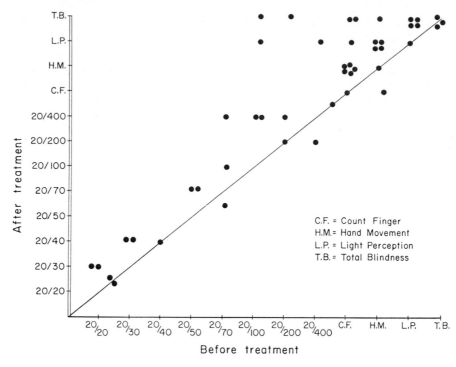

Fig. 6-21. Visual acuity before and after penicillin treatment of syphilitic optic atrophy. Note that patients with relatively good initial vision maintained good acuity, whereas those with poor initial vision progressed to severe visual impairment or total blindness. Therapy cannot be expected to improve vision. (Modified from Benton, C. D., and Harris, J. F.: Arch. Ophthalmol. **48:**449, 1952.)

types of crystalline penicillin.[155] These effects include ophthalmoscopically observable retinal edema (lasting up to 10 days), pigmentary migration, localized atrophic patches in the retina, irregularity and condensations in the vitreous, and blistering of the internal limiting membrane. Vacuolation of the nerve fiber layer, limited areas of neuroepithelial damage, and preretinal exudation were histologically demonstrated. Penicillin K produced neovascularization, while penicillin G was the least toxic. Obviously the interior of the eye will *not* tolerate the massive concentrations of penicillin that can be injected elsewhere in the body.

Clinically, the anterior chamber will tolerate irrigation with potassium penicillin G, 5000 units/ml. A penicillin solution of this concentration may be used for anterior chamber irrigation at the time of surgical closure

of an injury or if paracentesis of a severe hypopyon is performed (such a procedure has virtually become obsolete since the development of effective antibiotics).

Penicillin is extremely irritating to the central nervous system and may cause serious and permanent nerve damage. Accidental injection into the sciatic nerve may cause permanent sensory and motor loss. The importance of avoiding sciatic nerve damage warrants cautioning your nurse against injecting into any portion of the buttock other than the upper outer quadrant.[121]

Five percent of the population in the United States is said to be allergic to penicillin.[156] This is presumably related to the enormous amount of penicillin used (350 tons/year or 3,000,000 units/inhabitant). Eighty percent of all drug eruptions are caused by penicillin. With the advent of benzathine and the other types of repository penicillin, reactions have become even more violent and prolonged.

The commonest type of penicillin allergy is the delayed response that simulates serum sickness. After an incubation period, usually lasting 1 to 2 weeks, urticaria, fever, and joint pains appear. This response is a result of the development of antibodies after the injection, and therefore skin tests and the past history will not reveal penicillin sensitivity.

Sensitization may be caused by penicillin therapy, by penicillin in ingested food (dairy products), or by previous fungus disease of the skin. Preliminary skin or conjunctival testing may be positive or negative, even in patients who will later develop severe penicillin allergy. These sensitized individuals will manifest allergic reactions more promptly, even after incubation periods as brief as a few minutes. Death may occur from acute serum sickness, angioedema, or anaphylaxis.[157]

The incidence of allergic reactions to penicillin in patients can be reduced by routine inquiry as to previous drug allergy. (Asthmatic patients are more likely to become sensitive to penicillin.) Juries are said to take a dim view of severe drug reactions induced in patients who know they have previously been allergic to the medication. As previously stated, however, neither the history nor skin testing will detect all patients who are allergic to penicillin. Use penicillin only when it is needed and only after ascertaining that the patient has had no previous penicillin reaction.

Aside from avoiding penicillin use in patients known to be sensitive to penicillin or generally allergic, the best method of treating allergic reactions is with penicillinase. Penicillinase, a bacterial product, destroys penicillin enzymatically. One unit of penicillinase will destroy 1 unit of penicillin in 1 minute and is not itself broken down by the reaction. Penicillinase is relatively nontoxic. The only reported reactions are slight soreness at the site of injection, local erythema, and occasionally a pyrogenic effect after intravenous injection. It may be given intra-

muscularly or intravenously, depending on the severity of the penicillin allergy. The usual therapeutic dose is 800,000 units (1 vial) dissolved in 2 ml of sterile water. (The resulting solution is isotonic.) Penicillinase is supplied as a dry powder, which is indefinitely stable. However, when the powder is dissolved, potency is lost after a week.

In a study with human volunteers, 20 persons received 800,000 units of procaine penicillin intramuscularly twice daily.[158] After constant penicillin blood levels had been established over several days, a single intramuscular injection of 800,000 units of penicillinase was given. Within 1 hour no circulating penicillin could be detected in blood samples. The action of this single dose of penicillinase kept the bloodstream free of penicillin for periods from 4 to 7 days despite continuing injections of penicillin (800,000 units, every 12 hours).

The response of the penicillin-allergic patient to penicillinase is very good; symptoms disappear in 80% of patients within 12 to 96 hours. If there is no clinical response after 4 days, 800,000 units of penicillinase should again be injected. Failure to respond to the second injection within 4 days indicates that some other allergen should be considered as the cause of the allergic reaction. Response to penicillinase is so effective and specific that such a negative therapeutic test virtually rules out penicillin allergy as the cause of the current trouble. A recurrence of symptoms within a week of their disappearance suggests reexposure to penicillin, which could be medicinal, from fungus infection, or from food (some types of cheese contain *Penicillium* type molds, and 11% of American milk samples show measurable quantities of penicillin).

Obviously penicillinase destroys the therapeutic value of penicillin as an antibiotic.

In addition to penicillinase, steroids and antihistaminics are useful in treatment of penicillin reactions. For anaphylactic shock, 1 ml of a 1:1000 concentration of epinephrine should be immediately given subcutaneously.

Despite the relative infrequency of penicillin reactions, an attitude of complacency is unwarranted. Penicillin reactions are estimated to occur in 2% to 8% of patients receiving the drug. The incidence of death in severe reactions is from 9% to 13%.[121] Patients found to be allergic to penicillin (or any other medication, for that matter) should be cautioned against its further use and advised to inform their future medical attendants.

The local ocular use of penicillin may result in as high as a 16% incidence of allergic blepharitis.[159] For this reason, topical application for minor infections is in disrepute. Such promiscuous use of penicillin may sensitize the patient, thereby precluding later use of this valuable drug in time of need. Furthermore, the more widespread the use of an antibiotic, the more numerous will be the strains of resistant microorganisms in the community.

Summary

Penicillin is one of the antibiotics of first choice for treatment of ocular infections (excluding endophthalmitis) caused by sensitive organisms. A variety of new penicillin derivatives have quite different antimicrobic spectra; hence laboratory sensitivity studies are essential in the management of severe infections.

Penicillin penetration into aqueous, lens, and vitreous is very poor but is considerably increased by subconjunctival injection or by iontophoresis. Alternate drugs (for example, chloramphenicol) are preferable for treatment of endophthalmitis.

From 5% to 10% of the population are allergic to penicillin. Death may follow use of penicillin in an allergic patient. Before use of penicillin, the physician should specifically inquire as to the possibility of past allergy.

PIMARICIN

Pimaricin, a semisynthetic polyene antibiotic of the same general class as nystatin and amphotericin B, is perhaps the most effective antifungal drug currently available for treatment of corneal infections.

The drug is poorly soluble in water, is stable in suspension, is poorly absorbed from the gastrointestinal tract or other mucosal surfaces, and is well tolerated. Fifteen human volunteers used a 5% suspension of pimaricin, 1 drop every 2 hours while awake for 2 weeks.[160] No ocular toxicity was observed in any of these volunteers.

Clinical use

Seven patients with culture-proved fungal corneal ulcers were given 5% pimaricin every 2 hours.[160] Four patients were cured of the infection within 2 to 4 weeks of therapy, while the other three required keratoplasty subsequent to the medical treatment. However, no viable fungus was recovered from the surgical specimens. Potassium iodide, 1% solution, was also instilled at 1- to 2-hour intervals in these eyes in the belief that the potassium ion helps an injured cornea maintain its water pump system and glycolytic cycle. The iodide ion may not be helpful. Clinically, the corneal reaction to fungal infection is less with potassium iodide therapy than without it.

Fusarium solani is the most common cause of fungal keratitis in Florida. Pimaricin, in a 5% suspension applied hourly, cured 16 of 18 culture-proved *Fusarium* corneal ulcers.[161] The suspension is viscous and adheres well to the cornea. It is well tolerated and causes no pain or secondary corneal damage. Improvement in the appearance of the ulcers could be recognized within 2 days. Amphotericin B had been used in the treatment of 20 previous patients with *Fusarium* ulcers, achieving a cure in only seven cases. Also, the amphotericin B caused intense local pain and diffuse surface damage to the cornea and conjunctiva. This study stresses the differences in the antibiotic responses of different species and strains of fungi and raises objections to the validity of the grouping "mycotic keratitis."

Experimental combined therapy

In the hope that fungal inflammatory corneal damage could be diminished while fungus growth was inhibited by pimaricin, corticosteroid therapy was also used in the treatment of *Aspergillus* corneal ulcers in rabbits.[162] Pimaricin, 5%, and potassium iodide, 2%, were given every 2 to 3 hours. Also, different groups of rabbits were treated with dexamethasone, 0.1%, 0.01%, and 0.001%, four times daily. The eyes treated with the higher concentrations of dexamethasone showed the most improvement during the first week of treatment but subsequently showed deterioration, larger ulcers forming and severe intraocular infection developing. The animals receiving 0.001% dexamethasone had recognizably less inflammation and did not suffer exacerbation of the fungus infection. Quite clearly, *great* care is required in the use of corticosteroids for corneal fungal infections, if they are used at all.

The intravitreal use of pimaricin is apparently not practical. In rabbits 50 μg will destroy the retina. In one study a dosage of 25 μg was tolerated by the eye but was not sufficient to be effective against experimental fungus infection (*Aspergillus*).[163]

POLYMYXIN B

Polymyxin B is bactericidal against most gram-negative microorganisms. For example, *Escherichia coli*, *Pseudomonas aeruginosa*, *Aerobacter aerogenes*, *Klebsiella pneumoniae*, and *Haemophilus influenzae* may be sensitive to polymyxin B concentrations ranging from 0.05 to 2 μg/ml. Sensitive organisms are unlikely to develop resistance. *Proteus vulgaris* is usually resistant to polymyxin B.

Polymyxin B is not absorbed from the gastrointestinal tract, will not readily pass the blood-brain and blood-aqueous barriers, and does not penetrate the intact cornea after topical application. Renal tubular epithelial damage and neurotoxicity are caused by parenteral dosage in excess of 2.5 mg/kg/day. If systemic use is indicated, 1.5 to 2.5 mg/kg/day is given intramuscularly in divided doses every 8 hours. Laboratory tests subsequent to the administration of polymyxin B should include blood urea nitrogen and albuminuria determinations.

Polymyxin B solutions are stable for at least 6 months if refrigerated.

Ocular tolerance

Concentrations of 0.25% (2.5 mg/ml) are nonirritating and may be used for topical application. Hence polymyxin B can be applied to tissues in concentrations 1000 times greater than that required to destroy sensitive organisms. Concentrations as high as 1% cause ocular irritation. The subconjunctival injection of 10 mg of polymyxin B produced severe chemosis, localized necrosis, and bloody discharge in rabbits.[164] Subconjunctival injection of 0.5 mg was fairly well tolerated.

Currently available ophthalmic ointments contain 0.2% polymyxin B (1 mg of purified drug contains 10,000 units).

Ocular penetration

Although the intact corneal epithelium prevents penetration of polymyxin B into the corneal stroma, therapeutic concentrations do enter the stroma after epithelial damage.[165] Good stromal penetration occurs after epithelial abrasion whether drug application is by topical instillation, subconjunctival injection, or corneal bath. The greatly enhanced penetration seen after epithelial removal suggests such a step in the clinical treatment of infectious corneal ulcers. Tissue obtained by curettement of the loose epithelium surrounding a corneal ulcer would be most likely to contain the infecting organisms and would therefore be ideal material for culture and staining.

No significant polymyxin B penetration into the vitreous is demonstrable after parenteral or local administration of the drug.

Use in treatment of corneal ulcers due to Pseudomonas

Corneal ulcers resulting from *Pseudomonas* infection are rapidly progressive and highly destructive. In 96 such infections reviewed in the literature, 45 eyes were lost (evisceration or enucleation), and only 10 eyes retained vision better than 6/60.[165] (Most of these cases occurred before effective antibiotics became available.) Even if the infection is arrested, dense stromal scarring occurs unless treatment has been very prompt. With intensive polymyxin B treatment started within several days of infection, two patients with *Pseudomonas* corneal ulceration regained 6/9 vision.[165]

Treatment of experimental corneal ulcers caused by *Pseudomonas* infection with subconjunctival injections of polymyxin B gave good results, with relatively clear corneas, if therapy was started within 18 hours of infection. When therapy was delayed for 48 hours, the infection could be controlled, but dense stromal scarring resulted.[164] Comparable results are reported by other investigators.[166] Secondary bacterial contamination of ulcers resulting from *Pseudomonas* infection can readily occur.[165] The antibacterial spectrum of polymyxin B does not include many gram-positive organisms. Repeated cultures taken during the course of therapy will detect such secondary invaders and will serve as a check on the sterilization of the ulcer. The concomitant prophylactic use of other antibiotics effective against gram-positive bacteria (for example, bacitracin and neomycin) seems logical and desirable.

Because of the great importance of early treatment, serious corneal ulcers should be treated with broad-spectrum antibiotics immediately, before culture and sensitivity results are reported. A gram stain will help greatly in anticipating the diagnosis of *Pseudomonas* infection.

Polymyxin B, 0.2%, should be applied topically at least hourly. If intraocular involvement is probable, cautious parenteral administration may be tried, with due consideration of the toxic nature of this drug.

Atropinization and adequate cleaning of the eye with hot moist compresses are indicated, as in any other type of severe keratitis with associated iritis.

Summary

Polymyxin B is one of the most effective antibiotics available against gram-negative organisms. Topical application achieves effective corneal stromal concentrations if the epithelium is not intact. Adequate intraocular concentrations of polymyxin B cannot be produced by topical or parenteral administration. Parenteral administration may seriously damage the kidneys and the central nervous system.

PYRIMETHAMINE (DARAPRIM)

Pyrimethamine (2,4-diamino-5-[*p*-chlorophenyl]-6-ethylpyrimidine) is a potent folic acid antagonist that is used clinically in the treatment of toxoplasmosis and malaria.

Pharmacology

Blood serum levels of approximately 0.2 to 0.4 mg of pyrimethamine/100 ml may be attained clinically by giving two 100 mg doses of pyrimethamine on the first day of treatment, followed by doses of 25 mg twice daily thereafter (Fig. 6-22). If this high initial dose is not given, a period of about 21 weeks is required for the smaller daily doses to achieve the same blood level.[167]

The concentration of pyrimethamine in the uveal tract and retina is somewhat higher than that in the serum. It is fortunate that *Toxoplasma* organisms exist within these tissues and not in the intraocular fluids, for the blood-aqueous barrier is poorly permeated by pyrimethamine. Less than 0.005 mg/100 ml was found in the aqueous of patients with serum levels of 0.1 mg/100 ml or higher. This very low aqueous concentration of pyrimethamine existed despite the presence of cells and flare in the anterior chamber of these patients with active uveitis. Since *Toxoplasma* organisms multiply only within cells and are susceptible to the action of pyrimethamine only while actively multiplying, it is the tissue concentration that determines the efficacy of the drug.

Actually, it is not possible to make a single quantitative determination of the "penetration of a drug into the eye." Medications have a greater affinity for some tissues than for others and may be selectively concentrated. The concentration of drug found in intraocular fluids may be greatly different from that in adjacent tissue. When the tissue to be treated is the retina, as in toxoplasmic retinitis, the pharmacologic fact of importance is the *retinal* concentration of pyri-

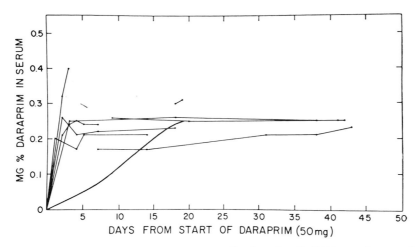

Fig. 6-22. Serum concentration in patients given a "loading dose" of 200 mg of pyrimethamine (Daraprim) the first day and 25 mg twice a day thereafter. Heavy line: mean curve for patients not given a loading dose showing the 2-week delay in reaching steady concentrations with smaller daily doses. (From Kaufman, H. E., and Caldwell, L. A.: Arch. Ophthalmol. **61:**885, 1959.)

methamine—not that in the aqueous or vitreous.

Measurement of pyrimethamine in various portions of the eye with the aid of radioactive labeling indicates a selective concentration of this drug within the retina.[168] Twelve hours after intramuscular injection of 2.5 mg/kg of labeled pyrimethamine in monkeys, the animals were killed by exsanguination (to minimize contamination of the tissues by blood radioactivity). The pyrimethamine concentrations 12 hours after this single dose were serum, 1.02 μg/ml; retina, 3.2 μg/ml; aqueous 0.03 μg/ml; and vitreous, no measurable radioactivity. For comparison, 2.5 μg/ml may be attained in human serum with a pyrimethamine dosage of 50 mg/day. *Toxoplasma* organisms in tissue culture may be killed by exposure to 0.25 μg/ml for 4 days.

Autoradiography was also performed with these monkey eyes.[169] Retinal radioactivity was three times and uveal radioactivity two times that of the blood. Sclera was not radioactive.

There is little chance that pyrimethamine alone will have a therapeutic effect on the eye. Subconjunctival injection of 0.05 mg of pyrimethamine in a 0.5 ml volume produced aqueous levels of 10 μg/ml (1 mg/100 ml) within 60 minutes in rabbits.[169] This aqueous level fell very rapidly (to 1 μg/ml in 2 hours). No measurable vitreous concentration was attained. Daily subconjunctival injection of 0.05 mg of pyrimethamine in rabbits was well tolerated for 2 months, causing only minimal cyclitis, which was evident on histopathologic examination. Retrobulbar injections of 0.1 mg in a 1 ml volume failed to introduce a measurable amount of pyrimethamine into the vitreous. Unfortunately pyrimethamine concentrations in the uveal tract after local injection were not measured. Injection of 0.5 to 5 mg (why so much?) into the aqueous or vitreous destroyed the eyes.

Response of Toxoplasma organisms

The sensitivity of *Toxoplasma* strains to pyrimethamine varies with their rate of growth. Experimental work is usually done with rapidly multiplying strains, which may be killed by 0.3 mg/100 ml of the drug. Clinical infection is usually caused by more slowly growing organisms that may be killed by 1 to 5 mg/100 ml in 5 days. Obviously the clinically attainable pyrimethamine concentrations are not high enough to kill resistant strains. Encysted and dormant *Toxoplasma* organisms are not affected by pyrimethamine, but then neither do they cause inflammation (although they may become active at some future time). Cure of a disease by an antibacterial drug does not require that all of the organisms be killed, but rather that their growth be slowed sufficiently to permit the body's defenses to control them. It has been demonstrated that pyrimethamine levels of 0.1 mg/100 ml inhibit the growth of *Toxoplasma* organisms in tissue culture.[170] This strain was killed by 1 mg/100 ml.

Because of considerable variations in the resistance and virulence of various strains of *Toxoplasma*, the clinical course and response to therapy will vary greatly. Because of the uncertainty of these variables, treatment should entail the highest drug dosage tolerated without toxic side effects.[171]

Two types of *Toxoplasma* infection have been described.[172] The *encysted form* is more common clinically and is characterized by acutely developing focal chorioretinitis with an exudative and often hemorrhagic appearance. Irritant or sensitizing material is believed to be discharged when the cysts rupture, resulting in intense, necrotizing inflammation. Organisms liberated from a ruptured cyst are usually destroyed in the ensuing inflammation. The episodes of cyst rupture are therefore usually self-limited, reach a maximum inflammatory size in 1 or 2 weeks, and subside slowly during the following several months, leaving a pigmented scar.

The *proliferative form* of toxoplasmosis is a chronic progressive inflammation resulting from active multiplication of the organisms in the retina. Ocular damage is more extensive in this form of the disease.

Differentiation of the two forms of toxoplasmosis is desirable because systemic corticosteroid treatment (in the same high dosage levels as used in the management of any other uveitis) may reduce the size of the final scar resulting from cyst rupture. Although there is no experimental evidence that corticosteroids promote *Toxoplasma* growth, it seems reasonable to assume that such growth might result from corticosteroid inhibition of defense mechanisms. The prophylactic use of pyrimethamine and sulfonamides is therefore advised during corticosteroid therapy for suspected toxoplasmosis. Some authors believe the proliferative form should not be treated with corticosteroids.

Immunity to toxoplasmosis involves restricting the parasite rather than destroying it. Vaccination of guinea pigs with formalin-killed *Toxoplasma* organisms plus an adjuvant resulted in high titers of complement fixing antibody (1:2048). Despite these high titers, the central nervous system can be readily infected, and living *Toxoplasma* organisms can subsequently be isolated. However, the immunized animals showed only mild clinical signs of illness in response to a standard inoculum that caused high fever, prostration, and death in control animals. Furthermore, immunization greatly reduced the infectivity of guinea pig tissue used for subsequent mouse inoculation. Only 23 of 120 mice were infected by tissue from immunized guinea pigs, while tissue from the controls infected 54 of 60 mice. Attempts to clinically control toxoplasmosis by active and passive immunization have not been reported.

Metabolic differences between Toxoplasma organisms and mammals

Intracellular folic acid and its subsequent active derivatives, as shown in Fig. 6-23, are derived from *p*-aminobenzoic acid by *Toxoplasma* and from folic acid by mammals.[173] Since the folic acid molecule contains a *p*-aminobenzoic acid structure, folic acid can be utilized (although less efficiently) by *Toxoplasma* and will interfere with the therapeutic effect of pyrimethamine, as does *p*-aminobenzoic acid. Folinic acid is poorly utilized by *Toxoplasma* but is effective in mammalian metabolism. Antitoxoplasmic therapy with 25 mg of pyrimethamine and 2 g of sulfadiazine is not weakened by 5 mg of folinic acid, which is sufficient to protect the patient

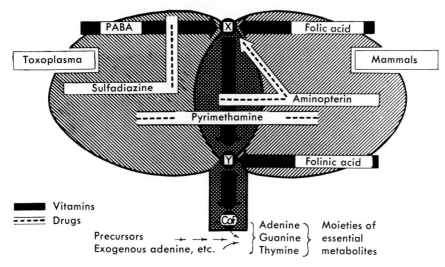

Fig. 6-23. Folic acid metabolism in *Toxoplasma* organisms and in mammals. Note synergistic effect of pyrimethamine and sulfadiazine, which act at two points in sequence on the same metabolic pathway. (From Frenkel, J. K.: Antibiot. Chemother. 7:630, 1957.)

against toxicity. Folinic acid may be given in one fifth the amount of pyrimethamine without inhibiting its therapeutic effect.

Combined sulfonamide and pyrimethamine therapy

Remarkably effective synergism between sulfadiazine and pyrimethamine has been demonstrated in studies of *Toxoplasma*-infected mice.[174] In these studies the median effective dose (MED) was designated as the amount of medication permitting a 50% survival for 10 days in mice given a standard lethal inoculum (1000 LD_{50}) of *Toxoplasma*. In their most efficient combination, $^1/_8$ MED of sulfadiazine combined with $^1/_{24}$ MED of pyrimethamine was the equivalent of 1 MED of either drug alone. Medication was administered via the diet and was expressed in terms of milligrams per 100 ml of diet. The MED of sulfadiazine was 40 mg% and of pyrimethamine, 9 mg%. The most efficient combination MED was 5 mg% of sulfadiazine with 0.37 mg% of pyrimethamine.

Although this sounds somewhat complicated, it clearly indicates powerful synergism between pyrimethamine and sulfadiazine when they are used in combination as therapy for toxoplasmosis. The simultaneous use

of these two drugs is therefore essential in the clinical management of patients with toxoplasmosis. Four grams per day of sulfapyrimidines are recommended.[172,175,176]

The sulfonamides vary in antitoxoplasmic potency; the most effective are the pyrimidine derivatives, sulfadiazine, sulfamerazine, and sulfamethazine.[177] The MED of sulfonamide (the pyrimidines), requires a blood level of 40 mg/100 ml, in contrast to 600 mg/100 ml for sulfanilamide and 450 mg/100 ml for sulfapyridine. The three sulfapyrimidines are best prescribed as a triple sulfonamide combination, for they are independently soluble in the urine and can be administered in higher dosage with less danger of crystalluria. The therapeutic effect of such a triple mixture is additive, being equivalent to the effect of an equal amount of only one sulfonamide compound. Alkalinization with 2 g of sodium bicarbonate daily further reduces the possibility of crystalluria.

The response of presumed toxoplasmic uveitis to pyrimethamine and sulfonamide, spiramycin, and corticosteroid therapies is shown in Fig. 6-24. The pyrimethamine- and sulfonamide-treated infections became inactive in half the time required for those treated with spiramycin.[178] Pyrimethamine

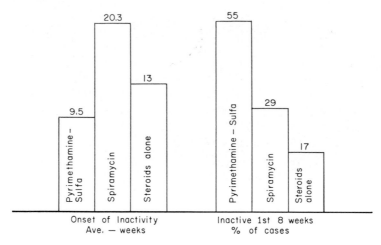

Fig. 6-24. Response of toxoplasmic uveitis to therapy. (From Fajardo, R. V., Furgiuele, F. P., and Leopold, I. H.: Arch. Ophthalmol. **67:**712, 1962.)

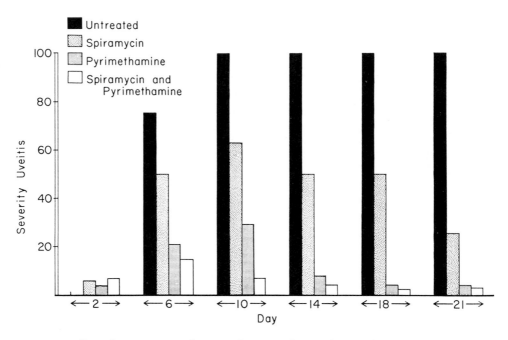

Fig. 6-25. Effect of spiramycin and pyrimethamine, alone and in combination, against experimental toxoplasmic anterior uveitis in rabbits. Vertical height represents severity of uveitis. Each treated group contained four rabbits. (Modified from Giles, C. L., Jacobs, L., and Melton, M. L.: Arch. Ophthalmol. **71:**119, 1964.)

dosage was 25 mg twice a day, following an initial primary dose of 100 mg; sulfadiazine, 1 g four times a day, was the sulfonamide first used and was accompanied by sodium bicarbonate, 2 g three times a day. Subse-quently, sulfamethoxypyridazine (Kynex) was given in dosage of 0.5 g daily. Spiramycin dosage was 1 g four times a day. Contrary to the impression given by the data in Fig. 6-24, the patients receiving pyrimethamine and sulfonamide and spiramycin also received methylprednisolone, 4 mg three times a day.

Tests of the toxicity and antitoxoplasmic effectiveness of spiramycin in rabbits indicate that a dose of 500 mg/kg is toxic.[179] Both 250 mg/kg and 125 mg/kg inhibited experimental anterior uveitis and did not cause systemic complications. The eyes of rabbits receiving 62.5 mg/kg were less inflamed than control eyes and yet had moderately severe uveitis. Experimental study of the possible additive effect of pyrimethamine and spiramycin indicates that combination therapy is slightly superior to the use of either drug alone (Fig. 6-25). However, the evidence of this increased effectiveness is not sufficient to recommend such combined therapy. Note that spiramycin alone is not nearly as effective as pyrimethamine.

Experimental toxoplasmosis in mice is not controlled by spiramycin in sublethal dosage.[180] Six of eight patients presumed to have toxoplasmic retinochoroiditis were not benefited by 2 weeks of spiramycin therapy.

Toxicity

The hematologic toxicity of pyrimethamine is related to the serum levels attained. Eleven patients who suffered no toxic effects had an average serum concentration of 0.25 mg/100 ml, as compared to an average of 0.33 mg/100 ml in eight patients who experienced bone marrow depression.[167] There are, of course, individual variations in sensitivity; one of the patients suffering from toxicity was reported to have a serum level of only 0.16 mg/100 ml. Obviously the therapeutic dose is quite close to the toxic dose, and it is therefore essential to count red cells, white cells, and platelets once or twice a week during pyrimethamine therapy. Please note that hematologic depression occurred in 8 of 19 patients given 200 mg of pyrimethamine the first day and 50 mg/day thereafter.

The hematologic toxicity of pyrimethamine has been studied in 87 patients treated for at least 5 weeks (doses ranging from 25 to 100 mg/day) for uveitis caused by *Toxoplasma* infection. Although bone marrow depres-

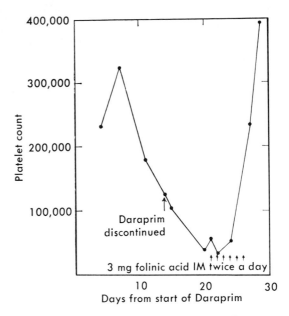

Fig. 6-26. Platelet counts during pyrimethamine (Daraprim) therapy. Drop in circulating platelets usually occurs after a week or more of therapy, continues to decline for a week or so after treatment is stopped, and returns to normal after another week, more or less (regardless of folinic acid). (From Kaufman, H. E., and Geisler, P. H.: Arch. Ophthalmol. **64:**140, 1960.)

sion caused a decrease in red cells, white cells, and platelets, thrombocytopenia was the most severe manifestation of pyrimethamine toxicity. When platelet suppression begins in a patient receiving pyrimethamine, the platelet count usually declines for 3 to 9 days after the drug is discontinued (Fig. 6-26).[181] Normal levels are regained in 1 to 2 weeks. Folinic acid did not hasten disappearance of the thrombocytopenia encountered in these patients.

More than half of the patients in this series developed thrombocytopenia, as evidenced by 150,000 or fewer cells per cubic millimeter. The toxicity of pyrimethamine is greater at higher dosage levels (Fig. 6-27). Ecchymoses and nosebleeds occurred when the platelet counts were below 50,000. Small retinal hemorrhages noted during the course of treatment were attributed to the natural course of the disease, since they are not symptomatic of platelet depression. Therapy

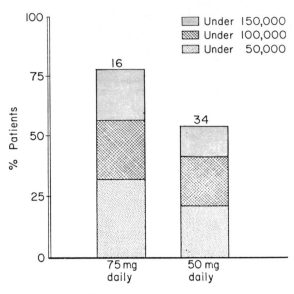

Fig. 6-27. Effect of pyrimethamine therapy on platelet counts. (Modified from Kaufman, H. E., and Geisler, P. H.: Arch. Ophthalmol. 64:140, 1960.)

should be discontinued or reduced when the platelet count drops to 80,000 or below; routine counts should be made twice weekly during treatment.

One of the earliest signs of hematologic depression (by any drug, including pyrimethamine) is hypersegmentation of the neutrophils.[182] Since this change is easily detected in stained blood smears, it is a useful warning sign of early toxicity. Therapy need not be discontinued when hypersegmented neutrophils appear, but the patient must be very closely observed lest the condition worsen. Reduction of dosage should be considered, depending on the clinical status of the retinochoroiditis.

Toxic manifestations of pyrimethamine also include convulsions, which have been described in monkeys and in accidentally poisoned children.[183] Two of these children, both approximately 2 years of age, died in convulsions within 2 hours after swallowing 400 mg of pyrimethamine. (Presumably, large doses of folic acid would be indicated as emergency treatment of accidental poisoning with pyrimethamine. One is again

reminded to caution patients against leaving potent medications within the reach of children.)

When administered to pregnant rhesus monkeys, pyrimethamine produces gross malformations of the fetal skull.[184] Since teratogenic drugs are particularly dangerous during early (and possibly unknown) pregnancy, the treatment of presumed toxoplasmic uveitis in young married women should be initiated only if effective contraceptive measures are being used. The importance of this precaution has been dramatized by the recent thalidomide tragedies, which are well known to both laymen and lawyers.

Folinic acid as antidote

Hematologic complications should be treated with folinic—*not* folic—acid (citrovorum factor [Leucovorin], formyl tetrahydropteroylglutamic acid), administered intramuscularly in amounts of 3 to 9 mg/day. Folinic acid should be used whenever the platelet count drops below 200,000. Pyrimethamine need not be discontinued if only mild cellular depression is observed. Folinic acid can be utilized by the human body and reduces the toxicity of pyrimethamine. *Toxoplasma* organisms, however, cannot utilize folinic acid, which therefore does not inhibit the toxoplasmacidal effect of pyrimethamine. Prophylactic use of folinic acid (3 mg/day) may be instituted when pyrimethamine therapy is started. Such prophylactic use does not impair the effectiveness of pyrimethamine in experimental mouse toxoplasmosis.[185] No toxic effects are reported with recommended doses of folinic acid. Vitamin B_{12} accentuates folinic acid deficiency[186] and should not be used during pyrimethamine therapy, as it will promote hematologic defects; this is a sufficiently marked effect to be of clinical significance. Multivitamin preparations containing folic acid or *p*-aminobenzoic acid will protect *Toxoplasma* organisms against pyrimethamine and therefore should not be used during a course of therapy.[187]

In a series of 14 patients treated with pyrimethamine (200 mg/day for 2 days followed by 25 mg orally twice a day) combined with sulfadiazine (1 g four times a day) and steroids, folinic acid (5 mg orally three times a day) was given from the start of therapy.[188] Only three of these patients (21%) developed thrombocytopenia of below 150,000 (lowest count 95,000). Without the protection of folinic acid, the platelet count in half the patients would have been expected to drop below 150,000 and, in one fourth of them, below 50,000. During the period of treatment the uveitis cleared completely in 12 patients and improved substantially in the remaining two.

The protective effect of folinic acid against pyrimethamine poisoning, without loss of antitoxoplasmic effect, was again demonstrated in experiments with mice.[189] Sixty mice were inoculated with a 100% fatal dose of *Toxoplasma* and were treated with a pyrimethamine dosage of approximately a 100% fatal amount. Of 20 mice treated with pyrimethamine alone, only two survived (deaths caused by drug toxicity). Of 20 mice treated with pyrimethamine and folinic acid (0.0006% of the diet), all survived.

Response of infection to treatment

Conflicting opinions exist as to the effectiveness of pyrimethamine for treatment of human ocular toxoplasmosis. The most difficult clinical problem is to establish whether a given case of chorioretinitis is a result of toxoplasmosis or has some other etiology. The diagnosis is usually presumptive. Also, variations in amount, frequency, and duration of pyrimethamine dosage are sufficiently great to account for differences of clinical opinion.

Experimental inoculation of the guinea pig vitreous with approximately 5000 *Toxoplasma* organisms was treated with the equivalent of a human dosage of 4 g of sulfadiazine and 75 mg of pyrimethamine administered daily.[190] All the infected animals developed chorioretinitis within 2 to 3 weeks despite treatment. Subsequent isolation studies demonstrated persistence of viable *Toxoplasma* organisms in all animals. No evaluation was made as to the relative severity of treated and control chorioretinitis.

Because of the tendency for cyst formation, it seems doubtful that a human infection can be eradicated. Clinical studies suggest that the severity of toxoplasmic chorioretinitis decreases after adequate therapy, which should be continued for at least a month. Typical of the published statistics is the report that 13 of 22 treated patients showed definite improvement, although only 4 patients were classified as being in "excellent condition."[191]

Alternate patients in a series of 164 patients with uveitis were treated with pyrimethamine, 25 mg/day, or with a placebo.[192] This was a "blind" study in that the physician did not know whether pyrimethamine or placebo was given. It was found that 50% of patients on pyrimethamine with a *negative* dye test and 50% of the control patients showed improvement within a month. This confirms that pyrimethamine has no nonspecific therapeutic effect against uveitis. Pyrimethamine is not known to have any effect on allergic conditions and has very slight antibacterial activity. In contrast, 76% of patients with positive dye tests treated with pyrimethamine improved within a month. There was no relationship between the height of dye test titer and therapeutic response, which supports the belief that a localized ocular infection may not cause a large rise in serum antibodies. A higher incidence of positive dye tests (and therefore of therapeutic response) was found for chorioretinitis than for iridocyclitis or panuveitis.

Corticosteroids and mydriatics were employed as usual in these cases, without regard to the dye test results. The distribution of corticosteroid usage was essentially the same for pyrimethamine and placebo groups and apparently did not influence the results.

Because of the significant improvement in many patients who had positive dye tests after pyrimethamine treatment of chorioretinitis, these authors advised a therapeutic trial with pyrimethamine. It is impossible to anticipate whether a given patient will respond to treatment. The current limited availability of the dye test leaves us in an unscientific quandary as to the best management of uveitis. Possibly as much as 25% of the cases of retinochoroiditis are caused by toxoplasmosis.[193]

Doubt is cast on the clinical value of pyrimethamine and sulfonamides by a double-blind study of 20 patients presumed to have active retinochoroiditis caused by *Toxoplasma* infection.[194] Pyrimethamine (200 and 100 mg on the first and second day, respectively, followed by 50 mg/day), triple sulfonamides (2 g/day), and prednisone (40 mg/day) were used in treatment of 10 patients. Prednisone and placebo capsules were used for the other 10 patients. All patients improved significantly within 3 weeks and were almost completely cured within 2 months. There was no significant difference in the response of the two groups to therapy.

Doses of pyrimethamine as low as 10 mg/kg and of sulfadiazine, 20 mg/kg, were ineffective in controlling experimental ocular toxoplasmosis in rabbits, whereas double this dosage was effective.[195] The clinical implication of this finding is that prolonged, very low-level dosage is not likely to be an effective prophylactic measure against recurrent toxoplasmic retinitis. If maintained for 7 days, a concentration of 3 to 4 μg/ml of pyrimethamine will clear *Toxoplasma* from tissue cultures; however, concentrations as high as 10 μg/ml will not clear the infection in less than 7 days. Obviously a clinically tolerated dosage of pyrimethamine will not destroy *Toxoplasma* rapidly (as a single large dose of penicillin might cure gonorrhea); rather, adequate blood levels must be maintained for a long time.

Summary

Without doubt, *Toxoplasma*-inhibiting concentrations of pyrimethamine and sulfonamide can be attained within the retina and choroid using clinically acceptable amounts of medication. The synergism of combined therapy *greatly* enhances the therapeutic effect; combined treatment requires only one eighth as much sulfonamide and one twenty-fourth as much pyrimethamine as would be necessary if either were used alone.

Simultaneously administered folinic—*not* folic—acid results in a 100% survival rate of animals given a lethal dose of pyrimethamine and yet does not decrease the therapeutic effect of the drug.

Platelet counts should be done at least once a week during the course of therapy. Counts below 80,000 require that pyrimethamine therapy be stopped.

Decision to use the drug is difficult because of the uncertainty as to the etiologic diagnosis. Treatment is decidedly unpleasant and not without danger. Prerequisites to pyrimethamine and sulfonamide therapy include a diagnosis of retinochoroiditis sufficiently severe to threaten central vision and a positive (in even the lowest titer) methylene blue dye test.

The role of associated corticosteroid therapy is not certain; nevertheless, simultaneous use of systemic corticosteroids is an accepted practice.

STREPTOMYCIN

Streptomycin is effective against a considerable number of organisms, both gram-negative and gram-positive. Unfortunately many resistant strains have developed; therefore it is not rational to use streptomycin without laboratory demonstration of bacterial sensitivity. Since most gram-positive organisms are much more sensitive to penicillin, it is ordinarily a preferable drug for such organisms. Development of the relatively nontoxic broad-spectrum antibiotics has further decreased the usefulness of streptomycin. Contributing greatly to the reluctance to use streptomycin is its tendency to cause serious damage to the eighth cranial nerve. Probably the most clear-cut indication for the use of streptomycin is the presence of tuberculosis.

Toxicity

I am describing the undesirable characteristics of streptomycin before discussing ocular penetration and dosage to emphasize that these toxic effects are so serious as to considerably limit the ophthalmologic use of the drug.

The selective toxic effects of streptomycin and dihydrostreptomycin are unusual in that they are delayed and may occur weeks or even as late as 6 months after use of the drug. Streptomycin destroys the cristae of the semicircular canals, resulting in vertigo, ataxia, and loss of postrotatory or caloric nystagmus. Dihydrostreptomycin destroys the organ of Corti, causing deafness. The degenerative changes produced by both of these drugs are irreversible. The prophylactic use of streptomycin in routine surgery or its prescription for minor and self-limited infections involve unwarranted risks. Often in such instances a shotgun combination of penicillin and streptomycin is prescribed "just to be on the safe side." The toxic effect of streptomycin is so reliable that 2 g/day for 2 weeks was used to relieve the vestibular symptoms of bilateral Meniere's disease.[196] The total loss of vestibular response in this patient within a 5-week period is illustrated in Fig. 6-28. Marked differences exist in individual susceptibility to these drugs. Because perma-

nent deafness is such a serious handicap, and since streptomycin is equally effective against gram-negative bacteria, dihydrostreptomycin should never be used in ophthalmology.

The frequency of damage to the eighth cranial nerve is extremely high. In a series of 82 patients receiving streptomycin, 1 g/day for 4 months, 30% had vestibular damage and 2.5% had auditory damage. Of 84 patients on the same dose of dihydrostreptomycin, 11% had vestibular damage, and 14% suffered deafness. As little as 1.5 g of dihydrostreptomycin can cause permanent, handicapping nerve deafness.[197]

Streptomycin may also cause the various well-known manifestations of drug allergy. Contact dermatitis is common and may affect nurses, pharmacists, and other personnel in frequent contact with streptomycin. Hence such personnel should be protected by rubber gloves and a mask while handling the drug.

Ocular penetration

After intramuscular injection, streptomycin penetrates the intact eye in therapeutic

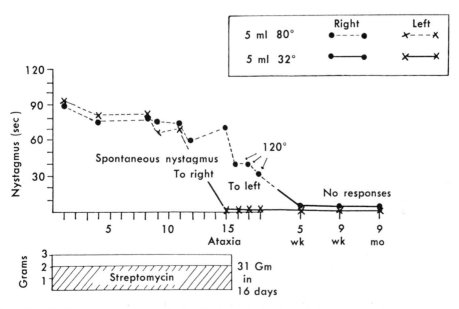

Fig. 6-28. Deliberate human vestibular destruction by 2 g of streptomycin/day, as measured by caloric nystagmus. (From McGee, T. M.: Trans. Am. Acad. Ophthalmol. **65:**222, 1961.)

concentrations. Administration of 10 mg/kg to rabbits (comparable to 0.7 g for a 70 kg patient) results in aqueous concentrations of 8 μg/ml and in vitreous concentrations of 3 μg/ml (Fig. 6-29).[198] Breakdown of the blood-aqueous barrier by paracentesis (presumably similar or greater changes would occur spontaneously in an infected eye) increases the streptomycin concentration to 20 μg/ml of aqueous.

Topically applied streptomycin does not penetrate the intact cornea sufficiently well to be of therapeutic value. Even after a 4-hour corneal bath with a 5% solution of streptomycin, no measurable quantity of drug (less than 6.25 μg/ml) was found in rabbit aqueous.[199]

Transcorneal penetration of streptomycin may be achieved by iontophoresis or by use of wetting agents. Iontophoresis with a 1% concentration of streptomycin hydrochloride for 30 minutes at 2 milliamperes and 22 volts (solution cup connected to anode) will produce a concentration of 25 μg/ml of aqueous. Similar concentrations are achieved with a 2-hour corneal bath with a 1% concentration of streptomycin plus an

effective wetting agent. If the corneal epithelium is experimentally abraded, a 2-hour corneal bath with a 1% solution of streptomycin hydrochloride will give aqueous values as high as 100 μg/ml. Hence therapeutic aqueous concentrations of streptomycin may be achieved by local application of the drug to an infected cornea.

A 1% streptomycin solution is well tolerated, is noninjurious to the conjunctiva and cornea, and does not delay healing of epithelial defects. In contrast, repeated instillation of 5% streptomycin solution delays healing of epithelial defects by at least twice the normal time and will cause corneal vascularization and scarring.

Effective streptomycin concentrations are not attained in the normal vitreous after parenteral injection. (Unfortunately this paper does not report vitreous penetration in the inflamed eye.) Twenty-four hours after intravitreal injection of 100 μg of streptomycin a therapeutic level of 12.5 to 25 μg/ml persists.

Intravitreal injections of 800 μg or less are satisfactorily tolerated by the rabbit eye.[200] However, larger intravitreal doses (as small

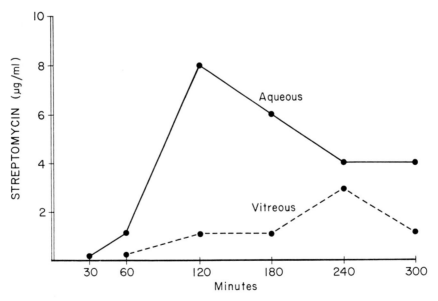

Fig. 6-29. Aqueous and vitreous concentrations of streptomycin after intramuscular injection of 10 mg/kg in rabbits. (Data from Leopold, I. H., and Nichols, A.: Arch. Ophthalmol. **35:** 33, 1946.)

as 1.5 mg) cause severe chorioretinal inflammation and degeneration. Prompt intravitreal injection of streptomycin will arrest vitreous infections caused by small numbers of susceptible organisms.

Dosage

For treatment of acute infections, doses of 1 to 4 g/day are given depending on the susceptibility of the organism and the severity of infection. These larger amounts of streptomycin cannot be given for more than a few days to a week without the risk of permanent vestibular damage.

The treatment of tuberculosis requires months of therapy with low dosage levels (1 g twice weekly). Para-aminosalicylic acid (3 to 4 g three times a day after meals) or isoniazid (100 mg three times a day) is given simultaneously.

Streptomycin is not absorbed from the gastrointestinal tract and therefore must be given intramuscularly.

For topical ocular use, ointments or solutions in a 0.5% concentration are usually tolerated satisfactorily.

Clinical use

In the past, tuberculosis was considered the predominant cause of uveitis. At the present time in the United States, tuberculosis is most certainly an infrequent, if not rare, cause of chorioretinitis.

Retinal perivasculitis has been considered (probably erroneously) to be characteristic of tuberculosis. In a series of 21 patients, antituberculous therapy (streptomycin, 1 g three times a week; isoniazid, 100 mg three times a day; and *p*-aminosalicylic acid, 10 to 12 g/day) did not alter the course of the disease.[201] None of these patients had clinical evidence of active tuberculosis, and only three had positive second-strength PPD skin tests. Pathologic examination of 19 additional eyes showed no evidence of tuberculous lesions or any acid-fast organisms. The response of other forms of clinically encountered uveitis to antituberculous therapy is usually likewise unremarkable.

When ocular infection is known to be the

Table 6-6. Sensitivity of bacteria to streptomycin*

Organism	Sensitivity range (μg/ml)
Aerobacter aerogenes	0.5-64
Escherichia coli	0.3-7.5
Haemophilus influenzae	1.5-5
Pasteurella tularensis	0.15-2
Pseudomonas	1-400
Staphylococcus aureus	0.5-120

*Data from Morgan, H. J., and associates: Streptomycin exhibit, Annual meeting, Medical Society of New Jersey, Atlantic City, 1947.

result of tuberculosis (as in experimental animals, in patients with generalized, active tuberculosis, and in the presence of lesions in which acid-fast bacilli are identified by culture or biopsy), specific therapy produces encouraging results, provided that preexisting destruction is not too severe. For instance, 10 of 14 patients with tuberculous eye infections (treated in 11 Veterans Administration Hospitals) improved after streptomycin treatment.[202] Six months of streptomycin treatment resulted in the cure of a solitary tuberculoma of the sclera (proved by biopsy) in a patient with generalized tuberculosis.[203]

Bacteria vary widely in their sensitivity to streptomycin. This variation exists not only between different species but also between strains of the same species (Table 6-6).[204] Because of this wide variation, rational clinical use of streptomycin requires bacterial isolation and sensitivity studies. This drug is not a first-choice medication for prophylactic or shotgun systemic use.

Summary

The prolonged use of streptomycin is justified only in the treatment of serious infections caused by organisms known to be sensitive to streptomycin and resistant to other less toxic antibiotics. The use of streptomycin is primarily indicated in the treatment of tuberculosis.

Permanent and disabling destruction of

the eighth cranial nerve not infrequently complicates streptomycin therapy.

SULFONAMIDES

The sulfonamide drugs are bacteriostatic by virtue of their ability to prevent bacterial utilization of *p*-aminobenzoic acid. Knowledge that many local anesthetics are esters of *p*-aminobenzoic acid is of practical value, since such drugs (procaine and tetracaine) will interfere with sulfonamide action. Purulent exudate also contains *p*-aminobenzoic acid and therefore interferes with the action of sulfonamides.

Generally, antibiotics have replaced sulfonamides as the first choice for the treatment of major infections. However, for topical treatment of minor ocular infections, sulfacetamide in a 10% to 30% concentration is still a valuable drug. Triple sulfonamides are used with pyrimethamine in the treatment of ocular toxoplasmosis.

Sulfonamides inhibit the growth of most gram-positive and a variety of gram-negative organisms, including *Pseudomonas*. Viral infections, including trachoma, may respond somewhat. Corneal infections by some types of fungi may be arrested by iontophoresis with sulfacetamide.[205] Microorganisms are not killed by sulfonamides, only inhibited.

Sulfacetamide is antagonistic to the inhibition of *Pseudomonas* by gentamicin. Gentamicin alone will inhibit *Pseudomonas* growth at levels of 7 μg/ml. In the presence of sulfacetamide, gentamicin levels of 15 μg/ml are required for inhibition.[206]

Toxic effects

Sulfonamides cause a variety of undesirable reactions. Renal complications are among the most common problems and include crystalluria, hematuria, and anuria. A fluid intake sufficient to produce at least 1000 ml of urine daily will help to avoid renal problems. Since sulfonamides are considerably more soluble in an alkaline pH, sodium bicarbonate greatly reduces the possibility of crystalluria.

Other complications include agranulocytosis, hemolytic anemia, toxic hepatitis, skin rashes and allergy, photosensitization, peripheral neuritis, drug fever, acute psychoses, and transitory myopia.[207,208] Four cases of transitory toxic amblyopia were attributed to moderate doses of sulfonamides.[209] Intravenous sulfonamide preparations are irritating and may cause local thrombophlebitis.

The topical application of sulfanilamide powder to the abraded cornea results in heavily vascularized scars. Epithelial regeneration is slowed greatly, requiring more than 13 days in treated rabbits as compared to 5 days for control rabbits (corneal epithelium completely removed).[210]

Topical use of sulfadiazine ointment for 1 year caused formation of multiple small white concretions within cysts of the palpebral conjunctiva. Spectroscopic studies identified these as being composed of sulfadiazine.[211]

Ocular penetration

The intraocular penetration of topically applied sulfonamides varies considerably in different species, being 5 to 15 times greater in rabbits than in dogs. Apparently the solubility and corneal penetrability of the various sulfonamides vary considerably. Topical application of sulfanilamide ointment (concentration not stated) every 30 minutes for 6 hours resulted in aqueous concentrations of 31 mg/100 ml (rabbit) and 6 mg/100 ml (dog). Corresponding aqueous sulfapyridine concentrations were 2.3 and 1.6 mg/100 ml. Sulfadiazine penetration into the aqueous approximates that of sulfapyridine. A human aqueous level of 22 mg/100 ml has been reported after topical sulfanilamide application.[212]

Intraocular penetration of topically applied sulfonamides seems directly related to their solubility characteristics and inversely related to their ability to combine with protein (Table 6-7).[213]

The intraocular penetration of sodium sulfadiazine is increased by as much as 15 times by iontophoresis, as contrasted to corneal bath. A 5-minute iontophoresis (2 milliamperes, 45-volt battery, cathode on cornea and anode on body) with a 5% solution of

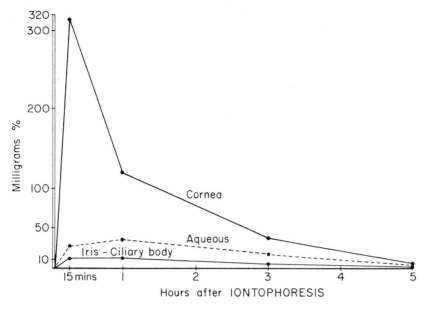

Fig. 6-30. Duration of sulfadiazine concentration attained by iontophoresis on normal rabbit corneas. (Modified from von Sallmann, L.: Am. J. Ophthalmol. **25**:1292, 1942.)

Table 6-7. Comparison of mean aqueous fluid levels with water solubility and albumin-combining capacity of four sulfonamide drugs*

Drug	Mean level in 45 min (mg%)	Water solubilities 37° C (g%)	Albumin-combining capacities (%)
Sulfanilamide	32.8	1.400	20
Sulfapyridine	3.5	0.05	40
Sulfathiazole	1.2	0.096	75
Sulfadiazine	Trace	0.0123	55

*From Gallardo, E., and Thompson, R.: Am. J. Ophthalmol. **25**:1210, 1942.

sodium sulfacetamide resulted in the following concentrations: cornea, 120 mg/100 ml; aqueous, 39 mg/100 ml; and ciliary body, 11.5 mg/100 ml. By contrast, a 5-minute corneal bath with the same solution achieved these concentrations: cornea, 9 mg/100 ml; aqueous, 2.5 mg/100 ml; and ciliary body, 1.7 mg/100 ml.[214] Considerably higher intraocular concentrations are attained if the corneal epithelium is absent (as high as 95 mg/100 ml in the aqueous). This iontophoretic technique was said not to cause biomicroscopically observable corneal damage. The rate of disappearance of sulfadiazine from a rabbit eye is shown in Fig. 6-30.

Similarly, corneal iontophoresis greatly increased the penetration of a 5% sulfathiazole solution into both the cornea (300 mg/100 ml) and aqueous (50 mg/100 ml). However, vitreous penetration of sulfathiazole by iontophoresis is too small to measure reliably.[215] Sulfathiazole penetration into the aqueous humor after oral administration is dependent on the blood levels achieved.[216] Aqueous levels in the normal eye are about one fifth of the blood levels. In contrast, sulfanilamide aqueous levels are about 80% of the blood levels.[217] Partial destruction of the blood-aqueous barrier by infection will increase the intraocular penetration of sulfathiazole in proportion to the severity of the inflammation. In the presence of an experimental vitreous abscess, the aqueous sulfathiazole levels will rise as high as 90% of the blood levels.[218] The penetration into the inflamed eye of other drugs and antibiotics as well as the normal constituents of the blood, such as protein, is similarly enhanced.

After paracentesis the concentrations of sulfanilamide, sulfapyridine, and sulfadiazine in the secondary aqueous are approximately equal to the sulfonamide concentration in the blood. Sulfathiazole penetration of the eye is considerably less than those of the other three sulfonamides and even after paracentesis reaches aqueous concentrations of less than half the blood level.[219]

Clinical use

As soon as the sulfonamides were introduced into clinical medicine, their value in controlling ocular infections caused by susceptible microorganisms became apparent.[220,221] However, the prognosis for salvage of eyes with really serious infections (for example, panophthalmitis after cataract extraction) remained poor despite the use of sulfonamides.[222]

In 26 cases of chronic staphylococcal blepharoconjunctivitis (identified by culture) all of the eyes healed within 25 days or less after treatment with 5% sulfathiazole ointment.[223] In contrast, the treatment of 22 patients with silver nitrate and mercury oxycyanide resulted in nine infections becoming chronic and persisting for many months. The cases of nonstaphylococcal acute conjunctivitis identified in this study were self-limited and healed rapidly whether treated with sulfonamides or silver nitrate. Not surprisingly, cases of conjunctivitis in which no significant bacteriologic pathogens were isolated failed to respond to sulfonamide therapy.

Although sulfonamides have largely been replaced by antibiotics, topical use of sulfacetamide (a 30% solution or a 10% ointment) is still a highly effective prophylaxis against corneal infection after abrasions or the entry of superficial foreign bodies and in the treatment of preexisting infections caused by susceptible organisms.[224] The sulfacetamide is instilled at the time of the first office visit and is dispensed to the patient to be used three or four times daily until epithelial healing has occurred. Although the 30% solution burns somewhat, this initial irritation is followed by an analgesic effect that is quite advantageous in the management of corneal epithelial defects. Such sulfacetamide prophylaxis was used over a 5-year period in a busy industrial practice and not a single case of drug sensitivity was encountered. No case progressed to corneal ulceration.[225] With the topical use of 30% sulfacetamide solution, intracorneal concentrations as high as 0.1% can be achieved within 5 minutes.

Sulfonamide therapy is an important supplement to pyrimethamine in the treatment of retinochoroiditis presumably caused by toxoplasmosis. The amount of pyrimethamine needed is greatly reduced by the synergistic effect of sulfonamides, thereby decreasing the risk of toxic side effects.[226] A total of 2 g is administered daily in four divided doses. Use of triple sulfonamides (sulfadiazine, sulfamerazine, and sulfamethazine) is said to reduce the danger of crystalluria.

Summary

The topical application of sodium sulfacetamide (30% solution and 10% ointment) is effective against surface ocular infections caused by a variety of microorganisms. For this purpose, sulfacetamide still compares favorably with the newer antibiotics.

Systemic administration of sulfonamides is no longer indicated in ophthalmic therapy, with the exception of the pyrimethamine and sulfonamide regiment for toxoplasmosis. Adequate intake of water and sodium bicarbonate will reduce the incidence of crystalluria.

TETRACYCLINES

The tetracycline group of antibiotics includes chlortetracycline (Aureomycin), demethylchlortetracycline (Declomycin), oxytetracycline (Terramycin), and tetracycline (Achromycin, Tetracyn). The tetracyclines are termed broad-spectrum antibiotics because of their ability to inhibit the activity of a wide variety of gram-positive organisms, many gram-negative organisms (including *Escherichia coli, Aerobacter, Klebsiella, Bacillus subtilis,* and *Neisseria gonorrhoeae*), *Rickettsia* sp., *Actinomyces, Spirochaeta* sp., and some of the large viruses (including those that cause inclusion conjunctivitis, trachoma, lymphogranuloma venereum, psittacosis, and molluscum contagiosum). Trichomonads, organisms causing tularemia, amebas, pinworms, and anthrax bacilli also respond to tetracycline therapy. Not all strains of these organisms are susceptible; for example, one third or more of staphylococcal strains may be highly resistant. *Pseudomonas aeruginosa* and *Proteus vulgaris* are rarely responsive to tetracycline. Herpetic infections are probably not benefited by tetracycline therapy.

Concentrations of the tetracyclines ranging from 1 to 8 μg/ml are usually adequate to inhibit growth of susceptible bacteria. Cross-resistance within the tetracycline group does not necessarily occur; however, there is little difference in therapeutic effectiveness among the tetracycline derivatives. Hence, if a patient fails to respond to one tetracycline, there is rarely any advantage in changing to another member of this same group of antibiotics.[227]

Dosage

From 1 to 4 g may be given daily in divided doses every 6 to 8 hours. Comparable amounts may be given intravenously if necessary, but therapy should be changed to the oral route as soon as practicable because of the possibility of phlebitis. For topical ocular use, 0.5% ointment is prescribed and the frequency of application is determined by the severity of the infection.

Significant serum concentrations are reached within an hour after oral dosage, reach a maximum level at 4 to 6 hours, and persist to some degree for as long as 24 hours. Dosage of 1 g every 6 hours will achieve minimal, sustained serum levels as high as 5 μg/ml.

Toxicity

Nausea, vomiting, and diarrhea may complicate oral dosage. Aluminum hydroxide gels markedly reduce absorption and therefore should not be used to relieve gastrointestinal symptoms. Thrombophlebitis may occur at the site of intravenous injection. Photosensitivity reactions, manifested by marked erythema after exposure to sunlight, have been reported. Overgrowth of nonsusceptible organisms (such as *Candida albicans*) may follow tetracycline therapy.

The intravenous LD_{50} of oxytetracycline in mice is 100 mg/kg. Daily oral doses of 500 mg/kg may be tolerated by dogs for as long as 2 months. Obviously there is a wide margin of safety between therapeutic and toxic doses.

In nine reported instances, death occurred late in pregnancy after prolonged intravenous use of high doses (up to 6 g/day) of tetracyclines. Autopsy revealed extensive fatty degeneration of the liver in all cases.[228]

Tetracycline that has deteriorated from aging in a moist environment may be highly nephrotoxic. Acute necrosis of the renal convoluted tubules may follow use of only a few such outdated capsules. Fortunately such a lesion is reversible.[229,230]

Intracranial hypertension with papilledema may follow tetracycline therapy in infants and children.[231]

Ocular penetration

When applied by corneal bath, oxytetracycline does not materially penetrate the intact rabbit cornea. If as much as one third of the corneal epithelium is abraded, a 5-minute bath with a 0.5% solution of oxytetracycline hydrochloride may produce aqueous levels of 28 μg/ml when measured 30 minutes after treatment. Similar application of chlortetracycline to the abraded cornea produced aqueous levels of 8 μg/ml.[232]

Oxytetracycline or chlortetracycline was

given intravenously to rabbits in a dosage of 30 mg/kg (dosage was comparable to 2.1 g in a 70 kg man). Aqueous samples withdrawn 100 minutes later contained 3 μg of oxytetracycline/ml. No measurable concentrations of chlortetracycline were achieved.[232]

Therapy of ocular infections

Surface ocular infections caused by susceptible microorganisms respond well to topical tetracycline application. The incidence of allergy and irritation is insignificant. Although intraocular penetration of tetracyclines is poor, large oral doses (6 to 8 g/day) produce demonstrable aqueous concentrations and may be advised for the treatment of intraocular infections.

Acute trachoma may be cured by topical application of the tetracyclines. An ointment vehicle is most effective. Treatment must be continued for 2 to 4 weeks.[233-236]

The prophylactic use of topical tetracycline antibiotics in the eyes of newborn children has been effective in several thousand patients.[237-240] The eyes of antibiotic-treated infants were open, clean, and noninflamed, in contrast to the reddened, irritated, closed eyes that characteristically persist for 3 to 4 days after use of silver nitrate. Secondary bacterial conjunctivitis (75% staphylococcal) was reported in 17% to 26% of the eyes treated with silver nitrate, in contrast to 2.3% to 5% of the eyes treated with tetracyclines. Because there is a wide spectrum of tetracycline antibiotics, which are safe, nonirritating, and reduce secondary infection, their use should replace the standard Credé prophylaxis of silver nitrate.

Identification of neoplasms

Oxytetracycline (Terramycin) is preferentially concentrated in rapidly growing neoplastic tissue.[241] The presence of oxytetracycline in tissue can be detected at the time of surgery by examination under ultraviolet light, which causes a brilliant yellow fluorescence. This method of tumor detection is applicable to the surgery of orbital neoplasms and will help to determine the completeness of malignant tissue removal. Intraocular neoplasms do not selectively

concentrate enough oxytetracycline to be diagnostically helpful. Possibly this is because of the inability of tetracyclines to penetrate the eye in high concentrations relative to its penetration of other tissues. Although a melanoma will not selectively fluoresce within the eye, it does so when it has extended extraocularly into the orbital tissue.

The dose of oxytetracycline required for the fluorescent detection of a neoplasm is 15 mg/kg/day for 3 days. (This is approximately 1 g/day for an adult.) No oxytetracycline is administered for at least 12 hours prior to surgery in order to permit high concentrations of the drug to leave normal structures.

Summary

The tetracycline derivatives are remarkably nontoxic antibiotics, highly effective against a wide variety of microorganisms. Unfortunately they penetrate poorly into the eye. At least 6 to 8 g/day should be given orally if these antibiotics are indicated for the treatment of an infection within the eye.

Pseudomonas, *Proteus*, and many strains of *Staphylococcus* are resistant to the tetracyclines.

TOBRAMYCIN

Tobramycin is yet another aminoglycoside antibiotic. Its actions closely resemble those of its better known relative, gentamicin. It is as effective as gentamicin against *Pseudomonas* and resistant staphylococci, as well as other gram-negative organisms.[242]

Tobramycin reaches an aqueous level of 5 μg/ml 1 hour after subconjunctival injection of 5 mg (rabbit).[243]

VANCOMYCIN

Vancomycin hydrochloride is a bactericidal antibiotic that is highly active against gram-positive cocci. Indeed, all clinically isolated strains of *Staphylococcus* tested as of 1962 were sensitive to vancomycin, which is therefore one of the drugs of choice in treating severe infections caused by resistant strains of this organism. Staphylococci are generally sensitive to less than 5 μg/ml (a plasma level of 60 μg/ml is still present 4

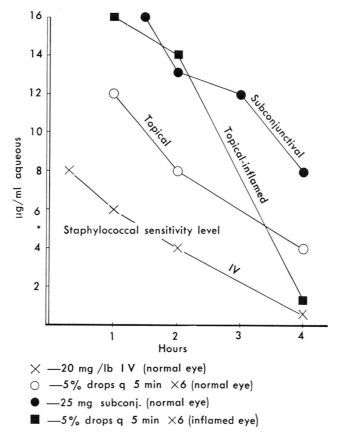

Fig. 6-31. Aqueous levels of vancomycin attained by various routes of administration in rabbits. (Modified from Pryor, J., Apt, L., and Leopold, I. H.: Arch. Ophthalmol. **67:**608, 1962.)

hours after intravenous administration of 20 mg/pound).

Streptococci, enterococci, corynebacteria, and clostridia are also sensitive to vancomycin.

Ocular penetration

The intraocular penetration of vancomycin is shown in Fig. 6-31.[244] Therapeutically effective aqueous levels of vancomycin were attained by topical, subconjunctival, or intravenous routes of administration in normal and inflamed eyes. No vancomycin was detected in most vitreous samples.

Dosage

Topical administration of 5% vancomycin solution is well tolerated, producing only occasional punctate corneal staining. Although vancomycin ophthalmic preparations are not commercially available, a 5% solution is easily made by adding 10 ml of sterile water to 500 mg of vancomycin prepared for intravenous use. Subconjunctival injection of 25 mg of vancomycin causes a slight chemosis lasting 48 hours. Tolerance of intraocular injections of vancomycin has not been evaluated.

Vancomycin is not absorbed from the gastrointestinal tract and is too irritating for intramuscular injection. Hence, for parenteral use, it must be given intravenously. The usual adult dose is 2 g daily in four divided doses. The infusion should be given in a 100 ml volume of isotonic solution over a period of 20 to 30 minutes.

Toxicity

The most serious complication of vancomycin therapy is deafness, which may be permanent. Ototoxicity is more likely to occur with high serum levels of the drug, which may result from excessive dosage or from decreased renal excretion (usually in patients with preexisting renal disease).

Summary

Vancomycin is one of the most effective antibiotics against resistant staphylococci. It penetrates the eye well. Ototoxicity limits its systemic use.

FUTURE ANTIBIOTICS OF CHOICE

The continuous development of new antibiotics and the changing susceptibility of microorganisms will surely modify the future choice of an individual antibiotic. However, the general facts of antibiotic use are so well established that a sound understanding of these principles will be helpful, regardless of the development of new drugs.

REFERENCES

1. Roberts, A. W., and Visconti, J. A.: The rational and irrational use of systemic antimicrobial drugs, Am. J. Hosp. Pharm. **29:** 823, October 1972.
2. Simmons, H. E., and Stolley, P. D.: Trends and consequences of antibiotic use in the United States, J.A.M.A. **227:**1023, March 4, 1974.
3. Karch, F. E., and Lasagna, L.: Adverse drug reactions, J.A.M.A. **234:**1236, December 22, 1975.
4. Suie, T., Havener, W. H., and Sroufe, S. A.: In vitro sensitivity of Micrococcus pyogenes to the commonly used antibiotics, Br. J. Ophthalmol. **40:**100, 1956.
5. Hallett, J. W., Wolkowicz, M. I., and Leopold, I. H.: Ophthalmic use of Neosporin, Am. J. Ophthalmol. **41:**850, 1956.
6. Leibowitz, H. M., Pratt, M. V., Flagstad, I. J., Berrospi, A. R., and Kundsin, R.: Human conjunctivitis. I. Diagnostic evaluation, Arch. Ophthalmol. **94:**1747, October 1976.
7. Leibowitz, H. M., Pratt, M. V., Flagstad, I. J., Berrospi, A. R., and Kundsin, R.: Human conjunctivitis. II. Treatment, Arch. Ophthalmol. **94:**1752, October 1976.
8. Locatcher-Khorazo, D., and Guiterrez, E.: Eye infections following cataract extractions, Am. J. Ophthalmol. **41:**981, 1956.
9. Hughes, W., Jr., and Owens, W. C.: Postoperative complications of cataract extraction, Arch. Ophthalmol. **38:**577, 1947.
10. Richards, R. D., and Catzen, M.: Statistics of eye collections, Ann. Ophthalmol. **7:** 221, February 1975.
11. Binder, P. S., and Worthen, D. M.: A continuous-wear hydrophilic lens, Arch. Ophthalmol. **94:**3109, December 1976.
12. Waring, G. O., III, and Flanagan, J. C.: Pneumocephalus, Arch. Ophthalmol. **93:** 847, September 1975.
13. Leopold, I. H.: Antibiotics and antifungal agents, Invest. Ophthalmol. **3:**504, 1964.
14. Marr, W. G.: Regeneration of corneal epithelium, Am. J. Ophthalmol. **34:**609, 1951.
15. Marr, W. G., Woods, R., and Grieves, M.: Regeneration of corneal epithelium, Am. J. Ophthalmol. **37:**544, 1954.
16. Fedukowicz, H., Wise, G. N., and Zaret, M. M.: Toxic conjunctivitis due to antibiotics, Am. J. Ophthalmol. **40:**849, 1955.
17. Halbert, S. P., Locatcher-Khorazo, D., Sonnkazar, C., and Swick, L.: Further studies on the incidence of antibiotic-producing microorganisms of the ocular flora, Arch. Ophthalmol. **58:**66, 1957.
18. Ley, A. P.: Experimental fungus infections of the cornea, Am. J. Ophthalmol. **42:**59, 1956.
19. Seligmann, E.: Virulence enhancing activities of aureomycin on Candida albicans, Proc. Soc. Exp. Biol. Med. **79:**481, 1952.
20. Rheins, M. S., Suie, T., and Van Winkle, M. G.: Further investigation of the effects of antibiotics, Am. J. Ophthalmol. **59:**221, 1965.
21. Naumann, G., Green, W. R., and Zimmerman, L. E.: Mycotic keratitis, Am. J. Ophthalmol. **64:**668, 1967.
22. Olson, C. L.: Fungal contamination of conjunctiva and lid margin, Arch. Ophthalmol. **81:**351, 1969.
23. Leopold, I. H.: The ophthalmologist and perinatal pharmacology, Arch. Ophthalmol. **77:**575, 1967.
24. Andriole, V. T., and Kravetz, H. M.: The use of amphotericin B in man, J.A.M.A. **180:**269, 1962.
25. Seabury, J. H., and Dascomb, H. E.: Results of the treatment of systemic mycoses, J.A.M.A. **188:**509, 1964.
26. Butler, W. T.: Pharmacology, toxicity, and therapeutic usefulness of amphotericin B, J.A.M.A. **195:**371, 1966.
27. Wood, T. O., and Williford, W.: Treatment of keratomycosis with amphotericin B 0.15%, Am. J. Ophthalmol. **81:**847, June 1976.

28. Brandriss, M. W., Wolff, S. M., Moores, R., and Stohlman, F., Jr.: Anemia induced by amphotericin B, J.A.M.A. **189:**663, 1964.

29. Green, W. R., Bennett, J. E., and Goos, R. D.: Ocular penetration of amphotericin B, Arch. Ophthalmol. **73:**769, 1965.

30. Foster, J. B. T., Almeda, E., Littman, M. L., and Wilson, M. E.: Some intraocular and conjunctival effects of amphotericin B in man and in rabbit, Arch. Ophthalmol. **60:** 555, 1958.

31. Axelrod, A. J., Peyman, G. A., and Apple, D. J.: Toxicity of intravitreal injection of amphotericin B, Am. J. Ophthalmol. **76:**578, October 1973.

32. Axelrod, A. J., and Peyman, G. A.: Intravitreal amphotericin B treatment of experimental fungal endophthalmitis, Am. J. Ophthalmol. **76:**584, October 1973.

33. Anderson, B., Roberts, S., Gonzalez, C., and Chick, E.: Mycotic ulcerative keratitis, Arch. Ophthalmol. **62:**169, 1959.

34. Gordon, M. A.: Corneal allescheriosis, Arch. Ophthalmol. **62:**758, 1959.

35. Montana, J. A., and Sery, T. W.: Effect of fungistatic agents on corneal infections with Candida albicans, Arch. Ophthalmol. **60:**1, 1958.

36. Barsky, D.: Keratomycosis, Arch. Ophthalmol. **61:**547, 1959.

37. Dudley, M. A., and Chick, E. W.: Corneal lesions produced in rabbits by an extract of Fusarium moniliforme, Arch. Ophthalmol. **72:**346, 1964.

38. Faulkner, R. F.: Ocular coccidioidomycosis, Am. J. Ophthalmol. **53:**822, 1962.

39. Falls, H., and Giles, C.: The use of amphotericin B in selected cases of chorioretinitis, Am. J. Ophthalmol. **49:**1288, 1960.

40. Sethi, K. K., and Schwartz, J.: Amphotericin B in ocular histoplasmosis of rabbits, Arch. Ophthalmol. **75:**818, 1966.

41. Olurin, O., Lucas, A. O., and Oyediran, A. B. O.: Orbital histoplasmosis due to Histoplasma duboisii, Am. J. Ophthalmol. **68:** 14, 1969.

42. Harrell, E. R., Wolter, J. R., and Gutow, R. F.: Localized aspergilloma of the eyelid, Arch. Ophthalmol **76:**322, 1966.

43. Meleney, F. L.: Bacitracin therapy, Am. J. Ophthalmol. **133:**675, 1947.

44. Bellows, J. G., and Farmer, C. J.: The use of bacitracin in ocular infection. Bacitracin therapy in experimental and clinical ocular infection, Am. J. Ophthalmol. **37:**1211, 1948.

45. Riley, F. C., Goyle, G. L., and Leopold, I.: Intraocular penetration of cephaloridine in humans, Am. J. Ophthalmol. **66:**1042, 1968.

46. Records, R. E.: Intraocular penetration of cephaloridine, Arch. Ophthalmol. **81:**331, 1969.

47. Moll, T. B., Crawford, J. R., and McPherson, S. D., Jr.: Ocular penetrance of cephaloridine after subconjunctival injection, Am. J. Ophthalmol. **71:**992, 1971.

48. Records, R. E.: Intraocular penetration of cephalothin. I. Animal studies, Am. J. Ophthalmol. **66:**436, 1968.

49. Records, R. E.: Intraocular penetration of cephalothin. II. Human studies, Am. J. Ophthalmol. **66:**441, 1968.

50. Boyle, G. L., Abel, R., Jr., Lazachek, G. W., and Leopold, I. H.: Intraocular penetration of sodium cephalothin in man after subconjunctival injection, Am. J. Ophthalmol. **74:**868, November 1972.

51. Uwaydah, M. M., and Faris, B. M.: Penetration of cephalothin in the aqueous humor of the rabbit, Arch. Ophthalmol. **83:**349, 1970.

52. Boyle G. L., Hein, H. F., and Leopold, I. H.: Intraocular penetration of cephalexin in man, Am. J. Ophthalmol. **69:**868, 1970.

53. Prisco, H. M., and Visconti, J. A.: Review of cephalosporins, Ohio State University Hosp. Pharm. Bull., January 1975.

54. Antimicrobial spectrum of chloromycetin, Therapeutic Notes **57:**168, 1950.

55. Bleeker, G. M., and Maas, E. H.: Penetration of penethamate, penicillin ester, into the tissues of the eye, Arch. Ophthalmol. **60:**1013, 1958.

56. Furgiuele, F. P., Sery, T. W., and Leopold, I. H.: Newer antibiotics: their intraocular penetration, Am. J. Ophthalmol. **50:**614, 1960.

57. Leopold, I. H., Nichols, A. C., and Bogel, A. W.: Penetration of chloramphenicol (Chloromycetin) into the eye, Arch. Ophthalmol. **44:**22, 1950.

58. Leopold, I. H.: Clinical trial with chloramphenicol in ocular infections, Arch. Ophthalmol. **45:**44, 1951.

59. Leopold, I. H.: Surgery of ocular trauma, Arch. Ophthalmol. **48:**738, 1952.

60. Broughton, W., and Goldman, J. N.: The intraocular penetration of chloramphenicol succinate in rabbits, Ann. Ophthalmol. **5:**71, 1973.

61. Beasley, H., Boltralik, J. J., and Baldwin, H. A.: Chloramphenicol in aqueous humor

after topical application, Arch. Ophthalmol. **93**:184, March 1975.

62. Weisberger, A. S., Wessler, S., and Aviolo, L. V.: Mechanisms of action of chloramphenicol, J.A.M.A. **209**:97, 1969.

63. Huguley, C. M., Jr.: Drug-induced blood dyscrasias, J.A.M.A. **188**:817, 1964.

64. Best, W. R.: Chloramphenicol-associated blood dyscrasias, J.A.M.A. **201**:181, 1967.

65. Wallerstein, R. O., Condit, P. K., Kasper, C. K., Brown, J. W., and Morrison, F. R.: Statewide study of chloramphenicol therapy and fatal aplastic anemia, J.A.M.A. **208**: 2045, 1969.

66. Stewart, G. T.: Clinical and epidemiologic impact of penicillins, old and new, Pediatr. Clin. North Am. **15**:24, 1968.

67. Edwards, M. H.: Chloromycetin: special report, Private Practice **3**:42, 1971.

68. Wong, V. G., and Collins, E.: Optic atrophy in cystic fibrosis of the pancreas, Am. J. Ophthalmol. **59**:763, 1965.

69. Lietman, P. S., Di Sant'Agnese, P. A., and Wong, V. G.: Optic neuritis in cystic fibrosis of the pancreas, J.A.M.A. **189**:924, 1964.

70. Harley, R. D., Huang, N. N., Macri, C. H., and Green, W. R.: Optic neuritis and optic atrophy following chloramphenicol in cystic fibrosis patients, Trans. Am. Acad. Ophthalmol. Otolaryngol. **74**:1011, 1970.

71. Council on Drugs, J.A.M.A. **178**:576, 1961.

72. Pico, G.: The management of endophthalmitis following cataract surgery, Arch. Ophthalmol. **59**:381, 1958.

73. Roberts, W.: Topical use of chloramphenicol in external ocular infections, Am. J. Ophthalmol. **34**:1081, 1951.

74. Aragones, J. V., and Eriksen, S. P.: Stable chloramphenicol solution for ocular infections, Am. J. Ophthalmol. **66**:104, 1968.

75. Chastain, J.: Intramuscular chloramphenicol therapy of trachoma, Rocky Mountain Med. J. **51**:191, 1953.

76. Thygeson, P.: Criteria of cure in trachoma, with special reference to provocative tests, Rev. Int. Trach. **30**:450, 1953.

77. Agarwal, L. P., Saxena, R. P., and Gupta, B. M. L.: Antibiotic and chemotherapeutic agents in treatment of trachoma, Am. J. Ophthalmol. **40**:553, 1955.

78. Huamonte, F., Refojo, M., and Banuelos, A.: Expandable silicone implants for scleral buckling. III. Experiments in vivo, Arch. Ophthalmol. **93**:354, May 1975.

79. Sugar, J., and Chandler, J. W.: Experimen-

tal corneal wound strength, Arch. Ophthalmol. **92**:248, September 1974.

80. Drapkin, M. S., Karchmer, A. W., and Moellering, R. C., Jr.: Bacteremic infections due to clindamycin-resistant streptococci, J.A.M.A. **236**:263, July 19, 1976.

81. Pryor, J. G., Apt, L., and Leopold, I. H.: Intraocular penetration of colistin, Arch. Ophthalmol. **67**:612, 1962.

82. Lund, M. H.: Colistin sulfate ophthalmic in the treatment of ocular infections, Arch. Ophthalmol. **81**:4, 1969.

83. Petersdorf, R. G., and Plorde, J. J.: Colistin —a reappraisal, J.A.M.A. **183**:123, 1963.

84. Perkins, R. L.: Apnea with intramuscular colistin therapy, J.A.M.A. **190**:421, 1964.

85. Roy, P. N., Mehra, K. S., and Sen, P. C.: Colistin and gentamicyn in the treatment of *Pseudomonas* corneal ulcer, Ann. Ophthalmol. **6**:1031, October 1974.

86. Jackson, G. G., Lepper, M. H., and Dowling, H. F.: Bacteriophage typing of staphylococci, J. Lab. Clin. Med. **44**:41, 1954.

87. Haight, T. H., and Finland, M.: Resistance of bacteria to erythromycin, Proc. Soc. Exp. Biol. Med. **81**:183, 1952.

88. Council on Drugs, J.A.M.A. **173**:1023, 1960.

89. Naib, K., Hallett, J. W., and Leopold, I. H.: Observations on the ocular effects of erythromycin, Am. J. Ophthalmol. **39**:395, 1955.

90. Jao, R. L., and Jackson, G. G.: Gentamicin sulfate: new antibiotic against gram-negative bacilli, J.A.M.A. **189**:814, 1964.

91. Furgiuele, F. P.: Ocular penetration and tolerance of gentamicin, Am. J. Ophthalmol. **64**:421, 1967.

92. Litwack, K. D., Pettit, T., and Johnson, B. L., Jr.: Penetration of gentamicin, Arch. Ophthalmol. **82**:687, 1969.

93. Golden, B., and Coppel, S. P.: Ocular tissue absorption of gentamicin, Arch. Ophthalmol. **84**:792, 1970.

94. Sloan, S.: Gentamicin penetration, Am. J. Ophthalmol. **73**:750, 1972.

95. Furgiuele, F. P.: Penetration of gentamicin into the aqueous humor of human eyes, Am. J. Ophthalmol. **73**:481, 1970.

96. Webster, J. C., McGee, T. M., Carroll, R., Benitez, J. T., and Williams, M. L.: Ototoxicity of gentamicin, Trans. Am. Acad. Ophthalmol. Otolaryngol. **74**:1155, 1970.

97. Zachary, I. G., and Forster, R. K.: Experimental intravitreal gentamicin, Am. J. Ophthalmol. **82**:604, October 1976.

98. Magnuson, R., and Suie, T.: Gentamicin

evaluation, Am. J. Ophthalmol. **70**:734, 1970.

99. Gordon, D. M.: Gentamicin sulfate in external eye infections, Am. J. Ophthalmol. **69**:300, 1970.

100. Records, R. E.: Gentamicin in ophthalmology, Surv. Ophthalmol. **21**:49, July-August 1976.

101. Knapp, P., and von Sallmann, L.: Treatment of experimental ocular tuberculosis with isoniazid, Am. J. Ophthalmol. **38**:199, 1954.

102. Kratka, W. H.: Isoniazid and ocular tuberculosis, Arch. Ophthalmol. **54**:330, 1955.

103. Coates, E.: Isonicotinic acid hydrazide resistant tubercle bacilli, N. Engl. J. Med. **248**:1081, 1953.

104. Jackson, H., Cooper, J., Mellinger, W. J., and Olsen, A. R.: Group A, B-hemolytic streptococcal pharyngitis—results of treatment with lincomycin, J.A.M.A. **194**:1189, 1965.

105. Becker, E. F.: The intraocular penetration of lincomycin, Am. J. Ophthalmol. **67**:963, 1969.

106. Boyle, G., Lichtig, M. L., and Leopold, I. H.: Lincomycin levels in human ocular fluids and serum following subconjunctival injection, Am. J. Ophthalmol. **71**:1303, 1971.

107. Coles, R. S., Boyle, G. L., Leopold, I. H., and Schneierson, S. S.: Lincomycin levels in rabbit ocular fluids and serum, Am. J. Ophthalmol. **72**:464, 1971.

108. Tabbara, K. F., and Salamoun, S. G.: Accidental intraocular injection of lincomycin, Am. J. Ophthalmol. **73**:596, 1972.

109. Galin, M. A., Davidson, R. A., Harris, L., and Best, M.: Experimental corneal infections, Am. J. Ophthalmol. **66**:447, 1968.

110. Einspruch, B. C., and Gonzalez, V. V.: Clinical and experimental nephropathy resulting from use of neomycin sulfate, J.A.M.A. **173**:809, 1960.

111. Lopez, S. P.: Topical use of neomycin in ophthalmology, Antibiot. Chemother. **4**:1189, 1954.

112. Brennon, J. W.: The use of furacin in ophthalmology, Am. J. Ophthalmol. **35**:1343, 1952.

113. Jeffords, J. V., and Hagertz, R. F.: The healing of donor sites, Ann. Surg. **145**:169, 1957.

114. Fajardo, R. V., Pryor, J., and Leopold, I.: Furaltadone in ophthalmology, Am. J. Ophthalmol. **54**:114, 1962.

115. Smith, J. L., and Creighton, J. B.: Sixth nerve palsy due to furaltadone (Altafur), Arch. Ophthalmol. **65**:61, 1961.

116. Loftus, L. R., and Wagner, A. W.: New allergic reaction to furaltadone, J.A.M.A. **173**:362, 1960.

117. Sery, T. W., Paul, S. D., and Leopold, I.: Novobiocin: new antibiotic, Arch. Ophthalmol. **57**:100, 1957.

118. Bailey, J. C., and Fulmer, J.: Aspergillosis of orbit, Am. J. Ophthalmol. **51**:671, 1961.

119. Fine, B., and Zimmerman, K.: Therapy of experimental intraocular Aspergillus infection, Arch. Ophthalmol. **64**:849, 1960.

120. Mangiaracine, A., and Liebman, S.: Fungus keratitis (Aspergillus fumigatus), Arch. Ophthalmol. **58**:695, 1957.

121. Hewitt, W. L.: The penicillins, J.A.M.A. **185**:264, 1963.

122. Rutenburg, A. M., and Greenberg, H. L.: Oxacillin in staphylococcal infections, J.A.M.A. **187**:281, 1964.

123. Anderson, K., Kennedy, R. P., and Plorde, J. J.: Effectiveness of Ampicillin against gram-negative bacteria, J.A.M.A. **187**:555, 1964.

124. Kurose, Y., and Leopold, I. H.: Intraocular penetration of ampicillin, Arch. Ophthalmol. **73**:361, 1965.

125. Rich, A. M., Dunlap, W. A., and Partridge, J. R.: The effectiveness, safety, and use of carbenicillin in ophthalmology, Am. J. Ophthalmol. **75**:490, 1973.

126. Faris, B. M., and Uwaydah, M. M.: Intraocular penetration of semisynthetic penicillins, Arch. Ophthalmol. **92**:501, December 1974.

127. Uwaydah, M. M., Faris, B. M., Samara, I. N., Shammas, H. F., and To'mey, K. F.: Cloxacillin penetration, Am. J. Ophthalmol. **82**:114, July 1976.

128. Faigenbaum, S. J., Boyle, G. L., Prywes, A. A., Abel, R., Jr., and Leopold, I. H.: Intraocular penetration of amoxicillin, Am. J. Ophthalmol. **82**:598, October 1976.

129. Sorsby, A., and Ungar, J.: Pure penicillin in ophthalmology, Br. Med. J. **114**:4480, 1946.

130. Sorsby, A., and Ungar, J.: Distribution of penicillin in the eye after injections of 1,000,000 units by the subconjunctival, retrobulbar, and intramuscular routes, Br. J. Ophthalmol. **32**:864, 1948.

131. Weimar, V.: Effect of amino acid, purine, and pyrimidine analogues on activation of

corneal stromal cells to take up neutral red, Invest. Ophthalmol. **1:**226, 1962.

132. von Sallmann, L., and Meyer, K.: Penetration of penicillin in the eye, Arch. Ophthalmol. **31:**1, 1944.

133. Boger, W. P., and Flippin, H. F.: Penicillin plasma concentrations, J.A.M.A. **139:**1131, 1949.

134. Bloome, M. A., Golden, B., and McKee, A. P.: Antibiotic concentration in ocular tissues, Arch. Ophthalmol. **83:**78, 1970.

135. Green, W. R., and Leopold, I. H.: Intraocular penetration of methicillin, Am. J. Ophthalmol. **60:**800, 1965.

136. Records, R. E.: The human intraocular penetration of methicillin, Arch. Ophthalmol. **76:**720, 1966.

137. Records, R. E.: Human intraocular penetration of sodium oxacillin, Arch. Ophthalmol. **77:**693, 1967.

138. Goldman, E. E., McLain, J. H., and Smith, J. L.: Penicillins and aqueous humor, Am. J. Ophthalmol. **65:**717, 1968.

139. Goldman, J. N., and Klein, J. O.: Penetration of ampicillin and penicillin G into the aqueous humor, Ann. Ophthalmol. **2:**35, April 1970.

140. McPherson, S. D., Jr., Presley, G. D., and Crawford, J. R.: Aqueous humor assays of subconjunctival antibiotics, Am. J. Ophthalmol. **66:**430, 1968.

141. Records, R. E., and Ellis, P. P.: The intraocular penetration of ampicillin, methicillin, and oxacillin, Am. J. Ophthalmol. **64:**135, 1967.

142. Records, R. E.: Intraocular penetration of dicloxacillin in experimental animals, Invest. Ophthalmol. **7:**663, 1968.

143. Barza, M., Baum, J., Birkby, B., and Weinstein, L.: Intraocular penetration of carbenicillin in the rabbit, Am. J. Ophthalmol. **75:**307, 1973.

144. Boyle, G. I., Gwon, A. E., Zinn, K. M., and Leopold, I. H.: Intraocular penetration of carbenicillin after subconjunctival injection in man, Am. J. Ophthalmol. **73:**754, 1972.

145. Sorsby, A., and Ungar, J.: The control of experimental infections of the anterior chamber and of the vitreous by subconjunctival and retrobulbar injections of crystalline penicillin in doses of 1,000,000 units, Br. J. Ophthalmol. **32:**873, 1948.

146. von Sallman, L., Meyer, K., and DiGrandi, J.: Experimental study on penicillin treatment of exogenous infection of vitreous, Arch. Ophthalmol. **32:**179, 1944.

147. Sorsby, A., and Ungar, J.: Preliminary note on the treatment of hypopyon ulcer by crystalline penicillin in adrenalin in doses in excess of 50,000 units injected by subconjunctival or retrobulbar routes, Br. J. Ophthalmol. **32:**878, 1948.

148. Leopold, I. H.: Recent advances in ocular therapy, N.Y. J. Med. **56:**2803, 1956.

149. Pearlman, M.: Prophylactic subconjunctival penicillin and streptomycin after cataract extraction, Arch. Ophthalmol. **55:**516, 1956.

150. Aronstam, R. H.: Pitfalls of prophylaxis, Am. J. Ophthalmol. **57:**312, 1964.

151. Hahn, R. D., Zellmann, H. E., Naquin, H., Cross, E. S., Jr., and Marcus, D.: Some observations on the course of treated syphilitic primary optic atrophy, J. Chronic Dis. **1:**601, 1955.

152. Kenney, J. A.: Treatment of syphilitic optic atrophy by penicillin, with and without therapy malaria, Am. J. Syph. **37:**449, 1953.

153. Benton, C. D., and Harris, J. F.: Syphilitic optic nerve atrophy treated with penicillin: observations to six years after treatment, Arch. Ophthalmol. **48:**449, 1952.

154. Bietti, G. B.: Repository drugs in the treatment of trachoma, Am. J. Ophthalmol. **47:**220, 1959.

155. Gardiner, P. A., Michaelson, I. C., Rees, R. J., and Robson, J. M.: Intravenous streptomycin: its toxicity and diffusion, Am. J. Ophthalmol. **32:**449, 1948.

156. Zimmerman, M. C.: The prophylaxis and treatment of penicillin reactions with penicillinase, Clin. Med. p. 305, 1958.

157. Waldbott, G. L.: Anaphylactic death from penicillin, J.A.M.A. **139:**526, 1949.

158. Becker, R. M.: Effect of penicillinase on circulating penicillin, N. Engl. J. Med. **254:**952, 1956.

159. Noe, C. A.: Penicillin treatment of eyelid infections, Am. J. Ophthalmol. **30:**477, 1947.

160. Newmark, E., Ellison, A. C., and Kaufman, H. E.: Pimaricin therapy of cephalosporium and fusarium keratitis, Am. J. Ophthalmol. **69:**458, 1970.

161. Jones, D. B., Forster, R. K., and Rebell, G.: Fusarium solani keratitis treated with natamycin (Pimaricin), Arch. Ophthalmol. **88:**147, 1972.

162. Newmark, E., Ellison, A. C., and Kaufman, H. E.: Combined pimaricin and dexamethasone therapy of keratomycosis, Am. J. Ophthalmol. **71**:718, 1971.

163. Ellison, A. C.: Intravitreal effects of pimaricin in experimental fungal endophthalmitis, Am. J. Ophthalmol. **81**:157, February 1976.

164. Williams, R. K., Hench, M. E., and Guerry, D.: Pyocyaneus ulcer, Am. J. Ophthalmol. **37**:538, 1954.

165. Moorman, L. T., and Harbert, F.: Treatment of Pseudomonas corneal ulcers, Arch. Ophthalmol. **53**:345, 1955.

166. McNeel, J. W., Wood, R. M., and Senterfit, L. B.: Effect of polymyxin B sulfate on Pseudomonas corneal ulcers, Arch. Ophthalmol. **66**:62, 1961.

167. Kaufman, H. E., and Caldwell, L. A.: Pharmacological studies of pyrimethamine (Daraprim) in man, Arch. Ophthalmol. **61**:885, 1959.

168. Kaufman, H. E.: The penetration of Daraprim (pyrimethamine) into the monkey, Am. J. Ophthalmol. **52**:402, 1961.

169. Chang, S. C.: Penetration of pyrimethamine (Daraprim) into ocular tissues of rabbits, Arch. Ophthalmol. **60**:603, 1958.

170. Cook, M. K., and Jacobs, L.: The effect of pyrimethamine and sulfadiazine on Toxoplasma in tissue culture, Am. J. Trop. Med. **5**:376, 1956.

171. Kaufman, H. E., Remington, J., Melton, M., and Jacobs, L.: Relative resistance of slow-growing strains of Toxoplasma gondii to pyrimethamine (Daraprim), Arch. Ophthalmol. **62**:611, 1959.

172. Frenkel, J. K., and Jacobs, L.: Ocular toxoplasmosis, Arch. Ophthalmol. **59**:260, 1959.

173. Frenkel, J. K.: A metabolic difference between toxoplasma and mammals, Antibiot. Chemother. **7**:630, 1957.

174. Eyles, D. E., and Coleman, N.: Synergistic effect of sulfadiazine and Daraprim against experimental toxoplasmosis in the mouse, Antibiot. Chemother. **3**:483, 1953.

175. Hogan, M. J.: Ocular toxoplasmosis, Arch. Ophthalmol. **55**:333, 1956.

176. Eyles, D. E.: Newer knowledge of the chemotherapy of toxoplasmosis, Ann. N.Y. Acad. Sci. **64**:252, 1956.

177. Eyles, D. E.: The relative activity of the common sulfonamides against experimental toxoplasmosis in the mouse, Am. J. Trop. Med. **2**:54, 1953.

178. Fajardo, R. V., Furgiuele, F. P., and Leopold, I. H.: Treatment of toxoplasmosis uveitis, Arch. Ophthalmol. **67**:712, 1962.

179. Giles, C. L., Jacobs, L., and Melton, M. L.: Chemotherapy of experimental toxoplasmosis, Arch. Ophthalmol. **71**:119, 1964.

180. Cassady, J. V., Bahler, J. W., and Hinken, M. V.: Spiramycin for toxoplasmosis, Am. J. Ophthalmol. **57**:227, 1964.

181. Kaufman, H. E., and Geisler, P. H.: The hematologic toxicity of pyrimethamine (Daraprim) in man, Arch. Ophthalmol. **64**:140, 1960.

182. McGowan, J. B., Lupovitch, A., and Katase, R. Y.: Daraprim: a folic acid antagonist, Am. J. Ophthalmol. **58**:608, 1964.

183. Grisham, R. S. C.: Central nervous system toxicity of pyrimethamine (Daraprim) in man, Am. J. Ophthalmol. **54**:1119, 1962.

184. Sand, B. J.: Teratogenesis from Daraprim, Am. J. Ophthalmol. **56**:1011, 1963.

185. Frenkel, J. K., and Hitchings, G. H.: Relative reversal by vitamin (p-amino-benzoic, folic, and folinic acids) on the effects of sulfadiazine and pyrimethamine on Toxoplasma, mouse and man, Antibiot. Chemother. **7**:630, 1957.

186. Harris, J. W.: Aggravation of clinical manifestations of folic acid deficiency by small daily doses of vitamin B_{12}, Am. J. Med. **21**:461, 1956.

187. Summer, W. A.: Antagonism of sulfonamide inhibition by para-aminobenzoic acid and folic acid in Toxoplasma infected mice, Proc. Soc. Exp. Biol. Med. **66**:509, 1947.

188. Giles, C. L.: The treatment of toxoplasma uveitis, Am. J. Ophthalmol. **58**:611, 1964.

189. Giles, C. L., Jacobs, L., and Melton, M.: Experimental use of folinic acid in the treatment of toxoplasmosis with pyrimethamine, Arch. Ophthalmol. **72**:882, 1964.

190. Hogan, M. J., Zweigart, P. A., and Lewis, A.: Experimental ocular toxoplasmosis (part II), Arch. Ophthalmol. **60**:448, 1958.

191. Jacobs, L., Naquin, H., Hoover, R., and Woods, A. C.: Comparison of the toxoplasmin skin tests, the Sabin-Feldman dye tests, and the complement fixation tests for toxoplasmosis in various forms of uveitis, Trans. Am. Acad. Ophthalmol. **60**:655, 1956.

192. Perkins, E. S., Smith, C. H., and Schofield, P. B.: Treatment of uveitis with pyrimethamine (Daraprim), Br. J. Ophthalmol. **40**:577, 1956.

193. Woods, A. C., Jacobs, L., Wood, R. M., and Cook, M. K.: A study of the role of toxoplasmosis in adult chorioretinitis, Am. J. Ophthalmol. 37:163, 1954.

194. Acers, T. E.: Toxoplasmic retinochoroiditis: a double-blind therapeutic study, Arch. Ophthalmol. 71:58, 1964.

195. Jacobs, L., Melton, M. L., and Kaufman, H. E.: Treatment of experimental ocular toxoplasmosis, Arch. Ophthalmol. 71:111, 1964.

196. McGee, T. M.: Streptomycin sulfate and dihydrostreptomycin toxicity, Trans. Am. Acad. Ophthalmol. 65:222, 1961.

197. Hawkins, J. E., Jr.: Antibiotics and the inner ear, Trans. Am. Acad. Ophthalmol. 63: 206, 1959.

198. Leopold, I. H., and Nichols, A.: Intraocular penetration of streptomycin following systemic and local administration, Arch. Ophthalmol. 35:33, 1946.

199. Bellows, J. G., and Farmer, C. J.: Streptomycin in ophthalmology, Am. J. Ophthalmol. 30:1215, 1947.

200. Leopold, I. H., Wiley, M., and Dennis, R.: Vitreous infections and streptomycin, Am. J. Ophthalmol. 30:1345, 1947.

201. Kimura, S. J., Carriker, F. R., and Hogan, M. J.: Retinal vasculitis with intraocular hemorrhage, Arch. Ophthalmol. 56:361, 1956.

202. Parisi, P. J.: Ocular tuberculosis treated with streptomycin, Am. J. Ophthalmol. 34:393, 1951.

203. Maiden, S. E.: Solitary tuberculoma of the sclera, Am. J. Ophthalmol. 34:387, 1951.

204. Morgan, H. J., Hunt, J. S., Kent, R., and Carlisle, J. M.: Streptomycin exhibit, Annual meeting, Medical Society of New Jersey, Atlantic City, 1947.

205. Gingrich, W. D.: Keratomycosis, J.A.M.A. 179:602, 1962.

206. Burger, L. M., Sanford, J. P., and Zweighaft, B. A.: The effect of sulfonamides on the anti-Pseudomonas activity of gentamicin in vitro, Am. J. Ophthalmol. 75:314, 1973.

207. Gailey, W. W.: Transient myopia from sulfanilamide, Am. J. Ophthalmol. 22:1399, 1939.

208. Rittenhouse, E. A.: Myopia after use of sulfanilamide, Arch. Ophthalmol. 24:1139, 1940.

209. Taub, R. G., and Hollenhorst, R. W.: Sulfonamides as a cause of toxic amblyopia, Am. J. Ophthalmol. 40:486, 1955.

210. Bellows, J. G.: Chemotherapy in ophthalmology, Arch. Ophthalmol. 29:888, 1943.

211. Boettner, E. A., Fralick, F. B., and Wolter, J. R.: Conjunctival concretions of sulfadiazine, Arch. Ophthalmol. 92:446, November 1974.

212. Chinn, H., and Bellows, J. G.: Corneal penetration of sulfanilamide and some of its derivatives, Arch. Ophthalmol. 27:34, 1942.

213. Gallardo, E., and Thompson, R.: Sulfonamide content of aqueous humor following conjunctival application of drug powders, Am. J. Ophthalmol. 25:1210, 1942.

214. von Sallmann, L.: Sulfadiazine iontophoresis in Pyocyaneus infection of rabbit cornea, Am. J. Ophthalmol. 25:1292, 1942.

215. Boyd, J. L.: Sodium sulfathiazole iontophoresis, Arch. Ophthalmol. 28:205, 1942.

216. Bellows, J. G., and Chinn, H.: Penetration of sulfathiazole in the eye, Arch. Ophthalmol. 25:294, 1941.

217. Scheie, H. G., and Souders, B.: Penetration of sulfanilamide and its derivatives into aqueous humor of eye, Arch. Ophthalmol. 25:1025, 1941.

218. Scheie, H. G., and Leopold, I. H.: Penetration of sulfathiazole into the eye, Arch. Ophthalmol. 27:997, 1942.

219. Liebman, S. D., and Newman, E. H.: Distribution of sulfanilamide and its derivatives between blood and aqueous, Arch. Ophthalmol. 26:472, 1941.

220. Guyton, J. S.: The use of sulfanilamide compounds in ophthalmology, Am. J. Ophthalmol. 22:833, 1939.

221. Thygeson, P.: Sulfonamide compounds in treatment of ocular infections, Arch. Ophthalmol. 29:1000, 1943.

222. Callahan, A.: Effect of sulfonamides and antibiotics on panophthalmitis complicating cataract extraction. Arch. Ophthalmol. 49: 212, 1953.

223. Thygeson, P., and Braley, A. E.: Local therapy of catarrhal conjunctivitis with sulfonamide compounds, Arch. Ophthalmol. 29:760, 1943.

224. Mayer, L. L.: Sodium sulfacetamide in ophthalmology, Arch. Ophthalmol. 39:232, 1948.

225. Kuhn, H. S.: Sodium sulfacetamide in ophthalmology, Trans. Am. Acad. Ophthalmol. 55:432, 1951.

226. Burnham, C. J., and Beuerman, V. A.:

Toxoplasmic uveitis, Am. J. Ophthalmol. **42:**217, 1956.

227. Ory, E. M., and Yow, E. M.: The use and abuse of the broad-spectrum antibiotics, J.A.M.A. **185:**273, 1963.

228. Dowling, H. F., and Lepper, M. H.: Hepatic reactions to tetracycline, J.A.M.A. **188:**307, 1964.

229. Kunin, C. M.: Nephrotoxicity of antibiotics, J.A.M.A. **202:**204, 1967.

230. Mavromatis, F.: Tetracycline nephropathy, J.A.M.A. **193:**91, 1965.

231. Giles, C. L., and Soble, A. R.: Intracranial hypertension and tetracycline therapy, Am. J. Ophthalmol. **72:**981, 1971.

232. Douvas, N. G., Featherstone, R. M., and Braley, A. E.: Role of terramycin in ophthalmology, Arch. Ophthalmol. **46:**57, 1951.

233. Thygeson, P.: Terramycin in ocular infections, Trans. Am. Ophthalmol. Soc. **49:**185, 1952.

234. Mitsui, Y., Tanaka, C., Toya, H., Iwashige, Y., and Yamashita, K.: Terramycin in the treatment of trachoma, Arch. Ophthalmol. **46:**235, 1951.

235. Naggache, R.: Topical use of terramycin ointment in trachoma, Br. J. Ophthalmol. **37:**106, 1953.

236. Bilger, I.: Terramycin therapy in trachoma, J.A.M.A. **149:**1667, 1952.

237. Willcockson, T. H., and Cox, C. D.: Bacteriological studies in newborns using terramycin, terramycin-polymyxin B, and silver nitrate, South Dakota J. Med. Pharm. **6:**147, 1953.

238. Kozinn, P. J., Minsky, A., and Solomons, E.: Oxytetracycline ophthalmic solution in the prophylaxis of ophthalmia neonatorum. In Antibiotics Annual, 1955-1956, New York, 1956, Medical Encyclopedia, Inc.

239. Clark, S. G., and Culler, A. M.: Aureomycin as prophylaxis against ophthalmia neonatorum, Am. J. Ophthalmol. **34:**840, 1951.

240. Musselman, M. M.: Terramycin, New York, 1956, Medical Encyclopedia, Inc.

241. Newell, F. W., Goren, S. B., Brizel, H. E., and Harper, P. V.: The use of iodine-125 as a diagnostic agent in ophthalmology, Trans. Am. Acad. Ophthalmol. Otolaryngol. **67:**177, 1963.

242. Smolin, G., Okumoto, M., and Wilson, F. M., II: The effect of tobramycin on *Pseudomonas* keratitis, Am. J. Ophthalmol. **76:**555, October 1973.

243. Uwaydah, M., and Faris, B. M.: Penetration of tobramycin sulfate in the aqueous humor of the rabbit, Arch. Ophthalmol. **94:**1173, July 1976.

244. Pryor, J., Apt, L., and Leopold, I. H.: Intraocular penetration of vancomycin, Arch. Ophthalmol. **67:**608, 1962.

7
ANTICOAGULANT DRUGS

Anticoagulant therapy has been advocated for diabetic retinopathy and for occlusion of the central retinal artery and vein. Rational or empirical support for anticoagulant treatment of diabetic retinal changes is lacking.[1] Such treatment of vascular occlusions of the eye may seem reasonable; however, the relative infrequency of these cases, their individual variations, and the difficulty of adequately controlling a significant series of patients seriously interfere with assessment of the value of anticoagulant treatment. Occlusions of the central retinal artery so rapidly destroy the retina that little benefit can be anticipated from anticoagulant therapy. Although venous occlusions are believed to result mainly from structural changes in the vessel wall, thrombi may block the remaining lumen. Whether anticoagulant therapy will prevent progressive thrombotic occlusion of an involved vein and permit additional time for collateral venous channels to develop is not clear to me.

HEPARIN

An immediate anticoagulant effect results from intravenous administration of heparin, which antagonizes the action of thrombin. The dosage is 5000 units (45 mg) intravenously every 4 hours. Oral administration is ineffective. The effect of heparin is measured by the clotting time, which should be maintained between 15 and 20 minutes and must be checked before each succeeding dose of heparin. Heparin does not dissolve existing blood clots, nor does it remove atherosclerotic or other abnormalities of the vessel wall.

Antidotes

Bleeding from overdosage of heparin may be almost immediately arrested by intravenous injection of hexadimethrine bromide or protamine sulfate. These drugs combine with heparin to neutralize its antithrombin activity. The dose of either drug is equivalent to the amount of heparin given within the past 3 to 4 hours; that is, 1 mg of protamine sulfate will neutralize 1 mg of heparin.

Hexadimethrine should be given in dilute solution (1 mg/ml) slowly (10- to 15-minute intravenous infusion). Mild and transient side effects include hypotension, dizziness, and generalized discomfort.

Protamine sulfate is injected in 1% solution over a period of a few minutes. The dosage should not exceed 50 mg of protamine every 2 to 4 hours. Protamine is a thromboplastin antagonist and itself prolongs clotting time. However, the affinity of protamine and heparin for each other is sufficiently great that their anticoagulant actions are mutually inactivated.

Tolonium chloride (toluidine blue) is an effective antiheparin medication when given orally, 100 mg three times a day. Obviously its onset of action will be less rapid than that of the intravenous drugs previously described.

Different brands of heparin come in concentrations that may vary from 1000 to 10,000 units per milliliter. This predisposes to serious errors if different vials are interchanged, since personnel may automatically give the same volume, not realizing the concentration differences.[2]

ANTIPROTHROMBIN DRUGS

Coumarin compounds and the phenylindandiones are chemically sufficiently similar to vitamin **K** to substitute for it in the enzyme structure responsible for prothrombin synthesis. By this mechanism, they block vitamin **K** action and prothrombin formation. This blocking effect is reversible and therefore can be overcome by providing an excess of vitamin **K**.

Because of the time required for disappearance of existing prothrombin supplies or for synthesis of new prothrombin, the response to these drugs or to their antidotes is much slower than the heparin anticoagulant effect. One to 3 days must elapse before effective anticoagulant levels are reached. The dosage is governed by prothrombin time determinations, with the intent of maintaining prothrombin activity at about 20% to 30% of normal. Considerable individual variation exists as to drug response; therefore close laboratory control is essential. Patients with liver and kidney disease are particularly likely to be sensitive to these anticoagulants.

Antidotes

If hemorrhage occurs, the vitamin **K** antagonist should be discontinued immediately. Vitamin **K** is given orally (250 mg) or intravenously (50 mg). Vitamin **K** analogues, menadiol sodium diphosphate and menadione sodium bisulfite, may be given intravenously in a dosage of 75 mg. Since formation of sufficient prothrombin to arrest bleeding may take 6 hours or more, plasma or blood transfusion is necessary to stop severe bleeding promptly.

Excessive dosage of vitamin **K** will restore prothrombin time to normal and will make the patient temporarily refractory to antiprothrombin drugs. If the thrombotic condition under treatment still persists, large doses of vitamin **K** will again create the hazard of intravascular clotting that existed before anticoagulant therapy. Hence, if the patient has an unduly low prothrombin time but is not bleeding, only small doses (5 to 15 mg) of vitamin **K** should be given.

COMPLICATIONS

The incidence of complications associated with anticoagulant therapy has been reported for a series of 978 patients whose prothrombin values were maintained at levels one and one half to two times normal.[3] Duration of treatment was longer than 1 year in 83% of patients. Minor bleeding episodes (epistaxis, hematuria, bruising, subconjunctival hemorrhage, menorrhagia, and melena) affected 22% of patients, but these patients did not require hospital care. Major hemorrhages requiring blood transfusions occurred in 1.5% of patients. Approximately half of these major hemorrhages occurred in patients with underlying organic disease (for example, active pulmonary tuberculosis, peptic ulcer, and carcinoma of the colon). Hence careful search for underlying disease is essential in every patient who develops serious bleeding while taking anticoagulants—it is not enough just to reduce or stop anticoagulant therapy. Fifty-five patients died during treatment. Four of these deaths may have been attributable to anticoagulant complications (one case of hematemesis, two cases of cerebral hemorrhage, and one case of myocardial hemorrhage).

CLINICAL USE
Occlusion of retinal vessels

In a study of 120 cases of arteriolar or venous occlusion, 51 were considered of hypertensive and/or arteriosclerotic etiology. Comparison was made between patients who had been treated with anticoagulants and vasodilators (basis for selection of treated or untreated patients not specified). Although the report advocates treatment, even if only for its psychologic value, it states, "On the basis of the therapeutic results which are reported here, one cannot develop any great enthusiasm for the treatment of retinal vascular occlusion."[4] Meaningful comparisons of the very small groups of patients are not possible, but the general impression is that there was little difference between treated and untreated patients.

A review of the literature[5] suggested that after anticoagulant treatment some improvement may be expected in 59% to 70% of eyes with occlusion of the central retinal vein. Of 33 treated patients, 48% improved, with a final average acuity of 0.76. Of 79 previously seen, untreated patients, 49% became worse, 35% were unchanged, and 15% improved. The literature review revealed great variation in reported prognosis after untreated central retinal vein occlusion, ranging from almost no good results to 20% almost normal vision.

The significance of this study is impossible to determine, since the patients selected for treatment were chosen on the basis of good prognosis. Those patients with extensive macular changes or secondary glaucoma were rejected, and individuals retaining fairly good vision were considered the best candidates for therapy. Conversely, patients with a poor prognosis were included in the untreated statistics. Interestingly, the results from a short period of heparin treatment were comparable to those of prolonged bishydroxycoumarin (Dicumarol) treatment. One is tempted to assume that this might mean that the natural course of events is unchanged by either form of anticoagulant therapy. The clinician should consider the fate of one 43-year-old patient whose prothrombin level suddenly dropped to 5% on the thirteenth day of treatment. Despite intravenous administration of vitamin K, she was dead of cerebral hemorrhage within 4 hours. Hemorrhagic complications, ranging from minor to troublesome, affected 28% of the patients in this series (prothrombin level maintained at 20% to 30%).

Rather sudden changes in the effects of drugs may result from interaction with other drugs. For example,[6] ingestion of salicylates by a patient on anticoagulant therapy may prolong prothrombin time enough to result in bleeding. They cite a startling statistic, if true. Extrapolation suggests that 1.5 million hospital admissions every year in the United States are because of disorders caused by drugs.

One of the most optimistic studies of central retinal venous occlusion reported good results in 46% of treated patients (0% of untreated), fair results in 23% treated (12% untreated), poor in 19% treated (12% untreated), and nil in 12% treated (76% untreated).[7] This series consisted of 26 patients and 17 control patients.

Regrettably, the method of selection of control and treated patients is not described in the study. Obviously, from the numerical discrepancy, the patients were not simply alternated. Since the treated patients responded much better and the control patients worse than usually reported, one wonders if some factor of prognostic significance entered into the choice of patients for anticoagulation therapy. Heparin was preferred for treatment and was given intravenously in 150 mg dosages. Details are somewhat vague, but apparently this dose was given four times a day for 10 to 21 days. Bishydroxycoumarin or phenindione was sometimes used during the first few weeks. After the initial intensive therapy, 100 mg heparin was given intravenously twice weekly for months or years as well as 100 mg vitamin E three times a day orally. Death of five control patients (no deaths in treated patients) from cerebral or coronary thrombosis suggested that anticoagulant therapy may have been of value to the general circulation as well as to the eye.

Histologic study of 21 eyes with occlusion of the central retinal vein showed all but two to have severe occlusive disease of the venous wall, either purely degenerative or apparently secondary to chronic inflammation.[8] The two cases resulting from thrombosis were both patients with severe malignant hypertension. Although this report further documents the belief that changes in the venous wall rather than thrombus formation are responsible for occlusion of the central retinal vein, one should recognize that these cases were presumably severe enough to require enucleation and therefore may not be representative of clinically encountered venous occlusions.

To quote from a study[9] of 221 eyes enucleated for hemorrhagic glaucoma: "In not one eye have I found that occlusion of the central retinal vein was due even in part to thrombosis."

If the basis of closure of the central retinal vein or its branches is a structural change in the wall rather than thrombosis, anticoagulant therapy would be of no value.

The spontaneous repair of retinal venous occlusions occurs through the formation of collateral channels. These new veins appear as early as 3 months or as late as a year or more after venous occlusion.[10] Continuance of anticoagulant therapy during this period of time until the new channels are established has been advocated for treatment of venous occlusion. The value of this recommendation is difficult to evaluate, since it is not clear that anticoagulant drugs encourage neovascularizaton. Presumably, prevention of further damage (if achieved) during this period of vascular repair would be beneficial. Nevertheless, I do not completely understand why completion of neovascularization is a better criterion for duration of therapy than would be, for instance, the length of time usually required for organization of a thrombus.

In a retrospective study of 179 patients with occlusion of the central retinal vein and 144 with branch vein occlusion, anticoagulant therapy seemed to have been of benefit.[11] Unfortunately evaluation of such a study is almost impossible. For instance, 25% of the patients with central vein occlusion developed hemorrhagic glaucoma, but only 15% of the anticoagulated patients developed this condition. However, half of the patients with hemorrhagic glaucoma already had this complication when first seen, but of course had not been treated with anticoagulants, and therefore were placed statistically in the untreated category. Obviously this represents a biased preselection of patients and cannot be considered as a control series. Opticociliary anastomoses were found in 15%

of 82 treated eyes and 10% of 41 untreated eyes—probably not a significant difference. In branch venous occlusion, no definite difference could be shown between the treated and untreated groups (about 75% achieved vision of 0.1 or better). In central vein occlusion, vision of 0.1 or better was achieved in 55% of treated and 40% of untreated eyes. Again, the significance of this data depends on the comparability of the groups. As an example of unfair selection, all patients "with malignant hypertension, polycythemia, etc." were placed in the untreated group. The prognosis should be substantially worse in these patients with major systemic disease.

The complications of therapy must also be considered. Anticoagulant therapy was stopped in 7% of these patients because of hemorrhagic complications. Two (0.5%) died of retroperitoneal and of cerebral hemorrhage.

A summary article[11] cited seven references to anticoagulant therapy of retinal vein occlusion: In three of these papers the treatment was found to be of no benefit; in four, favorable results were reported (but the selection of their patients was subject to weaknesses comparable to those of the previously discussed papers).

I incline toward the belief that anticoagulant therapy of retinal vein occlusion is certainly undramatic, at best does not greatly improve the statistical outcome, and at worst is fatal. Is it justified? I do not know, but I am more skeptical than I am convinced.

Senile macular degeneration

Biweekly intravenous injection of 100 mg heparin has been advocated for treatment of macular degeneration.[12] Of an uncontrolled series of 23 such patients, moderate to marked improvement was reported in more than half. Disciform degeneration was said to respond particularly favorably.

Unfortunately similar heparin or placebo treatment of a series of 34 patients showed no difference between treated and control groups over a 6-month period.[13] This controlled series showed that the natural course of senile macular degeneration is spontaneously variable. From month to month, visual acuity may improve and then decrease as much as two lines above or below the initial acuity. Such variability of the disease, combined with the psychologic effects of treatment, can easily be misinterpreted as therapeutic benefit unless the study is controlled.

Retinitis pigmentosa

After treatment with bishydroxycoumarin (Dicumarol) for vascular disease, a patient with retinitis pigmentosa was noted to have an increased visual field and acuity. A series of 37 patients were then treated with Dicumarol, with improvement reported in 33.[14] The prothrombin time was carried at 38 to 40 seconds for about 6 weeks. Improvement was reported as "rapid" without specification of time, and no relapse occurred on cessation of treatment.

Unfortunately further evaluation has not confirmed the response of retinitis pigmentosa to anticoagulant therapy.[15] Since there is no known rational basis for such treatment, and because observation of empirical use of anticoagulants shows no significant improvement, the hazard of anticoagulant therapy is certainly not warranted in treatment of retinitis pigmentosa.

Corneal ulceration

Destruction of corneal stroma by *Pseudomonas* infections may be a result of a bacterial collagenase. (Collagenases may also be of corneal epithelial origin.) Because of the rationale that heparin may inactivate collagenase, *Pseudomonas* corneal ulcers were treated with various combinations of antibiotics and heparin.[16] The heparin was applied topically every 2 hours in a concentration of 2500 units/ml. Fewer rabbit eyes developed descemetoceles in the heparin-treated group.

Ocular symptoms caused by cerebrovascular insufficiency

Intermittent blurring of vision, hemianopia, diplopia, and other cerebral manifesta-

tions may be caused by chronic occlusion of the carotid and vertebral arteries.[17] Of 183 patients with vertebral-basilar disease, 79% had related ocular problems. Two thirds of 124 patients with carotid insufficiency or occlusion had ocular abnormalities.[18] Both groups of patients were reported to respond very favorably to anticoagulants, with prompt relief of ocular symptoms in the great majority of treated patients.

Of a similar group of patients with cerebrovascular insufficiency, only 4% of 115 patients receiving anticoagulant therapy (prothrombin time two to two and one half times normal) developed cerebral infarction. In 40 untreated patients, 40% developed cerebral infarction. After cessation of anticoagulant treatment in 75 patients, 32% developed cerebral infarction.[19]

These reports (all from the Mayo Clinic) certainly encourage use of anticoagulant therapy for incipient vascular occlusions.

Since the development of effective surgical procedures for endarterectomy, mechanical removal of the obstructing material from the carotid artery has become popular.

The Joint Study of Extracranial Arterial Occlusion[20] reports on information derived from 1044 patients with carotid occlusion, registered between 1959 and 1973. Of these, 108 were randomized into a group treated with vascular surgery and 103 were treated medically (details not specified, other than that there was no surgery). Within 30 days after surgery, 43% of this group had suffered additional strokes or death. At the end of 66 months, only 34% of operated patients were still alive, as compared with 63% of unoperated patients still living. Of the total 1044 patients with carotid occlusion, 622 were operated on, indicating the enthusiasm of the surgeons for a procedure that was ultimately shown to reduce survival by one half! The moral I would draw from this is that physicians and patients prefer treatment, whether it works or not. This observation holds as true for medical therapy as for surgical therapy and results in dreadful bias in uncontrolled clinical studies.

Coronary disease in relation to ocular symptoms

Although patients with myocardial infarction have no directly related eye problems, a great deal of our information regarding anticoagulants is derived from such patients. Hence the findings of a recent and well-controlled study may bear some relevance to the treatment of ocular vascular disease.[21] Carefully balanced, but randomly chosen, treatment groups were selected from 178 patients receiving anticoagulant therapy. Most patients had coronary disease, but some had cerebral vascular disease or rheumatic embolic disease. Group 1 was maintained at prothrombin levels from 10% to 25%; group 2, at levels from 30% to 50%; and group 3, at levels over 60%. The study extended for 2 years.

During this time the mortality was the same in all three groups. Significant hemorrhage occurred in seven intensively treated patients—three of these died of cardiac complications within the month. The study suggested the possibility of rebound hypercoagulability when anticoagulant therapy is abruptly terminated. Only one control patient bled—from an ulcer.

The three groups differed greatly in the incidence of nonfatal thromboembolic complications, which numbered one, three, and fourteen in groups 1, 2, and 3, respectively. The rate of development of these complications is given in Fig. 7-1. Except for two emboli, a stroke, and one case of myocardial insufficiency, all of which occurred in group 3, these complications were nonfatal myocardial infarctions.

Group 2 (prothrombin 30% to 50%) fared best. Their incidence of nonfatal complications was only slightly greater than in the more intensively treated group; yet they were entirely free of hemorrhagic problems. Of great practical importance is the less frequent need for blood tests of prothrombin time when the patient is maintained at these safer levels. This is convenient, saves expense, and is psychologically beneficial.

To a certain extent, the rationale for anticoagulant therapy of vascular diseases of the

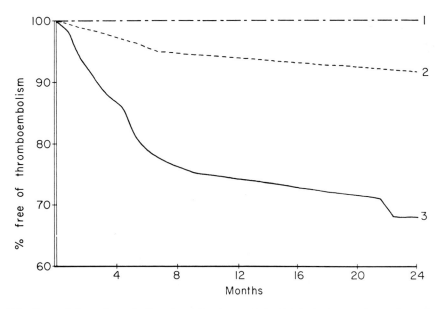

Fig. 7-1. Rate of thromboembolism in patients receiving high-dosage anticoagulant therapy *(1)*, moderate anticoagulant therapy *(2)*, and no anticoagulant therapy *(3)*. (From Moschos, C. B., Wong, P. C. Y., and Sise, H.: J.A.M.A. **190:**799, 1964.)

eye is based on the supposed success of this treatment in the management of other diseases. More recent reports, based on long-term controlled evaluation, cast some doubt on this premise. For instance, a 7-year, double-blind study of survival and complications in 196 patients on prophylactic anticoagulants after myocardial infarction showed no significant difference between treated and control patients with respect to survival and thromboembolic complications.[22]

SUMMARY

Anticoagulant therapy is the only treatment that might reasonably be expected to benefit chronic or incipient occlusion of retinal veins. Unfortunately the empirical results of such therapy suggests that the outcome is likely to be fortuitous rather than related to treatment.

Retinal death after occlusion of the central retinal artery is so rapid as to preclude benefit from any therapy in most patients.

Cerebrovascular insufficiency, commonly associated with transient visual symptoms, may respond to anticoagulant therapy. However, information about patients with occlusion of coronary, carotid, or vertebral arteries is not necessarily applicable to central retinal veins.

REFERENCES

1. Kronenberg, B.: Current status of the therapy of diabetic retinopathy, Guildcraft, p. 15, 1957.
2. Cranley, J. J.: Dosage errors with heparin, J.A.M.A. **231:**701, February 17, 1975.
3. Mosley, D. H., Schatz, I. J., Breneman, G. M., and Keyes, J. W.: Long-term anticoagulant therapy, J.A.M.A. **186:**914, 1963.
4. Anderson, B., and Vallotton, W.: Etiology and therapy of retinal vascular occlusions, Arch. Ophthalmol. **54:**6, 1955.
5. Duff, I. F., Falls, H. F., and Linman, J. W.: Anticoagulant therapy in occlusive vascular disease of the retina, Arch. Ophthalmol. **46:**601, 1951.
6. Sigell, L. T., and Flessa, H. C.: Drug interactions with anticoagulants, J.A.M.A. **214:**2035, 1970.
7. Vannas, S.: Treatment of retinal venous occlusion, Arch. Ophthalmol. **58:**812, 1957.
8. Klein, B. A., and Olwin, J. H.: A survey of the pathogenesis of retinal venous occlusion, Arch. Ophthalmol. **56:**207, 1956.
9. Mancall, I. T.: Occlusion of central retinal vein, Arch. Ophthalmol. **46:**668, 1951.
10. Klein, B. A.: Spontaneous vascular repair, Am. J. Ophthalmol. **50:**691, 1960.
11. Vannas, S., and Raitta, C.: Anticoagulant treatment of retinal venous occlusion, Am. J. Ophthalmol. **62:**874, 1966.
12. Rome, S.: Heparin in senile macular degeneration, Arch. Ophthalmol. **57:**190, 1957.
13. Havener, W. H., Sheets, J., and Cook, M. J.: Evaluation of heparin therapy of senile macular degeneration, Arch. Ophthalmol. **61:**390, 1959.
14. Leo, L. S., and Lidman, B.: Dicumarol in retinitis pigmentosa; resulting changes in visual acuity and visual field: preliminary report, Am. J. Ophthalmol. **39:**46, 1955.
15. Frell, A. C.: Dicumarol in retinitis pigmentosa, Watson Gailey Eye Digest **2:**32, 1959.
16. Ellison, A., and Poirier, R.: Therapeutic effects of heparin on *Pseudomonas*-induced corneal ulceration, Am. J. Ophthalmol. **82:**619, October 1976.
17. Minor, R. H., Kearns, T. P., Millikan, C. H., Siekert, R. G., and Sayre, G. P.: Ocular manifestations of occlusive disease of the vertebral basilar arterial system, Arch. Ophthalmol. **62:**84, 1959.
18. Hollenhorst, R. W.: Ocular manifestations of insufficiency or thrombosis of the internal carotid artery, Am. J. Ophthalmol. **47:**753, 1959.
19. Siekert, R. G., Millikan, C. H., and Whisnant, J. P.: Anticoagulant therapy in intermittent cerebrovascular insufficiency, J.A.M.A. **176:**19, 1961.
20. Fields, W. S., and Lemak, N. A.: Joint Study of Extracranial Arterial Occlusion, J.A.M.A. **235:**2734, June 21, 1976.
21. Moschos, G. B., Wong, P. C. Y., and Sise, H.: Controlled study of the effective level of long-term anticoagulation, J.A.M.A. **190:**799, 1964.
22. Seaman, A. J., Griswold, H. E., Reaume, R. B., and Ritzman, L. W.: Prophylactic anticoagulant therapy for coronary artery disease, J.A.M.A. **189:**183, 1964.

8
ANTHELMINTHIC THERAPY

Fortunately intraocular parasites are extremely rare. The larger larvae require surgical removal, since their death induces destructive intraocular inflammation. Smaller parasites such as microfilaria may be successfully destroyed by medical treatment.

THIABENDAZOLE

Thiabendazole is an effective anthelminthic and antifungal drug. Topically applied thiabendazole is effective against experimental infections with *Trichophyton*, *Epidermophyton*, and *Microsporum* species. *Aspergillus fumigatus*, an organism reported as causing human keratomycosis, is highly susceptible to thiabendazole, being inhibited by 2 to 4 μg/ml of drug. Greater concentrations are fungicidal.[1-3]

The corneal penetration of ^{14}C-labeled thiabendazole is shown in Fig. 8-1.[1] This was applied as a 4% suspension and maintained on the rabbit cornea for 1 hour. The peak corneal concentration of 52 μg/g far exceeds the necessary level for inhibition of *Aspergillus*. Deeper portions of the eye attain much lower drug concentrations; for example, lens, 4.0, and vitreous, 0.9. Some systemic absorption followed topical application, and peak plasma levels approached 0.5 μg/ml. An average of 1420 μg of thiabendazole was excreted via the urine in the 4-hour period.

Toxicity

Topically applied thiabendazole is well tolerated by the eye. Repeated ocular instil-lation of 10% solution of 4% ointment in rabbits caused no signs of eye irritation.[4] The drug is well tolerated when given systemically, and general poisoning from absorption during ocular use appears impossible unless some type of idiosyncrasy (unreported) is present. The acute LD_{50} for animals is greater than 3000 mg/kg. Chronic dosage of 400 mg/kg interferes with weight gain and causes normochromic anemia.

Clinical use

One day after administration of 2 g of thiabendazole orally, a previously visible intraretinal nematode (presumably *Toxocara*) disappeared, leaving a localized hemorrhage at its previous site.[5] Perhaps this resulted from death of the worm and body response to the dead tissue, but the possibility of escape of the worm from the eye cannot be excluded. The edematous and hemorrhagic response disappeared during the following month, leaving a permanent small scotoma.

Because of the possibility of increased reaction and retinal damage on death of the worm, a moving parasite might be permitted to leave the foveal area before thiabendazole administration. Although published photographs of two cases document presence of an actively motile parasite,[5] this condition is so rare that the effect of thiabendazole is not known with certainty.

In the treatment of a patient with keratitis caused by *Phialophora verrucosa*, thiabendazole, 0.3% solution, was applied topically

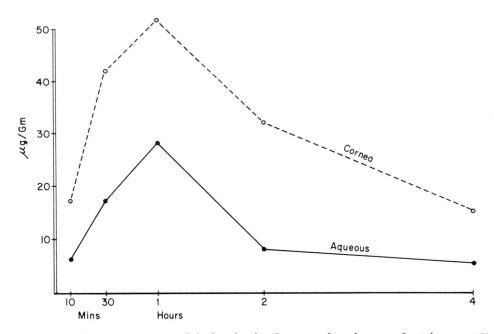

Fig. 8-1. Ocular concentrations of thiabendazole after topical applications for 1 hour as 4% suspension. (Based on data from Robinson, H. J., and associates: Am. J. Ophthalmol. **62:**710, 1966.)

every 30 minutes for 1 week without improvement. The organism was again isolated in culture after this treatment. (Incidentally, covering the cornea with a thin conjunctival flap cured the patient within 2 weeks.) The low concentration of thiabendazole was selected because of poor solubility of the drug in water. However, a 12% suspension can be prepared in 1% sodium carboxymethyl cellulose, and ointment may be made in any desired concentration.[6]

MEBENDAZOLE

This anthelminthic acts by blocking glucose uptake in nematodes but has no effect on blood glucose levels in animals or man. A dose of 100 mg morning and evening for 3 days in children over 2 years of age is highly effective against pinworms, whipworms, and roundworms[7] and is considered the drug of choice.

DIETHYLCARBAMAZINE (HETRAZAN)

Diethylcarbamazine, the anthelminthic drug of greatest value in treatment of on-

chocerciasis, will destroy microfilariae within the eye. The dosage is 2 to 3 mg/kg orally three times daily. Death of the microfilariae causes localized tissue inflammation that is manifested in the eye by increased severity of uveitis and conjunctivitis. Corticosteroid therapy will reduce this undesirable inflammatory response. Unfortunately the adult *Onchocerca* worms are not killed by diethylcarbamazine and remain as a source of new microfilariae. Repeated courses of diethylcarbamazine treatment are required over many years to control the disease.

Because ocular involvement is the most commonly disabling manifestation of onchocerciasis, the ocular penetration of an ophthalmic preparation of diethylcarbamazine was studied.[8] A single topical application of 2 drops of 5% diethylcarbamazine (a nonirritating concentration) results in aqueous concentrations of approximately 10 μg/ml at 30 minutes, falling to 0.5 μg/ml within 4 hours. Serum concentrations of 3 to 5 μg/ml after oral administration are therapeutically effective levels. These preliminary experiments suggest that some routine of topical prophylaxis might be evolved to control ocular microfilariae.

REFERENCES

1. Robinson, H. J., Graessle, O. E., Lehman, E. G., Kelley, K. L., Geoffroy, R. F., and Rosenblum, C.: Ocular absorption of thiabendazole-^{14}C by the rabbit, Am. J. Ophthalmol. **62:**710, 1966.
2. Robinson, H. J., Phares, H. F., and Graessle, O. E.: Antimycotic properties of thiabendazole, J. Invest. Dermatol. **42:**479, 1964.
3. Blank, H., and Rebell, G.: Thiabendazole activity against the fungi of dermatophytosis mycetomas and chromomycosis, J. Invest. Dermatol. **44:**219, 1965.
4. Robinson, H. J., Stoerk, H. C., and Graessle, O. E.: Studies on the toxicologic and pharmacologic properties of thiabendazole, Toxicol. Appl. Pharmacol. **7:**53, 1965.
5. Rubin, M. L., Kaufman, H. E., Tierney, J. P., and Lucas, H. C.: An intraretinal nematode (a case report), Trans. Am. Acad. Ophthalmol. Otolaryngol. **72:**855, 1968.
6. Wilson, L. A., Sexton, R. R., and Ahearn, D.: Keratochromomycosis, Arch. Ophthalmol. **76:** 811, 1966.
7. Wolfe, M. S., and Wershing, J. M.: Mebendazole: treatment of trichuriasis and ascariasis in Bavarian Children, J.A.M.A. **230:**1408-1411, December 4, 1974.
8. Lazar, M., Lieberman, T. W., Furman, M., and Leopold, I. H.: Ocular penetration of Hetrazan in rabbits, Am. J. Ophthalmol. **66:**215, 1968.

9
ANTIHISTAMINIC AGENTS

In the immediate-response type of allergy (such as hay fever), histamine-like substances released in the tissues are responsible for the symptoms. Drugs that are histamine antagonists will effectively relieve the allergic symptoms, including the ocular itching, redness, and tearing. The antihistamines should be taken systemically because they are relatively ineffective when used topically. Contact drug allergies and eczema are not histamine mediated and do not respond to antihistaminic agents. In these cases, corticosteroids, which have a nonspecific blocking action against inflammation, are much more generally effective than antihistaminics. However, the mild local anesthetic effect of the antihistamine drugs may give some symptomatic relief.[1]

SIDE EFFECTS

Sedation is the most common undesirable effect of antihistamines. Incoordination, dizziness, nervousness, insomnia, muscular weakness, gastrointestinal disturbances, dryness of the mouth, and a variety of other symptoms may be encountered. Many of these drugs effectively control nausea and vomiting. Narcotics and sedatives may be greatly potentiated by antihistaminic drugs; their effect is sometimes doubled.

DOSAGE

The prescribed dose varies with the particular antihistaminic drug employed. Representative doses include promethazine hydrochloride (Phenergan), 12.5 to 25 mg one to three times daily, tripelennamine citrate (Pyribenzamine), 75 mg four times a day, and pheniramine maleate (Trimeton), 25 mg three times a day. Dosage should be the smallest amount adequate to relieve symptoms.

CLINICAL USE
Allergic conjunctivitis

Antazoline (Antistine), 0.5% concentration, may benefit hay fever conjunctivitis. It is instilled as required to relieve allergic symptoms, perhaps every few hours in a severe case. This drug is said to cause less irritation than the other antihistaminic compounds, and it is the only ophthalmic preparation generally available in this class of medications.

The effect of 0.05% naphazoline (sympathomimetic), of 0.5% antazoline, of a combination of these two drugs, and of a placebo was studied in 51 patients with allergic conjunctivitis.[2] All patients were ragweed pollen sensitive, and the challenge consisted of topical instillation of ragweed pollen extract 15 minutes after medication. Lacrimation, redness, itching, photophobia, and pain were the 5 parameters studied. The combination of sympathomimetic and antihistaminic drugs was more effective than either component alone, and far superior to placebo alone.

Myokymia

The refractory period of muscle is prolonged by antihistaminic drugs. This property permits their use in treatment of myokymia (twitching of the lids).[3] The antihistaminic drug of choice may be given alone or together with quinine (0.32 g one to three times daily).

Cataract surgery

Constriction of the pupil occurs during cataract surgery despite the preoperative use of atropine and other mydriatics. That this constriction is a result of liberation of histamine from injured tissue is suggested by demonstration that preoperative antihistamine therapy can prevent pupilloconstriction.[4] The antihistamine may be administered orally (promethazine, 25 mg 2 hours before surgery) or topically (pyrilamine maleate, 0.1% solution every 10 minutes three times) with equal effect. Antihistamine therapy maintained a well-dilated pupil in 12 of 14 eyes in contrast to only 8 of 13 control eyes. Similar results obtained in experimental rabbit surgery suggest that antihistamine medication may facilitate the delivery of cataracts through a round pupil.

Wound healing after oral surgery has been reported to be accelerated by antihistamines. Healing of experimental corneal incisions in rabbit eyes seems to be delayed by antihistamine therapy, but numerical data to assess the significance of this finding were not given.[5]

Histaminic cephalalgia

Desensitization to histamine provides effective relief to more than 90% of patients with histamine cephalalgia.[6,7] This unusual syndrome includes excruciating unilateral headaches, commonly referred to the orbit. During an attack the eye is very red and congested, with miotic pupil. The condition almost exactly resembles a severe case of acute iritis except for the complete absence of aqueous flare or cells. Unilateral lacrimation and facial perspiration are conspicuous. Attacks of histaminic cephalalgia often occur at night and may be precipitated by alcohol. Histamine desensitization utilizes the commercial preparation of 0.175 mg/ml of histamine diphosphate (equivalent to 0.1 mg of histamine base). The initial dose is 0.05 ml subcutaneously. Injections are given every 12 hours. Each dose is increased by 0.05 ml until a dose of 0.5 ml is reached. Adequate dosage is determined by the relief of symptoms. Sometimes injections must be continued until a dose of 1 ml is given.

OCULAR TOLERANCE TO HISTAMINE

Histamine in a 1:1000 concentration was applied as often as every 10 minutes for 8 hours on an experimental rabbit corneal abrasion.[8] Healing of the abrasion was delayed only very slightly beyond that of the control. Intrastromal injection of 0.05 ml of a 1:1000 concentration of histamine causes transient corneal haze that lasts several hours. Conjunctival hyperemia and edema persist for 6 hours. Although histamine causes miosis, topical application has no therapeutic value.

REFERENCES

1. Theodore, F. H.: Drugs in ocular allergies, Am. J. Ophthalmol. **39**:97, 1955.
2. Miller, J., and Wolf, E. H.: Antazoline phosphate and naphazoline hydrochloride, singly and in combination for the treatment of allergic conjunctivitis—a controlled, double-blind clinical trial, Ann. Allergy **35**:81, August 1975.
3. Lowe, R.: Facial twitching, Trans. Ophthalmol. Soc. Aust. **11**:1, 1951.
4. File, T. M.: Studies on the use of antihistamines in cataract surgery, Am. J. Ophthalmol. **51**:1240, 1961.
5. Weil, V. J., Elisaoph, I., and Laval, J.: Cataract wound healing in the rabbit eye, Arch. Ophthalmol. **59**:551, 1958.
6. Horton, B. T.: Histaminic cephalalgia, J.A.M.A. **160**:468, 1956.
7. Horton, B. T.: The use of histamine in the treatment of specific types of headaches, J.A.M.A. **116**:377, 1941.
8. Hagedoorn, W. G., and Maas, E. R.: The effect of histamine on the rabbit's cornea, Am. J. Ophthalmol. **42**:89, 1956.

10
ANTIMITOTIC AGENTS

AZATHIOPRINE

Systemically administered immunosuppressive drugs such as the nucleic acid antimetabolites are used to permit acceptance of human renal homografts. At the present time use of these drugs is too dangerous to be acceptable in corneal transplantation. However, such drugs as azathioprine (Imuran), 24 mg/kg/day, have been shown experimentally to inhibit corneal graft rejection (calf cornea donor to rabbit recipient) in 100% of cases. In inadequate dosage, azathioprine seems to enhance graft rejection.[1]

Combined administration of azathioprine (48 mg/kg daily during the first 10 postoperative days) and 6α-methylprednisolone (0.1% topical ointment two times a day, starting on the eleventh postoperative day) was the most effective immunosuppressive regimen evaluated in a study that showed maintenance of clarity of calf-to-rabbit corneal grafts for 42 days.[2] The death of a number of these rabbits emphasizes that this technique is not yet ready for clinical use.

Thirty percent of cat-to-rabbit corneal heterografts remained clear for as long as 8 months in animals treated with an immunosuppressive regimen of azathioprine and prednisolone.[3]

Corneal wound healing is markedly retarded by azathioprine administered in the optimum dose required for suppression of the corneal heterograft reaction in rabbits (48 mg/kg daily). The tensile strength of a 5 mm wound strip at the eleventh postoperative day averaged 134 g in control rabbits and 59 g in azathioprine-treated rabbits. Such a large dose may not be necessary in clinical use; only 3 mg/kg/day is considered optimal for suppression of human renal transplantation reactions.[4]

Subconjunctival (rabbit) injection of 0.1 mg of radioactive azathioprine results in penetration into the aqueous of 5 μg/ml at 1 hour, 11 μg/ml at 4 hours, 7 μg/ml at 6 hours, and 2 μg/ml at 24 hours.[5]

6-MERCAPTOPURINE

The modification of corneal immunologic responses by radiation or "radiomimetic drugs" is apparently a systemic rather than a local effect. This is suggested by experimental study of the immune response produced by intralamellar corneal injections of bovine serum in rabbits. The typical corneal immune ring and the circulating antibody response were blocked by total body radiation but not by radiation of the head alone or by beta radiation of the cornea.[6] This finding indicates that the antibodies or cells producing the immune response originate outside the eye.

Similar results were obtained with 6-mercaptopurine.[7] Systemic treatment with 5 mg/kg/day with this drug does inhibit the corneal immune reaction to bovine albumin.[8] Topically applied 6-mercaptopurine did not inhibit the immune response except in doses so large as to produce a systemic effect resulting from drug absorption from the eye. These experimental findings cast doubt on the value of this class of drugs in local ocular therapy. (Incidentally, topical application four times daily of 1.5% hydrocortisone acetate ointment did prevent the corneal reaction to injected bovine albumin.)

METHOTREXATE

Use of methotrexate has been found to be an effective but highly dangerous treatment for severe uveitis. This drug, a potent folic acid antagonist, is capable of inhibiting antibody production and inflammatory reactions.

The dosage of methotrexate is approximately 25 mg/m^2 of body surface intravenously every 4 days. The treatment is suppressive rather than curative; hence it must be continued for the duration of the individual episode of uveitis—perhaps 2 to 10 months. Toxic effects occur in almost all patients, limit the acceptable dosage, and are sufficiently dangerous to require close supervision by an experienced physician. Toxic manifestations include anorexia, nausea and vomiting, stomatitis, alopecia, secondary infections, leukopenia, thrombocytopenia, and liver damage.

Because of the therapeutic hazards, methotrexate therapy is indicated only in sight-threatening uveitis that has not responded to standard uveitis therapy (for example, corticosteroids and cycloplegics). In a series of 17 such patients, 14 showed encouraging remissions.[9] Decreased uveitis activity was evident within 1 week after treatment was started. However, 11 of these 14 patients relapsed within 1 to 11 months after methotrexate was discontinued. The most dramatic results occurred in 2 patients with severe sympathetic ophthalmia (generally accepted to be an autoimmune disease). The response of cyclitis was better than that of posterior uveitis. A literature survey indicated improvement in 34 of 36 patients with cyclitis; in 8 of 10 patients with sympathetic ophthalmia; but in only 2 of 12 patients with presumed histoplasmic chorioretinitis.

In another series, 17 of 25 patients with severe chronic ocular inflammatory diseases improved with immunosuppressive therapy (methotrexate, 25 mg/m^2 body surface intravenously every 4 days, or cyclophosphamide, 1 g/m^2 intravenously once weekly). A 6-week course of treatment was chosen empirically.[10] In most cases, relapse followed discontinuation of immunosuppressive treatment. In a few cases, corticosteroid control of the inflammation seemed less difficult after immunosuppressive therapy.

Of practical significance is the finding that clinical improvement was unrelated to the extent of immunosuppression as measured by various immunologic tests. This means that such parameters are ineffective as guides to therapy and that treatment must be guided by the results of clinical improvement of the disease of development of drug toxicity.

A rather specific indication for immunosuppressive therapy might be protection of the eye with sympathetic ophthalmia from destructive postoperative inflammation after cataract extraction or glaucoma surgery. In 5 such cases the postoperative recovery period was uneventful. No delay in wound healing was encountered.

A particularly severe case of sympathetic ophthalmia, which had lasted for a year and caused dense bilateral cataract and secondary glaucoma, was treated successfully with methotrexate.[11] Within 48 hours of a single intravenous dose of 25 mg of methotrexate, the inflammatory signs had almost completely disappeared from both eyes, which remained clear for over a week. During the next 4 months the uveitis was controlled by varying doses of methotrexate, mostly 15 mg every 4 days. Thereafter dexamethasone, 2 mg/day, controlled the inflammation (no steroid was used during antimetabolite therapy).

It seems likely that antimetabolite therapy will be appropriate for treatment of exceptionally severe cases of sympathetic ophthalmia that do not respond to corticosteroid therapy. If such treatment is considered, the physician must justify the great risk of using such a toxic medication. Severe, indeed fatal, hematologic, gastrointestinal, or infectious complications may ensue. *Be careful!*

A patient with choriocarcinoma metastatic to the choroid in both eyes was treated with methotrexate. Remarkable improvement resulted, with restoration of vision and disappearance of pulmonary metastases.[12]

Methotrexate is teratogenic. A dosage of 2.5 mg daily for 5 days at the ninth week of gestation caused multiple severe skeletal and skull defects in the infant.[13]

THIO-TEPA

Corneal vascularization can be inhibited by topical application of antimitotic chemicals.[14] Triethylenethiophosphoramide (thio-tepa) is a nitrogen mustard derivative that will selectively inhibit rapidly growing normal or neoplastic tissues. The rate of ingrowth of new corneal vessels (induced by injection of alloxan into rabbit anterior chambers) was decreased by more than 80% by instillation three times a day of an oily suspension containing 10 mg/ml of thio-tepa. No systemic toxicity results from this dosage. Unfortunately new vessel growth began again as soon as inhibitor therapy was stopped, and the ultimate condition of the cornea was not greatly benefited by this treatment (Fig. 10-1).

Recurrence of pterygium has been prevented by instillation of a 1:2000 solution (15 mg in 30 ml of Ringer's solution) of thio-tepa every 3 hours (while awake). Instillations were started 2 days postoperatively and were continued for 6 weeks. No adverse effects on the eye resulted from this concentration and frequency of use. In a series of 19 patients so treated, no recurrence was encountered. No rebound vascularization occurred after thio-tepa was discontinued.[15]

Additional cases confirm thio-tepa inhibition of pterygium recurrence, but treatment must be continued for 6 to 8 weeks. If the drug is used only for 2 to 4 weeks, recurrence may develop. In a series of 17 patients treated postoperatively, there was not a single recurrence.[16] In another series of 26 patients, only a single recurrence was encountered.[17] Eleven patients with bilateral pterygia were treated with thio-tepa in only

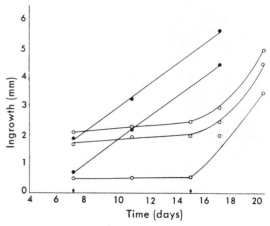

Fig. 10-1. Inhibition of corneal vascularization by thio-tepa. Closed circles: vascularization in two control series. Open circles: arrest of vascularization in three rabbits treated from the seventh to fifteenth day. Note recurrent vascular growth when treatment was stopped, with ultimate vascularization equivalent to untreated control eyes. (From Langham, M. E.: Am. J. Ophthalmol. **49:**1111, 1960.)

one eye after surgery. Three of the eleven untreated eyes developed recurrences, in contrast to none of the eleven treated eyes.[18] At room temperature, thio-tepa solutions maintain 100% potency for at least 2 weeks, and it is presumed the patient may be given a 6-week supply for home use after surgery.[17]

Although topical instillation of a 1% solution of thio-tepa slowed vascularization of experimental corneal transplants in alloxan-scarred rabbit corneas,[19] the final vascular invasion of the grafts was about the same with or without thio-tepa (Fig. 10-2). Faulty wound healing sufficiently severe to require resuturing occurred in several thio-tepa–treated eyes, presumably because of its antimitotic action on fibroblasts.

Topical instillation of a 1:445 solution of thio-tepa on the eyes of weanling rats eight times daily for 6 weeks caused cataract and corneal neovascularization. Both corneal and lens changes were dose related.[20]

In clinical use, thio-tepa is very irritating and of little value in preventing vascularization of corneal transplants.[21]

Permanent depigmentation of the lid skin

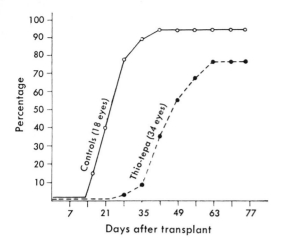

Fig. 10-2. Rate of complete vascularization of experimental corneal transplants with and without thio-tepa treatment. (From Rock, R. L.: Arch. Ophthalmol. **69:**330, 1963.)

of a black woman occurred after application of a 1% thio-tepa solution for a period of 23 days twice daily to prevent (successfully) vascularization of a corneal graft.[22] The depigmentation developed progressively during the 6-month period after use of thio-tepa; the lid-skin became chalky white and remained depigmented during the subsequent 5 years of observation. Two other cases of depigmentation had been seen, and a similar permanent local depigmentation developed almost a year after thio-tepa treatment of a Puerto Rican man for pterygium.[23]

Possibly this depigmentation represents a photosensitization phenomenon, inasmuch as it may occur more severely on exposure to sunlight during thio-tepa therapy.[24]

TRIETHYLENEMELAMINE (TEM)

Combined therapy with x-radiation and antimitotic drugs has been advocated in management of retinoblastoma.[25] As of 1957, 20 patients had been so treated, with apparent cure in about 70%. Whether these two forms of therapy are synergistic or merely additive is not certain; however, better results and control of more advanced retinoblastomas were reported with combined therapy.

Since emesis and irregular absorption complicate oral administration, TEM is given intramuscularly. The initial dose is 0.1 mg/kg given 24 hours before radiation. The second dose is given at the end of radiotherapy. The size of subsequent dosage of TEM is determined by the hematologic response and should be supervised by a competent internist. The empirical dosage used in this series was intramuscular administration of a total of 7.5 to 10 mg over 6 to 12 months.

Because of occasional unpredictable individual sensitivity, the initial dose of TEM was later reduced to 0.08 mg/kg.[26] The size and frequency of later doses was determined by the amount and duration of hematologic depression. Hematologic depression is a measure of therapeutic effect, and no beneficial result is obtained without it. Maximal depression to 3000 leukocytes or 100,000 platelets indicates adequate TEM dosage. Second and third doses are not given until the blood cell counts have returned to normal numbers. Prophylactic antibiotic therapy is advocated for leukopenia of less than 2000 cells. Although only one death has been attributable to TEM in a series of about 100 children, the physician must realize this is a highly dangerous drug.

Comparison of combined TEM and radiation therapy with radiation alone was attempted in a series of 12 alternate patients, matched as closely as possible as to severity of retinoblastoma.[7] Six received standard x-ray therapy (3250 rads); the other six received the same x-ray therapy plus TEM. Three of the six eyes treated with x-rays alone showed subsequent growth, which was then arrested by further x-ray therapy and TEM. The retinoblastoma within all six of the eyes treated with combined TEM and x-ray therapy was arrested.

Direct intracarotid injection of TEM in a concentration of 1 mg/ml is said to expose the tumor to a higher effective dose. The amount given is the same as by intramuscular injection, that is, 0.08 mg/kg. Intracarotid injection is the treatment of choice for large, recurrent, or otherwise difficult tumors. The intracarotid injection technique gives a cure rate of 60% even in difficult cases. Cure rates as high as 90% may be expected in less seriously involved eyes.

Other antimitotic agents such as cyclophosphamide (Cytoxan) may be substituted for TEM.

OTHER AGENTS

A variety of other immunosuppressive agents have been used in the treatment of assorted unpleasant eye conditions. For example, 11 patients with Behçet's disease were reported to respond favorably to chlorambucil.[27] Phenylalanine mustard and actinomycin D were used in five cases of orbital rhabdomyosarcoma, with results no better than would have been expected from exenteration alone.[28] Five patients with Wegener's granulomatosis showed significant improvement after treatment with cyclophosphamide (a sixth patient died of bone marrow depression).[29] All of 12 patients with peripheral uveitis showed improvement with cyclophosphamide therapy.[30]

REFERENCES

1. Leibowitz, H. M., and Elliott, J. H.: Chemotherapeutic immunosuppression of the corneal graft reaction, Arch. Ophthalmol. **75**:826, 1966.
2. Leibowitz, H. M., and Elliott, J. H.: Chemotherapeutic immunosuppression of the corneal graft reaction, Arch. Ophthalmol. **76**:338, 1966.
3. D'Amico, R. A., and Castroviejo, R.: Suppression of the immune response in keratoplasty, Am. J. Ophthalmol. **68**:829, 1969.
4. Elliott, J. H., and Leibowitz, H. M.: The influence of immunosuppressive agents upon corneal wound healing, Arch. Ophthalmol. **76**:334, 1966.
5. Polack, F. M.: Effect of azathioprine (Imuran) on corneal graft reaction, Am. J. Ophthalmol. **64**:233, 1967.
6. Sellyei, L. F., and Ellis, P. P.: Modification of corneal immune response, Am. J. Ophthalmol. **61**:702, 1966.
7. Leibowitz, H. M., and Elliott, J. H.: Antimetabolite suppression of corneal hypersensitivity, Arch. Ophthalmol. **73**:94, 1965.
8. Ellis, P. P., Sellyei, L. F., and Kurland, L. R.: Modification of corneal immune response, Am. J. Ophthalmol. **61**:709, 1966.
9. Lazar, M., Weiner, M. J., and Leopold, I. H.: Treatment of uveitis with methotrexate, Am. J. Ophthalmol. **67**:383, 1969.
10. Wong, V. G.: Immunosuppressive therapy of ocular inflammatory diseases, Arch. Ophthalmol. **81**:628, 1969.
11. Wong, V. G., Hersh, E. M., and McMaster, P. R. B.: Treatment of a presumed case of sympathetic ophthalmia with methotrexate, Arch. Ophthalmol. **76**:66, 1966.
12. Keates, R. H., and Billig, S. L.: Metastatic uveal choriocarcinoma, Arch. Ophthalmol. **84**:381, 1970.
13. Milunsky, A., Graef, J. W., and Gaynor, M. F., Jr.: Methotrexate-induced congenital malformation, J. Pediatr. **72**:790, 1968.
14. Langham, M. E.: The inhibition of corneal vascularization by triethylene thiophospharamide, Am. J. Ophthalmol. **49**:1111, 1960.
15. Meacham, C. T.: Triethylene thiophosphoramide, Am. J. Ophthalmol. **54**:751, 1962.
16. Cassady, J. R.: The inhibition of pterygium recurrence by thio-tepa, Am. J. Ophthalmol. **61**:886, 1966.
17. Liddy, B. St. L., and Morgan, J. F.: Triethylene thiophosphoramide (thio-tepa) and pterygium, Am. J. Ophthalmol. **61**:888, 1966.
18. Joselson, G. A., and Muller, P.: Incidence of pterygium recurrence, Am. J. Ophthalmol. **61**:891, 1966.
19. Rock, R. L.: Inhibition of corneal vascularization by triethylene thiophosphoramide (Thio-Tepa), Arch. Ophthalmol. **69**:330, 1963.
20. Robertson, D. M., and Creasman, J. P.: Effects of topical Thio-TEPA on rat eyes, Am. J. Ophthalmol. **73**:73, 1972.
21. King, J. H.: A symposium—present status of corneal transplant surgery, Trans. Am. Acad. Ophthalmol. **67**:309, 1963.
22. Berkow, J. W., Gills, J. P., Jr., and Wise, J. B.: Depigmentation of eyelids after topically administered thio-tepa, Arch. Ophthalmol. **82**:415, 1969.
23. Howitt, D., and Karp, E. J.: Side-effect of topical Thio-tepa, Am. J. Ophthalmol. **68**:473, 1969.
24. Asregadoo, E. R.: Surgery, thio-tepa, and corticosteroid in the treatment of pterygium, Am. J. Ophthalmol. **74**:960, November 1972.
25. Reese, A. B., Hyman, G. A., Merriam, G. R., and Forrest, A. W.: The treatment of retinoblastoma by radiation and triethylene melamine, Am. J. Ophthalmol. **43**:865, 1957.
26. Reese, A. B., Hyman, G. A., Tapley, N.

duV., and Forrest, A. W.: The treatment of retinoblastoma by x-ray and triethylene melamine, Arch. Ophthalmol. **60:**897, 1958.

27. Mamo, J. and Azzam, S. A.: Treatment of Behçet's disease with chlorambucil, Arch. Ophthalmol. **84:**446, 1970.

28. Dayton, G. O., Langdon, E., and Rochlin, D.: Management of orbital rhabdomyosarcoma, Am. J. Ophthalmol. **68:**906, 1969.

29. Raitt, J. W.: Wegener's granulomatosis: treatment with cytotoxic agents and adrenocorticoids, Ann. Intern. Med. **74:**344, 1971.

30. Gills, J. P., Jr., and Buckley, C. E.: Oral cyclophosphamide in the treatment of uveitis, Trans. Am. Acad. Ophthalmol. Otolaryngol. **74:**505, 1970.

11
ANTIVIRAL DRUGS

IDOXURIDINE (IDU)

Clinically useful selective metabolic inhibition of viruses was first achieved against herpes simplex infection of the cornea.[1] Before this was reported, no medication had ever been known to cure or improve an established virus infection without destroying the host cells.

Mechanism of action

Virus metabolism is closely akin to that of the nucleic structure within cells. One of the fundamental building blocks of which these nucleic acids are composed is thymidine. If the 5-methyl group of thymidine is replaced by an iodine atom, the molecule becomes 5-iodo-2′-deoxyuridine (IDU). IDU so closely resembles thymidine that it can substitute for thymidine in nuclear synthesis. IDU-containing molecules apparently cannot function as infection-producing viruses.

Related compounds

A number of antimetabolites were evaluated for their ability to inhibit virus multiplication.[2] The only antimetabolites found to be effective were those that block the final step of nucleotide (thymidine) incorporation into DNA. Blockade of earlier steps in synthesis was ineffective, presumably because of alternate metabolic pathways. The best drug was found to be 5-iodo-2′-deoxyuridine. Although also effective, 5-bromo-2′-deoxyuridine tends to produce chemical conjunctivitis and iritis. The chloro derivative was less effective, and the fluoro derivative was inactive. Since IDU is competitive with thymidine, addition of excess thymidine antagonizes the therapeutic effect of IDU.

Antiherpetic activity equivalent to that of IDU has been demonstrated for cytosine arabinoside. This latter compound blocks a step in nucleic acid metabolism but is not incorporated within the final molecule, as is IDU. The additive or synergistic action of IDU and cytosine arabinoside is suggested by preliminary experiments.[3]

Stability

IDU is a chemically stable drug, losing only 1% to 2% of its potency per month in solution at room temperature. Strangely, however, solutions of IDU several months old are more variable in therapeutic effect than are fresh solutions, and the old solutions are likely to cause ocular irritation and punctate corneal staining.[4] These facts suggested that substances resulting from IDU breakdown might antagonize the therapeutic effect and/or cause toxicity. Iodouracil, a major breakdown product, was found to antagonize the antiviral effect of IDU in tissue culture even when present in only 0.000,01% concentration. Irritation and punctate corneal staining were produced in human volunteers with a 0.01% concentration of iodouracil. In experimental rabbits, a 0.01% solution of iodouracil did not inhibit the antiviral effect of a 0.1% concentration of IDU.

The practical clinical recommendations derived from these findings included storage of solutions in dark bottles under refrigeration. Preparations that cause ocular burning may be considered old and should be replaced with fresh solutions. Failure of herpetic keratitis to respond as expected to IDU therapy should suggest the possibility of deterioration of the medication and may indicate trial of a fresh preparation.

Ocular penetration

The intraocular penetration of topically applied IDU is very poor. Radioactive iodine-labeled IDU was measured in the rabbit eye after 24 hours of instillation every 2 hours of a 0.1% solution of IDU.[5] Immediately after the last instillation of drug, the concentration (measured as micrograms of IDU per gram of tissue) was only 6.5 in epithelium, 2.2 in corneal stroma, 0.8 in aqueous, 1 in iris, and 0.2 in vitreous. Four hours after instillation these concentrations had decreased only slightly, to 5.3 in epithelium, 1 in corneal stroma, 0.4 in aqueous, 0.4 in iris, and 0.1 in vitreous.

Therapeutic concentration

In tissue cultures an IDU concentration of 1 μg/ml will inhibit herpes simplex and growth of vaccinia virus. Concentrations in excess of this minimum inhibitory concentration can be achieved in the cornea by topical application. As indicated in the preceding paragraph, the intraocular concentrations of IDU are therapeutically inadequate, a finding that probably explains the failure of herpetic iritis to respond to topical treatment.

Toxicity

Although inhibition of epithelial growth would be anticipated, IDU in a 0.1% concentration apparently is nontoxic to the corneal surface. Even if the corneal epithelium has been completely removed, healing is not inhibited by IDU. Stromal clarity is maintained and corneal edema does not occur. No ocular abnormalities have been observed in rabbits maintained on IDU for a month. Even if it were absorbed systemically after topical instillation, IDU should have no toxic

effect because it is rapidly metabolized. Within 4 hours after intravenous administration of radioactive iodine–labeled IDU, 75% of the labeled iodine had been excreted in the urine.

Idoxuridine may cause a severe local reaction characterized by edematous and follicular conjunctivitis. With continuing treatment despite the appearance of this toxic reaction, the lacrimal puncta will become occluded and permanently stenotic.[6]

Ocular tolerance

Hourly instillation of IDU does not retard the healing of corneal epithelial wounds as

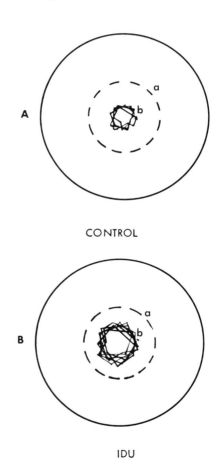

CONTROL

IDU

Fig. 11-1. Circles *a* represent size of experimental freezing injury of rabbit cornea. Circles *b* represent extent of keratocyte regeneration after 5 days in control eyes, **A**, and in IDU-treated eyes, **B**. (From Polack, F. M., and Rose, J.: Arch. Ophthalmol. **71:**520, 1964.)

compared to the healing of control injuries treated with sterile distilled water.[7] No lens damage has been reported to follow the use of IDU. The mitotic activity of lens epithelium is unchanged after 1 month of hourly IDU treatment of an eye.

The effect of 0.5% concentration of IDU ointment every 2 hours on the healing of corneal stromal wounds was studied by radioactive thymidine labeling of rabbit corneas that had been injured by freezing the central 6 mm portion.[8] As indicated in Fig. 11-1, at the end of 5 days the regeneration of corneal stromal cells was approximately twice as far advanced in the control eyes (treated with Neosporin ointment) as in the experimental eyes (IDU treated). Radioautograph counts indicated that the corneal stromal cell population in the injured area of the IDU-treated corneas was only half that in the control corneas.

The effect of IDU on stromal healing of the cornea was further studied by making a linear full-thickness incision across the center of rabbit corneas. A 0.1% solution of IDU was instilled into one eye every hour for 14 hours every day. The fellow eyes were treated with saline solution only. Wound strength was studied by excising a 5 mm strip of cornea perpendicularly oriented across the incision and measuring the grams of weight required to disrupt the incision. In a group of 23 rabbits sacrificed at 13 days, the average tensile strength of the IDU-treated eyes was 130 g, as contrasted with 244 g for the control eyes. Tensile strength at other time intervals was studied in isolated rabbits. Most noteworthy was the very low breaking strength of many treated eyes, in contrast to the uniformly strong control wounds (Table 11-1).[9]

These data suggest that IDU treatment is contraindicated during the healing period of ocular surgery (as, for instance, after corneal transplantation for herpetic keratitis).

Contraindications

Because of its inhibition of corneal stromal healing, use of IDU is probably not advisable during the first few weeks after corneal transplantation or other penetrating corneal incisions.

IDU is not helpful in the treatment of bacterial infections, degenerative changes, allergic keratitis, ocular trauma, and other nonviral conditions. Its use in these disorders is a waste of time and denies the patient specific therapy, if it is available. With the possible exception of vaccinia, insufficient evidence is available to recommend use of IDU for therapy of other virus infections of the cornea.

One case of IDU allergy has been reported.[10]

Dosage

Since continuing presence of IDU is required to inhibit virus growth, it is necessary that topical ocular instillation of a 0.1% concentration of IDU drops be given at least every 2 hours, *day* and *night*. It was initially recommended that drops be instilled hourly during the day and every 2 hours at night for 3 days. For the next 4 days the intervals were doubled, to every 2 hours during the day and every 4 hours at night. When grossly visible staining disappears, the frequency of drops may be reduced to every 2 hours during the day. Herpetic keratitis may relapse if IDU is discontinued before microscopic staining has cleared.

Table 11-1. Reduction of tensile strength of corneal wounds by treatment with IDU*

| Wound age (days) | Tensile strength† | |
	IDU (g/5 mm)	Control (g/5 mm)
7	0	35
9	10	510
11	95	160
12	45	120
14	15	300
15	200	205
17	205	240
19	50	250
21	210	745

*From Payrau, P., and Dohlman, C. H.: Am. J. Ophthalmol. **57**:999, 1964.
†IDU used in one eye and saline solution in control eye.

When prescribed as 0.5% ointment, IDU may be used five times a day (not at night). The therapeutic response to this frequency of application of ointment is reported to equal that of drops used hourly during the day and every 2 hours at night.[5]

Experimental use

The effect of a 0.1% concentration of IDU every 2 hours in treatment of experimental herpetic keratitis in rabbits is unequivocal. If it is given before virus inoculation, IDU will prevent keratitis.[1] When treatment was begun 2 hours after virus inoculation, only one fourth of the eyes developed dendritic keratitis, which appeared after 48 hours (all control eyes developed keratitis in 24 hours). The lesions in treated eyes remained small and disappeared with continuous treatment. Delay in treatment until 48 hours after virus inoculation permitted development of extensive dendritic lesions and several cases of associated herpetic iritis. After 48 hours of IDU treatment, even severely infected eyes were completely healed. Despite clinical cure, virus cultures were positive in one third of these eyes, which presumably could develop recurrences. Of 43 rabbit eyes

treated after infection was established, 27 had no recurrences.

To determine whether recurrences were a result of persistent corneal virus or of reinfection from the lacrimal gland or other adjacent structures, photographs of the original ulcers and of the recurrences were compared. In each case, recurrences appeared at the site of an original ulcer, even though the cornea had completely healed before the recurrence. This finding strongly suggests local survival of virus within the apparently healthy cornea. Recurrent herpetic keratitis was not prevented or reduced in incidence by active immunization induced by repeated intradermal injections of the same strain of herpes simplex virus.

Strains of herpes simplex virus isolated from three patients with very severe keratitis behaved quite differently from the milder stock strain already described, producing widespread keratitis, stromal infiltration, and encephalitis, with death of most rabbits within 2 weeks. IDU was not so effective against these virulent strains, curing only 7 of 17 eyes. However, in only 2 of the 17 treated eyes was keratitis as severe as in the 17 control eyes. Obviously these results indicate

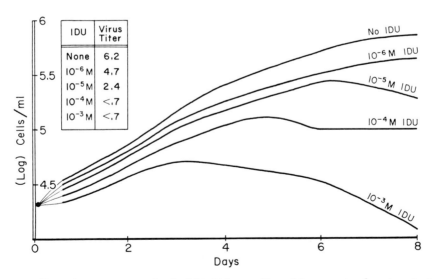

Fig. 11-2. Effect of IDU on growth of rabbit kidney cells and herpes simplex virus in tissue culture. (The 0.1% concentration of IDU used clinically corresponds to three times 10^{-3}M.) (Modified from Ey, R. C., and associates: Arch. Ophthalmol. **71:**325, 1964.)

that virus resistance to metabolic antagonists will present clinical problems comparable to those encountered in antibiotic therapy of bacterial infections.

Development of resistance to IDU has been demonstrated in culture propagation of herpes simplex virus.[11]

Herpes simplex infections of the chicken chorioallantoic membrane can be eradicated by hourly treatment with 0.1% solution of IDU.[12] At least 6 hourly doses of IDU were required before a measurable reduction in the virus concentration was demonstrable. At least 28 hourly doses of IDU were required before disappearance of the herpes virus. This experimental study further confirms the need for prolonged and intensive treatment of acute herpetic keratitis.

The existence of a specific antiviral effect of IDU has been questioned.[13] Multiplication of cells in tissue culture is completely inhibited by IDU in $10^{-3}M$ concentrations and is slowed by $10^{-6}M$ concentrations (Fig. 11-2). Virus growth is similarly blocked by IDU in concentrations of $10^{-4}M$ or greater and is partially inhibited by lesser concentrations. The degree of inhibition of virus multiplication parallels the inhibition of cell multiplication. This finding suggests that the beneficial effects of IDU therapy may be caused by a mild cauterizing action that affects both virus and tissue cells simultaneously.

This interpretation does not deny that IDU reduces virus titers in treated eyes, but doubts the therapeutic significance of such a reduction and attributes ultimate cure to the effect of natural immunity. Virus titers of IDU-treated and untreated eyes (Fig. 11-3) decrease to zero in about 3 weeks. The rapid drop in titer of the treated eye is attributed to slowing of cell and virus growth, not to a specific virucidal effect. This view is supported by the gradual rise of virus titer despite continued treatment.

Clinical use

Dendritic ulcer. Clinical experience with IDU has been as encouraging as the preliminary laboratory work.[14] In a series of 76 dendritic ulcers, all but 1 responded favorably, as follows. No increase in size of the dendritic figure occurred after the start of therapy. Subjective relief was marked within 12 to 24 hours. Conspicuous epithelial healing was already achieved within 3 days (Fig. 11-4), and residual punctate staining usually disappeared within 10 days. In the single

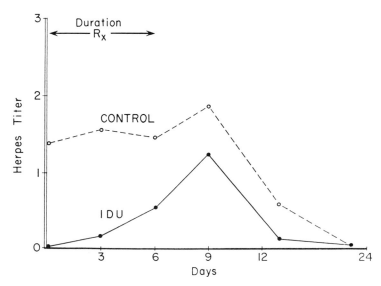

Fig. 11-3. Virus titers from eyes of IDU-treated and control rabbits. (Modified from Ey, R. C., and associates: Arch. Ophthalmol. **71:**325, 1964.)

case nonresponsive to IDU, debridement and continuation of IDU therapy resulted in cure.

Herpetic keratitis may relapse if IDU is discontinued before microscopic staining has cleared. However, when grossly visible staining has disappeared, the frequency of drops may be reduced to every 2 hours during the day and once during the night. Recurrence will respond to a repeat course of therapy.

During the first few weeks of healing, superficial stromal infiltrate in the pattern of a dendritic figure will persist beneath the healed epithelium. This dendritiform ghost figure is of no significance, will disappear completely, and does not in itself indicate a need for treatment to be continued.

Large and chronically active herpetic stromal ulcers with staining also respond rapidly to IDU therapy; the average healing time is 6.5 days (none more than 13 days). Herpetic iritis and deep keratitis, unassociated with surface disease, were not helped by IDU. Chronic disciform keratitis with marked corneal thickening did not respond well. Recurrent small epithelial defects overlying dense stromal scar became painful with IDU treatment, healed with use of a bland ointment every hour as needed, and were presumed to represent some type of noninfectious recurrent erosion.

This response to IDU may be compared with the course of 53 untreated patients[15] (this was another series and *not* a control series in the same study). The average period

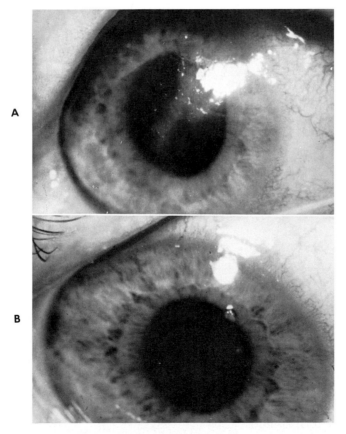

A

B

Fig. 11-4. Dendritic keratitis. **A,** Appearance of eye 2 days before IDU therapy. **B,** Appearance of eye 2 days after IDU therapy. (From Kaufman, H., Martola, E., and Dohlman, C.: Arch. Ophthalmol. **68:**235, 1962.)

of staining in these cases was 21 days, and the eyes remained red for an average of 41 days.

In three cases of ophthalmic cutaneous zoster, dendritic corneal figures were present. Virus cultures confirmed the presence of zoster virus (not simplex) in these dendritic figures. All three corneal lesions cleared promptly with corticosteroid therapy (which was combined with IDU in two cases).[16]

Since IDU is somewhat unstable, failure of a dendritic ulcer to respond promptly should arouse suspicion of faulty medication; this has been experienced, and retreatment with a potent drug has been shown to be effective. No IDU toxicity has appeared in 155 patients; however, allergy to the thiomersol preservative occurred three times. IDU is not irritating.

Stromal herpes. The initial evaluations of IDU consisted of uncontrolled treatment in a series of cases of herpetic keratitis.[12,17] These cases were generally divided into epithelial and stromal keratitis. About 80% of the epithelial cases and 50% of the stromal cases healed after IDU therapy. Average healing time for the epithelial cases was approximately 1 week and for the stromal cases 2 weeks. These results led to the conclusion that at last an effective treatment had been found for at least some cases of chronic herpetic keratitis, a condition that has been notoriously unresponsive to medical management. Unfortunately, time has not justified this conclusion.

Clinical evaluation of IDU by a group of practicing ophthalmologists showed healing of 21 of 26 dendritic ulcers in an average of 13 days.[18] Herpetic stromal involvement prolonged healing time to an average of 16 days, with good response in 14 of 21 cases.

Well-controlled double-blind studies of the effect of IDU on herpetic keratitis indicate that the spontaneous recovery rate is at least 25% and may be greater than 50%.[10,19,20] The combined number of IDU-treated patients with acute epithelial keratitis in these three studies was 57. Of these, 41 responded well to IDU. Placebo treatment of 53 patients with epithelial keratitis resulted in improvement in 19.

Only small numbers of patients with stromal keratitis were reported; however, a total of 34 eyes were given placebo therapy. Of these 34, 17 (50%!) improved spontaneously.

Other double-blind studies agree that IDU treatment significantly improves the course of acute epithelial herpetic keratitis.[21] However, chronic stromal herpes seems to do just as well with placebo treatment as with IDU treatment. Apparently the 50% improvement of stromal herpes reported in the earlier uncontrolled studies of IDU represents merely the spontaneous recovery rate of this disease.

IDU therapy does not seem to decrease the recurrence rate of herpetic keratitis. In 23 recurrences, 12 eyes had been treated with IDU therapy and 9 with placebo therapy.

Virtually all of the original clinical studies of IDU were uncontrolled. In a series of 28 cases of acute herpetic keratitis divided into placebo and IDU groups, excellent to good results were attained in 15 IDU-treated patients and in only 5 placebo-treated patients. This was said to be a statistically significant difference. In contrast, no difference could be noted between the result of IDU and placebo treatment of 43 patients presumed to have chronic herpetic keratitis.[19]

COMBINED CORTICOSTEROID AND IDU THERAPY

Having available in 5-iodo-2'-deoxyuridine a specific antiviral drug, can the ophthalmologist simultaneously treat herpes simplex keratitis with corticosteroids?[1] Clinically, the answer seems to be *yes.* Cases of chronic herpetic keratitis that have stubbornly persisted for months will often become quiet and comfortable after topical corticosteroid therapy. Unfortunately corticosteroids reactivate dendritic keratitis in some such patients. Such reactivation is much less likely when IDU and corticosteroids are simultaneously used to treat chronic herpetic keratitis.

Experimental use of hydrocortisone and IDU in the treatment of rabbit herpes simplex keratitis indicates that IDU does indeed protect the cornea against steroid activation of the disease.[22] The quality of protection is directly related to the frequency of IDU application, being greater when IDU is used every 2 hours than when it is used four times a day. Increasing the frequency of hydrocortisone treatment from four times a day to every 2 hours made the IDU-treated keratitis worse in one series of rabbits. Although the clinical appearance of the rabbits receiving combined IDU and hydrocortisone treatment was good, cultures of these eyes showed persistence of virus. Virus was recovered in 17 of 20 eyes receiving combined treatment, but in only 4 of 8 eyes receiving IDU only. It should further be noted that these studies lasted only 2 to 7 days and do not reveal possible late complications of corticosteroid therapy occurring thereafter. Hence indiscriminate use of steroids with IDU cannot be recommended, even though the danger of enhancement of virus by corticosteroids appears to be markedly lessened by use of IDU. If a patient with a stubborn case of metaherpetic keratitis is treated with steroids, simultaneous use of IDU every 2 hours is clearly indicated.

Although IDU is effective in the treatment of superficial corneal herpetic infection, its use is disappointing in deeper forms of infection such as disciform keratitis or herpetic iritis. This lack of effect may be because of poor penetration of the drug; however, several trials of irrigation of the anterior chamber with IDU did not enhance its effect.[23] Since these deeper infections respond to corticosteroid treatment, combined IDU and steroid treatment was used for 76 patients with disciform keratitis, geographic ulcers, and diffuse keratitis with iritis.[23]

Combined therapy is guided by experimental and clinical findings that corticosteroids worsen superficial herpetic infection and facilitate its spread, whereas IDU benefits surface infections. Combinations of the two drugs give results that depend on the intensity of treatment with each medication; hence corticosteroid dosage should be kept to the minimum amount required to benefit the deep herpetic reaction. One drop of corticosteroid three times a day was generally sufficient to suppress the deep inflammation.

Concentrations of 0.1% dexamethasone, 0.12% to 1% prednisolone, and 0.5% hydrocortisone were used without obvious difference in response to the different corticosteroid compounds. IDU drops were given every 1 to 2 hours during the day.

Duration of treatment depended on the spontaneous course of the disease, which commonly lasted 1 or 2 months. When the deep infection improved, the corticosteroid drops were gradually discontinued, but the IDU dosage was maintained constant until no more steroid was being used. IDU may be stopped abruptly without need to taper off when the eye is observed to remain quiet without corticosteroid treatment.

Clinically, the great majority of these 76 patients responded very favorably to combined treatment, which was definitely recommended for such cases of deep herpetic inflammation. Simultaneous use of corticosteroid therapy is *not* recommended for acute epithelial herpes, which is expected to respond to IDU alone.

CYTOSINE ARABINOSIDE

Culture of herpes simplex virus in media containing IDU results in development of virus strains resistant to IDU.[24] This experimental finding indicates that clinically troublesome resistant strains will emerge with continued use of this drug. In contrast, only slight resistance developed to cytosine arabinoside, an inhibitor of nucleic acid snythesis that is experimentally effective against herpetic and vaccinia infections of rabbit eyes.

Cytosine arabinoside has the following advantages over idoxuridine.

1. Virus resistance to cytosine arabinoside develops more slowly.
2. IDU-resistant viruses remain sensitive to cytosine arabinoside.
3. Cytosine arabinoside is quite soluble, which permits preparations of very potent concentrations.

The main disadvantage of cytosine arabinoside is its corneal toxicity. It causes corneal damage in doses comparable in antiviral effect to the IDU preparations now in clinical use. Beginning as punctate subepithelial opacities, cytosine arabinoside toxicity may progress to punctate staining or even corneal ulceration. Studies of tritiated thymidine uptake indicate inhibition of cellular metabolism of both corneal epithelium and stroma to a much greater degree than that caused by IDU.[25]

A fine punctate fluorescein staining of the corneal epithelium was reported to occur in human volunteers after instillation of 1% or 0.5% cytarabine six times daily for 2 days. These changes disappeared within 2 to 15 days after the drug was stopped. Similar use

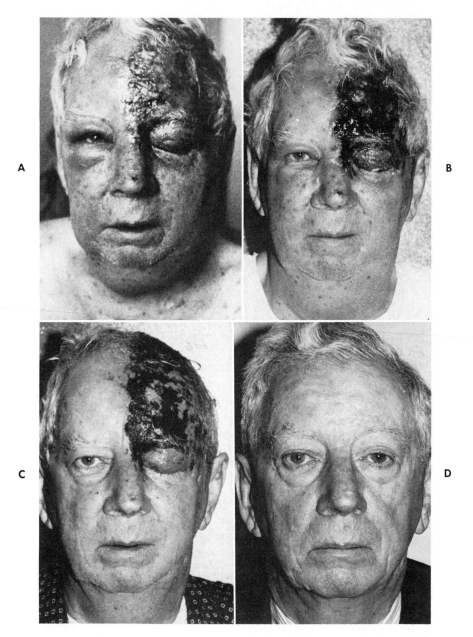

Fig. 11-5. **A,** Pretreatment appearance of herpes zoster. **B,** After 36 hours of cytarabine treatment. **C,** After 5 days of cytarabine treatment. **D,** Seven months later. (From Pierce, L. E., and Jenkins, R. B.: Arch Ophthalmol. **89:**21, 1973.)

of 0.1% cytarabine caused no corneal changes.[26]

A case report suggests that cytosine arabinoside therapy (1% ointment every 2 hours) combined with topical corticosteroids and a cycloplegic was responsible for curing acute vaccinial blepharitis and keratitis within several weeks.[27]

Intravenous cytarabine (100 mg/m^2/24 hours) caused prompt improvement (within 24 hours) of severe ophthalmic herpes zoster in three of four patients (Fig. 11-5).[28]

Apparently the high doses of cytarabine routinely advocated are unnecessary for herpes zoster ophthalmic infections. In seven cases of herpes zoster, cytarabine doses varying from 10 to 40 mg/m^2/day were found to be effective (usual recommendation, 100 mg). Toxic effects were insignificant with these low dosage schedules.[29]

VIDARABINE (ARA-A; ADENINE ARABINOSIDE)

This structural analogue of nucleic acid arrests the growth of the viral deoxynucleotide chain, a different mechanism from idoxuridine, which is incorporated into the deoxynucleotide chain, creating a fraudulent DNA. It is less toxic and more effective than idoxuridine and cytarabine and can be used effectively in treatment of patients who are allergic to idoxuridine or who are infected with herpetic strains resistant to idoxuridine.

In a double-masked study of 54 herpetic corneal epithelial ulcers, the responses to vidarabine 3% ointment or to idoxuridine 0.5% ointment, instilled 5 times daily, were virtually identical. The mean time for complete healing was 25 days for vidarabine and 20 days for idoxuridine. (The range of healing times was from 7 to 98 days.) Another group of 21 patients intolerant to idoxuridine and 37 patients nonresponsive to idoxuridine healed in a mean time of 10 days (range up to 192 days).[30]

Vidarabine was given as 3% ointment five times daily in the treatment of 56 cases of severe herpes simplex keratitis that had been resistant to IDU therapy. Eighty percent of cases of epithelial keratitis and 52% of cases

of stromal keratitis healed within 2 weeks of vidarabine therapy.[31]

In another series of 22 cases of herpes simplex keratitis uncontrolled by idoxuridine, the administration of vidarabine resulted in healing in an average of 8 days.[32]

In addition to the strain differences in herpes simplex, two distinct types are recognized. Type 1 causes the usual ocular or oral infection. Type 2 is the genital strain and is the commonest cause of neonatal viral conjunctivitis, as well as an increasingly frequent cause of adult keratoconjunctivitis. Type 2 causes more severe clinical and experimental disease. Both types may respond almost equally well to vidarabine or idoxuridine.[33]

Vidarabine can be given intravenously in dosage of 20 mg/kg, over an 8- to 12-hour period daily for a week, in the treatment of herpetic iridocyclitis.[34] Of 18 patients, 40% improved, as compared with only 10% improvement in the placebo group. Myalgia, nausea, and leukopenia were among the reactions encountered.

An important characteristic of vidarabine is that it does not interfere with the development of host immunity as does Ara-C (cytarabine; arabinosylcytosine). For this reason, it can be used in clinical antiviral therapy without the fear that it will inactivate the patient's own defense mechanisms.[35]

Comparison of topical therapy of experimental vaccinia keratitis with 0.1% idoxuridine or 5% vidarabine suspension in polyethylene glycol 4000 resulted in much superior response to the vidarabine. Idoxuridine is only weakly effective against the vaccinia virus. Vaccinia immune globulin may increase stromal scarring in vaccinia keratitis.[36]

Keratoconjunctivitis caused by adenoviruses types 3, 7, 8, and 19 does not respond to 3.3% vidarabine ointment instilled every 4 hours.[37] The typical subepithelial infiltrates developed in 81% of the vidarabine treated patients and in 63% of the controls.

Vidarabine adenine 5 phosphate (Ara-AMP) is a nucleotide form of this antiviral drug. It has the advantage of being much more soluble than vidarabine, and it possesses equal antiviral potency. Given intravenously in a dosage of 100 mg/kg, Ara-AMP will produce aqueous humor levels of 50 to 80 μg/ml lasting for 4 hours or more in rabbits. Unfortunately, topical administration of 3% Ara-AMP did not result in any detectable aqueous penetration of the drug.[38] Ara-AMP is metabolized to vidarabine, which in turn is metabolized to hypoxanthine arabinoside (Ara-Hx). Ara-Hx has about 20% of the antiviral effect of vidarabine and is sufficiently soluble to attain aqueous levels of 2 to 8 μg/ml following topical application.[39]

Neither 0.5% idoxuridine ointment nor 3% vidarabine ointment interferes with the rate of closure of corneal epithelial defects. Superficial punctate staining and epithelial edema may occur with idoxuridine but are less frequent with vidarabine. Both drugs interfere with stromal healing to the same degree. The rupture of control corneas occurred at 41 pounds per square inch of pressure at 3 weeks, in contrast to rupture of the antiviral-treated corneas at only 24 pounds per square inch. This decreased wound strength is correlated with a decrease in wound collagen content, as demonstrated by hydroxyproline assay. The therapeutic index (highest nontoxic dose/lowest effective dose) against herpes simplex keratitis is 60 for vidarabine, 4 for idoxuridine, and 4 for cytarabine.

TRIFLUOROTHYMIDINE

A new antiviral drug, trifluorothymidine (F_3TDR) has proved more potent than IDU both in vivo and in vitro. F_3TDR is not only twice as potent in antiherpetic activity but is also considerably more soluble. Concentrations of 1% are easily achieved with F_3TDR, whereas the maximum solubility of IDU is about 0.1%. No corneal toxicity was biomicroscopically evident in human volunteers receiving a 0.1% solution of F_3TDR every 2 hours for 1 week or a 1% ointment five times daily for 3 weeks.

The virus rebound phenomenon already known for IDU also occurs with F_3TDR. Treatment of experimental herpetic keratitis with F_3TDR will eliminate a recoverable virus within 2 days. However, if treatment is stopped at 1 week, the virus titer reappears and rapidly raises to values higher than those of untreated control corneas. In some animals, recurrent herpetic ulcers appear during this rise in virus titer. No such herpetic relapses occurred when treatment with either IDU or F_3TDR was continued for 2 weeks.[41]

In a double-blind trial of 40 patients with herpes simplex corneal ulcers the ulcers healed in a mean time of 6.3 days after treatment with 1.0% F_3TDR was begun, as compared to 8.2 days after treatment with 0.1% IDU was begun. Both drugs were administered by instilling 1 drop five times daily for 2 weeks, and both were nontoxic.[42]

Trifluorothymidine 0.5% every 4 hours will almost eradicate experimental vaccinia keratitis within a week. Used in 5% concentration, trifluorothymidine will sterilize the eye to viral culture and will clinically eradicate the ulcer. Trifluorothymidine is much more active against vaccinia than is idoxuridine and somewhat more active than is vidarabine.[43]

INTERFERON

An excellent review of antiviral drugs identifies a virus as having a core of either deoxyribonucleic acid (DNA) or ribonucleic acid (RNA).[44] A naturally occurring species-specific defense against viruses is the intracellular manufacture of interferon, a substance that increases resistance to virus infection. Since naturally occurring interferon is impractical to obtain, synthetic analogues such as polyinosinic acid–polycytidylic acid have been used to induce patients to form their own interferon. Much interest has been expressed in this therapeutic approach and it has been shown that interferon will increase host resistance to herpes simplex and vaccinia. Unfortunately no practical clinical value has yet resulted from these studies.[45-58]

GERMICIDES

Commonly used germicides such as cationic detergents, isopropyl alcohol, and ortho-phenol derivatives do not inactivate nonlipid-containing viruses (enterovirus, poliomyelitis, rhinovirus, encephalomyocarditis virus, and Coxsackie virus) but are active against the lipid-containing viruses (herpes simplex, vaccinia, influenza, and mumps). Three of the oldest used germicides do, however, inactivate all types of viruses. These are ethyl alcohol, 70% to 90%; carbolic acid, 5%; and sodium hypochlorite, 200 ppm. These concentrations should be observed for reliable virucidal activity.

REFERENCES

1. Kaufman, H., Nesburn, A. B., and Maloney, E. D.: IDU therapy of herpes simplex, Arch. Ophthalmol. **67**:583, 1962.
2. Kaufman, H. E., Maloney, E. D., and Nesburn, A.: Comparison of specific antiviral agents in herpes simplex keratitis, Invest. Ophthalmol. **1**:686, 1962.
3. Kaufman, H. E., and Maloney, E. D.: IDU and cytosine arabinoside in experimental herpetic keratitis, Arch. Ophthalmol. **69**:626, 1963.
4. Maloney, E. D., and Kaufman, H. E.: Antagonism and toxicity of IDU by its degradation products, Invest. Ophthalmol. **2**:55, 1963.
5. Kaufman, H. E.: Chemotherapy of herpes keratitis, Invest. Ophthalmol. **2**:205, 1963.
6. Cherry, P. M. H., and Falcon, M. G.: Punctal stenosis—caused by idoxuridine or acrodermatitis enteropathica? Arch. Ophthalmol. **94**:1632, September 1976.
7. Laibson, P. R., Sery, T. W., and Leopold, I.: The treatment of herpetic keratitis with 5-iodo-2'-deoxyuridine (IDU), Arch. Ophthalmol. **70**:52, 1963.
8. Polack, F. M., and Rose, J.: The effect of 5-iodo-2'-deoxyuridine (IDU) in corneal healing, Arch. Ophthalmol. **71**:520, 1964.
9. Payrau, P., and Dohlman, C. H.: IDU in corneal wound healing, Am. J. Ophthalmol. **57**:999, 1964.
10. Laibson, P. R., and Leopold, I. H.: An evaluation of double-blind IDU therapy in 100 cases of herpetic keratitis, Trans. Am. Acad. Ophthalmol. **68**:22, 1964.
11. Kobayashi, S., and Nakamura, T.: Herpes corneae and development of IDU resistance in herpes simplex virus, Jpn. Ophthalmol. **8**:14, 1964.
12. Maxwell, E., and Schleicher, J. B.: Experimental and clinical experiences with IDU, Eye Ear Nose Throat Mon. **43**:39, 1964.
13. Ey, R. C., Hughes, W. F., Holmes, A. W., and Deinhardt, F.: Clinical and laboratory evaluation of idoxuridine (IDU) therapy in herpes simplex keratitis, Arch. Ophthalmol. **71**:325, 1964.
14. Kaufman, H., Martola, E., and Dohlman, C.: Use of 5-iodo-2'-deoxyuridine (IDU) in treatment of herpes simplex keratitis, Arch. Ophthalmol. **68**:235, 1962.
15. Gundersen, T.: Herpes corneae: with special reference to its treatment with strong solution of iodine, Arch. Ophthalmol. **15**:225, 1936.
16. Pavan-Langston, D., and McCulley, J. P.: Herpes zoster dendritic keratitis, Arch. Ophthalmol. **89**:25, 1973.
17. Maxwell, E.: Treatment of herpes keratitis with 5-iodo-2'-deoxyuridine (IDU), Am. J. Ophthalmol. **56**:571, 1963.
18. Havener, W. H., and Wachtel, J.: IDU therapy of herpetic keratitis, Am. J. Ophthalmol. **55**:234, 1963.
19. Burns, R. P.: A double-blind study of IDU in human herpes simplex keratitis, Arch. Ophthalmol. **70**:381, 1963.
20. Jepson, C. N.: Treatment of herpes simplex of the cornea with IDU, Am. J. Ophthalmol. **57**:213, 1964.
21. Hart, D. R. L., Brightman, V. J. F., Readshaw, G. G., Porter, G. T. J., and Tully, M. J.: Treatment of human herpes simplex keratitis with idoxuridine, Arch. Ophthalmol. **73**:623, 1965.
22. Kaufman, E. H., and Maloney, E. D.: IDU and hydrocortisone in experimental herpes simplex keratitis, Arch. Ophthalmol. **68**:396, 1962.
23. Kaufman, H. E., Martola, E.-L., and Dohlman, C. H.: Herpes simplex treatment with IDU and corticosteroids, Arch. Ophthalmol. **69**:468, 1963.
24. Underood, G. E., Wisner, C. A., and Sheldon, D. W.: Cytosine arabinoside (CA) and other nucleosides in herpes virus infections, Arch. Ophthalmol. **72**:505, 1964.
25. Kaufman, H. E., Capella, J. A., Maloney, E. D., Robbins, J. E., Cooper, G. M., and Uotila, M. H.: Corneal toxicity of cytosine arabinoside, Arch. Ophthalmol. **72**:535, 1964.
26. Elliott, G. A., and Schut, A. L.: Studies with cytarabine HC1 (CA), Am. J. Ophthalmol. **60**:1074, 1965.
27. Gordon, D. M., and Advocate, S.: Vaccinial blepharokeratitis: treated with cytosine arabinoside, Am. J. Ophthalmol. **59**:480, 1965.

28. Pierce, L. E., and Jenkins, R. B.: Herpes zoster ophthalmicus treated with cytarabine, Arch. Ophthalmol. **89**:21, 1973.

29. Hryniuk, W., Foerster, J., Shojania, M., and Chow, A.: Cytarabine for herpes virus infections, J.A.M.A. **219**:715, 1972.

30. Pavan-Langston, D.: Clinical evaluation of adenine arabinoside and idoxuridine in the treatment of ocular herpes simplex, Am. J. Ophthalmol. **80**:495, September 1975.

31. O'Day, D. M., Poirier, R. H., Jones, D. B., and Elliott, J. H.: Vidarabine therapy of complicated herpes simplex keratitis, Am. J. Ophthalmol. **81**:642, May 1976.

32. Hyndiuk, R. A., Hull, D. S., Schultz, R. O., Chin, G. N., Laibson, P. R., and Krachmer, J. H.: Adenine arabinoside in idoxuridine unresponsive and intolerant herpetic keratitis, Am. J. Ophthalmol. **79**:655, April 1975.

33. North, R. D., Pavan-Langston, D., and Geary, P.: Herpes simplex virus types 1 and 2, Arch. Ophthalmol. **94**:1019, June 1976.

34. Abel, R. J., Kaufman, H. E., and Sugar, J.: Intravenous adenine arabinoside against herpes simplex keratouveitis in humans, Am. J. Ophthalmol. **79**:659, April 1975.

35. Sam, Z. S., Centifanto, Y. M., and Kaufman, H. E.: Failure of systemically administered adenine arabinoside to affect humoral and cell-mediated immunity, Am. J. Ophthalmol. **81**:502, April 1976.

36. Hyndiuk, R. A., Okumoto, M., Damiano, R. A., Valenton, M., and Smolin, G.: Treatment of vaccinial keratitis with vidarabine, Arch. Ophthalmol. **94**:1363, August 1976.

37. Waring, G. O., III, Laibson, P. R., Satz, J. E., and Joseph, N. H.: Use of vidarabine in epidemic keratoconjunctivitis due to adenovirus types 3, 7, 8, and 19, Am. J. Ophthalmol. **82**:781, November 1976.

38. Pavan-Langston, D., North, R. D., Jr., Geary, P. A., and Kinkel, A.: Intraocular penetration of the soluble antiviral, Ara AMP, Arch. Ophthalmol. **94**:1585, September 1976.

39. Pavan-Langston, D., Langston, R. H. S., and Geary, P. A.: Prophylaxis and therapy of experimental ocular herpes simplex, Arch. Ophthalmol. **92**:417, November 1974.

40. Langston, R. H. S., Pavan-Langston, D., and Dohlman, C. H.: Antiviral medication and corneal wound healing, Arch. Ophthalmol. **92**:509, December 1974.

41. Hyndiuk, R. A., and Kaufman, H. E.: Newer compounds in therapy of herpes simplex keratitis, Arch. Ophthalmol. **78**:600, 1967.

42. Wellings, P. C., Awdry, P. N., Bors, F. H., Jones, B. R., Brown, D. C., and Kaufman, H. E.: Clinical evaluation of trifluorothymidine in the treatment of herpes simplex corneal ulcers, Am. J. Ophthalmol. **73**:932, 1972.

43. Hyndiuk, R. A., Seideman, S., and Leibsohn, J. M.: Treatment of vaccinial keratitis with trifluorothymidine, Arch. Ophthalmol. **94**:1785, October 1976.

44. Proffitt, S. D., and Smith, M. F. W.: Antiviral drugs, Trans. Am. Acad. Ophthalmol. Otolaryngol. **74**:319, 1970.

45. McDonald, T. O., and Borgmann, A. R.: Polyinosinic acid—polycytidylic acid in ophthalmology, Ann. Ophthalmol. **3**:1135, 1971.

46. Weissenbacher, M., Schacter, N., Galin, M. A., and Baron, S.: Intraocular production of interferon, Arch. Ophthalmol. **84**:495, 1970.

47. Nesburn, A. B., and Zinith, P. J.: Long-term topical poly I:C in experimental chronic ocular herpes simplex infection, Am. J. Ophthalmol. **72**:821, 1971.

48. Centifanto, Y. M., Goorha, R. M., and Kaufman, H. E.: Interferon induction in rabbit and human tears, Am. J. Ophthalmol. **70**:1006, 1970.

49. Kaufman, H. E., Ellison, E. D., and Centifanto, Y. M.: Difference in interferon response and protection from ocular virus infection in rabbits and monkeys, Am. J. Ophthalmol. **74**:89, 1972.

50. Moschini, G. B., and Oh, J. O.: Experimental vaccinial keratoconjunctivitis, Arch. Ophthalmol. **87**:211, 1972.

51. Chowchuvech, E., Weissenbacher, M., Schmunis, G., Sawicki, L., Galin, M. A., and Baron, S.: The influence of polyinosinic-polycytidylic acid complex on experimental acute toxoplasmic retinochoroiditis in rabbits, Invest. Ophthalmol. **11**:182, 1972.

52. Weissenbacher, M., Galin, M. A., Chowchuvech, E., Schachter, N., and Baron, S.: Protection by polyinosinic-polycytidylic acid complex of rabbit eye tissue cultures infected with herpes simplex virus, Invest. Ophthalmol. **9**:857, 1970.

53. Kaufman, H. E., Ellison, E. D., and Waltman, S. R.: Double-stranded RNA, an interferon inducer, in herpes simplex keratitis, Am. J. Ophthalmol. **68**:486, 1969.

54. McDonald, T. O., Fox, L. G., Timberlake, G. M., Belluscio, P. R., and Borgmann, A. R.: Polyinosinic acid—polycytidylic acid in ophthalmology, Ann. Ophthalmol. **3**:371, 1971.

55. Schachter, N., Galin, M. A., Weissenbacher, M., Baron, S., and Billiau, A.: Comparison of antiviral action of interferon, interferon inducers, and IDU against herpes simplex and other viruses, Ann. Ophthalmol. **2:**795, 1970.

56. Chowchuvech, E., Weissenbacher, M., Galin, M., and Baron, S.: The influence of polyinosinic-polycytidylic acid complex on vaccinia keratitis in rabbits, Invest. Ophthalmol. **9:**716, 1970.

57. Pollikoff, R., Cannavale, P., Dixon, P., and DiPuppo, A.: Effect of complexed synthetic RNA analogues on herpes simplex virus infection in rabbit corneas, Am. J. Ophthalmol. **69:**650, 1970.

58. Interferon research report, Ann. Ophthalmol. **3:**1176, 1971.

12
AUTONOMIC DRUGS

The autonomic drugs, which include the miotic, mydriatic, and cycloplegic agents, include many of the most important and most commonly used drugs in ophthalmology.

The autonomic innervation of the eye and its effector chemicals are shown diagrammatically in Fig. 12-1. As indicated in the illustration, adrenergic impulses are transmitted to the muscle cell by norepinephrine (which is inactivated by catechol-O-methyl transferase), with the cholinergic mediator being acetylcholine (which is destroyed by acetylcholinesterase).[1]

The preganglionic fiber transmits impulses by a mechanism of progressive change in permeability, just as do all other nerve fibers. The internal resting potential of a nerve axon is about -70 mv. This potential results from a relatively low internal concentration of sodium ions, associated with a relatively high internal concentration of potassium ions (diagrammatically shown in Fig. 12-2). The mechanism of discharge of the nerve is a sudden increase in permeability of the neuronal membrane to sodium; the rapid entry of sodium changes the internal potential from negative to positive.[2] This membrane permeability change is self-propagating and is responsible for the progress of the nerve impulse. The mechanism of this progressive permeability change is unknown but probably is not caused by acetylcholine as has been postulated in the past.

When the nerve action potential reaches the end of the axon, it causes release of the neurohumoral transmitter chemical, the agent responsible for chemical propagation of the impulse across the synapse or neuroeffector junction. These neurochemicals are stored in synaptic vesicles, spherical structures about 500 Å in diameter, which are densely present at presynaptic terminals. After release, the neurochemical diffuses across the synaptic cleft, a distance of 100 to

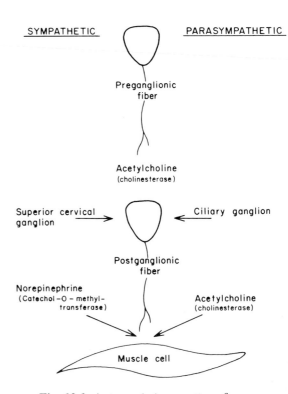

Fig. 12-1. Autonomic innervation of eye.

218

500 Å, and reacts with the receptor surface. This reaction can cause either excitation or inhibition, depending on whether membrane permeability is increased generally or only selectively. The extreme complexity of synaptic transmission is illustrated by electron microscopy, which shows that as many as 50,000 terminal boutons may connect with a single anterior horn cell.

The synaptic vesicle membranes of cholinergic axons contain concentrations of choline acetylase, the catalyst responsible for the final synthesis of acetylcholine. The synaptic vesicles apparently contain pockets of acetylcholine (estimated as 1000 molecules per vesicle) that are discharged as units. High concentrations of cholinesterase are present at all sites of cholinergic transmission.

Norepinephrine, the adrenergic transmitter, is found within the synaptic vesicles, in the terminal axonal cytoplasm, and in a reserve form that is bound to adenosine triphosphate. Two enzymes, monoamine oxidase and catechol-O-methyl transferase, are responsible for norepinephrine breakdown but do not terminate adrenergic effects in the same manner as acetylcholine. At adrenergic terminals the norepinephrine is dissipated partly by diffusion but mostly through active resorption by the adrenergic axon terminal. Apparently the resorbed norepinephrine reenters the storage granules.

The pathways of catecholamine metabolism are shown in greatly simplified form in Fig. 12-3. From the precursor tyrosine, the three functional catecholamines (dopamine, norepinephrine and epinephrine) are synthesized and ultimately metabolized to vanillylmandelic acid. The reader should be aware that many intermediate compounds occur, many specific enzymes function, and different parts of the body (for example, the liver, kidney,

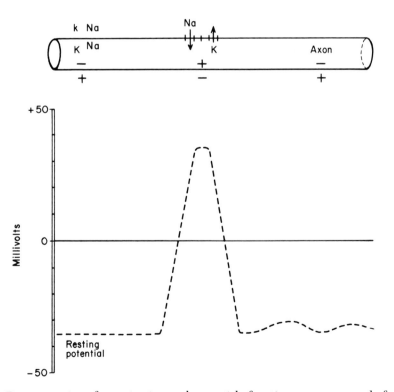

Fig. 12-2. Representation of negative internal potential of resting nerve axon and of positive electrical spike produced by localized increased membrane permeability to sodium as the nerve impulse progresses down the axon. After passage of impulse, membrane permeability and electrical balance rapidly return to resting state.

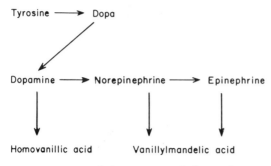

Fig. 12-3. Catecholamine metabolic pathways. (Data from Crout, J. R.: Anesthesiology **29**:661, 1968.)

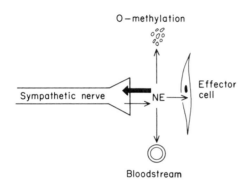

Fig. 12-4. Fate of norepinephrine, *NE*, after release from sympathetic terminal. (Modified from Kramer, S. G., and Potts, A. M.: Am. J. Ophthalmol. **67**:705, 1969.)

and adrenergic neuron) contribute differently to catecholamine metabolism.[3,4] As is suggested by the diagram, the major end metabolite of norepinephrine, vanillylmandelic acid, is a useful index of total catecholamine synthesis. For this reason, urinary assays of vanillylmandelic acid are useful in the diagnosis of pheochromocytoma and neuroblastoma, tumors that produce large amounts of catecholamines.

After release from the postganglionic sympathetic nerve terminal, norepinephrine may be absorbed by the effector cell, may diffuse into the bloodstream, may be broken down enzymatically (a relatively slow process), or may undergo uptake by the same sympathetic nerve terminal from which it was released —probably the most rapid and effective

route of norepinephrine removal. Fig. 12-4 schematically illustrates these four norepinephrine pathways.[5]

The phenomenon of denervation hypersensitivity is chronologically related to the progressive failure of the degenerating nerve to take up norepinephrine. Carotid infusion with radioactive norepinephrine results in a rapid and selective concentration of radioactivity in tissues rich in sympathetic innervation (for example, the iris and ciliary body). After superior cervical ganglionectomy in cats, this selective radioactive uptake is progressively lost (Fig. 12-5)[5] within a 2-week period as the sympathetic nerves degenerate.

This abolition of iris uptake of catecholamines closely corresponds in time to the development of maximal supersensitivity of denervation (Fig. 12-6).[5] Presumably the supersensitivity occurs because of the loss of uptake into the degenerating neurons, which represents a loss of the mechanism for inactivation of catecholamines.[6]

Blocking of the superior cervical ganglion with lidocaine does not cause denervation hypersensitivity and does not interfere with catecholamine uptake by the iris. In this experiment the radioactive norepinephrine was administered by right carotid infusion. Fig. 12-5 shows the great difference in norepinephrine uptake between the right and left iris. This may be construed to indicate that a medication that is rapidly absorbed from the blood can be given most effectively by intraarterial injection into the vessel nourishing the organ to be treated. A practical illustration of this method is the intracarotid injection of triethylenemelamine for retinoblastoma.

Transient mydriasis and iritis 15 to 24 hours after superior cervical ganglionectomy are of theoretical interest. The mydriasis is caused by release of norepinephrine from the degenerating sympathetic terminal.[7] The hyperemia is caused by prostaglandin synthesis, which is dependent on norepinephrine release. Indomethacin will inhibit prostaglandin synthesis and prevent denervation hyperemia.[8]

Differences in the effects produced by

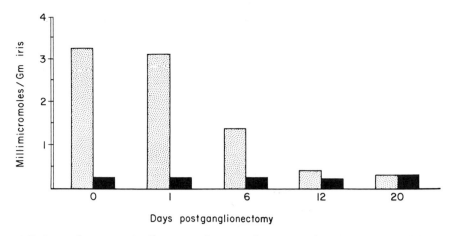

Fig. 12-5. Iris radioactivity (millimicromols tritiated norepinephrine) on specified days after right superior cervical ganglionectomy. Solid bars: left iris. Dotted bars: right iris. Norepinephrine administered by right carotid infusion. (From Kramer, S. G., and Potts, A. M.: Am. J. Ophthalmol. **67:**705, 1969.)

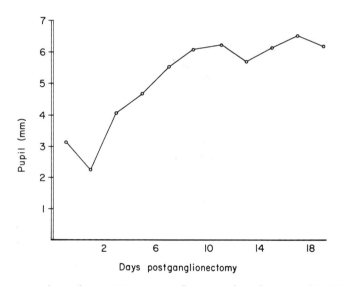

Fig. 12-6. Denervated pupil size 45 minutes after topical application of 0.1% epinephrine. (From Kramer, S. G., and Potts, A. M.: Am. J. Ophthalmol. **67:**705, 1969.)

adrenergic stimulation also vary with the receptor sites. Alpha receptors are excitatory; for example, they may mediate vasoconstriction. Beta receptors are inhibitory and may mediate vasodilation. Norepinephrine is primarily an alpha stimulator. Isoproterenol is primarily a beta stimulator. Epinephrine can act on either alpha or beta receptors. Compounds that block either alpha or beta receptors are available. Alpha blockers include

drugs such as ergotoxine and Dibenamine, Dechlor-isoproterenol is a beta blocker.[9,10]

In the human eye, alpha adrenergic stimulation (norepinephrine) decreases the resistance to aqueous outflow. Beta adrenergic stimulation (isoproterenol) decreases the rate of aqueous secretion. Epinephrine, having both alpha and beta activity, reduces intraocular pressure through both mechanisms.[11-15]

Experimental pharmacologic methods indicate that the intraocular muscles ordinarily have dual adrenergic receptor mechanisms. The relative distribution of these receptors in a given intraocular muscle varies in different species of animals; hence drug responses are different from one species to another. For example, the cat ciliary muscle has mostly beta adrenergic receptors, whereas that of the rabbit has mostly alpha receptors.[16] Furthermore, individual muscles, such as the cat iris dilator, may receive both sympathetic and parasympathetic innervation.[17,18]

Both autoradiographic[19] and fluorescent histochemical[20] studies show the presence of catecholamines throughout the uveal tract (iris, ciliary body, and choroid) and surrounding the retinal arterioles. These studies provide the anatomic basis for the expected responses to autonomic stimulation of uveal and retinal vessels (epinephrine constriction and acetylcholine dilation).[21] However, the evaluation of autonomic effects on intraocular hemodynamics is beset with difficulty, since other authors believe these changes are passive responses to alterations of the systemic blood pressure.[22]

Transmission of autonomic nerve impulses may be altered by drugs in a number of ways, depending on which portion of the system is involved. Mechanisms pertinent to ophthalmology include the following[2]:

Inhibition of enzymatic breakdown of transmitter
Physostigmine, isofluorophate
Blockade of transmitter at postsynaptic receptor
Atropine
Mimicry of transmitter at postsynaptic receptor
Phenylephrine (alpha adrenergic)
Isoproterenol (beta adrenergic)
Methacholine (muscarinic cholinergic)
Displacement of transmitter from axonal terminal
Carbachol (cholinergic)
Ephedrine (adrenergic, rapid)
Guanethidine (adrenergic, slow, depletes adrenergic effector)

Autonomic effects are termed direct when the drug acts on the muscle end plate in the same manner as norepinephrine or acetylcholine. The effect is termed indirect if the drug either inhibits destruction or liberates the natural effector chemical from nerve endings.

Since adrenergic and cholinergic actions are mutually antagonistic, it is evident that a comparable effect results from inhibition of the one (lytic effect) or stimulation of the other (mimetic effect). Accordingly, autonomic effects may be logically subdivided as follows.[23,24]

I. Adrenergic action (mydriasis and cycloplegia)
  A. Sympathomimetic (mydriasis)
    1. Direct acting
      a. Epinephrine
      b. Phenylephrine
    2. Indirect acting
      a. Hydroxyamphetamine
      b. Cocaine
      c. Ephedrine
  B. Parasympatholytic (cycloplegia)
    1. Atropine
    2. Homatropine
    3. Scopolamine
    4. Cyclopentolate
    5. Tropicamide
    6. Oxyphenonium
II. Cholinergic action (miosis and accommodation)
  A. Parasympathomimetic
    1. Direct acting
      a. Acetylcholine
      b. Methacholine
      c. Carbachol
      d. Pilocarpine
    2. Indirect acting
      a. Reversible
        (1) Eserine
        (2) Carbachol
        (3) Edrophonium
      b. "Irreversible"
        (1) Isoflurophate
        (2) Echothiophate
        (3) Demecarium
  B. Sympatholytic
    1. Guanethidine
    2. Dibenamine
    3. Dihydroergocornine
    4. Tolazoline
III. Ganglionic blocking agents
  A. Tetraethyl ammonium chloride
  B. Hexamethonium

Autonomically innervated muscles such as

Table 12-1. Miotic effect of parasympathomimetic drugs on normal and denervated iris sphincters*

Drug	Normal eye	Parasympathetic denervation
Pilocarpine, 1% solution	+	+ +
Methacholine, 2.5% solution	0	+
Isoflurophate, 0.1% solution	+ +	0

*Modified from Leopold, I. H.: Arch. Ophthalmol. **51:** 885, 1962.

the iris sphincter continue to respond to stimulation by appropriate direct-acting autonomic drugs even when their innervation is destroyed. Indeed, the denervated muscle becomes sensitized and will react to smaller concentrations of drug than will a normal muscle. However, indirect-acting miotics, which achieve their effect by inhibiting cholinesterase, will not stimulate a completely denervated sphincter. The response to miotics of a patient with paralytic mydriasis is outlined in Table 12-1.[25] It is apparent that pilocarpine will constrict the pupil of such a patient, thereby eliminating glare and cosmetic defect. Of course, if the mydriasis is a result of anatomic tearing or destruction of the sphincter, it will not respond to pilocarpine. Similarly, posterior synechiae immobilize the pupil to all drugs.

ADRENERGIC AGENTS
Epinephrine

In ophthalmology, epinephrine is useful because of its vasoconstrictor and ocular hypotensive effects.

Pharmacology

Epinephrine and norepinephrine are the naturally occurring sympathomimetic effector substances. They act directly on the effector cells; the cellular response is increased rather than blocked by autonomic denervation. Epinephrine is produced by the adrenal medulla and acts mainly as a neurohumoral agent. Norepinephrine (levarterenol) is the neurotransmitter of peripheral sympathetic nerves.

The adrenergic neurotransmitter chemicals are catecholamine derivatives. The three sympathomimetically active catecholamines (dopamine, norepinephrine, and epinephrine) are all derived from tyrosine in the chemical sequence tyrosine → dopamine → norepinephrine → epinephrine. Norepinephrine, the true sympathetic neurotransmitter, is stored in vesicles at the synaptic end of the axon. Apparently the release of norepinephrine is accomplished by extrusion of vesicle contents. Although norepinephrine may be inactivated by monoamine oxidase or by catechol-O-methyl transferase, inhibition of these enzymes does not greatly potentiate the effects of nerve stimulation.[26] Uptake by sympathetic neurons is a more important means of norepinephrine removal than either metabolism or diffusion. Sympathetic supersensitivity, as may be produced by cocaine administration or by chronic sympathetic denervation, is associated with a significant decrease in norepinephrine uptake by the sympathetic neuron.[27]*

Topical application of a monoamine oxidase inhibitor (pargyline) on rabbit eyes causes a 20% decrease in intraocular pressure within a 4-hour period. Since the outflow facility is unchanged, this effect is presumably a result of inhibition of aqueous secretion. This destruction of monoamine oxidase does not, however, permit a catecholamine accumulation sufficient to cause mydriasis.[28]

Pargyline 0.5% drops reduced intraocular pressure in glaucomatous human eyes by as much as 18 mm Hg, the effect beginning in about 1 hour and lasting for 5 hours. Pupil size was unchanged.[29]

Monoamine oxidase activity is histochemically demonstrable in the retina, optic nerve, ciliary body, iris, choroid, and cornea, but not in the sclera, vitreous, or lens substance.[30]

*An excellent symposium concerning the autonomic nervous system may be found in Anesthesiology **29:** 643, 1968.

Depletion of norepinephrine from the iris may be achieved by guanethidine, which may be administered by parenteral injection, intraocular injection, or topical ocular instillation. Comparable norepinephrine depletion results from postganglionic sympathectomy or from reserpine pretreatment. Norepinephrine depletion results in miosis and ptosis as well as in increased sensitivity (denervation hypersensitivity) to the directly acting catecholamines (for example, epinephrine and phenylephrine). However, norepinephrine depletion reduces or abolishes the mydriatic effect of indirectly acting sympathomimetic amines (amphetamine, hydroxyamphetamine, ephedrine, and tyramine). These findings have been confirmed in human patients receiving 10% guanethidine drops twice daily for treatment of thyroid lid retraction.[31]

Epinephrine and norepinephrine cause sympathomimetic effects in extremely minute doses. A concentration as dilute as 0.01 μg/ml (0.000,001%) will cause demonstrable relaxation of ciliary muscle.[32] Norepinephrine, an alpha stimulator, causes vasoconstriction of the cat ophthalmic artery with measurable (about 10%) reduction of the flow rate.[33] Tolazoline (Priscoline), an alpha blocker, inhibits this vasoconstriction. The remarkable sensitivity of this response requires a concentration of only 0.000,000,01% of norepinephrine and 0.000,000,1% of tolazoline. Beta-stimulating sympathomimetic agents in 0.000,001% concentration (isoproterenol, isoxsuprine, and nylidrin) have been demonstrated to counteract constriction of the ophthalmic artery caused by alpha stimulators. Pilocarpine (0.000,001%) dilated the ophthalmic artery.

Accommodation. It has been suggested that just as parasympathetic activity accommodates the eye for near vision, sympathetic activity adapts the eye for distant vision. If this were true, use of epinephrine and cocaine would be expected to alter the refraction of a fully atropinized eye. Subconjunctival injection of 0.2 ml of a 1:1000 solution of epinephrine following six instillations of a 4% concentration of cocaine at 10-minute inter-vals does not change the refraction of human eyes atropinized for 3 days.[34]

Negative accommodation (block of accommodation) of as much as 10 D could be produced in monkeys by beta sympathetic stimulation resulting from subconjunctival injection of isoproterenol. Propranolol, a beta blocker, inhibited this negative accommodation response.[35]

Clinical use

Vasoconstriction. The vasoconstricting effect of epinephrine helps to control bleeding from capillaries and small arterioles but is ineffective against hemorrhage from larger vessels. During most ophthalmic operations it is the oozing from these smaller vessels that obscures surgical details; hence preliminary use of epinephrine is of considerable value in eye surgery. It may be used in a 1:1000 solution for surface application to the conjunctiva or wound surface and in a 1:50,000 solution (combined with the anesthetic) for injection at the site of incision. Vasoconstriction occurs within 5 minutes but lasts for less than 1 hour.

Inclusion of a 1:50,000 concentration of epinephrine in solutions of anesthetics for local injection will cause vasoconstriction sufficient to delay the loss of anesthetic effect through absorption. Used in this way, epinephrine reduces possible systemic toxicity by allowing time for detoxification of the slowly absorbed anesthetic and by reducing the amount of anesthetic required for the procedure. No local ischemic damage results from the injection of this concentration of epinephrine about the eye.

Epinephrine enhances intraocular penetration of subconjunctivally injected medications. Presumably, vasoconstriction prevents rapid loss of the medication into the general circulation.[36]

Application of epinephrine in a 1:1000 solution has been suggested as a means of differentiation between superficial and deep inflammation. Epinephrine vasoconstriction primarily affects the superficial conjunctival vessels, but it also has an effect on the deep conjunctival vessels.[37] Repeated application of epinephrine will ultimately also constrict the episcleral vessels. Hence prompt blanching of a red eye suggests that conjunctivitis is a more likely diagnosis than is iritis. However, epinephrine blanching is a less reliable diagnostic criterion in the evaluation of a red eye than are the physical signs such as pupil size, intraocular pressure, and opacities of the media.[38]

A theoretically interesting effect of epinephrine blanching of the conjunctiva is the appearance of conspicuous aqueous veins, which were blood filled before the vasoconstriction. A single drop of 1:1000 epinephrine will reduce the blood component sufficiently to reveal the aqueous lamination.[39]

Because of their vasoconstricting effects, solutions of 1:1000 and 1:100 epinephrine may be used as decongestants to blanch conjunctival vessels that have become reddened because of nonspecific chronic irritation or allergy. This blanching effect usually lasts for less than an hour and may be followed by reactive hyperemia. Hence the longer acting sympathomimetic drugs such as phenylephrine are more commonly prescribed as nonspecific decongestants.

Mydriasis. Epinephrine in a 1:1000 concentration is not a very good mydriatic in the normal human eye, probably because of its rapid destruction. When the permeability of the eye is increased by trauma (as during surgery for strabismus), the pupil may become quite dilated from topical application of epinephrine. Prolonged contact with the eye (and probably minor trauma) may be achieved by placing a small cotton pack soaked with epinephrine in the lower cul-de-sac. This method of application will result in mydriasis and has been advocated for the breaking of posterior synechiae. The use of epinephrine together with miotics in glaucoma therapy will cause the pupil to be slightly larger than it is with miotics alone.

It is well recognized that mydriatics are less effective in dark-colored eyes than in light-colored ones. Epinephrine, an adrenergic mediator for the dilator system, is destroyed by dihydroxyphenylalanine (dopa), a link in melanin metabolism. Homogenates of dark-colored rabbit irides (but not of light-colored ones) will inactivate epinephrine.[40] Guinea pig irides that are pigmented will

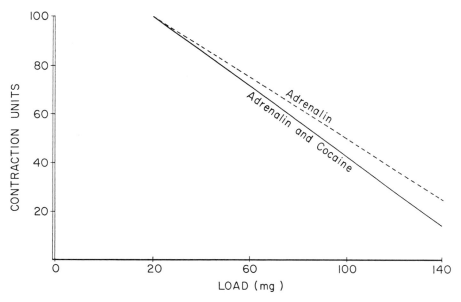

Fig. 12-7. Response of dilator muscle of albino rabbit to epinephrine and to epinephrine-cocaine combination. Note decreased strength of the cocainized muscle at any given level of contraction. (From Sachs, E., and Heath, P.: Am. J. Ophthalmol. **23:**1376, 1940.)

bind twice as much norepinephrine as will those that are nonpigmented.[41]

Although cocaine sensitizes the iris dilator muscle to respond to lesser amounts of epinephrine, the sensitization is not synonymous with increased strength of contraction. As shown in Fig. 12-7, the strength of a muscle at any given degree of contraction is greater in response to epinephrine alone than to a combination of epinephrine and cocaine (both drugs in a 1:500,000 concentration).[42] Clearly, cocaine decreases the working capacity of the dilator muscle. Hence the ancient combination of cocaine and epinephrine is an irrational approach to dilation of the pupil.

Glaucoma. Although it seems paradoxical to sue a pupil-dilating drug in the treatment of glaucoma, there is sound evidence to support such therapy. Clinicians have long known that sympathomimetic mydriatics are not useful in provocative testing for open-angle glaucoma, since they are more likely to reduce pressure than to cause elevation. Also for this reason, drugs such as phenylephrine and hydroxyamphetamine (Paredrine) have been advocated to aid the general practitioner in ophthalmoscopic examination. They do not cause dangerous pressure elevation in chronic simple glaucoma, produce minimal cycloplegia, and act for only a short period of time.

Sympathomimetic mydriatics reduce intraocular pressure by decreasing the rate of aqueous formation. In most patients the coefficient of outflow is at first unchanged by the use of sympathomimetics. Particularly important is the fact that the therapeutically effective increase in the coefficient of outflow produced in human glaucomatous eyes by miotics is *not* decreased when the pupils are dilated by simultaneous use of sympathomimetics such as phenylephrine.[43] An additive effect is produced by the simultaneous use of miotics and sympathomimetics (and also carbonic anhydrase inhibitors) in the treatment of glaucoma.

Clinical study of a number of sympathomimetic compounds showed that a 1% solution of levo-epinephrine occasionally helped control glaucoma.[44] A 10% solution of phenylephrine was slightly more effective than a 1% concentration of levo-epinephrine but was less effective than a 2% solution of levo-epinephrine. The 2% solution (Glaucon) was used predominantly in this study of 219 glaucoma patients. It was found to be stable for more than 6 months when refrigerated and was well tolerated by most patients. Topical application of a 2% solution of levoepinephrine to 44 glaucomatous eyes caused an average drop in pressure of 13.5 mm Hg (range, 3 to 38 mm Hg). A marked pressure drop was obtained within 1 hour, and pressure continued to fall slightly for 4 hours (Fig. 12-8). A slow rise followed, with a good effect lasting for 12 hours and a slight effect for as long as 24 hours. Eyes most likely to respond well to a 2% solution of levo-epinephrine were those with a coefficient of outflow better than 0.15, the pressures of which were maintained in the upper twenties with miotics. The pressure in most of these eyes could be dropped to the low twenties or below by instillation of a 2% solution of levo-epinephrine twice daily. Although in some instances glaucoma could be controlled by a 2% concentration of levo-epinephrine alone, the best results were obtained when this drug was used in combination with a miotic. Patients with early cataracts were particularly pleased by the improvement in vision resulting from partial dilatation of the pupil. Secondary, absolute, and congenital types of glaucoma were not controlled by a 2% solution of levo-epinephrine.

A pressure-lowering effect can be demonstrated with epinephrine concentrations as low as 0.125%; however, a substantially greater response occurs to 1%.[45]

There were few significant adverse effects from the topical use of a 2% solution of levo-epinephrine. Systemic effects such as tachycardia were not troublesome. Blanching of the conjunctival vessels caused the eyes to appear very white, which was cosmetically desirable. Several patients developed reactive hyperemia of the conjunctiva, which appeared about 5 hours after instillation. Two patients suffered intense orbital pain for

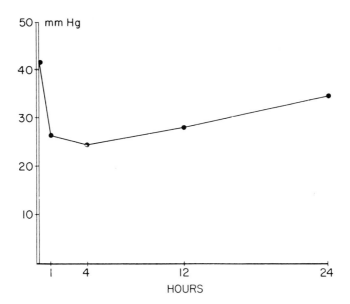

Fig. 12-8. Average response of 44 untreated glaucomatous eyes to 1 drop of a 2% solution of levo-epinephrine. (From Garner, L. L., and associates: Arch. Ophthalmol. **62:**230, 1959.)

several hours after treatment. However, the comment that any type of local medication resulted in considerable pain in these same two patients suggests that they were exceptionally sensitive individuals. Mydriasis, with photophobia and blurred vision, resulted from the use of a 2% solution of levo-epinephrine alone but was eliminated by simultaneous use of a 1% concentration of pilocarpine or some stronger miotic. Three cases of allergy were noted, but all were proved to result from the tetracaine used in the experimental solution.

The side effects of topical epinephrine therapy are quite annoying, however. In one series of 50 patients, only 20% could continue epinephrine drops for a 4-year period.[46] Reactive hyperemia, irritation, and tearing affected two thirds of the patients. Headaches affected 5 patients; cardiac palpitation, 4; blurred vision, 10; allergy, 6; and conjunctival pigmentation, 12. The epinephrine preparations originally available, which were used in this series of patients, were much more irritating than are the more recently developed commercial preparations. Thus ocular tolerance to currently dispensed

epinephrine drops is much greater than that indicated by these statistics.

The effect of single drops of three different epinephrine compounds—bitartrate (Epitrate), hydrochloride (Glaucon), and epinephryl borate (Eppy)—on intraocular pressure and outflow facility was evaluated in 24 patients. No significant difference was found.[47]

Gonioscopy is advised before use of sympathomimetic mydriatics to avoid precipitation of acute angle-block glaucoma. I have personally observed a patient with subacute angle-closure glaucoma (initial pressure, 30 mm Hg) in whom a 1% solution of hydroxyamphetamine precipitated an acute attack that could *not* be controlled medically. Particular caution is necessary if the anterior chamber is visibly shallow.

An additive effect occurs when epinephrine and acetazolamide (Diamox)[48] are used simultaneously to reduce the rate of aqueous secretion (Fig. 12-9). Forty-one glaucomatous eyes treated with azetazolamide, 250 mg every 6 hours, showed an average pressure drop of 13 mm Hg (range, 5 to 50 mm Hg). Addition of a 4.5% solution of epinephrine

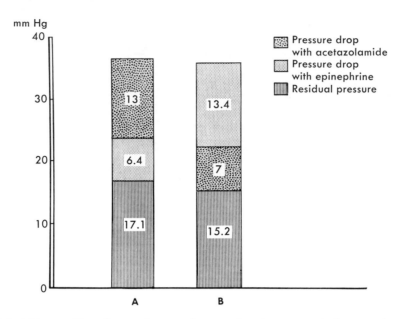

Fig. 12-9. Additive effect of epinephrine and acetazolamide in control of intraocular pressure. **A,** Acetazolamide first and then epinephrine. **B,** Epinephrine first and then acetazolamide. (Data from Becker, B.: Am. J. Ophthalmol. **45**:639, 1958.)

bitartrate at night (only *once* daily) further lowered intraocular pressure by an average of 6.4 mm Hg (range, 1 to 21 mm Hg). When epinephrine was used initially, the pressure in 20 eyes dropped an average of 13.4 mm Hg (range, 4 to 54 mm Hg). Addition of acetazolamide further lowered the pressure an average of 7 mm Hg (range, 2 to 15 mm Hg). These studies were carried out on known glaucomatous eyes that were continued on their regular miotic therapy throughout the experiment. The facility of aqueous outflow was unchanged by epinephrine or acetazolamide. In many of these patients the addition of epinephrine and/or acetazolamide made the difference between uncontrolled pressures and a good therapeutic response. The author concluded that aqueous secretion was suppressed approximately 37% by topical application of epinephrine and 50% by acetazolamide. Used together, the drugs have an additive effect, reducing secretion an average of 66%.

What is the mechanism whereby aqueous secretion is decreased by sympathomimetic amines? Tonometry and fluorometric measurement of outflow were employed in glau-

Table 12-2. Improvement of outflow facility in 72 patients with open-angle glaucoma after topical use of a 2% solution of epinephrine*

Duration of epinephrine therapy	Fifty percent increase in outflow facility†
6 months	62%
2 years	56%

* From Becker, B., Petitt, T. H., and Gay, A. J.: Arch. Ophthalmol. **66**:219, 1961.
† Percentages represent proportion of patients with improved outflow facility of 50% or more.

comatous eyes to evaluate the effect of levo-epinephrine, dextro-epinephrine, and isoproterenol (Aludrine).[49] (Isoproterenol inhibits smooth muscle and is *not* a vasoconstrictor.) The average pressure drop after administration of levo-epinephrine was 8.5 mm Hg; after dextro-epinephrine, 2.5 mm Hg; and after isoproterenol, 10.7 mm Hg. It was concluded that the sympathomimetic pressure-lowering effect is not caused by vasoconstriction, since isoproterenol is not a vasoconstrictor and since the pressure-lowering

Table 12-3. Improvement of outflow facility in 38 patients with open-angle glaucoma after use of a 2% solution of levo-epinephrine in one eye and other eye used as control*

Duration of epinephrine therapy	Percent of pretreatment outflow facility†	
	Eyes receiving therapy	Control eyes
3 months	145%	98%
6 months	163%	106%

*From Becker, B., Petitt, T. H., and Gay, A. J.: Arch. Ophthalmol. **66:**219, 1961.
†Percentages represent outflow facility values in terms of pretreatment average considered to be 100%.

effect lasted for 24 hours or more (longer than the duration of vasoconstriction). Nor is the increased tone of the dilator muscle responsible for the reduced aqueous production, since isoproterenol is not a mydriatic. Apparently a beta-stimulating sympathetic effect on the secretory mechanism is responsible for the hyposecretion.

A second mechanism of action by which epinephrine reduces intraocular pressure, namely, improvement of the facility of outflow, has been demonstrated. This improved facility is not immediate but may be observed after several months of topical epinephrine therapy. Evidence supporting this mechanism of action consists of a retrospective study of 72 patients and a controlled study of 38 patients.[50] The first group of patients had used a 2% solution of epinephrine topically twice a day for 6 to 24 months. All of the patients had proved open-angle glaucoma. In this series of 121 glaucomatous eyes, 62% showed increased facility of outflow by at least 50% over pretreatment levels at the end of 6 months. Of 55 eyes followed for over 2 years, 56% still maintained this 50% (or more) improvement in outflow (Table 12-2). Side effects forced discontinuance of epinephrine therapy in 27 of these 72 patients. Twenty had reactive hyperemia, and seven developed severe contact allergy of the lids. No corneal or lens opacities or other serious complications have been attributed to epinephrine therapy.

The second group, consisting of 38 patients, used a 2% levo-epinephrine solution in one eye only, the other eye serving as a control. The tonographically more abnormal eye was selected for treatment. At the end of 3 months the facility of outflow of the treated eyes averaged 145% of the pretreatment level, whereas the average facility of the control eyes was only 98% of the pretreatment value. At 6 months the facility of outflow of treated eyes averaged 163% of pretreatment values, compared with outflow facility of control eyes of 106% (Table 12-3). The improvement of outflow in the treated eyes is of a statistically significant magnitude and must be accepted as valid evidence of an epinephrine effect.

That the coefficient of outflow in glaucomatous eyes is improved after prolonged levo-epinephrine therapy has been confirmed by other studies.[51] In a series of 81 eyes with chronic simple glaucoma, 68% were found to attain an increase in outflow facility of at least 50% after levo-epinephrine therapy. This increase in outflow facility occurred only after prolonged therapy. In 40% of the treated eyes the response occurred within 1 month and in 63%, within 1 year (Fig. 12-10). In five eyes improved outflow was first noted only after more than a year of epinephrine therapy. Although the improved outflow was maintained by most eyes, it was subsequently lost in 10 eyes after intervals of 2 to 9 months. About 10% of this series of patients developed allergy to the epinephrine preparation. It was suggested that this sensitivity might be caused by antioxidants in the solution and not by epinephrine itself.

The outflow-increasing effect of epinephrine appears to result from its action on the innervation of the trabecular meshwork. Experimental work indicating this as the site of action may be summarized as follows[52]: Cer-

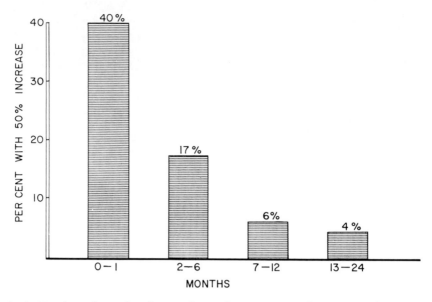

Fig. 12-10. Number of months of epinephrine therapy required to attain at least a 50% improvement of outflow facility. Percentage represents proportion of group of 81 eyes with chronic simple glaucoma that attained 50% improvement within the specified number of months. (Modified from Ballintine, E. J., and Garner, L.: Arch. Ophthalmol. 66:314, 1961.)

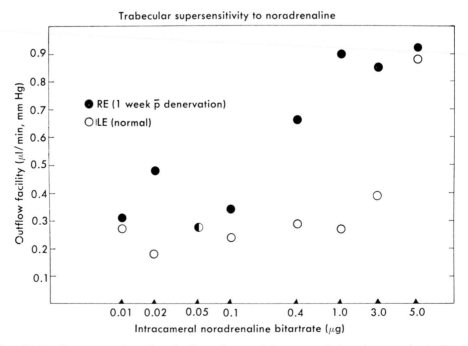

Fig. 12-11. Response of outflow facility of normal (open circles) and sympathetically denervated (black circles) rabbit eyes to injection of various amounts of norepinephrine. (From Sears, M. L., and Sherk, T. E.: Invest. Ophthalmol. 3:157, 1964.)

vical sympathectomy in rabbits increased the sensitivity of the outflow response to norepinephrine by about 150 times. (Intracameral injection of 0.02 μg/ml in the denervated eye produced an outflow increase comparable to that produced by 3 μg in normal eyes.) Complete sympathetic blockade (by intravenous phenoxybenzamine) eliminated all outflow response to norepinephrine. The increased facility of outflow is quite marked 1 hour after injection of norepinephrine into the anterior chamber (Fig. 12-11). Other sites of action that were ruled out included episcleral resistance (excluded by dissection away of surface tissue and by a lesser response to subconjunctival injection than to intracameral injection), ciliary muscle stimulation (excluded by lesser response to vitreous injections adjacent to the ciliary muscle), iris (excluded by absence of pupillary response at low levels and by absence of aqueous protein alterations), mechanical deepening of the anterior chamber (excluded by control injection of saline solution), nonspecific chemical effect (excluded by phenoxybenzamine block), and vascular responses (excluded by the variation in response to different sites of injection and by absence of aqueous protein changes).

In monkeys, an immediate increase in the true facility of outflow and in pseudofacility can be demonstrated after topical application of epinephrine.[53] Apparently the primate eye can respond to epinephrine by both immediate and delayed improvement of outflow. A comparable immediate increase in outflow facility has been demonstrated in some normal and glaucomatous human eyes.[54]

Topically applied epinephrine may have primarily a beta effect (decreased aqueous secretion) in low concentrations (0.06% to 0.50%), whereas higher concentrations (1.0% to 2.0%) activate the alpha mechanism (increased outflow facility).[55] However, such a supposition seems incompatible with the extreme sensitivity known to characterize autonomic responses. This study also indicated that epinephrine supplementation of 4% pilocarpine therapy of glaucomatous eyes was of no clinical value in concentrations of less

than 0.5%. An increasing hypotensive response was reported with epinephrine concentrations ranging from 0.5% to 2%. A 20% to 30% increase in the hypotensive effect was achieved by adding 2% epinephrine borate to the 4% pilocarpine.

Chemical sympathectomy with 6-hydroxydopamine sensitizes the eye to epinephrine. Subsequent epinephrine therapy (1% three times daily) maintained 29 of 36 eyes below 20 mm Hg for up to 29 weeks. This management was most effective in patients who had previously been well controlled with pilocarpine and epinephrine and was not very effective in patients who had not been well controlled medically prior to use of the 6-hydroxydopamine.[56] Chemical sympathectomy is not likely to supplant conventional medical therapy.

Contrary to current belief, the use of epinephrine in the treatment of glaucoma is not new, but was popular a generation ago.[57-60]

Diagnosis of sympathetic denervation. The sensitivity of the miotic pupil of Horner's syndrome of sympathetic denervation to dilation by a 1:1000 epinephrine solution is a well-known clinical diagnostic test.

Comparable epinephrine sensitization, but to a lesser degree, exists in Fuchs' heterochromic iritis. Instillation of 1% epinephrine (Eppy) increased the pupil diameter of the hypopigmented eye by 98% in four patients with heterochromia. In comparison the pupils of eight control patients were dilated only 1% by the epinephrine. An unexpected finding was the 72% dilation of the normally pigmented fellow eyes. Apparently, Fuchs' syndrome is a bilateral fault in the postganglionic sympathetic pathways, although more marked on the hypopigmented side.[61]

Toxicity

During surgery. Minor systemic side effects commonly occur after injection of solutions of epinephrine and anesthetic. These effects include nervousness and anxiety, tachycardia, tremors, headache, and pallor. Such symptoms may be quite alarming to the patient, who should be reassured that they are without significance and will soon disappear.

The frequency of these side effects is not surprising if one realizes that the average adult therapeutic dose of epinephrine, 0.25 mg, is contained in 12.5 ml of a 1:50,000 solution of epinephrine and anesthetic. Of course, this is not all absorbed at once, and the rapid systemic detoxification of the drug helps to reduce the frequency and severity of reactions.

Accidental intravenous injection of epinephrine may cause a transient rise in blood pressure as high as 400/300 mm Hg.[62] Measurement of such high pressures requires optical manometric methods, since they are too brief to record accurately with a mercury sphygmomanometer. To minimize the hazard of intravenous injection, the syringe should be aspirated prior to injection of solutions of epinephrine and anesthetic.

Pallor, perspiration, and faintness, associated with an increase in blood pressure to 230 mm Hg, were reported in two patients after topical use of 2 drops of 2% epinephrine (2.7 mg), for hemostasis during local surgery in one case and to relieve redness after tonometry in the other.[63] A number of similar reactions were cited in this paper. The toxic effects of epinephrine closely simulate adverse reactions to anesthetic agents. As a result, the local anesthetic is often wrongly blamed for what is really a complication of the vasoconstrictor. Prolonged and severe cardiac palpitations and headaches are almost pathognomonic of toxic reactions to vasoconstrictors. In contrast, topical application of 10% phenylephrine rarely elevates blood pressure. Nevertheless, a subarachnoid hemorrhage associated with a hypertensive episode has been reported to follow a conjunctival pack of 10% phenylephrine.[64]

Excessively large doses of epinephrine may cause cerebral hemorrhage and ventricular fibrillation. Patients with hypertension, hyperthyroidism, coronary artery disease, and advanced cerebral arteriosclerosis are more likely to suffer these serious complications.

During general anesthesia induced by cyclopropane or halothane, the myocardium is more susceptible to stimulation by epinephrine, which may precipitate ventricular fibrillation. The topical use of epinephrine is therefore contraindicated during anesthesia with these agents.

A number of sympathomimetic drugs interact with certain anesthetics to produce cardiac arrhythmias. The mechanisms of action involved are extremely complex.[65] The safe use of catecholamines for local hemostasis during general anesthesia requires minimal doses and avoidance of hypercarbia and hypoxia. The ophthalmologist should obtain the approval of the anesthesiologist before applying epinephrine to the operative field. In practice, I have entirely abandoned the use of topical epinephrine during general anesthesia and rely on diathermy applications to achieve hemostasis.

The effect of epinephrine on the sympathetic end organ depends on whether it activates alpha or beta adrenergic receptors. This concept of alpha and beta receptors has been devised as a functional explanation; however, no anatomic or chemical component has been identified for such receptors. Activation of alpha adrenergic receptors results in arteriolar constriction, whereas beta stimulation dilates arterioles. Alpha receptors are stimulated strongly by phenylephrine and are blocked by Dibenamine.

During glaucoma therapy. The usual systemic dose of epinephrine is 0.1 to 0.5 mg. One drop of 2% epinephrine contains approximately 0.1 mg of drug. Since such drops are usually instilled in both eyes, twice this dosage may be reached during glaucoma therapy. Extrasystoles can be recognized in tonograms as sudden downward deflections of the tonographic tracing. Analysis of tonograms of 535 patients indicated that extrasystoles occurred roughly twice as frequently in patients on epinephrine as in those not receiving this drug. Such objective evidence supports the occasional complaints of palpitations, tachycardia, and faintness encountered after epinephrine therapy. Because of the known cardiotoxic effects of epinephrine in doses comparable to those used in the eye, ophthalmologists should be aware of the cardiac status of patients for whom use of epinephrine is being considered.[66]

Actually, these extrasystoles are probably caused by the stress of tonography. Electrocardiographic monitoring showed that premature ventricular systoles were induced by tonography, or even by Goldmann applanation tonometry.[67]

Local irritation. The topical use of levoepinephrine is accompanied by a number of annoying side effects. Early commercial preparations produced a very severe burning sensation. It was often sufficiently marked to incapacitate the patient for a minute or so and required preliminary use of a local anesthetic in some patients. A boric acid and epinephrine complex, epinephryl borate (Eppy 1%), has been developed that is much less irritating. Because of improved stability, this preparation can be buffered to pH 7.4 (instead of the pH 3.5 previously necessary), which is more physiologic and which may result in better corneal penetration. Refrigeration is not required for preservation of this boric acid and epinephrine complex, as it maintains stability for at least 3 years in closed containers and for at least 1 month when kept open at room temperature.

Forty of 56 patients treated with epinephryl borate once or twice a day found it significantly less irritating than the previously available forms of epinephrine.[68] Its tension-lowering effect over a 10-month period seemed equal to that of other forms of epinephrine. However, as in the past, severe headaches, aching of the eyes, conjunctival hyperemia, and local allergy occur with this new form of epinephrine. It was used in two patients with narrow-angle glaucoma, and as expected, they developed acute angle-closure glaucoma.

Epinephrine inhibits mitosis and migration of corneal epithelial cells and doubles the time required for healing of corneal epithelial defects. Tissue cultures of human corneal epithelium develop vacuolation, granularity, and finally cell death when exposed to 0.001% concentrations of epinephrine. (This

is 10 μg/ml, the level at which an antibiotic would inhibit a moderately sensitive microorganism.)[69]

Unwisely, surgeons have instilled epinephrine in the anterior chamber to induce pupillary dilation at the time of cataract surgery. This practice may result in serious damage to the endothelial cells, causing transitory or irreversible corneal edema and opacification. The endothelial damage results from the toxic action of the 0.1% sodium bisulfite that is used as an antioxidant in commercially available epinephrine solutions. Pure epinephrine, 1:1000, does not cause endothelial damage even after 5 minutes of perfusion.[70]

Allergy. Prolonged topical use of levo-epinephrine may rarely cause a local conjunctival allergy but does cause tearing, burning, and ocular discomfort. The conjunctiva is slightly hyperemic (less so than in the usual allergy because of the vasoconstricting properties of epinephrine), follicles appear on the palpebral conjunctiva, and eosinophils may be demonstrated in scrapings. A case is reported in which allergic conjunctivitis caused by epinephrine persisted 7 months before it was diagnosed.[71] On a statistical basis, allergy to pilocarpine, eserine, and environmental factors should first be suspected and, if present, should be eliminated or treated with corticosteroids. This accounts for the delay in diagnosis, which is unavoidable as the ophthalmologist must evaluate the diagnostic possibilities. The patient in this case was not relieved by corticosteroid therapy but was asymptomatic within 5 days after epinephrine therapy was stopped. To rule out the possibility of reaction to other ingredients of the commercially prepared solution, chlorobutanol and sodium bisulfite were instilled and did not cause ocular irritation. At 2 weeks and 2 months after diagnosis, epinephrine was used, and the allergic conjunctivitis returned within 48 and 24 hours, respectively.

Although the pressure values that provided the basis for the diagnosis of galucoma in this case are not given, the disease was apparently of sufficient severity to require use

234   *Drugs in ophthalmic practice*

of an increasing strength of pilocarpine. After 4 years of treatment, despite use of a 4% solution of pilocarpine, it was necessary to add levo-epinephrine in a 2% solution twice a day to the treatment. Interestingly, when the diagnosis of epinephrine allergy was made, all antiglaucoma medication was discontinued; nevertheless, intraocular pressure and tonographic studies were within normal limits and remained so in the absence of treatment for at least the 5 months prior to submission of the report for publication. Recent reports on prolonged improvement of outflow facility after long-term use of epinephrine explain this apparent remission of glaucoma.

That epinephrine "allergy" truly represents a sensitization phenomenon was proved by demonstration of circulating antiepinephrine antibodies in a series of five patients with clinical evidence of epinephrine allergy. No cross-reactivity to phenylephrine or pilocarpine was demonstrated. In these patients the conjunctival allergy was manifested by diffuse vascular engorgement, follicular hypertrophy, and finally chemosis. Slight iritis developed in several cases, with fine deposits on the posterior cornea and lens surface, and 1+ aqueous cells and flare. Fine subepithelial infiltrates of the cornea were frequent.[72]

An experimental counterpart to this clinical epinephrine allergy was achieved by weekly injection of rabbits with Freund's adjuvant and polymerized epinephrine followed by topical ocular instillation of polymerized epinephrine.[73] Mild to very severe allergic responses were observed, including conjunctival and limbal hyperemia, subepithelial corneal infiltrates, aqueous flare and cells, chemosis, and disciform stromal opacities. Histologically, the reaction was characterized by polymorphonuclear leukocyte and lymphoid cell infiltrations. Two human cases of phenylephrine allergy in which high antibody titers to polymerized epinephrine suggested cross-reactivity were also reported.

Madarosis. Loss of eyelashes occurred in one patient who was being treated twice daily with 2% epinephrine hydrochloride.[74] This loss of lashes occurred gradually over a period of 15 months, following 5 years of uncomplicated epinephrine use. Following discontinuance of the epinephrine, lash regrowth occurred within 10 months. This article outlines a long differential diagnosis of the causes of madarosis but does not include self-inflicted epilation. No other similar cases are reported. Was it trichotillomania?

Epinephrine pigmentation. The prolonged use of epinephrine drops may result in localized conjunctival deposits of pigment.[75] A year or more of daily therapy is required for the development of such lesions. Presumably these deposits develop within the translucent conjunctival cysts commonly seen in older patients. Oxidation of the epinephrine results in a slow accumulation of black or dark brown pigment within these cysts.

Pigmented deposits of oxidized epinephrine may also accumulate within roughened and edematous corneal areas. Two such cases of circumscribed, black, nodular, superficial corneal deposits developed after use of a 2% solution of epinephrine three or four times daily for more than a year.[76] Epinephrine treatment of a patient with chronic secondary glaucoma for more than a year resulted in dense brown-black discoloration of the entire central corneal stroma, much like severe bloodstaining of the cornea.[77]

Corneal pigmentation caused by epinephrine is particularly likely to occur in eyes with a damaged epithelium and is enhanced by the use of old and discolored solutions of oxidized epinephrine.[78] The granules of pigment can be deposited intralamellarly throughout the stroma of a corneal graft.[79] In another patient an elevated, densely black plaque of oxidized epinephrine was deposited between the epithelium and Bowman's membrane, covering half of the corneal surface. This eye was enucleated following the mistaken diagnosis of malignant melanoma.[80]

Topical epinephrine therapy will also cause plastic artificial eyes to turn black. This was reported in two elderly patients with glaucoma and unilateral enucleation who were receiving drops in both eyes. Apparently this pigment deposit is superficial and can be scrubbed off the prosthesis with a toothbrush.[81]

The prolonged use of epinephrine in patients wearing soft contact lenses may cause the lens to turn almost jet black. Although one might think that such a lens is irreparably damaged, immersion in 3% hydrogen peroxide for 5 hours will bleach it back to its original state. Be sure to rinse out the peroxide in water before the lens is worn again.[82]

Conjunctival pigmentation somewhat similar in appearance to that produced by epinephrine may follow prolonged use of dark cosmetics applied to the conjunctival side of the eyelash margin. The black cosmetic pigment is deposited as multiple circumscribed dots within the center of conjunctival papillae. The upper margin of the superior tarsal conjunctiva is selectively involved. Although the associated symptom of conjunctival irritation disappears within a few weeks if the cosmetic is kept from the conjunctiva, the pigmentation itself persists as a permanent tattoo.[83]

Epinephrine maculopathy. Aphakic patients using epinephrine topically as treatment for glaucoma tend to develop a reversible maculopathy.[84] This epinephrine maculopathy affects at least 20% to 30% of aphakic eyes treated with epinephrine. The onset of symptoms may occur within a few weeks to many months after therapy is started. The affected patient complains initially of blurring and distortion of vision and later of progressively decreasing visual acuity. In some patients, visual acuity will drop to as low as 20/400 during prolonged epinephrine use.

Examination of the patient reveals an edematous appearance of the macula, most readily recognized with biomicroscopy. Occasionally small cysts or hemorrhages develop at the posterior pole.

Discontinuance of epinephrine therapy is followed by improvement in visual acuity and ophthalmoscopic appearance. Usually visual improvement is detectable within a month, but maximum return of vision often requires 6 months or more. If epinephrine maculopathy is unrecognized and continues for many months, some permanent loss of acuity may

result. For this reason, the ophthalmologist should be alert to the possibility of epinephrine maculopathy when the aphakic patient with treated glaucoma complains of changes in central vision. Do not immediately assume the condition is an untreatable senile macular degeneration or a problem with aphakic glasses.

It should be emphasized that the majority of aphakic glaucoma patients can be safely treated with epinephrine, which is highly effective in controlling pressure elevations. Even if epinephrine maculopathy occurs, the amount of visual impairment may be so slight as to be considered preferable to the hazards of the otherwise uncontrollable glaucoma. Since the maculopathy is dose related, it may be avoided by reducing the concentration of epinephrine from 2% to 1% or by reducing the frequency of administration. Good pressure control may be maintained when epinephrine therapy is decreased if miotic use is increased appropriately.

Substitution of another sympathomimetic drug such as 10% phenylephrine does not appear to be helpful. One patient developed maculopathy while using epinephrine only twice weekly and 10% phenylephrine four times daily.

Intravenous injection of 1 mg of epinephrine in rabbits will transiently abolish the c wave of the ERG. This wave disappears in 1 to 3 minutes and returns to normal in 10 to 20 minutes. Since the c wave originates from the pigment epithelium, this finding apparently indicates that epinephrine is selectively toxic to the pigment epithelium. (The other components of the ERG were unaffected.[85]) Perhaps this c wave change offers an explanation of the mechanism of epinephrine maculopathy.

The clinical and fluorescein photographic appearance of postcataract cystoid macular edema and epinephrine maculopathy are identical.[86,87] Presumably a similar predisposing factor underlies both conditions. However, there is no question but that alternating use and nonuse of epinephrine can result in correlated exacerbation and remission of maculopathy.[88]

Herpes simplex reactivation. Multiple factors alter the equilibrium between latent herpes simplex and active infection. Such physiologic insults as exposure, illness, fever, or corticosteroid application may activate herpes ulcers. Injected intramuscularly in rabbits on 3 consecutive days, epinephrine in oil, 0.5 ml of a 1:500 concentration, was reported to reactivate experimental corneal herpes simplex, as judged by virus recovery or corneal staining.[89]

Epinephrine has also been shown to enhance the intracerebral penetration of poliovirus in mice. This finding may explain the relationship between stress and susceptibility to poliomyelitis.[90]

Epinephrine-related compounds

Norepinephrine 2% has, as would be expected, an effect comparable to that of epinephrine when used in treatment of glaucomatous eyes. Norepinephrine acts on the alpha-adrenergic system to increase the facility of outflow and produces an effect additive to that of pilocarpine. It is less irritating to the eye than is epinephrine and does not produce beta-adrenergic effects such as tachycardia.[91]

Dipivalyl epinephrine is a lipophilic analogue of epinephrine that is better able to penetrate corneal barriers. It lowers intraocular pressure after topical application in concentrations as low as 0.025% and may be clinically useful in 0.1% concentrations. If further experience confirms the effectiveness of these low concentrations, perhaps this drug will be better tolerated than epinephrine.[92]

Isoproterenol, a beta-adrenergic stimulating drug, will reduce intraocular pressure for as long as 8 hours after topical instillation in the rabbit.[93]

Phenylephrine (Neo-Synephrine)

A 10% concentration of phenylephrine hydrochloride, a direct-acting sympathomimetic mydriatic that stimulates alpha receptors, is a valuable aid in ophthalmoscopy. It burns transiently on ocular instillation, causes several hours of light sensitivity (as do all dilating drops), may occlude structurally narrow angles, and usually produces no, or only minimal, systemic side effects after topical application of a few drops.

Three cases of severe acute hypertension (210/110 and higher) were reported to follow the use of 10% phenylephrine eye drops during surgery.[94] The authors point out that a single drop of a 10% solution contains 3.3 mg of drug. One patient, a 12-pound infant, received 6 drops of 10% phenylephrine and responded with a systolic pressure of 230. It was also postulated that systemic absorption may be enhanced by an inflamed or postsurgical eye and that some individuals may be more susceptible to the hypertensive effect.

Acute hypertension so severe as to cause subarachnoid hemorrhage followed insertion in the lower cul-de-sac of a cotton wick soaked in 10% phenylephrine.[64]

Even a drug as safe as phenylephrine requires some prudence in its use. We may become so preoccupied with our goal of wide mydriasis that we forget that systemic absorption occurs transconjunctivally.

What would you do if a 76-year-old man in your waiting room suddenly became agitated and confused, unable to stand, and unresponsive to verbal instructions? This happened 15 minutes after a patient received 3 drops of phenylephrine in each eye over a 12-minute period. His blood pressure was 270/170 (normally 150/100). Over a period of several hours, his blood pressure and mental state returned to normal.[95]

Clinical use

Mydriasis. Maximal mydriasis from a single instillation of phenylephrine occurs in 60 to 90 minutes. Recovery from mydriasis takes 5 to 7 hours. The dose-response curve for phenylephrine shows an increasing dilation as concentrations increase to about 5%. Little additional response is achieved by increasing the strength to 10%.[96] Repeated instillations of a mydriatic, either alone or in combination with a cycloplegic, will achieve greater dilation. Intense light stimulation, as in indirect ophthalmoscopy or fundus photography, will cause constriction of a pupil that has been dilated with only one instillation of phenyl-ephrine. Cycloplegic drops will prevent this response to illumination.

Sympathomimetic mydriatics are particularly useful as an aid to ophthalmoscopy. They act rapidly and do not have an excessively long duration. Virtual absence of cycloplegic effect spares the patient the inconvenience of being unable to read or see near details. Eight instillations of a 10% solution of phenylephrine, given at 2-minute intervals, caused recession of the near point averaging 0.66 D in five young subjects (Fig. 12-12).[97] This effect was produced within 30 minutes and disappeared within 2 hours. Mydriasis appeared within 30 minutes and lasted long after accommodation had returned to normal, thereby indicating that the demonstrated loss of accommodation was not simply an artifact resulting from a decrease in field depth.

Although the miosis of old age is commonly attributed to mechanical changes of the iris, it is most likely caused by decreased sympathetic tone. Comparison of the effect of 10% phenylephrine in young and old subjects resulted in an equal dilation of young and old pupils (average pupil diameter 8 mm), although the original pupil size was definitely smaller in the older patients. Hy-droxyamphetamine and cocaine, drugs with an indirect mechanism of action, were not nearly so effective in dilating older patients, indicating the decrease in sympathetic tonus.[98]

Phenylephrine mydriasis is slightly less than that produced by cycloplegic drugs. The comparative effects of these drugs, as measured 40 minutes after instillation of 3 drops of each medication tested, are illustrated in Fig. 12-13.[99] As expected, the eyes of black persons dilate with greater difficulty, especially when phenylephrine, cyclopentolate, and hydroxyamphetamine are used.

The mydriatic effect may be enhanced by use of a phenylephrine pack.[100] After instillation of a topical anesthetic, a small piece of cotton is placed in the lower conjunctival sac and moistened with about 3 drops of 10% phenylephrine. The patient then closes the lids for about 30 minutes. This method of treatment was used in 29 eyes with flat or shallow chambers after a cataract extraction. Within an hour, 27 of these eyes showed recognizable chamber deepening. The temptation to instill additional drops at frequent intervals should be resisted, lest systemic toxicity result from transconjunctival absorption.

Even in concentrations as small as 0.125%,

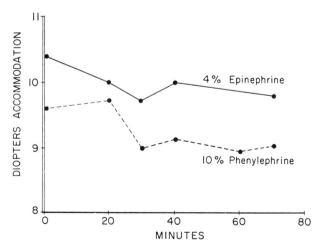

Fig. 12-12. Effect on accommodation of topical application of phenylephrine and epinephrine. (Modified from Biggs, R. A., Alpern, M., and Bennett, D. R.: Am. J. Ophthalmol. **48:**169, 1959.)

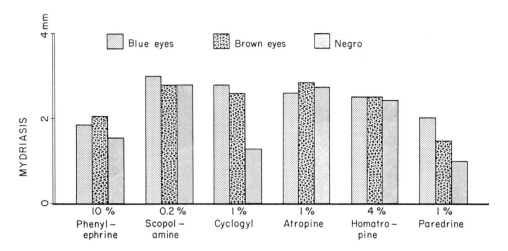

Fig. 12-13. Comparison of mydriasis produced by phenylephrine, scopolamine, cyclopentolate (Cyclogyl), atropine, homatropine, and hydroxyamphetamine (Paredrine). (Modified from Barbee, R. F., and Smith, W. O.: Am. J. Ophthalmol. **44:**617, 1957.)

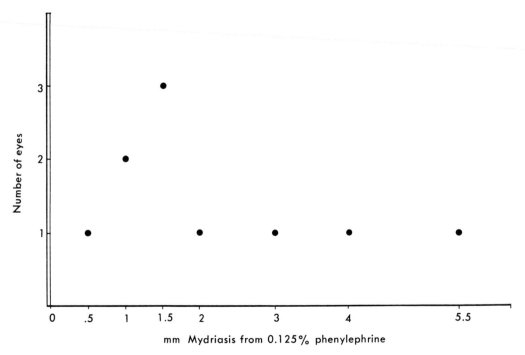

Fig. 12-14. Pupillary dilation produced in 45 minutes by a 0.125% solution of phenylephrine instilled after tonography. (Data from Weiss, D. I., and Shaffer, R. N.: Arch. Ophthalmol. **68:** 727, 1962.)

phenylephrine may cause mydriasis. The mydriatic effect is greater if the corneal epithelium is damaged, thereby increasing drug penetration. The effect of 2 drops of 0.125% solution of phenylephrine instilled in one eye of each of 10 patients with normal corneas was measured after 45 minutes.[101] (Race of the patients was not stated.) In only three patients was the pupil dilated 1 to 1.5 mm greater than its mate. Three eyes were dilated 0.5 mm, and four were unchanged. Similar phenylephrine instillation was done in 10 patients after routine tonography of both eyes. In all these patients who were not receiving miotic therapy, the test pupil was dilated and in several instances attained a diameter of 8 mm (Fig. 12-14).

This study of the mydriatic effect of a 0.125% concentration of phenylephrine was initiated because an attack of narrow-angle glaucoma had been precipitated by use of a

solution of 0.125% phenylephrine and 0.25% zinc sulfate. Fourteen years previously the patient had undergone an operation for acute glaucoma in the right eye. A 2% concentration of pilocarpine had been used twice a day in the left eye for 14 years. The zinc and phenylephrine medication had been prescribed for mild conjunctivitis in both eyes (intraocular pressure of the left eye was 16 mm Hg). Within 2 hours the left eye was painful. The next day, intraocular pressure of the left eye was 57 mm Hg and the angle was completely occluded. This acute glaucoma developed during use of pilocarpine (last installation of a 2% solution of pilocarpine was 8 hours prior to use of phenylephrine) and was not controlled by subsequent pilocarpine administration by the patient. The case history convincingly shows the 0.125% concentration of phenylephrine to be the cause of this attack of angle-closure glaucoma; however,

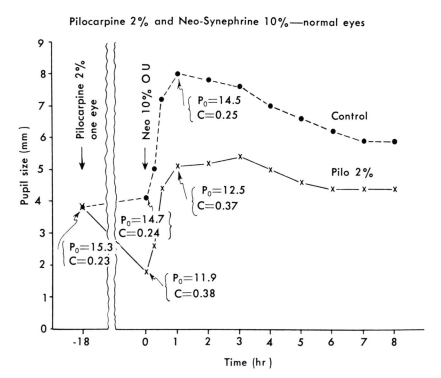

Fig. 12-15. Mydriatic effect of phenylephrine, 10% solution. Solid circles: response of normal pupil. Crosses: response of eye pretreated with 2% solution of pilocarpine. P_0, Intraocular pressure; C, facility of outflow. (From Becker, B., and associates: Am. J. Ophthalmol. **48**:313, 1959.)

the patient obviously was strongly predisposed to angle closure.

Phenylephrine in a 0.125% concentration is contained in numerous proprietary collyria designed to produce vasoconstriction and whiten the eye. These medications, usually prescribed freely, are potentially harmful in eyes predisposed to angle-closure glaucoma, especially if the corneal epithelium is abraded by tonometry or disease.

Competitive action with miotics. The effect of phenylephrine, 10% solution, on eyes pretreated with pilocarpine, 2% solution, is illustrated in Fig. 12-15. The data presented in this illustration represent the average response of 10 eyes. The untreated pupil dilates in response to phenylephrine, reaching a maximum diameter within 30 to 60 minutes. Maximum dilation persists for several hours and then gradually decreases. The pilocarpine-treated pupil also dilates in response to phenylephrine, although not as widely as the untreated pupil. Instillation of additional mydriatic or miotic drops would, of course, further alter the size of the pupil in the expected direction.

In a series of 16 patients with chronic simple glaucoma adequately controlled with demecarium, a 10% solution of phenylephrine dilated the pupil nicely (average increase in pupil size, 2.4 mm). Both before and after phenylephrine dilation, the mean coefficient of outflow in these patients was 0.22.[43] These findings imply that phenylephrine will partially overcome the miosis produced by even the strongest miotics and can therefore be used for periodic fundus examination in patients with chronic simple glaucoma. Furthermore, diagnostic dilation with phenylephrine does not jeopardize the control of chronic simple glaucoma. This is in contrast to parasympatholytic dilation, which does reduce the coefficient of outflow. Phenylephrine is *not* necessarily safe to use in patients with shallow angles, particularly if subacute angle closure already exists.

Infrequently phenylephrine or epinephrine may increase intraocular pressure in open-angle chronic simple glaucoma.[102] This is less likely to occur if the patient is simultaneously receiving miotic therapy. Because of this occasional pressure rise, it is prudent to recheck the intraocular pressure during the week following prescription of sympathomimetic supplements to glaucoma therapy.

Hazard in acute glaucoma. Caution is necessary when any dilating drop is used in an eye predisposed to acute angle-closure glaucoma. Precautions include the use of sympathomimetic mydriatics as well as parasympatholytic mydriatics (although the former are certainly safer). Particular care is necessary if the intraocular pressure is at a borderline level before dilation or if the eye has had a previous attack of acute glaucoma that was subsequently controlled by miotic therapy without surgery. Under such circumstances, dilation is justifiable only if the patient's symptoms suggest a melanoma, retinal detachment, or a similar major ocular disorder. Before dilation is started, the patient should be informed that the necessity for fundus examination outweighs the danger of surgery, which may well become necessary as an emergency procedure. Even with the aid of carbonic anhydrase inhibitors, intravenous osmotic agents, and miotics, attacks of acute glaucoma that are medically irreversible can be precipitated by sympathomimetic mydriatics. If dilation is necessary in the examination of an eye structurally predisposed to angle closure, the patient should remain in the office for several hours until good miosis is reestablished, the pressure has returned to normal, and the eye is comfortable.

Miotic cysts. Miotic cysts of the iris, sometimes the result of ocular drug therapy, can be prevented by the simultaneous administration of phenylephrine.[103] Commercially available phenylephrine solution may be used to dissolve echothiophate powder, and thereby both drugs can be dispensed in a single solution. Twenty patients with esotropia received a 0.125% concentration of echothiophate iodide alone in one eye every hour as needed. The other eye received a 0.125% solution of echothiophate combined with phenylephrine in solutions of 10%, 5%, or 2.5%. After 1 to 6 weeks of therapy, 11 of the eyes treated solely with echothiophate developed iris cysts,[103] but none of the eyes on combined medication did so. These cysts will disappear in 1 or 2 months if echothiophate is discontinued or if combined echothiophate and phenylephrine therapy is substituted. The 2.5% concentration of phenylephrine was as effective in preventing cyst formation as was the 10% solution. Phenylephrine did not interfere with the therapeutic effect of the echothiophate on the accommodative esotropia. The only undesirable effect of the phenylephrine was the slight burning it caused on application—this was less with the 2.5% solution than with the stronger concentrations.

The mechanism of cyst formation by echothiophate and cyst prevention by phenylephrine is not clearly understood. If a 10% solution of phenylephrine is used each morning, while echothiophate is instilled each night, iris cysts will develop. This observation suggests that prevention of the initial intense miosis is a more likely mechanism of action than is parasympathetic-sympathetic interaction.

Addition of a 2.5% solution of phenylephrine to a 0.125% solution of echothiophate iodide is recommended to prevent the development of miotic cysts during the treatment of accommodative esotropia.

Ptosis. Ptosis resulting from sympathetic denervation (Horner's or Raeder's syndrome) may be relieved by topical instillation of a 0.125% concentration of phenylephrine. The frequency of dosage depends on response but is usually three or four times daily. Such treatment will sometimes benefit other types of mild ptosis that are cosmetically undesirable because of the uneven palpebral apertures that accompany the condition. Ptosis seen after enucleation may be reduced by instillation of a 10% solution of phenylephrine if a proper fitting of the prosthesis does not correct it. Apparently the mechanism of response is direct action on Müller's muscle.*

The procedure of resection of Müller's muscle for ptosis may be selectively advised

for patients in whom instillation of 10% phenylephrine will elevate the lid to a normal level.[104]

Test for Horner's syndrome. Phenylephrine, 1%, causes minimal or no dilation of the normal pupil but will markedly dilate a pupil with postganglionic sympathetic denervation. If 10% phenylephrine is used, both the normal pupil and the Horner's pupil will dilate, but the denervated pupil will respond more rapidly and will tend to be 1 or 2 mm larger during the dilation process. Although such minimal differences are recognizable in photographs, they may be difficult to assess reliably in clinical practice. Unilateral corneal epithelial abrasions will permit entry of more phenylephrine, resulting in a misleading increase in dilation on the damaged side.[105]

Provocative test for sickle cell anemia. Vasoconstriction of conjunctival vessels by phenylephrine intensifies the typical slit-lamp appearance of these vessels in sickle cell disease and may be used as a diagnostic aid. Saccular venous dilatations, capillary microaneurysms, and readily visible sludging of blood flow are characteristic of sickle cell anemia, even in remission. Apparently the anoxia produced by vasoconstriction is responsible for intensifying these changes.[106]

Liberation of iris pigment

An interesting side effect of sympathomimetic mydriatics is the release of pigment granules from the iris neuroepithelium. This pigment debris may be confused with the biomicroscopic appearance of iritis, but it is readily differentiated by the absence of other inflammatory signs, including aqueous flare. In a series of 948 eyes examined with the slit lamp before and after dilation with a 5% solution of phenylephrine hydrochloride, 44 eyes showed a definite increase in aqueous floaters with dilation.[107] The subsequent response of these 44 eyes was evaluated after instillation of solutions of 5% phenylephrine, 0.1% epinephrine, 1% atropine, 1% homatropine, 3% cocaine, 1% pilocarpine, and 0.5% eserine. Aqueous floaters in varying numbers were produced in all cases in which phenyl-

---

*de la Motte, Walter: Personal communication, 1964.

ephrine and epinephrine were used. The other five drugs caused no floaters at all in most cases, and only a few scattered cells in the remainder. Direct stimulation of the dilator muscle (composed of pigmented epithelial cells) by the sympathomimetic drugs was postulated as the cause of rupture of some of these cells, with subsequent release of pigment granules. Microscopic examination of aspirated aqueous revealed these aqueous floaters to be pigment granules from the iris neuroepithelium. These mydriatic-induced particles were 1 to 1.5 μ in size and were brown with Giemsa stain—properties characteristic of pigment granules of iris neuroepithelium. This pigmentary response to dilation was found primarily in older patients and is considered a senile change.

In general, floaters first appear about 30 minutes after instillation of phenylephrine, increase in number for 1 to 2 hours, and disappear within 12 to 24 hours. Repeated dilations of the same eye will again produce pigment floaters, but not in as great a number. Gonioscopy shows that patients in whom mydriasis produces floaters have trabecular pigmentation considerably greater than normal. No reference was made to the presence or absence of glaucoma in these patients, who might be expected to show a predisposition to chronic trabecular blockage.

Postdilation miosis

In older patients, phenylephrine appears to alter the dilator muscle, resulting in a smaller pupil that is less responsive to subsequent dilation.[96] This change is of such a magnitude that the maximally dilated pupil area may be decreased by 30% to 40%. In a series of 12 patients over 50 years of age, electronic pupillography showed an average increase in pupil diameter of 2 mm 75 minutes after instillation of 2 drops of 10% phenylephrine. Twenty-four hours later the average pupil diameter was 0.73 mm smaller than it was before the use of phenylephrine. Repeated instillation of phenylephrine at this time resulted in a dilation of only 1.5 mm, as compared to the previous 2 mm. Whether this miosis and decreased response to mydriatic instillation lasted more than 1 day was

not reported. Cyclopentolate dilation did not cause such a postdilation miosis.

Endothelial toxicity

During the prolonged surgery of vitrectomy, the corneal epithelium may become hazy and the pupil small. One way of dealing with these problems is to scrape off the epithelium and instill 10% phenylephrine. Unfortunately, this results in rapid clouding of the cornea. The reason for this was first thought to be phenylephrine toxicity, but it actually is the fault of the vehicle. Commercial preparations of phenylephrine are dispensed at a low pH to maintain stability. When the epithelium is not present, the penetration of this acid pH is more rapid than can be neutralized by the buffering capacity of the cornea. Detailed pharmacologic and electron microscope studies have shown the consequence to be severe pH-related vacuolation of the endothelial cells.[108] This consequence could occur any time the epithelium is not present, as in corneal ulceration from any cause.

Hydroxyamphetamine (Paredrine)

Hydroxyamphetamine hydrobromide is an indirect-acting sympathomimetic drug.[31] Its effect is reduced or abolished by pretreatment with guanethidine, which depletes norepinephrine from the adrenergic nerve terminal. In a 1% solution, hydroxyamphetamine is an effective mydriatic when instilled on an eye with a normal adrenergic innervation.

The use of 1% hydroxyamphetamine in testing for defective postganglionic sympathetic innervation is more specific and subject to less error than the cocaine or epinephrine tests. Hydroxyamphetamine releases endogenous norepinephrine from the normal nerve terminal. In postganglionic Horner's syndrome, norepinephrine is absent; hence dilation cannot occur. Fig. 12-16 summarizes the responses to hydroxyamphetamine of 12 patients with unilateral Horner's syndrome.[105] In central and preganglionic lesions, endogenous epinephrine is present and dilation occurs. In postganglionic lesions the affected pupil actually becomes smaller

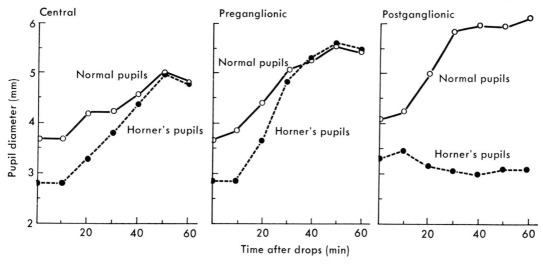

Fig. 12-16. Pupil responses to 1% hydroxyamphetamine in unilateral Horner's syndrome. (From Thompson, H. S., and Mensher, J. H.: Am. J. Ophthalmol. **72:**472, 1971.)

because more light enters the opposite dilated pupil.

In all such tests the drops should be instilled in both eyes to permit comparison of the normal and abnormal pupil responses. The cocaine, epinephrine, and phenylephrine tests are subject to error if one eye has an epithelial abrasion, permitting entry of a greater amount of drug. The hydroxyamphetamine test is not subject to errors due to somewhat uneven administration of drops, because the response depends primarily on the amount of norepinephrine available for release. One possible error should be avoided. Cocaine blocks the uptake of hydroxyamphetamine into the nerve endings; hence the hydroxyamphetamine test should not be performed within 2 days after a cocaine test. Incidentally, another possible source of error in testing for Horner's pupil occurs in patients with a heavily pigmented iris—cocaine dilation in such a dark iris is extremely slow and may take as long as 3 hours to become maximal.[105]

Because of the similarity of molecular structure between hydroxyamphetamine and norepinephrine, the possibility of direct action of hydroxyamphetamine on smooth muscle adrenergic receptors has been suggested. If this were to occur, perhaps the differentiation between preganglionic and postganglionic lesions might not be quite as certain as has been suggested.[109]

Cocaine

Because it was primarily used in ophthalmology as an anesthetic (now replaced by less toxic synthetic anesthetics), cocaine was described in the chapter on anesthesia. However, cocaine is also an indirect-acting sympathomimetic drug. Its mechanism of action has been postulated to be prevention of uptake of catecholamines by the adrenergic nerve terminal.[27]

Studies with radio-labeled cocaine incubated on the guinea pig iris showed that the pigmented iris had an uptake of eighteen times as much cocaine as did the nonpigmented iris. Furthermore, the cocaine was firmly bound to the pigmented iris, resisting the washout that easily occurred in the nonpigmented iris. Chemical sympathectomy with 6-hydroxydopamine did not alter cocaine binding by the iris, indicating that the effect was unrelated to sympathetic nerve terminals.[110]

Ephedrine

This indirect-acting sympathomimetic drug causes rapid displacement of norepinephrine from the adrenergic nerve terminal.[2] It is not currently used by ophthalmologists.

ANTICHOLINERGIC AGENTS
Atropine

Atropine is useful in the management of iridocyclitis and in the refraction of children with accommodative esotropia.

Pharmacology

Mechanism of action. Atropine acts directly on the smooth muscles and secretory glands innervated by postganglionic cholinergic nerves. It blocks the response to acetylcholine and related parasympathomimetic drugs at these sites. This blockage is relative and can be overcome by use of pilocarpine, physostigmine, isoflurophate, and the like, if these drugs are applied in sufficient concentration and frequency relative to the amount of atropine used.

The quantitative nature of atropinization is well illustrated by the response of a ciliary muscle, which was contracted by 1 μg/ml of acetylcholine, to different concentrations of atropine.[32] Contraction was not blocked by 0.01 to 0.1 μg/ml of atropine, was diminished by 1 μg/ml, was strongly reduced by 10 μg/ml, and was completely blocked by 100 μg/ml. Peculiarly, washing the atropine out of the muscle bath restored the responsiveness of the muscle to 1 μg/ml of acetylcholine. (Because of the clinically recognized long duration of atropine, one would have expected it to remain fixed to the muscle receptor. Although this work, dealing with the entire group of autonomic drugs, was very well done and in general confirmed the classic concepts of autonomic pharmacology, I suspect that some experimental artifact or a species peculiarity of the cat ciliary muscle accounted for the failure of the atropine to remain fixed to the muscle.)

Mydriatic and cycloplegic action. Atropine produces both mydriasis and cycloplegia. Additional mydriasis occurs if sympathomimetic drugs such as phenylephrine are used simultaneously. In clinical usage, such synergistic combinations are commonly prescribed to attain maximal dilation of the pupil. Cycloplegia is not enhanced by the simultaneous use of sympathomimetic drugs, as they have insignificant cycloplegic action.

The response of individual eyes to cycloplegic drugs varies greatly. Within 30 to 40

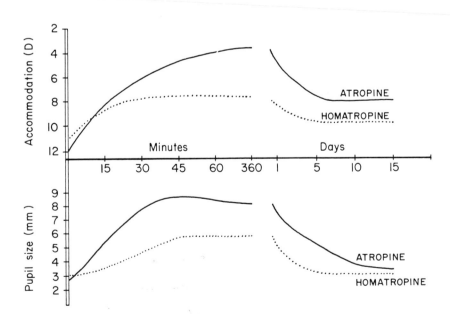

Fig. 12-17. Average cycloplegia and mydriasis achieved by 1 drop of a 1% solution of atropine or of a 1% solution of homatropine in young adult human eyes. (Modified from Wolfe, A. V., and Hodge, H. C.: Arch. Ophthalmol. **36:**293, 1946.)

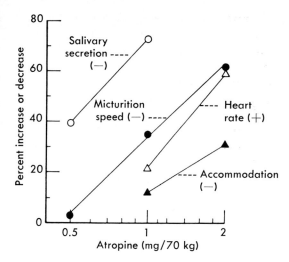

Fig. 12-18. Human response to subcutaneous injection of atropine sulfate. Plus signs indicate increase in function. Minus signs indicate decrease in function. (From Riker, W. F.: J.A.M.A. **179:** 355, 1962.)

minutes, atropine produces maximal mydriasis, which lasts for as long as 12 days. Atropine cycloplegia is attained within a few hours and may last 2 weeks or longer (Fig. 12-17).[111] In comparison, maximal mydriasis from homatropine is attained in 10 to 30 minutes, with recovery in from 6 hours to 4 days. Maximal homatropine cycloplegia (from a single instillation) is reached in 30 to 90 minutes, with recovery in 10 to 48 hours.

The systemic administration of many drugs, including atropine, evokes multiple responses. For instance, atropine inhibits salivation, increases heart rate (by vagus block), and decreases accommodation. Since the rate at which these responses change (in relationship to increasing atropinization) is essentially the same for all systems (Fig. 12-18),[112] this indicates a similar mechanism of action on all systems. However, the sensitivity of these different bodily functions to atro-

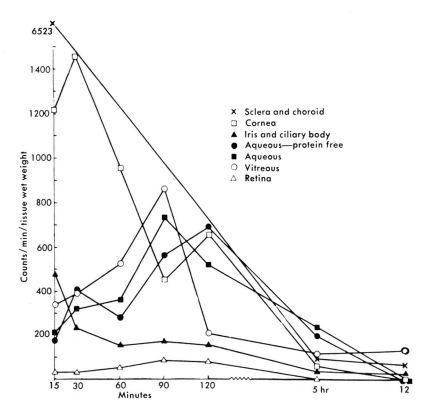

Fig. 12-19. Distribution of ^{14}C-labeled atropine after subconjunctival injection in rabbits. (From Janes, R. G., and Stiles, J. F.: Arch. Ophthalmol. **62:**69, 1959.)

pinization varies considerably. As illustrated, a 70% inhibition of salivation has already occurred at a dosage that reduces accommodation by only 10%. It is evident that a 0.5 mg dose of atropine used as preanesthetic medication will effectively reduce secretions and yet cause only minimal ocular response.

Absorption and excretion. Atropine is readily absorbed transconjunctivally and is distributed throughout the body. It is hydrolyzed in the liver or excreted in the urine, the latter of which was the basis for an interesting test in antiquity. Belladonna alkaloids were favorites of the professional poisoners of the Middle Ages. Such poisoning could be detected by placing a drop of the victim's urine in a cat's eye, which would dilate if as little as 0.0003 mg of atropine were present in the urine![62]

The intraocular distribution of atropine has been studied after subconjunctival injection of a radioactive drug.[113] The atropine content of various ocular tissues and fluids during a 12-hour period immediately after such injection in a rabbit is shown in Fig. 12-19. (As subsequently noted, rabbits destroy atropine rapidly; hence these values are not necessarily representative of the distribution and persistence of atropine in the human eye.) The very high values for sclera can be disregarded as surface contamination by the injection. Most interesting is the penetration of atropine into the retina. Since these retinal concentrations were low and transient, they most likely represent blood radioactivity. (The atropine was rapidly picked up by the bloodstream, and within 5 hours 95% of the radioactivity had already been excreted in the urine.) Although relatively persistent, the iris and ciliary body values are lower than I would expect—possibly this is related to the rabbit's ability to destroy atropine.

Species tolerance. Rabbits are tolerant to large doses of atropine and related alkaloids, presumably because of their ability to destroy these drugs rapidly. This fact must be considered in the interpretation of experimental ocular responses. The ability to destroy atropine is due to an enzyme, atropine esterase, which is inherited as a dominant gene.[114] Varying amounts of atropine esterase are found in serum obtained from 25% to 65% of strains of rabbit. Almost all chickens possess serum atropine esterase.[115]

Effect of pigment

When applied to a heavily pigmented eye, atropine exhibits an unusually slow onset of cycloplegic effect. Paradoxically, the same eye that responds only partially and slowly to atropine will then show a quite prolonged duration of cycloplegia. Specifically, the eyes of black patients will not dilate well, even with repeated doses of cycloplegic drugs; thereafter, they will complain of much longer-lasting inability to read and persistent dilation of the pupils. The explanation for this is the binding effect of melanin on many types of drugs. (For example, miotics are bound just as are cycloplegics. So are phenthiazines, accounting for the well-known ocular toxic effects of this type of drug compound.) Initially the melanin binding of atropine slows attainment of a therapeutic drug level in the iris. Later the melanin-bound drug reservoir slowly releases atropine, resulting in the prolonged cycloplegia. The magnitude of this effect has been studied in the rabbit.[116] The average duration of atropine pupil dilation in albino rabbits was 30 hours, as contrasted to over 90 hours in pigmented rabbits. These rabbits had been tested and found to be lacking serum atropinesterase activity. In another group of atropinesterase-positive rabbits, the duration of atropine dilation was 4 hours in albino rabbits and 12 hours in pigmented rabbits. The wide variations in drug effect in these various groups of rabbits, depending on the presence or absence of melanin and atropinesterase, illustrate how animal experiments may give surprising results that cannot be directly applied to the human eye.

Clinical use

Iridocyclitis. Atropine has long been one of the favorite drugs for the treatment of inflammation of the anterior segment of the eye. The mechanism of its anti-inflammatory effect probably includes the following three actions.

Atropinization reduces the pain characteristic of iridocyclitis, presumably because of relaxation of the inflamed musculature of the ciliary body and iris. Quite dramatic relief of severe ocular pain characteristically accompanies the onset of cycloplegia in the treatment of acute iritis; however, this is not a local anesthetic effect and will relieve the pain of a corneal abrasion only to the extent that it is compounded by iritis.

Among the most serious complications of iridocyclitis are those associated with posterior synechiae: seclusion of the pupil with subsequent iris bombé and acute glaucoma, occlusion of the pupil with loss of sight, and cataract formation. If started early enough, atropinization will break these adhesions and will decrease the possibility of serious complications resulting from synechiae. The peripheral lens is slightly farther back than the central portion, and the iris-lens contact is less intimate when the pupil is dilated. Furthermore, the greater circumference of a dilated pupil is less likely to be secluded, and its greater diameter is less likely to be occluded.

Finally, atropine tends to restore the permeability of inflamed vessels and thereby decreases the outpouring of protein and inflammatory cells into the aqueous. These components of the inflamed aqueous tend to clog up the chamber angle, with resultant secondary glaucoma and anterior synechiae. Characteristically, the rather abrupt rise of pressure associated with severe acute iritis will respond within hours to atropine and acetazolamide. Even hypopyon iritis may clear rapidly with adequate cycloplegia.

The eye with iridocyclitis is much more resistant to atropinization than is a normal eye. If posterior synechiae are present when the patient is first seen, an intensive effort should be made to break them while the patient is still in the office. This requires repeated instillation of atropine and phenylephrine or of similar drugs. If synechiae have been present for as long as a week, the iris may continue to break away from the lens for several days or more. During active inflammation, instillation of a 1% solution of atropine three times a day, supplemented by a 10% solution of phenylephrine three times a day, may be required to maintain good mydriasis. Less severe inflammation, such as follows cataract extraction, may be controlled by atropine administered once daily.

Slit-lamp evaluation of aqueous flare and cells is the very best guide to atropinization of the inflamed eye. The red-eyed patient without flare and cells will usually not benefit from cycloplegia and will be handicapped by the paralysis of accommodation. One of the mistakes commonly made by emergency room interns is to atropinize an eye with a minor corneal abrasion. This is an unnecessary nuisance to the patient. Cycloplegic therapy of iridocyclitis should not be discontinued until flare and cells have disappeared from the aqueous.

The effectiveness of atropine in reducing abnormal vascular permeability may be observed experimentally by the use of a fluorescein marker. In the normal cat eye, intravenous fluorescein does not leak from the ciliary processes. A marked leakage of fluorescein into the aqueous occurs if as little as 0.01 μg/ml of acetylcholine bathes the eserinized ciliary processes. Acetylcholine is believed to affect the blood-aqueous barrier by dilating blood vessels. Atropinization of the ciliary processes with 10 μg/ml of drug will completely block the acetylcholine-induced permeability increase.[117]

Refraction. Since accurate measurement of hyperopia is necessary to correct accommodative esotropia and to avoid a blurring of distance vision that will cause a child to refuse to wear glasses, maximum cycloplegia is important. This may be more reliably achieved by the 3-day routine of atropinization than by shorter courses with other medications. The parent is instructed to instill atropine three times a day in both eyes for the 3 days immediately preceding the next office visit unless toxicity occurs. This routine also has the practical advantage of the drops being instilled elsewhere; the child need not wait unhappily in the office.

Actually, this is more atropine than is really necessary for most patients. Repeated refraction during the course of atropine instillation indicates that maximum cycloplegia is usually reached during the second day, after the patient has received only 4 of the 9 drops.[118] The excess medication ensures that even the most resistant eyes will be completely cycloplegic and allows for the omission of one or more instillations, which so often happens.

Refraction of nonsquinting children does not require atropine. Because of its long duration, atropine is not useful for refraction of adults.

Occlusion. In the treatment of suppression amblyopia, atropine may be useful if cycloplegia will reduce the acuity of the good eye below that of the amblyopic one and thus force fixation with the amblyopic eye. The mechanical and cosmetic nuisance of patching may thereby be avoided. Prolonged occlusion is not of benefit if the amblyopic eye fixes eccentrically. Use of the visuscope to determine fixation behavior will spare the patient the considerable inconvenience of useless occlusion.[119]

Accommodative spasm. Rarely, patients exhibit a functional excess of accommodation and convergence. Atropinization will certainly stop their accommodation and will usually disrupt their visual habits enough to stop the convergence as well.

Treatment of myopia

Half a century ago, Walter Lancaster believed that atropinization would arrest the progress of myopia. There has been a general tendency to scoff at this, but periodically poorly controlled studies report such facts as that after 3 years untreated patients average a 1.22 D increase in myopia as compared to a 0.07 D average decrease in myopia in eyes treated with 1 drop of 1% atropine every night.[120] Because of uncertainties of selection of these patients and considerable variations in the duration of treatment, it is hard to interpret the validity of such studies.

However, I am not prepared to dismiss the possibility of autonomic control of ocular growth. Bear in mind that repeated instillation of echothiophate will cause growth of the anterior margin of the embryonic optic cup in a 5-year-old child (the well-known miotic cysts of the pupil margin).

Toxicity

Systemic reactions. The fatal dose of atropine is about 100 mg for adults and 10 mg for children. Since a drop of 1% atropine solution contains about 0.5 mg of drug (the usual preoperative dose for controlling secretions), simple calculation will reveal that an ordinary ophthalmic bottle of atropine may contain enough drug to kill several children. Patients should be warned to keep drugs such as atropine and isoflurophate safely out of the reach of children.

Minor but alarming toxic reactions may follow the use of atropine for refraction in children. Systemic absorption may be decreased by using ointment rather than drops, by wiping excess solution or ointment from the eye immediately after instillation (I sincerely doubt that "pressure over the sac," as commonly advocated, is of any value whatsoever in reducing systemic absorption), or by using 0.5% rather than 1% solutions. Parents should be instructed to skip prescribed drops in the atropine refraction routine if toxic symptoms are present at the time the medication is due. These symptoms include dryness of skin and mouth, fever (because of the inability to perspire), irritability or delirium (caused by stimulation of the central nervous system), tachycardia (resulting from vagal block), and flushing of the face (caused by cutaneous vasodilation in the blush area). Such symptoms have been misdiagnosed as scarlet fever or other childhood infections.

Should severe atropine poisoning occur, the patient may be treated with subcutaneous injection of 1 mg of physostigmine. Repeated 0.25 mg doses may be given every 15 minutes until salivation occurs or symptomatic relief is obtained.

Subcutaneous injection of 5 mg of methacholine has been suggested as a diagnostic test for parasympatholytic poisoning. This dose normally causes parasympathomimetic symptoms, which will be blocked if the patient has been poisoned by atropine. Actually, the ancient urine-in-cat's-eye test (p. 246) sounds easier and safer!

The naturally occurring belladonna alkaloids may be accidentally ingested or taken purposefully with the intent of achieving a hallucinogenic reaction. One such plant, the angel's trumpet, contains in a single flower more than the usual therapeutic dose of belladonna alkaloids (atropine, hyoscyamine, and scopolamine). The name, angel's trumpet, is derived from the fact that it is a beautiful white trumpet-shaped flower and also from the fact that if you eat enough of them the angels will call you to heaven. Ninety cases of intentional ingestion of this plant, with 7 deaths, were reported from the Brevard County Mental Health Center in Florida.[121] Remember, 1 mg of physostigmine is the antidote for parasympatholytic poisoning.

In glaucoma. Parasympatholytic drugs such as atropine will increase intraocular pressure in eyes with chronic simple glaucoma and should not be used to dilate such eyes. An intraocular pressure elevation of 6 mm Hg or more occurred in response to cycloplegia in 23% of 40 patients with known open-angle glaucoma but in only 2% of 100 nonglaucomatous patients.[122] Hence such a hypertensive response to cycloplegia is strongly indicative of chronic simple glaucoma. All of the potent cycloplegic agents produced this hypertensive response, which was not caused by noncycloplegic mydriatic drugs.

Eyes predisposed to acute glaucoma (shallow angle and shallow anterior chamber) may develop an acute attack if they are atropinized. Atropine is strongly contraindicated in such eyes.

Although atropine is advocated in the management of glaucoma secondary to acute anterior segment inflammation, an eye with old inflammatory scars may have enough trabecular damage to simulate chronic simple glaucoma and require miotic therapy.[123] Atropinization of such eyes increases pressure.

Will preoperative atropinization in general surgery be harmful to patients with chronic simple glaucoma? This question frequently causes concern among students. The answer clearly is *no*, for three reasons. First, the sensitivity of the eye to systemic atropine is relatively low. Second, the local effects of miotic therapy are far greater than can be overcome by systemic atropinization. (Of course, the miotic therapy should be continued at the usual frequency during the period of preoperative preparation, anesthesia, and recovery. Should control of pressure be borderline, the possibility of increasing the frequency of miotic instillation by several times a day might be worthwhile.) Third, even if intraocular pressure were slightly elevated for 1 or 2 days, no perceptible damage would result. However, in the unlikely event that a patient with untreated subacute angle-closure glaucoma is atropinized preoperatively, complete angle closure might well ensue. When ophthalmologists are treating patients with unilateral acute glaucoma, they must not forget miotic therapy for the "normal" eye.

Allergic reactions. Contact dermatitis confined to the lids of the treated eye is not uncommonly caused by atropine. This is recognized by the characteristic itching and by the reddened, swollen, weeping texture of the skin. Conjunctival redness, although present, is less conspicuous.

No treatment is satisfactory except discontinuance of the offending drug. Corticosteroids only postpone this necessary step. Fortunately, many effective atropine substitutes are readily available and usually do not cause sensitivity. These include scopolamine, cyclopentolate (Cyclogyl), and oxyphenonium (Antrenyl).

Even years later the use of atropine usually causes a prompt return of the allergic blepharitis.

In subluxated lens. A very rare contraindication to mydriasis is subluxation of the lens, which may occur after injury, in megalocornea, or in Marfan's syndrome. Although most such eyes may be dilated without consequence, several instances have been reported in which the lens slipped into the anterior chamber and caused acute pupillary block glaucoma.[124] However, dilation is clearly indicated in complete examination of an injured eye or of the periphery of an eye with Marfan's syndrome and should not be foregone because of the slight risk of anterior lens displacement.

Homatropine

Homatropine is a parasympatholytic drug quite similar to atropine except that it is weaker and has a much shorter duration of action. It is primarily used in cycloplegic refraction.

Maximum cycloplegia, induced by a 2% solution of homatropine, is reached within an hour after initial drug instillation (Fig. 12-20).[125] The cycloplegic effect is maintained for about 3 hours and then gradually decreases; some effect remains for more than 24 hours. The average recovery time from 2% homatropine solution is 32 hours, varying from 12 to 49 hours in a series of 23 eyes. The residual accommodation averages 1.00 D, varying from 0.50 to 2.00 D. These results were obtained after the instillation of 6 drops of a 2% solution of homatropine at 10-minute intervals in patients ranging from 17 to 39 years of age (average age 22 years).

During the onset and disappearance of cycloplegia, as caused by homatropine, the accommodative convergence/accommodation (AC/A) ratio changes. As shown in Fig. 12-21, this change in the AC/A ratio differs among individuals.[126] The practical implication of this change is that reliable measurements of muscle balance should be made before or after but not during cycloplegia.

In both the normal and glaucomatous human eye the resistance of the trabecular meshwork may be reduced by parasympathomimetic tonus and increased by parasympatholytic drugs. The average increase in outflow resistance 45 minutes after instillation of 2 drops of a 5% solution of homatropine in 64 normal human eyes and in 29 eyes with open-angle glaucoma is shown in Fig. 12-22.[127] As illustrated, the glaucomatous eyes showed a greater susceptibility to a cycloplegic-induced rise of outflow resistance than did the normal eyes.

The effect of a 5% concentration of homatropine hydrobromide on intraocular pressure was studied in 140 normal eyes and in 70 eyes with chronic simple glaucoma.[128] Forty-five minutes after medication the intraocular pressure had decreased in 50% of the normal eyes, had remained the same in

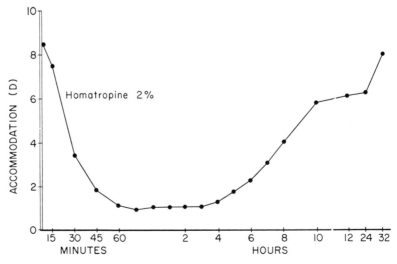

Fig. 12-20. Average cycloplegic response of 23 young adult eyes to homatropine hydrobromide solution, 1 drop every 10 minutes for 1 hour. (Modified from Thorne, F. H., and Murphey, H. S.: Arch. Ophthalmol. **22**:274, 1939.)

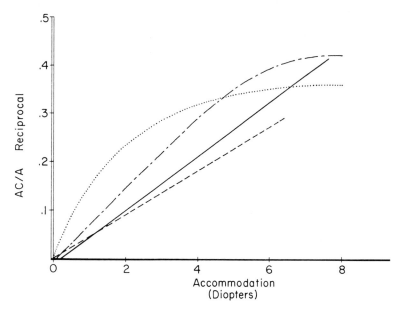

Fig. 12-21. Change in AC/A ratio during recovery from homatropine (four persons). (Modified from Fry, G. A.: Am. J. Optom. **36:**525, 1959.)

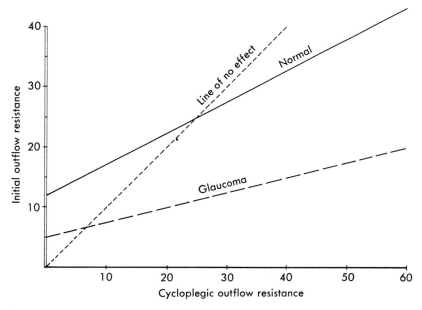

Fig. 12-22. Average change of outflow resistance after homatropine in normal and glaucomatous human eyes. Lines represent slopes of the least squares calculations to fit results in 64 normal and 29 glaucomatous eyes. (Modified from Bárány, E., and Christensen, R. E.: Arch. Ophthalmol. **77:**757, 1967.)

30%, and had increased in only 20%. In contrast, the pressure of 73% of the glaucomatous eyes increased, 10% remained the same, and 17% decreased. The increased pressure was because of a reduction in the facility of aqueous outflow, which dropped by an average of 28% in the glaucomatous eyes and by 15% in the normal eyes. There was no definite relationship between the amount of mydriasis and the decrease in outflow.

These findings have two clinically important implications. First, routine tonometric screening is more likely to detect increased intraocular pressure after parasympatholytic medication, and therefore tonometry should be done on the dilated eye, rather than before dilation. (Recall that sympathomimetic dilation does *not* regularly increase intraocular pressure but rather decreases it.) Second, since dilation commonly increases intraocular pressure in chronic simple glaucoma, a dilation-provocative test for angle-closure glaucoma is not to be interpreted as positive (requiring iridectomy) unless the angle is gonioscopically closed at the time of pressure elevation.

Scopolamine

Except for a much shorter duration of action, the effects of scopolamine are, for practical ophthalmic purposes, the same as those of atropine. In a 0.5% concentration, scopolamine is commonly used as an atropine substitute in the event of atropine allergy or when a shorter period for cycloplegia is required (for example, in mild iritis).

The cycloplegic strengths of 1% atropine and 0.2% scopolamine are comparable when they are administered for purposes of refraction.[129] The duration of scopolamine cycloplegia is less than that of atropine, however.

Instillation of a 0.5% solution of scopolamine causes a maximum cycloplegic effect within 40 minutes. Half this cycloplegic effect wears off within 3 to 4 hours, but more than a day is required for full restoration of accommodation (Fig. 12-23).[118]

Systemic toxicity

Seven cases of confusional psychosis were recognized in a series of several hundred patients whose eyes were dilated with several drops of 1% scopolamine hydrobromide.[130]

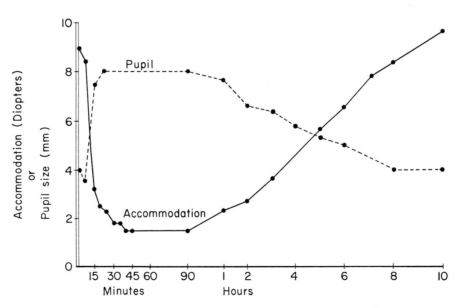

Fig. 12-23. Cycloplegic and mydriatic effect of 2 drops of a 0.5% solution of scopolamine hydrobromide (at 0 and 30 minutes) in 42 young adult eyes. (Modified from Marron, J.: Arch. Ophthalmol. **23**:340, 1940.)

These reactions included restlessness, confusion, hallucinations, incoherence, violence, amnesia, unconsciousness, spastic extremities, vomiting, and urinary incontinence. It was suggested that concentrations of scopolamine higher than 0.5% were not appropriate for ophthalmic use. Comparable symptoms occur with the other belladonna derivatives (atropine and homatropine) and with similar synthetic parasympatholytic drugs (cyclopentolate).

Antidote for scopolamine poisoning. Anticholinergic poisoning should not be regarded as being necessarily benign or transient and deserves treatment if it is at all severe. The central nervous system anticholinergic syndrome includes a variety of stimulant and depressant psychotic reactions. Depending on the level of toxicity, the symptoms may disappear within a few hours, may persist for days, or may be fatal.

Physostigmine is a specific antidote to central anticholinergic poisoning. It is lipid soluble and readily enters the central nervous system. In contrast, neostigmine and edrophonium do not cross the blood-brain barrier. Similarly, parasympathomimetic drugs such as pilocarpine combat only the peripheral nervous system effects of anticholinergic poisoning and do not alleviate central nervous system reactions.

The adult dose of physostigmine is 1 mg, which may be given intramuscularly, intravenously, or subcutaneously. Such a dose is entirely eliminated within 2 hours and therefore may need to be repeated if toxic symptoms recur. Should the initial dose fail to reverse toxic symptoms, it may safely be repeated in 15 to 30 minutes. The 1 mg dose of physostigmine is said to produce no or minimal parasympathomimetic effects in the normal individual even if an anticholinergic drug has not been given previously. The pediatric dose is 1 mg/m² of body surface.

Two cases of scopolamine poisoning were reported. In one, scopolamine, 0.25%, was instilled every 10 minutes for 2 hours in both eyes prior to retinal detachment surgery. The other case involved a 4-year-old boy who had ingested 0.25% scopolamine drops pre-

scribed for his father's traumatic iritis. Both patients responded well to the physostigmine antidote.[131]

Cyclopentolate (Cyclogyl)
Clinical use

Cyclopentolate is a potent parasympatholytic drug of great value in inducing cycloplegia and wide mydriasis. Its cycloplegic effect is superior to that of homatropine, having a more rapid onset, shorter duration, and greater intensity. A concentration of 0.5% cyclopentolate, instilled two times 10 minutes apart, will produce maximum cycloplegia in 40% of white patients in 15 minutes or less (Fig. 12-24). However, 22% of the eyes treated with cyclopentolate did not attain the maximum effect until 45 minutes or more after instillation. Note that 1.00 D or more of residual accommodation remains in many eyes. It is important to measure this remaining accommodation at the time of refraction; an anisometropic error in prescription may occur if an unequal cycloplegic effect in the two eyes is not recognized. The cycloplegic effect of a 0.5% solution of cyclopentolate is usually dissipated within 24 hours. However, some mydriasis may last for several days.

For comparison, the responses of opposite eyes of the same patients to instillation of a 5% solution of homatropine and a 1% solution of hydroxyamphetamine (Paredrine), repeated after 10 minutes, is shown in Fig. 12-25. The eyes treated with homatropine and hydroxyamphetamine attained the same level of cycloplegia as did the eyes treated with cyclopentolate, but more slowly. The homatropine cycloplegia often lasted more than 24 hours, and the patients were able to read with the cyclopentolate-treated eye sooner than with the opposite eye.

A single drop of a 1% solution (or 2 drops of a 0.5% solution, separated by a 5-minute interval) will provide sufficient cycloplegia for most refractive purposes. Within an hour, instillation of 3 drops at 10-minute intervals will give retinoscopic values comparable to those obtained by atropinization for 3 days in children. The eyes of black patients are resistant to cyclopentolate, just as they are to

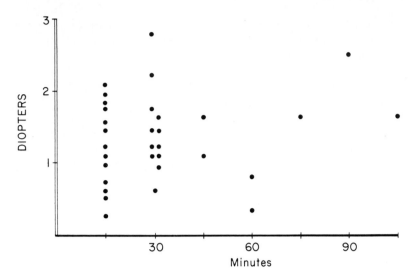

Fig. 12-24. Time of onset of maximum cycloplegia and residual accommodation at that time after 2 drops of a 0.5% solution of cyclopentolate in white patients. (Modified from Milder, B., and Riffinburgh, R. S.: Am. J. Ophthalmol. **36:**1724, 1953.)

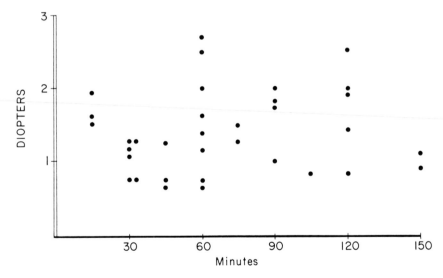

Fig. 12-25. Time of onset of maximum cycloplegia and residual accommodation at that time after instillation of 2 drops of a 5% solution of homatropine and of a 1% solution of hydroxyamphetamine (Paredrine) in white patients. (Modified from Milder, B., and Riffinburgh, R. S.: Am. J. Ophthalmol. **36:**1724, 1953.)

other cycloplegics, and may require repeated instillation of a 2% solution and a longer than usual time for dilation (Fig. 12-26).[132] As much as 5.00 to 6.00 D of accommodation may remain after two instillations of cyclopentolate in the eye of a black person.

Excellent mydriasis is produced by cyclopentolate. Pupils dilated with this drug do not constrict even when exposed to the prolonged, intense light of the indirect ophthalmoscope or during fundus photography. Dilation with the combination of cyclopentolate

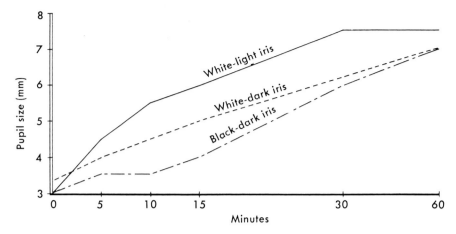

Fig. 12-26. Effect of iris pigmentation on cyclopentolate mydriasis. (Modified from Priestley, B. S., and Medine, M. M.: Am. J. Ophthalmol. 34:572, 1951.)

and phenylephrine provides maximal mydriasis, which, for instance, is of great value during the examination of patients with retinal detachment. Good mydriasis can be achieved within 20 minutes with cyclopentolate.

Cyclopentolate in a 0.5% solution is a more potent mydriatic and cycloplegic than is a 5% solution of homatropine. In 100 patients the average residual accommodation 1 hour after instillation of 2 drops of a 0.5% solution of cyclopentolate was 1.25 D, as compared to 2.00 D for 2 drops of a 5% solution of homatropine.[132]

Twenty patients with contact allergy to atropine were successfully treated with cyclopentolate, with no cross sensitivity.[133] If iridocyclitis is severe, it may be necessary to instill cyclopentolate as often as every 3 hours since its duration of action is not as long as that of atropine.

As would be expected, the keratometric measurement of corneal curvature is unaffected by the use of cycloplegics or anesthetics. In a series of 100 human eyes, keratometry was performed before and 30 to 60 minutes after instillation of solutions of either 1% cyclopentolate or 10% phenylephrine. Proparacaine followed by tonometry was also used in one third of the eyes.[134] There was no statistically significant difference between the readings taken before and after therapy. The clinical implication is that dilation of the pupils, if advantageous for the sequence of examination, does not interfere with subsequent keratometry.

Toxicity

A considerable burning sensation results from instillation of a 1% or 2% solution of cyclopentolate. The 0.5% solution is definitely less irritating. This burning sensation is transient and the patient should be assured that it is to be expected and will rapidly disappear. Children are especially distressed by such discomfort.

As is true of all parasympatholytic drugs, cyclopentolate will increase the intraocular pressure of most patients with chronic simple glaucoma.[135] Dilation with any drug, including cyclopentolate, may precipitate an attack of acute glaucoma in patients predisposed to this disorder because of the narrow angles.[136]

Even after prophylactic peripheral iridectomy, very few eyes with narrow angles may develop quite marked pressure elevations after cyclopentolate dilation.[137]

Disturbances of central nervous system. Ocular instillation of cyclopentolate may cause disturbances of the central nervous system in children. After instillation of 4 drops of a 1% solution of cyclopentolate, an 8-year-old child developed marked ataxia, visual hallucinations, and incoherent speech. Some days later the same child was given 6 drops of a 1% concentration of cyclopentolate during a 15-minute period. Twenty minutes later the previously described symptoms reappeared and persisted for 4 hours. There was no flushing or dryness of skin or mucous membranes. Temperature, pulse, and respiration were normal. One is reminded that each drop of a 1% solution contains 0.5 mg of the medication.[138]

Psychiatric evaluation of 40 children before and after use of a 2% solution of cyclopentolate for refraction detected an acute psychotic reaction in five of these children.[139] Symptoms develop about 30 to 45 minutes after instillation of the drops and include restlessness, aimless wandering, irrelevant talking, hallucinations, memory loss, and faulty orientation as to time and place. A solution of 1% cyclopentolate is much less likely to cause such reactions. Solutions of 1% homatropine and 1% hydroxyamphetamine (Paredrine) did not cause psychotic symptoms. Cyclopentolate contains a dimethylated group ($-N-[CH_3]_2$) that is also found in some hallucinogenic drugs.

Hallucinations and amnesia lasting 3 hours were produced in a 9-year-old boy by 1 drop of a 1% solution of cyclopentolate in each eye, followed in 15 minutes by a drop of a 2% solution of the same drug in both eyes.[140]

Rarely, adults may develop a comparable reaction. After the instillation of 1 drop of 2% cyclopentolate (Cyclogyl) in each eye, the 27-year-old wife of a physician developed an episode of hallucination lasting for an hour.[141]

An unusual case of addiction to cyclopentolate was described in a 25-year-old emotionally unstable man. He used from 100 to 200 drops of cyclopentolate daily. On withdrawal, he suffered from salivation, vomiting, anxiety, tremors, and other objective signs of physical withdrawal from the drug.[142]

In evaluation of retinal detachments, I routinely use 4 to 6 drops of 1% cyclopentolate (both eyes dilated). Infrequently a patient complains that "the drops make me woozy," but I have never recognized overt hallucinations.

Now that we know these facts, what do we do? How would you examine a premature child suspected of possibly having oxygen-induced retinopathy of prematurity? You might make the same mistake as I would—dilate his eyes with cyclopentolate and phenylephrine so that you could get a good look at the periphery. By now the suspicion that this might not be a good idea has entered your mind. Dilation of premature infants' eyes with 2.5% phenylephrine and 0.5% cyclopentolate has resulted in conspicuous periorbital blanching and lethargy lasting for 12 hours. Concentrations of 10% phenylephrine used as eye drops in the premature infant will result in systemic hypertension.[143] In an infant this small, an eye drop contains a toxic dosage of drug.

Allergy. A characteristic type of severe allergic response may follow the repeated use of cyclopentolate. Because of the circumstances of the drug's use and the unusual appearance of this allergy, the ophthalmologist almost always fails to recognize its presence.

Each of the three or four cases I have encountered was associated with the use of cyclopentolate during an office examination. Following the office visit the patient developed redness and discomfort of the eyes lasting a day or more. The physician is, of course, unaware of this subsequent allergic response. The patient assumes the irritation to be normal and is resigned to this fate. None of my patients have spontaneously presented a diagnostic history of cyclopentolate allergy, although such a history can easily be elicited by specific questioning. The history includes persistent irritation developing within minutes of instillation, rather severe watering, and stringy discharge. Vision is blurred and the eyes are red, while itching, the classic sign of allergy, is not a significant complaint. Comparable symptoms occur at each office visit, the allergic reactions sometimes extending over a period of 6 months or more.

In the presence of allergy the eyes are diffusely red after instillation of cyclopentolate. If only one eye is involved, the physician misinterprets the problem as being an exacerbation of whatever condition is under treatment—for example, unusually persistent redness following surgery. An annoying amount of stringy white mucus is present, enough to move over the cornea with blinking and to distort the image of the indirect ophthalmoscope. Such mucus is not uncommon in surface infection, so the physician simply wipes it away and continues with the examination. However, if within a few minutes the mucus strands have re-formed, this is the first indication of cyclopentolate allergy. Such rapid mucous secretion does not occur in the usual conjunctival infections.

The fundus view is diffusely hazy—not really bad, but enough to be annoying. The indistinctness is comparable to any opacity of the media, such as a moderate nuclear cataract or a diffuse vitreous condensation, except that it is a result of corneal changes.

Typically, biomicroscopy reveals innumerable tiny superficial punctate epithelial lesions scattered uniformly across the entire corneal surface.

I have devoted so much space to this uncommon allergy because its reasonably prompt detection may be very important to the patient. Not only is the acute stage annoying and uncomfortable, but following numerous insults, the lacrimal drainage system

may become occluded. In one of my patients, all four lacrimal punctae became so stenotic that they literally disappeared, resulting in continuing epiphora.

Tropicamide (Mydriacyl)

Tropicamide is a rapidly acting parasympatholytic drug useful in producing cycloplegia and mydriasis of short duration. The diopters of residual accommodation at various times after instillation of a single drop of a 1% solution of tropicamide are shown in Fig. 12-27. Assuming that residual accommodation should not exceed 2.00 D for a satisfactory cycloplegic refraction, it is evident that one instillation of tropicamide in a 1% solution is generally inadequate for such refraction. Even at the time of maximum effect, from 20 to 25 minutes after instillation, only half the patients were adequately cycloplegic. Because of the transient period of cycloplegia, by the time the second eye was examined its accommodation was frequently as much as 3.00 D greater than that of the first eye. Obviously a disparity of this magnitude may contribute to erroneous refractive findings.

Considerably better cycloplegia was obtained by a second instillation of a 1% solution of tropicamide 5 to 25 minutes after the

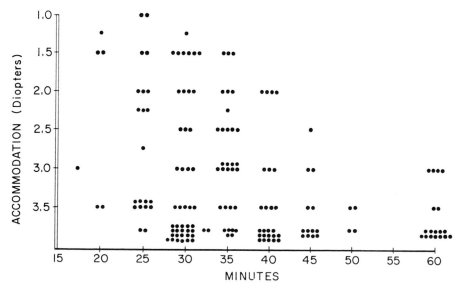

Fig. 12-27. Residual accommodation after instillation of 1 drop of a 1% solution of tropicamide. (Modified from Gettes, B.: Arch. Ophthalmol. **65:**632, 1961.)

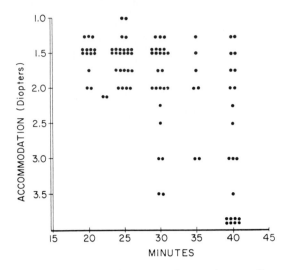

Fig. 12-28. Residual accommodation after instillation of a second drop of a 1% solution of tropicamide, instilled 5 to 25 minutes after the first. (Modified from Gettes, B.: Arch. Ophthalmol. **65:** 632, 1961.)

first (Fig. 12-28).[144] All patients had 2.00 D or less residual accommodation within 20 to 25 minutes after instillation of the second drop. After 35 minutes, cycloplegia was no longer reliable. All patients were able to read within 2 to 4 hours, with complete return of accommodation within 6 hours.

The mydriatic effect of a 0.5% solution of tropicamide was found to be more rapid than and at least as great as that of a 10% concentration of phenylephrine. Tropicamide in a 0.5% solution is not effective for cycloplegic examination.

Tropicamide tends to have a greater mydriatic than cycloplegic effect. This is clinically important because the presence of tropicamide-induced mydriasis does *not* necessarily indicate adequate cycloplegia. This mydriatic-cycloplegic dissociation is more characteristic of tropicamide than of cyclopentolate.

The effect of various mydriatics has been

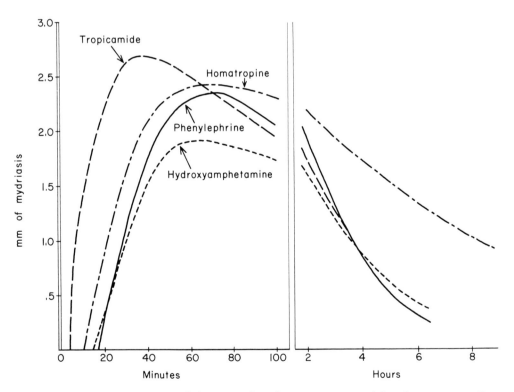

Fig. 12-29. Onset, intensity, and duration of mydriasis as measured by electronic pupillograph. (From Gambill, H. D., Ogle, K. N., and Kearns, T. P.: Arch. Ophthalmol. **77:**740, 1967.)

particularly accurately studied using the infrared electronic pupillograph. The mydriasis resulting from single instillations, of 0.5% tropicamide, 2% homatropine, 1% hydroxyamphetamine, and 10% phenylephrine is compared in Fig. 12-29.[145] The charted lines represent the computer-derived curves of the pupillographic values. Any given reading is the difference in size of the treated pupil and the fellow control pupil at the moment of peak response to a standard light flash. The subjects of this study were 15 white men and women ranging from 12 to 38 years of age (average age, 26 years). The method of measurement used in this study probably is the most accurate clinical determination available.

Although tropicamide is the shortest acting of our cycloplegic drugs, it also shares the capability of transiently increasing the intraocular pressure of open-angle glaucoma eyes. Used in 50 patients with open-angle glaucoma, 2 drops of 1% tropicamide caused varying pressure elevations, one of which

was as great as 10 mm Hg.[146] However, in most of these patients, there was less than a 5 mm elevation of pressure after 40 minutes. The effect is so small as to be clinically insignificant.

Comparison of cyclopentolate, tropicamide, and homatropine

The three short-acting cycloplegic drugs most commonly used for refraction are cyclopentolate hydrochloride, 1% solution; tropicamide, 1% solution; and homatropine, 4% solution. The effectiveness of these cycloplegics is compared in Fig. 12-30. Tropicamide is the most rapidly acting of the three and has the shortest duration of cycloplegia. Because of the very short duration of tropicamide's effect, it is necessary to instill a second drop 5 minutes after the first one. (The comparisons in Fig. 12-30 are of two instillations of tropicamide, 1 drop of cyclopentolate, and two instillations of homatropine.) After two instillations of tropicamide, excellent cycloplegia is obtained within 20 to 35 minutes.

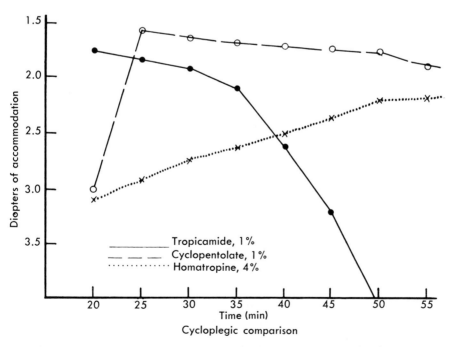

Fig. 12-30. Duration and effectiveness of cycloplegia induced by two instillations of tropicamide, 1% solution; 1 drop of cyclopentolate, 1% solution; and two instillations of homatropine, 4% solution. (From Gettes, B., and Belmont, O.: Arch. Ophthalmol. **66:**336, 1961.)

Table 12-4. Residual accommodation at specific time after two instillations of cycloplegic drug*

Age (yr)	No. of cases	Residual accommodation	
		Tropicamide at 30 min	Homatropine or cyclopentolate at 60 min
0-9	6	6.25 D	2.50 D
10-14	20	3.65 D	2.40 D
15-19	7	3.20 D	1.40 D
20-29	7	3.10 D	1.40 D
30-39	7	2.60 D	2.00 D
40+	3	1.70 D	1.10 D

*From Milder, B.: Arch. Ophthalmol. **66**:70, 1961.

After 35 minutes, accommodation returns rapidly. Only 60% of 193 patients could be examined during the interval between 20 and 35 minutes after instillation.[147] The authors emphasized the difficulty of maintaining a schedule of such precision. In clinical practice a third drop of tropicamide must be instilled if examination is delayed beyond 35 minutes. However, tropicamide has the advantage of permitting the patient to recover from cycloplegia within 2 to 6 hours.

Cyclopentolate was found to be an effective cycloplegic between 25 and 75 minutes after a single drop. Recovery time varied from 6 to 24 hours. The slowest acting of the three drugs, homatropine, required two instillations and was effective within 40 to 90 minutes, with residual cycloplegia lasting 36 to 48 hours. Less than 2.50 D of residual accommodation was achieved in 79% of white patients and 69% of black patients receiving tropicamide, in 83% of white patients receiving cyclopentolate, and in 59% of patients (racial breakdown unspecified) receiving homatropine.

In a series of 50 consecutive refractions, tropicamide (1% solution instilled twice, 5 minutes apart) was placed in one eye and compared with solutions of 5% homatropine and 1% cyclopentolate instilled in the other eye twice, 10 minutes apart.[148] Better cycloplegia was produced by homatropine in 20 of 25 patients and by cyclopentolate in 23 of 25 patients. In only seven patients was better

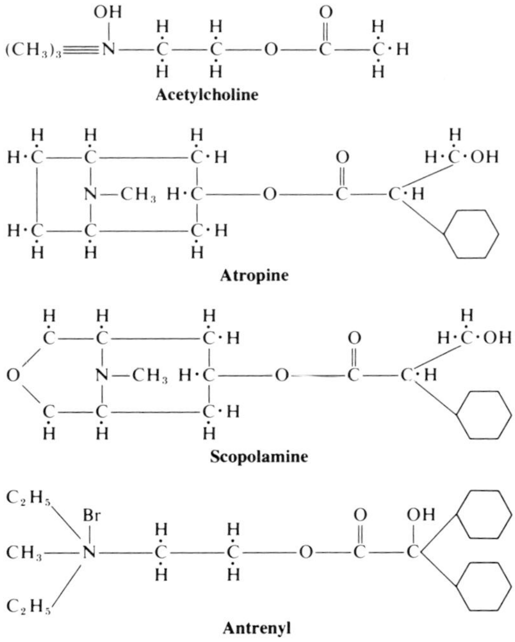

Fig. 12-31. Molecular structure of acetylcholine and several long-acting anticholinergic drugs. (From Havener, W. H., and Falls, H. F.: Arch. Ophthalmol. **52**:515, 1954.)

cycloplegia attained by tropicamide. The amount of residual accommodation remaining at the time of maximum effect of these drugs is recorded in Table 12-4. It is evident that tropicamide is a relatively inadequate cycloplegic drug, since an average of 6.00 D of accommodation remains in children

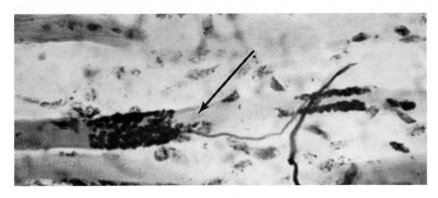

Fig. 12-32. Dense accumulation of cholinesterase (special enzyme stain of frozen section) distributed about ending of single nerve axon (arrow) on fiber of human extraocular muscle. (From Wolter, J. R., and O'Keefe, N. T.: Invest. Ophthalmol. **2:**558, 1963.)

younger than 10 years and 3.60 D in patients 10 to 14 years of age. The residual accommodation in the patients 10 to 14 years of age with cyclopentolate was 1.60 D and with homatropine, 2.60 D. However, the mydriatic effect of tropicamide was said to be equal to or better than any other available drug in terms of rapidity of onset, size of pupil, and brevity of duration. (My personal observations in paired eyes indicate that cyclopentolate produces equal or greater mydriasis as rapidly and of much longer duration than does tropicamide.)

In summary, the great advantage of tropicamide is its very short duration of action. I use a 1% solution of tropicamide as an aid in the teaching of ophthalmoscopy and find it to be very effective for this purpose. Students do not complain of the prolonged cycloplegia that bothers them considerably when other drugs are used.

Oxyphenonium (Antrenyl)

Oxyphenonium is a synthetic, potent, long-acting anticholinergic drug. The effect of a 1% solution of oxyphenonium bromide in a 1:5000 concentration of benzalkonium chloride is comparable in degree and duration to that of a 1% solution of atropine.[149] These two drugs may be used interchangeably in ophthalmic therapy. The structure of oxyphenonium differs from that of atropine much more than does that of scopolamine

(Fig. 12-31). During my experience with dozens of patients with atropine allergy, I have never encountered one in whom cross sensitivity to oxyphenonium existed. Oxyphenonium mydriasis is quite resistant to the effect of pilocarpine and isoflurophate.

Oxyphenonium is dispensed commercially as an antispasmodic for gastrointestinal use. A solution suitable for ophthalmic use may be made by preparing a 1% concentration in a 1:5000 solution of benzalkonium chloride.

Rabbit eyes dilate much better with oxyphenonium than with atropine.

CHOLINERGIC AGENTS
Acetylcholine

Acetylcholine is a chemical mediator that transfers nerve impulses from one neuron to another or from neurons to effector cells. It is formed at parasympathetic nerve endings, at skeletal muscle-nerve junctions (Fig. 12-32),[150] and at ganglion synapses. The actions of acetylcholine are classified as muscarinic and nicotinic.

Pharmacology

Muscarinic action is the stimulation of smooth muscle and glands that are innervated by postganglionic parasympathetic nerves. The muscarinic action of acetylcholine is blocked by atropine but not by curare.

The nicotinic action of acetylcholine entails its stimulation of skeletal muscle and autonomic ganglia. (The former is antagonized by curare and the latter by nicotine.) A practical application of this information is the simultaneous administration of prostigmine and atropine in testing for myasthenia gravis. Atropine blocks the undesirable muscarinic side effects of acetylcholine (for example, bowel evacuation), and yet it does not alter the desired response of skeletal muscle.

Acetylcholine is destroyed by cholinesterase, which is strategically located in the end-plate region. Within a few milliseconds after release of acetylcholine by the nerve impulse, this effector chemical is hydrolyzed, thereby permitting the end plate to repolarize and become receptive to the next impulse.[151]

The classic concepts of the effects of autonomic drugs have been confirmed by bathing isolated strips of cat ciliary muscle with these drugs.[32] These experiments are noteworthy because they provide quantitative data as to the sensitivity of the ciliary muscle to drug stimulation. A concentration of acetylcholine of only 1 μg/ml causes abrupt contraction of the ciliary muscle. Eserine, 1 μg/ml, potentiates the effect of acetylcholine by about 100 times, so that 0.01 μg/ml of acetylcholine will cause contraction of the eserinized ciliary muscle. (This is a concentration of only one-hundred millionth of a gram per milliliter, or 0.000,001%!)

Eserine sensitization of the iris sphincter to acetylcholine is quite different from cocaine sensitization of the dilator to epinephrine.[18] Whereas cocaine decreases the absolute strength of the muscle, eserine enhances the strength of contraction. In most experimental trials the combined effect of eserine and acetycholine is even greater than the sum of their separate effects. Fig. 12-33 shows the response to maximum effective concentrations of eserine and acetylcholine (1:50,000 for each drug) by a sphincter muscle supporting a very heavy load (sufficient so that almost no shortening response occurred). Addition of acetylcholine to the eserinized strip produced a much stronger contraction than the maximal response obtained by either drug alone.

Clinical use

Despite the extreme sensitivity of the iris to acetylcholine, topical ocular instillation causes no useful response. This is because cholinesterase destroys the molecule more rapidly than it can penetrate the cornea. Accelerated corneal transfer, as by iontophoresis, will produce miosis, as will direct application on the iris.

Instillation of a 1:100 concentration of acetylcholine directly on the iris after cataract extraction will cause prompt, marked (2 mm) miosis, which is helpful in keeping the iris temporarily away from the incision.[152] Irrigation of the anterior chamber with acetylcholine may also be of value dur-

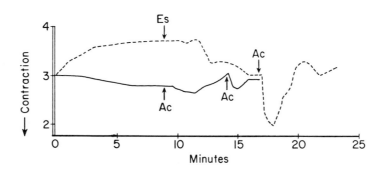

Fig. 12-33. Response of sphincter of albino rabbit to repeated applications of acetylcholine (solid line) and of the same preparation (after washing) to eserine (broken line) and then to acetylcholine (broken line). (Modified from Sachs, E., and Heath, P.: Am. J. Ophthalmol. **23:** 1376, 1940.)

ing keratoplasty, iridectomy, or cyclodialysis.[153-155] The miotic action of acetylcholine is very brief, lasting for only about 10 minutes. Use of acetylcholine at the time of surgery may be preferable to instillation of pilocarpine or eserine, since the prolonged miosis caused by these latter drugs is one of the principal causes of postoperative pain.

In the past, systemic or retrobulbar injection of acetylcholine has been advocated in the treatment of occlusion of the central retinal artery.[156] This treatment was based on the unproved supposition that beneficial vasodilation would result. In a series of 73 patients with retinal arterial occlusion treated by various means, only one regained any vision.[157] Twenty-two of these patients received retrobulbar injection of acetylcholine, 0.1 to 0.05 g. After injection, five patients developed extraocular muscle pareses, corneal anesthesia, and nonreactive fixed pupils. The fourth cranial nerve was never involved, presumably because its anatomic course is not readily accessible to the effect of retrobulbar injection. Trauma was excluded as a cause of this nerve damage, since the same physicians had never encountered such complications after retrobulbar injections for surgical anesthesia. Apparently, very high concentrations of acetylcholine have the ability to cause prolonged damage to nerve junctions. Almost all of the patients experiencing paralysis recovered after several months.

Toxicity

Since acetylcholine is so rapidly destroyed, its toxicity is very low and its therapeutic effects are very transient. As much as 100 mg/min can be tolerated intravenously by adult human beings. There is no evidence of cumulative action; as much as 1 g of acetylcholine has been given intravenously during a 10-minute period with only transient cholinergic effects. Intramuscular or subcutaneous injection of 500 mg does not alter pulse rate or blood pressure.[62]

A systemic reaction occurred after injection into the anterior chamber of 20 mg of acetylcholine (Miochol) subsequent to cataract extraction.[158] The patient's blood pressure immediately dropped to 75 mm Hg systolic and the pulse rate slowed to 48 beats per minute. The cardioscope showed transient ventricular bigeminy and sinus bradycardia. Intravenous atropine in two doses of 0.6 and 0.8 mg did not change the heart rate. The hypotension and bradycardia lasted for about 20 minutes. There were no untoward consequences of this episode.

Methacholine (Mecholyl)

Methacholine bromide has pharmacologic properties quite similar to those of acetylcholine,[159] except that it is considerably more resistant to cholinesterase and therefore has a more prolonged effect. It has been given by retrobulbar injection in an attempt to induce vasodilation and by iontophoresis to constrict the pupil. It has been used in the diagnosis of Adie's pupil as well.

Clinical use

Retrobulbar injection. Because it causes peripheral vasodilation, the retrobulbar injection of methacholine has been advocated to improve retinal circulation. The dosage of methacholine when given by subcutaneous injection varies from 2.5 to 40 mg. Apparently there is considerable individual variation in response, and trial of smaller doses is recommended before use of larger amounts. Methacholine should never be given intravenously.

Atropine blocks the effect of methacholine. All of the systemic muscarinic toxic effects of methacholine retrobulbar injection (as well as the therapeutic effects, if any) can immediately be abolished by the intravenous injection of 1 mg of atropine.

Toxic effects likely to be observed after retrobulbar injection are nausea and vomiting, involuntary evacuation of bladder and bowels, and transient heart block or cardiac arrest. The patient should be recumbent during injection and the period of methacholine's action, since fainting is common. Because the patient cannot safely stand to go to the toilet, a bedpan should be available. Eserine greatly enhances the effect of methacholine and should never be given before methacholine injection.

Since there is doubt as to its therapeutic value and because of its unpleasant systemic side effects, retrobulbar injection of methacholine is rare. Priscoline would be a better drug for such use.

Iontophoresis. Since all the choline esters are water soluble, they do not readily penetrate the corneal epithelium and are relatively ineffective when applied topically. Iontophoresis will enhance the corneal penetration of a 10% solution of methacholine, resulting in good miosis within a few minutes. Because of the relatively small amount of drug absorbed, bothersome systemic side effects do not accompany ocular iontophoresis. Methacholine iontophoresis has been advocated for treatment of acute glaucoma and is doubtless as effective as any other miotic; however, this drug seems less desirable than other potent miotics that readily penetrate the cornea unaided by iontophoresis.

Because of its poor corneal penetration and short duration of action (several hours), methacholine is not suitable for treatment of chronic simple glaucoma.

Diagnosis of Adie's pupil. Miosis usually is not produced by topical application of methacholine in concentrations lower than 10%. However, individual variations in sensitivity occur, and infrequently patients become miotic with a 1% solution. Since this failure of response is caused by the destruction of the drug being more rapid than its corneal penetration, miosis will result from lesser concentrations if the corneal epithelium is abraded or if a wetting agent is used.

Breakdown of the corneal epithelium (as in keratitis sicca or after anesthesia and tonometry) allows greater penetration of topical medications such as 2.5% methacholine, which under such circumstances may cause constriction of a normally innervated pupil.[160]

Partial parasympathetic denervation, as from Adie's pupil or in some cases of traumatic mydriasis, sensitizes the iris to cholinergic drugs. Such pupils can be made to constrict by a 2.5% aqueous solution of metha-

choline (without a wetting agent). Comparison of the drug response of the normal pupil with that of suspected Adie's pupil makes the diagnosis more valid.

The original patient with Adie's syndrome, on whom the observation of methacholine sensitization was first made, still showed the classic hypersensitivity to methacholine when observed 25 years later.[161]

Although hypersensitivity to 2.5% methacholine chloride has been considered characteristic of Adie's tonic pupil syndrome, such hypersensitivity may be absent at the onset of this disorder. Apparently the onset of Adie's syndrome may be fairly abrupt, with acute unilateral mydriasis and loss of accommodation. Only after periods of 8 and 11 months did two patients develop the typical sluggish reaction and the expected methacholine hypersensitivity.[162] (In this paper, five cases from a single pedigree were reported, indicating a genetic origin.)

A positive methacholine test also occurs in familial dysautonomia, a condition characterized by partial parasympathetic denervation. Sixteen of 18 dysautonomic patients developed miosis within 30 minutes after ocular instillation of 2.5% methacholine. (The ocular symptoms of this disease include deficient lacrimation and corneal anesthesia, with subsequent trophic damage to the cornea; 12 of the 15 patients also had exotropia.)[163]

Because methacholine is not easily available and is quite expensive, clinical testing for parasympathetic denervation is more easily performed with dilute solutions of pilocarpine (p. 286).

Carbachol (Carcholin)

Carbachol is an ingenious combination of portions of the molecules of acetylcholine and of physostigmine. Carbachol is not destroyed by cholinesterase; therefore its action is not increased by anticholinesterase drugs. Besides its direct parasympathomimetic action, carbachol is also believed to have an indirect mechanism of action whereby acetylcholine is displaced from the parasympathetic nerve terminal.[2] Carbachol is stable in solution.[157]

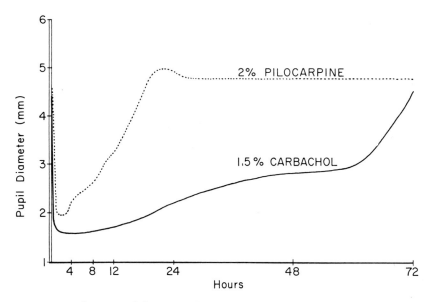

Fig. 12-34. Average degree and duration of miosis in 10 normal adults after single instillations of pilocarpine and of carbachol. (Modified from O'Brien, C. S., and Swan, K. C.: Arch. Ophthalmol. **27:**253, 1942.)

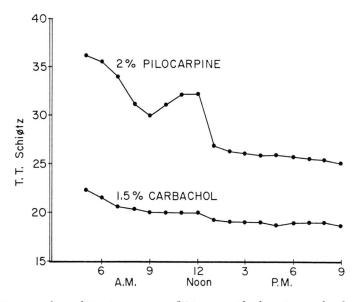

Fig. 12-35. Average diurnal tension curves of 34 eyes with chronic simple glaucoma when treated with a 2% solution of pilocarpine four times a day and with a 1.5% solution of carbachol three times a day. (Modified from O'Brien, C. S., and Swan, K. C.: Arch. Ophthalmol. **27:**253, 1942.)

Systemic toxicity is not caused by ocular use of carbachol in recommended dosages.

Clinical use

Glaucoma. Carbachol in a 1.5% solution produces more intense and considerably more prolonged miosis than does a 2% solution of pilocarpine. As shown in Fig. 12-34, a single instillation of carbachol in a normal eye causes miosis lasting more than 2 days.[164] Because of its prolonged action, carbachol is usually prescribed for use only two or three times daily.

Carbachol in a 0.75% solution is more effective than a 2% solution of pilocarpine in the control of pressure in chronic simple glaucoma. In 14 eyes adequately controlled by pilocarpine administered four times a day, the pressure was lowered an average of 5 mm Hg (measured by the Schiøtz tonometer) by the administration of carbachol three times a day. Pressure in another series of 34 eyes could not be maintained below 30 mm Hg with a 2% solution of pilocarpine; however, instillation of a 1.5% solution of carbachol three times a day kept the pressure in these eyes below 25 mm Hg (Fig. 12-35).[164] Car-

bachol decreases diurnal fluctuations in pressure more effectively than does pilocarpine. Because of the prolonged action of carbachol, pressure is less likely to rise if the patient misses the instillation of a drop.

Disadvantages

Carbachol causes more severe headache and accommodative spasms of the eye than does pilocarpine, but these symptoms decrease after several days of treatment. Its vasodilating effect may cause slight conjunctival hyperemia. Local allergic sensitivity to carbachol is uncommon, but it may occur. Carbachol is usually prescribed for patients who are allergic to pilocarpine or those whose condition cannot be quite adequately controlled by pilocarpine. Unlike the alkaloids commonly used in ophthalmology, carbachol is not lipid soluble at any pH. Hence it penetrates the intact corneal epithelium very poorly. To be clinically useful, carbachol must be dispensed in combination with a wetting agent such as benzalkonium chloride, 0.03%. The marked enhancement of carbachol action by benzalkonium is illustrated in Fig. 12-36. This enhanced action is

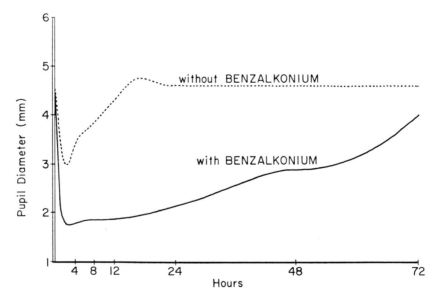

Fig. 12-36. Average degree and duration of miosis produced in 10 normal adult eyes by a single instillation of a 1.5% solution of carbachol, with and without a 0.03% concentration of benzalkonium. (Modified from O'Brien, C. S., and Swan, K. C.: Arch. Ophthalmol. **27:**253, 1942.)

not a result of potentiation of drug action by the benzalkonium but rather of increased corneal penetration. Mechanical damage to the corneal epithelium produces a penetration and miotic effect as great as that obtained with benzalkonium. Wetting agents do not greatly enhance the action of pilocarpine or other drugs that readily penetrate the cornea.

Intracameral administration

When applied directly on the iris through a corneal incision, carbachol is an intensely powerful miotic. It is 100 times more effective than acetylcholine and much longer lasting, and it is 200 times more effective than pilocarpine. For example, 0.01% carbachol instilled directly on the rabbit iris produced greater miosis than did 1% acetylcholine or 2% pilocarpine.[165] These findings indicate that carbachol would be an extremely effective miotic for use at the time of surgery. Comparable results were obtained on strips of bovine iris, on which carbachol was 30 times more effective than pilocarpine and 4800 times more effective than acetylcholine.[166]

Different concentrations of carbachol, from 0.01% to 1.0%, were placed into the rabbit anterior chamber daily for 3 weeks. No toxicity resulted, even from the 1% concentration. Apparently, carbachol is not only a potent miotic when administered by this route but is also nontoxic.[167]

Pilocarpine

Pilocarpine has long been the most popular medication for the treatment of primary glaucoma (both open angle and closed angle) and for neutralization of dilating drops used during eye examination.

Pharmacology

Pilocarpine is a direct-acting parasympathomimetic drug. Since it acts directly on the cells, it is effective even on denervated structures. Specifically, pilocarpine will constrict the pupil after cataract extraction under retrobulbar anesthesia. (Since retrobulbar anesthesia blocks acetylcholine liberation, the indirect-acting miotics such as eserine and isoflurophate will not constrict the anesthetized pupil.)

Pilocarpine duplicates the muscarinic ef-

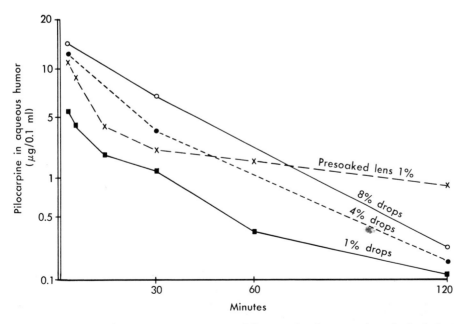

Fig. 12-37. Aqueous pilocarpine concentrations following the designated method of administration. (Modified from Asseff, C. F., and associates: Am. J. Ophthalmol. **75:**212, 1973.)

fect of acetylcholine but not its nicotinic effects. Hence it will stimulate smooth muscle and secretory glands but has no effect on striated muscle. It will cause lacrimation,[168] salivation, sweating, vomiting, and diarrhea. Unfortunately the parasympathomimetic stimulation of secretion, as by pilocarpine and neostigmine (Prostigmin), is of no benefit in keratoconjunctivitis sicca, since the pathologic process in this disease is parenchymatous atrophy of the lacrimal gland.[169]

Ocular penetration

Being an alkaloid with the differential solubility characteristics necessary to traverse the fat-water-fat corneal barrier, pilocarpine penetrates into the eye very well after topical application. By polarographic methods, a pilocarpine concentration of 0.2% was found in human aqueous 20 minutes after topical instillation of 2 drops of a 2% solution.[170,171]

Radioactive tracer studies in monkey eyes revealed the aqueous concentrations of pilocarpine shown in Fig. 12-37.[172] The drops were instilled only once, whereas the soft lens remained on the cornea until the time of paracentesis. In all instances the maximum aqueous concentration was found at the 5-

minute paracentesis. As expected, higher drug concentrations resulted in higher aqueous concentrations. The aqueous concentrations decreased rapidly with time, although the soft lens application maintained a detectable aqueous level for almost 4 hours. It must be recognized that aqueous assays do not reveal the amount of drug bound to the ocular tissues.

The importance of the parameter of frequency of application is usually overlooked. What happens if a drop of pilocarpine is instilled three times at 5-minute intervals in-

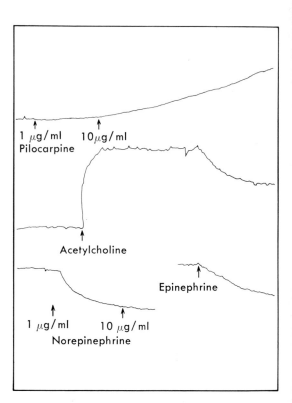

Fig. 12-39. Drug-induced responses of eserinized cat ciliary muscle. Small horizontal bar measures 20 seconds; small vertical bar, 20 mg of contraction (ciliary muscle strip was 6 mm wide). Upper curve shows effect of 1 and 10 μg/ml pilocarpine. Middle curve shows rapid contraction produced by 0.1 μg/ml acetylcholine. Relaxation of muscle after 1 and 10 μg/ml norepinephrine is shown. Arrow represents the time of application of epinephrine, 1 μg/ml, with subsequent muscle relaxation. (Modified from van Alphen, G. W., and associates: Arch. Ophthalmol. **68:**81, 1962.)

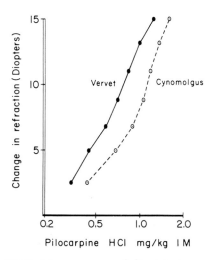

Fig. 12-38. Mean curves of dioptric increase of myopia with varying pilocarpine dosage in vervet and cynomolgus species of monkey. (From Törnqvist, G.: Invest. Ophthalmol. 4:211, 1965.)

stead of only once? Forty-five minutes after initial instillation the aqueous concentrations were, as you might expect, three times greater after the triple instillation than after the single instillation.[173] This increased concentration with repeated instillation is not unique to pilocarpine but would be expected for all types of drugs.

Action on intraocular muscles

The dose-response curve of the effect of intramuscularly injected pilocarpine on accommodation in monkeys is shown in Fig. 12-38.[174] Systemic effects occurred with the same general range of dosage. Salivation began after 0.1 mg pilocarpine/kg and became profuse with 0.5 mg/kg. Vomiting, defecation, and urination resulted after ad-

ministration of from 1 to 5 mg/kg. Topical pilocarpine causes half maximal miosis in doses about 100 times smaller than those necessary to produce half maximal accommodative change.[175,176]

A pilocarpine concentration of 1 μg/ml (0.001%) will cause contraction of the ciliary muscle. The response to pilocarpine is different from that to acetylcholine in several respects. As seen in the top curve in Fig. 12-39, pilocarpine induces a slowly increasing muscular contraction, which requires several minutes to reach its peak. This contrasts with the second curve (acetylcholine), which rises abruptly to a maximum within a few seconds. The effect of pilocarpine could not be reversed simply by washing it out of the muscle bath. This continuing ciliary contraction must

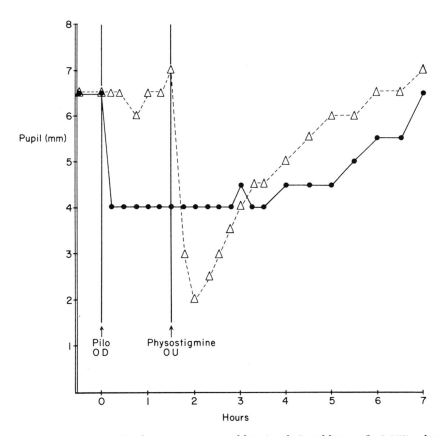

Fig. 12-40. Pilocarpine, 4% solution, miosis in rabbits (circles). Addition of a 0.25% solution of eserine does not change the pilocarpine miosis. Eserine, 0.25% solution, alone causes greater miosis (triangles). Eserine was instilled in both eyes at 1½ hours (average data from 22 rabbits). (Modified from Swan, K. C., and Gehrsitz, L.: Arch. Ophthalmol. **46:**477, 1951.)

be caused by persistent adherence of pilocarpine to the muscle receptors. Unlike pilocarpine, the acetylcholine effect promptly disappears when it is washed from the bath. Pretreatment with eserine reduces the response of the cat ciliary muscle to pilocarpine (whereas as previously mentioned, eserinization potentiates acetylcholine).

Further experimental data in support of a competitive rather than an additive relationship between pilocarpine and eserine (and also between pilocarpine and isoflurophate) are shown in Fig. 12-40.[177] Pretreatment with pilocarpine in rabbits substantially reduces the miosis resulting from eserine. An average miosis of 2 mm was attained with eserine alone, in contrast to 4 mm with both drugs.

Similar competitive results were obtained when pilocarpine preceded isoflurophate instillation in rabbits (Fig. 12-41).[177] The authors refer to their clinical experience as indicating that pilocarpine pretreatment in human beings reduces the subsequent response to eserine or isoflurophate.

Twice daily echothiophate instillation for 8 weeks caused the outflow response of monkey eyes to become markedly subsensitive to pilocarpine. This subsensitivity lasted several weeks to several months. The clinical implication of this finding relate to situations in which pilocarpine is substituted for echothiophate. For example, several weeks before cataract or glaucoma surgery, pilocarpine is often substituted for echothiophate with the intent of minimizing the inflammatory response. Quite probably this use of pilocarpine is ineffective.

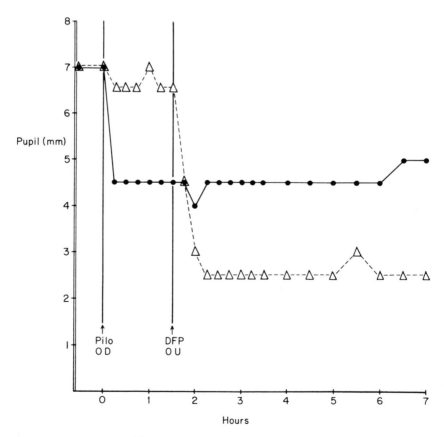

Fig. 12-41. DFP miosis in rabbit eyes (triangles). Preliminary miosis with pilocarpine (circles) blocks effect of isoflurophate (DFP). (Modified from Swan, K. C., and Gehrsitz, L.: Arch. Ophthalmol. **46:**477, 1951.)

Most clinicians simply assume that a direct-acting miotic such as pilocarpine and an indirect-acting miotic such as eserine have additive effects if administered together, since their mechanism of action is different. In cats and rabbits the effect of these miotic combinations is competitive, not additive.

Are pilocarpine and physostigmine additive or competitive in man? To study the miotic response to these drugs separately and in combination, it was necessary to use weak solutions (0.1% of each) to avoid maximal miosis. As shown in Fig. 12-42,[178] the combined administration of small doses of pilocarpine and physostigmine is more effective in producing miosis than is either drug alone.

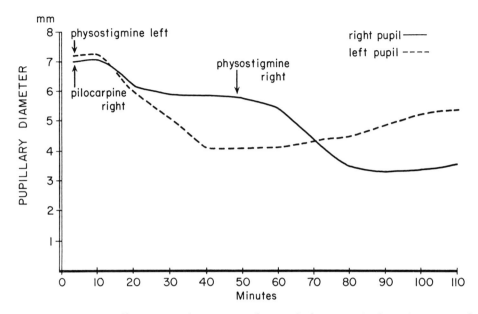

Fig. 12-42. Response of human pupil to a 0.1% solution of pilocarpine (right eye), a 0.1% solution of physostigmine (left eye), and both miotics combined (right eye). (Modified from Lowenstein, O., and Loewenfeld, I. E.: Arch. Ophthalmol. **50:**311, 1953.)

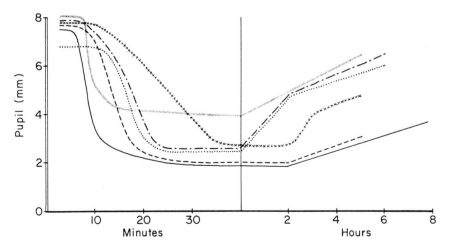

Fig. 12-43. Miotic response of six normal human eyes to 1 drop of a 1% solution of pilocarpine. (Modified from Lowenstein, O., and Loewenfeld, I. E.: Arch. Ophthalmol. **50:**311, 1953.)

These experiments on human subjects demonstrate an additive miotic effect of pilocarpine, physostigmine, and physiologic acetylcholine. These results also suggest, but do not prove, an additive effect of these drugs in reduction of intraocular pressure. Rather marked individual differences exist in the miotic response to pilocarpine. These differences of sensitivity occur in the latent period before miosis; in the rate, degree, and duration of contraction; and in the time required to redilate (Fig. 12-43).[178]

Pupillographic studies of the effect of a 1% solution of pilocarpine (Fig. 12-44) illustrate not only the progressive miosis that begins about 10 minutes after instillation, reaches a peak within 30 minutes, and gradually decreases over a period of at least 6 hours, but also the pupillary response to light at various stages of miosis.[179] The time relationships of the miotic response to a 0.1-second flash of light are unaltered, but the amount of change in pupillary diameter is greatly reduced by miosis. These findings are in accord with clinical observations that the light reflex becomes harder to recognize with increasing miosis and finally cannot even be recognized with the aid of slit-lamp magnification.

Inactivation

Human serum contains a heat-labile component capable of inactivating pilocarpine. Incubation of 500 mg of pilocarpine with 0.5

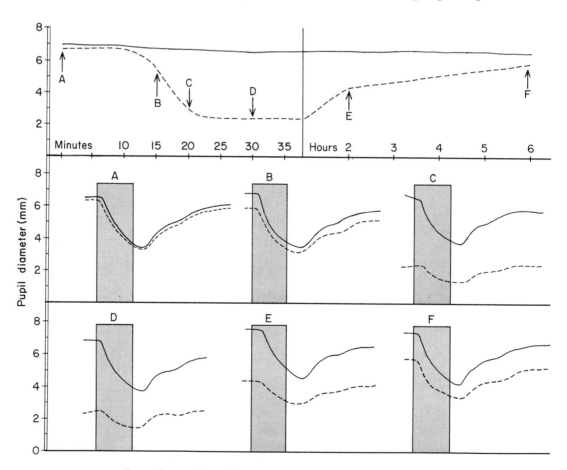

Fig. 12-44. Pupillographic study of pilocarpine miosis. Solid lines: size of normal pupil. Broken lines: pupil size after instillation of a 1% solution of pilocarpine. **A** to **F**, Response to a 0.1-second light flash at the designated times after pilocarpine instillation. (Modified from Lowenstein, O.: Am. J. Ophthalmol. **42:**105, 1956.)

ml of human serum at 37° C for 1 hour will inactivate 40% of the pilocarpine. Similar incubation with 0.2 ml of human secondary aqueous inactivates 10% of the pilocarpine.[180]

Ocular responses

Iris, ciliary body, and trabeculum. The structural changes of the iris and ciliary body resulting from miosis and mydriasis have been studied in monkey eyes.[181] As would be expected, the iris is much thicker during mydriasis, whereas the ciliary body is thicker during miosis (circular muscle contraction). The posterior pigment layer of the iris becomes four times as thick during the change from miosis to mydriasis. This increase in thickness is achieved by marked elongation of the cuboidal cells (Fig. 12-45). Such marked distortion of these cells probably explains why they may rupture and release pigment after phenylephrine dilation. The

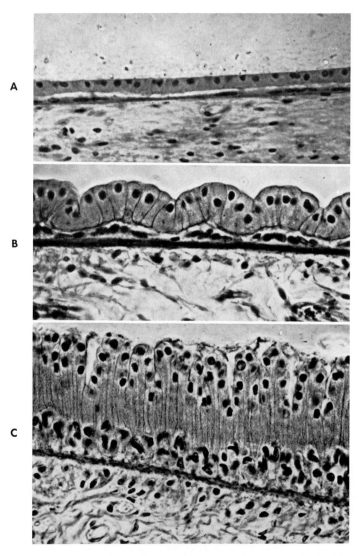

Fig. 12-45. Posterior pigment epithelium layer of iris. **A,** During miosis using isoflurophate (DFP). **B,** During dilation with atropine. **C,** During dilation with atropine and phenylephrine. (From van Alphen, G. W.: Arch. Ophthalmol. **69:**802, 1963.)

trabecular spaces are wider in miosis than in mydriasis.

Anatomically, the longitudinal fibers of the ciliary muscle attach directly to the trabecular meshwork and to the scleral spur.[182] By their contraction, these muscle bundles open the trabecular meshwork[183] and thereby enhance aqueous outflow.

The iris itself is not directly attached to the scleral spur or to the trabecular meshwork; hence its state of contraction or relaxation does not necessarily affect outflow facility. Rather, it is the ciliary body that primarily determines the trabecular patency. These anatomic facts are in accord with the following pharmacologic responses. Parasympathomimetic stimulation of the ciliary muscle increases outflow, the pupil being coincidentally miotic. Addition of a sympathomimetic drug (for example, phenylephrine) dilates the pupil but does not alter ciliary innervation and therefore does not reverse the parasympathomimetic enhancement of outflow. However, a parasympatholytic drug (for example, homatropine) blocks contraction of the ciliary muscle and decreases outflow, the pupil being coincidentally mydriatic. There is no direct relationship between pupil size and outflow facility.

The preceding paragraph is not intended to deny completely any relationship between the iris and the facility of aqueous outflow. A self-regulating pressure control mechanism is present at the chamber angle and is related to the depth of the anterior chamber.[184] The deeper the chamber, the easier the outflow of aqueous, and vice versa (Fig. 12-46). This effect is mechanically mediated by the patency of the trabecular meshwork of the open or shallow angle. Extreme miosis may alter this relationship by creating a physiologic iris bombé. Ordinarily minor forward displacement of the iris is more than compensated for by ciliary muscle contraction, but if the chamber angle is very narrow, its closure may rarely result from the physiologic iris bombé of miosis. Usually, of course, the withdrawal of iris mass from the angle by miosis reduces the tendency of a narrow angle to close.

Further descriptions of the trabeculum, the canal of Schlemm, and the collector chan-

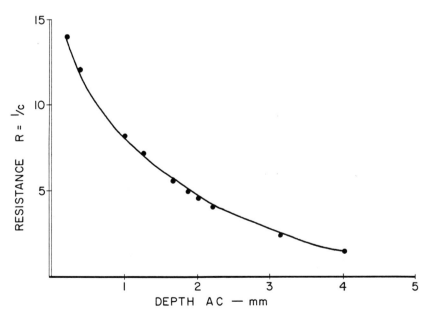

Fig. 12-46. Inverse relationship between resistance to aqueous outflow and depth of anterior chamber in perfused human eyes. (Modified from François, J., and associates: Arch. Ophthalmol. **59**:683, 1958.)

nels are in accord with the mechanisms of outflow described previously.[185-190]

Vacuoles, which may represent transendothelial channels, are demonstrable by electron microscopy in the endothelium of the inner wall of Schlemm's canal. In pilocarpine-treated monkey eyes the number of channels was reduced by half. It was hypothesized that pilocarpine straightens and shortens these channels, thereby reducing the chance of their existing in ultrathin sections. Unfortunately in this study there was no correlation between improved facility of outflow and the transendothelial channel count.[191]

Lens and anterior chamber. Ultrasonic measurements of axial length indicate that pilocarpine increases the thickness of the lens. This is a dose-related response, averaging 0.11 mm increased thickness with 1% pilocarpine in 20-year-old volunteers and 0.39 mm with 4% pilocarpine. The increased thickness occurs in the anterior part of the lens (as is known to be characteristic of accommodation), for the depth of the anterior chamber decreases by almost the exact amount of increase in lens thickness. The duration of this effect is longer with higher concentrations of pilocarpine, as is true of all its other pharmacologic effects (pupil, facility of outflow, intraocular pressure changes). This lens change is, of course, the basis of the myopia induced by pilocarpine.[192]

Even in 60-year-old patients with long-term pilocarpine treatment of open-angle glaucoma, pilocarpine causes increased lens thickness (average, 0.21 mm) and decreased depth of anterior chamber (average, 0.19 mm). An increased physiologic iris bombé is not the explanation of this phenomenon, as can be identified from these measurements. The lens does not become unresponsive to pilocarpine, either because of age or because of continuous therapeutic use of pilocarpine for as long as 10 years.[193]

Facility of outflow. A detailed study of the pilocarpine-induced reduction of outflow resistance has been carried out in monkeys.[194] Within 3 minutes after an anterior chamber injection of 1.5 µg of pilocarpine, the facility of outflow has already measurably increased (Fig. 12-47). To determine

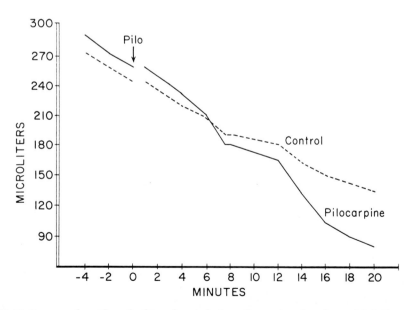

Fig. 12-47. Increased outflow facility after infusion of anterior chamber with 1.5 µg of pilocarpine. Ordinate represents microliters of saline solution remaining in perfusion reservoir—slope of fall, therefore, is related to outflow facility. (Modified from Bárány, E. H.: Invest. Ophthalmol. **1:**712, 1962.)

whether the pilocarpine affected smooth muscle, atropine was given intravenously after the pilocarpine effect had been attained. A rapid atropine reversal of the pilocarpine effect occurred (Fig. 12-48), almost completely blocking the pilocarpine effect within 10 minutes. This finding seems to prove that the improvement of outflow by pilocarpine is atropine reversible; hence it represents an effect on smooth muscles. Note that approximately 30 minutes elapse before the outflow facility has returned to that of the control eye. This suggests the possibility of a second mechanism, which is slowly reversed by atropine. A histamine-like action, causing leaking of the trabecular endothelium, has been postulated as possibly being the second mechanism of pilocarpine action.[194] Proof that

the parasympatholytic action of atropine would not be delayed for as long as 30 minutes is provided by atropine reversal of a pilocarpine-induced accommodative spasm, which occurs within 5 minutes (Fig. 12-49).

Intravenous administration of pilocarpine causes an immediate drop of resistance to aqueous outflow, reaching a maximum effect within 2 minutes. At this time the aqueous concentration of pilocarpine is too low to cause any outflow change. This finding is interpreted as excluding any direct action on the trabecular tissue or canal of Schlemm as the mechanism of action. Of course, the intravenous route delivers the pilocarpine to the ciliary body, the contraction of which is presumably responsible for the reduction of outflow resistance.[195]

Intraocular pressure. Pilocarpine in a 2% solution causes a decrease in intraocular pressure in both normal and glaucomatous eyes. The percentage decrease of pressure is comparable in both groups; the drop varies from 8% to 38% in normal subjects and from 12% to 40% in patients with glaucoma.[196] Diurnal pressure variations are considerably reduced (Fig. 12-50). Although the pressure-lowering effect of pilocarpine is usually associated with an increased coefficient of outflow, in seven eyes of this study the pressure drop occurred without any change in out-

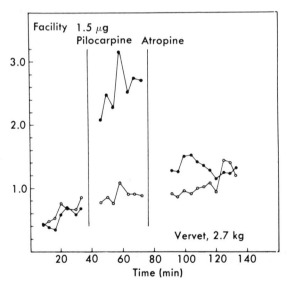

Fig. 12-48. Atropine reversal of pilocarpine-increased outflow facility. Facility of outflow is shown during constant pressure perfusion experiment. Open circles: control eyes show gradually increased facility attributed to slow trabecular damage from perfusion. Pilocarpine in anterior chamber rapidly and markedly increases outflow facility. Intravenous administration of 1 mg/kg of atropine rapidly blocks most of the pilocarpine effect. A slower component of atropine action requires about 30 minutes to return the outflow facility to that of the untreated control eyes. (From Bárány, E. H.: Invest. Ophthalmol. **1:**712, 1962.)

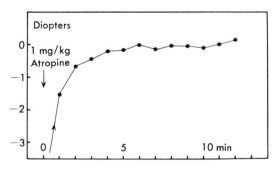

Fig. 12-49. Reversal by intravenous administration of atropine, 1 mg/kg, of pilocarpine-induced accommodative spasm (0.2 mg pilocarpine instilled on cornea 60 minutes before atropine was given). Parasympatholytic effect is complete within 5 minutes. (From Bárány, E. H.: Invest. Ophthalmol. **1:**712, 1962.)

flow. This effect was postulated to be caused by decreased aqueous formation.

The decrease in applanation pressure of normal eyes and of eyes with chronic simple glaucoma is first evident at 60 minutes and reaches a maximum at 75 minutes.[197]

A dose-response analysis of the hypotensive effect of pilocarpine on open-angle glaucoma suggested that the effect of a single drug instillation was virtually the same whether the drug concentration was 1% or 10%. This finding suggests that the mechanism of response is maximally stimulated by a 1% concentration and that higher concentrations do not evoke a greater response. Apparently there is another factor affecting duration of response: with chronic administration (four times daily for 1 week), a greater hypotensive effect was achieved with 4% than with 1% pilocarpine. Again, no greater effect was achieved with 8% pilocarpine

than with 4%.[198] No mention was made of the pigmentation of these eyes.

Pigment effect. Thirty-minute incubation of pigmented and albino rabbit irides in pilocarpine solution results in the absorption of 8 μg of pilocarpine/mg of pigmented iris but of only 3.9 μg of pilocarpine/mg of albino iris.[199] Experiments using melanin granules indicate that melanin is the specific binding site for drug absorption and presumably is responsible for the reduced drug effect on pigmented irides. Such melanin binding affects not only pilocarpine but also ephedrine, atropine, cocaine, and cyclopentolate. For example, the binding of cocaine by the pigmented iris is 18 times greater than by the nonpigmented iris.[200] Ephedrine mydriasis is three times greater in albino than in pigmented irides.[201]

The effect of ocular pigmentation is of significance in the therapy of glaucoma. A study of the response of chronic simple glaucoma to pilocarpine indicated that comparable hypotensive effects were obtained with 1% pilocarpine in blue-eyed patients, with 4% pilocarpine in brown-eyed patients, and with 8% pilocarpine in black patients.[202]

Secretory inhibition. Although the intraocular pressure–regulating effect of parasympathomimetic drugs is usually considered to occur via a change in outflow facility, this does not preclude an additional effect of secretory inhibition. A technique of determining secretion by measuring the rate of decrease in the volume of the ciliary process has been devised[203] and is used to study the effect of various autonomic drugs on aqueous secretion.[204] In vitro secretory inhibition was achieved by pilocarpine in a concentration of 10^{-9}M; physostigmine, 10^{-7}M; atropine, 10^{-7}M; acetazolamide, 10^{-6}M; carbachol, 10^{-5}M; acetylcholine, 10^{-5}M; and epinephrine, 10^{-4}M. Combination of acetazolamide and epinephrine was *not* synergistic.

Further evidence of the effect of pilocarpine on the metabolism of the ciliary epithelium is obtained by study of the spontaneous movement of iodide from the surrounding medium into the ciliary epithelium. This iodide accumulation is inhibited by 10^{-7}M

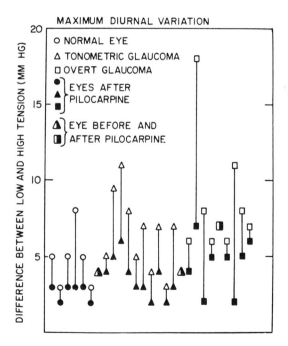

Fig. 12-50. Variations in reduction in diurnal tension in 27 eyes treated with pilocarpine. Open figures: pretreatment diurnal variation. Solid figures: diurnal variation of the same eye after pilocarpine administration. (From Krill, A. E., and Newell, F. W.: Am. J. Ophthalmol. **57:**34, 1964.)

pilocarpine. Oxygen uptake of the lens is markedly inhibited by 10^{-3}M pilocarpine. For reference, a 10^{-2}M concentration of pilocarpine is reached in human aqueous 20 minutes after conjunctival instillation of 2 drops of 2% pilocarpine.[205] The significance of these biochemical alterations is not entirely clear, but it is evident that pilocarpine has other than a purely mechanical effect on the anterior segment of the eye.

Pilocarpine in a 10^{-5}M concentration accelerates the loss of radioactive rubidium from isolated ciliary processes. Rubidium is a tracer substance with a metabolism comparable to that of potassium. While this find-

ing indicates that pilocarpine affects the electrolyte economy of the ciliary processes, it has not yet been correlated with secretory activity.[206]

Conjunctival vessels and aqueous veins. Initially, pilocarpine instillation causes vasodilation of the conjunctival vessels.[207] Within 30 minutes this vasodilation has disappeared, and in glaucomatous patients the aqueous content of aqueous veins may have increased.

The appearance of aqueous veins may remain changed for as long as 6 hours after topical instillation of concentrations of 2% pilocarpine and 1% eserine.[208] In addition, the rate of aqueous flow may increase, the caliber

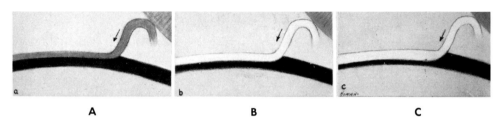

A   **B**   **C**

Fig. 12-51. Influence of pilocarpine on aqueous vein. **A,** Immediately after instillation. **B,** Twenty minutes after instillation. **C,** Thirty minutes after instillation. (From Ascher, K. W.: Am. J. Ophthalmol. **25:**1301, 1942.)

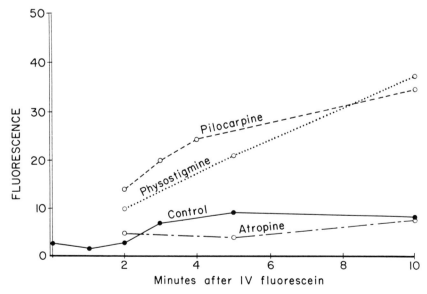

Fig. 12-52. Miotic and atropine effects on fluorescein penetration of blood-aqueous barrier. (Modified from Stocker, F. W.: Arch. Ophthalmol. **37:**583, 1947.)

of the aqueous veins may dilate, and the proportion of red blood cells in the aqueous veins and recipient vessels may decrease (Fig. 12-51). Obviously these changes are manifestations of increased aqueous outflow, which follows pilocarpine or eserine treatment.

Blood-aqueous barrier. The permeability of the blood-aqueous barrier is considerably increased by miotics.[209] Fig. 12-52 shows the increased penetration of fluorescein into the anterior chamber of rabbits after instillation of solutions of 2% pilocarpine nitrate, 0.5% physostigmine salicylate, and 1% atropine sulfate, three times daily for 2 days. Atropine does not significantly reduce the permeability of the normal blood-aqueous barrier, but it does restore toward normal the permeability of an inflamed eye.

The miotic-induced increase in permeability of the blood-aqueous barrier has also been demonstrated by the use of inulin, a polysaccharide molecule too large to penetrate the normal barrier.[210] After instillation of methacholine (Mecholyl), 0.75% solution, eserine, 1% solution, and carbachol, 0.75% solution, inulin does penetrate from blood into the aqueous. Inulin also crosses the blood-aqueous barrier during the stage of secondary vasodilation that occurs 2 to 3 hours after instillation of a 2% solution of epinephrine. Pilocarpine, 4% solution, does not increase the barrier permeability sufficiently to permit inulin passage, nor does it decrease the time required for intravenously administered fluorescein to appear in the aqueous. However, it does increase the total solid content of the aqueous; this indicates a slightly increased barrier permeability.

Atropine, 2% solution, does not alter the normal barrier to inulin and fluorescein and slightly decreases total solids in the vitreous.

Physiologic miosis (obtained with a bright light) and mydriasis (induced by darkness) produced no detectable changes in the blood-aqueous barrier, thereby indicating that these changes are independent of pupillary size and area of iris.

That this miotic-induced breakdown of the blood-aqueous barrier is of clinical importance is suggested by a study of the postoperative course of 38 glaucoma patients who were continued on miotic treatment to within 48 hours of surgery (group A), in comparison to a similar group of patients in whom miotic treatment was discontinued at least 72 hours before surgery (group B).[211] The method by which these two groups of patients were selected is not specified, but they were supposedly comparable in terms of severity of glaucoma and in other pertinent characteristics. The degree of inflammation in these eyes was determined by slit-lamp examination 2 months postoperatively. (Sclerectomy, iridectomy, and iridencleisis procedures were performed with approximately the same frequency in each group.) A zero reaction indicated that there had been virtually no preceding inflammation; a 2+ reaction was attained in the presence of extensive posterior and anterior synechiae, extensive pigment debris on the lens, and other evidence of preceding severe inflammation.

Scattergraph plotting shows a marked tendency for more severe inflammation in the eyes treated with miotics to within 48 hours of surgery (Fig. 12-53). In addition, further surgery was required to control 24% of the

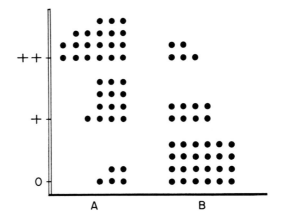

Fig. 12-53. Relationship of postoperative inflammation to use of miotics before surgery. Patients in group A continued miotic treatment to within 48 hours or less of surgery. Patients in group B discontinued miotics at least 72 hours before surgery. (Modified from Abraham, S. V.: Am. J. Ophthalmol. **48:**634, 1959.)

eyes in group A but only 5% of the eyes in group B. Twenty 2+ reactions occurred in group A and only five in group B. Ten postoperative hemorrhages occurred in group A and two in group B. Although this series of patients is not large enough to be of statistical significance, it is in accord with theoretical expectations based on the condition of the blood-aqueous barrier at the time of surgery.

Stability

When maintained in a buffered, slightly acid solution, pilocarpine is indefinitely stable, retaining full activity at 6 months. Neither summer temperatures nor freezing destroys its effectiveness.[159]

Commercial preparations

One hundred samples of 1% pilocarpine ophthalmic solution were obtained from various parts of the United States. These fresh, unopened containers were checked for sterility and drug concentration. Of the 100, 66 were prepared by local pharmacies and 34 by interstate commercial drug companies. Only one of the commercial preparations showed bacterial growth, in contrast to 79% of the samples prepared by local pharmacies. Eighteen of these samples showed *Pseudomonas* species! The range of 0.8% to 1.1% was met by 94% of the commercial preparations but only 53% of the local preparations, which varied from less than 0.5% to 3.0%.[212] Once again it is quite clear that generic equivalents are *not* equivalent.

Clinical use

Chronic simple glaucoma. Clinical management of glaucoma requires thorough evaluation of the individual case, followed by the trial use of one or more of an ever-increasing variety of drugs.

Pilocarpine is used in a 1% to 4% concentration, its frequency of instillation varying from two or three times daily to as often as every 2 hours. The more frequent courses of instillation tend to reduce the patient from a person with glaucoma to one who takes drops. If adequate control is not achieved

with reasonably frequent instillations of pilocarpine, the physician should supplement it with other types of medication (for example, acetazolamide or levoepinephrine) or switch to another miotic (for example, echothiophate) rather than simply increase the strength and frequency of pilocarpine.

Occasionally the clinician will simply use increasingly large concentrations of pilocarpine in an attempt to achieve better glaucoma control. This stratagem is not very effective beyond a concentration of 4%, since 6% or 8% will not additionally lower the intraocular pressure. Apparently all the tissue receptors are saturated with a 4% pilocarpine concentration and higher concentrations cannot increase the response. Higher concentrations of pilocarpine do have a longer duration of effect than do lower concentrations. For example, the pressure-reducing effect of 1% pilocarpine begins to wear off at 8 hours, whereas the effect of 4% or 8% pilocarpine will last for as long as 14 hours.[213] Since 6%, 8%, or 10% pilocarpine does not produce an enhanced therapeutic effect, but only increases toxicity, there is no logic in using pilocarpine stronger than 4%.

To illustrate the greater effect of drug combinations, the average untreated intraocular pressure of 19 glaucomatous eyes was 27 mm Hg; instillation of 2% pilocarpine four times daily reduced the average pressure to 21.8 mm Hg and instillation of 2% pilocarpine and 1% epinephrine four times daily reduced the pressure to 19.2 mm Hg.[214] The clinician should be aware that wide variations in the response of an individual patient to pilocarpine may occur from time to time.

The differences between the effects of 2% pilocarpine and 0.06% echothiophate are shown in Fig. 12-54.[215] Pilocarpine acts by improving the facility of outflow and by decreasing aqueous secretion. Echothiophate only improves outflow, but does so for a much longer time than does pilocarpine. Echothiophate and pilocarpine do not differ greatly in maximum hypotensive effect but have a marked difference in duration of action.

Although in the past, pilocarpine and other

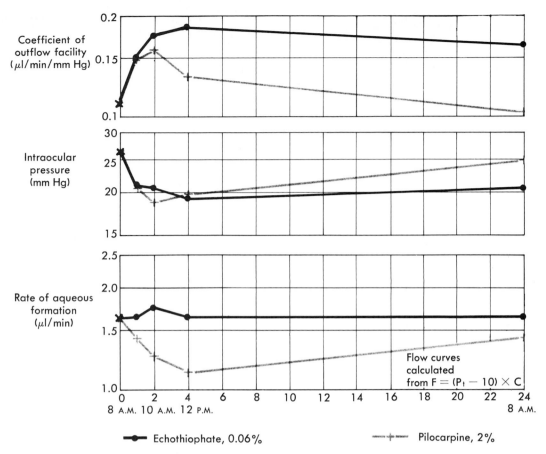

Fig. 12-54. Coefficient of outflow, intraocular pressure, and aqueous flow rate changes resulting from 2% pilocarpine and 0.06% echothiophate. (From Barsam, P. C.: Am. J. Ophthalmol. 73:742, 1972.)

miotics (for example, eserine) have been used in combination in the hope of achieving an additive effect, present information suggests that these relationships are more likely to be competitive. It is doubtful that any benefits result from the simultaneous use of different miotics, and the known disadvantages contraindicate such usage. These disadvantages include the higher cost of two medications, the nuisance and confusion arising from multiple bottles, the greater possibility of allergy and toxicity, as well as the likelihood of decreased therapeutic effect. Hence the traditional practice of alternating pilocarpine and eserine in the emergency treatment of acute glaucoma and the daytime use of pilocarpine combined with the bedtime use of eserine should not be encouraged.

Ophthalmologist and patient alike will be alarmed by the effect of pilocarpine on the visual field if they are unaware that this is a characteristic and harmless optical phenomenon. The effect of the miotic pupil is to reduce the intensity of the test object, thereby recording a smaller isopter. This effect is particularly marked if axial cataract is present. As compared with the original record of the nonmiotic field, the miotic field may simulate a considerable progression of typical glaucomatous field defects.[216]

Fig. 12-55 shows the apparent loss of visual field resulting from constriction of the pupil from 3.5 to 1 mm.[217] Obviously this explains

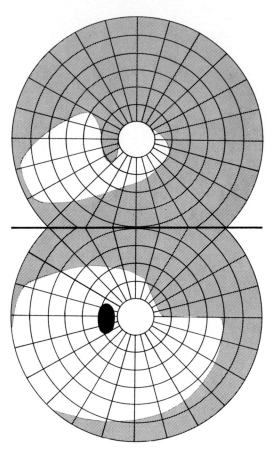

Fig. 12-55. Visual field in 65-year-old glaucoma patient with clear lens. Upper field recorded with 1 mm pupil; lower field, with 3.5 mm pupil. (Modified from Forbes, M.: Invest. Ophthalmol. **5:**139, 1966.)

the patient's complaint of dimness of vision when placed on miotic therapy. Perimetry should be performed soon after starting a new miotic. This will establish a base line to distinguish between subsequent true changes in the visual field and those due to pupillary variation. Alternatively, the field should be performed when the pupil is dilated with phenylephrine.

The response of glaucoma to miotics is of theoretical as well as of practical interest, for it further confirms that the site of resistance to outflow is sufficiently internal to respond to ciliary muscle pull. Histologic and experimental evidence indicate that the

block in chronic simple glaucoma is internal to the canal of Schlemm.[218]

Acute glaucoma. Intensive use of pilocarpine is part of the effective standard therapy of acute angle-closure glaucoma. Three or four instillations of several drops of a 4% solution of pilocarpine every 10 minutes will undoubtedly result in a great excess of the drug reaching the ciliary body and iris. Excess solution should be wiped promptly from the eye so that this therapeutically useless portion does not flow into the lacrimal system, where it would be absorbed systemically. After the first 30 minutes of treatment, no benefit results from applying pilocarpine more often than every 1 or 2 hours; only irritation and toxicity can be expected from continued intensive treatment. Because of the understandable concern and excitement inherent in an attack of acute glaucoma, such a patient commonly receives considerably more pilocarpine than is beneficial or desirable. The nausea and vomiting subsequent to pilocarpine toxicity is misinterpreted as resulting from the glaucoma and is "treated" with more pilocarpine.

The dilated pupil of acute glaucoma is often found to be completely refractory to all types of miotic drugs. The mechanism of this miotic-resistant pupil was studied by experimentally increasing the intraocular pressures of dogs (introduction of trochar into vitreous).[219] It was clearly demonstrated that above a critical level of approximately 60 mm Hg the sphincter dilated despite previous or continued use of miotics (or calcium, which acts directly on muscle). When pressure was reduced below this level, the sphincter once again responded to constricting stimuli. Parasympathetic and/or sympathetic denervation did not alter this response. It was concluded that the pressure rendered the sphincter musculature incapable of contraction.

The clinical implications of such findings are evident—when such a miotic-resistant pupil is dealt with, the pressure will first have to be lowered by other types of supplemental therapy such as administration of acetazolamide or intravenous injection of hypertonic solutions. Nevertheless, miotics

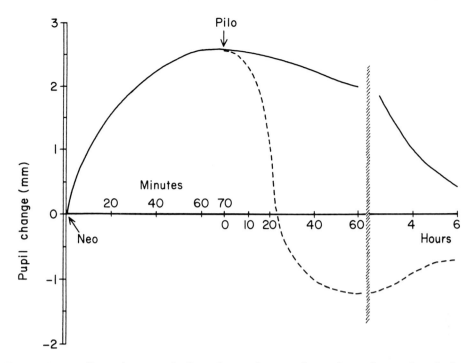

Fig. 12-56. Pupillographic record of pupil size changes after 1 drop of 10% phenylephrine (Neo-Synephrine) and after 1 drop of 1% pilocarpine at the time of maximal mydriasis. (Modified from Anastasi, L. M., Ogle, K. N., and Kearns, T. P.: Arch. Ophthalmol. **79:**710, 1968.)

should be instilled at the outset of treatment so that they can act promptly when the pressure drops.

During and after an attack of acute glaucoma, treatment of the second eye is often neglected. Evaluation of 47 cases indicates that 62% of the fellow eyes will develop acute glaucoma within 5 years of the original attack in the first eye.[220] This second eye may be involved hours or years later. Continuous prophylactic use of miotics will reduce the incidence of acute glaucoma in the second eye to 40%, in contrast to an incidence of 88% in untreated second eyes. If for some reason prophylactic iridectomy is not performed (as in an elderly patient), miotic treatment of the "normal" eye should be strongly considered.

To counteract mydriasis. Pilocarpine, 1%, is often routinely instilled at the close of a mydriatic or cycloplegic eye examination. The patient then leaves the office and the physician is unaware of the result of this mi-

otic installation. What happens? Fig. 12-56 shows the pupillary diameter changes in man after instillation of 1 drop of 10% phenylephrine.[221]

After a 20-minute delay, phenylephrine mydriasis rapidly increases to a maximum at 70 minutes. The solid line continues, representing the spontaneous rate of return to normal pupil size in about 7 hours. One drop of 1% pilocarpine was instilled at the time of maximal mydriasis, and the subsequent pupil size is represented by the interrupted line. The latent period for pilocarpine action was less than 10 minutes. Within 16 minutes after pilocarpine instillation, the pupil dilation had diminished by one half, and at 22 minutes the pupil had returned to normal size. Note that pilocarpine-induced miosis follows, lasting for 4 to 6 hours. A comparable experiment was performed with another sympathomimetic drug, 1% hydroxyamphetamine (Paredrine), with similar results.

Fig. 12-57 shows the pupillary diameter

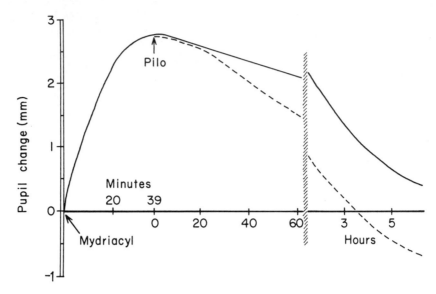

Fig. 12-57. Pupillographic record of pupil size changes after 1 drop of 0.5% tropicamide (Mydriacyl) and after 1 drop of 1% pilocarpine at the time of maximal dilation. (Modified from Anastasi, L. M., Ogle, K. N., and Kearns, T. P.: Arch. Ophthalmol. **79:**710, 1968.)

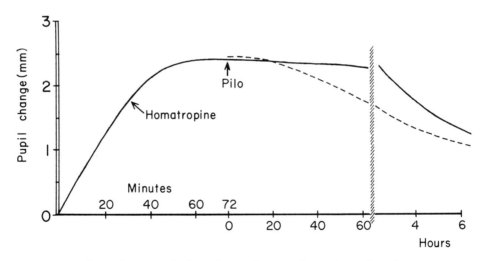

Fig. 12-58. Pupillographic record of pupil size changes after 1 drop of 2% homatropine, instilled at 0 time, and after 1 drop of 1% pilocarpine at the time of maximal dilation. (Modified from Anastasi, L. M., Ogle, K. N., and Kearns, T. P.: Arch. Ophthalmol. **79:**710, 1968.)

changes in man after instillation of 1 drop of 0.5% tropicamide.[221] After a 5-minute delay, tropicamide dilation rapidly increases to a maximum at 40 minutes. The solid line continues, representing the spontaneous rate of return to normal pupil size in about 7 hours. One drop of 1% pilocarpine was instilled at the time of maximal dilation; the subsequent

pupil size is represented by the dotted line. Within 1½ hours after pilocarpine instillation, dilation had decreased by 50%; full recovery required 3½ hours. Subsequent to this, some pilocarpine miosis occurred.

A comparable experiment with a longer lasting cycloplegic drug, 2% homatropine, is illustrated in Fig. 12-58.[221] Homatropine's latent period lasts about 10 minutes. Maximum dilation is reached in about 70 minutes. The pilocarpine-induced half-recovery time is 5½ hours, and full recovery requires 28 hours.

The implications of these pilocarpine reversal findings with respect to the choice of dilating drugs are apparent. If the clinician wishes to counteract mydriasis with pilocarpine (as in a patient with potential angle-closure glaucoma), a sympathomimetic dilating drug should be selected. Relatively little pilocarpine miosis will follow the use of a long-acting cycloplegic. Note that the pilocarpine accommodative spasm will last for many hours after phenylephrine mydriasis has been overcome. This spasm may be quite unpleasant—considerably more so than if the mydriasis were left to disappear spontaneously. I have discontinued the routine use of pilocarpine after phenylephrine or tropicamide examinations, except in glaucomatous eyes. The duration of cycloplegia is not greatly influenced by pilocarpine, although depth of focus is improved by miosis.

Accommodation. As would be expected, parasympathomimetic stimulation of the ciliary muscle results in accommodation. In a young eye this drug-induced accommodation may amount to several diopters, cannot be relaxed voluntarily, and therefore may cause myopia of several hours' duration.

Optical measurement[222] shows that the anterior chamber of a normal eye decreases in depth by about 12% after instillation of pilocarpine hydrochloride.[223] The method used (measurement of the distance between surfaces of the posterior cornea and anterior lens) could not differentiate between a forward movement of the entire lens or an increase in anteroposterior thickness of the lens, as occurs with accommodation.

Surprisingly, pilocarpine also induces accommodation in presbyopic lenses. Ultrasonic measurement of the eyes of 60- to 80-year-old patients indicated that 2% pilocarpine causes an average lens thickening of 0.25 mm and a 0.19 mm shallowing of the anterior chamber. The extent of pilocarpine-induced accommodative spasm in these 25 eyes ranged from 2.00 to 13.00 D, the average being 7.00 D.[224]

Examination of 21 eyes in patients 18 to 30 years of age by the same ultrasonic methods showed 2% pilocarpine to cause an average lens thickening of 0.32 mm and a 0.29 mm shallowing of the anterior chamber. Of theoretical interest in the mechanism of accommodation is the finding that the entire lens moves forward; in one third of the eyes the posterior surface of the lens was actually more anterior during pilocarpine-induced accommodative spasm than when the ciliary body was relaxed.[225]

Drug-induced accommodative spasm is quite annoying to young patients with glaucoma and to a lesser degree to presbyopic persons. Excessive concentrations of pilocarpine (for example, 4%) should not be used for miosis after a cycloplegic or mydriatic has been used during office examinations. Because its effect is longer lasting than that of the cycloplegic, the pilocarpine will subsequently cause severe discomfort resulting from accommodative spasm. Similarly, instillation of pilocarpine after cataract extraction seems to cause postoperative pain, presumably because of ciliary spasm. In a series of 151 patients who did not receive pilocarpine, 59% complained of postoperative discomfort. In contrast, 78% of 296 patients receiving pilocarpine postoperatively complained of subsequent pain.[226] In addition to its greater frequency, the pain experienced by the pilocarpine-treated patients was more severe and of longer duration.

Pilocarpine has been used with some effectiveness in the treatment of accommodative strabismus, but it is not nearly so well suited for this purpose as are the indirect-acting parasympathomimetic agents. The effect of the latter drugs varies with the amount of physiologically produced acetylcholine; hence in proper dosage they enhance the intensity of normal accommodation. Since convergence intensity is of central origin and is not affected by local application of indirect-acting parasympathomimetic drugs, their instillation alters the AC/A ratio. The pilocarpine effect, however, does not vary with accommodative effort and is thus comparable to the wearing of plus lenses.

Hyphema. Miosis will hasten the absorption of hyphema* by increasing the ease with which red blood cells exit via Schlemm's canal (Fig. 12-59). Formed clots cannot, of course, escape in this manner. If traumatic iritis is severe, cycloplegic therapy may be preferable.[227]

Differential diagnosis of dilated pupil. Neurologic disease causing a fixed, dilated pupil may be simulated by the accidental

---

*Bredemeyer, H. G.: Unpublished data, 1958.

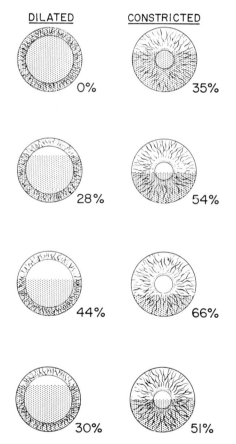

DILATED   CONSTRICTED

0%   35%

28%   54%

44%   66%

30%   51%

Fig. 12-59. Rate of disappearance of radioactive-labeled (^{51}Cr) red blood cells from anterior chamber of rabbit. Left eye was dilated (oxyphenonium) and right eye was constricted (pilocarpine). Data from four rabbits indicate much more rapid clearing of blood from miotic eye in each animal (24-hour experimental period). (From Bredemeyer, H. G.: Unpublished data, 1958.)

or intentional use of a cycloplegic or mydriatic drug. For example, the accidental self-inoculation with atropine by medical personnel or the dilation of a farmer's eye by Jimson weed may result in an alarming unilateral dilation of the eye.

Pharmacologic dilation can easily be recognized if the pupil fails to constrict after instillation of 0.5% pilocarpine. If a stronger solution is used, it may overcome minimal dilation, giving a confusing response. Patients with mydriasis of neurologic etiology will promptly respond to pilocarpine.

This technically simple and definitive test should be used as an office procedure any time a question arises as to the etiology of pupil dilation.[228]

Diagnosis of Adie's pupil. The well-known use of 2.5% methacholine to detect the hypersensitivity of partial parasympathetic denervation is no longer practical because of the commercial unavailability of methacholine. Evaluation of different concentrations of pilocarpine indicated that 0.0625% consistently constricted Adie's pupils yet had only minimal effect on normal pupils.[229] Use of 0.12% pilocarpine caused considerable miosis in normal pupils, and 0.03% did not consistently constrict Adie's pupils.

The methacholine test was positive in only 63% of 57 Adie's pupils.[230] Testing with 0.125% pilocarpine showed supersensitivity in 69% of these eyes and induced greater anisocoria than resulted from methacholine. Apparently pilocarpine is not only more readily available than methacholine but actually is a better test for Adie's supersensitivity.

After cataract extraction. Pilocarpine is instilled after cataract extraction to supposedly protect the vitreous face and to withdraw the iris from the wound area. However, it definitely increases postoperative pain. I have in recent years discontinued the use of pilocarpine after cataract extraction and have witnessed no particular complications in its absence.

Toxicity

Systemic reactions after the ocular use of pilocarpine are rare. Although poisonous, pilocarpine is much less toxic than the newer synthetic miotics such as echothiophate. A dose of 100 mg of pilocarpine (10 ml of a 1% solution) is considered a dangerous amount.[62] Symptoms include salivation, lacrimation, sweating, nausea, vomiting, and diarrhea. Bronchiolar spasm and pulmonary edema may cause death.

Pilocarpine allergy not uncommonly follows its prolonged use for glaucoma. In most such patients I have seen, the glaucoma was not well controlled by a pilocarpine regimen, and the change to another miotic benefited the glaucoma control as well as eliminated the allergy. The onset of this allergy may be rather insidious, and it becomes accepted by the patient as a necessary part of treatment. Part of every routine glaucoma check should be an inspection of the lids and conjunctiva for the characteristic signs of contact allergy. If allergy is present to any degree, a different miotic should be used.

Pilocarpine, 2% solution, was instilled every 10 minutes in the treatment of a patient with acute glaucoma.[231] After about 30 drops, the patient began to sweat profusely and to salivate. He was nauseated and retched. Severe muscular tremor and twitching developed. His blood pressure dropped, and the patient appeared to be in shock. The symptoms disappeared within 7 hours after intensive administration of pilocarpine was discontinued. Although at the time these symptoms were attributed to the acute glaucoma, in retrospect it was evident that they were caused by pilocarpine toxicity.

If one assumes that 20 drops contain 1 ml of pilocarpine, a solution of 2% pilocarpine contains 1 mg/drop. The diaphoretic dose (subcutaneous) of pilocarpine is 5 mg.

Miotic cysts may follow long-term use of pilocarpine but are practically never of clinical significance.

Furtrethonium (Furmethide)

Although furtrethonium iodide (Furmethide) is no longer used as a miotic, the characteristic toxicity that led to its abandonment is noteworthy, as it will again remind the clinician to be alert to the possibility of unexpected toxic side effects after the use of new medications. Of 21 patients using furtrethonium for longer than 3 months, 15 (71%) developed permanent occlusion of the lacrimal canaliculi.[232] Furtrethonium, 10% solution, was well tolerated and more effective than pilocarpine and eserine in the treatment of glaucoma.[233,234] Its relationship to dacryostenosis was recognized only after permanent damage had occurred in a small group of patients with glaucoma.

Aceclidine

Aceclidine is a synthetic cholinergic drug that acts directly on muscarinic end plates in a manner comparable to pilocarpine. In human eyes with open angles, the pressure-lowering affect of 4% aceclidine was found to be comparable to that of 2% pilocarpine. This drug was used in patients allergic to pilocarpine.[235]

Aceclidine produces far less accommodative spasm than does pilocarpine and may be the drug of choice for most glaucoma patients with considerable remaining accommodation. In patients ranging in age from 26 to 49 years of age, an average induced myopia of 2.96 D was present 45 minutes after instillation of 2% pilocarpine. At 45 minutes after 2% aceclidine, the induced myopia was only 0.34 D.[236]

Physostigmine (eserine)

Physostigmine is an indirect parasympathomimetic. Since it acts by preserving acetylcholine, physostigmine has no effect on denervated structures. For instance, physostigmine will not constrict the pupil during the period of retrobulbar anesthesia.

Pharmacology

Physostigmine does not destroy cholinesterase but inactivates it by forming a temporary chemical combination. In vivo, physostigmine is gradually destroyed, thereby liberating the cholinesterase. Physostigmine is therefore classified as a reversible cholinesterase inhibitor. Neostigmine is a very similar synthetic drug.

Since some acetylcholine is constantly

present in the normally innervated iris and ciliary body, miosis and accommodation result from physostigmine even when the eye is at rest. In response to the accommodative effort, additional acetylcholine is formed. Preservation of this acetylcholine results in the accommodative spasms typical of indirect parasympathomimetic drugs.

The electrical and motor activity of extraocular muscles are greatly enhanced by eserine. Fig. 12-60 shows the grams of force (solid line) exerted by the inferior oblique muscle of a cat and its electrical activity (oscillating line). The upper portion shows the activity without eserine and the lower portion shows the activity after eserine administration. In each instance the nerve to the inferior oblique muscle received a single electric stimulus. The normal response to such a stimulus is a single tetanic contraction, followed by relaxation. When acetylcholine destruction is prevented by eserine, however, a single stimulus causes prolonged and

forceful muscular contraction. Enormously intensified muscular responses such as this are responsible for the painful spasms of iris and ciliary muscles that are so distressing to the glaucomatous patient receiving anticholinesterase therapy.

Convergence-accommodation studies also demonstrate the similar effect of eserine on the ciliary muscle. Eserine enhances ciliary contraction and therefore alters the AC/A ratio, as shown in Fig. 12-61.[237] The clinical implications of this effect are evident. A nonpresbyopic patient will develop a myopic blur when eserinized. The eyes of a hyperopic child with accommodative esotropia may completely straighten under the effect of anticholinesterase medications.

As shown in Fig. 12-61, eserine not only increases the amount of accommodation induced by a given amount of convergence but also increases the total amount of accommodation to a greater than normal value. In this 30-year-old patient the maximum normal accommodation was 7.30 D, but it increased to 9.50 D with the aid of a 0.05% solution of eserine. (Accommodation was measured by an

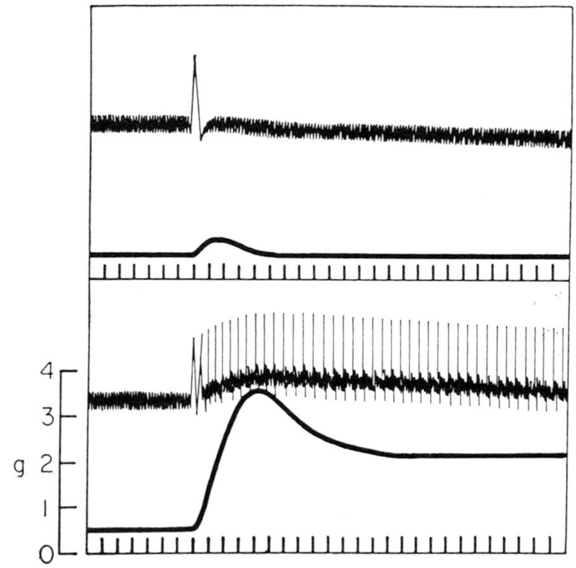

Fig. 12-60. Electrical action potential and myogram (solid line) of inferior oblique muscle of cat showing response to a single stimulus before (top) and after (bottom) administration of eserine. Vertical scale represents grams of muscular pull. (From Moses, R. A.: Adler's physiology of the eye, ed. 5, St. Louis, 1970, The C. V. Mosby Co.)

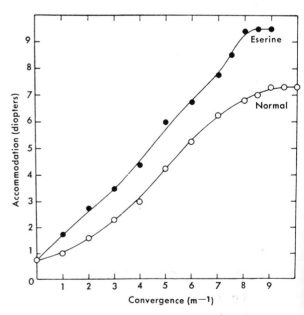

Fig. 12-61. Effect of a 0.05% solution of eserine on AC/A ratio of 30-year-old patient. (From Fincham, E. F.: J. Physiol. **128**:99, 1955.)

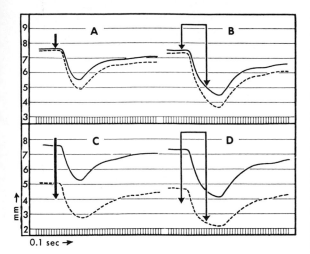

0.1 sec →

Fig. 12-62. Response of pupil to light 20 minutes after instillation of eserine. *A* and *B*, 0.1% solution; *C* and *D*, 1% solution. Arrows indicate duration of light stimulus. Solid line: diameter of normal right pupil. Broken line: diameter of eserinized left pupil. (From Loewenfeld, I. E.: Arch. Ophthalmol. **70:**42, 1963.)

optometer, thereby eliminating the effect of pupil size that would seem to increase subjectively measured accommodation through greater depth of field.)

Pupillographic records indicate that eserinization enhances the response of the pupil to light (Fig. 12-62).[238] Even when miosis in the dark has been induced by strong eserine solutions, further contraction results from light stimulation.

Clinical use

Physostigmine ointment, 0.5%, causes intense miosis within 30 minutes. This miosis lasts for 12 to 36 hours. During this period the facility of outflow is increased. Because of its long action, physostigmine ointment has often been prescribed for bedtime use to prevent nocturnal rises in tension. The alternating use of physostigmine and pilocarpine has been recommended for the treatment of acute glaucoma. However, the combined use of these two drugs, although theoretically additive in effect, is probably competitive. It has been definitely established that prior use of physostigmine greatly reduces the dura-

tion of action of isoflurophate. Present information suggests that glaucoma responds better to a single miotic than to combinations of miotics.

Topical application of physostigmine may be useful in the treatment of ocular myasthenia gravis. Although physostigmine may be used as a diagnostic test for myasthenia, neostigmine is more effective. Subcutaneous injection of 0.5 mg of neostigmine will relieve myasthenic symptoms within 15 minutes in a high percentage of cases. Diplopia and ptosis as well as general muscular strength may be greatly improved by such a diagnostic test. Simultaneous injection of atropine, 0.5 mg, blocks the undesirable muscarinic effect of neostigmine (for example, bowel evacuation) but does not impair the therapeutic response.

Familial dysautonomia (of Riley) is a rare condition presumably caused by an imbalance of the autonomic innervation. Defective lacrimation is the most common ocular finding and results in corneal ulceration in about one third of the patients. One such patient, with a Schirmer test of only 3 to 4 mm, formed grossly visible tears after subcutaneous injection of 0.25 mg of neostigmine.[239] Whether systemic parasympathomimetic medication would benefit the corneal ulcerations of whether artificial tears would be a more practical therapy was not stated in this study.

Antidote for anticholinergic toxicity. The potent anticholinergic drugs used in ophthalmology (for example, atropine, scopolamine, and cyclopentolate) may cause central nervous system toxicity with symptoms such as delirium, confusion, hallucinations, agitation, ataxia, and somnolence. Comparable anticholinergic effects may occur from a variety of antihistaminic, hypnotic, antidepressant, and tranquilizing agents. Overdosage of such drugs may occur during clinical use or when taken for suicidal or psychedelic purposes. Spontaneous recovery may require 1 to 5 days, or the overdose may be fatal.

Physostigmine salicylate, 1 to 4 mg given subcutaneously or intravenously, will inhibit cholinesterase throughout the body, including the central nervous system. Physostigmine readily crosses the blood-brain barrier and hence is effective against central nervous system anticholinergic toxicity.[240] Within minutes, such an injection will reverse the anticholinergic toxicity. The great specificity of this antidote is evidenced by the fact that 1 to 4 mg of physostigmine can completely reverse the delirium and coma produced by 200 mg or more of atropine! Since physostigmine is destroyed within 1½ to 2 hours, repeated doses may be necessary in the treatment of severe anticholinergic poisoning.[241]

Toxicity

Twitching of the eyelids is commonly noted after ocular use of the indirect parasympathomimetic agents. This minor but annoying side effect is caused by percutaneous absorption of the drugs and inactivation of the orbicularis cholinesterase.

Chronic conjunctival irritation is not uncommon after the use of physostigmine. Typical contact allergic dermatitis may develop after prolonged use.

The systemic parasympathomimetic toxicity resulting from physostigmine was the basis for its use as an ordeal poison in ancient Africa.[242,243]

A rather unusual toxic response is the depigmentation of lid skin in black patients allergic to eserine ointment.[244] This depigmentation was noted in four patients and occurred 10 months to 5 years after the beginning of eserine treatment. The characteristic itching and irritation of allergic blepharitis were present in two of these patients. The depigmentation gradually disappears when eserine is discontinued, but recognizable changes have persisted for as long as 3 years.

Eserine gradually oxidizes to a pink or rusty color. Since the decomposition products are quite irritating and are therapeutically ineffective, discolored preparations should be discarded.

Salicylate (this is dispensed as physostigmine salicylate) is incompatible with benzalkonium chloride (Zephiran).

Edrophonium (Tensilon)

Edrophonium chloride has both anticholinesterase and direct neuromuscular stimulating effects. Its effect is much greater at the neuromuscular junction than at other cholinergic sites; hence its undesirable muscarinic side effects are minimal and do not ordinarily require symptomatic reversal by atropine. (In the neostigmine test for myasthenia, pretreatment with atropine is advised to prevent involuntary bowel and bladder action.) Edrophonium does not increase the strength of normal muscle contraction, but it does counteract the effect of curare and improves the contraction of myasthenic muscles. In excess, edrophonium reverses its action and has a muscle-relaxing effect. This paralyzing action is particularly likely to occur in patients with myasthenia gravis. Bronchiolar spasm may follow its use in asthmatic patients.

The only ophthalmic use of edrophonium is as a test for myasthenia gravis, for which it is the drug of choice. Its effect is transient; therefore the drug-induced symptoms are brief and, if necessary, the test may be repeated during the same office visit. Bowel and bladder side effects are minimal. Edrophonium will evoke a positive response in some myasthenic patients whose condition is not detected by the neostigmine test.

The technique of the edrophonium test is as follows: Prepare a tuberculin syringe containing 1 ml (10 mg) of drug; 2 mg is injected intravenously during a 15-second period, and the needle is left in position within the vein. The remaining 8 mg is injected only if there is no response within 30 seconds after administration of the first 2 mg. If a cholinergic reaction occurs after 2 mg, the test should be discontinued and repeated with only 1 mg at least 30 minutes later.[245]

Myasthenic responses

Patients with myasthenia gravis will respond to edrophonium within 30 to 40 seconds as follows[246]:
1. Increased muscle strength as compared to previous weakness
2. Marked subjective improvement

3. Minimal or no muscarinic side reactions
4. No muscle fasciculations

It must be emphasized that positive edrophonium responses usually occur within the first 1 or 2 minutes and completely disappear within 5 minutes.

Normal patients do not experience increased muscle strength and are more likely to have side effects (sweating, lacrimation, ocular cramping sensations, and mild sensations of gastrointestinal motility). Fasciculations of the muscles are almost always caused by 10 mg of edrophonium in normal patients. Although muscle strength may be improved in hysterical patients as a result of this test, subsequent placebo testing with saline solution or nicotinic acid will differentiate such patients if the condition is suspected. Disorders of the central nervous system that may clinically mimic myasthenia do not give false positive responses to this test.

Diplopia resulting from glutethimide (Doriden) will disappear during therapeutic testing with edrophonium chloride. Since this diplopia also varies according to the blood level of the drug, the misdiagnosis of myasthenia gravis is possible.[247]

In a series of 110 patients with myasthenia gravis, eight patients given 10 mg of edrophonium gave a false negative response because of cholinergic overreaction. These patients exhibited typical cholinergic responses, with fasciculations, vomiting, salivation, and the like. Also, muscular weakness was accentuated. Use of 2 or 1 mg, as previously described, avoided this false negative response.[245] Simultaneous electromyography may make the test more sensitive, since increased electric potentials occur in some myasthenic patients who experience insignificant increases in muscular strength after injection of edrophonium.

Since more ophthalmologists have access to tonographic apparatus than to diagnostic electromyography, "edrophonium tonography" has been suggested as a useful diagnostic test for myasthenia gravis.[248] This test consists simply of the intravenous administration of 10 mg of edrophonium chloride during tonography. A positive response is a discrete rise in pressure of 2 to 5 mm, occurring within a minute of injection. This pressure rise is a result of a strengthening of the extraocular muscles.

All of 12 myasthenic patients tested in this manner gave positive responses, although in three instances only one eye gave a positive response.[249] For this reason, diagnostic edrophonium tonography should be done on both eyes, unless the first eye is positive (Fig. 12-63).[249] Nonmyasthenic patients do not respond to edrophonium injection with an increase of intraocular pressure even in

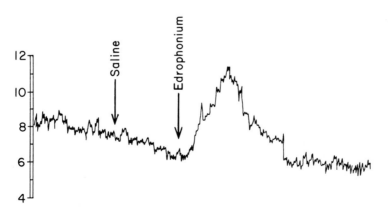

Fig. 12-63. Edrophonium tonography of patient with myasthenia showing diagnostic response. (Modified from Glaser, J. S., Miller, G. R., and Gass, D. M.: Arch. Ophthalmol. 76:368, 1966.)

the presence of other oculoparetic disorders.

In 8 of these 12 myasthenic patients the tonographic refinement of the edrophonium test was necessary for diagnosis. The subjective and objective response to the test dose was so subtle in these cases as to preclude unequivocal interpretation of a positive test. By contrast, the recorded and definite tonographic response was easily recognized as typical of myasthenia gravis.

The edrophonium tonography test is advised in evaluation of any unusual extraocular paresis. Three cases are reported that clinically simulated internuclear ophthalmoplegia but were proved to be myasthenia gravis by use of edrophonium tonography.[250]

The edrophonium test is also useful in the management of myasthenic patients in relapse. If they have been undertreated, the test causes improvement of symptoms; if overtreated, the symptoms become worse.

Isoflurophate (diisopropyl fluorophosphate, DFP; Floropryll)

Isoflurophate was useful in the management of chronic simple glaucoma that was uncontrolled by the shorter acting miotics and in the management of accommodative esotropia. Its use has been replaced by echothiophate; however, the following data on isoflurophate are of basic pharmacologic importance.

Pharmacology

Mechanism of action. The parasympathomimetic effect of isoflurophate is due to cholinesterase inactivation. Isoflurophate has no direct effect on the iris muscle itself and causes absolutely no miosis in an experimentally denervated iris. Clinically, therefore, isoflurophate would be ineffective in a patient with complete paralysis of the third cranial nerve and for the duration of action of a retrobulbar anesthetic injection.

Additive and competitive effects. Apparently, reversible and irreversible cholinesterase inhibitors have the same point of chemical activity. If eserine is first instilled into an eye, followed by isoflurophate, the duration of miosis will be the half-day ex-

pected from eserine and not the week produced by isoflurophate. Obviously the eserine has combined with available cholinesterase, rendering it inaccessible to the action of isoflurophate. If isoflurophate is instilled first, subsequent eserine administration does not alter its effect.

If two different anticholinesterase drugs are used in succession, they may produce either a potentiated or a competitive effect. These effects are outlined in Table 12-5.[25] As shown, eserine and demecarium (Humorsol) are additive no matter in which order they are administered. In the case of eserine and isoflurophate (or echothiophate) the drugs are competitive if eserine is given first but additive if it is given second. These differences are explained by the different durations of action of these drugs and by the existence of different types of cholinesterase. Eserine and demecarium combine primarily with acetylcholinesterase, whereas isoflurophate and echothiophate react predominantly with nonspecific cholinesterase and to a lesser degree with acetylcholinesterase. Prior use of eserine will block acetylcholinesterase until subsequently administered isoflurophate is hydrolyzed or lost by diffusion, so that the clinically observable miotic effect of this combination is the same as the short duration of eserine. If isoflurophate is given first, it incompletely blocks acetylcholinesterase, the remainder of which is inactivated by eserine to produce an additive effect.

Isoflurophate in a 0.05% concentration will overcome the effect of 5 drops of a 0.5% solution of atropine instilled during a 36-hour period. Not only is the pupil constricted but accommodation is also partially restored. If isoflurophate is used clinically to overcome atropinization, the physician should remember that the effect of the isoflurophate may last longer than the atropine effect.

Duration of action. Isoflurophate-induced miosis is of rapid onset and prolonged duration.[251] In the normal human eye, miosis begins within 5 to 10 minutes and is maximal within 15 to 20 minutes. The duration of miosis is from 2 to 4 weeks. Solutions of a 0.05% concentration produce maximum miosis,

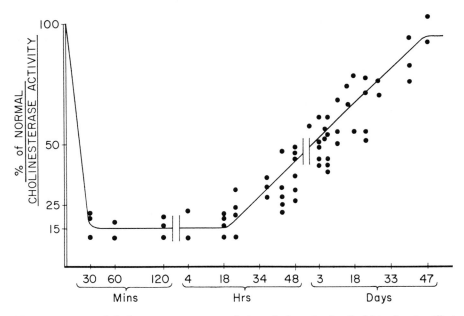

Fig. 12-64. Recovery of cholinesterase activity of iris and ciliary body of rabbit after instillation of 1 drop of a 0.2% solution of isoflurophate (DFP). (Modified from de Roetth, A., Jr.: Am. J. Ophthalmol. **34:**120, 1951.)

Table 12-5. Increase (+) or decrease (−) of anticholinesterase activity produced by topical use of two drugs*

First drug administered	Second drug administered			
	Eserine	Demecarium	Echothiophate	Isoflurophate
Eserine	+	+	−	−
Demecarium	+	+	−	−
Echothiophate	+	+	+	+
Isoflurophate	+	+	+	+

*Modified from Leopold, I. H.: Am. J. Ophthalmol. **51:**885, 1962.

whereas solutions of less than 0.01% are ineffective miotics. Isoflurophate reduces the intraocular pressure of the normal eye; the maximal depression is achieved within 24 hours. The return of normal intraocular pressure requires about 1 week. Isoflurophate-induced ciliary spasm induces myopia that is maximal in 1 hour and lasts for 3 to 7 days. The pain accompanying such spasm is worse with close work because of the greater production of acetylcholine during accommodation.

The duration of action of isoflurophate may be measured by analyzing the cholinesterase activity of a rabbit iris and ciliary body after the single instillation of 1 drop of a 0.2% solution of isoflurophate.[252] Within the first half hour, the cholinesterase activity drops to less than 15% of normal (Fig. 12-64). Activity remains at this level for 18 hours and then gradually rises. Fifty percent of normal activity returns within the first week, but full recovery takes up to 2 months. The miotic effect of isoflurophate is maximal for 18 hours in rabbits and is gone in 48 hours. It is interesting that a measurable effect of isoflurophate persists for so much longer than the visible miosis.

This phenomenon of transient miosis is demonstrable in rabbits, dogs, rats, mice, and monkeys but not in humans. Despite the continuing instillation of 0.1% isoflurophate or 0.25% echothiophate twice daily, monkey pupils redilate to near normal size by the fifth day of treatment and show normal pupil light reflexes. Peculiarly, these normal-sized pupils do not react with miosis to the instillation of pilocarpine or carbachol. After long-term isoflurophate treatment is discontinued, the insensitivity to pilocarpine remains for 3 to 7 days.[253] This report did not offer a pharmacologic explanation for these unexpected findings. This is another example of the fact that species differences preclude the uncritical transfer of animal data to human situations.

Effect on blood-aqueous barrier. The dilation of iris vessels caused by isoflurophate is easily demonstrated when preparations of normal and isoflurophate-treated iris are injected with India ink.[254] The isoflurophate-induced vasodilation is a true pharmacologic effect and is associated with increased permeability of the vessel walls. In contrast, the enlargement of vessels in the homatropine-treated iris is a mechanical change resulting from the shortening of radial iris vessels when the pupil is dilated and is not associated with increased permeability.

Topical ocular application of anticholinesterase drugs causes a breakdown of the blood-aqueous barrier, permitting protein and cells to enter the aqueous. The protein concentration in normal aqueous humor is about 50 mg/100 ml. Isoflurophate increases

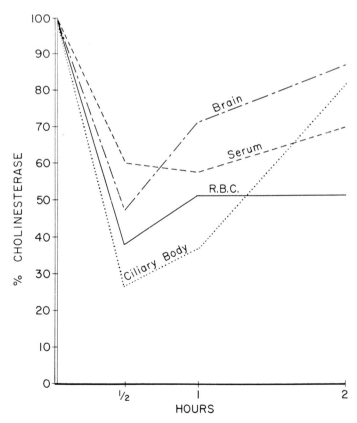

Fig. 12-65. Percent of normal cholinesterase activity remaining in various tissues after ocular instillation in rabbits of 1 drop of a 10% solution of Dipterex. (From Kadin, M.: Am. J. Ophthalmol. **53:**512, 1962.)

the protein concentration to as high as 1200 mg/100 ml.[255] Eserine causes a much lower increase in aqueous protein (maximum, 120 mg/100 ml) than do the organic phosphates. The increased levels of protein in primary aqueous humor persist for at least 2 weeks after isoflurophate therapy is stopped. There is considerable individual variation in the response of the blood-aqueous barrier to anticholinesterase drugs. (Aqueous protein values after isoflurophate may vary from 35 to 2253 mg/100 ml.)

The isoflurophate breakdown of the blood-aqueous barrier is incomplete, as indicated by the leakage of intravenously injected fluorescein (a substance of low molecular weight) into the aqueous, but not of inulin (a much larger molecule).[251] These findings have been interpreted to mean that isoflurophate causes arteriolar vasodilation but not an increase of capillary permeability (as occurs with histamine).

Systemic absorption. The systemic absorption of anticholinesterase drugs applied topically to the eye is rapid and of surprising magnitude. Systemic anticholinesterase activity is detectable within a few minutes of ocular instillation and approaches the levels produced by intravenous administration.[255] The amount of cholinesterase inhibition resulting from ocular instillation of a single drop of a 10% concentration of Dipterex in rabbits is shown in Fig. 12-65.[256] (Dipterex is an anticholinesterase insecticide about 100 times less toxic than isoflurophate.) This single drop reduced cholinesterase levels of the ciliary body to 26% of normal, red blood cell levels to 38%, brain levels to 48%, and serum levels to 58%. The therapeutic use of related medications (for example, isoflurophate) causes a similar marked drop of systemic cholinesterase. Fortunately the physiologic margin of safety in this enzyme function is so great that toxic symptoms do not occur even when more than half of the systemic cholinesterase activity has been inhibited. (The dose of Dipterex lethal to 50% of rabbits, 60 mg/kg, is approximately 1000 times greater than that contained in a drop of a 10% solution.)

Similar reductions of erythrocyte cholinesterase levels have been demonstrated in glaucomatous patients receiving topical therapy with the irreversible cholinesterase inhibitors.[257] The greatest systemic effect resulted from demecarium and the smallest from isoflurophate. The effect of echothiophate was considerably greater than that of isoflurophate but less than that of demecarium.

Stability

Aqueous solutions of isoflurophate deteriorate rapidly, having no effect within a week. In contrast, a solution in peanut oil will maintain maximum potency for more than 3 months. (However, allergy to peanut oil is not rare.) Contamination of the bottle with water (as from tears or washing the dropper) rapidly inactivates the isoflurophate. This possibility should be considered when previously well-controlled glaucoma suddenly fails to respond to isoflurophate. An ointment containing a 0.025% concentration of isoflurophate is more stable and less irritating than the drops. Only the smallest bit of this ointment should be placed in the eye, as a larger amount may cause greater irritation.

Clinical use

Glaucoma. Tonography indicates that isoflurophate increases aqueous outflow facility in both glaucomatous and normal human eyes, thereby reducing intraocular pressure.[258] This increased outflow facility is not dependent on miosis, because it is not lost when the pupil is partially dilated by simultaneous use of a 10% solution of phenylephrine.

A single daily instillation of a 0.1% solution of isoflurophate is suggested as the average starting dosage but should be adjusted as necessary to control individual cases of glaucoma. Bedtime use is recommended to minimize the severity of accommodative spasm. Instillation more than twice daily does not usually provide additional glaucoma control, may be toxic, and should rarely be prescribed. Some cases of aphakic glaucoma are well controlled by 1 drop of isoflurophate every 2 or 3 days. If the glaucoma patient's life has been reduced to a seemingly constant instillation of pilocarpine drops, serious consideration of the use of a longer acting miotic is in order. The strong miotics have the advantages of infrequent instillation and better control of pressure in borderline conditions.

In general, any case of glaucoma (except narrow angle) that can be controlled with miotic therapy may be treated with isoflurophate or echothiophate.[259] In practice, their use is reserved for patients with chronic simple glaucoma that have not responded well to weaker miotics and for those with aphakic glaucoma. Their use is so limited because of the rather severe ciliary spasm often encountered when these strong miotics are used in younger persons and also because of their greater toxicity.

Substantially better control of intraocular pressure is sometimes attained by changing to these stronger miotics. Statistical data to this effect are variable because of factors such as strength, frequency, and type of other medications being taken; severity of the glaucoma; and patient reliability.

The effect of pilocarpine and/or physostig-mine was compared with that of isoflurophate, 0.05% solution, in 78 glaucomatous eyes.[260] Although pilocarpine and/or physostigmine controlled the pressure in only 43.7% of these eyes, 89.5% of the same eyes were controlled by isoflurophate. Not only was isoflurophate more effective but it required much less frequent use, the majority of patients requiring only one instillation daily, if that often (Fig. 12-66). The proper frequency of use of isoflurophate is the minimum that will control intraocular pressure at the desired level, as determined by tonometry.

Occasionally better control is achieved by echothiophate than by isoflurophate and vice versa. Ordinarily, failure of isoflurophate to control glaucoma indicates either the trial use of other types of medication (for example, acetazolamide or levo-epinephrine) or the need for surgery.

After the clinical introduction of isoflurophate, patients were encountered in whom the drug increased intraocular pressure rather than controlled the glaucoma. In 1953 a literature survey cited 31 cases of marked pressure increase resulting from isofluro-

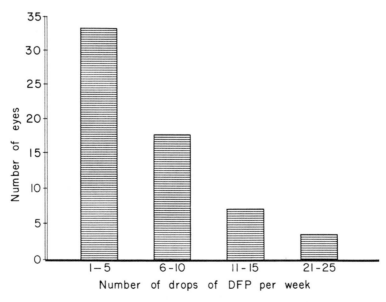

Fig. 12-66. Number of instillations of isoflurophate (DFP) required per week for control of intraocular pressure in glaucoma. (Modified from Leopold, I. H., and Comroe, J. H.: Arch. Ophthalmol. **36**:1, 1946.)

phate as well as two cases of isoflurophate-induced acute glaucoma of such severity that no medical control was possible and emergency surgery was necessary.[261] Initially, the mechanism of this paradoxical pressure rise was not understood, and the precaution of observing the patient for at least several hours after the first instillation of isoflurophate was recommended. Isoflurophate-induced acute glaucoma is now known to be caused by closure of an initially shallow angle, and its prevention requires gonioscopic confirmation of the presence of open angles before prescription of isoflurophate. The use of isoflurophate is contraindicated in narrow-angle glaucoma, because it is quite likely to precipitate a medically uncontrollable acute attack that will require immediate surgery. To maintain a patient with narrow-angle glaucoma on pilocarpine until pressures rise and then to employ isoflurophate would be poor surgical judgment, indeed.

The mechanism of isoflurophate-induced angle closure has not been established. Possibly, ciliary spasm shifts the iris-lens diaphragm forward; or vascular congestion may close the angle. The extreme miosis may increase the degree of physiologic iris bombé, with consequent deepening of the posterior chamber and closure of the chamber angle.

As would be expected, isoflurophate helps to open cyclodialysis clefts. In a series of 15 such patients the cleft was noted to appear or to become more widely open when the pupil was constricted with isoflurophate.[262] Daily postoperative use of isoflurophate was recommended, beginning on the first postoperative day, to separate the ciliary body widely from the sclera and decrease the tendency for closure of the cyclodialysis. It is important to note that patients in whom pressure is not controlled by surgery may thereafter respond to miotics, even though medical therapy had previously been ineffective. Before concluding that a second antiglaucoma operation is necessary, the physician should usually wait a reasonable period of time, during which isoflurophate, epinephrine, and carbonic anhydrase inhibitors are again tried.

Accommodative esotropia. The accommo-dative component of esotropia may be identified by the use of isoflurophate.[263] The nightly use for 2 weeks of a 0.025% solution (commercial strength solution diluted with *anhydrous* peanut oil) or ointment will eliminate the accommodative part of the deviation. A diagnostic trial of isoflurophate is recommended even for patients without a significant refractive error, since an occasional emmetropic patient is benefited, presumably because of a change in the AC/A ratio.

In the treatment of accommodative esotropia with isoflurophate the smallest effective amount should be used. Dosage is reduced by giving the medication less frequently rather than by decreasing the concentration. (In lower concentrations, isoflurophate becomes so unstable as to be clinically unreliable.) A dosage frequency of every other night, every third night, or even less often may maintain straightness of the eyes.

Thirty-three of a series of 145 patients with esotropia were satisfactorily controlled by isoflurophate.[263] Eight other patients were benefited by this medication after surgery. Isoflurophate treatment must be continued for 1 to 5 years, rarely longer, before the eyes will remain spontaneously straight. The duration of therapy is determined by the clinical response.

Twenty-eight of 32 children over 7 years of age showed continued improvement in their AC/A ratio even after isoflurophate was stopped.[264] Only 4 of 15 children less than 5 years of age continued to have a normal AC/A ratio when isoflurophate was stopped. These figures suggest that isoflurophate therapy of accommodative esotropia should be continued until the child approaches 7 years of age. Other variables such as fusion ability will modify this recommendation.

Ideally, under medication the eyes of a patient will remain straight for distant and near vision with or without glasses, will retain reasonably good distant vision, and will incur minimal side effects. In practice, the nonaccommodative portion of a squint will persist annoyingly (glasses will sometimes give additional help), some blurring of vision occurs (though surprisingly little), and parents note redness of the eyes and resistance to instillation of the medication. Miotic therapy is particularly useful for the patient who might otherwise need bifocal lenses because the accommodative esotropia is more marked for near work and for the child who wishes to swim without glasses during the summer.

Astigmatism is not corrected by isoflurophate and if it is great enough to cause symptoms requires the wearing of glasses. The need for hyperopic spherical corrections in esotropic children is virtually eliminated by isoflurophate. This avoids many of the nuisances of spectacles in childhood—resistance to wearing, problems in fitting frames, breakage, and the like.

Iris cysts, the main complication of isoflurophate therapy in children, may be avoided by reducing the frequency of dosage or by the concomitant use of a 10% solution of phenylephrine.

Parasitic infestation. Because it is closely related to commercial insecticides, isoflurophate can be used to destroy louse infestations of the eyelashes or eyebrows. After any encrustations of the lids have been removed by mechanical scrubbing, isoflurophate ointment, 0.025%, is carefully applied to the eyelashes or eyebrows, using caution to avoid ocular instillation if possible. A single such application will kill all parasites about the eye. Reinfection from other parts of the body, from clothing, and from other persons is not uncommon, and appropriate preventive measures should be undertaken. Since toxic amounts of isoflurophate can be absorbed through the skin, it should not be applied to large areas of the body such as the scalp. (DDT dust, for instance, is much safer for application to extensive body surfaces.[265])

Complications

Discomfort. Ciliary spasm is the most common and annoying side effect encountered in the use of all miotics. The indirect-acting miotics (and particularly the irreversible ones) produce a more severe ciliary spasm than does pilocarpine, because each accommodative or miotic effort results in a new supply of acetylcholine. This explains the in-

creased discomfort associated with near work and bright lights. Instillation at bedtime minimizes discomfort, because fewer acetylcholine-producing stimuli are encountered when the eyes are not in use. Younger persons are more severely affected by this ciliary spasm and may be totally disabled for several days by a single drop of a 0.1% solution of isoflurophate. The treated eye is congested, red, and painful, experiences sharp discomfort during light or accommodative effort, and is highly myopic from the accommodative spasm. These symptoms are minimized by the use of atropine and may be immediately neutralized by administration of pyridine-2-aldoxime methiodide. Fortunately the older glaucoma patient is less likely to experience such severe side effects. Aphakic patients often have no such complaints at all. Use of lower concentrations of miotic and instillation at bedtime will minimize discomfort. With prolonged usage, the glaucomatous patient develops a tolerance to these initially troublesome side effects and within a few weeks is bothered only for a few minutes after treatment or not at all. Forewarning patients of the possibility of such symptoms will reassure them that the pharmacist did not dispense the wrong drops and will result in better cooperation.

Iris cysts. Although miotic cysts of the pupillary pigment margin may occur in adults, they are much more frequent in children. Isoflurophate and echothiophate are more likely to cause these cysts than are the weaker miotics. Less frequent miotic use greatly reduces the incidence of cysts. Since children are particularly likely to develop cysts, it is suggested that isoflurophate be instilled every other night or even less frequently for treatment of accommodative strabismus.

These cysts are smoothly rounded, multiple nodules that appear on the pupil pigment margin. In one instance a child was blinded by bilateral total pupil occlusion by cysts. Fortunately they spontaneously disappear when miotics are discontinued; the aforementioned case of "blindness" was instantly cured by phenylephrine.

Apparently, prolonged and intense miosis

is required to produce these cysts. The daily use of isoflurophate caused 42 of 66 children (average age 7 years) to develop such cysts in an average of 10 weeks. In all patients the cysts disappeared when isoflurophate therapy was stopped, although they persisted for more than 2½ months in eight eyes. Small pigment tags persisted on the pupil margins for as long as 2 years. The cysts re-formed rapidly if isoflurophate was again used.[266]

In one tragic case, miotic cysts were erroneously diagnosed as melanoma and the child's eye was enucleated. (These cysts do not transilluminate well because of the density of pigmentation.) Subsequent histopathologic study showed the proliferation to be limited to the neuroepithelial layers of pigment, which extended beyond the pupil margin and contained cystic spaces between the two cell layers (Fig. 12-67).[267]

The possibility that this pigment proliferation is a selective response to parasympathetic stimulation tempts speculation as to whether the growth of an immature eye might be altered by autonomic drugs.

Occurrence of isoflurophate cysts during treatment of accommodative esotropia may be minimized by the simultaneous use of phenylephrine.[268]

Horopter alterations. Pilots spraying organic phosphorus insecticide from airplanes occasionally contaminate one eye with the solution with resultant parasympathomimetic effects. Occasionally these effects cause difficulty in judging distance. Experimental unilateral ocular instillation of tetraethyl pyrophosphate (an insecticide comparable to isoflurophate) in seven volunteers resulted in fumbling, stumbling, and clumsiness in six of them. Four of these individuals complained specifically of difficulty in judging distance. Binocular instillation did not cause problems of distance judgment.[269] When the strong miotics are used clinically, both eyes are ordinarily treated. If, however, only one eye is started on such treatment, the ophthalmologist should anticipate at least transitory complaints of space perception problems comparable to those of a patient with a new pair of glasses with considerable change of strength in one eye. (The concept of the horopter in physiologic optics provides the basis for these perceptual alterations.)

Systemic poisoning. Generalized parasympathomimetic toxicity is much more likely to complicate the use of echothiophate and demecarium than treatment with isoflurophate and is discussed in the consideration of these drugs.

Retinal detachment. Although retinal detachments are reported to follow the use of isoflurophate, they are probably but another complication that occurs in aphakic glaucomatous eyes. The horseshoe tears often seen in these detachments are clearly the result of vitreous traction bands and are unrelated to any hypothetical ciliary spasm, with resultant suprachoroidal traction. The statis-

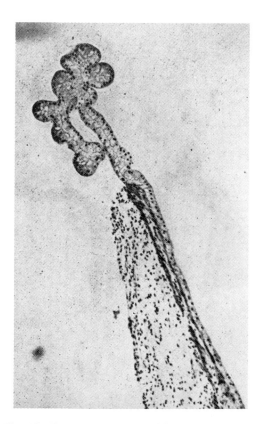

Fig. 12-67. Miotic cyst caused by pilocarpine and physostigmine therapy of 9-year-old boy with congenital glaucoma. (From Christensen, L., Swan, K. C., and Huggins, H.: Arch. Ophthalmol. **55:** 666, 1956.)

tician who correlates detachments with the use of strong miotics must take into account the popularity of their use in aphakic patients as well as the known higher incidence of *both* glaucoma and detachment after operative complications such as vitreous loss.

As an example, retinal detachment occurred in a 70-year-old woman after 2 years of miotic therapy, including 5 months of isoflurophate therapy.[270] The evidence presented suggests only a coincidental relationship between the use of isoflurophate and the retinal detachment.

Ostensibly, miotic detachments occur because of traction from the longitudinal portion of the ciliary muscle. This muscle originates from the suprachoroidal space, not from the retina. Most retinal tears appear to be caused by internal pull by the vitreous rather than by ciliary body activity. Based on my own personal experience with retinal detachments (up to 500 operations annually), I see no reason to believe that any causal relationship exists between use of isoflurophate and retinal detachment.

Cataract. A particularly serious consequence of the use of strong anticholinesterase drugs such as isoflurophate is the devel-

opment of cataract. A detailed description of such cataract formation is presented in the section on echothiophate.

Toxicity

Isoflurophate is a derivative of a class of chemicals used as insecticides and war gases. These drugs are extremely poisonous. The contents of a bottle of eye drops could easily kill a child.

Manifestations of cholinergic poisoning such as diarrhea, epigastric cramps, nausea and vomiting, cold sweats, and salivation are rarely observed under conditions of clinical usage. Although such symptoms may be reduced in severity by the administration of atropine, they indicate serious systemic depletion of cholinesterase and dictate a reduced frequency of medication or complete discontinuance. The specific etiology of these symptoms may be confirmed by laboratory testing of the patient's cholinesterase levels.

A fairly simple test strip method for determining plasma cholinesterase activity has been devised.[271] This method is suitable for use in glaucomatous patients suspected of having anticholinesterase poisoning.

A specific antidote exists for poisoning by

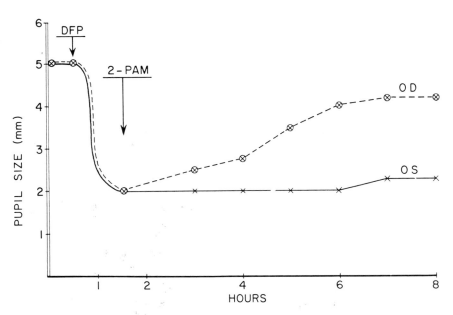

Fig. 12-68. Response of rabbit pupil to a 0.1% solution of isoflurophate (DFP) in both eyes and to P₂AM, 1% solution, every 10 minutes six times in the right eye. (Modified from Mamo, J. G., and Leopold, I. H.: Am. J. Ophthalmol. 46:724, 1958.)

cholinesterase inhibitors (Fig. 12-68).[272] Pyridine-2-aldoxime methyl iodide (P$_2$AM) promptly separates the bound cholinesterase from eserine and neostigmine (Prostigmin) and also from the irreversible inhibitors isoflurophate and echothiophate. P$_2$AM is a relatively nontoxic compound. By itself it produces no effect on the pupil or on outflow facility. Topical ocular application is relatively ineffective, but subconjunctival injection of 0.2 ml of a 4% solution of P$_2$AM will neutralize echothiophate or isoflurophate miosis within an hour.[258] Systemic anticholinesterase poisoning is also effectively counteracted by P$_2$AM. Either topical or systemic use of atropine is a quite effective antidote to poisoning by the strong miotics. However, atropine action is purely symptomatic, whereas P$_2$AM is a specific chemical antidote against phosphoryl inactivation of cholinesterase.[273] It is believed that hydrolysis of acetylcholine results in an intermediate formation of an acetylcholinesterase molecule that is highly unstable and breaks down rapidly, thereby freeing the cholinesterase for further enzymatic action. Phosphate inhibitors such as isoflurophate bind the enzyme in a stable phosphoryl-cholinesterase compound. P$_2$AM will reactivate phosphoryl-inhibited cholinesterase within minutes. Given in doses of 75 mg/kg body weight, P$_2$AM will protect all animals against an LD$_{100}$ dose of cholinesterase inhibitor. The minimal lethal dose of P$_2$AM is 100 mg/kg.

A thought-provoking report shows a statistical correlation between the incidence of myopia in Japanese schoolchildren and the amount of organophosphorous pesticides used in their agricultural districts. Increased pesticide usage in 1963, 1968, and 1972 coincided with peaks in myopia incidence.[274] Recall that atropine has been advocated to reduce myopic progress.

Echothiophate (Phospholine)

Echothiophate iodide is a relatively irreversible cholinesterase inhibitor. Its clinical characteristics and the indications for its use are almost identical to those of isoflurophate.

Echothiophate is indefinitely stable when dry; however, it must be kept in tightly sealed containers because the powdered form is hygroscopic. Assay of refrigerated aqueous solutions of echothiophate shows a drop to 90% of the original potency within 4 weeks. At room temperature this drop is to 83% of the original potency within 4 weeks and to 76% in 8 weeks.[275] Solutions should probably be discarded after 2 months at room temperature.

Echothiophate is destroyed by autoclaving. Benzalkonium is incompatible with iodides and may not be used as a preservative. Chlorobutanol, 0.5% solution, is a satisfactory and compatible preservative.

Echothiophate is marketed as a powder and accompanied by a diluent sufficient to prepare a 0.125% solution (the strength most commonly employed for treatment of chronic simple glaucoma and accommodative esotropia). In many instances a 0.06% solution gives satisfactory therapeutic results and causes less irritation. Pure echothiophate powder should *not* under any circumstances be applied directly to a patient's eye. Transconjunctival absorption is rapid, and serious systemic poisoning will result. The experiment of placing pure echothiophate powder on a rabbit's eye will create an unending respect for the potency of this drug. (The rabbit drops dead!)

Ocular penetration

The entry of the organophosphorous anticholinesterase agents into the rabbit eye was studied with the use of tritium-labeled isoflurophate and by histochemical demonstration of cholinesterase inhibition by echothiophate.[276] Within 2 hours after the topical application of 2 drops of 0.06% echothiophate, profound inhibition of cholinesterase staining was observed over almost the entire anterior segment of the eye. Cholinesterase activity was abolished in the cornea and conjunctiva, greatly reduced throughout the iris, abolished in the subcapsular lens epithelium in the region of the pupil, and reduced in the lens equator. The iris appeared to act as a chemical trap, protecting the peripheral lens but not the pupillary zone from the topically applied drug.

Cholinesterase inhibition in the ciliary

body appeared to penetrate through the sclera, being most marked near the sclera and least apparent in the interior of the eye. This distribution rules out transcorneal penetration via the aqueous into the posterior chamber to the internal aspect of the ciliary body.

In reduced amounts the radioactively labeled isoflurophate was found in all parts of the eye within a few hours. Because all ocular sites in the experimental eye contained more radioactivity than the fellow eye, systemic perfusion alone did not account for drug penetration, even into the posterior segment of the eye.

These studies also indicated that the cholinesterase of the lens epithelium is of the nonspecific, or pseudo, variety and is diffusely distributed throughout the cytoplasm of the epithelial cells. In contrast, the corneal epithelium cholinesterase is of the true variety and is distributed external to the cells, apparently within a plexus of branching fibers that could occasionally be traced to a branch of a corneal nerve fiber. The function of nonspecific cholinesterase, such as is found in the lens epithelium, has not been established but may be related to a sodium pump mechanism.

Pharmacology

Two types of cholinesterase exist. The true cholinesterase, acetylcholinesterase, is extracellular, comprises only 10% to 20% of the total tissue cholinesterase activity, and is the enzyme pool involved in regulating responses to cholinergic drugs. The pseudo- or nonspecific cholinesterase, butyrylcholinesterase, is intracellular, comprises 80% to 90% of total tissue cholinesterase activity, and plays no pharmacologic role in the cholinergic responses to the various cholinesterase inhibitors.

True acetylcholinesterase inhibition can be achieved by echothiophate in concentrations as weak as 10^{-8}M, whereas no detectable inhibition results from isoflurophate below concentrations of 10^{-6}M. It should be noted that 100% of enzyme inhibition is not produced by echothiophate concentrations as strong as 10^{-3}M. True cholinesterase inhibition by such concentrations of echothiophate may be reversed within 15 minutes by 10^{-3}M pralidoxime. Pralidoxime has poor lipid solubility, does not penetrate all membranes, and does not reactivate the inhibited intracellular pseudocholinesterase.

It is a prevalent misconception that there are strong and weak miotics. A response of maximum contractile strength can be obtained from an iris sphincter strip with any cholinergic drug providing a sufficiently high dose is used. Echothiophate is not a "stronger" miotic and does not, in fact, cause any contraction of the iris sphincter at all. However, by inhibition of cholinesterase, echothiophate renders the affected muscle sensitive to lower concentrations of cholinergic drugs. Another concept of strength may be related to duration. The clinical effect of echothiophate is, indeed, of long duration.[277]

Dose-response analysis of echothiophate with respect to intraocular pressure and outflow facility indicates that little additional pharmacologic response is obtained by increasing the drug concentration above 0.06% (Fig. 12-69).[278] Prolonged maintenance of intraocular pressure at or below 21 mm Hg, another parameter of drug effectiveness, was best achieved by a concentration of 0.125% echothiophate. The parameter of patient complaint included decreased visual acuity and decreased night vision (related to increasing miosis), accommodative spasm, brow ache, and headache. Few complaints were encountered with the 0.03% concentration, 3 of 15 patients noted acuity problems with 0.06%, and half the patients had multiple complaints with 0.25%. The toxic parameters of cholinesterase inhibitor-induced cataracts and systemic poisoning are also dose dependent. Consideration of all these parameters suggests that there is little rationale for the use of echothiophate concentrations in excess of 0.06%. If adequate clinical control is not achieved by the use of 0.06% echothiophate twice a day, the next logical step would be to add epinephrine to the regimen or to change to another miotic. The use of a higher concentration of echothiophate is more likely

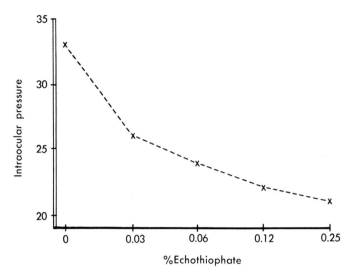

Fig. 12-69. Mean intraocular pressure in 15 patients with open-angle glaucoma treated with the specified concentrations of echothiophate. (Data from Harris, L. S.: Arch. Ophthalmol. **86:** 502, 1971.)

to produce toxic manifestations than benefits. However, consideration of mean statistical values can be deceptive and consideration of the individual patient's problem is always necessary.

Clinical use

Open-angle glaucoma. Echothiophate benefits glaucomatous eyes by increasing the facility of outflow.[279] An average improvement in outflow facility of 127% was achieved in 28 glaucomatous eyes with a 0.25% or 0.1% solution of echothiophate. Most of these eyes had not been controlled by conventional miotics. Echothiophate also increases the facility of outflow in normal eyes. The improvement in outflow facility in 86 glaucomatous eyes is illustrated in Fig. 12-70.[258]

The considerable diurnal variations in intraocular pressure that are characteristic of chronic simple glaucoma are well known to clinicians and are considered to be a primary cause of continuing field loss in patients who are "controlled" at the time of daytime office checks. These diurnal variations are reduced by pilocarpine therapy but not to the extent that may be achieved with a longer acting miotic. In 24 of 32 eyes receiving pilocarpine

therapy for chronic simple glaucoma, measurement of pressure every 3 hours during the night showed tension rises to 25 mm Hg or more.[280] When treated with a 0.06% solution of echothiophate, none of the pressures rose above 20 mm Hg during the night. Thus it appears that the long-acting miotics not only require less frequent instillation but also produce better 24-hour control of pressure.

Daytime measurements also confirm the greater effectiveness of a 0.06% echothiophate solution in controlling chronic simple glaucoma.[281] This concentration of echothiophate, given once or twice daily and supplemented as required by acetazolamide and epinephrine, maintained pressure at 20 mm Hg or less in 83% of 54 glaucomatous eyes. The pressure in all of these eyes had been above 20 mm Hg when pilocarpine, supplemented by acetazolamide and epinephrine, was given. While receiving pilocarpine therapy, the pressures of 78% of these eyes ranged from 21 to 30 mm Hg, and 22% were higher than 30 mm Hg. In a 0.06% concentration, echothiophate is well tolerated, causing much less irritation than 0.25% or 0.125% concentrations.

The effect of a 4% solution of pilocarpine given four times a day as compared to that of

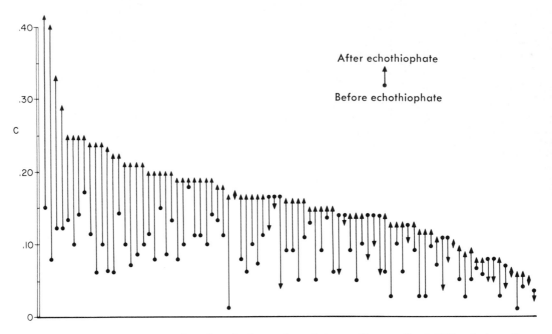

Fig. 12-70. Improvement of outflow facility with nightly instillation of a 0.25% solution of echothiophate (Phospholine) in 86 eyes with chronic simple glaucoma inadequately controlled by pilocarpine, epinephrine, and acetazolamide. (Modified from Becker, B., Pyle, G. C., and Drew, R. C.: Am. J. Ophthalmol. 47:635, 1959.)

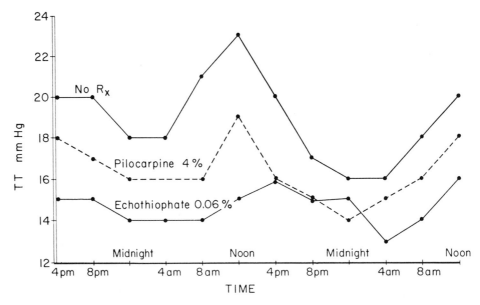

Fig. 12-71. Mean diurnal tension curves of 20 glaucomatous eyes—untreated, receiving a 4% pilocarpine solution four times a day, and receiving a 0.06% echothiophate solution twice a day. (Modified from Pratt-Johnson, J. A., Drance, S. M., and Innes, R.: Arch. Ophthalmol. **72:**485, 1964.)

a 0.06% solution of echothiophate iodide given twice a day was studied in 20 glaucomatous eyes in 13 patients.[282] During pilocarpine treatment, 40% of the eyes showed diurnal peaks of pressure above 24 mm Hg, while only 10% of the eyes exceeded 24 mm Hg pressure during echothiophate therapy. The mean diurnal tension curves of these 20 eyes (untreated, receiving pilocarpine, and receiving echothiophate) are shown in Fig. 12-71.

The side effects of the 4% solution of pilocarpine and those of the 0.06% solution of echothiophate (a lower concentration than normally used) were almost equal. Four patients preferred echothiophate, six preferred pilocarpine, and three noted no difference. One patient suffered severe headaches and gastrointestinal upsets during echothiophate therapy.

Clinical results such as these indicate that the frequent use of the stronger concentrations of pilocarpine is no longer the method of choice in controlling difficult cases of chronic simple glaucoma. Substantially better control of pressure, greater convenience, and almost equal side effects recommend the use of echothiophate, 0.06% solution, for such patients. However, solutions of 4% pilocarpine and 0.06% echothiophate are considerably more irritating than a solution of 1% pilocarpine; hence easily controlled cases of glaucoma should be treated with a 1% solution of pilocarpine.

Comparison of echothiophate therapy alone with intensive standard treatment (pilocarpine, eserine, epinephrine, or acetazolamide) shows the greater effectiveness of treatment with several medications, which have different but additive effects (Table 12-6).[283]

Obviously more patients were controlled by intensive therapy than by echothiophate therapy alone; however, it should be noted that 11 patients did better with echothiophate therapy. There is, of course, no reason why echothiophate therapy should not be supplemented as necessary with epinephrine and acetazolamide.

From the practical standpoint, the long duration of echothiophate action is a great convenience to the patient, who needs only to instill drops once at night instead of repeatedly during the day.

Concentrations of echothiophate as dilute as 0.01% have been reported to satisfactorily control more than half of patients with open-angle glaucoma. Side effects of this concentration were considered comparable to those of 2% pilocarpine; however, all patients had used other miotics before starting the 0.01% echothiophate.[284]

Use of 0.03% echothiophate once daily in 50 patients with chronic simple glaucoma established good control in 20 patients.[285] Perhaps a reasonable concept in the use of this drug is to begin with the most dilute concentration (0.03%) likely to control an appreciable proportion of cases and gradually to increase the strength and frequency of dosage until reaching the minimum amount necessary to control the individual case of glaucoma. This approach seems more reasonable than to start immediately with a 0.25% concentration. Use of the minimum effective amount will also improve patient tolerance and reduce toxic side effects.

Closed-angle glaucoma. Twenty-two eyes with angle-closure glaucoma were treated with echothiophate for intervals varying from a few days to several years.[286] Nine of these eyes had been operated on previously (either iridectomy or iridencleisis) without achieving satisfactory pressure control. Five of these postoperative eyes were controlled with echothiophate. In eight cases of acute angle closure, temporary control of pressure was achieved with echothiophate. From 1 to 7

Table 12-6. Comparative effect of echothiophate and standard therapy*

	Intensive standard therapy	
Echothiophate	*Controlled*	*Uncontrolled*
Controlled	23	11
Uncontrolled	20	6

*Data based on Giardini, A., and Paliaga, G. P.: Boll. Oculist. 38:683, 1959.

weeks later, when the eye had become quiet, iridectomy or iridencleisis was performed. In none of these eight acute eyes was the condition made worse by "strong" miotic treatment. In only 2 of the 22 eyes was the drug discontinued because of pain, and in these patients medication had been continued for 5 and for 8 weeks. There was no instance of echothiophate precipitating a more severe acute attack.

These facts are at variance with the belief that narrow-angle glaucoma contraindicates the use of the organic phosphate miotics. However, surgery was ultimately performed on all but three of these patients, which indicates that echothiophate therapy is at best of only temporary benefit in angle-closure glaucoma.

Accommodative esotropia. Most articles dealing with echothiophate treatment of accommodative esotropia state that a 0.1% solution of echothiophate gives results comparable to those of a 0.025% concentration of isoflurophate.[287]

A weaker concentration (0.06%) of echothiophate was found to be of benefit in 23 of 32 cases of accommodative esotropia.[288] Medication was required nightly or every other night. Iris cysts developed in only three patients, in contrast to the much higher incidence when stronger concentrations of miotics are used.

Presbyopia. Miosis does have the optical advantage of increasing field depth. In a series of 65 presbyopic eyes, 0.06% echothiophate used twice daily permitted 80% of the patients to avoid the use of bifocals for reading.[289] However, I would consider the known hazards of this drug to outweigh the advantage of avoiding bifocals.

Complications

Systemic toxicity. The use of long-acting anticholinesterase drugs for the treatment of glaucoma may result in systemic toxicity. The incidence of such toxicity is particularly high with echothiophate iodide. Of 24 patients taking echothiophate, 9 had systemic symptoms.[290] Frequency of dosage is an important factor in toxicity. All nine patients with

symptoms were using 4 drops/day, whereas the asymptomatic patients were receiving medication less frequently.

The systemic toxic effects caused by echothiophate drops include diarrhea, nausea, abdominal cramps, and general fatigue and weakness. One patient required hospitalization for evaluation of severe, persistent diarrhea of undetermined etiology. Respiratory symptoms simulating pulmonary infection may be caused by anticholinesterase poisoning but are more characteristic of the inhalation route of absorption (as by persons using insecticide sprays). Anticholinesterase toxic symptoms may simulate an acute gastrointestinal upset or an upper respiratory infection.

If such symptoms appear in a patient receiving echothiophate therapy, determination of the cholinesterase values in red blood cells may indicate whether the symptoms can be attributed to this drug. The normal range of cholinesterase in red blood cells is between 0.6 and 1.1 units. Values below 0.4 are usually associated with moderately severe exposure to anticholinesterase chemicals. The nine symptomatic patients using 4 drops of echothiophate/day had an average cholinesterase value of 0.26 in their red blood cells.

Low cholinesterase values were also found in 12 asymptomatic patients using 2 drops of echothiophate/day. Their average value was 0.38, but some individual values were much lower. A cholinesterase value of 0.68 was found in two patients receiving only 1 drop of echothiophate/day. Apparently, low cholinesterase values do not necessarily mean that the symptoms are drug induced, while normal values do rule out drug toxicity.

Plasma and red cell cholinesterase levels were measured in glaucoma patients after the use of 1 drop of echothiophate in both eyes twice a day. Within a month, 75% to 80% inhibition of the enzyme resulted from the use of 0.25% echothiophate. From 35% to 40% inhibition resulted from the use of 0.06% or 0.03% concentrations (Fig. 12-72).[291] As would be expected, there was no relationship between the degree of glaucoma control and the extent of cholinesterase inhibition, since

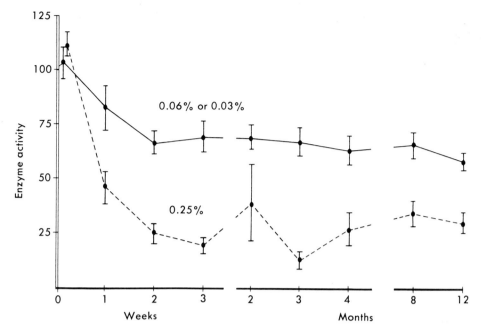

Fig. 12-72. Plasma cholinesterase activity measured after use of echothiophate in both eyes two times a day for specified times and drug concentrations. (Modified from de Roetth, A., Jr., and associates: Am. J. Ophthalmol. **62:**834, 1966.)

the severity of glaucoma results from a different factor, namely, trabecular anatomy.

Although adverse local symptoms may be decreased by use of 0.0625% echothiophate iodide (instead of 0.25%), red cell cholinesterase values were below normal in all patients receiving 0.0625% drops once daily for longer than 2½ months, and more than half of these patients had systemic side effects (gastrointestinal disorders, sweating, salivation, nasal congestion, and weakness).[292] Obviously the same precautions against systemic toxicity are necessary with either concentration of this potent drug.[293]

Since long-acting anticholinesterase drugs may reduce red cell cholinesterase for as long as 4 months, treatment with a specific antidote may be desirable in patients with severe toxicity. P₂AM (pyridine-2-aldoxime methyl iodide), 25 mg/kg, may be given intravenously in 500 ml of a 5% solution of dextrose and water over a 2-hour period. P₂AM neutralizes both the systemic toxicity and the ocular therapeutic effect.

Variable paresthesias severe enough to re-

quire hospitalization for neurologic investigation were caused by the use of a 0.25% solution of echothiophate iodide twice daily in each eye for treatment of chronic simple glaucoma.[294] Cholinesterase levels in red blood cells were determined in eight consecutive echothiophate-treated patients, seven of whom showed marked cholinesterase reduction. Five of the eight patients had values below the level (0.5 ᐞph units/hour) that requires removal of industrial workers from further chemical exposure. In one patient the oral use of atropine failed to reverse the inhibition of cholinesterase. Not only did the atropine fail to reverse the cholinesterase drop but it also caused an elevation of intraocular pressure. The authors of this study advised routine blood anticholinesterase determinations for patients receiving echothiophate or demecarium therapy, but a frequency for such blood tests was not specified. I would infer that blood cholinesterase measurements might be performed 1 month after therapy with these drugs is instituted or increased.

Because echothiophate poisoning is cumulative, toxic systemic symptoms do not appear for weeks or months after the start of therapy. For this reason, the relationship between symptoms and ocular therapy may not be recognized.[295] Frequently symptoms are discovered only by direct questioning.

Since plasma cholinesterase hydrolyzes succinylcholine and procaine, patients with low blood cholinesterase resulting from anticholinesterase therapy for glaucoma are more susceptible to the toxic effects of these anesthetic drugs. Death has been reported from the use of succinylcholine during anesthesia in a patient with low blood cholinesterase.[295] It might be wise to inform the patient's general physician when strong anticholinesterase therapy is in use.

One case is reported in which the administration of 0.125% echothiophate three times a day resulted in circulatory collapse with periods of cardiac arrest.[296] Given intravenously, atropine caused prompt recovery.

Of possible clinical significance is the tendency of alcoholic beverages to increase the severity of poisoning by organic phosphate parasympathomimetic drugs.[297] Of great importance is the vulnerability of patients to additional medication once their systemic cholinesterase levels have been greatly reduced. Deprived of their normal cholinesterase reserves, such patients may suffer severe toxic effects from a small amount of an anticholinesterase drug. This toxic response may be out of all proportion to the small size of the last dose of medication. Hence echothiophate should be discontinued or at least drastically reduced if a patient has symptoms suggesting a toxic reaction.

After ocular instillation of echothiophate in rabbits, the most marked extraocular site of cholinesterase inhibition is the gastrointestinal tract.[298] This finding is compatible with the clinical knowledge that gastrointestinal disturbances are the most common side effects observed after use of echothiophate eye drops. In contrast to echothiophate, after ocular instillation, isoflurophate does not inhibit cholinesterase in any of the extraocular tissues. Presumably this is explained by the ease with which nonenzymatic hydrolysis destroys isoflurophate.

Cornea. In excessive dosage, echothiophate apparently is toxic to the cornea. In two patients receiving 0.25% echothiophate four times a day, pain, corneal bedewing, and fine endothelial deposits developed. These abnormalities disappeared when the dosage was reduced.[299] This excessive dose frequency was due to patient error; apparently they confused the instillation frequency of echothiophate with that of pilocarpine, which they had previously been using four times a day. When changing to the use of echothiophate, the physician should emphasize the reduced frequency of drop instillation and the hazards of overdosage.

Iritis. Unexpected toxic manifestations are not infrequently encountered during the clinical trial use of potent new drugs. Three patients are reported to have developed severe fibrinous iritis after several days of echothiophate therapy.[258] This iritis was prolonged, despite use of mydriatics, steroids, and P_2AM and the cessation of echothiophate, and resulted in formation of posterior synechiae. However, this is the only report of such a complication.

Iris cysts. There is no question that iris cysts may result from the excessive use of either echothiophate or isoflurophate. Similarly, either drug in a smaller dosage can control accommodative esotropia without extensive cyst formation, especially when phenylephrine is used simultaneously. Whether the therapeutic index is better for one of these drugs than for the other has not been established, but in practical clinical usage, there seems to be no significant difference.

Use of phenylephrine, 2.5% to 10% solution, in combination with echothiophate in treatment of accommodative esotropia will prevent the formation of miotic cysts and yet will not impair the therapeutic effect.

A combination of echothiophate, 0.125% solution, and phenylephrine, 2.5% solution, was used in 22 patients with esotropia for varying periods of time (average 3.25 months). In most patients, instillation was nightly in each eye, but some patients required treatment twice a day. Iris cysts occurred in only 4 of these 44 eyes. Fourteen of the 22 patients benefited from miotic treatment.[300]

Cataract. The most serious ocular complication of echothiophate therapy appears to be cataract formation.

Evidence that clinical use of the strong anticholinesterase agents (echothiophate, isoflurophate, and demecarium) causes cataract seems conclusive.[301-303] The typical anticholinesterase cataract begins in the form of anterior subcapsular vacuoles, which are characteristic but not pathognomonic (Fig. 12-73).[302] Typical anterior subcapsular vacuoles were found in 51% of anticholinesterase-treated eyes, in 16% of pilocarpine-treated eyes, and in 15% of the cataracts in nonglaucomatous eyes. In their early stage these vacuoles can be seen only by retroillumination, but they progress to incapacitating density.

The prevalence of cataract formation is greater with treatment of longer duration, with use of higher drug concentration, with greater frequency of dosage, and in older eyes, especially those with preexisting early cataractous changes. Once established, the cataract progresses even if the drug is discontinued. Patients differ in their susceptibility to anticholinesterase cataract, possibly on a genetic basis.

A composite graph illustrating the data from three clinics shows a much higher incidence of cataract in groups of patients treated with strong anticholinesterase agents as compared with normal control patients of comparable age or with patients treated with parasympathomimetic drugs (Fig. 12-74).[301-303] However, these studies are subject to the criticism of having been retrospective.

In a prospective study of the cataractogenic effect of echothiophate therapy, *monocular* treatment of 16 glaucomatous patients was evaluated for periods varying from 7 to 21 months.[304] Three patients were treated with 0.06% echothiophate twice daily. During the study no lens changes were noted in either the treated or fellow control eyes. Three patients were treated with 0.125% echothiophate twice daily. One of these eyes (a *control* eye) developed nuclear cataract during the study.

Ten patients were treated with 0.25% echothiophate in one eye twice daily. Two of

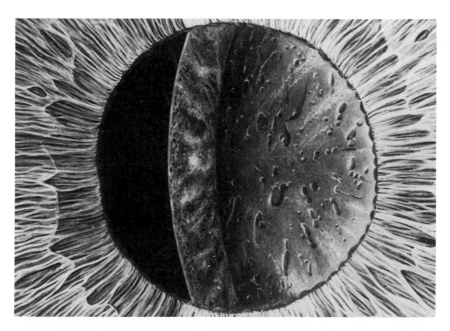

Fig. 12-73. Anterior subcapsular vacuoles characteristic of anticholinesterase cataract. (From Shaffer, R. N., and Hetherington, J. M.: Am. J. Ophthalmol. **62:**613, 1966.)

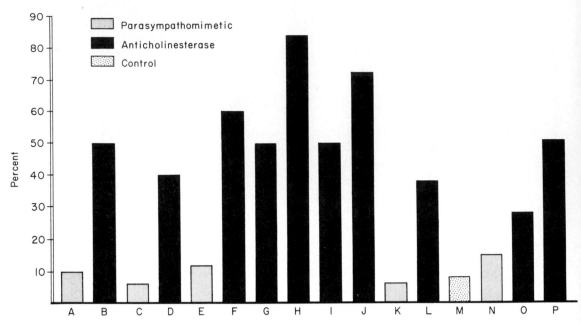

Fig. 12-74. Percent cataract formation reported in three studies. **A,** One hundred and three eyes treated with pilocarpine after 22 months mean use. **B,** Seventy-eight eyes treated with echothiophate after 12 months mean use. **C,** Forty-seven eyes without previous cataract treated with pilocarpine. **D,** Forty eyes without previous cataract treated with echothiophate. **E,** Eyes with previous cataract treated with pilocarpine. **F,** Eyes with previous cataract treated with echothiophate. **G,** Twenty eyes treated with 0.06% echothiophate two times a day for 1 year. **H,** Thirteen eyes treated with 0.25% echothiophate two times a day for 1 year. **I,** Thirty-eight eyes treated with echothiophate for 1 year. **J,** Eighteen eyes treated with echothiophate for 2 years. **K,** Two hundred forty-five eyes treated with pilocarpine or carbachol for 3 years. **L,** Sixty eyes treated with echothiophate, isoflurophate, and demecarium for 6 months to 3 years. **M,** Three hundred and five eyes of comparable age groups followed for 3 years as a control. **N,** Seventy-nine eyes treated with pilocarpine or carbachol for 3 years (clinical patients). **O,** Fifty eyes treated with anticholinesterase for 6 months to 3 years (clinical patients). **P,** Eighty-five eyes treated with 0.25% isoflurophate two times a day for 6 months to 6 years. (Data for **A** to **J** from Axelsson, U., and Holmberg, A.: Acta Ophthalmol. **44:**421, 1966; data for **K** to **O** from Shaffer, R. N., and Hetherington, J. M.: Am. J. Ophthalmol. **62:**613, 1966; data for **P** from de Roetth, A., Jr.: Am. J. Ophthalmol. **62:**619, 1966.)

these patients developed significant cataracts but equally in both eyes. Three patients did not develop cataracts. Five patients showed more severe lens changes in the echothiophate-treated eye. However, this 50% incidence of "echothiophate-induced" cataract becomes much less convincing when the author notes that two of the five patients had decreased vision from monocular cataract before beginning echothiophate treatment. Two others had much more severe glaucoma in the echothiophate-treated eye,

presumably indicating its greater susceptibility to degenerative disease. Hence in only 1 of the 10 patients treated with 0.025% echothiophate could unqualified suspicion be directed against the drug. (Remember that a control eye developed cataract.) Incidentally, the cataractous changes noted in these patients were nuclear and posterior cortical opacities such as are commonly seen in older untreated patients. In addition, previously described anterior subcapsular vacuoles or "mossy" anterior cortical cataracts, supposedly "typical" of echothiophate cataracts, were found in many untreated patients.

The inability of a large clinic (the Massachusetts Eye and Ear Infirmary) to convincingly demonstrate the cataractogenic effect of echothiophate over a 21-month study period is indeed testimony of the difficulty of this problem.

In another prospective study, 35 previously untreated patients with ocular hypertension were given various concentrations of echothiophate in one eye twice daily for 3 years. The fellow eyes served as untreated controls. In another group of patients, one eye was treated with 4% pilocarpine 4 times daily for 3 years.[305] Half of the patients receiving 0.25%, 0.125%, or 0.06% echothiophate showed progressive visual deterioration in the treated eyes. This visual loss was attributed to anterior and posterior subcapsular opacities. No such vision loss occurred in the eyes treated with 0.03% echothiophate or 4% pilocarpine. In two patients the visual loss gradually improved during the 6-month period following discontinuance of echothiophate therapy. Two other patients developed extensive posterior synechiae despite dilation every 2 months for examination of the lens.

In another prospective study group of 10 patients using 0.25% echothiophate twice daily, five developed early posterior subcapsular cataracts after 4 months of therapy.[306] In the same study, no lens opacities were found in children treated for accommodative esotropia with echothiophate (dose unspecified) for as long as 6 years. One posterior subcapsular cataract was found in 60 pesticide users (farmers, exterminators, and distributors).

Reversible miotic-induced cataract has been described in two patients. One was a 13-year-old patient with esotropia who developed anterior subcapsular cataract after 3 months of daily instillation of 0.025% isoflurophate. The other patient was a 59-year-old glaucoma patient who had used isoflurophate daily for several weeks. These cataracts disappeared completely 3 weeks after miotic therapy was discontinued.[307]

Another study of 175 miotic-treated glaucoma patients suggested that lens damage follows echothiophate use. Pilocarpine treatment of 170 eyes (average duration, 29 months) was accompanied by at least two lines loss of acuity in 17% of the eyes attributable to lens changes. The average age of these patients was 76 years. No cataract extractions were performed in this pilocarpine series.

Demecarium treatment of 51 eyes (average duration, 14 months) was accompanied by the same amount of visual loss in 33% of the eyes. The average age of the patients was 74 years. Two cataract extractions were performed.

Echothiophate treatment of 81 eyes (average duration, 11 months) was accompanied by the same visual loss in 43% of the eyes. The average age of the patients was 73 years. Six patients required cataract extraction.[308]

The high frequency of spontaneous cataract development must be considered in any evaluation of a potentially cataractogenic agent. To ascertain the "normal" incidence of lens opacities, 327 eyes were examined. The subjects of this study were all over 40 years of age, did not have glaucoma or congenital cataract, and were not taking glaucoma medication. Only 19% of these lenses were completely clear. The incidence of anterior subcapsular vacuoles was 28%; posterior subcapsular opacities, 20%; cortical spokes, 20%; and nuclear sclerosis, 16%. The incidence of clear lenses dropped from 40% at age 50 to 0% at age 80.[309]

Experimental anticholinesterase cataract. Intracarotid injection of near-lethal doses of isoflurophate in guinea pigs causes rapidly developing and often irreversible cataract.[310]

Critical evaluation of this type of cataract indicates that the lens opacity is the result of a nonspecific hyperosmolar mechanism. Such a dose of isoflurophate resulted in lethargic animals whose eyes remained open and became dehydrated. Apparently this causes a hyperosmolar aqueous and the osmotic removal of lens water, resulting in a cataract that may develop within an hour. Comparable cataract develops in guinea pigs rendered unconscious by pentobarbital if the eyelid is taped open. The fellow eye, taped closed, does not develop cataract. Similar cataracts can be produced by drying of the eyes of rats, mice, and hamsters and may be misinterpreted as "drug-induced" cataracts if the researcher is unaware of the true mechanism.[311,312]

If a relationship exists between the use of anticholinesterase agents and cataract, one would expect to find cholinesterase activity in the lens. Analysis reveals that the lens capsule does have a true cholinesterase activity, comparable in amount to that of the iris.[313] Cholinesterase enzymatic activity is demonstrable in the lens epithelium by histochemical and biochemical methods.[303] The complete elimination of this cholinesterase activity by topical instillation of anticholinesterase drugs (such as echothiophate) in clinical dosage has been demonstrated in humans and animals. In vitro incubation of the calf and rabbit lens in $10^{-3}M$ concentrations of echothiophate will cause cataract.[302]

Under experimental in vitro conditions, demecarium bromide ($10^{-4}M$) and echothiophate iodide ($10^{-3}M$) cause a marked increase in lens permeability to positive cations.[314] Similar alterations of lens permeability occur with ionizing irradiation and steroid treatment, which also may cause subcapsular lens vacuoles. Demecarium blocks aerobic lens metabolism, shifting lens metabolism exclusively to anaerobic pathways, whereas echothiophate does not block aerobic lens metabolism. Hence, whatever the mechanism of miotic-induced cataract, it is not necessarily unique to parasympathomimetic drugs, nor do all parasympathomimetic drugs necessarily have the same effect on the lens.

Additional studies confirm this in vitro cataractogenesis, which is related to the concentration of anticholinesterase drug in the culture medium.[315] However, the mechanism of action might not be cholinesterase inhibition, since recognizable cataractogenesis does not occur until drug levels are reached that are 1000 times greater than those required for total inhibition of cho-

linesterase. Inasmuch as these in vitro experiments only last 24 to 48 hours, they may not accurately reproduce the response of an in vivo lens exposed to far smaller concentrations of a drug for a much longer period of time.

Implications of anticholinesterase cataractogenesis. The skeptic may still raise the question of patient preselection in retrospective studies. Could a relationship exist between severity of glaucoma and the likelihood of cataract development? Were only eyes with a poor prognosis chosen for therapy with the stronger agents, which are themselves innocent of cataractogenesis? Despite these doubts, the evidence for anticholinesterase cataractogenesis seems reasonably acceptable and should be considered in making clinical decisions.

The strong anticholinesterase drugs probably should not be used in the management of glaucoma that can be adequately controlled by reasonable doses of direct-acting parasympathomimetic agents, either alone or in combination with epinephrine. Inadequately controlled glaucoma necessitates a choice between irreversible blindness and possible miotic cataract, an operable condition. Clearly, a strong anticholinesterase drug is the obvious choice when lesser drugs fail. Obviously the least concentration and frequency of use required for control should be prescribed, which holds true for all medications.

Is the hazard of echothiophate-induced cataract, which occurs in perhaps 50% of patients so treated, greater than the risk of glaucoma surgery? In comparing the relative dangers, one should realize that cataract extraction was necessary in 30% of 60 patients within 2½ years after filtering surgery for open-angle glaucoma.[316] Postoperative medical therapy was still necessary to control pressure in about one third of these patients. I would rather take the risk of echothiophate therapy.

Demecarium (Humorsol)

Demecarium bromide is an extremely potent long-acting cholinesterase inhibitor synthesized by connecting two neostigmine molecules with a carbon chain. It is water soluble and indefinitely stable in solution. Demecarium is the most toxic of the clinically available anticholinesterase drugs.

Pharmacology

Pharmacologically, demecarium bromide differs from isoflurophate in that it inactivates both true cholinesterase (found in erythrocytes) and pseudocholinesterase (found in plasma). (Isoflurophate primarily inactivates pseudocholinesterase. Eserine inhibits both true cholinesterase and pseudocholinesterase.[317])

Within 45 to 60 minutes, a single instillation of demecarium in human eyes produces miosis that becomes maximum within 2 to 4 hours. Miosis persists for 3 to 10 days. Rarely, slight miosis may persist for as long as 3 or 4 weeks. The rapidity of onset and duration of miosis are directly related to the concentration used (0.1% or 0.25%). Reduction of intraocular pressure by 3 to 11 mm Hg occurs in normal eyes, is first recorded in about 30 minutes, is maximum at 24 hours, and persists for 9 days or more after a single instillation. This pressure lowering is achieved by increasing the facility of outflow.[318]

Sympathomimetic dilation (as with a 10% solution of phenylephrine) does not decrease outflow facility or increase intraocular pressure when used in combination with demecarium in treatment of chronic simple glaucoma.

Human eyes maximally dilated with atropine become miotic after instillation of a 0.5% solution of demecarium. This miosis is maintained for 5 to 7 days, just as if there had been no atropinization. Surprisingly, a single instillation of a 1% solution of atropine will reverse the maximal miosis attained 6 hours after instillation of a 0.5% solution of demecarium. The action of eserine and demecarium is additive rather than competitive, regardless of the order of instillation. (This is in contrast to the blocking effect of eserine when used *before* isoflurophate or echothiophate.[319])

Toxic effects

After instillation of demecarium in normal human eyes, the unpleasant side effects of ciliary spasm are uniformly encountered. These include brow ache and blurred vision caused by the induced myopia of accommodative spasm. Superficial and deep vascular congestion lasting 1 to 3 days affects almost all eyes. These local side effects rarely persist beyond the first week.

Histologic sections in rabbits after demecarium treatment showed vascular congestion not only in the conjunctiva but also in the iris and ciliary body. Apparently because of this vascular congestion, several human eyes showed transient rises of intraocular pressure during the first hour. Permeability of the blood-aqueous barrier is increased. Two of eight patients were nauseated by 2 drops of a 0.5% solution of demecarium instilled on the eyes. Ocular instillation of 1 ml/5 pounds body weight of a 0.25% solution of demecarium killed all of six rabbits in an average time of 2 hours.[318]

Systemic side effects include nausea, vomiting, diarrhea, salivation, sweating, and bradycardia. Systemic parasympatholytic medication (such as atropine) may provide prompt relief. Apparently, unnecessary extensive medical and x-ray studies and even exploratory laparotomy have been done on patients suffering systemic anticholinesterase side effects. These unfortunate occurrences should be averted by the ophthalmologist by inquiring as to the presence of such symptoms. The patient should be instructed to instill only 1 drop (not multiple drops, as some patients are prone to do) and not to use the medication more frequently than advised.

Clinical use

Glaucoma. Use of demecarium in 40 eyes with chronic simple glaucoma, mostly uncontrolled by other unspecified miotics, caused a satisfactory pressure drop in 38 eyes (Fig. 12-75).[320] The average pressure fall in these eyes was 48%. An average time of 34 hours was required for the maximal fall of intraocular pressure to occur. The average

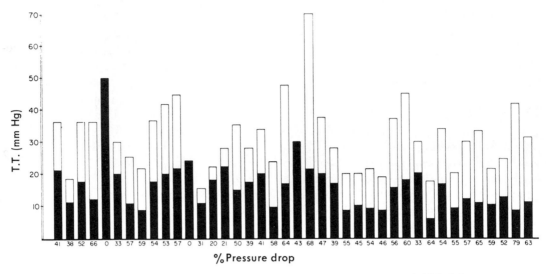

Fig. 12-75. Drop in intraocular pressure after demecarium treatment. Solid black bars: pressures after treatment. (Modified from Drance, S. M.: Arch. Ophthalmol. **62**:673, 1959.)

increase in facility of outflow was 121%. The effect of demecarium in glaucoma was studied in 76 patients whose glaucoma had not been controlled by *short*-acting miotics, carbonic anhydrase inhibitors, and epinephrine.[321] Criteria for successful demecarium therapy were very rigid, including pressures less than 24 mm Hg and outflow of more than 0.10, tolerable side effects, a minimum of 6 months' regularly evaluated therapy, and no field loss. Demecarium, 0.25% solution (once or twice daily or less often), met these criteria for successful control in approximately one half of this group of problem patients (most had chronic simple glaucoma). In some patients, control was maintained without the aid of secretory inhibitors. Supplementary epinephrine and acetazolamide were used in most cases, however.

Comparison of demecarium with echothiophate indicates that in about 25% of cases one may result in effective glaucoma control where the other had failed. It is therefore considered advisable to try a different long-acting cholinesterase inhibitor if one has failed.

Demecarium as well as echothiophate and other miotics may cause significant decreases in scleral rigidity. This results in underesti-

mation of intraocular pressure by Schiøtz tonometry and unwarranted optimism as to the degree of glaucoma control. Such errors may be avoided by applanation tonometry.[321]

ANTICHOLINESTERASE ANTIDOTE
Pralidoxime (Protopam)

The oximes are of ophthalmologic interest because of their ability to neutralize anticholinesterase activity. The action of isoflurophate, echothiophate, demecarium, and physostigmine may be reversed by pralidoxime.[322]

Pharmacology

Mechanism of action. Physiologically, acetylcholine and its specific enzyme, cholinesterase, form a chemical bond that lasts for only a few microseconds. This evanescent compound then hydrolyzes into free intact cholinesterase and broken remnants of the acetylcholine molecule. When cholinesterase inhibitors such as organic phosphates (for example, isoflurophate) react with cholinesterase, a nonhydrolyzable phosphorylated enzyme results. This molecular combination does not destroy the cholinesterase structure but effectively inhibits its enzymatic function.

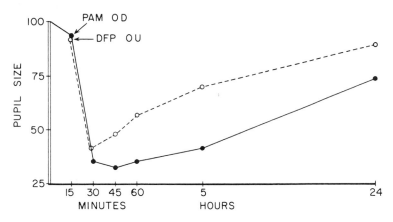

Fig. 12-76. Pupil size (expressed as percent of initial size) after bilateral instillation of isofluro-phate (DFP) in rabbit eyes. Pyridine-2-aldoxime, 5%, in a 1:10,000 solution of benzalkonium was instilled in the right eye only. The oxime effect occurs when it is used within 30 minutes before isoflurophate instillation or any time subsequent to isoflurophate. (Modified from Hunter, W. S., and McCulloch, C.: Am. J. Ophthalmol. **52:**841, 1961.)

The use of pyridine-2-aldoxime methyl iodide (P₂AM) (the chloride is less irritating than the iodide and is therefore used clinically) proves that the organic phosphates are not irreversible inhibitors of cholinesterase. The oximes act by separating the phosphoryl group from the enzyme, releasing the cholinesterase molecule intact. Within 1 minute, P₂AM in a 10⁻⁵M concentration may reactivate 80% of phosphate-inhibited cholinesterase.[323] If isoflurophate is chosen as the enzyme inhibitor, its reversibility slowly decreases with time because of the gradual formation of a more stable chemical bond.

Pralidoxime does not have a parasympatholytic effect, and its mechanism of action is not like that of atropine. Atropinization of a pupil that is miotic because of use of isoflurophate results in a dilated and nonreactive pupil. Intravenous injection of pralidoxime abolishes the miosis, leaving a pupil of normal size and with intact light reaction.

As would be expected, pralidoxime inactivation of echothiophate nullifies the therapeutic effect of the miotic on the facility of aqueous outflow.[258] This was demonstrated by subconjunctival injection of 0.2 ml of a 4% solution of pralidoxime in seven echothiophate-treated glaucomatous eyes. Topical application of a 5% solution of pralidoxime was usually ineffective in neutralizing the echothiophate effect.

Administration. Because topical ocular instillation of oxime solutions is ineffective, subconjunctival injection is advocated. The dose is 0.1 to 0.2 ml of a 5% aqueous solution of pralidoxime. This is an effective antidote to the otherwise prolonged ocular effects of isoflurophate or echothiophate.

Actually, the failure of topical pralidoxime to neutralize the action of cholinesterase inhibitors on the iris sphincter is a result of inadequate transcorneal penetration. Preparation of the drug in a 1:10,000 concentration of benzalkonium enhances penetration, making its topical administration clinically effective (Fig. 12-76).[324]

If applied to the eye before isoflurophate, oximes will protect against miotic action for about 30 minutes. Presumably, after this time the drug is no longer present in a therapeutic concentration. The neutralizing action against isoflurophate is greatest when the oxime is used within 30 minutes after miotic instillation but is demonstrable after a longer period of time. The neutralizing action of oximes does not wear off and does not permit recurrent miosis from the original instillation of isoflurophate.[325]

Stability

As a dry powder, pralidoxime is indefinitely stable at room temperature if the room is kept dark. Aqueous solutions remain effective for 2 weeks at room temperature and for several months under refrigeration.

Clinical use

Pralidoxime may be used to reverse the ocular effects of cholinesterase inhibitors and as an antidote to systemic poisoning by these parasympathomimetic agents.

Neutralization of ocular anticholinesterase effects. The prolonged discomfort resulting from accidental instillation of isoflurophate, echothiophate, and demecarium may be promptly relieved by pralidoxime. Ophthalmoscopic examination of the glaucomatous patient is desirable at periodic intervals or when symptoms referable to the posterior segment of the eye develop. Such fundus examination is aided by miotic neutralization.

Although parasympatholytic drugs such as atropine will also relieve ciliary spasm and mydriasis, these drugs have the disadvantage of causing prolonged cycloplegia and impairing facility of outflow.

Prophylaxis during glaucoma therapy. Theoretically, oral administration of pralidoxime could reverse systemic anticholinesterase toxicity without affecting glaucoma control. This supposition is based on the poor intraocular penetration of pralidoxime. Twenty patients treated with echothiophate for open-angle glaucoma were given 500 mg of pralidoxime three times a day for 3 weeks or every other day for 4 weeks.[326] In no patient did this result in a significant rise of intraocular pressure or in a significant decrease in aqueous outflow. Blood cholinesterase levels increased after therapy by an average of 0.07 unit. The pretreatment cholinesterase levels ranged from 0.18 to 0.87 unit. Except for one patient who developed a rash from the pralidoxime, no toxic effects were identified.

From the clinical viewpoint, the results achieved with this medication do not warrant the bother and expense to the patient. If anticholinesterase toxicity is recognized in any glaucoma patient, the therapy should be stopped or reduced.

As antidote for systemic anticholinesterase poisoning. Since accidental swallowing of eye drops (as by children) could easily be lethal, a brief outline of treatment is in order.[327,328] Comparable therapy is appropriate for insecticide poisoning.

1. Gastric lavage will prevent further absorption of any chemical remaining in the stomach. Since percutaneous absorption occurs, contaminated skin should be washed with water.

2. In severe poisoning, artificial respiration and maintenance of an open airway are essential. Nasopharyngeal and bronchial secretions are increased by parasympathomimetic stimulation and may require removal by suction.

3. Atropine should be given intravenously in the dosage of 2 mg every 5 minutes until the symptoms of parasympathomimetic overdosage disappear and should be repeated whenever such symptoms recur. As much as 50 mg of atropine may be required the first day. Full dilation of the pupils may be used as a criterion in achieving an optimum dose of atropine.

4. Pralidoxime chloride, 1000 mg, should be given slowly intravenously, in not less than 2 to 5 minutes. An additional 500 mg may be given in 30 minutes if muscular weakness is not relieved. Pralidoxime is effective orally, but this route is usually not feasible because of vomiting. In the case of insecticide poisoning, pralidoxime is *not* an effective substitute for atropine.

5. If convulsions block respiration, intravenous administration of barbiturates is recommended. Diazepam (Valium) may be even more effective than barbiturates and is recommended as the drug of choice.

6. Do not use morphine, theophylline, or aminophylline. These drugs accentuate symptoms.

For improved mydriasis. Better dilation of resistant pupils has been reported by a constriction-dilation approach.[329] Miosis resulting from isoflurophate was neutralized by subconjunctival injection of 0.1 to 0.2 ml of a

5% solution of pralidoxime. Subsequent instillation of a 10% solution of phenylephrine and of a 1% solution of atropine caused greater dilation of resistant pupils than could be achieved prior to the isoflurophate and pralidoxime treatment. This greater dilation may be caused by lysis of posterior synechiae by sphincter action or could result from enhanced penetration of the mydriatic into the eye after the trauma of subconjunctival injection.

Toxicity

Intravenous injection of as much as 1800 mg of pralidoxime in normal human adults results in only minor and transient side effects such as dizziness, blurred vision and diplopia, headache, and nausea. These symptoms last for less than 45 minutes. Within an hour after intravenous injection, half of the pralidoxime has already been eliminated, mostly via the urine. Since these doses far exceed the amount used in ocular therapy, no systemic toxicity need be feared after local ophthalmologic use.

The minimal lethal dose of P_2AM is about 100 mg/kg. The LD_{50} dose is 137 mg/kg.[323]

No local toxicity results from subconjunctival injection of 0.2 ml of a 5% solution of pralidoxime chloride, other than the expected mechanical trauma.

SYMPATHOLYTIC AGENTS
Guanethidine (Ismelin)

Guanethidine is a sympatholytic drug that acts by displacing norepinephrine from the sympathetic nerve terminals. For the first few hours after topical ocular administration of 10% guanethidine sulfate, intraocular liberation of norepinephrine occurs. This causes mydriasis and a transitory increase of facility of aqueous outflow. Thereafter the tissue stores of norepinephrine are depleted, resulting in miosis and reduced secretion of aqueous humor. Both of these guanethidine effects lower intraocular pressure.[330,331]

Topical instillation of 10% guanethidine produced significant cosmetic and symptomatic improvement in seven patients with lid retraction associated with thyroid dis-

order. The dosage was 1 to 4 drops daily. The lid-lowering effect of 1 drop appeared about 6 to 8 hours after instillation and lasted for about 1½ days. Apparently the action of guanethidine is cumulative, since a greater effect is achieved after 2 to 3 days of treatment. Miosis occurs in the treated eye.

Horner's syndrome was produced in human eyes by the topical instillation of 10% guanethidine monosulfate three times daily for 1 week. This chemical syndrome is entirely analogous to postganglionic cervical sympathetic denervation in respect to pupillography and testing with cocaine and epinephrine. Horner's syndrome disappeared a week after the guanethidine was discontinued.[332]

6-Hydroxydopamine

6-Hydroxydopamine, an isomer of norepinephrine, has the unique capability of causing selective degeneration of adrenergic nerve terminals without affecting other nerves. It can be used to perform chemical sympathectomy.

The technique of treatment is simply subconjunctival injection, special care being taken to avoid blood vessels—an operating microscope is advised for this purpose. Following injection, a cotton-tipped applicator is used to massage the fluid around the circumference of the limbus. Injection is not made at the 12 o'clock position in order to avoid ptosis from denervation of Müller's muscle.

Only 0.2 ml of a 2% solution is required. The chemical is very unstable and must be freshly dissolved in a 0.045M solution of sodium bisulfite at pH 6.9. Oxidation results in a faint pink discoloration, at which time the solution should be discarded.

Epinephrine therapy should be discontinued 2 days before 6-hydroxydopamine injection, since these drugs are competitive for uptake at the sympathetic terminal.

The local reaction to injection is a moderately severe conjunctival hyperemia, sometimes associated with mild chemosis and lid edema, which persist for several days to a week. The pupil dilates for 2 or 3 hours and then becomes miotic during the first day.

Systemic side effects do not occur, but enough drug enters the general circulation to cause demonstrable but minimal sympathetic supersensitivity in the other eye.

The day following injection a hydroxyamphetamine (Paredrine) test is performed to check the completeness of denervation. Five drops of 1% hydroxyamphetamine given over a period of 1 hour should cause less than 0.5 mm dilation of the pupil if sympathetic denervation is complete. If the sympathectomy is incomplete, glaucoma will not be controlled and another injection need be given.

Sympathetic denervation does not in itself have any effect on glaucoma control. Its only purpose is to induce sympathetic supersensitivity and thereby enhance the pressure-lowering effect of epinephrine. Both the alpha effect (increased outflow) and the beta effect (decreased aqueous secretion) are enhanced.

The effects of treatment in 128 eyes (92 patients) were reported. These patients were selected because their pressures could not be controlled by maximal medical therapy or because they could not tolerate the necessary drugs. The study extended over a 2-year period. Up to 70% of these patients could be controlled (pressures below 20 mm Hg) following sympathectomy. It must be emphasized that while topical epinephrine and pilocarpine therapy was still necessary, it resulted in much better control than before 6-hydroxydopamine injection.

As would be expected, sympathetic terminal regeneration occurs. Chemical sympathectomy must be repeated three or four times a year. The duration of effect varies from a few weeks to 6 months or more.

In general, the authors of the study believe that 6-hydroxydopamine chemical sympathectomy is a reasonable alternative to surgery in the management of glaucoma that is difficult to control.[333-335]

REFERENCES

1. Moses, R. A.: Adler's physiology of the eye, ed. 6, St. Louis, 1975, The C. V. Mosby Co.
2. Koelle, G. B.: Functional anatomy of synaptic transmission, Anesthesiology **29**:643, 1968.
3. Crout, J. R.: Sampling and analysis of catecholamines and metabolites, Anesthesiology **29**:661, 1968.
4. Hanna, C.: Metabolism of catecholamines, Invest. Ophthalmol. **4**:1095, 1965.
5. Kramer, S. G., and Potts, A. M.: Iris uptake of catecholamines in experimental Horner's syndrome, Am. J. Ophthalmol. **67**:705, 1969.
6. Kramer, S. G., and Potts, A. M.: Intraocular pressure and ciliary body norepinephrine uptake in experimental Horner's syndrome, Am. J. Ophthalmol. **68**:1076, 1969.
7. Treister, G., and Bárány, E. H.: Degeneration mydriasis and hyperemia of the iris after superior cervical ganglionectomy in the rabbit, Invest. Ophthalmol. **9**:873, 1970.
8. Neufeld, A. H., Chavis, R. M., and Sears, M. L.: Degeneration release of norepinephrine causes transient ocular hyperemia mediated by prostaglandins, Invest. Ophthalmol. **12**:167, 1973.
9. Leopold, I. H.: Trends in ocular therapy, Am. J. Ophthalmol. **65**:297, 1968.
10. Sears, M. L.: Adrenergic receptors, Arch. Ophthalmol. **74**:150, 1965.
11. Kitazawa, Y.: Topical adrenergic potentiators in primary open-angle glaucoma, Am. J. Ophthalmol. **74**:588, 1972.
12. Gaasterland, D., Kupfer, C., Ross, K., and Gabelnick, H. L.: Studies of aqueous humor dynamics in man, Invest. Ophthalmol. **12**:267, 1973.
13. Macri, F. J.: Local ganglion-like stimulating properties of some adrenergic amines which affect blood vessels of the anterior segment of the eye, Invest. Ophthalmol. **11**:838, 1972.
14. Ross, R. A., and Drance, S. M.: Effects of topically applied isoproterenol on aqueous dynamics in man, Arch. Ophthalmol. **83**:39, 1970.
15. Kronfeld, P. C.: Early effects of single and repeated doses of L-epinephrine in man, Am. J. Ophthalmol. **72**:1058, 1971.
16. van Alphen, G. W. H. M., Kern, R., and Robinette, S. L.: Adrenergic receptors of the intraocular muscles, Arch. Ophthalmol. **74**:253, 1965.
17. Ehinger, B.: Double innervation of the feline iris dilator, Arch. Ophthalmol. **77**:541, 1967.
18. Geltzer, A. I.: Autonomic innervation, Arch. Ophthalmol. **81**:70, 1969.

19. Kramer, S. G., Potts, A. M., and Mangnall, Y.: Autoradiographic localization of catecholamines in the uveal tract, Am. J. Ophthalmol. **74:**129, 1972.

20. Fukuda, M.: Presence of adrenergic innervation to the retinal vessels: a histochemical study, Jpn. J. Ophthalmol. **14:**91, 1970.

21. Chandra, S. R., and Friedman, E.: Choroidal blood flow, Arch. Ophthalmol. **87:**67, 1972.

22. Best, M., Masket, S., and Rabinovitz, A. Z.: Effect of sympathetic stimulation on ocular hemodynamics, Invest. Ophthalmol. **11:** 211, 1972.

23. Van Dyke, H. B.: Autonomic nervous system and action of drugs important in ophthalmology, Arch. Ophthalmol. **38:**145, 1947.

24. Guyton, J. S.: Pharmacodynamics of the intraocular muscles, Arch. Ophthalmol. **24:** 555, 1940.

25. Leopold, I. H.: Ocular cholinesterase and cholinesterase inhibitors, Am. J. Ophthalmol. **51:**885, 1962.

26. Nickerson, M.: Adrenergic mediators, Invest. Ophthalmol. **4:**1085, 1965.

27. Kopin, I.: Biosynthesis and metabolism of catecholamines, Anesthesiology **29:**654, 1968.

28. Zeller, E. A., Shoch, D., Cooperman, S. G., and Schnipper, R. I.: Enzymology of the refractory media of the eye, Invest. Ophthalmol. **6:**618, 1967.

29. Mehra, K. S., Roy, P. N., and Singh, R.: Pargyline drops in glaucoma, Arch. Ophthalmol. **92:**453, December 1974.

30. Mustakallio, A.: Monoamine oxidase activity in the various structures of the mammalian eye, Acta Ophthalmol. **93**(suppl.):1, 1967.

31. Sneddon, J. M., and Turner, P.: The interactions of local guanethidine and sympathomimetic amines in the human eye, Arch. Ophthalmol. **81:**622, 1969.

32. van Alphen, G. W. H. M., Robinette, S. L., and Macri, F. J.:Drug effects on ciliary muscle and choroid preparations in vitro, Arch. Ophthalmol. **68:**81, 1962.

33. Morgan, W. E., III, and Macri, F. J.: Vascular responses of the posterior segment of the cat eye, Arch. Ophthalmol. **79:**779, 1968.

34. Hartgraves, H., and Kronfeld, P. C.: The synergistic action of atropine and epinephrine on the intrinsic muscles of the eye, Arch. Ophthalmol. **5:**212, 1931.

35. Hurwitz, B. S., Davidowitz, J., Chin, N. B., and Breinin, G. M.: The effects of the sympathetic nervous system on accommodation, Arch. Ophthalmol. **67:**668, 1972.

36. Swan, K. C.: Ocular penetration of procaine following subconjunctival injection, Arch. Ophthalmol. **52:**774, 1954.

37. Feldman, L. A., and Sherman, H.: Hypersensitiveness of mucous membranes: slit lamp studies of conjunctival reactions induced in normal and in atopic persons with histamine, ethylmorphine, and atopens, Arch. Ophthalmol. **29:**989, 1943.

38. Havener, W. H.: Differential diagnosis of the red eye, Ohio Med. J. **52:**836, 1956.

39. Gazala, J. R., and Guerry, D., III: On the definition of the aqueous veins, Am. J. Ophthalmol. **66:**532, 1968.

40. Angenent, W.: Destruction of epinephrine by the dopa-oxidase system of ocular tissue, Science **116:**543, 1953.

41. Patil, P. N., and Jacobowitz, D.: Unequal accumulation of adrenergic drugs by pigmented and nonpigmented iris, Am. J. Ophthalmol. **78:**470, September 1974.

42. Sachs, E., and Heath, P.: The pharmacological behavior of the intraocular muscles, Am. J. Ophthalmol. **23:**1376, 1940.

43. Becker, B., Gage, T., Kolker, A. E., and Gay, A. J.: The effect of phenylephrine hydrochloride on the miotic-treated eye, Am. J. Ophthalmol. **48:**313, 1959.

44. Garner, L. L., Johnstone, W. W., Ballintine, E., and Carroll, M. E.: Effect of 2% levorotary epinephrine on the intraocular pressure of the glaucomatous eye, Arch. Ophthalmol. **62:**230, 1959.

45. Obstbaum, S. A., Kolker, A. E., and Phelps, C. D.: Low-dose epinephrine, Arch. Ophthalmol. **92:**118, August 1974.

46. Becker, B., and Morton, W. R.: Topical epinephrine in glaucoma suspects, Am. J. Ophthalmol. **62:**272, 1966.

47. Criswick, F. G., and Drance, S. M.: Comparative study of four different epinephrine salts on intraocular pressure, Arch. Ophthalmol. **75:**768, 1966.

48. Becker, B.: Additive effect of epinephrine and acetazolamide in control of intraocular pressure, Am. J. Ophthalmol. **45:**639, 1958.

49. Weekers, R., Dilmarcelle, Y., and Gustin, J.: Treatment of ocular hypertension by adrenaline and diverse sympathomimetic amines, Am. J. Ophthalmol. **40:**666, 1955.

50. Becker, B., Petitt, T. H., and Gay, A. J.: Topical epinephrine therapy of open-angle glaucoma, Arch. Ophthalmol. **66:**219, 1961.

51. Ballintine, E. J., and Garner, L.: Improve-

ment of the coefficient of outflow in glaucomatous eyes, Arch. Ophthalmol. 66:314, 1961.

52. Sears, M. L., and Sherk, T. E.: The trabecular effect of noradrenalin in the rabbit eye, Invest. Ophthalmol. 3:157, 1964.

53. Bárány, E. H.: Topical epinephrine effects on true outflow resistance and pseudofacility in vervet monkeys studied by a new anterior chamber perfusion technique, Invest. Ophthalmol. 7:88, 1968.

54. Krill, A. E., Newell, F. W., and Novak, M.: Early and long-term effects of levo-epinephrine, Am. J. Ophthalmol. 59:833, 1965.

55. Harris, L. S., Mittag, T. W., and Galin, M. A.: Aqueous dynamics of pilocarpine-treated eyes, Arch. Ophthalmol. 86:1, 1971.

56. Kitazawa, Y., Nose, H., and Horie, T.: Chemical sympathectomy with 6-hydroxydopamine in the treatment of primary open-angle glaucoma, Am. J. Ophthalmol. 79:98, January 1975.

57. Green, J.: Two percent epinephrine solutions as substitutes for levo-glaukosan, Arch. Ophthalmol. 5:350, 1931.

58. Post, L. T.: Levo-glaukosan and epinephrine bitartrate in the treatment of glaucoma, Arch. Ophthalmol. 11:187, 1934.

59. Howell, S. C.: Action of epinephrine on the normal human eye, Arch. Ophthalmol. 12:833, 1934.

60. Howell, S. C.: Action of epinephrine on the diseased human eye, Arch. Ophthalmol. 16:1018, 1936.

61. Jammes, J. L., and Nigam, M. P.: Pupillary autonomic functions in heterochromia iridis, Arch. Ophthalmol. 89:291, 1973.

62. Goodman, L., and Gilman, A.: The pharmacological basis of therapeutics, ed. 4, New York, 1970, Macmillan Publishing Co., Inc.

63. Lansche, R. K.: Systemic reactions: to topical epinephrine and phenylephrine, Am. J. Ophthalmol. 61:95, 1966.

64. McReynolds, W. U., Havener, W. H., and Henderson, J. W.: Hazards of use of sympathomimetic drugs in ophthalmology, Arch. Ophthalmol. 56:176, 1956.

65. Katz, R. L.: The interaction of anesthetic agents and adrenergic drugs to produce cardiac arrhythmias, Anesthesiology 29:763, 1968.

66. Ballin, N., Becker, B., and Goldman, M.: Systemic effects of epinephrine applied topically to the eye, Invest. Ophthalmol. 5:125, 1966.

67. Lichter, P. R., and Bergstrom, T. J.: Premature ventricular systole detection by applanation tonometry, Am. J. Ophthalmol. 81:797, June 1976.

68. Vaughan, D., Shaffer, R., and Riegelman, S.: A new stabilized form of epinephrine for the treatment of open-angle glaucoma, Arch. Ophthalmol. 66:232, 1961.

69. Krejci, L., and Harrison, R.: Epinephrine effects on corneal cells in tissue culture, Arch. Ophthalmol. 83:451, 1970.

70. Hull, D. S., Chemotti, T., Edelhauser, H. F., Van Horn, D. L., and Hyndiuk, R. A.: Effect of epinephrine on the corneal endothelium, Am. J. Ophthalmol. 79:245, February 1975.

71. Byron, H. M.: Conjunctival reaction due to 1-epinephrine bitartrate (Epitrate), Arch. Ophthalmol. 63:567, 1960.

72. Aronson, S. B., and Yamamoto, E. A.: Ocular hypersensitivity to epinephrine, Invest. Ophthalmol. 5:75, 1966.

73. Aronson, S. B., and Sassetti, R.: Experimental ocular hypersensitivity to polyepinephrine and its analogues, Invest. Ophthalmol. 9:12, 1970.

74. Kass, M. A., Stamper, R. L., and Becker, B.: Madarosis in chronic epinephrine therapy, Arch. Ophthalmol. 88:429, 1972.

75. Corwin, M. E., and Spencer, W. H.: Conjunctival melanin depositions, Arch. Ophthalmol. 69:317, 1963.

76. Reinecke, R. D., and Kuwabara, T.: Corneal deposits secondary to topical epinephrine, Arch. Ophthalmol. 70:170, 1963.

77. Donaldson, D. D.: Epinephrine pigmentation of the cornea, Arch. Ophthalmol. 78:74, 1967.

78. Krejci, L., and Harrison, R.: Corneal pigment deposits from topically administered epinephrine, Arch. Ophthalmol. 82:836, 1969.

79. Madge, G. E., Geeraets, W. J., and Guerry, D., III: Black cornea secondary to topical epinephrine, Am. J. Ophthalmol. 71:402, 1971.

80. Ferry, A. P., and Zimmerman, L. E.: Black cornea: a complication of topical use of epinephrine, Am. J. Ophthalmol. 58:205, 1964.

81. Ferry, J. F.: Black prosthesis, Am. J. Ophthalmol. 64:162, 1967.

82. Miller, D., Brooks, S. M., and Mobilia, E.: Adrenochrome staining of soft contact lenses, Ann. Ophthalmol. 8:65, January 1976.

83. Zuckerman, B. D.: Conjunctiva pigmentation due to cosmetics, Am. J. Ophthalmol. **62:**672, 1966.

84. Kolker, A. E., and Becker, B.: Epinephrine maculopathy, Arch. Ophthalmol. **79:**552, 1968.

85. François, J., Jonsas, C., and DeRouck, A.: Studies of the effect of levorenine, Am. J. Ophthalmol. **68:**119, 1969.

86. Irvine, A. R.: Cystoid maculopathy, Surv. Ophthalmol. **21:**1, July-August 1976.

87. Obstbaum, S. A., Galin, M. A., and Poole, T. A.: Topical epinephrine and cystoid macular edema, Ann. Ophthalmol. **8:**455, April 1976.

88. Michels, R. G., and Maumenee, A. E.: Cystoid macular edema associated with topically applied epinephrine in aphakic eyes, Am. J. Ophthalmol. **80:**379, September 1975.

89. Laibson, P. R., and Kibrick, S.: Reactivation of herpetic keratitis by epinephrine in rabbit, Arch. Ophthalmol. **75:**254, 1966.

90. Sellers, M. I.: Medical Tribune, Monday, July 14, 1961.

91. Pollack, I. P., and Rossi, H.: Norepinephrine in treatment of ocular hypertension and glaucoma, Arch. Ophthalmol. **93:**173, March 1975.

92. Kaback, M. B., Podos, S. M., Harbin, T. S., Jr., Mandell, A., and Becker, B.: The effects of dipivalyl epinephrine on the eye, Am. J. Ophthalmol. **81:**768, June 1976.

93. Bietti, G., Virno, M., Pecori-Giraldi, J., Pellegrino, N., and Motolese, E.: Possibility of isoproterenol therapy with soft contact lenses: ocular hypotension without systemic effects, Ann. Ophthalmol. **8:**819, July 1976.

94. Solosko, D., and Smith, R. B.: Hypertension following 10 percent phenylephrine ophthalmic, Anesthesiology **36:**187, 1972.

95. Wilensky, J. T., and Woodward, H. J.: Acute systemic hypertension after conjunctival instillation of phenylephrine hydrochloride, Am. J. Ophthalmol. **76:**156, 1973.

96. Haddad, N. J., Moyer, N. J., and Riley, F. C., Jr.: Mydriatic effect of phenylephrine hydrochloride, Am. J. Ophthalmol. **70:**729, 1970.

97. Biggs, R. A., Alpern, M., and Bennett, D. R.: The effect of sympathomimetic drugs upon the amplitude of accommodation, Am. J. Ophthalmol. **48:**169, 1959.

98. Korczyn, A. D., Laor, N., and Nemet, P.: Sympathetic pupillary tone in old age, Arch. Ophthalmol. **94:**1905, November 1976.

99. Barbee, R. F., and Smith, W. O.: A comparative study of mydriatic and cycloplegic agents, Am. J. Ophthalmol. **44:**617, 1957.

100. De Ocampo, G., and Lim-Catipon, P.: Phenylephrine pack for flat anterior chamber following cataract extraction, Am. J. Ophthalmol. **66:**881, 1968.

101. Weiss, D. I., and Shaffer, R. N.: Mydriatic effects of one-eighth percent phenylephrine, Arch. Ophthalmol. **68:**727, 1962.

102. Lee, P. F.: The influence of epinephrine and phenylephrine on intraocular pressure, Arch. Ophthalmol. **60:**863, 1958.

103. Chin, N. B., Gold, A. A., and Breinin, G.: Iris cysts and miotics, Arch. Ophthalmol. **71:**611, 1964.

104. Putterman, A. M., and Urist, M. J.: Müller muscle-conjunctiva resection, Arch. Ophthalmol. **93:**619, August 1975.

105. Thompson, H. S., and Mensher, J. H.: Adrenergic mydriasis in Horner's syndrome, Am. J. Ophthalmol. **72:**472, 1971.

106. Fink, A. I., Funahashi, T., Robinson, M., and Watson, R.: Conjunctival blood flow in sickle cell disease, Arch. Ophthalmol. **66:**824, 1961.

107. Mitsui, Y., Takagi, Y., and Machi, K.: Nature of aqueous floaters due to sympathomimetic mydriatics, Arch. Ophthalmol. **65:**626, 1961.

108. Edelhauser, H., and Van Horn, D.: Personal communication.

109. Mindel, J. S.: Hydroxyamphetamine test in Horner's syndrome, Am. J. Ophthalmol. **79:**523, March 1975.

110. Patil, P. N.: Cocaine binding by the pigmented and the nonpigmented iris and its relevance to the mydriatic effect, from the College of Pharmacy, Ohio State University (experimental work).

111. Wolfe, A. V., and Hodge, H. C.: Effects of atropine sulfate, methylatropine nitrate (Metropine) and homatropine hydrobromide on adult human eyes, Arch. Ophthalmol. **36:**293, 1946.

112. Riker, W. F.: Contributions to medicine by research in pharmacology, J.A.M.A. **179:**355, 1962.

113. Janes, R. G., and Stiles, J. F.: The penetration of C^{14} labeled atropine into the eye, Arch. Ophthalmol. **62:**69, 1959.

114. Duke-Elder, S., editor: System of ophthal-

mology, vol. 7, St. Louis, 1962, The C. V. Mosby Co.

115. Sharon, I. M.: The clinical significance of atropinesterase, Invest. Ophthalmol. 3:461, 1964.

116. Patil, P. N.: Iris pigmentation and atropine mydriasis, Pharmacologist 16:311, 1974.

117. van Alphen, G. W. H. M., and Macri, F. J.: Entrance of fluorescein into aqueous humor of cat eye, Arch. Ophthalmol. 75:247, 1966.

118. Marron, J.: Cycloplegia and mydriasis by use of atropine, scopolamine, and homatropineparedrine, Arch. Ophthalmol. 23:340, 1940.

119. Havener, W. H., and Harris, W. R.: The management of suppression amblyopia, Am. Orthopt. J. 2:5, 1961.

120. Gimbel, H. V.: The control of myopia with atropine, Can. J. Ophthalmol. 8:527, 1973.

121. Popkin, M. K.: 'Angel's trumpet' provides deadly thrills for youth, J.A.M.A. 236:249, July 19, 1976.

122. Harris, L. S.: Cycloplegic-induced intraocular pressure elevations, Arch. Ophthalmol. 79:242, 1968.

123. Gorin, G.: Glaucoma induced by prolonged use of atropine, Am. J. Ophthalmol. 56:639, 1963.

124. Hilding, A. C.: Pupillary blockage by a subluxated lens, causing glaucoma, Am. J. Ophthalmol. 57:33, 1957.

125. Thorne, F. H., and Murphey, H. S.: Cycloplegics, Arch. Ophthalmol. 22:274, 1939.

126. Fry, G. A.: The effect of homatropine upon accommodation/convergence relations, Am. J. Optom. 36:525, 1959.

127. Bárány, E., and Christensen, R. E.: Cycloplegia and outflow resistance in normal human and monkey eyes and in primary open-angle glaucoma, Arch. Ophthalmol. 77:757, 1967.

128. Christensen, R. E., and Pearce, I.: Homatropine hydrobromide, Arch. Ophthalmol. 70:376, 1963.

129. Doczy, L.: A comparison of the action of atropine and scopolamine producing cycloplegia, Klin. Monatbl. Augenheilkd. 138:398, 1961.

130. Freund, M., and Merin, S.: Toxic effects of scopolamine eye drops, Am. J. Ophthalmol. 70:637, 1970.

131. Young, S. E., Ruiz, R. S., and Falletta, J.: Reversal of systemic toxic effects of scopolamine with physostigmine salicylate, Am. J. Ophthalmol. 72:1136, 1971.

132. Priestley, B. S., and Medine, M. M.: A new mydriatic and cycloplegic drug, Am. J. Ophthalmol. 34:572, 1951.

133. Gettes, B. C.: Three new cycloplegic drugs, Arch. Ophthalmol. 51:467, 1954.

134. Daily, L., and Coe, R.: Lack of effect of anesthetic and mydriatic solutions on the curvature of the cornea, Am. J. Ophthalmol. 53:49, 1962.

135. Schimek, R. A., and Lieberman, W. J.: The influence of Cyclogyl and Neo-Synephrine on tonographic studies of miotic control in open-angle glaucoma, Am. J. Ophthalmol. 51:871, 1961.

136. Gartner, S., and Billet, E.: Mydriatic glaucoma, Am. J. Ophthalmol. 43:975, 1957.

137. Lipsich, M. P.: Effect of cyclopentolate on the aqueous dynamics of iridectomized eyes, Am. J. Ophthalmol. 66:543, 1968.

138. Simcoe, C. W.: Cyclopentolate (Cyclogyl) toxicity, Arch. Ophthalmol. 67:406, 1962.

139. Binkhorst, R. D., Weinstein, G. W., Baretz, R. M., and Clahane, A. C.: Psychotic reaction induced by cyclopentolate (Cyclogyl), Am. J. Ophthalmol. 55:1243, 1963.

140. Beswick, J. A.: Psychosis from cyclopentolate, Am. J. Ophthalmol. 53:879, 1962.

141. Awan, K. J.: Systemic toxicity of cyclopentolate hydrochloride in adults following topical ocular instillation, Ann. Ophthalmol. 8:803, July 1976.

142. Ostler, H. B.: Cycloplegics and mydriatics, Arch. Ophthalmol. 93:432, June 1975.

143. Kingham, J. D.: Acute retrolental fibroplasia, Arch. Ophthalmol. 95:39, January 1977.

144. Gettes, B.: Tropicamide, a new cycloplegic mydriatic, Arch. Ophthalmol. 65:632, 1961.

145. Gambill, H. D., Ogle, K. N., and Kearns, T. P.: Mydriatic effect of four drugs determined with pupillograph, Arch. Ophthalmol. 77:740, 1967.

146. Portney, G. L., and Purcell, T. W.: The influence of tropicamide on intraocular pressure, Ann. Ophthalmol. 7:31, January 1975.

147. Gettes, B., and Belmont, O.: Tropicamide: comparative cycloplegic effects, Arch. Ophthalmol. 66:336, 1961.

148. Milder, B.: Tropicamide as a cycloplegic agent, Arch. Ophthalmol. 66:70, 1961.

149. Havener, W. H., and Falls, H. F.: Oxyphenonium (Antrenyl), Arch. Ophthalmol. 52:515, 1954.

150. Wolter, J. R., and O'Keefe, N. T.: Localization of nerve endings in relation to cholines-

terase deposits in normal human eye muscles, Invest. Ophthalmol. **2**:558, 1963.

151. Leopold, I. H.: Cholinesterases, Am. J. Ophthalmol. **62**:771, 1966.
152. Barraquer, J. I.: Acetylcholine as a miotic agent for use in surgery, Am. J. Ophthalmol. **57**:406, 1964.
153. Rizzuti, A. B.: Acetylcholine in surgery of the lens, iris and cornea, Am. J. Ophthalmol. **63**:484, 1967.
154. Ray, R. R.: Use of acetylcholine in peripheral iridectomy, Am. J. Ophthalmol. **60**:728, 1965.
155. Harley, R. D., and Mishler, J. E.: Acetylcholine in cataract surgery, Br. J. Ophthalmol. **50**:429, 1966.
156. Hartmann, E.: Acetylcholine in ophthalmology and the treatment of ocular pain, Arch. Ophthalmol. **28**:599, 1942.
157. Payne, I. W., and Reed, H.: Ocular palsies following retrobulbar injection of acetylcholine for retinal arterial occlusion, Br. J. Ophthalmol. **38**:46, 1954.
158. Babinski, M., Smith, R. B., and Wickerham, E. P.: Hypotension and bradycardia following intraocular acetylcholine injection, Arch. Ophthalmol. **94**:675, April 1976.
159. Morrison, W. H.: Stability of aqueous solutions commonly employed in the treatment of primary glaucoma, Am. J. Ophthalmol. **37**:391, 557, 744, 1954.
160. Gay, A. J.: Comments on Goldberg et al.'s article in December, 1968 issue, Arch. Ophthalmol. **81**:601, 1969.
161. Laties, A. M., and Scheie, H. G.: Adie's syndrome: duration of methacholine sensitivity, Arch. Ophthalmol. **74**:458, 1965.
162. Hedges, T. R., Jr.: The tonic pupil, Arch. Ophthalmol. **80**:21, 1968.
163. Smith, A. A., Dancis, J., and Breinin, G.: Ocular responses to autonomic drugs in familial dysautonomia, Invest. Ophthalmol. **4**:358, 1965.
164. O'Brien, C. S., and Swan, K. C.: Carbaminoylcholine chloride in the treatment of glaucoma simplex, Arch. Ophthalmol. **27**:253, 1942.
165. McDonald, T. O., Beasley, C., Borgmann, A., and Roberts, D.: Intraocular administration of carbamylcholine chloride, Ann. Ophthalmol. **1**:232, 1969.
166. Yamauchi, D. N., DeSantis, L., and Path, P. N.: Relative potency of cholinomimetic drugs on the bovine iris sphincter strips, Invest. Ophthalmol. **12**:80, 1973.
167. McDonald, T. O., Roberts, M. D., and

168. Borgmann, A. R.: Intraocular safety of carbamylcholine chloride (carbachol) in rabbit eyes, Ann. Ophthalmol. **2**:878, 1970.
168. Goldstein, A. M., dePalau, A., and Botelho, S. Y.: Inhibition and facilitation of pilocarpine-induced lacrimal flow by norepinephrine. Invest. Ophthalmol. **6**:498, 1967.
169. Sjögren, H.: Some problems concerning keratoconjunctivitis sicca and sicca-syndrome, Acta Ophthalmol. **29**:33, 1951.
170. Potts, A.: Physiological chemistry of the eye, Arch. Ophthalmol. **66**:578, 1961.
171. Müller, H. K., Hockwin, O., and Kleifeld, O.: Die Bestimmung von Pilocarpin in menschlichen Kammerwasser mit Hilfe der Polarographie, Graefes Arch. Klin. Exp. Ophthalmol. **162**:107, 1960.
172. Asseff, C. F., Weisman, R. L., Podos, S. M., and Becker, B.: Ocular penetration of pilocarpine in primates, Am. J. Ophthalmol. **75**:212, 1973.
173. Ramer, R. M., and Gasset, A. R.: Ocular penetration of pilocarpine: the effect of multiple doses on the ocular penetration of pilocarpine, Ann. Ophthalmol. **7**:25, January 1975.
174. Törnqvist, G.: Effect on refraction of intramuscular pilocarpine in two species of monkey (Cercopithecus aethiops and Macaca irus), Invest. Ophthalmol. **4**:211, 1965.
175. Törnqvist, G.: Accommodation in monkeys, Acta Ophthalmol. **45**:429, 1967.
176. Törnqvist, G.: Comparative studies of the effect of pilocarpine on the pupil and on the refraction in two species of monkey (Cercopithecus ethiops and Macaca irus), Invest. Ophthalmol. **3**:388, 1964.
177. Swan, K. C., and Gehrsitz, L.: Competitive action of miotics on the iris sphincter, Arch. Ophthalmol. **46**:477, 1951.
178. Lowenstein, O., and Loewenfeld, I. E.: Effect of physostigmine and pilocarpine on iris sphincter of normal man, Arch. Ophthalmol. **50**:311, 1953.
179. Lowenstein, O.: The Argyll Robertson pupillary syndrome, Am. J. Ophthalmol. **42**:105, 1956.
180. Schonberg, S. S., and Ellis, P. P.: Pilocarpine inactivation, Arch. Ophthalmol. **82**:351, 1969.
181. van Alphen, G. W. H. M.: The structural changes in miosis and mydriasis of the monkey eye, Arch. Ophthalmol. **69**:802, 1963.
182. Rones, B.: A mechanistic element in trabecular function, Am. J. Ophthalmol. **45**:189, 1958.

183. Flocks, M., and Zweng, H. C.: Studies on the mode of action of pilocarpine on aqueous outflow, Am. J. Ophthalmol. **44**:380, 1957.

184. François, J., Rabaey, M., Neetens, A., and Evens, L.: Further perfusion studies on the outflow of aqueous humor in human eyes, Arch. Ophthalmol. **59**:683, 1958.

185. Ashton, N.: Anatomical study of Schlemm's canal and aqueous veins by means of neoprene casts. I. Aqueous veins, Br. J. Ophthalmol. **35**:291, 1951.

186. Ashton, N.: Anatomical study of Schlemm's canal and aqueous veins by means of neoprene casts. II. Aqueous veins, Br. J. Ophthalmol. **36**:265, 1952.

187. Ashton, N., Brini, A., and Smith, R.: Anatomical studies of the trabecular meshwork of the normal human eye, Br. J. Ophthalmol. **40**:257, 1956.

188. Theobald, G. D.: Further studies on the canal of Schlemm, Am. J. Ophthalmol. **39**:65, 1955.

189. François, J., Neetens, A., and Collette, J. M.: Microradiographic study of the inner wall of Schlemm's canal, Am. J. Ophthalmol. **40**:491, 1955.

190. Flocks, M.: The anatomy of the trabecular meshwork as seen in tangential section, Arch. Ophthalmol. **56**:708, 1956.

191. Holmberg, A., and Bárány, E. H.: The effect of pilocarpine on the endothelium forming the inner wall of Schlemm's canal: an electronmicroscope study in the monkey Cercopithecus aethiops, Invest. Ophthalmol. **5**:53, 1966.

192. Abramson, D. H., Chang, S., Coleman, J., and Smith, M. E.: Pilocarpine-induced lens changes, Arch. Ophthalmol. **92**:464, December 1974.

193. Abramson, D. H., Chang, S., and Coleman, J.: Pilocarpine therapy in glaucoma, Arch. Ophthalmol. **94**:914, June 1976.

194. Bárány, E. H.: The mode of action of pilocarpine on outflow resistance in the eye of a primate (Cercopithecus ethiops), Invest. Ophthalmol. **1**:712, 1962.

195. Bárány, E. H.: The immediate effect on outflow resistance of intravenous pilocarpine in the vervet monkey, Cercopithecus ethiops, Invest. Ophthalmol. **6**:373, 1967.

196. Krill, A. E., and Newell, F. W.: Effects of pilocarpine on ocular tension dynamics, Am. J. Ophthalmol. **57**:34, 1964.

197. Fenton, R. H., and Schwartz, B.: The effect of 2% pilocarpine on the normal and glaucomatous eye. I. The time response of pressure, Invest. Ophthalmol. **2**:289, 1963.

198. Harris, L. S., and Galin, M. A.: Dose response analysis of pilocarpine-induced ocular hypotension, Arch. Ophthalmol. **84**:605, 1970.

199. Lyons, J. S., and Krohn, D. L.: Pilocarpine uptake by pigmented uveal tissue, Am. J. Ophthalmol. **75**:885, 1973.

200. Patil, P. N.: Cocaine binding by the pigmented and nonpigmented iris and its relevance to the mydriatic effect, Invest. Ophthalmol. **11**:739, 1972.

201. Seidehamel, R. J., Tye, A., and Patil, P. N.: An analysis of ephedrine in relationship to iris pigmentation in the guinea pig eye in vitro, J. Pharmacol. Exp. Ther. **171**:205, 1970.

202. Harris, L. S., and Galin, M. A.: Effect of ocular pigmentation on hypotensive response to pilocarpine, Am. J. Ophthalmol. **72**:923, 1971.

203. Berggren, L.: Effect of composition of medium and of metabolic inhibitors on secretion in vitro by the ciliary processes of the rabbit eye, Invest. Ophthalmol. **4**:83, 1965.

204. Berggren, L.: Effect of parasympathomimetic and sympathomimetic drugs on secretion in vitro by the ciliary processes of the rabbit eye, Invest. Ophthalmol. **4**:91, 1965.

205. Walinder, P.: Influence of pilocarpine on iodopyracet and iodide accumulation by rabbit ciliary body-iris preparations, Invest. Ophthalmol. **5**:378, 1966.

206. Vale, J., and Bárány, E. H.: Effects of phenylephrine, butylsympatol, pilocarpine, and lithium on runout of ^{86}Rb from isolated rabbit ciliary processes, Invest. Ophthalmol. **8**:422, 1969.

207. Gartner, S.: Blood vessels of conjunctiva, Arch. Ophthalmol. **32**:464, 1944.

208. Ascher, K. W.: Aqueous veins, Am. J. Ophthalmol. **25**:1301, 1942.

209. Stocker, F. W.: Experimental studies on the blood-aqueous barrier, Arch. Ophthalmol. **37**:583, 1947.

210. Swan, K., and Hart, W.: A comparative study of the effects of Mecholyl, Doryl, eserine, pilocarpine, atropine, and epinephrine on the blood-aqueous barrier, Am. J. Ophthalmol. **23**:1311, 1940.

211. Abraham, S. V.: Miotic iridocyclitis: its role in the surgical treatment of glaucoma, Am. J. Ophthalmol. **48**:634, 1959.

212. MacDonald, R., Jr., Keller, K. F., Blatt, M.

M., and Cox, H. B.: Sterility and concentration of pilocarpine solutions, Am. J. Ophthalmol. **68:**1099, 1969.

213. Drance, S. M., and Bensted, M.: Pilocarpine and intraocular pressure, Arch. Ophthalmol. **91:**104, February 1974.

214. Brounley, D. W.: A comparison of pilocarpine hydrochloride and epinephrine bitartrate, Ann. Ophthalmol. **3:**970, 1971.

215. Barsam, P. C.: Comparison of the effect of pilocarpine and echothiophate on intraocular pressure and outflow facility, Am. J. Ophthalmol. **73:**742, 1972.

216. Scheie, H., and Day, R. M.: Simulated progression of visual field defects of glaucoma, Arch. Ophthalmol. **50:**418, 1953.

217. Forbes, M.: Influence of miotics on visual fields in glaucoma, Invest. Ophthalmol. **5:**139, 1966.

218. Flocks, M.: The pathology of the trabecular meshwork in primary open-angle glaucoma, Am. J. Ophthalmol. **47:**519, 1959.

219. Tyner, G., and Scheie, H.: Mechanism of the miotic-resistant pupil with increased intraocular pressure, Arch. Ophthalmol. **50:**572, 1953.

220. Winter, F. C.: The second eye in acute, primary, shallow-chamber angle glaucoma, Am. J. Ophthalmol. **40:**557, 1955.

221. Anastasi, L. M., Ogle, K. N., and Kearns, T. P.: Effect of pilocarpine in counteracting mydriasis, Arch. Ophthalmol. **79:**710, 1968.

222. Bleeker, G. M.: Evaluation of three methods of recording the anterior chamber depth of the eye, Arch. Ophthalmol. **65:**369, 1961.

223. Wilkie, J.: Miotics and chamber depth, Am. J. Ophthalmol. **68:**78, 1969.

224. Abramson, D. H., Franzen, L. A., and Coleman, D. J.: Pilocarpine in the presbyope, Arch. Ophthalmol. **89:**100, 1973.

225. Abramson, D. H., Coleman, D., Forbes, M., and Franzen, L. A.: Pilocarpine effect on the anterior chamber and lens thickness, Arch. Ophthalmol. **87:**615, 1972.

226. Scheie, H. G., and Williams, N. S.: Comparative studies on anesthetic properties of primacaine HCl, Arch. Ophthalmol. **59:**81, 1958.

227. Chan, P. H., and Havener, W. H.: Factors of importance in traumatic hyphema, Am. J. Ophthalmol. **55:**591, 1963.

228. Thompson, H. S., Newsome, D. A., and Loewenfeld, I. E.: The fixed dilated pupil, Arch. Ophthalmol. **86:**21, 1971.

229. Cohen, D. N., and Zakov, Z. N.: The diagnosis of Adie's pupil using 0.0625% pilocarpine solution, Am. J. Ophthalmol. **79:**883, May 1975.

230. Pilley, S. F. J., and Thompson, H. S.: Cholinergic supersensitivity in Adie's syndrome: pilocarpine vs. Mecholyl, Am. J. Ophthalmol. **80:**955, November 1975.

231. Epstein, E., and Kaufman, I.: Systemic pilocarpine toxicity from overdosage, Am. J. Ophthalmol. **59:**109, 1965.

232. Shaffer, R. N., and Ridgway, W. L.: Furmethide iodide in the production of dacryostenosis, Am. J. Ophthalmol. **34:**718, 1951.

233. Owens, E. U., and Woods, A. C.: The use of Furmethide in comparison with pilocarpine and eserine for the treatment of glaucoma, Am. J. Ophthalmol. **30:**995, 1947.

234. Goodwin, R. C.: Changes in the intraocular pressure in normal and glaucomatous eyes following Furmethide, Am. J. Ophthalmol. **34:**1139, 1951.

235. Drance, S. M., Fairclough, M., and Schulzer, M.: Response of human intraocular pressure to aceclidine, Arch. Ophthalmol. **88:**394, 1972.

236. Fechner, P. U., Teichmann, K. D., and Weyrauch, W.: Accommodative effects of aceclidine in the treatment of glaucoma, Am. J. Ophthalmol. **79:**104, January 1975.

237. Fincham, E. F.: The proportion of ciliary muscular force required for accommodation, J. Physiol. **128:**99, 1955.

238. Loewenfeld, I. E.: The iris as pharmacologic indicator, Arch. Ophthalmol. **70:**42, 1963.

239. Pilger, I. S.: Familial dysautonomia, Am. J. Ophthalmol. **43:**285, 1957.

240. Hussey, H. H.: Physostigmine: value in treatment of central toxic effects of anticholinergic drugs, J.A.M.A. **231:**1066, March 10, 1975.

241. Duvoisin, R. C., and Katz, R.: Reversal of central anticholinergic syndrome in man by physostigmine, J.A.M.A. **206:**1963, 1968.

242. Rodin, F. H.: Eserine: its history in the practice of ophthalmology, Am. J. Ophthalmol. **30:**19, 1947.

243. Lebensohn, J. E.: The first miotic, Am. J. Ophthalmol. **55:**657, 1963.

244. Jacklin, H. N.: Depigmentation of the eyelids in eserine allergy, Am. J. Ophthalmol. **59:**89, 1964.

245. Osserman, K. E., and Teng, P.: Studies in myasthenia gravis—a rapid diagnostic test, J.A.M.A. **160:**153, 1956.

246. Borucho, S. A., and Goldberg, B.: Edrophonium (Tensilon) in diagnosis of ocular myasthenia gravis, Arch. Ophthalmol. **53:**718, 1955.

247. Kearns, T. P.: Neuro-ophthalmology, Arch. Ophthalmol. **76:**746, 1966.

248. Glaser, J. S.: Tensilon tonography in the diagnosis of myasthenia gravis, Invest. Ophthalmol. **6:**135, 1967.

249. Glaser, J. S., Miller, G. R., and Gass, D. M.: The edrophonium tonogram test in myasthenia gravis, Arch. Ophthalmol. **76:**368, 1966.

250. Glaser, J. S.: Myasthenic pseudo-internuclear ophthalmoplegia, Arch. Ophthalmol. **75:**363, 1966.

251. Leopold, I. H., and Comroe, J. H., Jr.: Effect of diisopropyl fluorophosphate (DFP) on the normal eye, Arch. Ophthalmol. **36:**17, 1946.

252. de Roetth, A., Jr.: Further studies on cholinesterase activity in ocular tissues, Am. J. Ophthalmol. **34:**120, 1951.

253. Bito, L. Z., and Banks, N.: Effects of chronic cholinesterase inhibitor treatment, Arch. Ophthalmol. **82:**681, 1969.

254. Janes, R. G., and Calkins, J. P.: Effect of certain drugs on the iris vessels, Arch. Ophthalmol. **57:**414, 1957.

255. Kadin, M.: Studies of total protein and radioiodinated serum albumin (Risa) content of primary aqueous humor, Am. J. Ophthalmol. **55:**93, 1963.

256. Kadin, M.: Studies on the toxicity and effect of Dipterex in rabbits, Am. J. Ophthalmol. **53:**512, 1962.

257. Leopold, I. H., Krishna, N., and Lehman, R. A.: The effects of anticholinesterase agents on the blood cholinesterases levels of normal and glaucoma subjects, Trans. Am. Ophthalmol. Soc. **57:**63, 1959.

258. Becker, B., Pyle, G. C., and Drew, R. C.: The tonographic effects of echothiophate (Phospholine) iodide: Reversal by pyridine-2-aldoxime methiodide (P₂AM), Am. J. Ophthalmol. **47:**635, 1959.

259. Leopold, I. H., Gold, P., and Gold, D.: Use of a thiophosphinyl quaternary compound (217-MI) in treatment of glaucoma, Arch. Ophthalmol. **58:**363, 1957.

260. Leopold, I. H., and Comroe, J. H.: Use of diisopropyl fluorophosphate (DFP) in treatment of glaucoma, Arch. Ophthalmol. **36:**1, 1946.

261. Zekman, T. N., and Snydacker, D.: Increased intraocular pressure produced by diisopropyl fluorophosphate (DFP), Am. J. Ophthalmol. **36:**1709, 1953.

262. Gorin, G.: Action of di-isopropyl-fluorophosphate on cyclodialysis clefts, Am. J. Ophthalmol. **50:**789, 1960.

263. Wheeler, M. C.: Isoflurophate (DFP) in the handling of esotropia, Arch. Ophthalmol. **71:**298, 1964.

264. Parks, M. M.: Abnormal accommodative convergence in squint, Arch. Ophthalmol. **59:**364, 1958.

265. Caccamise, W. C.: Phthiriasis palpebrarum, Am. J. Ophthalmol. **43:**305, 1956.

266. Abraham, S. V.: Intraepithelial cysts of the iris, Am. J. Ophthalmol. **37:**327, 1954.

267. Christensen, L., Swan, K. C., and Huggins, H.: The histopathology of iris pigment changes induced by miotics, Arch. Ophthalmol. **55:**666, 1956.

268. Newell, F. W.: Editorial, Am. J. Ophthalmol. **56:**311, 1963.

269. Upholt, W. M., Quinby, G., Batchelor, G. S., and Thompson, J. P.: Visual effects accompanying TEPP-induced miosis, Arch. Ophthalmol. **56:**128, 1956.

270. Westsmith, R. A., and Abernethy, R. E.: Detachment of retina with use of diisopropyl fluorophosphate in treatment of glaucoma, Arch. Ophthalmol. **52:**779, 1954.

271. Wang, R. I. H.: Determining cholinesterase activity in human plasma, J.A.M.A. **183:**792, 1963.

272. Mamo, J. G., and Leopold, I. H.: Oximes in ophthalmology, Am. J. Ophthalmol. **46:**724, 1958.

273. Kewitz, H., and Wilson, I. B.: A specific antidote against lethal alkylphosphate intoxication, Arch. Biochem. **60:**26, 1956.

274. Tamura, O., and Mitsui, Y.: Organophosphorous pesticides as a cause of myopia in school children: an epidemiological study, Jpn. J. Ophthalmol. **19:**250, 1975.

275. Lawlor, R. C., and Lee, P.: Use of echothiophate (Phospholine iodide) in the treatment of glaucoma, Am. J. Ophthalmol. **49:**808, 1960.

276. Laties, A. M.: Localization in cornea and lens of topically-applied irreversible cholinesterase inhibitors, Am. J. Ophthalmol. **68:**848, 1969.

277. Harris, L. S., Shimmyo, M., and Mittag, T. W.: Cholinesterases and contractility of cat irides, Arch. Ophthalmol. **89:**49, 1973.

278. Harris, L. S.: Dose-response analysis of

echothiophate iodide, Arch. Ophthalmol. **86:**502, 1971.

279. Drance, S. M., and Carr, F.: Effects of phospholine-iodide (217MI) on intraocular pressure in man, Am. J. Ophthalmol. **49:**470, 1960.

280. Barsam, P. C., and Vogel, H. P.: The effect of Phospholine iodide on the diurnal variations of intraocular pressure in glaucoma, Am. J. Ophthalmol. **57:**241, 1964.

281. Klayman, J., and Taffet, S.: Low-concentration Phospholine iodide therapy in open-angle glaucoma, Am. J. Ophthalmol. **55:**1233, 1963.

282. Pratt-Johnson, J. A., Drance, S. M., and Innes, R.: Comparison between pilocarpine and echothiophate for chronic simple glaucoma, Arch. Ophthalmol. **72:**485, 1964.

283. Giardini, A., and Paliaga, G. P.: Concerning the treatment of glaucoma with 2-diethoxyphenylthioethyltrimethylammonium iodide (Phospholine iodide), Boll. Oculist. **38:**683, 1959.

284. Kellerman, L., and King, A. D.: Preliminary observations on the use of new concentrations of echothiophate iodide in the treatment of glaucoma, Am. J. Ophthalmol. **62:**278, 1966.

285. Atchoo, P. D., and Vogel, H. P.: Phospholine iodide (0.03%) in the therapy of glaucoma, Am. J. Ophthalmol. **62:**1044, 1966.

286. Lloyd, J. P. F.: Phospholine iodide (217-MI) (echothiophate iodide) in the treatment of glaucoma, Br. J. Ophthalmol. **47:**469, 1963.

287. Miller, J. E.: A comparison of miotics in accommodative estropia, Am. J. Ophthalmol. **49:**1350, 1960.

288. Abrahamson, I. A., Jr., and Abrahamson, I. A., Sr.: Preliminary report on 0.06 percent phospholine (echothiophate) iodide in the management of estropia, Am. J. Ophthalmol. **57:**290, 1964.

289. Cohen, S. W.: Management of errors of refraction with echothiophate iodide, Am. J. Ophthalmol. **62:**303, 1966.

290. Humphreys, J. A., and Holmes, J. H.: Systemic effects produced by echothiophate iodide in treatment of glaucoma, Arch. Ophthalmol. **69:**737, 1963.

291. de Roetth, A., Jr., Wong, A., Dettbarn, W.-D., Rosenberg, P., and Wilensky, J. G.: Blood cholinesterase activity of glaucoma patients treated with phospholine iodide, Am. J. Ophthalmol. **62:**834, 1966.

292. Wahl, J. W., and Tyner, G. S.: Echothiophate iodide, Am. J. Ophthalmol. **60:**419, 1965.

293. de Roetth, A., Jr., Dettbarn, W.-D., Rosenberg, P., Wilensky, J. G., and Wong, A.: Effect of phospholine iodide on blood cholinesterase levels of normal and glaucoma subjects, Am. J. Ophthalmol. **59:**586, 1965.

294. Klendshoj, N., and Olmsted, E.: Observation of dangerous side-effect of phospholine iodide in glaucoma therapy, Am. J. Ophthalmol. **56:**247, 1963.

295. Ellis, P. P.: Systemic effects of locally applied anticholinesterase agents, Invest. Ophthalmol. **5:**146, 1966.

296. Hiscox, P. E. A., and McCulloch, C.: Cardiac arrest occurring in a patient on echothiophate iodide therapy, Am. J. Ophthalmol. **60:**425, 1965.

297. Williams, J. W., Griffiths, J. T., Jr., and Sterns, C. R.: Parathion poisoning in citrus grove operations in 1951, J. Fla. Med. Assoc. **39:**655, 1953.

298. Wilensky, J. G., Dettbarn, W.-D., Rosenberg, P., and de Roetth, A., Jr.: Effect of ocular instillation of echothiophate iodide and isoflurophate on cholinesterase activity of various rabbit tissues, Am. J. Ophthalmol. **64:**398, 1967.

299. Klayman, J.: Use of long-acting cholinesterase agents in glaucoma, Invest. Ophthalmol. **5:**136, 1966.

300. Abraham, S. V.: The use of an echothiophate phenylephrine formulation (echophenyline-B-3) in the treatment of convergent strabismus and amblyopia—with special emphasis on iris cysts, J. Pediatr. Ophthalmol. **1:**68, 1964.

301. Axelsson, U., and Holmberg, A.: The frequency of cataract after miotic therapy, Acta Ophthalmol. **44:**421, 1966.

302. Shaffer, R. N., and Hetherington, J. M.: Anticholinesterase drugs and cataracts, Am. J. Ophthalmol. **62:**613, 1966.

303. de Roetth, A., Jr.: Lens opacities in glaucoma patients on phospholine iodide therapy, Am. J. Ophthalmol. **62:**619, 1966.

304. Thoft, R. A.: Incidence of lens changes in patients treated with echothiophate iodide, Arch. Ophthalmol. **80:**317, 1968.

305. Morton, W. R., Drance, S. M., and Fairclough, M.: Effect of echothiophate iodide on the lens, Am. J. Ophthalmol. **68:**1003, 1969.

306. Pietsch, R. L., Bobo, C. B., Finklea, J. F.,

and Vallotton, W. W.: Lens opacities and organophosphate cholinesterase-inhibiting agents, Am. J. Ophthalmol. **73:**236, 1972.

307. Harrison, R.: Bilateral lens opacities, Am. J. Ophthalmol. **50:**153, 1960.

308. Tarkkanen, A., and Karjalainen, K.: Cataract formation during miotic treatment for chronic open-angle glaucoma, Acta Ophthalmol. **44:**932, 1966.

309. Cinotti, A. A., and Patti, J. C.: Lens abnormalities in an aging population of nonglaucomatous patients, Am. J. Ophthalmol. **65:**25, 1968.

310. Diamant, H.: Cataract due to cholinesterase inhibitors in the guinea pig, Acta Ophthalmol. **32:**357, 1954.

311. Bronson, L. J., and Lazar, M.: The role of corneal exposure in cataract formation in DFP-treated guinea pigs, Am. J. Ophthalmol. **69:**858, 1970.

312. Leopold, I. H.: Problems in ophthalmic drug therapy, Trans. Am. Acad. Ophthalmol. Otolaryngol. **76:**81, 1972.

313. Michon, J., Jr., and Kinoshita, J. H.: Cholinesterase in the lens, Arch. Ophthalmol. **77:**804, 1967.

314. Michon, J., Jr., and Kinoshita, J. H.: Experimental miotic cataract, Arch. Ophthalmol. **79:**611, 1968.

315. Michon, J., Jr., and Kinoshita, J. H.: Experimental miotic cataract, Arch. Ophthalmol. **79:**79, 1968.

316. Allen, J. C.: Delayed anterior chamber formation after filtering operations, Am. J. Ophthalmol. **62:**640, 1966.

317. Terner, I., Linn, J., and Goldstrohm, R.: Clinical experiences with demecarium bromide (BC-48) in the treatment of glaucoma, Am. J. Ophthalmol. **52:**553, 1961.

318. Krishna, N., and Leopold, I. H.: The effect of BC-48 (demecarium bromide) on normal rabbit and human eyes, Am. J. Ophthalmol. **49:**270, 1960.

319. Krishna, N., and Leopold, I. H.: Use of BC-48 (demecarium bromide) in treatment of glaucoma, Am. J. Ophthalmol. **49:**554, 1960.

320. Drance, S. M.: Effect of demecarium bromide (BC-48) on intraocular pressure in man, Arch. Ophthalmol. **62:**673, 1959.

321. Becker, B., and Gage, T.: Demecarium bromide and echothiophate iodide in chronic glaucoma, Arch. Ophthalmol. **63:**126, 1960.

322. Krishna, N., and Leopold, I. H.: Effect of protopam on the rabbit pupil, Am. J. Ophthalmol. **52:**565, 1961.

323. Kewitz, H., Wilson, I. B., and Nachmansohn, D.: A specific antidote against lethal alkyl phosphate intoxication. II. Antidotal properties, Arch. Biochem. **64:**456, 1956.

324. Hunter, W. S., and McCulloch, C.: The neutralization of cholinesterase inhibition by various oximes and by atropine, Am. J. Ophthalmol. **52:**841, 1961.

325. Harris, G., and McCulloch, C.: Neutralization of the action of diisopropylfluorophosphate by an oxime (monosionitrosoacetone), Am. J. Ophthalmol. **50:**414, 1960.

326. Lipson, M. L., Holmes, J. H., and Ellis, P. P.: Oral administration of pralidoxime chloride in echothiophate iodide therapy, Arch. Ophthalmol. **82:**830, 1969.

327. Grob, D., and Johns, R. J.: Use of oximes in the treatment of intoxication by anticholinesterase compounds in normal subjects, Am. J. Med. **24:**497, 1958.

328. Quinby, G. E.: Further therapeutic experience with pralidoximes in organic phosphorus poisoning, J.A.M.A. **187:**202, 1964.

329. Byron, H. M., and Posner, I.: Clinical evaluation of protopan, Am. J. Ophthalmol. **57:**409, 1964.

330. Bonomi, L., and DiComite, P.: Outflow facility after guanethidine sulfate administration, Arch. Ophthalmol. **78:**337, 1967.

331. Bonomi, L., and DiComite, P.: Effect of guanethidine and other sympatholytic drugs, Am. J. Ophthalmol. **59:**544, 1965.

332. Riley, F. C., and Moyer, N. J.: Experimental Horner's syndrome: a pupillographic evaluation of guanethidine-induced adrenergic blockade in humans, Am. J. Ophthalmol. **69:**442, 1970.

333. Holland, M. G., Wei, C.-P., and Gupta, S.: Review and evaluation of 6-hydroxydopamine (6-HD): chemical sympathectomy for the treatment of glaucoma, Ann. Ophthalmol. **5:**539, 1973.

334. Holland, M. G.: Treatment of glaucoma by chemical sympathectomy with 6-hydroxydopamine, Trans. Am. Acad. Ophthalmol. Otolaryngol. **76:**437, 1972.

335. Holland, M. G., and Mims, J. L.: Anterior segment chemical sympathectomy by 6-hydroxydopamine, Invest. Ophthalmol. **10:**130, 1971.

13
BIOLOGIC DRUGS

ANTILYMPHOCYTE SERUM

Homograft reactions may be effectively prevented by use of antilymphocyte serum. This agent successfully blocks immunologic reactions against either lamellar or penetrating corneal transplants. However, the prolonged series of daily injections necessary for successful treatment of graft reactions may be associated with serious side effects such as serum sickness and anaphylactic reactions. For this reason, use of antihuman lymphocyte serum does not seem justified in routine corneal transplant surgery.[1,2]

Because the mechanism of action of antilymphocyte serum is a reduction of the immunologic defenses of the entire body, local use of the drug by subconjunctival injection or topical instillation is an ineffective method of suppressing homograft reactions. Such local use failed to prevent experimental corneal graft reactions in rabbits.[3,4]

Systemic administration of antilymphocyte serum reduces resistance to experimental keratitis produced by *Candida albicans.* The infection is more prolonged and severe in treated animals than in controls.[5] This immunosuppressive medication increases the risk of infection in the treated patient.

ENZYMES USED AS DRUGS
Fibrinolysin

Enzymatic dissolution of fibrin is of value in the removal of blood from the anterior chamber and may be of benefit in the treatment of various inflammatory and traumatic disorders.

Mechanism of action

The human fibrinolytic mechanisms are outlined briefly in Table 13-1.[6] Profibrinolysin is the enzyme precursor found in circulating blood. When activated by tissue factors or artificially by streptokinase, it is converted into the active proteolytic enzyme, fibrinolysin. Fibrinolysin will dissolve fibrin clots. Inhibitors (antifibrinolysin) exist in normal blood and inactivate fibrinolysin.

Human fibrinolysin

Commercially available fibrinolysin is produced by streptokinase activation of purified human profibrinolysin. A small amount of residual streptokinase remains in this product and accounts for its variable toxicity. Activated fibrinolysin is antigenic and may provoke allergic responses, especially on repeated use. Intravenous administration causes febrile reactions in about two thirds of patients.

Fibrinolysin breaks fibrin into noncoagulable polypeptides. It also inactivates fibrinogen and other related proteins. Fibrinolysin treatment is suggested for thromboembolic disorders, on the premise that it may hasten intravascular dissolution of clots. (This action is differentiated from that of anticoagulants, which prevent thrombus formation but do not dissolve clots.) By inactivating fibrino-

Table 13-1. Human fibrinolytic mechanisms*

Profibrinolysin + Activator ⟶ Fibrinolysin
Fibrinolysin + Fibrin ⟶ Proteolysis
Fibrinolysin + Antifibrinolysin ⟶ Inactivation

*Modified from Scheie, H. G., Ashley, B. J., and Weiner, A.: Arch. Ophthalmol. **66:**226, 1961.

gen, fibrinolysin also has an anticoagulant action.

Ocular tolerance

Irrigation of the anterior chamber with 10 to 15 ml of 1250 units/ml of fibrinolysin over a period of 20 to 30 minutes is well tolerated by rabbit corneas.[7] Half of eyes so treated had mild striate keratitis for 1 or 2 days only. Histologic examination showed stromal and endothelial edema for 4 days or less. Thereafter the corneas were normal during a follow-up period for as long as 18 months. Irrigation with 5000 units/ml destroyed 60% of endothelial cells; the use of 10,000 units/ml destroyed 95%. Corneal edema was still visible on slit-lamp examination 6 months after irrigation with 5000 units/ml and was grossly visible 6 months after use of 10,000 units. Obviously these higher concentrations of fibrinolysin are not suitable for clinical treatment of hyphema.

Clinical use

Hyphema. The effect of anterior chamber irrigation with 2000 units/ml of human fibrinolysin was studied in 30 rabbits with total hyphema produced by injection of human blood. Irrigation with fibrinolysin resulted in slightly more rapid improvement of the eyes than did irrigation with saline solution; however, the differences appear to be so slight as to be of doubtful statistical significance. Removal of the blood by irrigation with either a saline or enzyme solution resulted in less corneal cloudiness than if the blood had been allowed to remain in the anterior chamber.[8]

Fibrinolysin-induced clearing of experimental hyphema is most effective against relatively fresh clots. The effect of fibrinolysin on human blood clots (in rabbit anterior chambers) 7, 35, and 60 hours old was studied in 60 eyes.[9] Irrigation with fibrinolysin was demonstrably superior to irrigation with saline solution at 7 hours, slightly better at 35 hours, and no better at 60 hours. These findings do not necessarily mean that fibrinolysin irrigation will fail in treatment of 5-day-old hyphemas, since many continue to bleed and may contain a considerable amount of fresh fibrin.

Lysis of clots is apparently greatly enhanced by the movement of irrigating fluid. When kept stationary in an incubator, blood clots 0.5 ml thick are lysed completely in 2 hours by 12,500 units of fibrinolysin/ml, in 16 hours by 3125 units/ml, and not at all by 1500 units/ml. Single injections of 6250 units/ml did not clear experimental hyphemas of rabbit anterior chambers any more rapidly than did control injections of saline solution. However, continuous irrigation with 1250 units/ml permits removal of almost all anterior chamber clots within 15 to 90 minutes. Irrigation with saline solution is not nearly so effective. Stronger solutions than 1250 units/ml do not materially improve clot lysis.

Fibrinolysin irrigation is useful in treatment of traumatic total hyphema with secondary glaucoma. The solution (1250 units/ml) is introduced via a blunt cannula inserted through a 3 mm beveled corneal incision. Gentle back-and-forth irrigation gradually breaks up the clot and permits complete removal within 15 to 30 minutes. Actually, complete removal of all small clots is not recommended, since scattered small remnants will spontaneously absorb. These findings have been substantiated in eight human eyes treated by the author of the article[10] and in 56 additional eyes reported to him by other ophthalmologists.

No complications were specifically attributed to the use of fibrinolysin. Cataract and corneal damage occurred infrequently and were considered caused by the original injury. Postoperative glaucoma or retinal injury did not seem to be related to fibrinolysin irrigation. Subsequent bleeding was infrequent. If secondary glaucoma complicates recurrent bleeding, repeated fibrinolysin irrigation is indicated.

Occlusion of central retinal artery. Because of the rapid death of the retina following arteriolar occlusion, I am doubtful of the value of any therapy. Furthermore, the great majority of retinal arteriolar occlusions are embolic, not fibrin, clots and therapeutic attention should be directed to the internal carotid origin of these emboli, which may be multiple.

Purified human fibrinolysin (Thrombolysin) has been used in the treatment of thromboembolic disease and may effectively lyse intravascular clots less than 48 hours old.[11] Since only the fibrin component of a clot is affected by fibrinolysin, older organized thrombi respond poorly to treatment.

After base-line blood samples are obtained, the patient is given 200,000 units of fibrinolysin intravenously. The prothrombin time is determined 30 to 40 minutes later. If the prothrombin time is greater than 40% of normal, additional fibrinolysin is given until the prothrombin time is between 35% and 40%. This level is maintained by a constant infusion of fibrinolysin, usually requiring 150,000 to 200,000 units every 4 hours. Hourly prothrombin measurements guide the rate of administration. Fibrinolysin therapy should be maintained for about 30 to 48 hours.

Since the damaged vessel has a tendency toward recurrent thrombosis, heparinization is recommended during the following week. The initial subcutaneous injection of heparin is 50 mg, followed by 25 to 35 mg every 4 hours, provided that the clotting time is not more than 25 minutes just preceding each heparin injection. (The authors of this study did not specify why they preferred heparin to longer acting drugs such as bishydroxycoumarin [Dicumarol], which would seem more convenient.)

In this series of 37 patients with thromboembolic problems there was one case of thrombosis of the central retinal artery. Within 24 hours the retinal blood flow was restored completely to normal. Unfortunately the patient had been blind for 6 hours before therapy was started, and vision did not return.

If fibrinolysin proves to be effective in lysing fresh occlusions of the central retinal artery, the use of 95% oxygen and 5% carbon dioxide to prolong survival time of the retina might become clinically valuable as an emergency measure. Available evidence suggests that combined therapy with fibrinolysin and anticoagulants is beneficial in various fresh thromboembolic conditions.[12] (Because fibrinolysin itself has an anticoagulant effect, and because its administration is controlled by prothrombin measurements, anticoagulant therapy should not commence until the fibrinolysin treatment is concluded.)

A detailed report on fibrinolysin treatment of a 62-year-old diabetic patient with incomplete occlusion of the central retinal artery strongly suggests that this medication is effective.[13] During a 3-day period, vasodilators (nitroglycerin, nicotinic acid, tolazoline, and stellate block), anticoagulants (heparin and sodium warfarin [Coumadin]), and repeated paracenteses were without effect. He was then given fibrinolysin (Thrombolysin) intravenously at a rate of 50,000 units/hour for 6 hours. Fresh solutions were prepared hourly. Immediately after this treatment, 75 mg of heparin was given intramuscularly, and Coumadin therapy was resumed. Vision—originally counts fingers at 3 feet—began to improve within 2 hours and was counts fingers at 6 feet at 18 hours, 20/200 at 24 hours, 20/80 three weeks later, and 20/40 four months later. Retinal edema was recognizably decreased at 24 hours posttreatment.

Three additional patients with arterial occlusion were treated similarly. Complete restoration of vision was achieved in a case of 7 hours' duration. Blood flow was restored but blindness persisted in a case of 24 hours' duration. Neither blood flow nor vision improved in a patient treated 72 hours after onset of symptoms.

Daily intravenous administration of fibrinolysin, 2500 units, was reported to hasten collateral vessel formation, absorption of hemorrhage, and disappearance of retinal edema in rabbits with experimental occlusion of branches of the central retinal vein.[14] The data given in the report are insufficient to judge with certainty the validity of these observations.

Streptokinase

Streptokinase, an enzyme derived from hemolytic *Streptococcus*, can activate profibrinolysin and will effectively lyse blood clots. In contrast to the use of fibrinolysin itself, the profibrinolysin activators have the disadvantage of requiring a source of profibrinolysin, either from the clot or from the circulating blood. Streptokinase is highly toxic, particularly when given intraocularly. Intraocular streptokinase injection has been studied with the intent of hastening absorption of hyphema.[15] Results are not dramatic. Intracameral injection of 0.2 ml streptokinase, 50,000 units/ml, reduced clearing time of experimental rabbit hyphema to about two thirds that of controls. Increased aqueous fibrinolytic function could be demonstrated for only 3 hours after injection, which suggests that normal aqueous flow carries away streptokinase. (Angle blockage by viscous solutions prolonged the aqueous fibrinolytic activity for as much as 7 hours.)

Toxic responses such as corneal edema and iritis were produced in the rabbit eye by concentrations of streptokinase in excess of 50,000 units/ml. Such reactions were not observed after intracameral injection of lesser concentrations. Streptokinase is antigenic, and antistreptokinase factors can be demonstrated in the aqueous within 12 days of the initial injection. No antistreptokinase is present in the aqueous of animals previously unexposed to streptokinase.

Clinical trials of streptokinase treatment for infection and for hemorrhage indicate that this drug is most toxic to the human eye. The human reaction to streptokinase is so severe as to preclude its use by intraocular injection.

Injection of 5000 units of streptokinase in five human eyes produced severe, intractable secondary glaucoma and corneal opacity.[16] (It should be noted that these eyes were selected because associated disease processes indicated enucleation.) Irrigation of the lacrimal sac with streptokinase in treatment of a fibrinous dacryocystitis resulted in acute exacerbation of the dacryocystitis.

Intravitreal injection of a streptokinase-streptodornase mixture was performed in two patients with vitreous hemorrhage.[17] Severe inflammatory reaction followed all injections. Some clearing of the vitreous was noted in the patient receiving 100 units. The second patient received two intravitreal injections of 200 and 500 units. Marked inflammatory response followed these injections and resulted in phthisis bulbi. Another patient received anterior chamber injections of streptokinase-streptodornase for hyphema. Severe iridocyclitis and secondary glaucoma resulted. (Streptodornase is deoxyribonuclease. It acts on nucleoprotein, which comprises 30% to 70% of purulent sediment, and is therefore effective in lysing pus.)

Streptokinase is also available in 10,000-unit tablets, which are to be held in the mouth until absorption presumably occurs across the buccal mucosa. This is supposed to activate fibrinolysin, which in turn removes fibrinous debris from sites of inflammation. Clinical evaluation of whether vascular, inflammatory, and traumatic ocular disorders respond to such treatment is almost impossible because of the variable course of these conditions. Of 41 assorted patients with such eye disorders, 13 improved after a 2-week course of 10,000 units of buccally administered streptokinase four times a day.[18] Obviously this is far from being a consistent and dramatic response.

Anti-inflammatory effect (?) of enzymes

Evaluation of the anti-inflammatory effect of proteolytic enzymes as used in ophthalmology is difficult. In a series of 115 consecutive eye operations (41 on muscles, 28 plastic surgical procedures, 39 for cataracts, and 7 corneal transplants), 1 ml of aqueous chymotrypsin (5000 units) was given intramuscularly at the close of surgery, and the dose was repeated the following day.[19] Less than the expected amount of postsurgical reaction was found in two thirds of the muscle operations, one half of the plastic procedures, one third of the cataract operations, and none of the corneal transplants. The "control" was stated to consist of the amount of reaction normally expected to occur by the same surgeon using the same technique over the past 30 years. The fact that my own judgment would be entirely inadequate in assessing a series of cases in this manner has been established in various controlled studies we have undertaken.

Also inconclusive are those studies of inadequate numbers of patients, such as a series of five treated and three untreated patients with strabismus.[20] The published photographs do not convincingly document the benefit claimed for chymotrypsin injection.

Intramuscular injection of 10 mg of trypsin in oil did not benefit experimental horse serum iridocyclitis in rabbits.[21]

Daily intramuscular injection of 0.5 to 7.5 mg of trypsin for 6 weeks did not recognizably alter the rate of absorption of blood injected into the vitreous cavity of rabbits.[22]

Absorption of experimental hyphema in the guinea pig is not hastened by intramuscular injection of trypsin (5 mg/kg) twice a day for 1 week. Subconjunctival injections of 4 mg of trypsin did not hasten absorption of hyphema. Increasing the subconjunctival dosage to 8 mg of trypsin caused severe chemosis and in several instances resulted in necrosis of the eyelid.[23]

The use of proteolytic enzymes to reduce inflammation after trauma or surgery has met with skepticism because most of the articles supporting its use cite uncontrolled clinical impressions, because individual responses to injuries of variable severity are hard to evaluate, and because no treatment can be expected to eliminate all inflammation. However, some well-controlled clinical studies suggest that a clinically recognizable anti-inflammatory effect results from the use of chymotrypsin.

Perhaps the best clinical evaluation of chymotrypsin was a study that utilized 500 episiotomy patients, alternately assigned to chymotrypsin or control groups.[24] (While an episiotomy is hardly ophthalmologic in nature, it is certainly a more standard lesion than the variable injuries produced by accidents or by more complex operations.) Factors such as multiparity, hemorrhoids, and the like were approximately the same for both groups. Treated patients received two enzyme tablets four times a day for 3 days after episiotomy. Each enteric-coated tablet (Chymoral) contained 50,000 Armour units of trypsin and chymotrypsin in a 6:1 ratio. Edema, local pain, analgesic effect, and walking pain were recorded.

The statistical evaluation of these episiotomy patients showed no dramatic differences between most patients in the two groups, but did indicate more rapid subsidence of edema and less pain in many patients receiving chymotrypsin. Selection of the most marked differences exaggerates the effect of chymotrypsin but illustrates the recognizable clinical response. On the third postpartum day, severe edema affected 11 control patients but no chymotrypsin-treated patients. On the first postpartum day, 39 patients receiving chymotrypsin but no control patients were free of local pain. On the third postpartum day, analgesics were still dispensed to 15 patients receiving chymotrypsin and 40 control patients. Pain on walking during the third day affected 57 patients receiving chymotrypsin and 112 control patients.

I think that careful surgery and a pressure dressing will more effectively reduce edema than will any presently available enzyme therapy.

HUMAN IMMUNE GLOBULINS
Gamma globulin

Gamma globulin obtained from human blood has been advocated for treatment or prophylaxis of ocular virus infections, including herpes simplex, herpes zoster, rubella, and vaccinia. The response of herpetic infections is uncertain. The improvement of vaccinia ocular lesions seems to be well established.

Clinical use

Herpes simplex. Human gamma globulin has been used topically and parenterally in

334 Drugs in ophthalmic practice

the treatment of herpetic keratitis, generally with disappointing results. Such failures have been attributed to the inability of the antibody proteins to penetrate the avascular cornea and the inaccessibility of the intracellular virus. To determine whether immune globulin could penetrate to the iris and ciliary body, the severity of herpetic iridocyclitis was studied in control rabbits and in rabbits preinoculated with 5 ml of gamma globulin.[25] During the first 4 days after virus inoculation and after 8 days, the iridocyclitis was equal in treated and control groups. No treated animals were protected against infection. From the fifth through the seventh day, the eyes of treated animals were less inflamed than those of control animals (chance alone could have caused this result five times in one hundred).

In the treatment of experimental rabbit herpes simplex keratitis, gamma globulin with a specific antibody titer of 1:512 was not of value during the acute epithelial stage of infection.[26] However, gamma globulin seemed to reduce the severity of inflammation during the chronic stromal stage of the disease.

Active and/or passive immunization of rabbits, even when very high titers of serum antibodies were achieved, did not protect the animals against herpes simplex keratitis, nor was the course of the disease modified.[27] Treatment with topical application of serum antibody to the infected corneas was of absolutely no benefit. However, the immune rabbits were completely protected against an intravenous dose of virus sufficient to cause death from encephalomyelitis in three of four normal rabbits. Presumably this indicates that circulating or locally applied antibodies cannot penetrate the cornea in therapeutic amounts.

The available evidence seems to indicate that immune globulin treatment of herpes simplex ocular infections is ineffective.

Herpes zoster. Administration of 250 ml of serum obtained from patients previously infected with herpes zoster were reported to improve the course of ocular herpes zoster.[28] Of 22 treated patients, 83% retained vision better than 6/18. In comparison, 60% of 39 untreated patients maintained 6/18 or better vision. These series of patients were uncontrolled and subject to some variables in selection; hence the value of herpes zoster immunotherapy is difficult to assess.

Herpes zoster occurs with selective frequency in patients with blood dyscrasia.[29] One might speculate that this indicates reduced immunologic resistance, possibly replaceable by administration of immune serum.

Infection in leukemic patients. A controlled study of the therapeutic effect of gamma globulin was made with a series of 46 patients with acute leukemia and superimposed acute infections (mostly bacterial). All patients received antibiotics, but random choice determined whether immune globulin or placebo was given. The therapeutic response of both groups was comparable, with no significant benefit resulting from the gamma globulin treatment.

Measles (rubella) immune globulin

Passive protection against German measles is conferred by intravenous injection of 30 ml of human serum obtained from volunteers approximately 3 weeks after disappearance of their rubella rash. To be effective, this serum must be injected within 5 days after exposure to rubella infection.[30]

Rubella prophylaxis may be indicated during the first trimester of pregnancy. The incidence of serious congenital malformations after rubella in the first trimester is about 17%.[31,32] The results of rubella prophylaxis are unfortunately equivocal.

Vaccinia immune serum globulin

Vaccinia immune globulin (VIG) is gamma globulin fractionated from the serum of patients vaccinated 1 to 2 months before blood donation. It is available from American Red Cross Regional Blood Centers. Vaccinia immune globulin is effective in arresting the complications of vaccinia such as generalized spread and ocular involvement. It is also effective in the treatment or prophylaxis of smallpox.

Dosage of VIG is 0.3 ml/pound by intramuscular injection for treatment of vaccinia or variola and 0.03 ml/pound for prophylaxis of an exposed patient. No more than 5 ml is injected at any one site and the total dose need not exceed 20 ml in any case. If response is not evident in 24 to 48 hours, the same dose may be repeated several times. VIG does not impair immunity resulting from a vaccination take. Concomitant treatment for ocular vaccinia includes gentle cleaning, avoidance of corneal trauma, and antibiotic control of secondary bacterial invaders. No antibiotic is known to have any effect on the vaccinia virus. Steroid therapy should be avoided, since it may reduce resistance.

Six patients with ocular vaccinia treated with VIG are reported to have shown good response, with freedom from serious scarring.[33] Reference is made to two brothers with accidental corneal inoculation with vaccinia. The corneal lesions were identical in the two brothers. One eye, untreated with VIG, required 4 weeks to recover and had slight permanent scarring. The other eye, treated with VIG, subsided within 24 hours and left no scar.

In another reported case, obvious improvement was evident within 24 hours of VIG treatment.[33]

OTHER IMMUNOLOGIC AGENTS
Autogenous staphylococcal vaccine

Since the advent of antibiotics, most cases of chronic staphylococcal blepharoconjunctivitis have been found to respond well to appropriate chemotherapy. In stubborn cases, culture and sensitivity studies help in selection of the most effective antibiotic. However, even the most ardent advocate of antibiotic therapy must admit the problem of reinfection from organisms harbored elsewhere on the patient's body. Furthermore, some difference in individual resistance seems to be the most likely explanation of why one patient becomes infected whereas another does not. Advocates of vaccine therapy report excellent results, presumably because of increased immunity or resistance. For instance, of 60 patients with staphylococcal in-

fection, vaccine therapy cured 44, improved the condition of 11, and failed in only 5.[34] Many of these patients had already been treated unsuccessfully with antibiotics.

Preparation of autogenous vaccine is fairly simple. The organism is obtained from the purest source. Ideally, if a small pustule exists, its surface is cleaned with a 1:1000 concentration of benzalkonium chloride. With sterile technique, the pustule is opened and inoculated generously on a trypticase soy-agar slant. After 18 to 24 hours' incubation at 37° C, the staphylococci are harvested by adding 5 ml of sterile isotonic saline solution and rotating the tube between the palms. The resulting suspension is aspirated and diluted with saline solution to a concentration of 600 million organisms/ml. Nephelometric standardization is employed. After standardization, 15 ml of suspension is transferred to a sterile vaccine vial. Add 2.5 ml of a 1:1000 solution of benzalkonium chloride, shake, and incubate at 37° C for 30 minutes. Agitate two or three times at intervals during the incubation. Test for sterility by 7-day culture of 1 ml in 6 ml of thioglycollate broth. Refrigerate at 4° C until ready for use.

For immunization, inject the vaccine intracutaneously, usually in the forearm. Injections are given at intervals of 2 to 3 days for a total of ten injections. The dosage for the first three injections is 0.01, 0.03, and 0.05 ml, and the remaining seven injections contain 0.08 ml each. If the infection has not responded, five additional injections may be given at intervals of 4 to 7 days.

The vaccine does not cause systemic reactions. Even the most severe local reactions do not exceed a 12 to 15 mm area of erythema.

Autogenous vaccine therapy is indicated when staphylococcal infection persists despite adequate antibiotic therapy, general measures such as hot compresses and improved hygiene, and environmental sanitation. Almost three fourths of such resistant cases are said to respond to autogenous vaccine. Stock vaccines are often not of benefit. Indeed, if reinfection occurs, it is commonly because of a new strain of *Staphylococcus,* nonresponsive to the original vaccine and requiring preparation of a new autogenous vaccine.

Good results are said to require effectively antigenic vaccines. Crucial points in preparation include killing with benzalkonium (rather than denaturation by heat), use of the original culture (not subcultures that may be changed by the artificial media), and standardization before killing (more reliable than standardization after cell death). The vaccine must be shaken before use.

In a series of 83 patients with blepharoconjunctivitis caused by hemolytic *Staphylococcus aureus*, 22 patients were cured by immunization with *Staphylococcus* toxoid and 53 patients' conditions were improved.[35] The course of treatment consisted of 12 to 14 weekly injections of commercial toxoid, beginning with 0.02 ml and increasing to 1 ml. The method of assay of this material was not specified. Eight patients had rather severe local reactions to the injections. Monthly injections were suggested as maintenance therapy in patients with stubbornly recurrent disease. This series of patients was accumulated before antibiotic therapy became available.

Tetanus toxoid and antitoxin

Wounds about the eye, just as those elsewhere in the body, may be the site of entry of *Clostridium tetani*. The management of each ocular wound therefore requires consideration of specific prophylactic measures against tetanus. The physician's task in management of these cases is considerably more involved than making a decision between use of antitoxin and toxoid booster simply on the basis of prior immunization. Proper judgment of the management of potential cases of tetanus (every patient with an unsterile wound has a potential case of tetanus) requires knowledge of the following facts.[36-39]

The tetanus organism is widespread, developing in the gastrointestinal tract of man and animal and existing in spore form in soil and dust. Development of the spores requires anaerobic conditions such as exist in wounds that are contaminated by foreign material or contain devitalized tissue. The symptoms of tetanus result from toxemia and not from spread of infection through the body. Tetanus produces one of the most potent neurotoxins known. A lethal amount of tetanus toxin is too small to induce immunity, which accounts for the well-established fact that a patient who has survived a tetanus infection has no resistance against reinfection and must be immunized just as anyone else. Once the toxin has reached the nerve fibers, it cannot be removed by antitoxins.

A wound contaminated with tetanus does not suppurate unless there is associated infection with other bacteria. An apparently trivial or already well-healed wound may contain viable tetanus organisms. The incubation period varies from 2 to 30 days, depending on the nature of the wound and the severity of contamination, and may be prolonged if antitoxin has been given. Signs of local tetanus about the wound precede systemic manifestations in the great majority of patients. Dirty wounds, extensive wounds, or wounds for which treatment has been delayed should be considered more dangerous potential sources of tetanus. Thorough cleaning with soap and water, careful removal of foreign material, and debridement of severely injured tissue that may be sacrificed without functional or cosmetic loss are of importance in minimizing the possibility of tetanus infection of such a wound.

Tetanus antitoxin is a biologic product obtained from horses or cows (or human beings) that have been immunized against tetanus toxin. One unit of tetanus antitoxin will protect a 350-g guinea pig against 1000 lethal doses of tetanus toxin. Obviously it is not possible to state what constitutes a protective level of antitoxin in man, since the amount of toxin produced by the microorganisms is the deciding factor. A single intramuscular dose of 1500 units of tetanus antitoxin will produce a gradually rising blood titer, which is detectable within minutes and which reaches a level of 0.1 unit of antitoxin/ml of serum by the fourth day. This level may be maintained until the tenth day and then decreases, until by the end of the third week no demonstrable antitoxin remains. It is generally agreed that any injured person who really needs tetanus antitoxin (dirty, extensive, or neglected wound) needs a dose as large as 5000 or 10,000 units. Children may be given proportionately smaller doses.

The value of administration of antitoxin to a patient sensitive to horse serum is doubtful. Such a sensitized patient has antibodies that will destroy the antitoxin, thereby decreasing or completely nullifying the expected therapeutic effect of passive immunity. This acceleration of antitoxin destruction by the sensitized patient must be realized by the physician when deciding on treatment. Furthermore, the risk of acute anaphylactic reaction, delayed serum sickness, damage to the central nervous system, and similar allergic complications may far outweigh the possible benefit to be obtained from prophylactic use of antitoxin.

Determination of sensitivity to horse serum is through intradermal injection of 0.1 ml of a 1:10 dilution of antitoxin. Before this injection, the patient should be questioned carefully about previous allergic conditions, especially asthma, urticaria, known sensitivity to horses, and reactions to past injections of sera. Epinephrine should be available for instant injection should it be needed. If the antitoxin test dose is placed peripherally on an extremity, a tourniquet may be applied in the event of a reaction, temporarily arresting further absorption. If no reaction appears within 30 minutes, the test is repeated with 0.1 ml of undiluted antitoxin. If this test is also negative, then the antitoxin may be given intramuscularly or subcutaneously. A positive skin reaction consists of a wheal, which is supposed to be larger in size in more sensitive individuals. A wheal less than 5 mm in diameter may represent a nonspecific reaction to injury, which may be determined by a control test with normal saline solution (use different syringe and needle). If an equal reaction occurs to the saline solution, the tetanus antitoxin reaction is considered negative. Negative skin tests do not exclude the possibility of later severe serum sickness.

Human tetanus immune globulin is now generally available. This preparation has the great advantage of being virtually free of the risk of inducing hypersensitivity. The half-life of human tetanus immune globulin in the patient is 3 to 4 weeks, much longer than the few days for which foreign globulins remain circulating within the body. The dosage is 4 units/kg body weight, given intramuscularly (250 units adult dose).[40]

Because of the inherent dangers of passive immunization, and because of the transient and possibly inadequate protection attained thereby, active immunization is far preferable and is advised for all persons, beginning in infancy. Inoculation with tetanus toxoid is virtually free of significant side effects and is highly effective. During World War II only 12 cases of tetanus occurred among members of the United States Armed Forces (only one case was fatal), and six of these were in patients who had not yet been properly immunized. Anyone who has been in the army will suspect that some of the other six patients may have evaded their shots in some way. Hospital admissions for service injuries numbered 2,735,000 during this period. In contrast to this military record, 500 to 600 civilians die of tetanus in the United States each year.

Active immunity is attained by giving three subcutaneous injections of 0.5 ml of alum-precipitated tetanus toxoid (Fig. 13-1).[39] The second injection is given 1 month after the first and the third, 6 to 12 months later. Booster doses are recommended at 4-year intervals. During the first month of immunization the antitoxin titer is very low, and the patient cannot be considered protected. Very soon after the second injection, satisfactory titers are attained and last for about a year, but not reliably longer. The third injection (at 1 year) is a vital part of the basic immunization and should not be considered only an optional booster. After the third injection, a rapid and prolonged elevation of antitoxin titer occurs, averaging 10 units/ml 1 month after injection. Once this basic level of immunization has been attained, subsequent booster doses will stimulate an adequate and prompt antibody response for as long as 15 years and possibly for

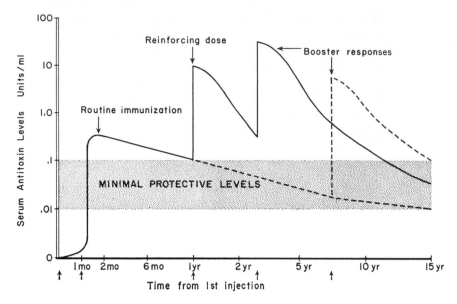

Fig. 13-1. Average response to tetanus toxoid injections. Arrows indicate times of injection of 0.5 ml of toxoid. Solid line: rise in circulating antitoxin levels attained by initial, 1-month, 1-year, and booster injections. Broken line: drop in titer in patients who did not receive subsequent injections. (Modified from Filler, R. M., and Ellerbeck, W.: J.A.M.A. **174:**1, 1960.)

a lifetime. In fact, the immunity attained from booster doses is so effective that a repeat booster is not recommended for a wound incurred less than a year after the last booster injection—unless the wound is exceptionally contaminated.

The duration of effective tetanus immunization is much longer than generally realized.[41] Approximately 90% of individuals immunized to tetanus during World War II still had protective levels of antibody 20 years later. Twelve years after immunization in infancy, only 4% of 190 children had antibody levels below the threshold of protection. Of 45 immunized children encountered in routine pediatric practice for the purpose of receiving a booster shot (for summer camp, a wound, etc.), all were found to have tetanus antibody levels from 40 to 2500 times higher than the minumum protective level. Some hyperimmunized individuals may develop exaggerated local reactions to tetanus toxoid.

At the time of an injury all patients who have not previously been immunized should begin active immunization. Tetanus antitoxin should be considered a medication to be administered only once in a lifetime. If it is used, simultaneous or subsequent active immunization should be mandatory and is the responsibility of the physician giving the antitoxin. Active and passive immunization may be initiated simultaneously, provided that the injections are made into different extremities with separate syringes. Alum-precipitated (*not* fluid) toxoid must be used if antitoxin is to be given simultaneously. (It is not definitely established that fluid toxoid is superior to alum-precipitated toxoid for any purpose, including attaining a more rapid effect from a booster dose.) The second and third toxoid injections should subsequently be given at the usual intervals of 1 month and 1 year.

The vegetative form of *Clostridium tetani* (not the spores) is very sensitive to penicillin, chloramphenicol, and the tetracyclines, responding to concentrations of 0.045 to 0.6 μg/ml. These antibiotics may be employed to kill the organisms before toxin is produced. (Antitoxin neutralizes toxin but has no effect on the organisms in the local wound.)

Antibiotics should not be used as a substitute for active immunization nor for clearly indicated passive immunization. If antibiotic prophylaxis for tetanus is employed, blood levels must be maintained for 3 weeks to protect against late germinating spores. A single injection of 1,200,000 units of benzathine penicillin G will maintain blood levels between 0.04 and 0.21 unit/ml for at least a month, killing the organisms as they emerge from the spore state. About a 1.5% incidence of penicillin allergy is reported after such injections. Broad-spectrum antibiotics may be used for patients known to be allergic to penicillin.

In view of the preceding facts, the principles of tetanus prophylaxis may be summarized as follows:

1. All wounds must receive accepted local surgical care.
2. Immunized patients must receive 0.5 ml of toxoid at the time of injury.
   a. For minor wounds sustained within a year of a known booster dose, an additional booster dose is unnecessary.
   b. For dirty, large, or neglected wounds, antibiotic prophylaxis should be used.
3. All nonimmunized patients should begin active immunization with alum-precipitated toxoid at the time of injury.
   a. For minor superficial injuries that can be adequately cleaned, no further tetanus prophylaxis is necessary.
   b. For dirty, large, or neglected wounds, 250 units of human antitoxin should be given.
   c. There is a difference of opinion as to whether wounds intermediate between trivial and severe in nonimmunized and nonsensitive patients should receive prophylactic antitoxin or prophylactic antibiotics. Traditionally, antitoxin has been given, but a logical presentation can be made in favor of antibiotics.

Two serious errors are commonly made in the prophylaxis of tetanus after penetrating ocular wounds.[42] The first error is routine administration of antitoxin and the second is failure to give toxoid routinely.

Five percent of patients receiving tetanus antitoxin experience complications, which may be as serious as anaphylactic death and encephalomyelitis. The usual doses of antitoxin are ineffective; from 5000 to 10,000 units is required for a month's protection. Destruction of antitoxin is accelerated if the patient has previously received horse serum. Not only may antitoxin be toxic and ineffective, but it is also usually unnecessary—because penicillin and tetracyclines destroy tetanus bacilli in the vegetative form (not spores). (Toxoid and antitoxin do not kill the organisms but neutralize the toxin.) Antitoxin administration is indicated, however, in management of a dirty, neglected wound suffered by a nonimmunized patient.

All wounded patients (except those who have had a booster toxoid dose within a year) should receive toxoid. Many patients are unaware that they have been immunized in childhood, and the toxoid will serve as a booster injection. Nonimmunized patients receiving toxoid will be protected against future injuries (and should receive second and third doses at 6 weeks and 6 months). It is the physician's responsibility to encourage patients to be immunized.

Gas gangrene antitoxin

Panophthalmitis caused by anaerobic bacilli closely related to tetanus is particularly destructive. Gas gangrene panophthalmitis (*Clostridium perfringens*) typically causes rapid purulent ocular destruction, usually with loss of vision within 12 hours after injury. Review of 53 cases indicates that the eye has invariably been lost despite treatment with penicillin and/or gas gangrene antitoxin.[43] The characteristics of intraocular *Clostridium* infection include unusually severe pain, early rise in tension, coffee-colored discharge (hemolysis), gas bubbles in the anterior chamber, and rapid loss of vision. Unfortunately destruction of the eye is so rapid that cultural diagnosis of the organism is of no value in guiding antibiotic selection.

BIOGENIC STIMULATORS

Included only to express my skepticism are the cure-all biogenic stimulators of Filatov.[44]

Tissue therapy with biogenic stimulators is advocated by Filatov for all degenerative or inflammatory eye disorders. These biogenic stimulators are supposedly formed by all living tissues under adverse circumstances but have not been chemically identified. Their administration enhances the resistance and regenerative powers of the patient. Daily injections for a month or more are claimed to double the visual acuity of patients with retinitis pigmentosa, for instance. The most effective biogenic stimulator is a mixture of extract of aloes, placental extract, and extract of mud from a lagoon near Filatov's laboratory.[45]

Although it is unscientific of me to reject these claims summarily, they are too reminiscent of the legendary witch's brew: eye of toad, bat wings, and three centipede tails. I have not encountered any convincing controlled studies supporting the use of biogenic stimulators in eye disease.

REFERENCES

1. Waltman, S. R., Faulkner, H. W., and Burde, R. M.: Modification of the ocular immune response, Invest. Ophthalmol. **8:**196, 1969.
2. Smolin, G.: Suppression of the corneal homograft reaction by antilymphocyte serum, Arch. Ophthalmol. **81:**571, 1969.
3. Smolin, G.: Corneal homograft reaction following subconjunctival antilymphocyte serum, Am. J. Ophthalmol. **67:**137, 1969.
4. Smolin, G.: Suppression of corneal graft reaction by antilymphocyte serum, Arch. Ophthalmol. **79:**603, 1968.
5. Smolin, G., and Okumoto, M.: Antilymphocyte serum potentiation of Candida keratitis, Am. J. Ophthalmol. **66:**804, 1968.
6. Scheie, H. G., Ashley, B. J., and Weiner, A.: The treatment of total hyphema with fibrinolysin (plasmin), Arch. Ophthalmol. **66:**226, 1961.
7. Morton, W. R., and Turnbull, W.: The effect of intracameral fibrinolysin on the rabbit cornea, Am. J. Ophthalmol. **57:**280, 1964.
8. Liebman, S., Pollen, A., and Podas, S. M.: Treatment of experimental total hyphema with intraocular fibrinolytic agents, Arch. Ophthalmol. **68:**72, 1962.
9. Podos, S., Liebman, S., and Pollen, A.: Treatment of experimental total hyphemas with intraocular fibrinolytic agents, Arch. Ophthalmol. **71:**537, 1964.
10. Scheie, H. G., Ashley, B. J., and Burns, D. T.: Treatment of total hyphema with fibrinolysin, Arch. Ophthalmol. **69:**147, 1963.
11. Anlyan, W. G., Silver, D., Deaton, H. L., Fort, L., and Webster, J. L.: Fibrinolytic agents in surgical practice, J.A.M.A. **175:**290, 1961.
12. Brinkhous, K. M., and Roberts, H. R.: Thrombolysis and thrombolytic agents, J.A.M.A. **175:**284, 1961.
13. Hecker, S. P., and Zweng, H. C.: Central retinal artery occlusion successfully treated with plasmin, J.A.M.A. **176:**1067, 1961.
14. Mutlu, F.: Experimental retinal vein occlusion and treatment with fibrinolysin, Am. J. Ophthalmol. **62::**282, 1966.
15. O'Rourke, J. F.: An evaluation of intraocular streptokinase, Am. J. Ophthalmol. **39:**119, 1955.
16. Braley, A. E.: Discussion of O'Rourke: an evaluation of intraocular streptokinase, Am. J. Ophthalmol. **39:**136, 1955.
17. Sacks-Wilner, A., Sinclair, S., and Boyes, T.: Streptokinase and streptodornase, Am. J. Ophthalmol. **39:**730, 1955.
18. Hurwitz, P.: Buccal varidase in ophthalmology, Am. J. Ophthalmol. **48:**823, 1959.
19. Hughes, W. L., Lewis, E. L., and Amdur, J.: Chymotrypsin in various ophthalmic surgical procedures, Am. J. Ophthalmol. **51:**103, 1961.
20. Fortier, E. G.: Chymotrypsin in strabismus surgery, Am. J. Ophthalmol. **51:**106, 1961.
21. Wood, R. M., and Bick, M. W.: A comparison of the influence of parenteral trypsin, cortisone, and heparin on acute inflammation, Arch. Ophthalmol. **62:**112, 1959.
22. Chandler, M. R., and Rosenthal, E.: The effect of intramuscularly administered trypsin on blood injected into the vitreous of rabbits, Arch. Ophthalmol. **59:**706, 1958.
23. Keeney, A. H., and Zaki, H. A.: The role of trypsin in experimentally induced Hyphema, Am. J. Ophthalmol. **43:**275, 1957.
24. Schmitz, H. E., and Pavlic, R. S.: Control of edema and pain in episiotomy, Obstet. Gynecol. **17:**260, 1961.
25. Howard, J., and Allen, H. F.: Treatment of experimental herpes simplex iridocyclitis with human serum gamma globulin, Arch. Ophthalmol. **59:**68, 1958.
26. Hudnell, A. B., and Osterhout, S.: The effect of gamma globulin on experimental herpes simplex keratitis, Invest. Ophthalmol. **2:**295, 1963.

27. Gispen, R.: Immunization against herpes keratitis in rabbits, Am. J. Ophthalmol. **44:** 88, 1957.

28. Gundersen, T.: Convalescent blood for treatment of herpes zoster ophthalmicus, Arch. Ophthalmol. **24:**132, 1940.

29. Wechsler, H. F., and Wolf, M. J.: Agammaglobulinemia, J.A.M.A. **161:**526, 1956.

30. Ward, H., and Parker, G.: Passive protection against rubella, Med. J. Aust. **1:**81, 1956.

31. Rauh, L. W.: Rubella and pregnancy, Ohio Med. J. **51:**875, 1955.

32. Cotlier, E.: Effective vaccines for rubella, Am. J. Ophthalmol. **67:**424, 1969.

33. Ellis, P. P., and Winograd, L. A.: Ocular vaccinia, Arch. Ophthalmol. **68:**600, 1962.

34. McCory, K. L., and Kennedy, E. R.: Autogenous vaccine therapy in staphylococcic infections, J.A.M.A. **174:**35, 1960.

35. Thygeson, P.: Treatment of staphylococcic blepharoconjunctivitis with staphylococcus toxoid, Arch. Ophthalmol. **26:**430, 1941.

36. Edsall, G.: Specific prophylaxis of tetanus, J.A.M.A. **171:**417, 1959.

37. Hampton, O. P., Altemeier, W. A., Edsall, G., Hampton, S. F., Snydern, H. E., and Stafford, E. S.: Principles of prophylaxis against tetanus, Ohio Med. J. **57:**164, 1961.

38. Stafford, E. S.: Active and passive antitetanus immunization, J.A.M.A. **173:**539, 1960.

39. Filler, R. M., and Ellerbeck, W.: Tetanus prophylaxis, J.A.M.A. **174:**1, 1960.

40. Council on Drugs: A new agent for prophylaxis of tetanus, J.A.M.A. **192:**471, 1965.

41. Edsall, G., Elliott, M. W., Peebles, T. C., Levine, L., and Eldred, M. C.: Excessive use of tetanus toxoid boosters, J.A.M.A. **202:**17, 1967.

42. Bettman, J. W.: The prophylaxis of tetanus, Am. J. Ophthalmol. **56:**806, 1963.

43. Leavelle, R. B.: Gas gangrene panophthalmitis, Arch. Ophthalmol. **53:**634, 1955.

44. Vail, D.: Biogenic stimulators (editorial), Am. J. Ophthalmol. **30:**635, 1947.

45. Kamel, S.: Ophthalmology in the Soviet Union, Am. J. Ophthalmol. **55:**953, 1963.

14
CHELATING AGENTS

BRITISH ANTI-LEWISITE

British anti-lewisite (BAL, 2,3-dimercap-to-1-propanol) is an effective antiarsenic agent that is of definite value in the treatment of various types of arsenic poisoning encountered in civilian practice as well as in treatment of war gas casualties.[1] When used within 5 minutes after doses of lewisite sufficient to cause corneal perforation in 11 days, BAL treatment reduces corneal damage to only slight residual scarring. The longer the interval between lewisite burn and BAL application, the less effective is the therapeutic effect. Some benefit results from treatment as late as 30 minutes after the burn, but treatment after 1 hour is useless.[2]

Two drops of a 5% solution or 0.1 ml of 5% ointment provides a large excess of BAL over that required to react with whatever arsenic is likely to be in the eye. Three percent concentration is as effective as 5%. Ten percent preparations and prolonged irrigations have no demonstrable additional therapeutic effect. A second BAL instillation is desirable, however, to be certain that an adequate amount of medication actually enters the eye.

BAL is itself most irritating to the eye. A 5% solution or ointment will produce severe lacrimation and blepharospasm lasting from 2 to 5 minutes. Marked conjunctival injection lasts for an hour after the use of 5% solution of BAL. Ten percent preparations are more irritating but cause no permanent rabbit cor-

neal damage. Concentrations of 20% or higher cause irreparable corneal scarring.

BAL is unstable in aqueous solution but is quite stable (no loss of therapeutic efficiency at room temperature for 6 weeks) in ethylene glycol solution or in ointment bases. Ointment and liquid preparations are equally effective therapeutically; however, from the practical standpoint, a gassed soldier can rub ointment into his eye much easier than he can instill drops (for example, ointment can even be rubbed into an eye while lying face down).[3] BAL is rapidly oxidized by iron or copper; hence it cannot be dispensed in ordinary metal tubes.

Aqueous chamber concentrations of BAL as high as 0.1% may be attained within 5 minutes after the repeated application of a 5% BAL solution to the surface of rabbit eyes.[4] Aqueous solutions penetrate two to four times more effectively than do ointment preparations. Unfortunately aqueous solutions are too unstable to be of practical value.

The arsenical war gas lewisite rapidly penetrates the cornea and can be demonstrated in the aqueous within 2 minutes. Ten minutes after exposure, irreversible corneal changes can already be detected. A single instillation of a 5% BAL solution or ointment within 2 to 5 minutes after exposure to lewisite will prevent this corneal destruction.[5]

Two percent sodium bicarbonate solution (1 teaspoon in a glass of water) is said to be helpful as an immediate first-aid treatment for eye burns by war gases such as lewisite or phosgene.[6] This is, of course, not nearly so effective as a specific antidote such as BAL but has the advantage of availability.

Hydrogen peroxide and potassium permanganate have also been recommended for lewisite poisoning but are definitely less effective than BAL.

DESFERRIOXAMINE

Desferrioxamine mesylate (Desferal) is a potent and specific iron-chelating agent capable of forming a highly stable bond with ferric ions. Since it is a relatively nontoxic chemical, it may be used clinically for selective removal of pathologic iron deposits from the tissues of the body.

Mechanism of action

Apparently intraocular iron is toxic by liberation of iron ions that diffuse to the cells, combine with vital enzymes, and thereby destroy the more sensitive cells (for example, of the retina). More resistant cells (for example, uveal cells) may detoxify and store the iron. Ultimately the iron becomes firmly bound in the form of nontoxic siderin pigments.

Desferrioxamine acts by chelating free iron ions or those that may be loosely attached to the acid mucopolysaccharides of the vitreous. Such chelation of free (toxic) iron will prevent inactivation of vital intracellular enzymes. Desferrioxamine cannot liberate iron from the secure binding of hemosiderin, hemoglobin, or siderin pigments (nontoxic). Cells already dead from enzyme destruction will not be revived by desferrioxamine.

Ocular toxicity

No toxic effects result from topical ocular application of 10% desferrioxamine in 0.5% methylcellulose. Solutions of 20% or greater strength are irritating and cause conjunctival chemosis.[7]

Subconjunctival injection of as much as 100 mg does not damage the rabbit eye, but a dose of 200 mg causes uveal congestion and exudative detachment of the retina. Daily subconjunctival injection of 50 mg to a total of 2000 mg did not cause intraocular damage.[8]

As much as 6 mg may safely be injected into the anterior chamber; however, as little as 3 mg injected intravitreally causes retinal necrosis and hemorrhagic destruction of the uveal tract.

Ocular penetration

The transcorneal penetration of desferrioxamine B is poor, producing an aqueous concentration of less than 30 ppm after topical instillation of 25% solution. Although higher levels are reached by subconjunctival injection, this route of administration is difficult for a drug requiring frequent dosage. Actually, since the prognosis of ocular siderosis is primarily dependent on the toxic effect of iron on the retina, and because intramuscular injection is the only practical method of obtaining therapeutically effective retinal drug concentrations, intraocular siderosis probably cannot be treated by topical application of desferrioxamine. In contrast, an effective drug concentration can easily be achieved on the corneal surface, as would be needed to remove rust staining from superficial foreign bodies.

Clinical use

Nonsurgical chemical removal of iron stains is applicable to the treatment of small corneal rust stains.[7] Experimental corneal rust stains were produced binocularly in 50 rabbits by embedding a 500 mg iron filing for 10 hours in each cornea. Ten percent desferrioxamine was instilled in the right eye of each animal 4 times daily. In all but one rabbit, visible rust staining was eliminated within 2 weeks. The rust stains of 95% of the control eyes persisted unchanged for periods up to 40 days.

Another obvious application of this drug would seem to be in the treatment of corneal bloodstaining. However, unpublished data indicate that experimental iron staining of the rabbit cornea does not clear more rapidly with desferrioxamine treatment.[9]

Therapeutic results

Experimental vitreous hemorrhage was not benefited by subconjunctival injection of 25 mg of desferrioxamine every 3 days for 10 weeks. There was no difference in rate of clearing of the vitreous or in the incidence of retinal detachment in treated or untreated eyes.[8] The problem of a ferrous intraocular foreign body was studied by introduction of a 2 mm iron wire into the rabbit vitreous, with subsequent treatment by subconjunctival injection of 25 mg of desferrioxamine every 3 days for 6 months. Desferrioxamine treatment prevented the development of siderosis, as evidenced by normal clinical appearance, absence of rust, normal ERG findings, and minimal histologic evidence of stainable iron.

A case report outlines the course of a patient with ocular siderosis treated with systemic desferrioxamine for almost a year.[10] The foreign body was deeply embedded and could not be removed surgically. The average daily dosage of desferrioxamine B was 500 mg given intramuscularly. The effectiveness of the drug was demonstrated by measuring urinary iron excretion, which was 366 μg daily without treatment but increased to 2266 μg daily with treatment. Topical application only of 5% desferrioxamine ointment four times a day increased iron excretion to 1100 μg daily. Both systemic and topical routes of administration were used. Visual acuity remained approximately 20/50 during the period of treatment and the already subnormal ERG findings did not indicate further deterioration. The dark brown siderotic iris became normal in color and the dilated pupil returned to normal size.

If the cause of a discolored and possibly siderotic iris is uncertain, a diagnostic "Desferal test" may be of value. Apparently, intramuscular injection of 500 mg of desferrioxamine greatly increases urinary iron excretion if pathologic amounts of iron exist anywhere in the body. Normally the daily urinary excretion of iron after such an injection will not exceed 1 mg. Higher values would indicate the iris discoloration was siderotic,

providing no other iron abnormality was present in the patient.

Perhaps a period of desferrioxamine B treatment should be considered after surgical removal of a foreign body if recognizable siderosis is present. Such therapy might prevent further retinal damage from the action of ferric salts remaining within the eye. Although of considerable theoretical interest, desferrioxamine seems of limited value in ocular therapy. The removal of a magnetic intraocular foreign body is more practicable than long-term repeated injections.

Solutions of desferrioxamine B lose their chelating properties rapidly; however, ointments are stable for at least 6 months.

ETHYLENEDIAMINE TETRAACETATE

Ethylenediamine tetraacetate (EDTA, edathamil) is a chelating agent with a high affinity for many metals. This affinity may be clinically useful in the removal of toxic alkalies from the cornea.[11] In Fig. 14-1 is given the periodic chart of the metallic elements, which have been evaluated for their toxicity to the rabbit cornea by means of 10-minute exposures of the cornea to 0.1M solutions of these metals. The results are recorded as 0 to 4+ (4+ represents complete permanent opacity). The initial reaction seems to be a binding of the metal cation to the corneal tissue. After a latent period, which may be as long as several hours, the cornea gradually becomes opaque. Subsequently, permanent scarring, necrosis, or even perforation may develop. Fortunately, if the initial binding of the metal ions can be undone promptly, corneal opacification may be significantly reduced.

Irrigation of the human cornea for periods of 15 to 20 minutes with a 0.01M solution of sodium EDTA at pH 8.0 does not cause recognizable ocular damage. As much as 100 ml or more may be used during this period of irrigation. The corneal epithelium should be mechanically scraped off before irrigation with EDTA. Concentrations as strong as 0.1M, pH 7.5, are definitely irritating, caus-

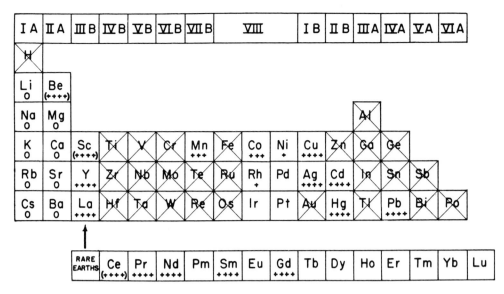

Fig. 14-1. Periodic chart of metallic elements, with corneal toxicity indicated as 0 to 4+. Crossed out elements were insufficiently soluble to test at the 0.1M concentration selected. (From Grant, W. M., and Kern, H. L.: Am. J. Ophthalmol. **42:**167, 1956.)

ing stromal edema, which lasts for several days. Experimentally, this treatment demonstrably reduces the toxic effect of beryllium, yttrium, lanthanum, thorium, nickel, copper, silver, and mercury. Evidence that metal has actually been removed from the cornea by EDTA treatment has been obtained by assay. For instance, EDTA-bathed corneas retained only one fourth as much yttrium as corneas bathed in the same manner with physiologic saline solution.[11]

This evidence seems to indicate strongly that prompt irrigation of the epithelium-denuded cornea with EDTA should be part of the emergency treatment of alkali burns, especially if discrete particles of alkali are superficially embedded within the tissues.

The disodium salt of ethylenediamine tetraacetic acid may also be used to dissolve calcific deposits within Bowman's membrane (for example, band keratopathy). Since EDTA does not penetrate the intact corneal epithelium, it must be mechanically scraped off before application of the chelating agent. Prolonged irrigation (20 minutes) with 0.37% solution will visibly dissolve these calcific changes. Since no delayed benefit accrues,

the desired amount of clearing must be achieved at the time of treatment.[12-15]

Zinc chloride, the flux used in soldering, causes severe corneal damage by rapid tissue fixation. Chelation with EDTA will bind zinc ions and minimize tissue damage, but only if applied within 2 minutes. Beyond this time, chelation is no more effective than washing with normal saline.[16]

The only chelating preparation listed in *New Drugs* is calcium disodium edathamil. This drug is the end product of calcium chelation and would be entirely ineffective in removing corneal calcium. It is useful in treatment of lead poisoning, since the lead chelate is more stable than that of calcium. However, to avoid confusion, I repeat that the disodium salt of ethylenediamine tetraacetic acid is used for removal of band keratopathy.

REFERENCES

1. Leopold, I. H., and Adler, F. H.: Specific treatment of ocular burns due to Lewisite (β-chlorovinyldichloroarsine), Arch. Ophthalmol. **38:**174, 1947.
2. Adler, F. H., Fry, W. E., and Leopold, I. H.: Patholgic study of ocular lesions due to lewis-

ite (β-cholorovinyldichloroarsine), Arch. Ophthalmol. **38:**89, 1947.

3. Mann, I., Pirie, A., and Pullinger, B. D.: The treatment of Lewisite and other arsenical vesicant lesions of the eyes of rabbits with British anti-Lewisite (BAL), Am. J. Ophthalmol. **30:**421, 1947.

4. Leopold, I. H., and Steele, W. H.: Penetration of locally applied BAL into the anterior chamber of the rabbit eye, Arch. Ophthalmol. **38:**192, 1947.

5. Hughes, W. F.: Treatment of Lewisite burns of the eye with dimercaprol (BAL), Arch. Ophthalmol. **37:**25, 1947.

6. Cordes, F. C.: Nonsurgical aspects of ocular war injuries, Am. J. Ophthalmol. **26:**1062, 1943.

7. Galin, M. A., Harris, L. S., and Papariello, G. J.: Nonsurgical removal of corneal rust stains, Arch. Ophthalmol. **74:**674, 1965.

8. Wise, J. B.: Treatment of experimental siderosis bulbi, vitreous hemorrhage and corneal bloodstaining with deferoxamine, Arch. Ophthalmol. **75:**698, 1966.

9. Bollheimer, D.: Personal communication, 1965.

10. Valvo, A.: Desferrioxamine B in ophthalmology, Am. J. Ophthalmol. **63:**98, 1967.

11. Grant, W. M., and Kern, H. L.: Cations and the cornea, Am. J. Ophthalmol. **42:**167, 1956.

12. Grant, W. M.: A new treatment for calcific corneal opacities, Arch. Ophthalmol. **48:**681, 1952.

13. Grant, W. M., and Kern, H. L.: Action of alkalies on the corneal stroma, Arch. Ophthalmol. **54:**931, 1955.

14. Breinin, G. M.: Correction, Arch. Ophthalmol. **53:**618, 1955.

15. Breinin, G. M., and DeVoe, A. G.: Chelation of calcium with edathamil calcium-disodium in band keratopathy and corneal calcium affection, Arch. Ophthalmol. **52:**846, 1954.

16. Johnstone, M. A., Sullivan, W. R., and Grant, W. M.: Experimental zinc chloride ocular injury and treatment with disodium edetate, Am. J. Ophthalmol. **76:**137, July 1973.

15
CORTICOSTEROID THERAPY

Before the advent of corticosteroids, their synthetic derivatives, and adrenocorticotropic hormone (ACTH), ophthalmologists achieved similar, although less intense, effects by means of foreign protein injection or anterior chamber paracentesis.[1] Fever therapy induced by foreign protein injection is believed to stimulate pituitary production of ACTH.[2]

In Fig. 15-1 the correlation between the febrile response after two injections of 5 million killed typhoid organisms and the plasma levels of 17-hydroxycorticosteroids is demonstrated.[3] As illustrated, the maximum steroid level coincides fairly closely with the peak of the febrile response. Normal plasma steroid levels by the author's method ranged from 4 to 28 μg and were increased to values ranging from 32 to 59 μg/100 ml of plasma. These peak steroid levels are comparable to those obtained clinically with intravenous ACTH.

The adrenal cortex response to foreign protein therapy does not occur if aminopyrine is used to block the febrile response (Fig. 15-2).[3] This is true even though other constitutional symptoms (malaise and nausea) are present. The clinical implications are clear—antipyretics will nullify the effectiveness of foreign protein therapy.

Secondary aqueous has been demonstrated to contain increased amounts of corticosteroids and antibodies, to which have been attributed the beneficial results of paracentesis in anterior uveitis.[1]

Discovery of ACTH made it possible to obtain the desirable effects of fever therapy without the accompanying unpleasant and sometimes dangerous fever, aching, and generalized illness. Another serious limitation to long-term use of foreign proteins is the rather rapid development of a refractory state that precludes obtaining a therapeutic response even with high doses of typhoid organisms. Although fever therapy might produce other beneficial effects besides production of corticosteroids, most clinicians agree that corticosteroids cause a therapeutic response equal or superior to that obtained with foreign proteins. An occasional case of uveitis is cited that has failed to respond to corticosteroids and subsequently has quieted during a course of fever therapy. I personally doubt that this relationship has been substantiated beyond the level of coincidence and spontaneous improvement.

Periodic references to the use of typhoid therapy in recalcitrant uveitis are still encountered. The author of the annual review of the uvea in the 1969 *Archives of Ophthalmology*[4] believes typhoid therapy is of historic interest only and that its use in treatment of uveitis is unwarranted. He cites the death from anaphylactoid reaction of a young girl after two intravenous injections of typhoid and quotes a fatality rate of three out of 2500 patients treated with typhoid.

As is well known, ACTH is not an unmixed blessing, and in addition to the desired anti-inflammatory effects, it causes profound metabolic derangements. ACTH itself has no

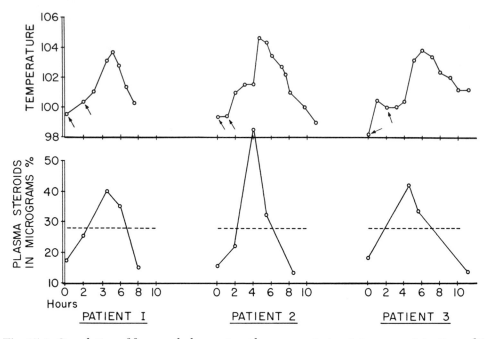

Fig. 15-1. Correlation of fever and plasma steroid responses to two intravenous injections of 5 million killed typhoid organisms (arrows). Broken line at 28 represents normal upper limit of steroid concentration. (Modified from Donn, A., and Christy, N.: Am. J. Ophthalmol. **42:**132, 1956.)

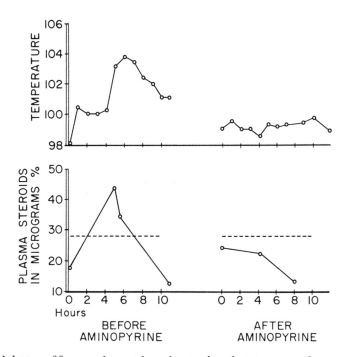

Fig. 15-2. Inhibition of fever and steroid production by administration of aminopyrine, 0.66 g, every 4 hours. Intravenous injection of 5 million killed typhoid organisms was given at zero time in each instance. (Modified from Donn, A., and Christy, N.: Am. J. Ophthalmol. **42:**132, 1956.)

anti-inflammatory or metabolic effects and achieves these through stimulation of the adrenal cortex to produce corticosteroids. Topical application of ACTH to an inflamed eye is therefore irrational and valueless. Oral administration of ACTH is also ineffective, since it is destroyed in the gastrointestinal tract.

The advantages of tablet and topical therapy were achieved with cortisone. Almost immediately hydrocortisone was found to be biologically more active and more potent and has been demonstrated to be more effective than cortisone against certain superficial eye conditions—for example, vernal conjunctivitis, sclerokeratitis, episcleritis, and superficial punctate keratitis. Iridocyclitis responds equally well to cortisone or hydrocortisone, possibly because of the better solubility and penetration of cortisone. A significant disadvantage of cortisone as compared with ACTH is the marked adrenal atrophy that results from prolonged therapy.

Of course, the body manufactures its own daily dose of adrenal steroids. The normal daily output is 25 mg of hydrocortisone and 5 mg of corticosterone.[5] The normal plasma concentrations of 11-hydroxycorticoids average approximately 20 μg/100 ml.[6] One day after a single oral dose of 0.75 mg dexamethasone, the average cortisol concentrations had dropped from 20 to 15.

A further advance in the field of corticosteroid therapy was the synthesis of prednisone and prednisolone. Not only are these drugs 5 to 10 times as potent as cortisone, but more important, their anti-inflammatory effect is relatively greater than their metabolic side effects. This should not be interpreted to mean that prednisone will be effective in cases where cortisone is not, but simply that prednisone requires a smaller (one fifth) dose. The results of treatment of experimental horse serum uveitis in rabbits with different steroids is illustrated in Fig. 15-3.[7] The amounts used in this program of experimental therapy are listed in Table 15-1. Note that prednisone therapy was only one fifth the amount of cortisone or hydrocortisone.

Even newer derivatives are evolving, ever more potent and specific in their anti-inflammatory activity. One of the most potent synthetic corticosteroid derivatives is dexamethasone, which has an anti-inflammatory effect 30 to 50 times that of cortisone (measured in activity by weight). Clinical administration of

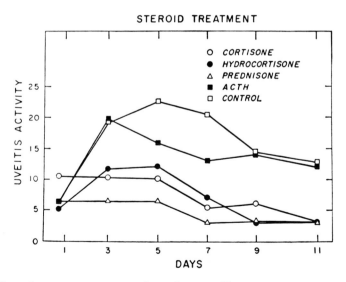

Fig. 15-3. Effect of various corticosteroids in therapy of horse serum uveitis in rabbits. Note the latent period before ACTH effect. Prednisone was given in one fifth the dose of cortisone or hydrocortisone. (From O'Rourke, J. F., Iser, G., and Ryan, R.: Arch. Ophthalmol. 55:323, 1956.)

dexamethasone employs dosages of 4 to 10 mg/day; 10 mg of dexamethasone is the anti-inflammatory equivalent of 100 mg of prednisolone. Most ocular diseases responsive to corticosteroids may be treated successfully with 4 mg dexamethasone/day. As is true for all other corticosteroids, higher doses are required for treatment of exceptionally severe cases of uveitis. The most important charac-

teristic of dexamethasone is not its extraordinary potency but its improved therapeutic ratio. Effective anti-inflammatory doses of dexamethasone are less likely to produce systemic side effects than are equivalent amounts of other corticosteroids. Sodium and water retention, potassium loss, and abnormal sugar metabolism are minimal with use of dexamethasone. Negative nitrogen, phosphorus, and calcium balances are produced, however. Peptic ulceration, tuberculosis, mental disease, and dendritic keratitis are still contraindications to its use.[8,9]

Reference to Table 15-2 will indicate that all corticosteroid derivatives still have some undesirable side effects, although they vary considerably in intensity.[10] The newer corticosteroids only change the proportionate risk of such side effects but do not eliminate them.[11] Interestingly, therapeutic response to locally applied corticosteroid seems to require approximately the same amount or concentration no matter which corticosteroid is used. This seems to confirm the hypothesis that at least one reason for the increased po-

Table 15-1. Dosage schedule of different steroids used in treatment of experimental horse serum uveitis in rabbits*†

Drug	Daily intramuscular dose
Cortisone	25 mg/kg
Hydrocortisone	25 mg/kg
Prednisone	5 mg/kg
Corticotropin	10 units/kg
Saline solution	1 ml/kg

*From O'Rourke, J. F., Iser, G., and Ryan, R.: Arch. Ophthalmol. **55**:323, 1956.
†Data presented in Fig. 15-3 based on this dosage schedule. Note that only one fifth as much prednisone was used.

Table 15-2. Comparative effects of corticosteroids*

	Cortisone	Hydro-cortisone	Pred-nisone	Pred-nisolone	Methyl-prednisolone	Triam-cinolone	Dexa-methasone
Equivalent daily dose (mg)	75	60	15	15	12	12	3
Edema, sodium retention	++++	+++	+	++	+	0	+
Weakness or potassium depletion	+++	++	+	+	+	++	+
Hypertension	++	+	+	++	+	+	+
Mental stimulation	+++	+	++	++	+	0 to −	++++
Increased appetite and weight gain	++	++	++	++	+	−	++++
Peptic ulcer	++	+	+++	+++	++	+++	++
Purpura	+	+	+++	+++	++	+++	++
Moon face	+++	++	++	++	++	+++	++
Hirsutism	++	++	++	++	++	++++	+
Skin effects	+	+	+	+	+	++++	+
Osteoporosis	+++	++	+++	+++	+++	+++	++
Diabetes	++	++	+++	++++	+++	++	+
Infections	++	++	++	++	++	++	++
Topical effect	+	+++	+	+++	++	+++	++
Adrenal atrophy	+++	+++	+++	+++	+++	+++	+++

*From Hollander, J. L.: J.A.M.A. **172**:306, 1960.

tency of newer derivatives is their slower destruction within the body.

The most recent derivatives, medrysone and fluorometholone, are claimed to be much less likely to cause an elevation of intraocular pressure. Medrysone does not penetrate into the eye and is recommended only for treatment of surface disorders. Fluorometholone is poorly soluble in both lipid and water vehicles and is dispensed as a microsuspension. As expected, it penetrates much less well than do the more soluble corticosteroids. Thirty minutes after instillation of 0.1% fluorometholone, corneal concentrations are only 1.45 μg/g and aqueous levels are 0.137. Remarkably, these concentrations do not increase with removal of the corneal epithelium or with inflammation of the eye, presumably because the drug remains relatively insoluble under all circumstances.[12] Not only does fluorometholone achieve only

low tissue concentrations, it is also eliminated more rapidly than prednisolone and dexamethasone.[13] Hence the reduced tendency to cause glaucoma appears to be related more to concentration and potency differences than to dissociation of therapeutic and toxic effects.

Widespread clinical use has kept pace with the evolution of all these new drugs, and their behavior, indications, and contraindications can be stated precisely.[14-17]

In a manner somewhat reminiscent of the Detroit horsepower race, the relative potencies of commercially available corticosteroid ophthalmic preparations can be compared graphically (Fig. 15-4).[18] Such comparison emphasizes the fact that concentration of a preparation as well as absolute strength of a drug affects its potency.

Table 15-3 shows relative anti-inflammatory potency of corticosteroids expressed in equivalent dosages.[19]

ANTI-INFLAMMATORY EFFECTS

Corticosteroids decrease cellular and fibrinous exudation and tissue infiltration, in-

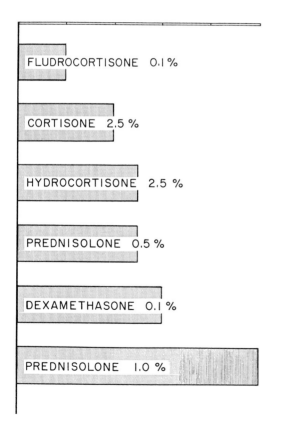

Fig. 15-4. Relative anti-inflammatory action of various corticosteroid preparations. (Modified from a commercial by Allergan Pharmaceuticals.)

Table 15-3. Relative potency of corticosteroids

	Anti-inflammatory potency	Sodium retention
Desoxycortico-sterone	0.0	100.0
Cortisone	0.8	0.8
Hydrocorti-sone	1	1.0
Prednisone	4	0.8
Prednisolone	4	0.8
Methylpredni-solone	5	0.5
Triamcinolone	5	0.0
Fludrocorti-sone	10	125.0
Betametha-sone	25	0.0
Dexametha-sone	25	0.0

From Kreines, K., and Weinberg, I. C.: The selection of adrenocorticosteroid preparations, Ohio State Med. J. **71:**698, October 1975.

hibit fibroblastic and collagen-forming activity, retard epithelial and endothelial regeneration, diminish postinflammatory neovascularization, and restore toward normal the excessive permeability of inflamed capillaries.[20] The biologic mechanisms whereby steroids produce these effects are not established. Failure of cortisone to inhibit epithelial or fibroblastic proliferation in vitro suggests the probability of an indirect action such as suppression of the substances that induce tissue activity in response to inflammation or trauma. The anti-inflammatory effects of steroids are nonspecific, occurring whether the etiology is allergic, traumatic, or infectious. The degree of response is related to dosage, and therefore corticosteroid therapy must be titrated against the severity of the individual disease. Subject to the limitations of toxic side effects, *enough* steroid is given to obtain a therapeutic response. It must be emphasized that an infectious or allergic cause of inflammation is *not* eliminated by corticosteroid therapy but continues to be present even though the inflammatory response of the body is inhibited. The clinical implication is that treatment must be continued after apparent cure, and dosage must be tapered off gradually to avoid relapse.

The anti-inflammatory effects of corticosteroids have been most useful to ophthalmologists because the delicate and transparent ocular structures are particularly susceptible to functional damage by inflammation and scarring. Properly used, corticosteroids will markedly reduce the amount of permanent scarring and may make the difference between useful vision and its loss. In general, therapeutic responses are obtained in clinically nonpyogenic inflammations such as uveitis and scleritis and in all forms of ocular allergy. Although pyogenic inflammations are initially reduced in severity, the ultimate tissue destruction will be more extensive because of the loss of bodily defense mechanisms. Corticosteroids reduce resistance to many types of invading microorganisms—bacteria, viruses, fungi, and the like—and should not be used in the presence of such infections except simultaneously with an *effective* antibiotic or other antibacterial medication. Degenerative diseases are completely refractory to corticosteroids. These facts indicate the great practical significance of accurate differential diagnosis. As an illustration, the similar-appearing lesions of idiopathic paramacular chorioretinitis, tuberculous choroiditis, and senile macular degeneration will, respectively, be greatly improved, be made considerably worse, and be unaffected at great expense to the patient through corticosteroid therapy.

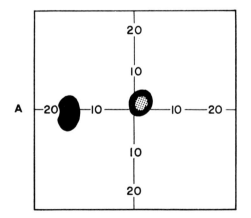 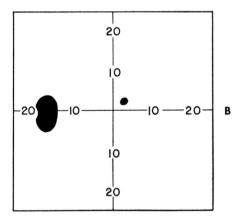

Fig. 15-5. **A,** Scotoma of acute chorioretinitis in a 33-year-old woman whose other macula had been destroyed by old inflammation. **B,** Greatly reduced scotoma in same eye after 4 days of intensive corticosteroid therapy (20 mg dexamethasone/day) given in hospital under supervision of endocrinologist. Vision has been restored to 20/20.

Additional details of the anti-inflammatory effects of corticosteroids are as follows. Normally the intraocular capillaries are relatively impermeable, and for this reason the transfer of fluorescein across the blood-aqueous barrier measures primarily capillary permeability rather than rate of blood flow. By this measure, corticosteroids do not alter the permeability of normal intraocular capillaries. Inflammation breaks down the normal blood-aqueous barrier, permitting leakage into the aqueous of protein and cells, a fact easily demonstrated biomicroscopically. Both clinically and experimentally, cortisone will reduce toward normal the increased capillary permeability characteristic of inflammation. The therapeutic benefit of stopping this abnormal cellular and protein leakage into the aqueous is evident.

The tissue infiltration and surface exudation of polymorphonuclear leukocytes, lymphocytes, and mononuclear cells are markedly inhibited by corticosteroids. Edema is also reduced. The dramatic corticosteroid-induced decrease in size and intensity of a scotoma caused by chorioretinitis is shown in Fig. 15-5. Such an improvement of function is accompanied by an ophthalmoscopically observable decrease in the activity of the lesion.

Formation of collagen and fibroblastic activity are definitely inhibited by cortisone. Although this is desirable in the prevention of corneal scarring, it is disadvantageous during the healing of surgical wounds. That scarring from corneal burns may be minimized by cortisone therapy is clearly indicated by experimental studies.[21] Standard corneal alkali, acid, and thermal burns were produced in 90 rabbits (30 for each type of burn). Cortisone therapy was administered by drops, subconjunctival injection, or intramuscular injection and adequate controls were left untreated. The data given in Table 15-4 leave no doubt that the final density of the corneal scars were significantly less in the eyes treated with cortisone. It can be inferred from this article that the topical instillation of cortisone drops is an effective route for the treatment of corneal burns, and that subconjunctival or systemic administration will not produce added benefits. Incidentally, not one of these eyes developed a secondary infection even though no antibiotics were used. This fact should be interpreted in light of the knowledge that rabbit corneas have an inherent resistance to infection that is far greater than that of human eyes. Certainly antibiotics are indicated in the management of human corneal burns.

A similar experimental study of alkali burns also concluded that cortisone therapy was very effective in minimizing scarring (Fig. 15-6).[22] In addition, this study reports four human alkali burns that responded rapidly to topical cortisone. No satisfactory human controls exist, which is understandable since such clinically sustained injuries are not of standard severity.

In contrast, chemical burns of rat eyes are reported not to respond to corticosteroid therapy.[23] Topical and subconjunctival routes were used; however, in most experiments corticosteroid treatment was given only once daily. Failure to obtain results from this rather homeopathic frequency cannot be interpreted to mean that properly used corticosteroids will not inhibit scarring.

Table 15-4. Severity of corneal scarring resulting from standardized acid, thermal, and alkali burns in cortisone-treated and control rabbit eyes*

Eyes	Density of corneal scar			
	1	*2*	*3*	*4*
Acid burns				
Cortisone treated	31	8	1	
Control		13	7	
Thermal burns				
Cortisone treated	29	11		
Control		20		
Alkali burns				
Cortisone treated			35	50
Control			4	16

*Data from Leopold, I. H., and Maylath, F.: Am. J. Ophthalmol. 35:1125, 1952.

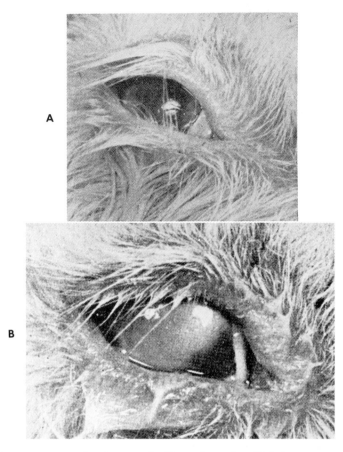

Fig. 15-6. A, Cortisone-treated right eye of rabbit 9 days after alkali burn. **B,** Control left eye of same rabbit 9 days after burn of same severity. No cortisone therapy given. (From Rundles, W., and Quinn, J.: Am. J. Ophthalmol. **37:**209, 1954.)

Collagenase augmentation

Although corneal scarring can be reduced by corticosteroid therapy, in some cases of corneal alkali burn or infection the use of corticosteroids results in a rapid destruction of the corneal stroma, so dramatic that it has been referred to as "melting." This destruction of the corneal stroma is a result of the enzyme collagenase, which may be produced by damaged corneal epithelial cells.

In vitro demonstration of the effect of hydrocortisone on collagenase utilized a substrate of collagen gel lysed by collagenase obtained from alkali-burned corneas. The area of collagen lysis was 42% greater in diameter in the presence of 10^{-2}M hydrocortisone than without it.[24] In the presence of 10^{-5}M dexamethasone the diameter of the area of ly-sis was 13% greater than without it. Cysteine, 0.01M, and EDTA, 0.01M, were both able to inhibit completely the lytic effect of collagenase, with or without corticosteroids.

Inhibition of wound healing

Inhibition of fibroblastic activity by corticosteroids significantly interferes with the healing of corneal incisions. The amount of inhibition is related to the dosage. Although small doses alter the histologic course of healing, the final wound closure is adequate. Large doses may greatly impair corneal healing (Fig. 15-7).[25] Corneal wound healing normally proceeds as follows:

1. *First day:* sealing of wound with fibrinous coagulum; epithelial regeneration rapid

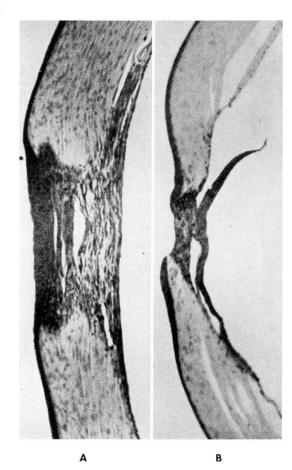

A   **B**

Fig. 15-7. A, Normal healing of corneal incision 10 days postoperatively in control rabbit. Epithelial healing is complete, normal corneal thickness is restored, and the wound is bridged by a mass of fibrocytes. **B,** Impaired healing of corneal incision 10 days postoperatively. This rabbit received 15 mg of cortisone subconjunctivally daily, beginning 2 days preoperatively. Note thinness of fibrous union and failure of epithelium and endothelium to regenerate. (From Ashton, N., and Cook, C.: Br. J. Ophthalmol. **35:**708, 1951.)

   2. *Second day:* considerable polymorphonuclear and macrophage infiltration of wound edges
   3. *Third day:* conversion of keratocytes to fibroblasts
   4. *Fifth day:* evident fibroblastic activity; endothelial proliferation visible
   5. *Seventh day:* fibroblastic closure of outer half of wound, with displacement of the previously inverted epithelium

   6. *Tenth day:* normal corneal thickness restored by fibroblastic bridge

Cortisone therapy, even in small amounts, inhibits *all* of the reparative activity just described.[25]

Study of the traction force required to disrupt rabbit corneal wounds of less than 2 weeks' duration indicated a high incidence of decreased tensile strength secondary to use of topical cortisone.[26] The strength of cortisone-treated wounds was, in some cases, less than half that of the untreated controls. Great individual variation existed, however, and several cortisone-treated wounds were stronger than their controls. Administration of cortisone was identical with presently accepted clinical usage—0.5% suspension six times daily or subconjunctival injection of 1.5 mg.

The impairment of wound healing resulting from corticosteroid treatment is dose related. Weak concentrations of corticosteroids and/or infrequent drug application cause little or no impairment of healing of experimental corneal wounds. For example, 0.1% dexamethasone four times daily or 0.01% 12 times daily did not impair corneal wound strength. However, 0.1% dexamethasone applied topically 12 times daily reduced wound strength to approximately half the normal.[27]

Dexamethasone ointment, 0.05%, applied twice daily for 21 days after experimental rabbit corneal incisions, did not alter the tensile strength of the wound when tested 21 days postoperatively.[28]

Not only the type and concentration of corticosteroid but also its molecular form may substantially alter clinical effectiveness. For example, equal molar concentrations of dexamethasone in the form of 0.1% alcohol, 21-acetate, or 21-phosphate were applied in dosages of 2 drops five times daily to rabbit eyes with 180-degree limbal incisions. The eyes were subsequently ruptured with oxygen under increasing pressures. Fig. 15-8 shows that dexamethasone alcohol completely inhibited the fibroblastic component of healing between 3 and 6 days.[29] Even 2 weeks later the average bursting strength of the treated eyes was 18 psi as compared to 24 psi for the

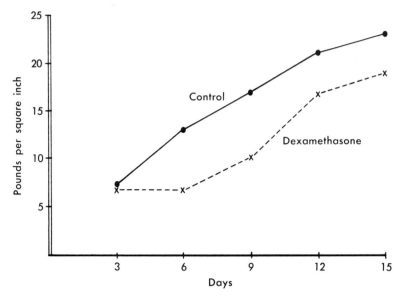

Fig. 15-8. Effect of 0.1% dexamethasone alcohol, 2 drops five times daily, on bursting strength of 180-degree limbal incision in rabbit eyes. (Modified from McDonald, T. O., and associates: Invest. Ophthalmol. **9:**703, 1970.)

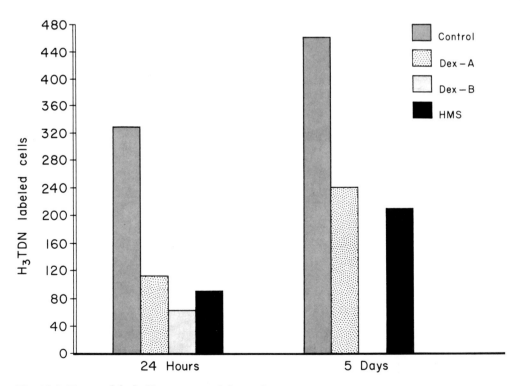

Fig. 15-9. Tritium-labeled keratocyte inhibition by corticosteroid therapy. *Dex-A,* 0.05% dexamethasone ointment three times a day after freezing; *Dex-B,* dexamethasone three times a day 1 day before and 1 day after freezing; *HMS,* 1% medrysone solution three times a day. (From Polack, F. M., and Rosen, P. N.: Arch. Ophthalmol. **77:**400, 1967.)

control. Although inhibition of wound healing was also demonstrated for the acetate and phosphate forms of dexamethasone, the amount of inhibition was only half as great as for the alcohol form. Even in 0.001% concentration, dexamethasone alcohol reduced the 6-day wound strength by 3 psi. Sufficient systemic absorption occurred in the animals receiving 2 drops of 0.1% dexamethasone alcohol to reduce the 6-day bursting strength of the untreated opposite control eye by 4 psi.[29] In comparable experiments, indomethacin, 0.5%, and phenylbutazone, 1%, did not impair wound healing.

A particularly sensitive experimental measure of the effect of corticosteroids on wound healing is the cellular uptake of tritiated thymidine after a freezing injury. Tritiated thymidine selectively enters cellular deoxyribonucleic acid (DNA) prior to mitosis and remains there during the life of the cell. Hence this method will demonstrate the number of cells undergoing active multiplication. The number of labeled keratocytes 1 and 5 days after a 1-minute freezing injury is shown in Fig. 15-9.[30] Obvious and marked inhibition of cellular multiplication by corticosteroid therapy is apparent.

Despite the general agreement that corticosteroids tend to inhibit experimental wound healing, clinical experience indicates that ocular surgery can be performed with impunity during corticosteroid therapy in moderate dosage. Unless required by severe uveitis or some similar medical indication, corticosteroid therapy is best postponed until 1 week postoperatively, by which time fibroblastic activity is already well advanced. The ophthalmologist will encounter, however, occasional cases that seem to incriminate corticosteroid therapy as the cause of serious wound disruptions. I am inclined to believe that an occasional case of wound disruption is contributed to by corticosteroid therapy. At any rate, delay in removal of sutures is prudent in patients receiving corticosteroids.

In fairness to the opposite point of view, it should be stated that the tensile strength of healing corneal incisions has been reported as completely unaffected by cortisone, 15

mg/kg, in rabbits.[31] Similarly, topical and subconjunctival application of corticosteroids are reported to cause no alteration in the healing of thermal corneal burns.[32] Biologic experiments have a perplexing way of giving different results in the hands of different investigators.

Inhibition of neovascularization

One of the most useful therapeutic actions of cortisone is inhibition of neovascularization. This effect is readily reproduced experimentally, provided that minimal lesions are studied. Naturally a sufficiently severe injury will heal with neovascularization despite use of corticosteroids. The rate of development of alloxan-induced corneal vascularization in cortisone-treated and control rabbits is shown in Fig. 15-10.[33] Cortisone has a nonspecific vasoconstrictor effect that may contribute to this inhibition of neovascularization and that may induce regression of existing vessels.[34]

Inhibition of epithelial regeneration

A relatively minor disadvantage of corticosteroids is the inhibition of epithelial and endothelial regeneration. The data given in Table 15-5 indicate that epithelial regeneration following standard thermal corneal burns occurred in 3 days in control animals but was delayed until the fourth day in three fifths of the cortisone-treated rabbits. This was not only an effect of topical administration but also occurred with intramuscular injection of cortisone. Similar slight retardation

Table 15-5. Retardation of epithelial regeneration by cortisone in standard corneal thermal burns in rabbits*

Eyes	Days required for epithelization			
	1	*2*	*3*	*4*
Cortisone treated			16	24
Control			19	1

*Data from Leopold, I. H., and Maylath, F.: Am. J. Ophthalmol. **35:**1125, 1952.

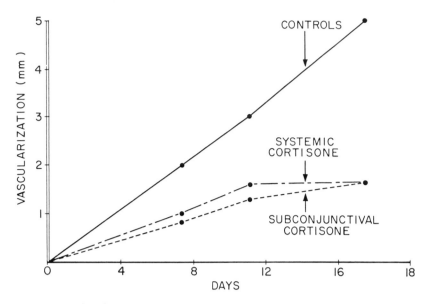

Fig. 15-10. Rate of development of alloxan-induced corneal neovascularization in control and cortisone-treated rabbits. (From Ashton, N., Cook, C., and Langham, M.: Br. J. Ophthalmol. **35:**718, 1951.)

of epithelial regeneration is reported in experimental wound healing and is observed clinically as persistent fluorescein staining.

Scanning electron microscopy shows loss of corneal microvilli subsequent to topical prednisolone therapy. Continuing therapy destroys the cytoplasmic membrane of the epithelial cells, eroding downward layer after layer into the corneal epithelium.[35]

INTRAOCULAR PENETRATION

Radioactive carbon–labeled cortisone acetate has been used to study the penetration of this substance into the eye.[36] One milliliter of a 0.25% suspension of this radioactive cortisone acetate was applied to rabbit corneas with a special stirring applicator. After 20 minutes, the eyes were thoroughly washed, enucleated, divided into their various portions, and subjected to chromatography and radioactivity counting. Cortisone acetate concentrations were extremely minute, being measured in millimicrograms (Table 15-6). Although only cortisone acetate was used, measurable quantities of radioactive cortisone and hydrocortisone were found in the tissues, indicating rapid metabolic trans-

Table 15-6. Range of concentration (mμg) of some steroid derivatives in specific tissues after 20-minute application of 0.25% solution of cortisone acetate to rabbit corneas*

Derivative	Cornea	Aque-ous	Iris and ciliary body	Choroid and sclera
Cortisone acetate	70-99	28-90	6-10	13
Cortisone	29-69	5-6	5-12	66
Hydrocor-tisone	14-26	6-30	—	8

*Data from Hamashige, S., and Potts, A.: Am. J. Ophthalmol. **40:**211, 1955.

formation of these substances. Highest concentrations were found in the cornea and aqueous, considerably lower concentrations in the iris, and no measurable quantity in the lens, vitreous, and retina. Considerable activity in the sclera and choroid might have been caused by posterior venous drainage or possibly by contamination, although the latter was believed unlikely. Since it is known

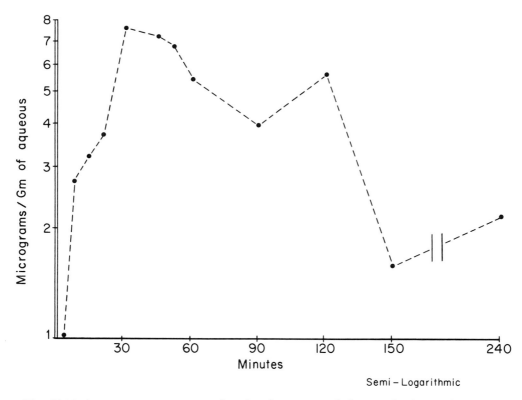

Fig. 15-11. Aqueous concentrations of prednisolone at specified intervals after ocular instillation of a drop of 1% suspension. (From Murdick, P. W., and associates: Arch. Ophthalmol. **76:** 602, 1966.)

that clinical response occurs to applications of corticosteroids of this concentration, it is apparent that these substances are biologically effective in extraordinarily dilute concentrations (for example, five billionths of a gram in the entire iris!).

Radioactive labeling permits identification of the distribution of cortisone after topical ocular instillation. An astonishing amount of corticosteroid is rapidly distributed throughout the body. Thirty minutes after instillation into rabbit eyes, only 1.6% of the radioactive corticosteroid was present within eye tissue.[37] Twenty-nine percent was still present in the conjunctival sac and was recovered by surface washing. The unusually long persistence of medication in the conjunctival sac resulted from the method of application—namely, pooling of 0.25 ml of solution between the lids that were held open by sutures. Nasal washings contained only 0.5%, suggesting that relatively little absorption occurred by this route (or that it was very rapidly absorbed into the general circulation and therefore did not accumulate within the nose). Liver, kidneys, adrenals, and gallbladder contained 21.4% of the radioactivity. The remaining 47.5% was presumably distributed throughout the other body tissues.

All parts of the eye contained radioactivity 30 minutes after cortisone application; however, the highest counts were obtained from cornea and conjunctiva. Counts-per-minute values for various eye tissues were as follows: cornea, 70; iris and ciliary body, 30; sclera and choroid, 20; retina, 16; aqueous, 8; lens, 4; vitreous, 1. (The total dose instilled on the eye was 10,000 counts/min of radioactivity.)

The corticosteroids present in the normal primary aqueous humor of the rabbit have been analyzed by chromatography.[38] No cortisone was found by a method capable of detecting as little as 60 mμg/ml. The only corticosteroid present had characteristics identical with those of crystalline hydrocortisone and was found in a concentration of 0.17 mμg/ml.

The aqueous concentrations of prednisolone alcohol after topical ocular instillation of a drop of 1% prednisolone (labeled with radioactive tritium) are shown in Fig. 15-11.[39]

As is true of all medications applied to the cornea, penetration of hydrocortisone compounds is also determined by differential solubility characteristics. It is pointed out in Table 15-7 that the water-soluble succinate and phosphate compounds of hydrocortisone did not penetrate the normal cornea enough to elevate the aqueous steroid concentration significantly above the normal control level.[40] In contrast, the lipoid-soluble acetate compound penetrated in effective concentration. Obviously the fact that a given corticosteroid preparation is a clear solution rather than a suspension does not necessarily indi-

cate that it will penetrate to the interior of the eye.

Does cortisone or hydrocortisone penetrate more readily into the aqueous? Is subconjunctival injection more effective than topical drops? These questions are answered by the information given in Table 15-8.[41] After subconjunctival injection of 50 mg of cortisone, aqueous steroid levels (Porter-Silber analytic method) were detectable within 30 minutes and persisted for at least 3 hours. Topical applications of a 2.5% suspension of cortisone or hydrocortisone drops were made every 15 minutes for 1 hour, at which time aqueous steroid levels were determined. Both normal rabbit eyes and eyes with rather severe corneal sodium hydroxide burns were used. Results may be summarized as follows:

1. Aqueous levels of cortisone were much higher than those of hydrocortisone.
2. Cortisone entered the aqueous readily via both topical and subconjunctival administration. Although the tabulated values are similar, they were obtained by subconjunctival injection of 50 mg of cortisone and by only 6 mg topically (4 drops of a 2.5% solution).
3. Higher aqueous levels were obtained in the presence of corneal damage.

Repeated topical applications of cortisone acetate will produce progressively higher aqueous cortisone levels, reaching a plateau after 3 days of therapy. Aqueous concentrations of 50 mμg/ml may be attained by topical application of cortisone acetate suspension nine times a day (Fig. 15-12).[21] A similar concentration was attained (but within 1 day rather than 3 days) by subconjunctival injection of 1.25 mg every 12 hours and by intra-

Table 15-7. Hydrocortisone (mμg/ml) recovered from rabbit aqueous after topical application every 5 minutes for six times of 0.5% solutions of some hydrocortisone compounds*

Hydrocortisone compound	Test eye	Control eye
Acetate	6.0	0.52
Succinate	0.48	0.65
Phosphate	0.9	0.70

*Data from Fleming, T. C., and Merrill, D. L.: Research report No. 5, Alcon Laboratories, Inc.

Table 15-8. Aqueous levels of steroid (μg/ml) after subconjunctival injection or topical use of drops of cortisone or hydrocortisone in normal and alkali-burned rabbit eyes*

Steroid	Normal eye	Burned eye
Subconjunctival injection of cortisone (50 mg)	5-10	15-17
Topical use of 2.5% cortisone (6 mg)	5-8	13-22
Subconjunctival injection of hydrocortisone (50 mg)	Not measurable	2-5
Topical use of 2.5% hydrocortisone (6 mg)	2	3-5

*Data from Leopold, I. H.: Arch. Ophthalmol. **52:**769, 1954.

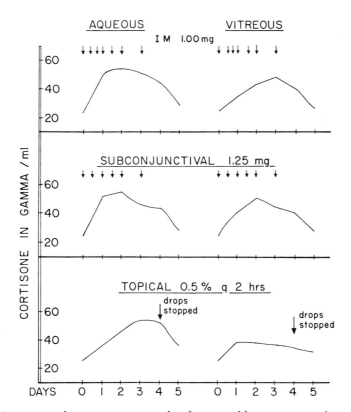

Fig. 15-12. Aqueous and vitreous cortisone levels attained by systemic, subconjunctival, and topical routes of administration. Drops were instilled nine times daily, subconjunctival injections were given every 12 hours, and intramuscular injections were given every 8 hours. (Modified from Leopold, I. H., and Maylath, F.: Am. J. Ophthalmol. **35:**1125, 1952.)

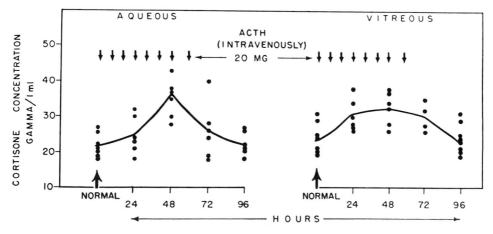

Fig. 15-13. Aqueous and vitreous cortisone concentrations after repeated intravenous injections of ACTH. (From Leopold, I. H., and Maylath, F.: Am. J. Ophthalmol. **35:**1125, 1952.)

muscular injection of 100 mg every 8 hours. Twenty-five milligrams of cortisone acetate by retrobulbar injection every day reached a peak of 35 mμg/ml. (This was a relatively early study, and the absolute values may be a little high.) By all routes, cortisone penetrated in appreciable quantity to the vitreous, although never quite attaining the aqueous concentrations. Topical applications gave the smallest vitreous concentrations. Cortisone was rapidly cleared from the aqueous, being virtually gone within 24 hours after the last of the series of applications by any route. Aqueous cortisone determinations done after ACTH injection indicated that a delay of 2 to 3 days occurred between injection and elevation of steroid levels (Fig. 15-13). From these penetration studies it would appear that anterior segment lesions could be treated equally well by topical, subconjunctival, or systemic routes, and that posterior lesions would be reached by systemic administration or subconjunctival injections.

Considerable variance exists in the intraocular penetration of prednisone and prednisolone, depending on whether free alcohol or acetate forms are employed and whether the cornea is normal or abraded. In Fig. 15-14 are shown aqueous concentrations of prednisone and prednisolone, in alcohol or acetate form, attained by topical instillation in rabbit eyes of 0.5% suspension every 15 minutes for an hour; aspiration of aqueous was done 15 minutes after the last drop.[42]

Prednisolone sodium phosphate is a highly water-soluble compound and is almost lipid insoluble. Theoretically it should not penetrate the intact corneal epithelium. Nevertheless, 30 minutes after instillation of a drop of 1% drug, corneal concentrations of 10 μg/g and aqueous levels of 0.5 μg/g are attained. If the epithelium is removed, corneal concentrations reach 235 μg/g and aqueous levels 17 μg/g.[43]

The intraocular penetration of topically applied prednisolone derivatives varies considerably. The aqueous concentration of corticosteroids attained by placing 1 drop of a 0.5% suspension into a rabbit cul-de-sac every 15 minutes for 1 hour is shown in Fig. 15-15; the sample was drawn 15 minutes after the last drop.[44] It is apparent that triamcinolone is present in far lower aqueous concentrations than are dexamethasone and methylprednisolone.

The blood-aqueous barrier definitely limits

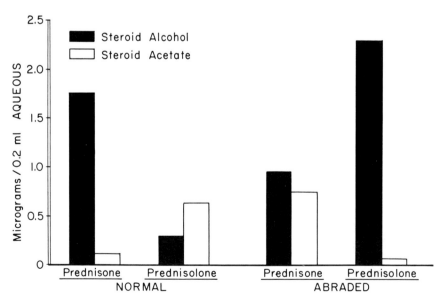

Fig. 15-14. Penetration of topically applied steroids, 0.5% suspension, given four times at 15-minute intervals. (Data from Leopold, I. H., Kroman, H., and Green, H.: Trans. Am. Acad. Ophthalmol. **59:**771, 1955.)

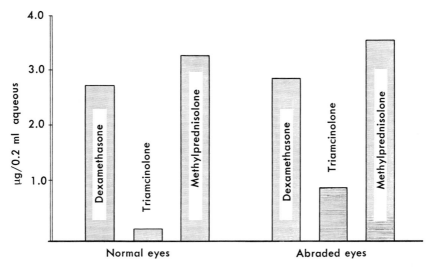

Fig. 15-15. Aqueous concentrations of corticosteroids 15 minutes after topical application of 0.5% suspension four times at 15-minute intervals. (Modified from Leopold, I. H., and Kroman, H. S.: Arch. Ophthalmol. **63:**943, 1960.)

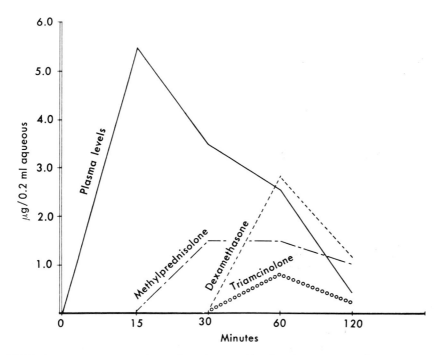

Fig. 15-16. Aqueous concentrations of corticosteroids after intravenous administration of 25 mg in rabbit. (Modified from Leopold, I. H., and Kroman, H. S.: Arch. Ophthalmol. **63:**943, 1960.)

the intraocular penetration of intravenously administered corticosteroids. After intravenous administration of 25 mg of dexamethasone (Fig. 15-16), no corticosteroid is demonstrable in the aqueous humor during the first 30 minutes. By 1 hour, a peak level is reached that is only slightly higher than that attained by topical application. Within 2 hours, the aqueous level of dexamethasone has fallen to half its peak value. (Triamcinolone given intravenously was found to penetrate much less well than dexamethasone, just as happened via the topical route.)

It was concluded from these studies (blue tetrazolium technique for determining steroids) that triamcinolone penetrates poorly into the aqueous humor of rabbits, as compared with dexamethasone and methylprednisolone.

The following year the same investigators, using a paper chromatography technique (stated to be more sensitive than the blue tetrazolium method), concluded that the prednisolone derivatives (dexamethasone [methylfluoroprednisolone], triamcinolone [fluorohydroxyprednisolone], and methylprednisolone) appeared to have equal ability to penetrate into the aqueous humor. Concentrations between 1 and 1.5 μg/1.5 ml of aqueous could be attained in 4- to 6-pound rabbits by intravenous injection of 25 mg of corticosteroid 1 hour before sampling, or by topical instillation of 0.5% suspension of corticosteroid every 15 minutes for 1 hour. Slightly higher concentrations were attained by the topical route of administration in these experiments.[45]

After reading about the endless variations of ocular penetration and therapeutic effect resulting from different corticosteroid derivatives and vehicles, it is reassuring to find that reputable manufacturers produce consistently effective products. For example, comparison of two brands (Pred Mild Suspension and Econopred—both 0.125% prednisolone acetate) showed no differences in concentration of drug in cornea and anterior chamber or in their anti-inflammatory effect against experimental clove oil keratitis.[46]

Indomethacin

Although indomethacin is not a corticosteroid, it does have anti-inflammatory action, and for convenience, its ability to penetrate the anterior chamber will be described here. One hour after instillation of a 1% aqueous suspension of radioactive indomethacin on the rabbit cornea, 0.4% of the applied radioactivity was found to be within the aqueous. This indicates that indomethacin, a lipid-soluble drug, penetrates the cornea well.[47]

ROUTES OF ADMINISTRATION AND DOSAGE
Topical application

The route of administration of corticosteroids depends primarily on the site of involvement. Topical therapy is effective in anterior segment disease, including disorders of lids, conjunctiva, cornea, iris, and ciliary body. Ease of application, relatively low cost, and absence of systemic complications strongly favor local routes whenever they are effective. Unusually stubborn anterior segment disease may require supplementary systemic or subconjunctival medications, if drops alone have failed to control the inflammation.

The course of posterior segment disease (chorioretinitis, optic neuritis, and posterior scleritis) is not appreciably affected by topical corticosteroids and requires systemic therapy. Patients prefer oral administration of corticosteroids to injections. Since the peak concentration of plasma steroids occurs within 1 hour after oral administration, it is unnecessary to resort to intravenous injections for faster results. Four to eight hours after an oral dose, plasma steroid levels have returned to normal; therefore one dosage regimen is to divide the total daily dose into equal amounts to be taken every 4 to 6 hours.

Dosage will vary with the severity of disease. For most topical purposes, 0.5% suspensions of cortisone, hydrocortisone, prednisone, and prednisolone are adequate.[48] For more severe disease processes, 2.5% suspensions may be desirable. Increased frequency of application is usually equal to or more effective than use of a stronger concentration. In unusually severe cases, hourly instillations may be employed until some response is obtained; then frequency may be tapered off. Chronic allergy (for example, vernal conjunctivitis) may require long-term (dangerous) treatment several times daily to maintain the patient symptom free. The possibility of relapse exists if therapy is prematurely stopped in a disease such as iritis, and topical usage should be tapered off over several days to a week, depending on the response of a given eye. Usually little difference is noted clinically between cortisone, hydrocortisone, prednisone, and other newer corticosteroid derivatives. Should a disappointing result be obtained from one of these medications, change to another is sometimes suggested. In general, hydrocortisone effects are similar to those of cortisone, but hydrocortisone is more potent against surface inflammations. Intramuscular hydrocortisone acetate is relatively inert, presumably because it is only one seventh as soluble in body fluids as is cortisone. This insolubility may reduce the effect of hydrocortisone on iritis as compared with cortisone.

The basic pharmacologic principle that drugs have dose-response relationships is, of course, of great practical importance. Not only therapeutic efficacy but also toxicity follows dose-response relationships. However, the amount of a clinically useful drug required for a therapeutic response will usually not induce a toxic response. From a practical standpoint, therefore, the smallest amount of drug that will achieve the desired therapeutic response should always be used.

As a specific example, 0.001% dexamethasone drops five times daily will reliably prevent experimental corneal graft reactions, whereas smaller doses fail to do so. Tensile strength of healing corneal wounds is impaired by 0.1% dexamethasone drops twelve times daily but not by smaller doses. If delayed until the seventh postoperative day, corticosteroid therapy does not impair corneal wound healing. The clinical implications of

these dose relationships are obvious insofar as they relate to avoidance of toxicity.[49] A less apparent implication is that corticosteroid overtreatment is probably the clinical rule rather than the exception, to the detriment of the patient. "More is not necessarily better" applies not only to vitamins but also to corticosteroids.

As a reminder, topical ocular medications *are* absorbed systemically. The only difference between topical and systemic routes of administration is the lesser amount of drug usually given topically. For example, adrenal gland atrophy occurs in rabbits given 1 drop of dexamethasone five times daily for 21 days. (Of course, a rabbit is smaller than a human being and this is a proportionately much higher dose.[50])

The typical dose-response curve describing the effect of corticosteroid therapy of keratitis would show an increasing response to greater concentrations of drug. This response is not limitless, however, since increments of response to further increases of dosage become smaller as a maximum value is reached. Theoretically, such a curve is somewhat S-shaped. There will also be a toxic response curve, which will be located somewhere to the right of the therapeutic curve, depending on the therapeutic index of the given drug. Ideally, a dose C (Fig. 15-17) would give a substantial therapeutic response, yet almost no toxic response. Unfortunately, variations in disease and host do not permit exact choice of this ideal dose C.

Dose D gives the maximal response possible—knowledge of this level is useful, since there is no benefit from further dosage increase.

Can a maximal corticosteroid response dose be established? Measurement of the radioactively labeled polymorphonuclear leukocyte response to the intracorneal injection of clove oil permits exact measurements that may be used to formulate a dose-response curve applicable to this specific toxic keratitis (not necessarily applicable to any given disease, though). Using this experimental technique, the maximal attainable therapeu-

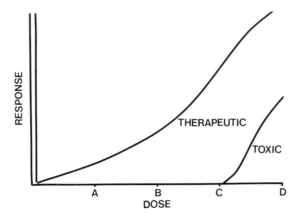

Fig. 15-17. Theoretical dose-response curve, indicating both therapeutic and toxic responses.

tic response was reduction of the leukocytes invading the cornea to 40% of their untreated number. This was achieved with 1% prednisolone acetate, topically applied (rabbits). Increasing the strength of the prednisolone to 3% did not significantly further decrease the number of leukocytes. The use of 0.125% prednisolone reduced the leukocytes to only 70% of their untreated number.[51]

Systemic therapy

Although the early literature advocated a standard oral cortisone dosage of 300 mg the first day, 200 mg the second day, and 100 mg every day thereafter, ophthalmologists now recognize that each diseased eye must be considered individually, just as there is no standard amount of insulin to be used in treating a diabetic. Highest doses are reserved for severe inflammations that threaten loss of sight (for example, macular chorioretinitis). In the presence of such severe inflammations the physician should immediately prescribe daily doses of the magnitude of 60 to 80 mg of prednisone. Initially, daily observations should include ophthalmoscopy and perimetry, and if the lesion progresses, dosage should be increased rapidly as high as the consulting internist believes to be safe. (As much as three times this dose may safely be given to healthy persons under careful expert supervision.) The minimum acceptable response is arrest of further progress of the disease; however, in many cases of acute chorioretinitis, clinical improvement will be clearly evident within the first few days or week. When improvement is noted, physicians may choose to reduce corticosteroid dosage stepwise to the minimum level necessary to produce steady, measurable regression of the lesion, or they may prefer to maintain high dosage in an attempt to restore the vital macular area to normal as rapidly as possible. Less critical inflammations will tend to be treated by the first choice and more critical ones by the second choice. Reduction in dosage should be accomplished in gradual steps, guided by ophthalmoscopic and perimetric findings, and will usually require more than a month before therapy can be stopped. If a given reduction is followed by exacerbation of the inflammation, therapy must immediately be raised to the high initial doses (Fig. 15-18).[52] Such escape of the disease from therapeutic control is a serious complication and should be avoided if at all possible by slow and gradual reduction of dosage. So long as any evidence of active inflammation persists, it is hazardous to discontinue therapy. Many patients will require months of treatment at fairly high dosage levels. Persistence of old retinal hemorrhage, hard whitish edema residues, and the irregular reflections of preretinal gliosis are not to be construed as continuing inflammation and do not constitute an indication for therapy.

Although it is to be expected that some patients with uveitis will not respond to cortico-

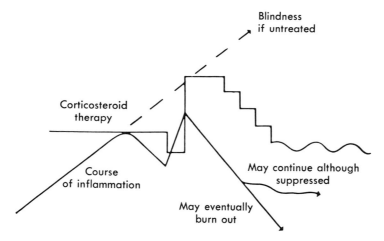

Fig. 15-18. Modification of course of chronic intraocular inflammation by corticosteroid therapy. Diagram is designed to illustrate the prevention of blindness by treatment, relapse with reduction of treatment, control by higher level treatment, and final quiescence. (From Gordon, D.: Arch. Ophthalmol. **62:**400, 1959.)

steroid therapy, many such patients are found to have received inadequate treatment and will respond to increased dosage. Uveitis made worse by properly intensive and continued corticosteroid treatment is uncommon.

Naturally, less severe inflammations will be treated less vigorously; the treatment is adjusted to control the symptoms and to prevent significant permanent scarring. Not all patients with chorioretinitis require treatment—witness the commonly observed asymptomatic scars of peripheral chorioretinitis, many of which were not even recognized by the patient during their acute stage.

Alternate-day therapy

The undesirable side effects of systemic corticosteroid therapy can be substantially reduced by using alternate-day therapy rather than divided dosage. Briefly stated, the entire total dose of corticosteroid that would have been given during a 2-day period is administered as a single dose every other morning. Such alternate-day dosage causes less suppression of the adrenals and other endocrine glands, minimizes growth alterations, and does not completely suppress cell-mediated immune responses, for example, those

measured by skin testing with histoplasmosis antigen.

How effective is this alternate-day regimen in the control of disease? Apparently in the control of systemic diseases (such as asthma and arthritis) this therapeutic ratio of 2:1 (double dose on alternate days) is effective. Evaluation of a corneal graft rejection model in rabbits indicated that the therapeutically equivalent ratio was 2.6:1 (two and a half times the daily dose given every other morning).[53] Inasmuch as we do not know in the individual case how large a corticosteroid dosage will be required on a daily basis, we then do not know how large a dose is 2 to 2.6 times as great. This corneal graft rejection model does demonstrate, however, that if the appropriate level of alternate-day corticosteroid dosage is empirically determined, it should control ocular inflammation (or at least corneal rejection) as well as the more toxic method of multiple daily dosage.

Alternate-day systemic corticosteroid therapy in children will minimize growth suppression and appears to be a worthwhile method. In adults there may be slightly less adrenal suppression, but this is counterbalanced by a lesser clinical response to the same total drug dosage. Hence, alternate-day systemic corticosteroid therapy is of doubtful value in adults.[54]

Repository injection

The ophthalmologist who wishes to administer corticosteroids by "subconjunctival" injection should consider use of the repository form of methylprednisolone acetate (Depo-Medrol). This suspension form of prednisolone provides a constant source of corticosteroid that lasts for 2 to 4 weeks. The technique is to inject (after topical anesthesia) 0.5 ml (20 mg) beneath Tenon's capsule at about the equator, in the upper temporal quadrant. Other quadrants may be used for subsequent injections. Pain and tenderness will be present for 6 to 12 hours, requiring analgesia and an ice bag. Transient conjunctival chemosis may occur.

Such injections were given to more than 200 patients suffering from a variety of ocular conditions responsive to corticosteroid therapy.[55] This clinical experience confirmed the effectiveness of such injections in anterior segment inflammations (acute iridocyclitis, scleritis and episcleritis, corneal transplant allergy, and the like). The main advantage of injection seemed to be elimination of the need for frequent topical medication. (Particularly during the night, continuous liberation of corticosteroid via repository injection should be therapeutically more effective than topical administration.) Naturally, injection should be limited to the treatment of the more severe inflammation and would be inappropriate for management of mild hay fever, for instance.

A long-term repository vehicle of triamcinolone acetonide is also available (Kenalog, administered parenterally). Injection beneath Tenon's capsule of 0.5 ml of this corticosteroid has been reported to benefit a variety of chronic inflammatory ocular diseases.[56]

Does retrobulbar injection of a depot-type corticosteroid really result in prolonged effective concentrations of medication in the intraocular tissues? To evaluate this, 0.3 ml of radioactive tritium–labeled Depo-Medrol with 0.2 ml of 1% lidocaine was given via retrobulbar injection to six monkeys.[57] At 2 days quite high concentrations of methylprednisolone were measured within the eye (Fig. 15-19). At 9 days after injection the concentrations were greatly reduced; however, 0.5 μg/100 mg of tissue persisted within the choroid-retina portion of the eye and 1.33 μg/100 ml within the optic nerve. An identical 0.3 ml dose of Depo-Medrol was given intramuscularly in four monkeys. Two days after this intramuscular injection, no radioactivity was demonstrable in the posterior portions of the eye. These experiments indicate that retrobulbar injection of a repository form of corticosteroid can be expected to deliver high concentrations of medication to the optic nerve, sclera, choroid, and retina for a period of a week or longer.

That a clinically significant anti-inflammatory response can be obtained from retrobulbar corticosteroid injection was demonstrated in a rabbit model of herpetic chorioretinitis.[58] A reproducible hemorrhagic chorioretinitis and optic neuritis appear in rabbit eyes 7 to 12 days after injection of herpes simplex virus into the anterior chamber of the opposite eye. Eyes with inflammations of comparable severity were matched in pairs and treated with retrobulbar injections of either 4 mg of dexamethasone (Decadron) in 1 ml or a control solution. Injections were given the first day of recognizable inflammation and were repeated once 48 hours later. Various inflammatory parameters were evaluated—all indicated improvement in the dexamethasone-treated eyes. For example, vitreous opacity sufficient to obscure the disc was present in all control eyes at 5 days but in only half of the dexamethasone-treated eyes. Virus was recoverable in more treated than control eyes and a higher titer of viruses (up to 1000 times greater) was found in the dexamethasone-treated eyes. At the end of 1 month the condition of treated and untreated eyes was comparable—apparently extensive retinal detachments were grossly visible with flashlight in almost all eyes. This experiment does not permit the inference that corticosteroid therapy is desirable for herpes simplex infections but does establish that a retrobul-

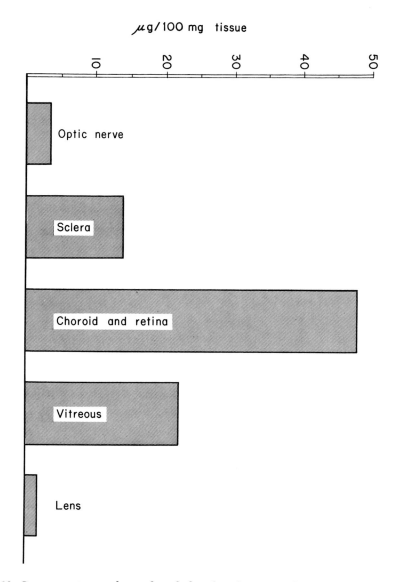

Fig. 15-19. Concentration gradient of methylprednisolone in ocular tissues 2 days after retrobulbar injection. (Modified from Hyndiuk, R. A., and Reagan, M. G.: Arch. Ophthalmol. **80:** 499, 1968.)

bar corticosteroid injection has a measurable intraocular effect.

The physician using corticosteroid injections in the area of the eye should be aware of the possibility of scleral perforation. The small, sharp needles used to permit comfortable injection will also enter the eye with minimal resistance. During 1 year I saw three such cases because of retinal detachment from the iatrogenic retinal hole and the vitreoretinal contraction secondary to trauma. In one eye a bead of vitreous projected from the scleral perforation even though the injection had been given several months earlier. This delayed healing was probably attributable to the corticosteroid effect. These cases do not respond well to detachment surgery because of progressive contraction of intraocular scar tissue.

Of a series of 6 cases of accidental intraocular injection of depot corticosteroids, 3 eyes developed irreparable organized retinal detachment.[59]

In treatment of pars planitis, methylprednisolone (Depo-Medrol), 0.4 ml, was injected into the choroid. The whitish material was seen in the choroidal vessels and dissected forward into the anterior chamber, where it appeared as white flocculent debris. This disappeared uneventfully after 2 months. The pars planitis did not improve.[60]

Permanent paralysis of the superior rectus muscle, found to be thin and atrophic on surgical exploration, followed injection of 1 ml of Depo-Medrol into the sub-Tenon's space superiorly.[61]

Following 6 subconjunctival injections of corticosteroid for persistent uveitis, atrophy of subcutaneous tissue over the inferior orbital rim resulted. A depression of the lower lid was cosmetically visible, but no enophthalmos was present.[62]

I deplore the advice that orbital injections should be made by stabbing a sharp needle through the lid, in a manner comparable to throwing a dart at the eye. A much safer approach is to cross the conjunctiva and Tenon's capsule at about the equator, with the needle held tangent to the globe and the tip directed slightly away from the sclera. Follow the curve of the eye with the needle, with a constant, slight side-to-side movement. If the tip engages the sclera, this sideways movement will abruptly become impossible. If previous injections or surgery have scarred the area, such lateral movement is impossible. *Never* point a needle at the eye. (This is also true in surgery—advance a needle through the sclera tangent to the curvature of the eye, adjusting the depth of passage by the amount of side pressure directed against the eye.)

The injection of repository corticosteroid may cause a susceptible eye to develop persistent glaucoma. Experimental infections are enhanced by such corticosteroid pretreatment. A considerable amount of scarring and fibrosis of Tenon's capsule is evident on surgical exploration of an injected area.

I agree with the conclusions of a review article[63] that, ". . . on balance, injection of repository forms of steroids are fraught with more complications than their potential benefits could justify."

ACTH injection

Being destroyed in the gastrointestinal tract, corticotropin must be administered parenterally. Its action is via adrenal cortical stimulation, and therefore topical usage is ineffective and irrational. Long-acting gel preparations should be injected every 12 hours to a total of 50 to 150 mg/day. Intravenous administration of corticotropin is stated to be 8 to 12 times as effective as intramuscular injection, but this method requires an 8 hours' continuous drip of 25 mg in 1 liter of 5% glucose solution. It has been advocated as a possibility in stubborn cases.

Intravitreal injection

In the treatment of experimental *Pseudomonas* endophthalmitis, gentamicin, 500 μg, and dexamethasone, 400 μg, were injected intravitreally. Within 3 hours after injection, half of the dexamethasone had disappeared from the eye (radioactive measurement). Four days after injection, a residual level of 0.05 μg/ml remained.

In the eyes treated 1 to 5 hours after infection, the dexamethasone-gentamicin treated eyes were less inflamed than were the eyes treated with gentamicin alone. However, in the 10-hour-old infections, extensive destruction occurred, with loss of sight in all eyes despite treatment.[65] Clinically, no physician is going to inject intravitreally an eye free of signs of infection. For practical purposes, we cannot duplicate this rabbit experiment clinically. Also, corticosteroid penetration into the inflamed eye can be achieved without intravitreal injection.

Controlled release vehicles

Ocusert devices delivering 10 μg of hydrocortisone acetate/hr were used to treat allergic conjunctivitis (to bovine albumin) in rabbits. The response to the continuous low-level drug delivery was as good as or better than that obtained by five times daily instillation of eye drops. This response establishes that the very high level of medication briefly attained with an eye drop is not necessary for successful treatment of allergic conjunctivitis.[66]

INDICATIONS

In general, corticosteroid therapy may be helpful for all allergic ocular diseases (vernal conjunctivitis, drug or contact sensitivity, and so forth), for most nonpyogenic inflammations (episcleritis, scleritis, uveitis, interstitial keratitis, sclerokeratitis, rosacea keratitis, optic neuritis, and the like), and for the reduction of scarring from certain types of severe injury (chemical or thermal corneal burns). The preceding discussion of the antiinflammatory actions of cortisone indicates what can be expected from such therapy.

For example, hourly instillation of 0.1% fluorometholone for 2 days reduced by 20% to 30% the number of radiolabeled polymorphonuclear leukocytes invading the cornea after intracorneal injection of 0.03 ml of clove oil.[64] Armchair contemplation suggests this response would be undesirable in the presence of infection but might be helpful to reduce nonspecific inflammatory reaction.

The effect of various corticosteroid derivatives on uveitis is essentially the same, differing only in the dosage level required to achieve a given amount of suppression of inflammation. This similar effect is shown in Fig. 15-20, compiled from the results of treatment of experimental horse serum uveitis in rabbits.[67] Differences in response are caused by relative potency of the drugs and could be altered by changing the dosage. In-

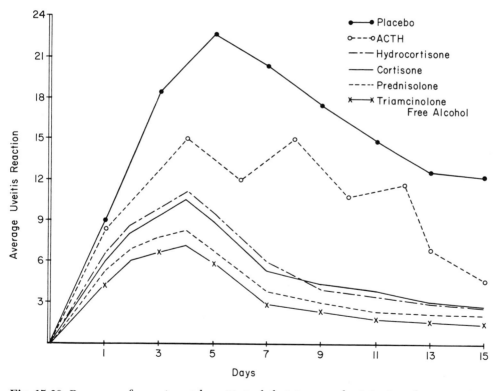

Fig. 15-20. Response of experimental uveitis to daily intramuscular injection of cortisone acetate, 25 mg/kg (Cortone); hydrocortisone sodium succinate, 25 mg/kg (Solu-Cortef); prednisolone phosphate, 5 mg/kg (Hydeltrasol); triamcinolone alcohol, 2.5 mg/kg (Aristocort); corticotropin, 10 units/kg (ACTH); and placebo (saline solution). (From Chavan, S. B., and Cummings, E. J.: Am. J. Ophthalmol. 49:55, 1960.)

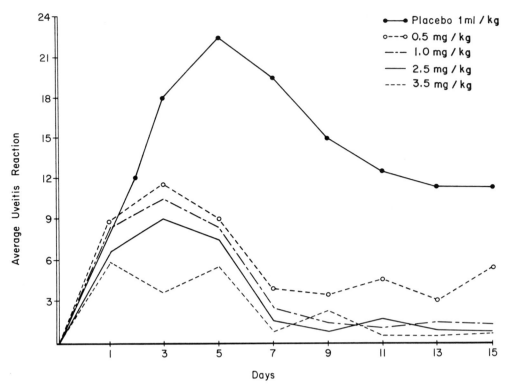

Fig. 15-21. Response of experimental uveitis to daily intramuscular injection of triamcinolone in different dosage levels. (Modified from Chavan, S. B., and Cummings, E. J.: Am. J. Ophthalmol. **49:**55, 1960.)

jections of triamcinolone varying from 0.5 to 3.5 mg/kg caused the increasing anti-inflammatory effect shown in Fig. 15-21.[67]

Corticosteroid therapy is of no benefit whatsoever in degenerative diseases (senile macular degeneration, cataract, corneal dystrophies, primary glaucoma, keratoconjunctivitis sicca, and the like).[68] Old scars (old inactive chorioretinitis, band keratopathy, traumatic corneal scars, and such) are not altered by cortisone. Most infections should not be treated with corticosteroids unless an effective antibiotic is used before and simultaneously.

As we learn more about the undesirable effects of corticosteroid therapy, perhaps we should question the traditional indications for such treatment and explore the possibilities of alternate methods of management. For example, in a double-blind study of the effect of 30 mg/day of prednisolone compared with 600 mg/day of oxyphenbutazone, 60 patients with nodular episcleritis or scleritis (most common etiology, rheumatoid arthritis) were evaluated.[69] There was very little difference in the effects of these two drugs. The prednisolone gave a more prompt initial response, but when treatment was discontinued, relapse was more frequent with prednisolone. Because of the toxic effects of corticosteroids, I do not believe they should be used for relatively benign conditions such as allergic conjunctivitis, contact lens irritation, or surface injuries.

Infrequently encountered diseases

Boeck's sarcoid. The response of Boeck's sarcoid uveitis (as well as the general manifestations) to corticosteroid therapy may be very gratifying. In our limited experience, topical use of corticosteroids and mydriatics has been insufficient to arrest the disease.

Addition of systemic corticosteroid therapy has in some cases given prompt subjective relief, followed within a few weeks by considerable objective improvement. Long-term, low-dose therapy may be necessary to maintain remission. A case report describes almost complete disappearance within 2 weeks of a huge (4 × 6 mm) iris nodule and moderately severe granulomatous iritis with prednisone treatment (average dosage level of 40 mg every 6 hours).[70] Apparently no serious side effects resulted from use of this tremendous amount of corticosteroid.

These impressions are confirmed by a report of treatment of 36 patients with rather severe sarcoid (four had uveitis) with cortisone.[71] Up to 200 mg daily was used and produced a consistently favorable symptomatic effect. Ocular and parotid involvement was notably responsive to treatment. In contrast, pulmonary lesions were quite variable in their response. Despite prompt initial symptomatic response, the chronic, long-term characteristics of sarcoidosis were not eradicated. Not one of these 36 patients developed tuberculosis during or after cortisone therapy. Reference is made to instances of explosive appearance of tuberculosis several weeks after cortisone therapy of supposed sarcoidosis. Such cases are attributed to mistaken diagnosis and are cited to demonstrate the unhappy effect of cortisone treatment of tuberculosis.

Endocrine exophthalmos. The malignant exophthalmos of thyrotropic disease is difficult to control by any means and is best avoided by refraining from thyroid surgery in the presence of congested eyes. Fairly high doses of systemic corticosteroids are sometimes effective in reducing the severity of exophthalmos. Topical instillations do not favorably alter the orbital contents, although surface redness may decrease. One case is reported in which the exophthalmos decreased from 30 to 27 mm during 2 months of treatment with ACTH.[72] The most effective response seems to be obtained in the patient with rather rapid onset of a watery edema, possibly related to rubbing and injuring the exposed conjunctiva. Such patients may respond surprisingly well to tarsorrhaphy, lubrication, and systemic administration of corticosteroids. A trial of such medical treatment should certainly be employed before orbital decompression surgery is undertaken. Decompression procedures in these nervous patients are unforgettably unpleasant experiences.

Temporal arteritis. Fortunately temporal arteritis is a rare disease, for it is visually disastrous. Of 32 patients, 11 became blind in both eyes and 7 in one eye.[73] Occlusion of the central retinal artery or of the vessels supplying the optic nerve may lead to blindness even during the course of corticosteroid therapy. Insufficient material exists to establish whether corticosteroids have any effect whatsoever on the visual prognosis in temporal arteritis. Nevertheless, use of corticosteroids is definitely indicated in this disease because of the resultant dramatic relief from pain. For purposes of prognosis, it is helpful to know that temporal arteritis in these 32 patients had an average duration of 4½ months (from 2 to 12 months) and that no patient suffered a recurrence after the active phase of the disease subsided.

Scleromalacia perforans. Another collagen disease that is at least partially helped by cortisone is scleromalacia perforans. Histologic study of a single such cortisone-treated eye has been compared with the findings in six untreated eyes.[74] It is pertinent to state that this eye was treated when supplies of cortisone were limited and received what would now be considered relatively light treatment, namely 100 mg of cortisone every day for several weeks. Thereafter, cortisone drops were administered every 4 hours for some months. Clinically, reduction in redness, nodule formation, and photophobia were attributed to the cortisone. Histologically, the treated eye showed a much less severe inflammatory reaction and had almost no polymorphonuclear cells and eosinophils, in contrast to the large numbers of these cells found in the six untreated eyes. Surprisingly, fibroblastic regeneration over the ulcerated areas of sclera and uniformly palisaded arrangement of the new fibroblasts were much more definite in the cortisone-treated eye. Apparently, corticosteroids prevent further inflammatory activity in scleromalacia perforans, thereby creating suitable conditions for fibrous regeneration. Excessive corticosteroid therapy may, however, inhibit the regenerative process, and in some cases scleral thinning seems to be accelerated by such treatment.

In another case the clinical response of scleromalacia perforans to corticotropin therapy was not significant.[75] This patient suffered onset and progression of scleromalacia during a 13-month course of corticosteroid therapy for rheumatoid arthritis. Dosage was 100 mg of cortisone every day for 4 months and then 40 mg of ACTH twice weekly. This patient also had retinitis pigmentosa and suffered progressive loss of field and acuity during the 13 months of cortisone therapy.

Rheumatoid arthritis. In a series of nine rheumatoid patients with peripheral corneal furrows, two developed peripheral corneal perforations after corticosteroid use.[76] None of these nine patients with rheumatoid corneal disease were helped by corticosteroid therapy. Five additional cases of central corneal perforations after corticosteroid therapy were reported in this paper.

A possible explanation for this untoward effect of corticosteroid therapy is reduction of corneal fibroblast metabolism by these drugs. The combined effect of a disease and a drug, both damaging the corneal stroma, may account for corneal thinning and perforation. A relevant fact is that the skin of a rheumatoid patient (but not of a normal patient) thins when corticosteroids are applied topically.[77]

In general, corticosteroid therapy of corneal or scleral disease in patients with rheumatoid arthritis is more likely to be harmful than to be beneficial.

Sjögren's syndrome. A report from the Wills Eye Hospital indicates that even in this huge patient population corneal perforation does not occur from untreated keratoconjunctivitis sicca.[78] However, over a 2-year period 4 patients were seen who had suffered corneal perforation following corticosteroid treatment of keratoconjunctivitis sicca. I

have seen one such patient who perforated both corneas. There is no rational reason to treat keratoconjunctivitis sicca with corticosteroids, and it is evident that some type of collagenase activation or fibroblastic repair inhibition may result in corneal melting from corticosteroids in such cases.

Congenital syphilis. In the past, atropinization has been a most important part of the treatment of interstitial keratitis and its associated iridocyclitis. The resulting prolonged cycloplegia interferes with a child's schoolwork (although temporary use of bifocal or reading glasses would help). Management of 16 patients with interstitial keratitis with topical hydrocortisone alone or with atropine briefly in the beginning gave a therapeutic response equally as good as that obtained with prolonged cycloplegia.[79] Goniosynechiae seemed to occur less frequently when hydrocortisone was used. Since months or even years of treatment may be required in some cases, it is of practical importance to know that topical application of corticosteroids alone will satisfactorily control chronic interstitial keratitis.

Vernal conjunctivitis. In a series of 400 cases of vernal conjunctivitis the effects of topical cortisone, hydrocortisone, and prednisone were evaluated.[80] Although statistics were not presented, prednisone was reported to be the most effective therapy. Corticosteroids do *not* cure vernal conjunctivitis, and relapse is to be expected when therapy stops. Oral supplements of prednisone were found to be valuable in severe cases, particularly in the presence of corneal ulceration.

Objective quantitation of conjunctival allergic response is possible with refractometric measurement of the protein concentration of tears.[81] Using this method and employing as a subject a patient with known conjunctival allergy to timothy grass pollen, the response to various medications was studied. As shown in Fig. 15-22, the allergic response cleared within 15 minutes after instillation of 0.12% phenylephrine or 1% epinephryl borate but required an hour to respond to 1% prednisolone. Prednisolone 0.1% was

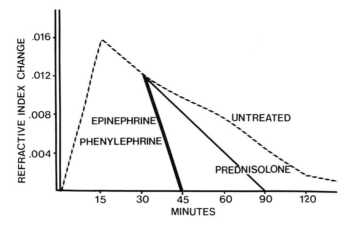

Fig. 15-22. The response of pollen-induced allergic conjunctivitis to 0.12% phenylephrine, 1% epinephryl borate, and 1% prednisolone, all instilled 30 minutes after the pollen was applied to the conjunctiva. (Data from Stegman, R., and Miller, D.: Arch. Ophthalmol. **93:**1354, December 1975. Copyright 1975, American Medical Association.)

also used but did not at all hasten the spontaneous rate of improvement.

I have seen bilateral aphakia and advanced glaucomatous visual field loss in a 30-year-old woman treated over a period of many years with topical corticosteroids for allergic conjunctivitis. Long-term use of corticosteroids for a relatively minor condition such as conjunctival allergy does not really make much therapeutic sense when sympathomimetic drugs actually give a more prompt response.

Herpes zoster. In a small series of 11 patients with herpes zoster, very favorable results are reported from the systemic administration of cortisone or ACTH.[82] Representative dosages were 20 mg of ACTH intravenously every day, 40 mg of ACTHAR gel intramuscularly every day, or 100 mg of cortisone every day (may be preceded by initial 300 mg on first day). Herpetic manifestations that were favorably influenced included the severe neuralgic pains, the characteristic iridocyclitis, keratitis, and occasional secondary glaucoma. Within several days these inflammatory manifestations underwent rather dramatic improvement, which was especially notable since most patients had suffered symptoms for about a week before treatment was instituted. Further in-

crease in the treatment level is helpful in resistant cases.

Corticosteroid treatment was considered suppressive but not curative, and it was necessary to continue it for weeks to a month or more before the eye disease was completely cleared. No evidence of exacerbation of this virus infection resulting from the use of cortisone or ACTH was noted.

Subsequently, a report of a total of 36 patients with herpes zoster ophthalmicus treated with ACTH or cortisone came to the same conclusions.[83] Only 16% of these 36 patients suffered permanent visual loss, in contrast to 58% of an untreated series.

Adenopharyngeal conjunctival virus. Study of 171 cases has delineated the clinical characteristics of A-P-C virus, type 3.[84] This virus produces conjunctivitis and pharyngitis, with mild fever and malaise. Antibiotics are ineffectual. The majority of patients treated with topical application of cortisone or hydrocortisone enjoyed rapid clearing of symptoms and signs of conjunctivitis. No patient's condition was made worse by corticosteroid treatment. It should be emphasized that laboratory confirmation of the diagnosis of type 3 A-P-C virus had been made in those patients who responded well to cortisone.

Neoplasms. Quite a dramatic decrease in the size of three hemangiomas resulted within 1 or 2 months following systemic therapy with prednisone in a dosage varying from 10 to 30 mg/day. This dosage was continued for 3 to 6 weeks and then tapered downward. In each case a rebound in the size of the hemangioma occurred when the treatment was discontinued.[85]

Since infants are particularly susceptible to the hazards of corticosteroid therapy, careful pediatric management is appropriate during such treatment. Avoid corticosteroid treatment during childhood infections, especially chickenpox. Measure body weight weekly and be sure the child is eating a proper diet.

When alternate-day corticosteroid treatment was used in these three cases, reduction in tumor size occurred only on the days the drug was given. Repository corticosteroid injection into the hemangioma was not mentioned.

Because of the spontaneous involution of hemangiomas beginning when the patient is about 1 year of age, any treatment (especially x-ray!) with significantly detrimental side effects is of doubtful wisdom and should be reserved for unusually severe cases.

Optic neuritis. This is really a hard diagnosis to make. Furthermore, even a true "neuritis" may be caused by a variety of etiologies, only some of which may be corticosteroid responsive. Even worse, a therapeutic trial of corticosteroids may cause temporary improvement of a brain tumor, thereby "confirming" the erroneous diagnosis of optic neuritis. In a case such as this, the visual acuity of a 32-year-old man improved from 20/200 to 20/20. The true diagnosis of a chromophobe adenoma was delayed 18 months by this presumed response of optic neuritis to corticosteroids.[86]

Not only hemangiomas[87] but also other tumors, for example, an intracranial plasmacytoma[88] respond to systemic corticosteroids. In the case of the plasmacytoma, the mistaken diagnosis of steroid responsive optic neuritis was initially made. Neurosurgical removal was ultimately necessary.

Neuralgia. Greater occipital neuralgia, a cause of severe radiating unilateral head pain that may be referred to the eye, may respond to corticosteroid injection (dexamethasone, 2 mg) at the site of maximum tenderness just beneath the occipital protuberance. Injections may have to be repeated at weekly intervals before the pain relief is maintained. Actually, the report indicates that 1 ml of 2% xylocaine is equally effective with or without the dexamethasone.[89]

Anterior segment ischemia. Following vertical muscle transplantation to correct paralysis of the lateral rectus muscle (Jensen procedure) combined with medial rectus recession in a 66-year-old woman, mild anterior segment ischemia resulted.[90] Prednisolone 1% was used four times daily, with gradual clearing of the corneal edema and anterior chamber cellular reaction. Although the time sequence of resolution is not stated clearly, I suspect that the improvement was simply the spontaneous course of the condition, unaffected by corticosteroid therapy.

Pseudotumor cerebri. This syndrome undoubtedly results from many etiologies and must be differentiated from intracranial neoplasms. It may be treated with fluid and salt restriction, with acetazolamide, or with corticosteroid. In a 5-year-old girl, administration of dexamethasone (Decadron), 0.5 mg, three times daily resulted in improvement starting on the first day of treatment. This dose was continued for 3 weeks and then gradually reduced until the patient was asymptomatic.[91]

NONRESPONSIVE CONDITIONS

Prophylactic use of corticosteroids for minor corneal abrasions and wounds must be frowned on, since no benefit can be anticipated and susceptibility to infection is increased. Only if the injury is severe enough (for example, chemical burn) so that significant scarring is anticipated does the potential benefit warrant the small but definite risk (and cost) of corticosteroid therapy.

For some illogical reason, prescription of combined corticosteroid-antibiotic ointments seems popular with general practitioners in the management of seborrheic blepharitis and chronic marginal blepharitis. Almost all chronic marginal blepharitis is of infectious origin and responds best to mechanical cleaning and antibiotics. Corticosteroids do not benefit such cases, may reduce resistance to infection, and are inevitably more expensive.

The entity of Fuchs' heterochromic cyclitis, said to represent 5% of cases of anterior uveitis, does not respond to corticosteroids, mydriatics, or other forms of therapy. Several times I have seen in consultation such patients who, misdiagnosed as having idiopathic uveitis, have spent considerable money on ill-advised corticosteroid therapy and have suffered some systemic side effects.

Gutter dystrophy of the periphery of the cornea is a peculiar disease of obscure etiology. "There is no doubt in my mind that excess local steroid therapy has a deleterious effect on these corneas and has led to perforation in several cases." This statement was made by Gundersen.[92] I personally am certain corticosteroids do not help gutter dystrophy and am inclined to agree that they may hasten further corneal thinning. At any rate, gutter dystrophy is not a disease that responds to medical therapy; it requires a conjunctival flap or lamellar corneal transplant if progressive thinning threatens the integrity of the eye.

USE IN OCULAR SURGERY

Most patients who have cataract extraction experience remarkably little discomfort and inflammation and do not require corticosteroid therapy. Theoretically, wound disruption and increased susceptibility to infection might result from topical use of corticosteroids after cataract extraction, but in practice these complications do not seem to occur. I have not used corticosteroids routinely after cataract extraction because this does not seem to make a great deal of difference in the average patient. Occasionally a postoperative eye will be far more red, swollen, and uncomfortable than usual. Such an eye should be observed most carefully for evidence of infection—which would indicate maximal antibiotic therapy. Repeated instil-

lation of atropine and other mydriatics is helpful. It may be prudent to watch such an irritable eye for 1 or 2 days to rule out infection, especially if this occurs within the first several days after surgery. Usually the difficulty is attributed to postoperative iridocyclitis, and when topical corticosteroids are used, the eye clears rapidly. Since postoperative iridocyclitis can produce secondary membranes of sight-impairing density, undue delay in starting corticosteroid therapy should be avoided.

Betamethasone phosphate 0.1% was instilled five times daily for 2 weeks in postoperative cataract eyes that had moderate or severe inflammation on their first postoperative day.[93] The inflammation was graded on a 0 to 3 scale, and a double-masked technique with placebo was used. The betamethasone group contained 56 patients; the placebo group, 51. During the 2-week treatment period the treated eyes averaged about 0.5 scale unit better than the placebo group. No complications in healing of the incision occurred. The discussion of this paper concluded that the corticosteroid effectiveness was a result of selection of inflamed eyes for treatment and the use of more frequent instillation of corticosteroid. Previous publications have showed that routine use three times daily of corticosteroid following cataract extraction does not reduce postoperative inflammation and is unjustified.[94,95] I advise against routine use of corticosteroids following cataract surgery.

Iridocyclitis is more likely after extracapsular extraction, and under these conditions, posterior synechiae and dense secondary membranes are particularly likely to form and create an almost inoperable condition. Since these inflammatory membranes and adhesions are far worse complications than retained cortical material alone, it is clear that corticosteroid therapy of iridocyclitis is indicated even though it may delay absorption of retained cortex. I believe that the worst of these conditions, where massive amounts of cortex have been permitted to remain within the eye, can rightly be blamed on an inexperienced surgeon who timorously refrains from taking the necessary steps to remove this material, or who is unskilled in extracapsular maneuvering and cannot accomplish the removal. This is not to say that the surgeon should persist until vitreous is lost, which may be an even more serious complication.

Clarity of homologous corneal transplants in rabbits is decidedly improved by cortisone, 6 mg/kg intramuscularly.[96] Of 18 treated transplants. 90% remained clear, in contrast to 50% of 34 control eyes. Unfortunately such improvement does not always occur when cortisone is used in human transplants; nevertheless, many surgeons routinely use topical corticosteroid therapy beginning 2 weeks postoperatively in transplants. Occasional human cases will be seen in which incipient clouding of the graft is arrested or reversed by corticosteroids. Quite often, the cases that develop cloudiness in the graft progress despite all therapy.

The fibrosis-inhibiting effect of cortisone might logically be expected to increase the success of filtering operations for glaucoma. Reference to this hypothesis is often heard in clinical discussions, but I cannot cite a reference to any adequately controlled study. Forty-nine rabbits were operated on with keratome or trephine incisions and were treated with cortisone subconjunctivally or intramuscularly.[97] Photomicrographs suggest, as expected, that scleral healing and fibroblastic activity were inhibited by intramuscular injection of cortisone. Unfortunately no reference whatsoever was made to whether or not the wound filtered aqueous, which would seem to be the critical factor in such an experiment. I am of the opinion that the success or failure of a filtering operation is more closely correlated with the quality of surgical technique than with the use of corticosteroids.

Modern scleral infolding and encircling tube operations for retinal detachment may result in a considerable amount of postoperative inflammatory reaction. Topical corticosteroid therapy seems to reduce the severity of swelling and discomfort and may be used after detachment procedures. I suggest that you handle the tissues gently rather than use corticosteroids.

The lesser trauma of strabismus surgery does not ordinarily require corticosteroid therapy. Reoperations are more difficult and may incite additional traumatic reaction. Furthermore, allergy to catgut has been documented as a cause of fulminating and severe local reactions in those children for whom reoperation was done.[98] Certainly corticosteroid therapy may be used in such cases.

Retraction of conjunctival flaps (placed for corneal ulcers) spontaneously occurs, and its rate is accelerated by technical factors such as excessive tension, tying sutures too tightly, and failure to separate Tenon's capsule from conjunctiva. Patient factors such as friable or infected tissues also accelerate flap retraction. It is probable that topical use of corticosteroid medications will retard healing enough to be a significant factor in premature retraction of conjunctival flaps.

Intraocular foreign body

Daily subconjunctival injection of dexamethasone slowed the inflammatory encapsulation of intraocular copper foreign bodies in rabbits.[99] Untreated, 92% of foreign bodies were enveloped in cellular response within 5 days, as compared to 63% in 9 days with treatment. Clearly, corticosteroid therapy is not an effective substitute for surgical removal of a reactive foreign body and will not clear existing inflammation sufficiently to permit a better view. Because of the tissue reaction to the corticosteroid injection itself, surgery would be easier without previous corticosteroid injection. Corticosteroids are of no practical value in management of intraocular foreign bodies and may well promote development of infection.

CONTRAINDICATIONS AND COMPLICATIONS

Undesirable effects of corticosteroids are most conveniently discussed when they are divided into systemic and local manifestations. The greatest contraindication to corticosteroid therapy, however, holds for both systemic and topical routes of administration; it is the *lack of a specific indication for corticosteroid use.* A drug so expensive and potent as cortisone should never be used as a placebo or a shotgun remedy. Do not use corticosteroids as a routine after cataract extraction, for Fuchs' heterochromic cyclitis, for all types of chronic cyclitis (especially in children, who are susceptible to corticosteroid side effects), or for presumed histoplasmic choroiditis as a long-term therapy.[100]

Systemic complications

Undesirable systemic side effects of corticosteroids do not ordinarily occur from topical use, even of long duration. Frequent topical use of concentrated preparations of potent corticosteroids can cause measurable systemic effects, however. Study of four volunteers receiving 1 drop of 0.01% dexamethasone in both eyes every 2 hours (24-hour dexamethasone dosage, 0.75 mg) for 4 days showed a reduction of urinary excretion of 17-hydroxycorticosteroids to a range of 19% to 72% of normal. Endogenous cortisol production rate was decreased to 11% to 43% of normal.[101] Because of this not inconsiderable physiologic effect, the same precautions should be observed in patients receiving frequent topical corticosteroids as in patients receiving small doses of systemic corticosteroids. The relative vulnerability of patients with some types of disease will be reviewed subsequently. Also, the ophthalmologist should realize that as little as 10 mg of prednisone or the equivalent daily for 4 weeks may suppress normal growth in children.

One drop of 0.1% dexamethasone sodium phosphate in each eye four times daily is a systemic dosage of 0.25 mg/day. Six weeks of such medication resulted in a lowering of plasma cortisol level from 22 μg/100 ml to 17 μg/100 ml. However, testing showed the hypothalamic-pituitary-adrenal function to be normal (metyrapone test).[102]

Daily orbital injections of 4 mg of dexamethasone for 6 days reduced plasma cortisol levels from an average of 19 μg/100 ml to 6.0 μg/100 ml, indicating that prolonged injection therapy can have systemic side effects.[103]

With systemic administration, the following complications may arise[104]:

1. Mental changes, ranging from euphoria to psychosis
2. Activation of infection, notably serious in tuberculosis
3. Temporary increase in severity of diabetes and hypertension
4. Peptic ulceration of duodenum or stomach
5. Osteoporotic changes, sometimes leading to pathologic fracture
6. Electrolyte imbalance, causing edema and the like
7. Delay in wound healing, infrequently noted with high dosage
8. Moon face and other manifestations of Cushing's syndrome

Relative contraindications to corticosteroid therapy, therefore, are present in patients with preexisting disease of the types just mentioned. Low-level dosage (for example, 5 mg of prednisolone four times a day) in the average healthy patient can be safely carried out with minimum supervision, including weekly weight and blood pressure readings, urinalysis, and a brief talk to detect gastrointestinal disorders and early evidence of psychotic manifestations. A chest x-ray film should be obtained at the onset of therapy and should be repeated monthly in long-term treatment. If high dosage is required, it is well to enlist the aid of an internist in supervision of the patient. (The internist may, for example, recommend such additional medication as thyroid or potassium.)

Peptic ulceration

The physician must know that the newer corticosteroids such as prednisone and prednisolone, although they produce less electrolytic imbalance, still may cause other serious systemic complications. In a series of 18 patients with rheumatoid arthritis treated for as long as 7 months with prednisone or prednisolone, three patients developed radiologic evidence of peptic ulcer and one developed severe depressive psychosis.[105] The ulcers were asymptomatic, and it is emphasized that perforation or severe hemorrhage may occur without previous warning in patients on corticosteroid therapy. One of my uveitis patients once required emergency surgery for a perforated ulcer. Routine administration of aluminum hydroxide gel or similar antacids may minimize peptic ulceration in corticosteroid-treated patients.

Cortisone not only enhances the formation of peptic ulcers but also increases the severity of ulceration. Experimental surgical anastomosis of stomach to colon greatly predisposes dogs to peptic ulceration. In a control group of 13 such dogs, 31% developed ulcers and 15% developed perforations. Of 10 dogs similarly operated on and treated with cortisone (200 mg daily injections), all developed ulcers, and perforation occurred in 80%.[106]

Drug-induced hypokalemia may result from use of thiazide diuretics or from corticosteroid therapy. Administration of potassium chloride in enteric-coated tablets has been frequently advocated to prevent such hypokalemia. Unfortunately enteric-coated potassium chloride has been responsible for a definite increase in ulcerative lesions and stenosis of the small intestine (300 reported cases). These lesions are not the result of

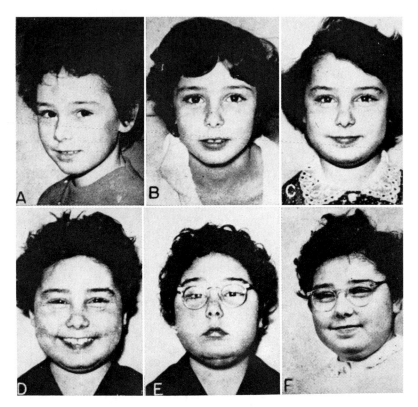

Fig. 15-23. Serial photographs made during prolonged prednisolone therapy. **A,** Patient at 7 years of age. **B,** Patient at 8½ years of age. **C,** Patient after 1 month of prednisolone therapy, 30 to 75 mg/day. **D,** Patient after 2 months of prednisolone therapy (20 mg/day was given during the second month). **E,** Patient after 6 months of prednisolone therapy. **F,** Patient after 1½ years of prednisolone therapy (still takes 20 mg/day). (From Sudarsky, R. D.: Arch. Ophthalmol. **62:**5, 1959.)

surface irritation but seem to result from rapid release of potassium chloride and its absorption over a short segment of intestine. This high concentration causes vasospasm and subsequent infarction. A typical, virtually pathognomonic circumferential ulceration and stenosis result.[107,108] To prevent potassium chloride intestinal lesions, an attempt should be made to supply potassium by dietary means (for example, orange juice); or if absolutely necessary, supplemental potassium should be given with meals rather than on an empty stomach. Potassium administration should immediately be discontinued if any unusual gastrointestinal symptoms develop during treatment.[109]

Osteoporosis

Pathologic vertebral fractures may spontaneously develop as a result of osteoporosis induced by prolonged systemic corticosteroid therapy.[110]

Pediatric problems

Being infrequently confronted with uveitis in growing children, the ophthalmologist is relatively unfamiliar with the response of persons in this age group to prolonged corticosteroid therapy. In general, the response of the disease and the side effects in the patient are comparable to what would be expected in adults. In addition, growth may be retarded. Rather serious changes in the appearance of the child that adversely affect the child's entire future life may be produced, as seen in Fig. 15-23.[111] This series of pictures documents the development of a most unsightly moon face and buffalo hump during the course of 1½ years' treatment with prednisone. The patient suffered from a severe case of Harada's syndrome of exudative retinal detachment and, through this therapy, achieved a final vision of 20/50. Clearly, the necessity for preservation of vision will warrant prolonged prednisone therapy with its associated side effects. Obviously such treatment can be justified only by the existence of serious disease known to be responsive to corticosteroids and is not to be undertaken lightly.

Pseudotumor cerebri. The syndrome of pseudotumor cerebri may develop rather suddenly if long-term corticosteroid therapy in children is abruptly discontinued or reduced. Twenty-eight such cases of corticosteroid-associated pseudotumor cerebri have been reviewed and reported.[112] Bilateral papilledema, headache, and vomiting were present in almost all patients. There was generalized abnormality of the electroencephalograms and increased pressure of the cerebrospinal fluid. Eight of the 28 patients had paresis of the sixth cranial nerve.

Treatment of this type of pseudotumor cerebri is fairly simple. An increase in the corticosteroid dosage will alleviate the symptoms. Dosage should then be reduced gradually. If the condition does not improve within a few weeks, a more thorough neurosurgical evaluation is in order.

Although pseudotumor cerebri after abrupt cessation of prolonged corticosteroid therapy has been thought to be peculiar to children only, several comparable cases have been cited in adults. Withdrawal of corticosteroid in such patients must be very gradual, requiring as long as several months.[113]

Exophthalmos

Exophthalmos as great as 25 mm may be caused by long-term corticosteroid therapy in patients with no demonstrable thyroid disease. This will subside only slowly and incompletely when the medication is discontinued.[114]

Possible teratogenic effect

Although no clinical evidence indicates that corticosteroids are teratogenic when administered to pregnant women, caution should be observed in administration of all potent drugs during pregnancy. Maternal treatment with cortisone did cause adverse effects in hybrid mice; the offspring of parents with recessive albinism were mated to those with dominant pigmentation. No such control hybrids were albino, but 62 of 520 (12%) hybrid offspring were albino after maternal treatment with cortisone (12.5% solution, 3 minims of which was injected subcutaneously on the seventh, eighth, and ninth days of gestation). In this experiment, maternal treatment with cortisone uncovered a normally recessive trait, albinism.[115]

Local contraindications and complications

Transient irritation is not infrequent during topical ocular use of cortisone and has been ascribed to the mechanical effect of clumps of steroid particles.[116] Apparently the manufacture and dispensing of tiny particles are difficult, since they tend to adhere and form larger clumps. Fortunately most patients do not seem to object to this minor discomfort.

Corticosteroid activation of infections

Since corticosteroids reduce the resistance of the body to most types of infection, their use should be avoided in ocular infections. Exceptions to this rule may arise if the infection is controlled by antibiotics and the physician wishes to reduce the ocular inflammatory reaction and in herpes zoster, which seems to be benefited by corticosteroid therapy.

Adverse effects in herpes simplex infection. General agreement exists that cortisone treatment of the typical dendritic keratitis caused by herpes simplex infection leads to more severe corneal scarring than would otherwise be expected. When a severe case of metaherpetic keratitis or chronic geographic ulceration is seen, the patient will usually give a history compatible with dendritic keratitis that was treated with cortisone by an unwary physician.

That such observations are not merely clinical impressions of doubtful validity is established by controlled experimentation. Forty-eight rabbits were inoculated with herpes simplex virus by corneal scratch or sub-Tenon's capsule injection.[117] Half were treated by subconjunctival injection of 20 to 50 mg (quite a large dose) of hydrocortisone or prednisolone every third day. Unequivocally, corticosteroid therapy caused the virus infection to become *much worse.* *All* 25 control rabbits recovered within 14 days, with corneal scarring so faint as to be visible only with magnification. Thirteen treated rabbits died of encephalitis, five were killed when signs of encephalitis were recognized (herpes simplex virus was recovered from the brains of four of these rabbits), three survived but developed corneal perforation, and the remaining two showed marked corneal scarring. The appearance of treated and untreated eyes 8 days after inoculation is shown in Fig. 15-24. Such experimental results are reproducible.[118]

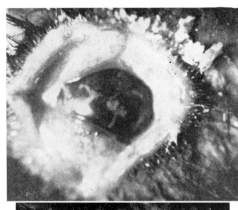

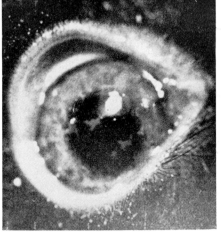

Fig. 15-24. A, Prednisolone-treated experimental herpes simplex infection 8 days after inoculation of sub-Tenon's space with virus. B, Untreated control rabbit eye 8 days after inoculation of sub-Tenon's space with herpes simplex virus in the same manner as in A. The severe exacerbation produced by corticosteroid therapy is shown in A. (From Kimura, S. J., and Okumoto, M.: Am. J. Ophthalmol. **43:**131, 1957.)

The literature is filled with such experiments indicating that corticosteroids potentiate herpes simplex infections. Another typical study, including clinical, pathologic, and histochemical evaluation, reported the effect of prednisolone, 5 mg, injected subconjunctivally every other day in rabbits.[119] Herpes simplex inoculation was by injection beneath Tenon's capsule. All rabbits, treated and control, developed keratoconjunctivitis; however, it was of earlier onset, greater severity, and longer duration in the prednisolone-treated groups. The incidence of uveitis was twice as great in the treated animals. Half the treated rabbits but no control rabbits developed disciform keratitis. Inclusion bodies could be found for 19 days in the prednisolone-treated rabbits and for 12 days in the control rabbits. Pathologic sections showed more severe damage, including stromal necrosis, in the treated rabbits.

The virus-enhancing effect of cortisone is also a property of the newer corticosteroid derivatives. Triamcinolone, methylprednisolone, and dexamethasone in 1% solutions were instilled three times a day topically on rabbit corneas inoculated with herpes simplex virus.[120] As illustrated in Fig. 15-25, the healing time of control corneas varied from 10 to 13 days; of triamcinolone-treated corneas, from 12 to 17 days; of methylprednisolone-treated corneas, from 14 to 24 days; and of dexamethasone-treated corneas, from 17 to 25 days.

Since the initial stages of herpetic keratoconjunctivitis may not be recognized without slit-lamp examination, the prudent physician will not prescribe corticosteroids indiscriminately for red eyes. Unfortunately shotgun therapy of red eyes with the commercially available and advertised antibiotic-corticosteroid mixtures is relatively common and has produced many cases of serious metaherpetic keratitis.

Adverse effects in other viral infections. Corticosteroids adversely influence the course of vaccinia infections. Experimental corneal inoculations in rabbits were made appreciably worse by subconjunctival or topical administration of cortisone.[121] Dis-

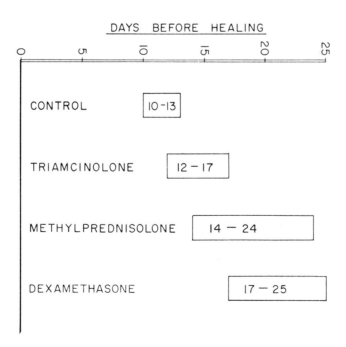

Fig. 15-25. Retardation of healing of experimental herpes simplex corneal infections by corticosteroids. Bars represent time span between minimum and maximum times required for healing. (Data from McCoy, G., and Leopold, I. H.: Am. J. Ophthalmol. **49:**1355, 1960.)

semination of the vaccinia virus, with more severe keratoconjunctivitis and several cases of encephalitis, occurred with cortisone treatment.

A clinical case of fatal human generalized vaccinia associated with systemic cortisone therapy has been reported.[122]

Trachoma virus is activated by topical cortisone therapy.[123] In old chronic cases, which no longer show characteristic inclusion bodies in scrapings, corticosteroid therapy may incite formation of typical inclusion bodies. This finding has been suggested as a provocative test for trachoma.

Behçet's syndrome of hypopyon iritis, aphthous oral lesions, and genital ulceration is reported to be caused by a virus.[124] Cortisone treatment is contraindicated, since it worsens the clinical manifestations and decreases the titer of circulating specific antibodies.

Fungus-promoting effect. Many able ophthalmologists are in agreement that the topical use of corticosteroids increases ocular susceptibility to fungus infection. Clinical reports of cases of fungus keratitis typically describe minor injuries treated with corticosteroid or corticosteroid-antibiotic medications.[125] Gradually progressive, gray-white corneal infiltrates develop and result in extensive corneal scarring or total loss of the eye. Since virtually all chronic corneal inflammations sooner or later receive a trial of corticosteroid therapy, it is doubtful that such reports alone establish a relationship between corticosteroids and fungus growth.

Fungi have been cultured from the eyes of 67% of patients receiving topical corticosteroids for 3 weeks or more compared to 18% of untreated control subjects.[126] Of 18 patients with negative cultures for fungus, 9 became positive for fungi after 3 weeks of topical use of corticosteroids. It is relevant to note that another author was able to culture fungi from 25% of normal eyes and 35% of diseased eyes.[127] No reference was made to corticosteroid therapy; however, this report helps to establish the existence of fungi about the eyes.

A report from India states that 71 fungus-free eyes were treated with topical 1% hydrocortisone three times daily for a month; at the end of this period, repeat cultures were positive for fungi in 41% of cases.[128]

Experimental fungus keratitis was produced in 80% of corticosteroid-treated rabbit eyes, but in only 20% of untreated control eyes.[129]

Candida albicans inoculation of abraded rabbit corneas resulted in keratitis in 37% of untreated eyes and in 75% of eyes treated with 1% hydrocortisone, 1 drop every 6 hours.[130]

The combined weight of clinical and experimental evidence strongly indicates that corticosteroid therapy decreases human resistance to ocular fungus infections. Fortunately the incidence of major infections is low. In material from the Armed Forces Institute of Pathology, fungus infection was found in 1 of every 727 cases of perforated ulcers or posttraumatic vitreous abscesses. However, before the advent of corticosteroids, fungi were found in only one of every 11,329 such eyes. I have the clinical impression that fungus infections are a great deal more common than these pathologic statistics indicate. Review of Birge's excellent 30-page article will convince one that fungus infection is frequent (for example, *Candida albicans* in 20% of women) and must be considered in the differential diagnosis of persistent eye inflammation.[131]

Consideration of the foregoing facts suggests that corticosteroid therapy of minor corneal abrasions is unwise. Corticosteroid therapy may promote serious infections, is certainly of no benefit in healing, and is always expensive.

Response of bacterial infection. Not only viral and fungal but also bacterial corneal infections may be made worse by cortisone. Experimental *Pseudomonas* corneal ulcers were demonstrated to produce much more extensive ulcerations and scarring when treated with cortisone (Fig. 15-26).[132] Fifty-four percent of cortisone-treated corneas and only 9% of control corneas showed extensive and deep ulceration and scarring. Simultaneous treatment with polymyxin B, however,

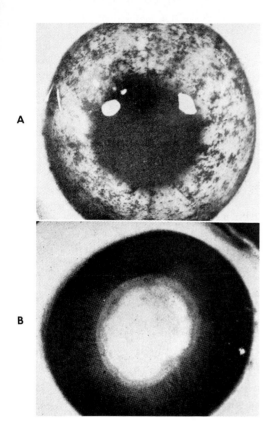

A

B

Fig. 15-26. A, Minimal superficial corneal involvement in control rabbit inoculated with *Pseudomonas* organisms in the same manner as shown in **B.** No cortisone therapy was given. **B,** Typical *Pseudomonas* corneal ulcer in cortisone-treated rabbit. (From Suie, T., and Taylor, F. W.: Arch. Ophthalmol. **56:**53, 1956.)

prevented extension of corneal involvement whether or not cortisone was used.

There seems to be a current belief that combined corticosteroid and antibiotic therapy is indicated in the treatment of severely infected eyes (for example, endophthalmitis after a penetrating injury). I know of no convincing controlled clinical or experimental evidence that this use of corticosteroids is of benefit to the eye. Such therapy must assume that the antibiotic is known to be effective against the infecting microorganism, that adequate amounts of antibiotic are constantly present throughout the infected eye, and that other contaminating organisms are not present. Unfortunately such assumptions can never be proved during the clinical treatment of an infected eye. I believe that the possible advantage of reducing scarring through such corticosteroid therapy of severe infections is clearly outweighed by the hazard of increasing the severity and extent of the infection. When systemic corticosteroid therapy is used, the danger of side effects also exists.

Can information derived from therapy of generalized severe infections help to determine whether corticosteroid therapy is beneficial to patients with eye infections? A series of 194 seriously infected patients (meningitis, pneumonia, and bacteremia) were treated with placebo or hydrocortisone in daily dosage of 300, 250, 200, 150, 100, and 50 mg for a period of 6 days. A double-blind technique of evaluation was employed.[133] No benefit resulted from the hydrocortisone treatment; 42% of the treated patients died, in comparison with 37% of the control group (not a significant difference). Five corticosteroid-treated patients had peptic ulceration (one perforated), in contrast to one such complication in the placebo-treated group.

I have seen several cases of unusually severe acute marginal blepharitis that were said to have become worse after treatment with corticosteroid-antibiotic ointment. Recovery was prompt when an effective antibiotic was prescribed and the corticosteroid was discontinued.

Activation of tuberculosis. Clinicians are quite familiar with the hazard of activating tuberculous infections with cortisone therapy. Presence of such infection is generally considered to be a strong contraindication to corticosteroid use. If corticosteroids are essential for the treatment of another condition, coexisting tuberculosis can ordinarily be controlled by simultaneous streptomycin or isoniazid therapy. Studies of experimental ocular tuberculosis indicate that the apparent initial cortisone-induced improvement of inflammatory signs is transient and is followed by severe caseating disease that destroys a high proportion of cortisone-treated eyes.[134] The long-term results of various types of therapy are illustrated in Fig. 15-27.

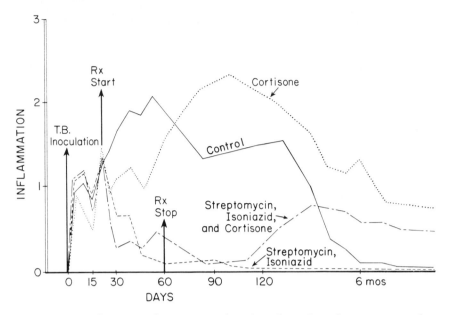

Fig. 15-27. Degree of activity of experimental ocular tuberculosis during a 6-month period. Note that cortisone treatment causes an initial favorable response, but at the cost of much more severe disease later. Even when simultaneous streptomycin and isoniazid treatment was given, cortisone caused late exacerbation. Note, however, that all therapy was discontinued after 1 month. (Data from Woods, A. C.: Arch. Ophthalmol. **59:**559, 1958.)

This study concludes that cortisone therapy of ocular tuberculosis is specifically contraindicated, even when accompanied by antituberculous medications. It is only fair to point out that treatment of these rabbits was for just 1 month, during which period no real difference existed between those streptomycin-treated rabbits that received cortisone and those that did not. Clinically, treatment would not have been stopped arbitrarily while activity of the uveitis persisted. This study does not permit conclusions as to the ultimate outcome had therapy continued. As seen in Table 15-9, treatment was insufficient to sterilize these eyes in the majority of any group of rabbits. Expert opinion on tuberculosis therapy recommends at least 3 to 6 months of continuing treatment because of the characteristic slow growth and susceptibility of these organisms.

Since it is impossible to prove the etiology of most cases of human uveitis, and because ultimate intraocular scarring in many cases can unquestionably be reduced by corticosteroid therapy, corticosteroids should be

Table 15-9. Demonstration of tuberculosis bacilli by culture and by acid-fast stain at end of 6-month experimental period*

	Culture positive for tuberculosis bacilli	Acid-fast stains positive for tuberculosis bacilli
Untreated controls	100%	38%
Cortisone treated only	100%	50%
Streptomycin and isoniazid therapy	60%	0%
Streptomycin, isoniazid, and cortisone therapy	57%	30%

Data from Woods, A. C.: Arch. Ophthalmol. **59:**559, 1958.
*It is obvious that bacteria persisted within all groups of eyes, despite treatment.

used in the management of endogenous uveitis. If tuberculosis is suspected, simultaneous specific therapy is prudent.

Prolonged corticosteroid administration may activate latent systemic tuberculous infection and adversely affect the course of active tuberculosis. These facts have been established by animal experimentation[135] and by clinical observation.[136] To prevent such exacerbation of tuberculosis, all patients requiring corticosteroid treatment for a period of 2 weeks or more should first be examined for tuberculosis (history of past symptoms or treatment, chest x-ray films, and tuberculin skin test). Prophylactic isoniazid (300 mg/day for adults; 8 mg/kg for children) should be prescribed during corticosteroid treatment of all patients with evidence of previous tuberculosis. A chest x-ray film at the close of therapy is advised to be sure that reactivation of infection has not occurred.

In summary, the physician must be aware that the intensive use of local corticosteroids will render the eye immunologically incompetent and hence unable to resist normally the invasion of microorganisms of all types.

Corticosteroid-induced glaucoma

A decade elapsed between the introduction of cortisone into ophthalmology and the recognition and acceptance of the fact that corticosteroids can produce the clinical picture of chronic simple glaucoma and that they do so with a frequency of undeniable clinical importance. A chronologic outline of these discoveries may be more interesting than a simple presentation of the facts.

Originally it was believed that ACTH and cortisone did not elevate intraocular pressure or cause positive glaucoma provocative tests in normal persons. In occasional patients with severe uveitis treated with corticosteroids a hypertensive response was noted.[137] This secondary type of glaucoma occurred only in eyes damaged so extensively as to hinder the normal aqueous outflow. Two explanations of this phenomenon were suggested:

1. Aqueous production is greatly reduced by the cyclitis and is permitted to return to normal levels by the corticosteroid therapy.
2. Increased permeability of inflamed iris

vessels destroys the blood-aqueous barrier, thereby eliminating the osmotic differential responsible for maintaining intraocular pressure. Corticosteroid-induced return to normal permeability blocks this abnormal leakage, thereby producing the hypertensive response.

Prolonged use of topical corticosteroids was subsequently incriminated as a cause of chronic glaucoma.[138] This form of glaucoma is characterized by painless increased pressure in a white eye. Optic atrophy and visual field loss occur, but glaucomatous cupping is absent and the field defects are said to be "uncharacteristic" of glaucoma. The published fields showed irregular constriction. Outflow facility is severely decreased. Despite discontinuance of corticosteroid therapy, surgery and antiglaucoma medications were necessary in treatment of these eyes. The five cases reported included one patient with malignant myopia with retinal detachment and corneal infiltrates of unstated etiology, one patient with recurrent iritis and severe diabetes with neuropathy, a 57-year-old woman whose visual field appeared to have a typical nasal step, one patient with recurrent uveitis of such severity as to cause extensive synechiae, iris atrophy, and band keratopathy, and a 34-year-old woman whose mother had glaucoma simplex. The descriptions of these cases certainly suggested that the patients were predisposed to glaucoma whether or not corticosteroid therapy was employed. If anyone but Goldmann had presented these cases, they would have been dismissed as pure coincidence. However, there could be no quarrel with his recommendation for periodic tonometry in eyes sufficiently diseased to require prolonged corticosteroid therapy.

Whether long-term systemic corticosteroid therapy might induce glaucomatous change was studied in 48 patients under treatment for rheumatoid arthritis and skin and collagen diseases.[139] The mean applanation pressure of the treated group was found to be statistically significantly increased and the facility of outflow to be decreased. Mean applanation pressure was higher (18.8 mm Hg) in patients receiving corticosteroid therapy for more than 4 years than in patients treated less than 1 year (15.9 mm Hg). The authors concluded that corticosteroid therapy was responsible for these changes. Although this conclusion may be justified, it must be recognized that the normal control group did not suffer from severe arthritis or collagen disease, although the group was matched for age, sex, race, and refractive error. Furthermore, examination of the data suggests that the control and corticosteroid-treated patients were very similar, with the exception of about a half dozen individuals in the corticosteroid-treated group who appeared predisposed to glaucoma.

The concept of corticosteroid-induced glaucoma was further substantiated by sporadic case reports. In two such cases of structurally normal eyes, pressures of 40 to 60 mm Hg developed after daily use of dexamethasone drops for 4 to 6 months.[140] The glaucoma disappeared in each case within a few days after the dexamethasone was discontinued.

Systemic or topical corticosteroid therapy was found to cause a decrease in facility of outflow and a corresponding increase of intraocular pressure.[141] This glaucomatous change may affect one eye alone in the case of topical therapy. The corticosteroid effect may be completely reversible within a month's time.

Conclusive proof of the glaucoma-producing effect of corticosteroids was pro-

vided by patients in whom intraocular pressure could be reversibly elevated again and again by topical use of corticosteroids. The data in Table 15-10 illustrate the magnitude of changes in coefficient of outflow and intraocular pressure resulting from instillation three times a day of a 0.1% solution of dexamethasone in the left eye. (The right eye was an untreated control.) This 42-year-old patient developed glaucoma during treatment of uveitis of the left eye. He had no family history of glaucoma, and for 29 months of follow-up care after the last use of dexamethasone his intraocular pressures remained normal.

In a group of 19 patients with untreated chronic simple glaucoma, administration three times a day of a 1.0% solution of dexamethasone for 2 to 3 weeks caused pressure elevations of 11 mm Hg or more in 18 of these patients.[142] These pressures returned to their original levels within 1 to 3 weeks after corticosteroid instillations were discontinued. The pressure and outflow facility values in a representative patient are shown in Fig. 15-28.

Dexamethasone-induced hypertension is markedly greater in a glaucomatous eye than in a normal eye. Fig. 15-29 gives the pressure increases resulting from topical use of dexamethasone three times a day in the right eye in four groups of patients (young normal patients, old normal patients, patients with known glaucoma with relatively low pressure elevations, and patients with un-

Table 15-10. Reversible glaucoma produced in normal human eyes by topical use three times a day of 0.1% solution of dexamethasone in left eye*

	Right eye		Left eye	
	Ocular pressure	*Outflow facility*	*Ocular pressure*	*Outflow facility*
3 months with drug	16	0.28	29	0.10
3 months without drug	17	0.26	16	0.28
3 weeks with drug	17	0.24	33	0.08
3 weeks without drug	15	0.30	17	0.25
4 weeks with drug	16	0.26	36	0.06
2 weeks without drug	17	0.26	17	0.27

*From Armaly, M. F.: Arch. Ophthalmol. **70:**482, 1963.

treated chronic simple glaucoma). The lines represent the ratio of intraocular pressure in the right eye (treated) to that in the left eye (untreated). Note that pressure increased even in normal young eyes, but the increase was much greater and more rapid in the glaucomatous eyes.

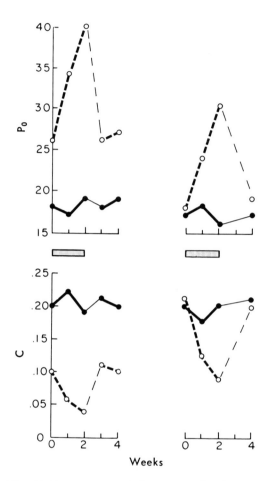

Fig. 15-28. Response of chronic simple glaucoma to a 0.1% suspension of dexamethasone three times a day. Solid line: pilocarpine-treated left eye. Broken lines: corticosteroid-treated right eye. Heavy bars: dexamethasone treatment for 2 weeks in right eye. Left-hand response was obtained without miotic treatment of right eye and right-hand response with a 2% solution of pilocarpine four times a day in right eye. Note that pilocarpine decreases but does not abolish the hypertensive effect of dexamethasone. P_o = initial intraocular pressure; C = coefficient of aqueous outflow. (From Armaly, M. F.: Arch. Ophthalmol. **70:**482, 1963.)

Dexamethasone glaucoma is only partly reversed by miotic, epinephrine, and carbonic anhydrase inhibitor therapy. Since corticosteroids are commonly used medications, inquiry should be made as to their use in all patients found to have glaucoma.

Further confirmation of the hypertensive effect of topical use of corticosteroids was provided by a study of 44 glaucoma patients (average rise in pressure, 15.2 mm Hg), 32 persons suspected of having glaucoma (average rise in pressure, 11.2 mm Hg), and 30 normal persons (average rise in pressure, 4.6 mm Hg).[143] This hypertensive response resulted after 3 to 8 weeks of treatment with betamethasone, prednisolone, dexamethasone, hydrocortisone, or triamcinolone. The outflow and pressure changes were completely reversible when treatment was discontinued.

Dexamethasone-induced glaucoma will cause visual field defects measurable with a 1/1000 white stimulus.[144] These field defects are similar to those typical of chronic simple glaucoma and include an enlarged blind spot,

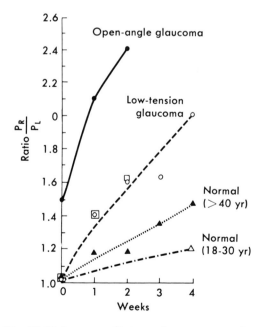

Fig. 15-29. Increase of intraocular pressure in dexamethasone-treated right eyes compared with untreated left eyes. (From Armaly, M. F.: Arch. Ophthalmol. **70:**482, 1963.)

arcuate scotomas, and peripheral constriction. The field defects are not related to the duration of corticosteroid therapy but to the elevation of intraocular pressure. Although these field defects may be slowly reversible when dexamethasone therapy is discontinued, as long as 2 months are required for disappearance of the field defect. Dexamethasone-induced pressure rise in eyes with chronic simple glaucoma will cause an increase in size of preexisting field defects (Fig. 15-30).

The clinical importance of corticosteroid-induced glaucoma is emphasized by a report of 26 patients seen during a 6-month period.[145] All were threatened by a progressive loss of visual fields, and several had been subjected to glaucoma surgery. All 26 were using corticosteroid topically—sometimes without the knowledge of their ophthalmologist. In some instances the corticosteroid had been prescribed to counteract the red-

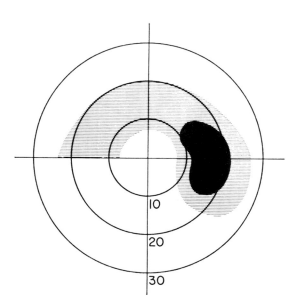

Fig. 15-30. Dexamethasone-induced increase in field defect. Black area indicates pretreatment scotoma in well-controlled glaucoma (intraocular pressure, 14 mm Hg). After 4 weeks of dexamethasone, 0.1% solution three times a day, the arcuate scotoma increased as represented by the stippled area (intraocular pressure, 29 mm Hg). (From Armaly, M. F.: Arch. Ophthalmol. **71:**636, 1964.)

ness caused by irritation from miotics. When the corticosteroid drops were discontinued, control of the glaucoma was easily achieved in all cases—indeed, a few eyes required no glaucoma therapy at all! Without doubt, these cases of glaucoma had been induced or made worse by the topical use of corticosteroids.[146]

Corticosteroid therapy after cataract extraction, a not uncommon practice, may cause glaucoma in the recently operated eye.[147] One of my own patients developed glaucoma in both eyes (each eye operated on at a separate time) during the first month after surgery, with pressures rising to 50 mm Hg. When corticosteroid therapy was discontinued, pressure dropped to normal, with no need for subsequent glaucoma treatment.

Statistical analysis of the corticosteroid hypertensive response indicates the existence of three separate groups of individuals within the general population. The largest group, 66.2% of the study, responded with an average rise in pressure of 1.6 mm Hg after 4 weeks of 0.1% dexamethasone three times a day.[148] The second group, 28.8%, responded with an average rise of 10 mm Hg. A pressure rise greater than 16 mm Hg occurred only in the third group (5% of sample). Although these three groups were differentiated on the basis of the magnitude of pressure rise, the time of pressure rise was also different and is of clinical significance. Fig. 15-31 shows that group 1 patients (66%) responded with only a slight pressure rise at the end of several weeks and that the pressure did not continue to rise. In contrast, during the month of study, group 2 and 3 pressures continued to rise at a steady rate that presumably would continue with further treatment. The clinical implication is that a patient who has received corticosteroid treatment for a month but still has pressure below 21 mm Hg is unlikely to have glaucomatous complications from such treatment. Should the pressure be above 21 mm Hg at the end of a month, subsequent corticosteroid therapy should include careful supervision of intraocular pressure.

The genotypic basis for these three groups of steroid responsiveness has been confirmed by a study of parents of individuals who were or were not corticosteroid responsive. The expected proportion of parental and offspring genotypes was found in this study of 109 families.[149]

The glaucomatous response to corticosteroids is a dominant trait found in one third of the population.[150] The homozygous state (double dose) of this gene causes chronic simple glaucoma. Hence the glaucomatous response to corticosteroids will be found in all patients with chronic simple glaucoma, in both their parents, and in all offspring. Eyes with angle-closure or secondary glaucoma will not respond to corticosteroids with increased pressure (unless the patient happens to carry this genetic trait, which occurs in one third of cases). A positive correlation has been noted between the presumably genetic traits of corticosteroid-induced glaucoma, inability to taste phenylthiocarbamide,[151] plasma cortisol suppression by oral dexamethasone,[152] and absence of proliferative retinopathy in diabetic patients.[153]

To confirm this theory of recessive inheritance of glaucoma, both parents of a glaucoma patient and all the children of a glaucoma patient should show a positive corticosteroid provocative test. Betamethasone, 0.1% three times a day for 3 to 6 weeks, caused a positive response in only 1 of 6 parents and only 29 of 87 children of glaucoma patients.[154] The authors concluded that a positive corticosteroid test indicates a predisposition to develop the disease, but that these data did not confirm the theory of recessive inheritance. Of considerable interest is the fact that 6 of 210 positive reactors to the corticosteroid test continued to have glaucoma (previously absent) after betamethasone was discontinued. Prolonged miotic therapy was required in these patients, who developed early perimetric defects. That these patients would have developed glaucoma anyway could be proposed as an explanation, but I suspect this would be received skeptically by previously normal patients who must use drops permanently after an "experiment."

In a study of 63 twins it was found that the pressure response to topical dexamethasone was more consistent between dizygotic twins than monozygotic twins. The significance of this unexpected finding is unclear.[155]

Although 100% of monozygotic twins would be expected to show the same corticosteroid pressure response, this actually

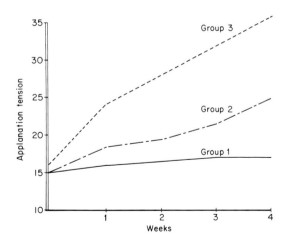

Fig. 15-31. Mean weekly applanation pressures after dexamethasone administration, three times a day, showing different rates of rise for the three groups previously separated by magnitude of corticosteroid response. (Modified from Armaly, M. F.: Invest. Ophthalmol. **4:**187, 1965.)

occurs in only 65%.[156,157] A possible explanation for this discrepancy is that the pressure response is not consistently reproducible in the same individual—it is, in fact, only 73% reproducible.[158]

Should eyes with secondary glaucoma be treated with corticosteroid? Will this control inflammation and reduce pressure or is this group of patients genetically predisposed to corticosteroid glaucoma as is true in the case of contusion-angle glaucoma?

Corticosteroid provocative testing caused a glaucomatous response in approximately one third of 28 eyes with secondary glaucoma. This incidence is the same as in the general population of nonglaucomatous patients; therefore it indicates that the response is a result of a genetic trait rather than a characteristic of eyes with damaged outflow channels.[159]

What is the relationship between retinal detachment and open-angle glaucoma? Of 20 patients with nontraumatic rhegmatogenous retinal detachment, 20% were high steroid responders (5% expected) and 53% had a C/D ratio greater than 0.3 (18% expected). Patients with recognizable open-angle glaucoma were excluded from the study group.[160] The practical application of this genetic relationship is that postoperative use of corticosteroids can be expected to increase pressure in one of every 5 detachment patients. I never use postoperative corticosteroids in my own detachment patients. Gentle surgery, not corticosteroids, is the key to quiet eyes. Furthermore, this supports my belief that "miotic-induced detachment" is simply a genetically associated coincidence of glaucoma, aphakia, and detachment.

Pigmentary glaucoma apparently has a different etiology than does primary open-angle glaucoma, for it does not show the same corticosteroid response.[161]

One should not conclude that the eyes respond uniquely to corticosteroids. Genetically determined differences in corticosteroid responsiveness occur in many tissues, including circulating lymphocytes and skin fibroblasts.[162]

Corticosteroid provocative testing for glaucoma is a far more sensitive examination than is the water-drinking tonography test. Evaluation of offspring of glaucomatous patients by the latter test showed 47% to be positive, in contrast to 97% positive to the betamethasone test.[150] This provocative test requires instillation four times a day of a 0.1% solution of betamethasone for 3 weeks. The tonographic and pressure criteria for a positive test are comparable to those for positive water-drinking tonography. Obviously corticosteroid provocative testing is impractical for diagnosis of glaucoma—it takes too long and is too much of a nuisance. Furthermore, it is positive for 30% of the population, diagnosing this genetic trait as well as cases of glaucoma.

As would be expected, glaucoma may also be induced by subconjunctival injection of corticosteroids in susceptible individuals. One of the particular hazards of this route of administration is that the depot will continue to release corticosteroid for some months, during which time pressure elevation will continue. The clinician should exercise appropriate judgment before giving such an injection. Was it indicated, for example, to give subconjunctival corticosteroids to four patients reported to have developed glaucoma from this treatment?[163] Their diagnoses were macular degeneration, vascularized corneal scar, pars planitis (all three conditions nonresponsive to corticosteroids), and episcleritis (easily controlled by corticosteroid drops).

Surgical excision of the subconjunctival corticosteroid depot may be necessary before the glaucoma can be controlled.[164] Such a dissection is not a minor matter such as is removal of a pterygium, for the repository mass diffuses within the tissues and requires painstaking dissection, with concern to avoid vital structural damage.

The potential seriousness of corticosteroid-induced glaucoma is illustrated by the tragedy of a 15-year-old boy who used prednisolone drops several times daily for hay fever. When first seen by the ophthalmologist, this boy had advanced glaucomatous cupping, 20/70 vision, a pressure of 50 mm Hg, and field loss to within 5 degrees of fixation.[165] This irreversible damage apparently occurred within a 6-month period.

The mineralocorticoids are much less likely to cause increased intraocular pressure than are the glucocorticoids. Of 17 glaucomatous patients receiving parenteral desoxycorticosterone (30 mg intramuscularly every day for 3 to 6 days) or aldosterone D (2 mg intravenously), only two patients showed elevation of intraocular pressure.[166] A pressure rise occurred despite unchanged coefficient of outflow, indicating that increased aqueous production (presumably on the basis of electrolyte alteration) was the mechanism of action.

The intensity of the glaucomatous response in a given individual depends on the potency of the corticosteroid compound used and the frequency and duration of administration. For instance, use four times a day of suspensions of 0.1% prednisolone or 0.1% triamcinolone will elevate intraocular pressure about as much as use once daily of

0.1% solutions of dexamethasone or betamethasone. The less effective corticosteroids also require a much longer period of use before they cause pressure elevation.

Attempts have been made to develop anti-inflammatory corticosteroids without the property of increasing intraocular pressure.[167] One such drug, hydroxymethylprogesterone (medrysone) is reported to have topical anti-inflammatory effects comparable to that of prednisolone. Topical instillation of hydroxymethylprogesterone, 1% three times a day for 1 month, in 23 patients caused no increase of intraocular pressure. These patients were chosen because they had previously shown an average increase of 6.7 mm Hg after use of 0.1% dexamethasone.[168]

Hydroxymethylprogesterone was used in a variety of eye conditions in 61 patients.[169] No increased intraocular pressure was noted. Furthermore, no reactivation of herpetic ulcers occurred.

The relative pressure-elevating potency

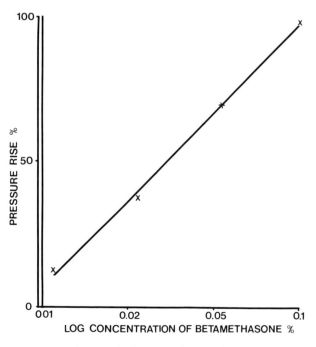

Fig. 15-32. Dose-response relationship between betamethasone and increased intraocular pressure in known high responders. (Data from Kitazawa, Y.: Am. J. Ophthalmol. **82:**492, September 1976.)

and anti-inflammatory effect of hydroxy-methylprogesterone and dexamethasone have been determined. In a selected group of 28 high responders the pressure elevations caused by 1% hydroxymethylprogesterone and by 0.001% dexamethasone were found to be virtually identical. In a rabbit corneal graft rejection model the protection resulting from 1% hydroxymethylprogesterone and 0.001% dexamethasone was comparable for both drugs. The clear implication from this data is not that hydroxymethylprogesterone has a better therapeutic index with respect to causing glaucoma; rather, hydroxymethylprogesterone is simply 1000-fold less strong than dexamethasone in its capability both to cause glaucoma and to suppress inflammation.[170]

This concept of dose-related pressure response to corticosteroids is, of course, of practical clinical significance. Use the least amount of corticosteroid necessary to achieve the therapeutic goal and the least amount of glaucoma will result. Fig. 15-32 shows clearly this dose-response relationship as measured in 24 eyes known to be high responders to corticosteroid.[171]

Animal experiments. An experimental glaucomatous response to corticosteroids may be produced in rabbits. Greater than a 10 mm Hg rise of intraocular pressure was induced in two of five rabbits receiving subconjunctival betamethasone (1.6 mg/day) for 6 weeks.[172]

Lethal intramuscular doses of cortisone (6 mg/kg/day intramuscularly) and prednisolone (7 mg/kg/week intramuscularly) did not increase intraocular pressure or change tonographic values in 11 rabbits during their average survival time of 4 weeks.[173]

Corticosteroid resistance (tachyphylaxis) develops in the rabbit, with return to normal pressure levels despite continuation of the same corticosteroid dosage that originally induced a glaucomatous response. Human tachyphylaxis to corticosteroids is suspected in the treatment of hematologic diseases.[174]

Intravenous hydrocortisone in cats causes a dose-related increase in intraocular pressure mediated by a decrease in outflow facility. At a dose of 0.1 mg/kg the average decrease of outflow was 23%.[175]

Summary. The implications of this information are clear. Topical administration of corticosteroids should be used only for limited periods of time and under adequate tonometric supervision in patients with chronic simple glaucoma and in their relatives. The possibility of pressure elevation should be considered in all patients receiving long-term corticosteroid therapy.

Corneal thickness

After 4 weeks of treatment with topical dexamethasone, 35% of patients developed a 3% increase in corneal thickness. This may be related to the effects of increased intraocular pressure.[176]

"Corticosteroid" mydriasis

Experimental use of topical corticosteroids to provoke a glaucomatous response has disclosed another effect, dilation of the pupil. For instance, all of 39 volunteers receiving dexamethasone, 0.1% four to five times daily in one eye, showed dilation of the treated pupil. Dilation occurred as early as the first week of treatment, averaged 1 mm, and disappeared in all cases promptly after dexamethasone was stopped. The amount of dilation bears no relationship to the ocular hypertensive response.[177] This author also questions the possible unreliability of volunteers: "If patients who know they are ill fail to take a medication designed to make them well, it seems even more likely that normal individuals would be likely to cheat when told to take a drug designed to make them ill. It may be more than intriguing that the percentage of individuals previously reported to be nonresponders to topically administered corticosteroids is about equal to the percentage of patients (about one third) who fail to take their required medications."[177]

The mydriatic effect of corticosteroids was studied on isolated monkey intraocular muscle preparations.[178] As expected, the tonus of the dilator muscle was increased and that of the sphincter was decreased. More careful analysis, however, revealed that the specific steroid components of these medications did *not* alter the muscle status. Rather, the response was caused by some effect of the vehicle (preservatives or surface tension–reducing agents).

Also in living monkeys, ptosis and mydriasis resulted from instillation of dexamethasone in its commercial vehicle and from use of the vehicle alone, but not from dexamethasone in saline solution. The vehicle contains various preservatives, antioxidants, and surface-active agents. The combination of surface-active agents (polysorbate 80, phenylethanol, and disodium edetate) appeared to be responsible for a direct myopathic effect.[179]

Exposure of the dilator, sphincter, and ciliary muscle preparations to the vehicles of corticosteroid eye drops (no corticosteroid) inhibited muscle responses to both acetylcholine and epinephrine as well as to potassium chloride. (Potassium chloride bypasses specific receptor sites and induces muscle contractions by direct depolarization of cell membranes.) Apparently these vehicles disturb the selective semipermeability of the cell membrane, thereby altering the ability of the muscle to respond.

Inasmuch as altered response of intraocular smooth muscle might be responsible for such clinically observed "corticosteroid-induced" (?) side effects as mydriasis, difficulty of accommodation, and increased resistance to aqueous outflow (glaucomatous response), the demonstration that such smooth muscle changes are a result of the eye drop vehicle rather than of the corticosteroid may be of great significance. Possibly other of our existing concepts as to "corticosteroid-induced complications" will need to be changed to "vehicle-induced" changes. Such speculation is presently premature.

Corticosteroid-induced cataract

Posterior subcapsular cataract formation has been reported as a complication of long-term, high-dosage systemic corticosteroid therapy.[180] This report evaluated 72 patients receiving long-term corticosteroid therapy and 23 control patients with rheumatoid arthritis not treated by corticosteroids. Posterior subcapsular cataracts were found in no patients receiving corticosteroids for less than a year, in 42% of those treated for

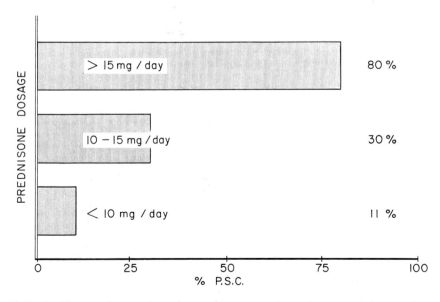

Fig. 15-33. Incidence of posterior subcapsular cataract in patients receiving corticosteroid therapy. (Data from Oglesby, R., and associates: Arch. Ophthalmol. **66:**625, 1961.)

1 to 3 years, and in 58% treated for 4 years or more. As shown in Fig. 15-33, cataract incidence was also closely related to corticosteroid dosage. Only 11% of patients receiving less than 10 mg daily of prednisone (or the equivalents) developed cataract, in comparison with 30% receiving 10 to 15 mg and 80% receiving more than 15 mg/day. Most of these cataracts were clinically insignificant, since they did not interfere with vision.

The dosage and duration of systemic corticosteroid administration appeared to be the primary determining factor in the production of posterior subcapsular cataracts in a series of 38 patients with rheumatic arthritis.[181] Fourteen (37%) of these patients receiving long-term corticosteroid therapy had such cataracts; these patients had no history of previous eye disease, injury, or radiation exposure. A control group of 24 arthritic patients had no cataracts. The duration and severity of the arthritis were comparable in the two groups. In addition, 2 of 12 asthmatic patients receiving corticosteroid therapy had characteristic posterior subcapsular cataracts.

The frequency of posterior subcapsular cataract was determined in 159 control patients, in 65 patients with rheumatoid arthritis who were not corticosteroid treated, and in 76 patients with corticosteroid-treated rheumatoid arthritis. In the patients under 55 years of age in these groups, the frequency of cataract was 2%, 4.5%, and 16.6%, respectively.[182]

The appearance of the presumably corticosteroid-induced cataract is shown in Fig. 15-34.[183] This cataract cannot be differentiated biomicroscopically from early complicated cataract, radiation cataract, cataract associated with ocular disease, and senile posterior subcapsular cataract.

Progression of these cataracts occured in three of five patients whose corticosteroid dosage was reduced. In one patient the cataract worsened 2 months after therapy was discontinued.[183]

It should be recognized that patients with rheumatoid arthritis not receiving corticosteroid treatment have an unusually high incidence of posterior subcapsular cataract. In a series of 43 patients with rheumatoid arthritis (not treated with corticosteroids) who had posterior subcapsular cataract requiring

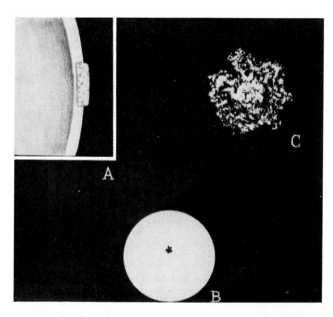

Fig. 15-34. Corticosteroid-induced posterior subcapsular cataract. (Modified from Oglesby, R., and associates: Arch. Ophthalmol. **66:**97, 1961.)

surgery, 19 were under 50 years of age at the time of operation. The youngest was only 27 years old.[184]

No posterior subcapsular cataracts were found in a group of 48 asthmatic patients who had been receiving corticosteroid therapy for many years.[185] Nineteen of these patients had used 16 mg or more of methylprednisolone equivalent for 2 to 7 years. In a control group of 148 patients without corticosteroid therapy, nine patients had cataract, two of these being posterior subcapsular.

In another series of 40 patients with rheumatoid arthritis receiving corticosteroid therapy, only two cases of posterior subcapsular cataract were found.[186] Both of these patients had a family history of cataract, a fact with obvious implications. Ten of these patients had received the equivalent of 10 to 15 mg of prednisone for 1 to 4 years, and 11 had been receiving this dosage for more than 4 years. One of the cataract patients had been treated for less than a year and the other for more than 4 years.

Three of 14 children on long-term corticosteroid therapy (more than a year) were found to have bilateral asymptomatic posterior subcapsular cataract.[187] The corticosteroid dosage was sufficiently high to cause typical cushinoid obesity.

Further documentation of the cataractogenic potential of prolonged systemic corticosteroid therapy appears in a report of 15 children so treated for 2 years or more.[188] Eight of these 15 children had posterior subcapsular cataracts. Three months after corticosteroid therapy was discontinued in three children, no regression of the cataracts was recognizable.

Of 109 children on long-term (more than 6 months) corticosteroid therapy, 22% developed posterior subcapsular cataract.[189]

A single case has been reported in which a posterior subcapsular cataract developed unilaterally in a 20-year-old man after a year's treatment of chronic herpetic keratitis with IDU and topical use of corticosteroids.[190]

Two other cases of cataract following topical use of corticosteroids seem especially tragic. These young girls, aged 17 and 20, used corticosteroid drops for the redness resulting from contact lens wearing. One used prednisolone daily for almost 2 years. The other used dexamethasone or prednisolone twice daily for 4 years. Both girls had posterior subcapsular cataract and glaucoma so resistant to medical therapy that sclerectomy was required for control. Both had also lost about half of their visual fields.[191] Millions of patients wear contact lenses and may gain access to corticosteroid drops to alleviate ocular irritation. Characteristically, these drops will be used for long periods of time without medical supervision. *Do not grant* contact lens wearers access to corticosteroids!

Experimentally induced cataract. Thirty-five 5-week-old rats were treated for 4 months with varying doses of dexamethasone up to 20 μg/g of body weight/day. The rats weighed between 100 and 200 g at the start of the experiment and therefore received up to 2 to 4 mg/day of dexamethasone—obviously a high dose for a baby rat. The growth rate of treated animals was less than half that of the control rats, showing that corticosteroid dosage was of toxic magnitude; nevertheless, there were no cataracts.[192]

Even when given in doses sufficiently large to cause weight loss and occasional death, prednisolone did not cause cataract in rats, rabbits, or chickens and did not potentiate the cataractogenic action of dinitrophenol, xylose, triparanol, or irradiation.[193] However, systemic prednisolone did accelerate the formation of galactose cataracts in rats.[194]

Topical cortisone (1.5%) and hydrocortisone (0.2%) three times daily for a 6-month period caused anterior subcapsular lens opacities in 50% of the cortisone-treated and 30% of the hydrocortisone-treated rabbits.[195] Comparable treatment with prednisolone (0.25%) caused opacities in 20% of rabbits.

Cataract was present in one third of mouse fetuses histologically examined on the eighteenth day of gestation after maternal subcutaneous injection of 1 mg hydrocortisone acetate on the ninth and tenth day of gestation.[196]

Seven adult albino rabbits weighing 2.5 to 3 kg were given daily subconjunctival injections in the left eye.[197] Four rabbits survived this treatment for 41 weeks. Two of these rabbits had bilateral axial posterior subcapsular cataracts sufficiently large to be grossly visible. Presumably the corticosteroid effect was mediated by systemic absorption, since both eyes were about equally affected.

A possible mechanism of cataract formation might be biochemical changes in the aqueous humor resulting from corticosteroid exposure. Prolonged topical use of methylprednisolone in rabbits causes quite marked chemical changes in the aqueous to occur. For example, ascorbic acid is lowered from 36 to 25 mg/100 ml; potassium is lowered from 6 to 4 milliequivalents/l, and pH increases from 7.6 to 7.8.[198]

Both clinical and experimental data strongly suggest a relationship between prolonged corticosteroid therapy and cataract. The risk increases proportionally to the duration and amount of therapy. In most cases the cataract causes minimal, if any, visual complaints.[199] Clinical perspective will identify situations where the risk of withholding beneficial treatment is a consideration at least as important as the possibility of cataract formation.

Uveitis

Two patients developed mild anterior uveitis of 2 to 3 weeks' duration after provocative testing for responsiveness to topical corticosteroids. The uveitis responded promptly to dexamethasone (the same drug used for the provocative testing). Whether this was a coincidental finding in a series of 2000 patients or related in some way to a corticosteroid reduction of ocular resistance was impossible to determine.[200]

Subsequently, 17 more patients (15 of whom were black) developed severe anterior nongranulomatous uveitis during or subsequent to corticosteroid testing for glaucoma. A positive FTA-ABS serologic test was found in 82% of these patients (14), although only

4 had positive VDRL tests. This suggests the possibility that corticosteroids may activate latent spirochetal ocular infection.[201]

Teratogenicity

Triamcinolone given during any trimester of pregnancy causes hypoplastic thymus glands and generalized defects of the lymphatic system in infant baboons.[202]

SUMMARY

Corticosteroid therapy is here to stay—for use *when indicated.* It is a two-edged sword, however, and can cause serious complications and side effects if it is used unwisely.

In clinical practice corticosteroids are often used as shotgun therapy, as a placebo when all is not going well, because empathy is felt for the patient, or just because everyone else does. This must stop.[203]

REFERENCES

1. Leopold, I.: Corticosteroids in aqueous, Am. J. Ophthalmol. **38**:101, 1954.
2. Arendshorst, W., and Falls, H.: Role of the adrenal cortex in treatment of ocular diseases with pyrogenic substances, Arch. Ophthalmol. **44**:635, 1950.
3. Donn, A., and Christy, N.: Plasma steroids after intravenous typhoid vaccine, Am. J. Ophthalmol. **42**:132, 1956.
4. Annual review: The uvea, Arch. Ophthalmol. **81**:730, 1969.
5. Leopold, I. H.: The steroid shield in ophthalmology, Trans. Am. Acad. Ophthalmol. Otolaryngol. **71**:273, 1967.
6. Levene, R. Z., and Schwartz, B.: Depression of plasma cortisol and the steroid ocular pressure response, Arch. Ophthalmol. **80**:461, 1968.
7. O'Rourke, J. F., Iser, G., and Ryan, R.: An initial evaluation of prednisone therapy in ocular inflammation, Arch. Ophthalmol. **55**:323, 1956.
8. Neilson, R. H.: The use of dexamethasone in ophthalmologic steroid therapy, Arch. Ophthalmol. **62**:438, 1959.
9. Gordon, D.: Dexamethasone in ophthalmology, Am. J. Ophthalmol. **48**:656, 1959.
10. Hollander, J. L.: Clinical use of dexamethasone, J.A.M.A. **172**:306, 1960.
11. Boland, E. W.: Chemically modified adrenocortical steroid, J.A.M.A. **174**:835, 1960.

12. Kupferman, A., and Leibowitz, H. M.: Penetration of fluorometholone into the cornea and aqueous humor, Arch. Ophthalmol. 93:425, June 1975.

13. Yamauchi, H., Kito, H., and Uda, K.: Studies on intraocular penetration and metabolism of fluorometholone in rabbits: a comparison between dexamethasone and prednisolone acetate, Jpn. J. Ophthalmol. 19:339, 1975.

14. Hogan, M. J., Thygeson, P., and Kimura, S.: Effects of prednisone and prednisolone in ocular inflammation, Trans. Am. Acad. Ophthalmol. 59:779, 1955.

15. Gordon, D.: Prednisone and prednisolone in ocular disease, Am. J. Ophthalmol. 41:593, 1956.

16. King, J. H., Jr., Passmore, J. W., Skeehan, R. A., Jr., and Weimer, J. R.: Prednisone and prednisolone in ophthalmology, Trans. Am. Acad. Ophthalmol. 59:759, 1955.

17. Woods, A.: The present status of ACTG and cortisone in clinical ophthalmology, Am. J. Ophthalmol. 34:945, 1951.

18. Commercial, Allergan Pharmaceuticals, Santa Ana, Calif.

19. Kreines, K., and Weinberg, I. C.: The selection of adrenocorticosteroid preparations, Ohio State Med. J. 71:698, October 1975.

20. Duke-Elder, S., and Ashton, N.: Action of cortisone on tissue reactions of inflammation and repair with special reference to the eye, Br. J. Ophthalmol. 35:695, 1951.

21. Leopold, I. H., and Maylath, F.: Intraocular penetration of cortisone and its effectiveness against experimental corneal burns, Am. J. Ophthalmol. 35:1125, 1952.

22. Rundles, W., and Quinn, J.: Management of acute ocular lime burns, Am. J. Ophthalmol. 37:209, 1954.

23. Bahn, G. C., Sonnier, E., and Allen, J. H.: Therapeutic studies in experimental chemical injury of the cornea, Am. J. Ophthalmol. 48:253, 1959.

24. Brown, S. I., Weller, C. A., and Vidrich, A.: Effect of corticosteroids on corneal collagenase of rabbits, Am. J. Ophthalmol. 70:744, 1970.

25. Ashton, N., and Cook, C.: Effect of cortisone on healing of corneal wounds, Br. J. Ophthalmol. 35:708, 1951.

26. Palmerton, E. S.: The effect of local cortisone on wound healing in rabbit corneas, Am. J. Ophthalmol. 40:344, 1955.

27. Gasset, A. R., Lorenzetti, D. W. C., Elli-son, E. M., and Kaufman, H. E.: Quantitative corticosteroid effect on corneal wound healing, Arch. Ophthalmol. 81:589, 1969.

28. Beams, R., Linabery, L., and Grayson, M.: Effect of topical corticosteroids on corneal wound strength, Am. J. Ophthalmol. 66:1131, 1968.

29. McDonald, T. O., Borgmann, A. R., Roberts, M. D., and Fox, L. G.: Corneal wound healing, Invest. Ophthalmol. 9:703, 1970.

30. Polack, F. M., and Rosen, P. N.: Topical steroids and tritiated thymidine uptake, Arch. Ophthalmol. 77:400, 1967.

31. Fink, A., and Baras, I.: Effect of steroids on tensile strength of corneal wounds, Am. J. Ophthalmol. 42:759, 1956.

32. Basu, P. K.: Effect of different steroids on the healing of nonperforating corneal wounds in rabbits, Arch. Ophthalmol. 59:657, 1958.

33. Ashton, N., Cook, C., and Langham, M.: Effect of cortisone on vascularization and opacification of the cornea induced by alloxan, Br. J. Ophthalmol. 35:718, 1951.

34. Ashton, N., and Cook, C.: In vivo observations of the effects of cortisone upon the blood vessels in the rabbit ear chambers Br. J. Exp. Pathol. 33:32, 1952.

35. Takashima, R.: Corticosteroid effects on the corneal surface of rabbits studied by scanning electron microscopy, Jpn. J. Ophthalmol. 19:393, 1975.

36. Hamashige, S., and Potts, A.: The penetration of cortisone and hydrocortisone into the ocular structures, Am. J. Ophthalmol. 40:211, 1955.

37. Janes, R. G., and Stiles, J. F.: The penetration of cortisol into normal and pathologic rabbit eyes, Am. J. Ophthalmol. 56:84, 1963.

38. Green, H., Kroman, H., and Leopold, I. H.: Corticosteroids in the aqueous humor of the rabbit, Arch. Ophthalmol. 54:853, 1955.

39. Murdick, P. W., Keates, R. H., Donovan, E. F., Wyman, M., and Short, C.: Ocular penetration studies, Arch. Ophthalmol. 76:602, 1966.

40. Fleming, T. C., and Merrill, D. L.: Water soluble and non-water soluble hydrocortisone, Research report No. 5, Alcon Laboratories, Inc., Fort Worth, Texas.

41. Leopold, I. H.: Intraocular penetration of local hydrocortisone and cortisone, Arch. Ophthalmol. 52:769, 1954.

42. Leopold, I. H., Kroman, H., and Green H.: Intraocular penetration of prednisone and prednisolone, Trans. Am. Acad. Ophthalmol. **59:**771, 1955.

43. Kupferman, A., and Leibowitz, H. M.: Topically applied steroids in corneal disease, Arch. Ophthalmol. **92:**331, October 1974.

44. Leopold, I. H., and Kroman, H. S.: Methyl and fluoro-substituted prednisolones in the blood and aqueous humor of the rabbit, Arch. Ophthalmol. **63:**943, 1960.

45. Kroman, H. S., and Leopold, I. H.: Studies upon methyl- and fluoro-substituted prednisolones in the aqueous humor of the rabbit, Am. J. Ophthalmol. **52:**77, 1961.

46. Kupferman, A., and Leibowitz, H. M.: Biological equivalence of ophthalmic prednisolone acetate suspensions, Am. J. Ophthalmol. **82:**109, July 1976.

47. Hanna, C., and Sharp, J. D.: Ocular absorption of indomethacin by the rabbit, Arch. Ophthalmol. **88:**196, 1972.

48. Havener, W. H.: Management of conjunctivitis, Ohio Med. J. **52:**40, 1956.

49. Kaufman, H. E.: Ocular anti-inflammatory therapy, Springfield, Ill., 1970, Charles C Thomas, Publisher.

50. McDonald, T. O., Kasten, K., Hervey, R., Gregg, S., Smith, D., and Robb, C. A.: Comparative toxicity of dexamethasone and its tertiary butyl acetate ester after topical ocular instillation in rabbits, Am. J. Ophthalmol. **76:**117, July 1973.

51. Leibowitz, H. M., and Kupferman, A.: Kinetics of topically administered prednisolone acetate, Arch. Ophthalmol. **94:**1387, August 1976.

52. Gordon, D.: The treatment of chronic uveitis, Arch. Ophthalmol. **62:**400, 1959.

53. Sugar, A., Benson, W., Burde, R. M., and Waltman, S. R.: Alternate-day versus daily systemic corticosteroids in corneal homograft rejection, Am. J. Ophthalmol. **75:**486, 1973.

54. Kaufman, H. E.: Practical considerations in the selection of anti-inflammatory agents, Trans. Am. Acad. Ophthalmol. Otolaryngol. **79:**OP-89, January-February 1975.

55. Cloes, R. S., Krohn, D. L., Breslin, H., and Braunstein, R.: Depo-Medrol in treatment of inflammatory diseases, Am. J. Ophthalmol. **54:**407, 1962.

56. Sturman, R. M., Laval, J., and Sturman, M. F.: Subconjunctival triamcinolone acetonide, Am. J. Ophthalmol. **61:**155, 1966.

57. Hyndiuk, R. A., and Reagan, M. G.: Radio-active depot-corticosteroid penetration into monkey ocular tissue, Arch. Ophthalmol. **80:**499, 1968.

58. Bohigian, G., Dawson, C., and Coleman, V.: Retrobulbar administration of steroids in herpes simplex uveitis, Arch. Ophthalmol. **85:**320, 1971.

59. Schlaegel, T. F., Jr., and Wilson, F. M.: Accidental intraocular injection of depot corticosteroids, Trans. Am. Acad. Ophthalmol. Otolaryngol. **78:**OP-847, November-December 1974.

60. McLean, E. B.: Inadvertent injection of corticosteroid into the choroidal vasculature, Am. J. Ophthalmol. **81:**835, March 1976.

61. Raab, E. L.: Limitation of motility after periocular corticosteroid injection, Am. J. Ophthalmol. **78:**996, December 1974.

62. Nozik, R. A.: Orbital rim fat atrophy after repository periocular corticosteroid injection, Am. J., Ophthalmol. **82:**928, December 1976.

63. O'Connor, G. R.: Periocular corticosteroid injections: uses and abuses, Eye Ear Nose Throat Mon. **55:**83, March 1976.

64. Kupferman, A., and Leibowitz, H. M.: Therapeutic effectiveness of fluorometholone in inflammatory keratitis, Arch. Ophthalmol. **93:**1011, October 1975.

65. Graham, R. O., and Peyman, G. A.: Intravitreal injection of dexamethasone, Arch. Ophthalmol. **92:**149, August 1974.

66. Keller, N., Longwell, A. M., and Birss, S. A.: Intermittent vs. continuous steroid administration, Arch. Ophthalmol. **94:**644, April 1976.

67. Chavan, S. B., and Cummings, E. J.: An initial evaluation of (aristocort) triamcinolone in the therapy of ocular inflammation (part I), Am. J. Ophthalmol. **49:**55, 1960.

68. Ganehofer, W.: The effect of cortisone on Sjögen's syndrome, Acta Med. Scand. **149:**441, 1954.

69. Watson, P. G., Lobascher, D. J., Sabiston, D. W., Lewis-Faning, E., Fowler, P. D., and Jones, B. R.: Double-blind trial of the treatment of episcleritis-scleritis with oxyphenbutazone or prednisolone, Br. J. Ophthalmol. **50:**463, 1966.

70. Herzog, F., Jr.: Absorption of Boeck's sarcoid iris nodule with systemic prednisone, Arch. Ophthalmol. **56:**135, 1956.

71. Israel, H., Sones, M., and Harrel, D.: Cortisone treatment of sarcoidosis, J.A.M.A. **156:**461, 1954.

72. Collier, R.: Corticotropic treatment of pro-

gressive exophthalmos of hyperthyroidism, Arch. Ophthalmol. **51:**402, 1954.

73. Mosher, H. A.: The prognosis of temporal arteritis, Arch. Ophthalmol. **62:**641, 1959.

74. Ashton, N., and Hobbs, H. E.: Effect of cortisone on rheumatoid nodules of the sclera, Br. J. Ophthalmol. **36:**373, 1952.

75. Mathias, D.: Scleromalacia perforans, Am. J. Ophthalmol. **39:**161, 1955.

76. Brown, S. I., and Grayson, M.: Marginal furrows, Arch. Ophthalmol. **79:**563, 1968.

77. Greenwood, B. M.: Capillary resistance and skin-fold thickness in patients with rheumatoid arthritis: effect of corticosteroid therapy, Ann. Rheum. Dis. **25:**272, 1966.

78. Krachmer, J. H., and Laibson, P. R.: Corneal thinning and perforation in Sjögren's syndrome, Am. J. Ophthalmol. **78:**917, December 1974.

79. Oksala, A.: Interstitial keratitis, Am. J. Ophthalmol. **44:**217, 1957.

80. Neumann, E., Gutmann, M. J., Blumenkrantz, N., and Michaelson, I. C.: A review of 400 cases of vernal conjunctivitis, Am. J. Ophthalmol. **47:**166, 1959.

81. Stegman, R., and Miller, D.: A human model of allergic conjunctivitis, Arch. Ophthalmol. **93:**1354, December 1975.

82. Scheie, H.: Treatment of herpes zoster ophthalmicus with cortisone or corticotropin, Arch. Ophthalmol. **53:**38, 1955.

83. Scheie, H. G., and McLellan, T.: Treatment of herpes zoster ophthalmicus with corticotropin and corticosteroids, Arch. Ophthalmol. **62:**579, 1959.

84. Ryan, R., O'Rourke, J. F., and Iser, G.: Conjunctivitis in adenoidal-pharyngeal-conjunctival virus infection, Arch. Ophthalmol. **54:**211, 1955.

85. Hiles, D. A., and Pilchard, W.: Corticosteroid control of neonatal hemangiomas of the orbit and ocular adnexa, Am. J. Ophthalmol. **71:**1003, 1971.

86. Senelick, R. C., and Van Dyk, H. J. L.: Chromophobe adenoma masquerading as corticosteroid-responsive optic neuritis, Am. J. Ophthalmol. **78:**485, September 1974.

87. McLean, E. B.: Untreated hemangioma of the eyelid, Arch. Ophthalmol. **94:**1422, August 1976.

88. Kennerdell, J. S., Jannetta, P. J., and Johnson, B. L.: A steroid-sensitive solitary intracranial plasmacytoma, Arch. Ophthalmol. **92:**393, November 1974.

89. Knox, D. L., and Mustonen, E.: Greater occipital neuralgia: an ocular pain syndrome with multiple etiologies, Trans. Am. Acad. Ophthalmol. Otolaryngol. **79:**OP-513, May-June 1975.

90. von Noorden, G. K.: Anterior segment ischemia following the Jensen procedure, Arch. Ophthalmol. **94:**845, May 1976.

91. Karakashian, N. A.: Pseudotumor cerebri, Ann. Ophthalmol. **7:**247, 1975.

92. Gundersen, T.: Conjunctival flaps in the treatment of corneal disease with reference to a new technique of application, Arch. Ophthalmol. **60:**880, 1958.

93. Corboy, J. M.: Corticosteroid therapy for the reduction of postoperative inflammation after cataract extraction, Am. J. Ophthalmol. **82:**923, December 1976.

94. Burde, R. M., and Waltman, S. R.: Topical corticosteroids after cataract surgery, Ann. Ophthalmol. **4:**290, 1972.

95. Mustakallio, A., Kaufman, H. E., Johnston, G., Wilson, R. S., Roberts, M. D., and Harter, J. C.: Corticosteroid efficacy in postoperative uveitis, Ann. Ophthalmol. **6:**719-730, 1973.

96. Ojers, G., Yasuna, J., and Scheie, H.: Cortisone in experimental homologous keratoplasty in the rabbit, Am. J. Ophthalmol. **36:**120, 1953.

97. Laval, J., and Coles, R.: Role of cortisone in glaucoma surgery, Arch. Ophthalmol. **49:**168, 1953.

98. Apt, L.: Catgut allergy in eye muscle surgery, Arch, Ophthalmol. **63:**30, 1960.

99. Rosenthal, A. R., Appleton, B., Zimmerman, R., and Hopkins, J. L.: Intraocular copper foreign bodies, Arch. Ophthalmol. **94:**1571, September 1976.

100. Kaufman, H. E.: Practical considerations in the selection of anti-inflammatory agents, Trans. Am. Acad. Ophthalmol. Otolaryngol. **79:**OP-89, January-February 1975.

101. Burch, P. G., and Migeon, C. J.: Systemic absorption of topical steroids, Arch. Ophthalmol. **79:**174, 1968.

102. Krupin, T., Mandell, A. I., Podos, S. M., and Becker, B.: Topical corticosteroid therapy and pituitary-adrenal function, Arch. Ophthalmol. **94:**919, June 1976.

103. O'Day, D. M., McKenna, T. J., and Elliott, J. H.: Ocular corticosteroid therapy: systemic hormonal effects, Trans. Am. Acad. Ophthalmol. Otolaryngol. **79:**OP-71, January-February 1975.

104. Hogan, M., Thygeson, P., and Kimura, S.: Uses and abuses of adrenal steroids and

corticotropin, Arch. Ophthalmol. **53:**165, 1955.

105. Ballet, A. J., Black, R., and Bunim, J.: Major undesirable side effects from prednisolone and prednisone, J.A.M.A. **158:** 459, 1955.

106. Nicoloff, D. M., Soisin, H., Peter, E. T., Leonard, A. S., and Wangensteen, O. H.: The effect of cortisone on peptic ulcer formation, J.A.M.A. **183:**1019, 1963.

107. Boley, S. J., Allen, A. C., Schultz, L., and Schwartz, S.: Potassium-induced lesions of the small bowel, J.A.M.A. **193:**997, 1965.

108. Allen, A. C., Boley, S. J., Schultz, L., and Schwartz, S.: Potassium-induced lesions of the small bowel, J.A.M.A. **193:**1001, 1965.

109. Lawrason, F. D., Albert, E., Mohr, F. L., and McMahon, F. G.: Ulcerative-obstructive lesions of the small intestine, J.A.M.A. **191:**641, 1965.

110. Curtiss, P. H., Clark, W. S., and Herndon, C.: Vertebral fractures resulting from prolonged cortisone and corticotropin therapy, J.A.M.A. **156:**467, 1954.

111. Sudarsky, R. D.: Exudative type of retinal separation, Arch. Ophthalmol. **62:**5,1959.

112. Walker, A. E., and Adamkiewicz, J. J.: Pseudotumor cerebri associated with prolonged corticosteroid therapy, J.A.M.A. **188:**779, 1964.

113. Ivey, K. J., and DenBesten, L.: Pseudotumor cerebri associated with corticosteroid therapy in an adult, J.A.M.A. **208:**1698, 1969.

114. Slansky, H. H., Kolbert, G., and Gartner, S.: Exophthalmos induced by steroids, Arch. Ophthalmol. **77:**579, 1967.

115. Barber, A. N., Afeman, C., and Willis, J.: Inheritance of congenital anophthalmia in mice, Am. J. Ophthalmol. **48:**763, 1959.

116. Lippman, O.: Local irritating effect caused by topical use of steroids in the eye, Arch. Ophthalmol. **57:**339, 1957.

117. Kimura, S. J., and Okumoto, M.: The effect of corticosteroids on experimental herpes simplex keratoconjunctivitis in the rabbit, Am. J. Ophthalmol. **43:**131, 1957.

118. Thygeson, P., Geller, H. O., and Schwartz, A.: Effect of cortisone on experimental herpes simplex keratitis of the rabbit, Am. J. Ophthalmol. **34:**885, 1951.

119. Kimura, S. J., Bonnet, V., Okumoto, M., and Hogan, M.: The effect of corticosteroid hormones on experimental herpes simplex keratitis, Am. J. Ophthalmol. **51:**945, 1961.

120. McCoy, G., and Leopold, I. H.: Simplex infections of the cornea, Am. J. Ophthalmol. **49:**1355, 1960.

121. Kimura, S., Thygeson, P., and Geller, H. O.: Observations on the effect of adrenal steroids on vaccinia virus. I. The effects of cortisone in experimental vaccinavirus keratoconjunctivitis of the rabbit, Am. J. Ophthalmol. **36:**116, 1953.

122. Olansky, S.: Fatal vaccinia associated with cortisone therapy, J.A.M.A. **162:**887, 1956.

123. Thygeson, P.: Criteria of cure in trachoma, with special reference to provocative tests, Rev. Int. Trach. **30:**450, 1953; abstracted in Am. J. Ophthalmol. **37:**821, 1954.

124. Sezer, N.: Further investigation on the virus of Behçet's disease, Am. J. Ophthalmol. **41:**41, 1956.

125. Anderson, B., Shaler, S. R., and Cesar, G.: Mycotic ulcerative keratitis, Arch. Ophthalmol. **62:**169, 1959.

126. Mitsui, Y.: Corneal infections after cortisone therapy, Br. J. Ophthalmol. **39:**244, 1955.

127. Fazakas: Magyar Orvosi A. **35:**325, 1934. K. M. Aug. **96:**227, 1936. Cited in Duke-Elder, S.: Textbook of ophthalmology, vol. 5, St. Louis, 1952, The C. V. Mosby Co., p. 5299.

128. Nema, H. V., Ahuja, O. P., Bal, A., and Mohapatra, L. N.: Effects of topical corticosteroids and antibiotics on mycotic flora of conjunctiva, Am. J. Ophthalmol. **65:**747, 1968.

129. Ley, A. P.: Fungus keratitis, Arch. Ophthalmol. **56:**877, 1956.

130. Berson, E. L., Kobayashi, G. S., Becker, B., and Rosenbaum, L.: Topical corticosteroids and fungal keratitis, Invest. Ophthalmol. **6:**512, 1967.

131. Birge, H. L.: Ocular aspects of mycotic infections, Arch. Ophthalmol. **47:**354, 1952.

132. Suie, T., and Taylor, F. W.: The effect of cortisone on experimental pseudomonas corneal ulcers, Arch. Ophthalmol. **56:**53, 1956.

133. Cooperative Study Group: The effectiveness of hydrocortisone in the management of severe infections, J.A.M.A. **183:**462, 1963.

134. Woods, A. C.: Studies in experimental ocular tuberculosis, Arch. Ophthalmol. **59:**559, 1958.

135. Laboratory Subcommittee of the Committee on Medical Research: The effect of cortisone and/or corticotropin on experimental tuberculosis infection in animals (statement pre-

pared by the Subcommittee), Am. Rev. Tuberc. **66:**257, 1952.

136. Committee on Therapy: The effect of cortisone and/or corticotropin on tuberculosis infection in man (statement prepared by the Committee), Am. Rev. Tuberc. **66:**254, 1952.

137. Laval, J., and Collier, R.: Elevation of intraocular pressure due to hormonal steroid therapy in uveitis, Am. J. Ophthalmol. **39:**175, 1955.

138. Goldman, H.: Cortisone glaucoma, Arch. Ophthalmol. **68:**621, 1962.

139. Bernstein, H. N., and Schwartz, B.: Effects of long-term systemic steroids on ocular pressure and tonographic values, Arch. Ophthalmol. **68:**742, 1962.

140. Briggs, H. H.: Glaucoma associated with the use of topical corticosteroid, Arch. Ophthalmol. **70:**312, 1963.

141. Bernstein, H. N., Mills, D. W., and Becker, B.: Steroid-induced elevation of intraocular pressure, Arch. Ophthalmol. **70:**15, 1963.

142. Armaly, M. F.: Effect of corticosteroids on intraocular pressure and fluid dynamics, Arch. Ophthalmol. **70:**482, 1963.

143. Becker, B., and Mills, D. W.: Corticosteroids and intraocular pressure, Arch. Ophthalmol. **70:**500, 1963.

144. Armaly, M. F.: Effect of corticosteroids on intraocular pressure and fluid dynamics, Arch. Ophthalmol. **71:**636, 1964.

145. Becker, B., and Mills, D. W.: Corticosteroid eye drops and intraocular pressure, Sight Sav. Rev. **33:**130, 1963.

146. Becker, B., and Mills, D. W.: Elevated intraocular pressure following corticosteroid eye drops, J.A.M.A. **185:**170, 1963.

147. Lerman, S.: Steroid therapy and secondary glaucoma, Am. J. Ophthalmol. **56:**31, 1963.

148. Armaly, M. F.: Statistical attributes of the steroid hypertensive response in the clinically normal eye, Invest. Ophthalmol. **4:**187, 1965.

149. Armaly, M. F.: The heritable nature of dexamethasone-induced ocular hypertension, Arch. Ophthalmol. **75:**32, 1966.

150. Becker, B., and Hahn, K. A.: Topical corticosteroids and heredity in primary open-angle glaucoma, Am. J. Ophthalmol. **57:**543, 1964.

151. Becker, B., and Ballin, N.: Glaucoma and corticosteroid provocative testing, Arch. Ophthalmol. **74:**621, 1965.

152. Rosenbaum, L. J., Alton, E., and Becker,

B.: Dexamethasone testing in Southwestern Indians, Invest. Ophthalmol. **9:**325, 1970.

153. Becker, B., Bresnick, G., Chevrette, L., Kolker, A. E., Oaks, M. C., and Cibis, A.: Intraocular pressure and its response to topical corticosteroids in diabetes, Arch. Ophthalmol. **76:**477, 1966.

154. François, J., Heintz-DeBree, C., and Tripathi, R. C.: The cortisone test and the heredity of primary open-angle glaucoma, Am. J. Ophthalmol. **62:**844, 1966.

155. Schwartz, J. T., Reuling, F. H., Jr., Feinleib, M., Garrison, R. J., and Collie, D. J.: Twin heritability study of the corticosteroid response, Trans. Am. Acad. Ophthalmol. Otolaryngol. **77:**126, 1973.

156. Schwartz, J. T., Reuling, F. H., Feinleib, M., Garrison, R. J., and Collie, D. J.: Twin study on ocular pressure following topically applied dexamethasone. II. Inheritance of variation in pressure response, Arch. Ophthalmol. **90:**281, October 1973.

157. Schwartz, J. T., Reuling, F. H., Feinleib, M., Garrison, R. J., and Collie, D. J.: Twin study on ocular pressure after topical dexamethasone. I. Frequency distribution of pressure response, Am. J. Ophthalmol. **76:**126, July 1973.

158. Palmberg, P. F., Mandell, A., Wilensky, J. T., Podos, S. M., and Becker, B.: The reproducibility of the intraocular pressure response to dexamethasone, Am. J. Ophthalmol. **80:**844, November 1975.

159. Becker, B.: The effect of topical corticosteroid in secondary glaucomas, Arch. Ophthalmol. **72:**769, 1964.

160. Shammas, H. F., Halasa, A. H., and Faris, B. M.: Intraocular pressure, cup-disc ratio, and steroid responsiveness in retinal detachment, Arch. Ophthalmol. **94:**1108, July 1976.

161. Zink, H. A., Palmberg, P. F., Sugar, A., Sugar, H. S., Cantrill, H. L., Becker, B., and Bigger, J. F.: Comparison of in vitro corticosteroid response in pigmentary glaucoma and primary open-angle glaucoma, Am. J. Ophthalmol. **80:**478, September 1975.

162. Bigger, J. F., Palmberg, P. F., and Zink, H. A.: In vitro corticosteroid: correlation response with primary open-angle glaucoma and ocular corticosteroid sensitivity, Am. J. Ophthalmol. **72:**92, January 1975.

163. Kalina, R. E.: Increased intraocular pressure following subconjunctival corticoste-

roid administration, Arch. Ophthalmol. **81:** 788, 1969.

164. Herschler, J.: Increased intraocular pressure induced by repository corticosteroids, Am. J. Ophthalmol. **82:**90, July 1976.

165. Roberts, W.: Raid progression of cupping in glaucoma, Am. J. Ophthalmol. **66:**520, 1968.

166. Frenkel, M., and Krill, A. E.: Effects of two mineralocorticoids on ocular tension, Arch. Ophthalmol. **72:**315, 1964.

167. Dorsch, W., and Thygeson, P.: The clinical efficacy of medrysone, a new ophthalmic steroid, Am. J. Ophthalmol. **65:**74, 1968.

168. Spaeth, G. L.: Hydroxymethylprogesterone, Arch. Ophthalmol. **75:**783, 1966.

169. Bedrossian, R. H., and Eriksen, S. P.: The treatment of ocular inflammation with medrysone, Arch. Ophthalmol. **81:**184, 1969.

170. Podos, S. M., Krupin, T., Asseff, C., and Becker, B.: Topically administered corticosteroid preparations, Arch. Ophthalmol. **86:**251, 1971.

171. Kitazawa, Y.: Increased intraocular pressure induced by corticosteroids, Am. J. Ophthalmol. **82:**492, September 1976.

172. Tuovienen, E., Liesmaa, M., and Esila, R.: The influence of corticosteroids on intraocular pressure in rabbits, Acta Ophthalmol. **44:**901, 1966.

173. Tuovienen, E., Esila, R., and Liesmaa, M.: The influence of corticosteroids on intraocular pressure in rabbits, Acta Ophthamol. **44:**581, 1966.

174. Levene, R. Z., Rothberger, M., and Rosenberg, S.: Corticosteroid glaucoma in the rabbit, Am. J. Ophthalmol. **78:**505, September 1974.

175. Oppelt, W. W., White, E. D., Jr., and Halpert, E. S.: The effect of corticosteroids on aqueous humor formation rate and outflow facility, Invest. Ophthalmol. **8:**535, 1969.

176. Baum, J. L., and Levene, R. Z.: Corneal thickness after topical corticosteroid therapy, Arch. Ophthalmol. **79:**366, 1968.

177. Spaeth, G. L.: Effects of topical dexamethasone on intraocular pressure and the water drinking test, Arch. Ophthalmol. **76:**772, 1966.

178. Kern, R., and Macri, F. J.: Steroid eye drops and effect on isolated intraocular muscles of monkeys, Arch. Ophthalmol. **78:** 794, 1967.

179. Newsome, D. A., Wong, V. G., Cameron, T. P., and Anderson, R. R.: "Steroid-induced" mydriasis and ptosis, Invest. Ophthalmol. **10:**424, 1971.

180. Oglesby, R., Black, R., von Sallmann, L., and Bunim, J.: Cataracts in patients with rheumatic diseases treated with corticosteroids, Arch. Ophthalmol. **66:**625, 1961.

181. Giles, C. L., Mason, G. L., Duff, I. F., and McLean, J. A.: The association of cataract formation and systemic corticosteroid therapy, J.A.M.A. **182:**719, 1962.

182. Wiesinger, H., and Irby, R.: Posterior subcapsular cataract (PSC) in patients with rheumatoid arthritis treated with corticosteroids, Invest. Ophthalmol. **2:**294, 1963.

183. Oglesby, R. B., Black, R. L., von Sallmann, L., and Bunim, J. J.: Cataracts in rheumatoid arthritis patients treated with corticosteroids, Arch. Ophthalmol. **66:**97, 1961.

184. Gordon, D. M., Kammerer, W. H., and Freyberg, R. H.: Examination for posterior subcapsular cataracts, J.A.M.A. **175:**127, 1961.

185. Leibold, J. E., and Itkin, I. H.: Cataracts in asthmatics treated with corticosteroids, J.A.M.A. **185:**448, 1963.

186. Pfahl, S. B., Makley, T. A., Rothermich, N., and McCoy, F. W.: The relationship of steroid therapy and cataracts in patients with rheumatoid arthritis, Am. J. Ophthalmol. **52:**831, 1961.

187. Havre, D. C.: Cataracts in children on long-term corticosteroid therapy, Arch. Ophthalmol. **73:**818, 1965.

188. Braver, D. A., Richards, R. D., and Good, T. A.: Posterior subcapsular cataracts in steroid treated children, Arch. Ophthalmol. **77:**161, 1967.

189. Ohguchi, M., Ohno, S., Shiono, H., Kadowaki, J., and Okuno, A.: Posterior subcapsular cataracts in children on long-term corticosteroid therapy, Jpn. J. Ophthalmol. **19:**254-260, 1975.

190. Cronin, T. P.: Cataract with topical use of corticosteroid and idoxuridine, Arch. Ophthalmol. **72:**198, 1964.

191. Burde, R. M., and Becker, B.: Corticosteroid-induced glaucoma and cataracts in contact lens wearers, J.A.M.A. **213:**2075, 1970.

192. von Sallmann, L., Caravaggio, L. L., Collins, E. M., and Weaver, K.: Examination of lenses of steroid-treated rats, Am. J. Ophthalmol. **50:**1147, 1960.

193. Bettman, J. W., Fund, W. E., Webster,

R. G., Noyes, P. P., and Vincent, N. J.: Cataractogenic effect of corticosteroids on animals, Am. J. Ophthalmol. **65:**581, 1968.

194. Cotlier, E., and Becker, B.: Topical corticosteroids and galactose cataracts, Invest. Ophthalmol. **4:**806, 1965.

195. Wood, D. C., Contaxis, I., Sweet, D., Smith, J. C., and Van Dolah, J.: Response of rabbits to corticosteroids, Am. J. Ophthalmol. **63:**841, 1967.

196. Rogoyski, A., and Trzcinska-Dabrowska, Z.: Corticosteroid-induced cataract and palatoschisis in the mouse fetus, Am. J. Ophthalmol. **68:**128, 1969.

197. Tarkkanen, A., Esilia, R., and Liesmaa, M.: Experimental cataracts following long-term administration of corticosteroids, Acta Ophthalmol. **44:**665, 1966.

198. Virno, M., Schirru, A., Pecori-Giraldi, J., and Pellegrino, N.: Aqueous humor alkalosis and marked reduction in ocular ascorbic acid content following long-term topical cortisone (9a-fluoro-16a-methylprednisolone), Ann. Ophthalmol. **6:**983, October 1974.

199. Sundmark, E.: The cataract-inducing effect of systemic corticosteroid therapy, Acta Ophthalmol. **44:**291, 1966.

200. Krupin, T., LeBlanc, R. P., Becker, B., Kolker, A. E., and Podos, S. M.: Uveitis in association with topically administered corticosteroid, Am. J. Ophthalmol. **70:**883, 1970.

201. Shin, D. H., Kass, M. A., Kolker, A. E., Becker, B., Marr, J. J., and Bell, C.: Positive FTA-ABS tests in subjects with corticosteroid-induced uveitis, Am. J. Ophthalmol. **82:**259, August 1976.

202. Anonymous: There's no "safe trimester" with teratogenic drugs, J.A.M.A. **234:**264-265, October 1975.

203. Havener, W. H.: Corticosteroid misuse. In Leopold, I., and Burns, R., editors: Symposium on ocular therapy, vol. 8, New York, 1975, John Wiley & Sons, Inc.

16
ETHANOL

Ethyl alcohol is uniquely valuable in oph-thalmology because it is specifically able to counteract the visual toxicity of wood alcohol. It may also be used safely as a sedative for elderly patients.

USE IN TREATMENT OF METHANOL POISONING

Characteristically, primates (monkey and human) respond to a minimum lethal dose of methanol (3 g/kg) with mild intoxication during the first day. Only with double the minimum lethal dose does semicoma appear on the first day. By the morning of the second day the victim seems to have recovered and is apparently normal for a brief latent period; this period is followed later in the day by progressive weakening, respiratory failure, and death. Pupillary dilation and horizontal nystagmus are common. Severe acidosis characteristically appears during this period; carbon dioxide–combining powers of as low as 15 vol% (normal 40 to 55 vol%) are recorded terminally.[1]

When acidosis was prevented by adequate dosage of sodium bicarbonate (dosage determined by carbon dioxide–combining power), it was possible to avoid death in four of eight monkeys given 6 g/kg of methanol (twice the certain lethal dose). Despite maintenance of normal carbon dioxide–combining power, half of the eight animals died of damage to the central nervous system. Retinal edema occurred in about 36 hours despite the alkali therapy. In these large dosages of methanol (twice lethal), retinal damage was not prevented by use of sodium bicarbonate.[2]

Evidence that formaldehyde is the proximal toxic agent in methanol poisoning is derived from ERG studies of the relative toxicities of methanol, formate, and formaldehyde. The b wave of the ERG was abolished by 0.0007 mol/kg of formaldehyde, 0.025 mol/kg of formate, and 0.03 mol/kg of methanol.[3] This closely parallels concentrations required for inhibition of retinal glycolysis.[4]

The reduction of retinene to vitamin A is mediated by the enzyme alcohol dehydrogenase.[5] Perhaps the existence of such alcohol-metabolizing enzymes in the retina is one reason for the selective damage suffered by the eye in methanol poisoning. (Vitamin A is itself an alcohol.)

Methanol poisoning of human beings and of monkeys can be divided into three components.[6] The first component is the narcotic action that methanol manifests, as do other alcohols and organic solvents. The lethal dosage required for narcotic death is about 10 g/kg, which may be all methanol, all ethanol, or a combination of the two. The second component is an uncompensated metabolic acidosis, caused indirectly by toxic metabolic products of methanol. It is characterized by a latent period and is probably caused by tissue damage by formaldehyde. The minimum lethal dose of methanol is between 2 and 3 g/kg; 4 g/kg or more (untreated) was fatal to all monkeys in this series. Death usually occurs about a day after an untreated fatal dose, although one monkey survived for 18 days. The third component of methanol poisoning occurs only if survival for 30 hours or more is permitted by treatment or because the methanol dose was just sublethal. It is characterized by ocular and central nervous system necrosis—death of retinal ganglion cells and the basal ganglia.[7]

Methanol is metabolized by an alcohol dehydrogenase, which is also utilized for ethanol metabolism. The two alcohols compete for this enzyme, ethanol having a marked selective advantage to the extent that inhibition of methanol metabolism is already demonstrable when the ethanol concentration is only one sixteenth that of methanol. Repeated administration of ethanol is capable of blocking completely the methanol breakdown. Evidence of this is the increased amount of methanol in the urine and the absence of formate (methanol metabolite) when ethanol is given repeatedly.

Urinary and pulmonary excretion of unchanged methanol will occur if sufficient ethanol is given for a long enough period. If ethanol treatment is begun early, acidosis and central nervous system and eye damage may be completely prevented. The initial dose of ethanol should be 0.75 g/kg; another 0.50 g/kg is given every 4 hours for about 2 to 3 days. (For a 150-pound man this would be an initial dose of 4.5 ounces of 100-proof whiskey, followed every 4 hours by 3 ounces more.)

Treatment of a patient suspected of receiving a toxic dose of methanol should be guided by blood determinations of carbon dioxide–combining capacity, methanol, and ethanol, repeated every 4 hours. Oral or intravenous alkali and ethanol therapy are governed by these blood levels (Fig. 16-1).

As would be expected, prompt treatment with ethanol is essential if the toxic effects of methanol are to be minimized. In a series of nine monkeys receiving 6 g/kg of methanol, the poisoning was reversible if ethanol

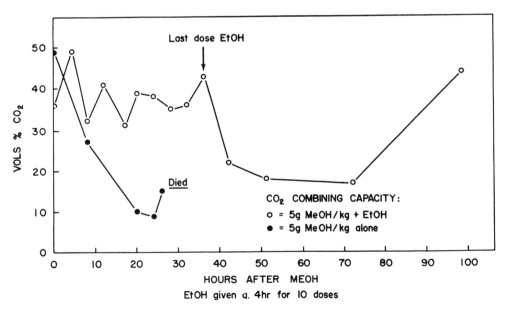

Fig. 16-1. Effect of ethanol on acute methanol toxicity in monkeys. Upper curve: course when treated every 4 hours with ethanol. Note onset of acidosis after the last dose of ethanol given 40 hours after poisoning showing persistence of toxic amounts of methanol. Lower curve: development of severe acidosis and death when the same dose of methanol without ethanol was given subsequent to recovery. (From Gilger, A. P., Potts, A. M., and Farkas, I. S.: Am. J. Ophthalmol. **42:**244, 1956.)

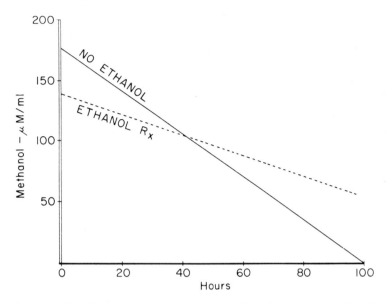

Fig. 16-2. Plasma methanol concentrations in monkey after administration of 6 g/kg methanol, with and without ethanol treatment. Note that ethanol therapy protects methanol from destruction, thereby prolonging methanol plasma levels. Ethanol Rx: average of ten monkeys. No ethanol: average of seven monkeys. (Modified from Gilger, A. P., Farkas, I. S., and Potts, A. M.: Am. J. Ophthalmol. **48:**153, 1959.)

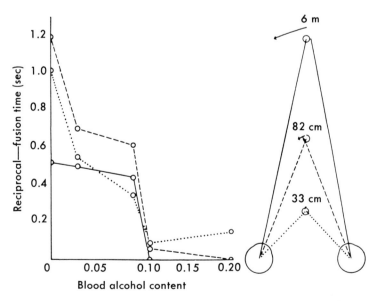

Fig. 16-3. Effect of ethanol on fusion time (expressed as reciprocal; therefore the lower the curve, the longer the fusion time). Blood alcohol levels expressed in percentage. (From Brecher, G. A., Hartman, A. P., and Leonard, D. D.: Am. J. Ophthalmol. **39:**44, 1955.)

treatment was begun within 8 to 12 hours. After a 16-hour delay in starting ethanol treatment, death was postponed but not prevented.[8] Since methanol is demonstrable in the plasma for as long as 4 days (Fig. 16-2), ethanol treatment of human poisoning would seem rational even if the patient were first seen several days after methanol ingestion. At least the damage resulting from metabolism of the remaining methanol could be prevented. Because the outcome varies with dosage, the previously mentioned 16-hour time should not be considered to contraindicate subsequent therapy.

USE IN ETHYLENE GLYCOL POISONING

Poisoning from antifreeze (ethylene glycol) ingestion closely parallels methanol poisoning. Ethylene glycol is not itself poisonous, but 100 ml is a lethal dose for an adult human. Death results from renal occlusion by the metabolite oxalic acid, which precipitates in the kidney as calcium oxalate. Alcohol dehydrogenase blockade by administration of ethyl alcohol (titrate to maintain moderate inebriation) prevents metabolism of ethylene glycol, which is excreted unchanged in 3 to 5 days (during which time the patient should remain constantly in a drunken state).[9]

SEDATIVE USE

Restlessness and unhappiness, perhaps even confusion and disorientation, may complicate the hospitalization of an elderly person. Sometimes barbiturates and anesthetics increase these problems. If the patient is accustomed to a nightly drink of whiskey or brandy, continuance of this habit in the hospital is said to be helpful.[10]

CAUSE OF DIPLOPIA

The well-known diplopia characteristic of alcoholism is caused by progressive impairment of the binocular fusion mechanism.[11] As shown in Fig. 16-3, the time required for fusion increases with rising levels of blood ethanol, and binocular function finally becomes impossible.

Careful haploscopic studies of the effect of alcohol on binocular function indicate that even quite small amounts of this drug will substantially reduce accommodative convergence, thereby lowering the AC/A ratio.[12] An increment of blood ethanol of only 0.01 g/100 ml will cause, on the average, a 5% decrease in the AC/A ratio. At the same time, increasing ethanol concentrations causes an increase of tonic convergence. Although these effects of ethanol would seem appropriate in the treatment of accommodative esotropia, convergence excess, and distance exotropia, the intoxicating properties of this drug render it unsuitable for medicinal use in children. The main significance of the effects of ethanol on muscle balance is to reveal that such physiologic changes may result from a systemic medication. This should inspire some enthusiastic ophthalmologist to undertake a systematic search for other drugs with a comparable therapeutic effect but without undesirable side effects. If the portions of the molecule that modify the convergence responses can be identified, doubtless an effective drug could be synthesized for treatment of tropias and phorias.

RESPONSE OF GLAUCOMA TO ETHANOL INTAKE

Ethanol intake is not harmful to glaucomatous patients. Indeed, 50 ml of alcohol (contained in whiskey or beer) caused a transitory decrease of intraocular pressure in 32 of 33 eyes of normal and glaucomatous subjects.[13] The intraocular pressure drop begins during the first hour and returns to normal after 4 or 5 hours. In general the patients with higher pressure showed greater pressure drops, which averaged 9 mm Hg in the glaucoma patients. Facility of outflow was not increased. An osmotic mechanism of action seems likely.

Although ethyl alcohol itself increases serum osmotic pressure, this effect is not prolonged because of the rapid intraocular penetration of alcohol. Alcohol enters the eye at nearly half the rate of water. A more potent osmotic mechanism is suppression of endogenous antidiuretic hormone formation by ethanol. The decrease in this hormone permits water loss and consequent increase of serum osmotic pressure. Support for this explanation of the antiglaucomatous action of ethanol is derived from the experimental finding that administration of vasopressin (the antidiuretic hormone) will partially or completely block the reduction of intraocular pressure by ethanol.[14]

ALCOHOL RETROBULBAR INJECTION

Prolonged local anesthesia is sometimes desirable in the treatment of painful blind eyes, particularly in elderly or seriously ill patients with an anticipated short life-span. Retrobulbar injection of absolute or 95% alcohol has most often been advocated for such treatment. Being initially painful, alcohol injection must be preceded by injection of lidocaine or procaine. After this, 0.5 to 1 ml of alcohol is injected through the same needle, which is left in position while the syringes are changed. The retrobulbar needle tip should be inserted with care to be certain that it is within the muscle cone and as far anterior as possible. Although destruction of the sensory nerves may be accomplished by injection anywhere within the muscle cone, undesirable paralysis of the extraocular muscles occurs only if their motor nerves are damaged by infiltration of the posterior orbit. Because of its thickness and surrounding protective sheaths, the optic nerve is less likely to be damaged than are the smaller ciliary nerves. The patient will usually experience no further decrease in light perception when retrobulbar alcohol injection is employed in eyes with severely impaired vision. Obviously, however, the risk of severe and permanent damage to the optic nerve or its blood supply is too great to permit this treatment of eyes with useful vision. Breakdown of corneal epithelium as seen in neuroparalytic keratitis is not a common complication of retrobulbar alcohol injection. For several days after injection, quite disturbing orbital edema and chemosis with moderate discomfort are present in some patients and may be relieved by cold compresses. More often, the patient will

experience less pain after injection than was caused by the preexisting eye disease. Apparently the sensory fibers of the ciliary nerves are capable of regeneration, for after some months, pain may recur, requiring reinjection.

Postinjection discomfort and conjunctival chemosis can be reduced or eliminated by taking care to prevent the anterior diffusion of alcohol into the subconjunctival tissues. This may be avoided by being certain that the needle tip is within the muscle cone. Gentle aspiration as the needle is withdrawn prevents escape of residual alcohol from the syringe and needle into the anterior tissues.

Irrigation of the orbit with absolute alcohol during the operative procedure of removal of a hydatid cyst has resulted in optic atrophy, ptosis, and multiple extraocular muscle pareses. Several muscle operations and a ptosis sling procedure were necessary to correct the cosmetic appearance.[15]

Retrobulbar injection of 2.5% benzocaine with 0.5% quinine urea hydrochloride in the treatment of painful blind eyes was suggested by complications in the use of this drug when employed as an anesthetic for cataract extraction. As long as 1½ years after cataract surgery, patients (in India) were observed to have complete facial paralysis (O'Brien akinesia), corneal insensitivity, and exposure keratopathy. After this prolonged effect was noted, 50 patients with painful useless eyes were treated with retrobulbar injection of benzocaine and compared with 20 similar patients treated with 0.5 ml of absolute alcohol given 5 minutes after 1.5 ml of a 2% solution of procaine.[16] Benzocaine injection was found to be superior to alcohol because of its more lasting effect and because it produced less local irritation. Six of the alcohol-injected eyes required repeated injection (time intervals not stated), whereas only one of the benzocaine-treated eyes required reinjection. Eleven of the alcohol injections caused transitory proptosis and chemosis, and one of these eyes developed retrobulbar fibrosis with limited ocular movement. Benzocaine was reported not to cause chemosis and proptosis, although local tissue necrosis can be produced by doses in excess of 1 ml.

The technique of benzocaine injection does not require preliminary use of procaine, since benzocaine is itself an effective anesthetic. The syringe and needle must be completely dry, since moisture will cause precipitation of benzocaine that will block the needle. (Within the tissues, this precipitation of microcrystalline benzocaine results in long-lasting "depot" action.) Injection into the skin, the needle tract, or intravenously must be avoided. One milliliter is an adequate amount for therapeutic effect. Larger volumes may cause tissue necrosis.

Destroying the sensation of painful blind eyes is not a technique to be used indiscriminately. Unsuspected malignant melanoma will exist in 4% of such eyes with opaque media.[17] If the underlying etiology is traumatic, the hazard of sympathetic ophthalmia should be considered. Of course, no cosmetic improvement is provided by retrobulbar injection of long-lasting anesthetics. Despite these objections, retrobulbar injection may clearly be the treatment of choice in such cases as a blind eye with hemorrhagic glaucoma in a seriously ill diabetic patient.

In a series of 25 seeing eyes, 1 to 2 ml of ethanol in 25% to 50% concentrations was injected retrobulbarly for the relief of chronic pain. As a rule, such injections were followed by temporary ptosis, proptosis, chemosis, and extraocular muscle paresis, lasting for several weeks. No instance of permanent damage to muscle innervation or the optic nerve was seen. Severe photophobia and pain as might result from a chemical burn may be effectively relieved by the retrobulbar injection of alcohol. Pain relief may be permanent.[18]

USE IN CRYOSURGERY

The use of 70% ethanol, an effective antifreeze, will prevent adhesion of a cryoprobe to tissue, although it permits heat transfer and freezing. Wiping the cryoprobe tip with an alcohol-soaked sponge applies sufficient alcohol to block adhesion to tissue.[19] No comment is made as to the absence of tissue irritation from this small amount of alcohol.

When applying cryotherapy under ophthalmoscopic control, I find the cryoprobe-sclera adhesion of great value in positioning the eye and indicating the location for the next cryoapplication. However, when cryotherapy is applied under surface control, the prevention of adhesion by silicone or alcohol might eliminate the defrost cycle.

REFERENCES

1. Gilger, A. P., and Potts, A. M.: Studies on visual toxicity of methanol; role of acidosis in experimental methanol poisoning, Am. J. Ophthalmol. **39**:63, 1955.
2. Potts, A. M.: Visual toxicity of methanol; clinical aspects of experimental methanol poisoning treated with base, Am. J. Ophthalmol. **39**:86, 1955.
3. Praglin, J., Spurney, R., and Potts, A. M.: Experimental study of electroretinography in experimental animals under influence of methanol and its oxidative products, Am. J. Ophthalmol. **39**:52, 1955.
4. Potts, A. M., and Johnson, L. V.: Studies on visual toxicity of methanol: effect of methanol and its degradation products on retinal metabolism, Am. J. Ophthalmol. **35**:107, 1952.
5. Moses, R. A.: Adler's physiology of the eye, ed. 6, St. Louis, 1975, The C. V. Mosby Co.
6. Gilger, A. P., Potts, A. M., and Farkas, I. S.: Studies on visual toxicity of methanol; effect of ethanol on methanol poisoning in rhesus monkey, Am. J. Ophthalmol. **42**:244, 1956.
7. Potts, A. M., Praglin, J., Farkas, I. S., Orbison, L., and Chickering, D.: Studies on visual toxicity of methanol; additional observations on methanol poisoning in primate test object, Am. J. Ophthalmol. **40**:76, 1955.
8. Gilger, A. P., Farkas, I. S., and Potts, A. M.: Studies on visual toxicity of methanol, Am. J. Ophthalmol. **48**:153, 1959.
9. Wacker, W. E. C., Haynes, H., Druyan, R., Fisher, W., and Coleman, J. E.: Treatment of ethylene glycol poisoning with ethyl alcohol, J.A.M.A. **194**:1231, 1965.
10. Litin, E. M.: Mental reaction to trauma and hospitalization in the aged, J.A.M.A. **161**:1522, 1956.
11. Brecher, G. A., Hartman, A. P., and Leonard, D. D.: Effect of alcohol on binocular vision, Am. J. Ophthalmol. **39**:44, 1955.
12. Cohen, M. M., and Alpern, M.: Vergence and accommodation, Arch. Ophthalmol. **81**:518, 1969.

13. Peczon, J. D., and Grant, W. M.: Glaucoma, alcohol, and intraocular pressure, Arch. Ophthalmol. **73**:495, 1965.

14. Houle, R. E., and Grant, W. M.: Alcohol, vasopressin, and intraocular pressure, Invest. Ophthalmol. **6**:145, 1967.

15. Baghdassarian, S. A., and Zakharia, H.: Report of three cases of hydatid cyst of the orbit, Am. J. Ophthalmol. **71**:1081, 1971.

16. Mathur, S. P.: Ciliary block with benzocaine, Am. J. Ophthalmol. **47**:867, 1959.

17. Makley, T. A., and Teed, R. W.: Unsuspected intraocular malignant melanomas, Arch. Ophthalmol. **60**:475, 1958.

18. Michels, R. G., and Maumenee, A. E.: Retrobulbar alcohol injection in seeing eyes, Trans. Am. Acad. Ophthalmol. Otolaryngol. **77**:164, 1973.

19. Becker, S. C.: Alcohol in cryosurgery, Arch. Ophthalmol. **79**:803, 1968.

17
FLUORESCEIN AND OTHER DYES

FLUORESCEIN

Sodium fluorescein is a water-soluble dye that produces an intense green fluorescent color in alkaline (above pH 5.0) solution. This color is detectable in concentrations as dilute as 1 ppm. Two percent solutions of fluorescein are nonirritating to the eye, even when it is injured. Fluorescein is used to demonstrate defects of the corneal epithelium in the fitting of contact lenses, for applanation tonometry, as an aid in corneal surgery, to demonstrate patency of the lacrimal drainage system, to show the rate of aqueous secretion, in measuring arm-to-retina circulation time, in fundus photography, and as an antidote to poisoning by aniline dyes.[1]

Mechanism of staining effect

Fluorescein does not actually stain tissues, but it is useful as an indicator dye by virtue of its visibility in very high dilutions. Being somewhat acid, the normal precorneal tear film appears yellow or orange with fluorescein. The more alkaline aqueous humor colors fluorescein green. The intact corneal epithelium, having a high lipid content, resists penetration of water-soluble fluorescein and is not colored by it. Any break in the epithelial barrier permits rapid fluorescein penetration into Bowman's membrane, into stroma, or even into the anterior chamber. Being accessible to aqueous in these locations, the fluorescein assumes a bright green color. Whether resulting from trauma, infec-

tion, or other cause, epithelial defects of the cornea appear bright green with fluorescein and are thereby easily visualized. When the epithelial surface has regenerated, the green color disappears, regardless of whether the underlying stroma is thickened, thinned, scarred, or irregular.

If epithelial loss is extensive, topically applied fluorescein will penetrate into the aqueous and is readily visible biomicroscopically as a green flare. As a practical point, slit-lamp observation of large corneal defects is best performed before fluorescein staining. This will permit identification of the aqueous flare that indicates early traumatic iritis and suggests a need for cycloplegic therapy. More advanced traumatic iritis is readily recognized by aqueous cells, miosis, marked discomfort, and photophobia and will not be obscured by the fluorescein flare.

Methods of use

Fluorescein may be applied as a drop of 0.5% to 2% solution or by placing a strip of fluorescein-impregnated filter paper[2] in the conjunctival sac until it is moistened by tears. If the purpose of fluorescein use is detection of epithelial defects, excess surface dye should be irrigated away with saline solution. Since inadequate irrigation lessens the contrast between stained pathologic lesions and adjacent normal areas, irrigation should continue until the tear film is entirely colorless. Blinking between irrigations helps to remove excess fluorescein beneath the lids.

Fluorescein staining of the eye is transient, disappearing within 30 minutes, and is therefore not cosmetically objectionable to the patient. Stains of the lid skin are easily removed with a tissue moistened with water.

If more fluorescein is desired than can readily be obtained by touching a fluorescein paper to the conjunctiva, the paper strip should be creased longitudinally before it is removed from the sterile wrapper. A drop of sterile solution can then conveniently be placed in the crease and conveyed to the patient's eye. (An anesthetic should not be used, since it tends to quench the fluorescence, and because it may cause misleading punctate corneal defects.)

Since the aqueous humor is more alkaline than tears, an aqueous leak (as after surgery or penetrating ocular trauma) is readily demonstrable with fluorescein. In this examination several drops of fluorescein are instilled and are *not* irrigated out. The lids are held widely apart, and the eye is observed under good illumination. If there is an aqueous leak of any magnitude, a tiny rivulet of green will be seen flowing downward from the perforating wound. If this is not evident at first, gentle pressure on the globe may cause visible aqueous outflow. Inasmuch as this test is usually employed to help determine the cause of shallow anterior chamber in recently operated cataracts, only the most gentle pressure is permissible. Sometimes the aqueous leak is diffuse through the area of a large wound, and no rivulet is visible. This situation is identified by the immediate bright green color change of the instilled fluorescein, as contrasted with the yellow-orange color in a nonleaking eye.

Contamination

Iatrogenic spread of ocular infections via contaminated eye drops is unfortunately all too common. Fluorescein is a major offender when used diagnostically in such lesions as corneal abrasions—natural portals of infection. Cultures of 50 samples of fluorescein from ophthalmologists' offices and hospitals showed 54% to be contaminated.[3] *Pseudomonas aeruginosa* was the contaminant in six of these samples.

The common preservatives of ophthalmic solutions (benzalkonium and chlorobutanol) are inactivated by fluorescein. Phenylmercuric nitrate in a 1:25,000 concentration, used as a fluorescein preservative, seems to kill bacteria, including *Pseudomonas*. This is actually a reversible inactivation, since culture in thioglycollate medium neutralizes the mercurial compound and permits bacterial growth.

Since fluorescein is heat stable, repeated autoclaving is an effective method of sterilization—until the container is again contaminated through use. A considerably more convenient and safer method is the use of individually packaged and sterilized fluorescein-impregnated filter paper strips, which are commercially available. Expense (about 5 cents per strip) is the main objection to this dispensing form.

I would recommend that fluorescein be used more sparingly than is the current practice. Epithelial defects can be readily recognized in the specular reflections from oblique, moving illumination with a flashlight. Certainly a wound will exist if a corneal foreign body has just been removed. Little if any additional information is derived from staining in such cases; the procedure is time-consuming, and some hazard of infection may exist unless the solutions are kept scrupulously sterile. It should be emphasized that meticulous care must be exercised by the physician to avoid contaminating the eye medications by touching the patient's lids with the container.

Uses

Fitting of contact lenses. One of the major uses of fluorescein is as an aid in the fitting of hard contact lenses. Staining renders visible the fluid layer between the cornea and the contact lens. Areas of lens-cornea contact are recognized by thinness or absence of this fluorescein-stained layer. Characteristic patterns of fluorescein distribution identify various faults in fitting of the lens (Fig. 17-1).[4] Observation of the fluorescein layer is greatly enhanced by use of ultraviolet light or by a dark blue filter to modify a white light source.

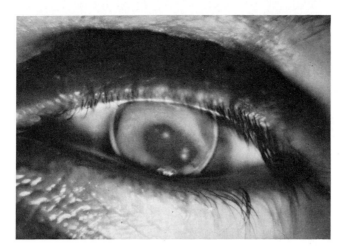

Fig. 17-1. Fluorescein pattern picture taken with cobalt blue filter over electron flash tube. Fluorescein pattern, peripheral bevel, and apical contact area are very noticeable. This patient is an Egyptian who had trachoma (the scars are evident) and now has an irregular cornea. (From Bitonte, J. L.: Contact Lens Society of America Reports, 1962.)

Fluorescein cannot be used in the fitting of soft contact lenses because it enters the pore structure of the hydrogel and remains within the lens for many hours. Such a stained lens is indistinguishable from the tear film. A larger molecular stain, Fluorexon, has the same staining properties as does fluorescein but will not readily enter the pores of the lens. Should study of fluid exchange or corneal apposition of the lens be desirable, this dye is available.[5]

Detection of foreign particles. Fluorescein may be helpful in detecting alkali particles (as in a lime burn) that may be embedded between folds of inflamed conjunctiva. Meticulous mechanical removal of all such particles is most important to prevent further chemical damage.

Recognition of filamentary keratitis may be aided by fluorescein staining of the filaments.

Study of lacrimal patency. Although the mechanical flow of irrigating solution usually proves to the physician and patient whether the nasolacrimal drainage system is open or not, addition of fluorescein to the irrigating solution provides visible evidence that the solution has indeed entered the throat. The patient may be asked to spit out this green material as a convincing demonstration of the success of the procedure.

Fluorescein testing of the patency of the lacrimal drainage system does not necessarily require mechanical irrigation. Several drops of a 2% solution may be instilled into one eye; after this, the patient blinks forcibly at least four times. At the end of 6 minutes the patient blows his nose and clears his throat into paper tissues. Traces of fluorescein are visible in these nasal and oral secretions in normal patients. The test is made much more sensitive with the aid of an ultraviolet lamp, such as the illumination of a Harrington perimeter. Fluorescence under ultraviolet illumination will occur in essentially all patients with functionally patent lacrimal passages. This test has the advantages of simplicity, comfort, and safety and is a more physiologic measure of lacrimal function than are probing and irrigation. It permits study of only one eye per visit.[6,7]

Applanation tonometry. The visibility of fluorescence assumes practical significance in applanation tonometry. The purpose of the fluorescein is to delineate the margin of the applanated area. On cross section, the fluorescein pool between the cornea and the tonometer will be triangular, with its apex directed toward the applanated area (Fig. 17-2).[8] This fluid apex may be invisible if the fluorescein concentration is too low or if the fluorescence is destroyed by acid solutions. Since unstained fluid cannot be differen-

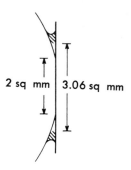

Fig. 17-2. Cornea partially flattened by applanation tonometer. Above and below flattened area are wedges of fluorescein-stained solution, the apices of which are too dilute and therefore invisible. The 3.06 mm² end point of applanation appears to have been reached, but in reality is composed of an erroneously small flattened area surrounded by the invisible apex of inadequately stained fluid. (From Moses, R. A.: Am. J. Ophthalmol. 49:1149, 1960.)

tiated from applanated cornea, the applanation end point of 3.06 mm² will be made up of these two factors rather than of applanated corneal area alone. This error causes underestimation of intraocular pressure.

Visibility of fluorescein varies with its concentration, the thickness of the fluid layer, and the solvent (Fig. 17-3). Note that fluorescence is least impaired by a 0.1% solution of benoxinate (Novesine), which is the anesthetic recommended by Goldmann. Proparacaine in a 0.5% solution is commonly used in the United States and markedly reduces fluorescence. The extent to which invisibility of the fluorescein apex could cause underestimation of intraocular pressure is shown in Fig. 17-4. A maximum error would give an apparent reading of 15.5 when intraocular pressure was actually 25! Such a potential error is invited by understaining the tear fluid with too small an amount of fluorescein or by moistening the fluorescein paper with anesthetic solution, which destroys fluorescence. Error may be avoided by moistening the fluorescein paper with saline solution or

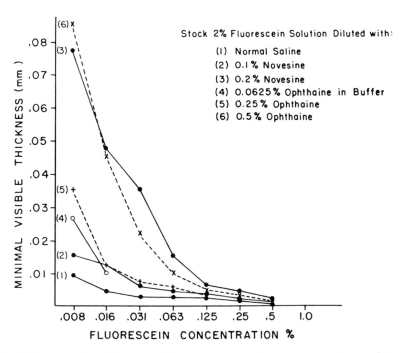

Fig. 17-3. Minimal visible thickness of fluorescein at various concentrations and in different solvents. (From Moses, R. A.: Am. J. Ophthalmol. 49:1149, 1960.)

water to transfer an adequate amount of stain to the eye. Previous anesthetization with proparacaine does not matter, provided an excess of this fluid is not present in the cul-de-sac. Additional proparacaine instilled after staining will, of course, destroy fluorescence and contribute to this source of error.

The technique of applanation tonometry is simplified by use of 0.25% fluorescein solution.[9] Instillation of a drop of this concentration just before measurement produces distinct and easily matched lines. More dilute fluorescein (0.125%) produces faint lines, whereas more concentrated solutions (0.5%) discolor the contact area and leave residual stain on the epithelium. A 2% solution is much too strong for use in applanation tonometry. With experience, the proper amount of fluorescein may be obtained from sterile fluorescein paper strips.

Combination of 0.25% fluorescein and 0.44% proparacaine in the same solution further simplifies the procedure of applanation tonometry. Instillation of this combined medication simultaneously anesthetizes the eye and supplies the proper concentration of dye for accurate reading.[10]

Although a considerable mythology is current in legislative circles about generic "equivalents," the formulation of a drug in a specifically designed vehicle will endow it with many desirable characteristics absent in the supposed "equivalent." A good example of this is a fluorescein-anesthetic combination (Fluress) specifically prepared for use in applanation tonometry.[11] In this preparation, 0.25% sodium fluorescein is combined with 0.4% benoxinate hydrochloride. This anesthetic was chosen because of effectiveness, stability, and patient comfort. A single drop of solution provides adequate anesthesia for applanation tonometry, with an onset within 15 seconds and a duration of 15 minutes. Benoxinate does not induce sufficient tearing to dilute the fluorescein undesirably.

A wetting and stabilizing agent, povidone,

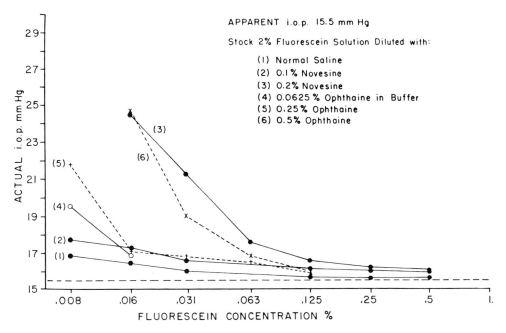

Fig. 17-4. Actual intraocular pressures (i.o.p.) corresponding to an apparent applanation reading of 15.5, in error because of inadequate concentrations of fluorescein or quenching of fluorescence by anesthetic solutions. Note that the error is insignificant if the tear concentration of fluorescein is not permitted to drop below 0.1%. (From Moses, R. A.: Am. J. Ophthalmol. 49:1149, 1960.)

is incorporated in the solution to prevent precipitation of the relatively insoluble benoxinate-fluorescein combination and to permit incorporation of 1% chlorobutanol in the preparation. Povidone also increases the duration of fluorescein-corneal contact in the tear film. Unlike methylcellulose and polyvinyl alcohol, povidone does not blur the definition of the margin of fluorescence at the applanation edge.

The notorious tendency for fluorescein solutions to become dangerously contaminated has been eliminated by the formulation with 1% chlorobutanol. Deliberate heavy contamination with many types of organisms (including *Escherichia coli*, *Staphylococcus aureus*, and *Candida albicans*) was self-sterilized within 15 to 180 minutes (Fig. 17-5).[11]

In other studies, opened bottles of Fluress were found to remain sterile in the clinical area for periods of a month or more. The solution was self-sterilizing even when

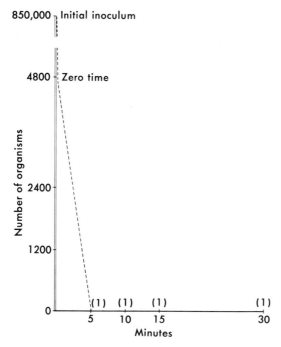

Fig. 17-5. Rate of destruction of *Pseudomonas aeruginosa* by Fluress (850,000 organisms in 2 ml of solution). (From Quickert, M. H.: Arch. Ophthalmol. **77:**734, 1967.)

deliberately contaminated with *Pseudomonas*.[12]

The 0.25% fluorescein concentration was selected because it provides adequate fluorescence to avoid applanation reading errors, yet it does not cause objectionable residual lid staining. The pH adjustment to 5.0 was selected to provide stability for the benoxinate.

In summary, Fluress is a carefully designed, stable, bacteriostatic, nontoxic, and nonirritating solution useful in applanation tonometry because the anesthetic and stain are efficiently applied as a single drop. It can also be used for simultaneous staining and anesthetization of injured corneas.

Corneal surgery. Use of fluorescein during corneal surgery can be most helpful. The green color change of previously instilled fluorescein indicates immediately when the corneal transplant trephine enters the anterior chamber—this is particularly informative in cases where the surrounding cornea is too opaque to permit the surgeon to see the iris.

The raw and the epithelial surfaces of a free conjunctival graft look very much alike and may become accidentally reversed. In case of doubt, fluorescein may be used to identify the raw surface, since only this side will stain.[13]

Should a persistent postoperative flat anterior chamber require surgical re-formation, fluorescein solution may be injected into the anterior chamber at the time of surgery. A stream of this colored solution will identify the site of a wound leak, if it is present.[14]

The rare condition of extensive stripping of Descemet's membrane from the stroma (as a surgical misadventure) is difficult to evaluate because of the transparency of the membrane lying against the iris and the overlying hazy corneal stroma. Intravenous fluorescein appears in the aqueous chamber, and the color difference on the two sides of the detached Descemet membrane aids in evaluation of the condition. Placement of a large air bubble behind the membrane will reappose it to the stroma, with return of corneal transparency.[15]

Detection of aqueous leak. The evaluation of a flat or shallow anterior chamber following surgery or penetrating injury may include fluorescein instillation on the surface of the eye. Use a generous amount of fluorescein and hold the eyelid open during biomicroscopic observation. The normal appearance of such an application is a uniform tear film of somewhat yellowish color. If an aqueous leak is present, the surface color will very rapidly turn green. The first green coloration will usually appear along the tear pool above the margin of the lower lid. Even a subtle leak will show this color change, which is caused by the pH indicator property of fluorescein. Note that the property of fluorescence is *not* used in seeking an aqueous leak.

Larger leaks may cause a tiny rivulet of green to flow downward across the cornea from the leak site. Leaks will commonly be hidden beneath the conjunctival flap—in such cases the green color change will ooze diffusely out from under the cut conjunctival edge.

Fundus photography. Intravenous fluorescein may be used to aid in the diagnosis of fundus lesions. A dose of 10 ml of a 5% fluorescein solution is injected rapidly into an arm vein. The dye appears in the central retinal artery after about 13 seconds and persists for about 20 seconds.[16] Slow injection of the fluorescein over a 2-minute period will prolong the duration of fluorescence.[17]

Abnormal fluorescence of the fundus may be explained by three mechanisms[18]:

1. The normal fluorescence of the choriocapillaris may become more apparent as a result of thinning of the retinal pigment epithelium.
2. Neovascularization may produce new vascular channels that contain the circulating fluorescein.
3. Any abnormality that increases capillary permeability may permit fluorescein to leak into the lesion.

These three mechanisms may be differentiated by the time of onset of the fluorescence. Choriocapillaris fluorescence appears as early as the arteriolar phase. Neovascularization fluorescence coincides with the arteriolar or venous phase, depending on the origin of the new vessels. Fluorescence resulting from abnormal capillary permeability appears later and slowly increases as the injected fluorescein recirculates and further stains the affected tissues.

Fluorescein angiography may be quite helpful in the examination of a variety of relatively subtle types of fundus pathology. For example, intravenous fluorescein injection is a valuable aid in the diagnosis of the cystoid macular edema-papilledema syndrome occurring after cataract extraction. This lesion may be difficult to see with the usual methods of examination, but it shows a very typical fluorescent pattern. Several minutes after injection the eye begins to leak into the cystic spaces surrounding the fovea. About an hour after injection a characteristic dark stellate macular pattern is clearly visible, surrounded by fluorescein-filled cystic spaces extending as much as a disc diameter or more in area. Although characteristic, this fluorescein pattern is not pathognomonic, since it may be found in macular degenerative changes secondary to chronic chorioretinitis, retinal venous occlusion, retinal vasculitis, chronic papilledema, and disciform macular degeneration.[19] Special camera equipment is not necessary to observe this fluorescein leakage into the macular cystic spaces. Ophthalmoscopy through a cobalt blue filter is an equally effective method of recognizing the typical defect.

Fluorescein angiography will also differentiate early papilledema from anatomic pseudopapilledema. In papilledema the fluorescein leaks into the extravascular tissues of the disc and the surrounding retina. This abnormal fluorescence may persist for several hours. In contrast, no leakage of fluorescein occurs in pseudopapilledema, and residual disc fluorescence is insignificant after 10 minutes. Papilledema resulting from malignant hypertension shows the same abnormal fluorescence as does that caused by brain tumor.[20] This staining persists long enough to be interpreted ophthalmoscopically when viewed through a cobalt blue filter.

Fluorescence occurs in hemangiomas,

amelanotic melanomas, disciform macular degeneration, and other chorioretinal lesions in which the choroidal vessels are exposed. Heavily pigmented melanomas fluoresce only slightly, and the absence of fluorescence is said to exclude choroidal hemangioma. Although this test was devised for the diagnosis of choroidal angioma, it is unfortunately nonspecific. Because of the similarity of their fluorescence patterns, choroidal melanoma and hemangioma of the choroid cannot be differentiated by fluorescein photography.[21] Subretinal fluid leakage from a hemangioma, which results in retinal detachment, may be reduced by photocoagulation, cryotherapy, or diathermy. Fluorescein photography will disclose the position of residual subretinal fluid leakage following such treatment and may help guide further therapy.

Properly chosen filters will greatly enhance the quality of photographs obtained in fluorescent angiography. The peak wavelength for excitation of fluorescence is between 4700 and 4900 Å. The fluorescent spectrum itself has peaks at 5250 and 6150 Å. For best detail the illuminating light should pass through a filter that will not transmit wavelengths longer than 5000 Å (for example, Baird-Atomic B-5), and the film should be screened by a filter that will not transmit wavelengths shorter than 5000 Å (for example, Ilford 109). In this way scattered illuminating light will not be photographed and will not blur the fluorescent detail. The quality of photographs obtained with these filters is far better than that obtained with a single blue filter.[22]

Summary. Study of the fundus by fluorescein fundus photography will provide three types of information:

1. Exceptionally good retroillumination of abnormally opaque or transparent areas
2. Delineation and measurement of abnormal capillary permeability
3. The time relationship of retinal blood flow

Study of circulation time. Fluorescein may be used to determine the arm-to-retina circulation time. This technique is a useful supplement to ophthalmodynamometry in selecting patients whose conditions warrant the risk of angiography.[23] Three physicians are required to perform this test. One injects 5% fluorescein solution rapidly into an arm vein. The other two simultaneously observe the optic discs with indirect ophthalmoscopes and record the fluorescein appearance time with stopwatches. A blue filter (Kodak Wratten 45) is required to see the fluorescein easily.

The normal arm-to-retina circulation time is 11 to 13 seconds and should not differ more than 1 second between the two eyes. Occlusive carotid disease may prolong the circulation time of the involved side to 16 to 30 seconds. Detection of prolonged arm-to-retina circulation time on one side is a practical and safe way of diagnosing carotid disease and selecting cases for angiography.[24]

Intravenous fluorescein caused nausea in five of 150 patients. Extravasation of the dye was quite painful for several minutes. No other adverse reactions were reported.

Study of aqueous flow. The appearance time of fluorescein in the anterior chamber may be used as a rough measure of the rate at which aqueous enters the eye. However, this appearance time is variable and is especially unreliable when capillary permeability is increased. For this purpose, 10 ml of a 5% fluorescein solution is injected intravenously over a 2-minute period. In normal eyes, visible green pupillary discoloration appears about 8 minutes after completion of the injection.[25]

Iris examination. Vascular abnormalities of the iris may be rendered more conspicuous by photography or observation through a blue filter immediately after intravenous injection of fluorescein.[26,27]

Antidote to poisoning by aniline dyes. A rather unusual use of fluorescein is in the detoxification of aniline dyes such as are used for indelible pencils.[28] Indelible pencils consist of 30% methylrosaniline chloride (methyl violet) in a graphite and gum tragacanth base. These compounds are highly dissociated salts, and the cations are protoplasmic poisons (triphenylmethane dyes). They will readily combine with the anion of sodium fluorescein to produce a slightly dissociated salt, methylrosaniline fluoresceinate. Precipitation of this insoluble compound effectively removes the toxic cation from the tissues.

Methyl violet is very toxic, spreads rapidly through ocular tissues and the lids, produces intense purple staining, and causes severe edema and rapid necrosis (within several hours) of involved tissue. Ocular injuries by indelible pencils, if significant amounts of dye are retained, may lead to loss of an eye after only relatively minor trauma.

Treatment requires prompt surgical removal of the pencil point and as much of the dye as possible without sacrificing essential structures. After this, the eye is irrigated with a 2% sodium fluorescein solution every 10 minutes until a blue-black precipitate no longer forms. Thereafter, fluorescein irrigation should be repeated every 30 minutes for 12 to 24 hours, at which time the eye may be completely free of purple staining. Healing will be slower than normal after such a chemical injury. A 2% fluorescein solution must be used since the commonly available ophthalmic 0.5% solution is not strong enough (NOTE!) for maximum therapeutic effect.

An unusual opportunity for the study of crystal violet ocular burns was presented by a series of 119 self-inflicted eye injuries occurring in a Polish prison.[29] Corticosteroid therapy was of little benefit; indeed, it seemed to predispose to corneal perforation. Glaucoma, a severe complication, failed to respond to pilocarpine or atropine and was best controlled by acetazolamide. Irrigation with a saline solution of vitamin C and 2% tannin was recommended, although it is stated that this was ineffectual in removing the dye. Fluorescein was not used.

Experimental studies. Because fluorescein is visible, it is an excellent tracer substance for physiologic studies of the penetration of a water-soluble molecule into the eye. For example, in a study of iontophoresis an electric current was found to drive fluorescein rapidly into the aqueous. After a 4-minute period of iontophoresis, 20 times as much fluorescein had entered the eye as when no current was used. Incidentally, this report notes that distilled water should be used as the vehicle rather than saline solution, presumably because the salt ions preferentially carry the current.[30]

Complications of fluorescein injection

About 10% to 20% of patients receiving intravenous fluorescein complain of moderate nausea and headache for a few minutes. Actual vomiting uncommonly occurs and may last for several minutes. Hives have developed in several of my patients and have been reported in three other patients.[31] An ampule of 1:1000 epinephrine should be available for intramuscular use in case the patient develops an allergic response. Unless the patient is warned that the dye is excreted by the kidneys, he may be alarmed when it appears in the urine.

An alarming and unusual allergic reaction to fluorescein occurred in an ophthalmologist after intravenous injection of 5 ml of 10% solution.* Within 10 minutes this physician became very faint and developed laryngeal edema, marked cutaneous and conjunctival vasodilation, and swelling of the face, hands, and feet. Hospitalization and systemic corticosteroid therapy for several days were required to control these manifestations. This individual had frequently used fluorescein over an 8-year period, was known to have other allergies, and had experienced a comparable severe allergic reaction to a penicillin injection some years earlier.

A survey of the literature and of other institutions revealed 55 cases of reaction to intravenous fluorescein.[32] Two thirds of these were of an allergic type and were characterized by urticaria. Seven of the cases were severe and included cardiac arrest, laryngeal edema, convulsive seizure, shock, and myocardial infarction. Only the patient who developed the infarction died. Since this coronary occlusion developed several hours after the fluorescein injection, the relationship to fluorescein is doubtful. The prevalence rate of these problems varied from 0.1% to 1.1% in the different institutions reporting.

---

*Keates, R.: Personal communication, 1967.

Antibody levels to fluorescein could not be detected in three patients with presumed allergic reactions. The possibility of a contaminant exists. In some batches of fluorescein, mercury has been detected and in other batches an unknown pyrogen has been present.

Three separate batches of fluorescein meeting USP specifications were evaluated by thin-layer chromatography.[33] Two of these batches contained several additional peaks, indicating presence of extraneous impurities. The third batch was specially prepared by the pharmaceutical manufacturer. Once again, this proves that generic equivalents may significantly differ in their purity, with nausea following injection varying from 2% to 20% depending on the preparation given.

Concentration of fluorescein is the most significant factor related to post-injection nausea. Following intravenous injection of 25% fluorescein, nausea occurred in 23% of patients. Only 11% were nauseated with 10% fluorescein; only 2% with 5% fluorescein.[34]

Recommended safety precautions include a positive pressure ventilation device, an airway, an indwelling venous catheter, a 1:1000 solution of epinephrine, and hydrocortisone sodium succinate (Solu-Cortef).

The patient should be aware that the skin and urine will be discolored by the fluorescein and should be reassured that this is a transient change that will disappear as soon as the dye is excreted. Within an hour after fluorescein injection, routine urinalysis will give a false positive test for protein (heating, 10% acetic acid) and will be positive for reducing substances (Benedict's test). The false positive sugar test may persist for 4 to 5 days.[35]

ROSE BENGAL

Unlike fluorescein, rose bengal actually stains cells and their nuclei. It selectively stains devitalized corneal and conjunctival epithelium a readily visible red color, which lasts for many hours. Characteristic triangular staining patterns are found in the interpalpebral conjunctiva of eyes with kera-toconjunctivitis sicca. This triangular conjunctival distribution of staining is less likely to occur in neuroparalytic keratitis, where extensive staining commonly affects the exposed portions of both cornea and conjunctiva.[36] Other conditions causing epithelial damage (for example, the punctate corneal staining associated with staphylococcal blepharoconjunctivitis, allergic keratoconjunctivitis, and devitalization after instillation of local anesthetics) will also result in staining by rose bengal.[37]

The main clinical use of rose bengal is identification of the conjunctival lesions of keratoconjunctivitis sicca. These lesions cause interpalpebral, limbus-based triangles of staining associated with relatively minor corneal staining. Typical rose bengal staining is a somewhat more sensitive and reliable test for keratoconjunctivitis sicca than is the Schirmer filter paper test for tear secretion. However, this diagnosis should not be made on the basis of insignificant punctate staining.

Rose bengal is instilled as 1% aqueous solution.[38] Irritation and discomfort are more marked with rose bengal than with fluorescein but usually do not require preliminary use of a local anesthetic. Local anesthetics, particularly cocaine, may cause enough surface damage to result in false positive staining. Excess rose bengal is removed by irrigation as in fluorescein staining. Discoloration of the skin of the patient's lids and the examiner's fingers as well as the ocular staining is more persistent than is fluorescein coloring.

METHYLENE BLUE

Vital staining of nerve tissue may be achieved with a 0.5% solution of methylene blue, which stains the corneal nerves as delicate blue filaments. Methylene blue is more irritating than rose bengal, and topical anesthesia is recommended before its use. Vital staining of corneal nerves requires at least three instillations at 5-minute intervals. Bluish ocular discoloration may persist for as long as a day after methylene blue staining.

Methylene blue irrigation of the lacrimal

sac before dacryocystorhinostomy will stain the mucosal lining a readily identified blue color. The dye should remain in the sac for several minutes. Before starting the operation, the surgeon should wash the sac free of excess methylene blue, since this solution would otherwise spill out on incision of the sac and stain the surrounding tissues.

In the "tract suture" technique, a methylene blue–stained suture is placed intracorneally across the site of the planned incision. The corneal incision is then performed, cutting this suture. The permanent suture is then passed through the blue-stained path of the temporary suture.

Some surgeons re-form the anterior chamber postoperatively by introducing air or saline solution through a previously prepared knife-needle incision in the lower cornea. Such an incision may be difficult to find unless the knife-needle has been dipped in methylene blue just before the incision is made.

Prolonged ingestion of methylene blue will cause the fundus to turn visibly blue.[39]

ALCIAN BLUE

Counterstaining with alcian blue may be used to differentiate mucous deposits from diseased cells.[40] A 1% solution of alcian blue is employed. With this dye, mucus and connective tissue stain blue, but diseased epithelial cells do not stain. Rose bengal stains both diseased epithelial cells and mucus.

Since mucus strands may usually be irrigated away and because their shape is recognizable, alcian blue counterstaining is rarely necessary. Alcian blue should not be used if the cornea is deeply eroded because it causes prolonged discoloration of exposed connective tissue.

Blue-stained flecks of mucus are normally found to line the conjunctival edge of the lid borders and to lie within the lacrimal canaliculus.[41] In ocular pemphigus, no mucus is demonstrable by alcian blue staining.

INDOCYANINE GREEN

Indocyanine green is well tolerated intravenously and can be used in humans for infrared angiography of the choroidal vessels as a clinical procedure. As an example of the type of information that can be obtained with the use of indocyanine green, the author demonstrated that the perfusion pressure of the choroidal circulation is higher than that of the retinal circulation and that choroidal circulation persisted after closure of the retinal circulation by artificially increased intraocular pressure.[42]

ARGYROL

Instilled in the conjunctival sac prior to surgical scrub of the eye, Argyrol serves as an excellent indicator of the adequacy of the preparation. Mucous strands and debris on the lid margin and the skin surface appear discolored by the dark stain lying on the surface. The tissues themselves are not stained and the Argyrol readily washes off—*if* the preparation is complete. Because of the great importance of thorough and complete washing of the field before intraocular surgery, such use of Argyrol or a comparable marker is highly advisable.

Argyrol also has considerable antimicrobial activity, but this is not the primary purpose for its use.

REFERENCES

1. Maurice, D. M.: The use of fluorescein in ophthalmological research, Invest. Ophthalmol. **6:**464, 1967.
2. Kimura, S. J.: Fluorescein paper; a simple means of insuring the use of sterile fluorescein, Am. J. Ophthalmol. **34:**446, 1951.
3. Valghan, D. G.: The contamination of fluorescein solutions, Am. J. Ophthalmol. **39:**55, 1955.
4. Bitonte, J. L.: Fluorescein pattern and biomicroscopy photography in contact lens fitting, Contact Lens Society of America Reports, 1962, p. 1.
5. Refojo, M. F., Miller, D., and Fiore, A. S.: A new fluorescent stain for soft hydrophilic lens fitting, Arch. Ophthalmol. **87:**275, 1972.
6. Campbell, H., Smith, J. L., Richmond, D. W., and Anderson, W. B., Jr.: A simple test for lacrimal obstruction, Am. J. Ophthalmol. **53:**611, 1962.
7. Flach, A.: Fluorescein oropharyngoscopy, Am. J. Ophthalmol. **82:**940, December 1976.

8. Moses, R. A.: Fluorescein in applanation tonometry, Am. J. Ophthalmol. **49:**1149, 1960.

9. Grant, W. M.: Fluorescein for applanation tonometry, Am. J. Ophthalmol. **55:**1252, 1963.

10. Tanton, J. H.: Fluorescein-proparacaine hydrochloride, Am. J. Ophthalmol. **58:**1055, 1964.

11. Quickert, M. H.: A fluorescein-anesthetic solution for applanation tonometry, Arch. Ophthalmol. **77:**734, 1967.

12. Stewart, H. L.: Prolonged antibacterial activity of a fluorescein-anesthetic solution, Arch. Ophthalmol. **88:**385, 1972.

13. Fox, S.: Ophthalmic plastic surgery, ed. 3, New York, 1963, Grune & Stratton, Inc.

14. Shaffer, R. N.: Open angle glaucoma, Trans. Am. Acad. Ophthalmol. **67:**467, 1963.

15. Hecht, S. D.: The use of intravenous fluorescein to estimate the extent of planar Descemet's membrane detachment, Eye Ear Nose Throat Mon. **54:**375, October 1975.

16. Smith, J., Lawton, D., Noble, J., Hart, L. M., Levenson, D. S., and Tillett, C. W.: Hemangioma of the choroid, Arch. Ophthalmol. **69:**51, 1963.

17. MacLean, A. L., and Maumenee, A. E.: Hemangioma of the choroid, Am. J. Ophthalmol. **50:**3, 1960.

18. Kearns, T. P., and Hollenhorst, R. W.: Chloroquine retinopathy, Arch. Ophthalmol. **76:**378, 1966.

19. Gass, J. D. M., and Norton, E. W. D.: Cystoid macular edema and papilledema following cataract extraction, Arch. Ophthalmol. **76:**646, 1966.

20. Kearns, T. P.: Neuro-ophthalmology, Arch. Ophthalmol. **76:**733, 1966.

21. Norton, E. W. D., and Gutman, F.: Fluorescein angiography and hemangiomas of the choroid, Arch. Ophthalmol. **78:**121, 1967.

22. Hodge, J. V., and Clemett, R. S.: Improved method for fluorescence angiography of the retina, Am. J. Ophthalmol. **61:**1400, 1966.

23. Pemberton, J. W., and Britton, W. A.: The arm-retina circulation time, Arch. Ophthalmol. **71:**364, 1964.

24. Winkelman, J. Z., Zappia, R. J., and Gay, A. J.: Human arm to retina circulation time, Arch. Ophthalmol. **86:**626, 1971.

25. Dobbie, J. G.: A study of the intraocular fluid dynamics in retinal detachment, Arch. Ophthalmol. **69:**159, 1963.

26. Rosen, E., and Lyons, D.: Microhemangio-

mas at the pupillary border, Am. J. Ophthalmol. **67:**846, 1969.

27. Bergstrom, T. J., Roth, M., and Martonyi, C. L.: Pigmented iris angiography, Arch. Ophthalmol. **94:**1180, July 1976.

28. Hosford, G.: Treatment of ocular methylrosaniline poisoning with fluorescein, J.A.M.A. **150:**1482, 1952.

29. Segal, P., Mrzyglod, S., Alichniewicz-Czaplicka, H., Dunin-Horkawicz, W., and Zwyrzkowski, E.: Self-inflicted eye injuries, Am. J. Ophthalmol. **55:**349, 1963.

30. Tonjum, A. M., and Green, K.: Quantitative study of fluorescein iontophoresis through the cornea, Am. J. Ophthalmol. **71:**1328, 1971.

31. Maumenee, A. E.: Further advances in the study of the macula, Arch. Ophthalmol. **78:**151, 1967.

32 Stein, M. R., and Parker, C. W.: Reactions following intravenous fluorescein, Am. J. Ophthalmol. **72:**861, 1971.

33. Yannuzzi, L. A., Justice, J., Jr., and Baldwin, H. A.: Effective differences in the formulation of intravenous fluorescein and related side effects, Am. J. Ophthalmol. **78:**217, August 1974.

34. Willerson, D., Tate, G. W., Jr., Baldwin, H. A., and Hearnsberger, P. L.: Clinical evaluation of fluorescein 25%, Ann. Ophthalmol. **8:**833, July 1976.

35. Weiter, J. J.: Intravenous fluorescein effects, Am. J. Ophthalmol. **71:**771, 1971.

36. de Haas, E. B.: Desiccation of cornea and conjunctiva; neuroparalytic keratitis, Arch. Ophthalmol. **67:**439, 1962.

37. Sjögren, H.: Keratoconjunctivitis sicca and the sicca syndrome: some actual problems, Trans. Ophthalmol. Soc. Aust. **11:**27, 1951.

38. Passmore, J. W., and King, J. H., Jr.: Vital staining of conjunctiva and cornea, Arch. Ophthalmol. **53:**568, 1955.

39. Gerber, A., and Lambert, R. K.: Blue appearance of the fundus caused by prolonged ingestion of methylthionine chloride, Arch. Ophthalmol. **16:**443, 1936.

40. Norn, M. S.: Vital staining of the cornea and conjunctiva, Am. J. Ophthalmol. **64:**1078, 1967.

41. Norn, M. S.: Vital staining of the canaliculus lacrimalis and the palpebral border (Marx' line), Acta Ophthalmol. **44:**948, 1966.

42. Flower, R. W.: Infrared absorption angiography of the choroid and some observations on the effects of high intraocular pressures, Am. J. Ophthalmol. **74:**600, 1972.

18
GERMICIDES

The choice of chemical antiseptics used to disinfect living tissue (such as the conjunctiva) is based on a number of factors. Of primary importance is the *toxicity* of the antiseptic, which determines the concentration that may be applied to the tissue.

The highest nonirritating concentrations of a number of antiseptic compounds are given in Table 18-1. This nonirritating concentration is the highest concentration that will produce not more than a slight inflammation of a rabbit eye 1 hour after the last of six instillations of 2 drops each, 5 minutes apart. These concentrations should be entirely safe to apply to the human eye.

The *rate of destruction* of bacteria by a germicide depends on the kind of organism, the degree of dispersion of the organisms (presence or absence of clumps), the amount of other organic matter present, the temperature, and the pH. Complete sterilization of a living tissue such as the conjunctiva is impossible from the practical standpoint; however, the number of microorganisms present can be greatly reduced by chemical germicides. The bactericidal effectiveness of the highest nonirritating concentration of a number of antiseptics is shown in Table 18-1. This germicidal activity was determined against a strain of *Staphylococcus aureus* suspended in a mixture of 10% serum in physiologic saline solution (intended to approximate tear fluid).[1]

Experimental increase of the organic matter by use of 20% serum reduces the rate of destruction of staphylococci by these germi-cides. This inactivation of the germicide is a variable characteristic of different chemicals, as tabulated in Table 18-2. Presence of conjunctival discharge would cause such inactivation.

Another pertinent characteristic (Table 18-2) of germicides is the effect of dilution on disinfectant action. Progressive dilution by tears of the antiseptics introduced into the conjunctival sac may rapidly destroy germicidal activity. The tabulated dilution effect is a 1:1 dilution from the highest nonirritating concentration.

Injurious effects on the natural defense factors may occur from germicide concentrations too dilute to affect bacteria. Phagocytosis by leukocytes and lysozyme activity are inhibited by most of these germicides in such dilution (Table 18-2).

Obviously the circumstances under which a germicide is to be used will determine the "best" agent. For instance, leukocytic damage (relatively little with iodine) would be of little consequence if the chemical were used once for preoperative cleansing but might impair resistance if the chemical were used repeatedly in treatment of an infection. Other properties might be of value, such as the coloring effect of Argyrol that is used to stain and identify mucous debris during the preoperative cleaning of an eye. Note that Argyrol is one of the poorest germicides. The rapid killing effect and the surface-active cleaning properties of the quaternary ammonium compounds suggest their use to flush the conjunctival sac before surgery. Unfortunate-

Table 18-1. Bactericidal effect of nonirritating concentrations of antiseptics*

Antiseptic	Maximum nonirritating concentration (%)	Original number of organisms surviving (%)	
		After 1 minute	After 10 minutes
Merthiolate	0.1	84.7	70.9
Argyrol	50 + } 12.5 used	55.2	19.8
Phenyl mercuric nitrate	0.01	53.2	2.9
Gentian violet	0.01	45.4	0.01
Chlorazene	0.1	22.8	2.3
Acriflavine	0.05	19.8	0.46
Mercurochrome	2.0	6.5	0.25
Silver nitrate	0.25	5.5	5.5
Iodine	0.025	1.0	0.39
Alba†	0.04	0.0	

*From Thompson, R., Isaacs, M. L., and Khorazo, D.: Am. J. Ophthalmol. **20:**1087, 1937.
† Proprietary quaternary ammonium surface-active germicide.

Table 18-2. Summary of characteristics of chemical germicides*

Antiseptic	Relative disinfectant action	Persistency of action	Drop in action with 1:1 dilution	Drop in action by increase of organic matter	Bacteriostatic concentration (leukocytic injury concentration)	Usable concentration (leukocytic injury concentration)	Usable concentration (lysozyme injury concentration)
Alba	Best	Good	50%	Slow, but marked	10	40.0	10.0
Iodine	Very good	Poor	75%	Marked	4	0.4	50.0
Silver nitrate	Good	Least persistent		Very marked			
Mercurochrome	Good	Very good	75%	Slight	8	33.0	1000.0
Acriflavine	Moderate	Very good	50%	Marked	No injury		12.5
Chlorazene	Moderate	Good	75%	Slight	2	0.4	100.0
Gentian violet	Fair	Best	75%	Very slight	4	166.0	1.6
Phenyl mercuric nitrate	Fair	Very good	10%	Slight	No bacteriostasis	1.4	8.3
Argyrol	Fair	Good	0	Slight	4	40.0	1040.0
Merthiolate	Poor	Good	0		4	3.3	0.16

*From Thompson, R., Isaacs, M. L., and Khorazo, D.: Am. J. Ophthalmol. **20:**1087, 1937.

ly, they are rapidly absorbed to fabric surfaces (such as cotton balls) or organic material, thereby being rendered useless. It is interesting that silver nitrate, historically valuable in prophylaxis of ophthalmia neonatorum, is rapidly inactivated by organic matter (such as the vernix caseosa on an in-

fant's skin). Gentian violet kills bacteria slowly but has a much more persistent germicidal effect that is only slightly diminished by organic matter. No doubt this accounts for its usefulness in treatment of chronic marginal blepharitis during the preantibiotic era.

The evaluation of the effectiveness of an

antiseptic is not simply a matter of determining a phenol coefficient or some comparable measurement. A given in vitro measurement may be entirely different from the clinical in vivo effect. The factors responsible for such differences include (1) drug absorption, (2) tissue affinities for the drug, (3) ability of the drug to diffuse or spread on surfaces and through tissues, (4) concentrations that are safe and practicable, (5) stability under adverse conditions, (6) rate of destruction or elimination of the drug, (7) difference of effect of the pH of tissues as compared with experimental conditions, (8) binding of drug to proteins or other constituents of body fluids and discharges, (9) presence of drug inhibitors, and (10) factors of resistance and metabolism of the microorganism.[2]

SURFACE-ACTIVE GERMICIDES

Surface-active agents are substances that alter the relationship of interfaces. These chemicals may be anionic (possess a negatively charged structure, for example, sulfonate), cationic (possess a positively charged structure, for example, quaternary ammonium), or nonionic (possess no ionized groups, for example, alcoholic esters). Such chemicals are useful as wetting agents, detergents, and emulsifying agents; however, their bactericidal properties are of most value in ophthalmology.

The mechanism of the bactericidal action of surface-active chemicals is not positively established but may result from partial disruption of the cellular membranes. The consequent increase in permeability may permit loss of vital intracellular constituents. A direct toxic effect against enzymes and other proteins is also possible.

The germicidal activity of a representative surface-active agent, cetyl pyridinium chloride aqueous solution (Ceepryn), is shown in Table 18-3. The critical killing dilution is defined as the highest dilution of germicide that kills in 10 minutes but not in 5 minutes.[3] It is evident that many common pathogenic microorganisms are destroyed by concentrations far more dilute than are employed for the usual germicidal purposes. However,

some *Pseudomonas* strains may be very resistant. Spores may be highly resistant. Fungi and viruses vary in susceptibility; some, such as the psittacosis virus, are extremely resistant.

Surface-active germicides such as the quaternary ammonium compounds are valuable in disinfecting tissue surfaces (or instruments such as the tonometer that will contact the corneal surface) because their toxicity index (ratio of bacterial toxicity to tissue toxicity) is more favorable than that of germicides containing chlorine, alcohol, and other irritant chemicals. The quaternary ammonium compounds have low toxicity on oral administration, are relatively nonirritating to skin, and are virtually odorless and tasteless. As chemical compounds, they are stable, noncorrosive, and neutral.

Disadvantages of quaternary ammonium compounds include their incompatibilities. They are inactivated by soap, anionic surface-active compounds, proteins, fats, and other organic matter. Although these compounds penetrate and wet surfaces by virtue of their surface activity, clumping of organisms and their adherence to instrument surfaces reduce germicidal effectiveness. Also, bacteria contained within clotted blood adherent to an instrument may be protected against destruction.

Benzalkonium (Zephiran)

One of the most popular cationic detergents is benzalkonium chloride. This drug is useful in ophthalmology for the preservation of eye drops, to enhance corneal penetration of drugs, for instrument sterilization, and for cleaning of skin and mucous membranes.

Use as preservative

Benzalkonium is well suited to use as a preservative for eye drops, since a 1:5000 solution is well tolerated by the eye. No irritation or sensitization results from use of this concentration. Solutions as strong as 1:750 begin to irritate the eye. Accidental use of the 12.8% concentrated stock solution for tonometer sterilization has resulted in almost immediate complete desquamation of the

Table 18-3. Germicidal activity of cetyl pyridinium chloride aqueous solution*

Organism	No. of strains tested	Average critical killing dilution in terms of active ingredients at 37° C†	
		No serum	10% bovine serum
Staphylococcus aureus	5	1:83,000	1:12,500
Staphylococcus albus	1	1:73,000	1:12,000
Streptococcus viridans	1	1:42,500	1:12,000
Streptococcus haemolyticus	2	1:127,500	1:17,000
Neisseria catarrhalis	2	1:84,000	1:13,000
Diplococcus pneumoniae I	1	1:95,000	1:14,000
Diplococcus pneumoniae III	1		1:20,000
Pseudomonas aeruginosa	2	1:5800	<1:1000
Klebsiella pneumoniae	2	1:49,000	1:5500
Corynebacterium diphtheriae	1	1:64,000	1:14,000
Mycobacterium phlei	1	1:1500	1:1000
Eberthella typhosa	5	1:48,000	1:3000
Escherichia coli	2	1:66,000	<1:1000
Proteus vulgaris	2	1:34,000	1:2000
Shigella dysenteriae	1	1:60,000	1:5000
Shigella paradysenteriae	2	1:52,000	1:3500
Shigella paradysenteriae	1	1:49,000	1:2000
Shigella sonne	2	1:68,000	1:6500
Lactobacillus acidophilis	1		1:16,500
Brucella abortus	1		1:19,500
Trichomonas vaginalis	1		1:3000‡
Candida albicans	1	1:37,000	1:3500
Cryptococcus neoformans	1	1:61,000	1:6000
Trichophyton mentagrophytes	1	1:36,000	1:3000
Microsporum canis	1	1:34,000	1:5000

*From Glassman, H. N.: Bacteriol. Rev. **12**:105, 1948.
†The critical killing dilution is defined as the highest dilution of germicide that will kill in 10 minutes but not in 5 minutes.
‡Twenty-five percent human serum.

corneal epithelium. Fortunately, in several cases where this misfortune occurred, healing was rapid with no residual stromal scarring.*

The ophthalmologist should be aware that eye medications formulated with antiseptic "preservatives" contain bacteriostatic rather than bactericidal concentrations of these drugs. Hence appropriate precautions against contamination of the solution during use are still necessary. When evaluated by in vitro cultures without proper neutralization, benzalkonium chloride appears to sterilize a solution contaminated with *Pseudomonas* af-

*Personal observation.

ter 5 minutes of contact. However, injection of these supposedly sterilized solutions into a rabbit cornea almost invariably results in *Pseudomonas* ulceration. The actual sterilizing time for *Pseudomonas* is 3 days for a 1:5000 concentration of benzalkonium chloride (1 day for a 0.5% chlorobutanol solution and 30 minutes for polymyxin B, 1000 units/ml).[4] The reason for the difference between in vivo and in vitro testing is persistence of the antiseptic in the culture medium.

Benzalkonium is incompatible with some anions, including nitrate, salicylate, fluorescein, and sulfonamides. Although pilocarpine nitrate and physostigmine salicylate cannot be preserved with benzalkonium, the hydrochloride salts of these alkaloids are entirely compatible with benzalkonium.

Wetting agents such as benzalkonium enhance the transcorneal penetration of drugs. This enhanced penetration is necessary for some medications to be effective. A notable example is carbachol, which is a rather unreliable miotic in aqueous solution because of its poor penetration.

Use as instrument disinfectant

Equipment that would be damaged by heat may be disinfected by immersion in a 1:750 aqueous solution of benzalkonium chloride. Thirty minutes of exposure to the 1:750 solution is advised. Inactivators of cationic detergents (soap, blood clots, and the like) must be completely removed from the equipment prior to immersion by mechanical scrubbing or wiping and thorough rinsing in water. The common practice of placing cotton gauze in the bottom of the sterilizing tray to protect delicate instruments from mechanical injury actually destroys the germicidal effect of benzalkonium through absorption of the chemical on the cotton fibers. Similarly, the soaking of cotton balls in benzalkonium solution is useless, since the germicidal effect is rapidly inactivated. Since benzalkonium does not reliably kill spores, fungi, and viruses, soaking of instruments in this solution is not a dependable means of sterilization.

A popular method of tonometer sterilization is suspension of the footplate assembly in a solution of 1:5000 benzalkonium between uses. The efficacy of this procedure was studied by contamination of the footplate with *Pseudomonas* organisms and culture of the footplate on trypticase soy agar at intervals.[5] In only 25% of the trials was the footplate sterilized within 1 minute of immersion in the 1:5000 benzalkonium solution. After 5 minutes, 56% of the footplate cultures still showed contamination with viable organisms. Obviously this is less than a foolproof method of sterilization. The ophthalmologist must avoid gross contamination of the instrument, which should never be used on a recognizably infected eye.

Ultrasonic energy has been used to enhance the benzalkonium effect by achieving more effective cleaning and contact.[5] The device used was a 500-watt ultrasound generator specifically devised to support the tonometer. This machine produces sufficient energy to cause visible dispersion of the water surface into a fine mist. Ultrasonic agitation of the 1:5000 benzalkonium solution sterilized 75% of the *Pseudomonas*-contaminated tonometers within 1 minute and 100% within 3 minutes. Ultrasonic vibration in distilled water does not destroy *Pseudomonas* organisms.

When used for instrument sterilization, benzalkonium solutions contain 0.5% sodium nitrate as a rust inhibitor. This solution should not be applied to skin or mucous membranes. Methemoglobinemia may result from nitrate absorption if a sufficiently large body area is treated with this instrument solution. Sodium nitrate may damage aluminum instruments.

Optical instruments with lenses fastened by cement may be damaged by the solvent action of benzalkonium.

Use in skin preparation

The germicidal and detergent properties of benzalkonium are useful in cleaning skin and mucous membranes. Normal skin will tolerate a 1:750 solution without irritation. Mechanical rubbing is essential in skin preparation with any solution to remove dirt, desquamating epithelium, skin fats, and superficial bacteria.

Anionic detergents such as soap or pHisoHex must be removed thoroughly with water and alcohol before use of benzalkonium, which is inactivated by these substances. Skin preparation techniques using such a combination of anionic and cationic detergents are irrational and ineffective and should be discontinued.

In a 1:5000 concentration, quaternary ammonium compounds comparable to benzalkonium may be used as germicidal detergents for eye irrigation before surgery.[6] Prior to the antibiotic era, irrigations with a 1:5000 benzalkonium solution were advised for the treatment of acute catarrhal conjunctivitis and acute blepharoconjunctivitis.[7]

Unfortunately, despite all this literature describing the effectiveness of quaternary ammonium compounds, they do not work very well clinically. For example, after routine preoperative eye preparation with benzalkonium chloride, 40% of skin cultures were still positive (compared to 12% prepared with povidone-iodine).[8]

Fifty-four cases of *Pseudomonas* infection followed inadequate disinfection of cystoscopes and bronchoscopes with 1:750 benzalkonium chloride. The epidemic strain was isolated from the basin used to "disinfect" the instruments.[9] An outbreak of *Pseudomonas* septicemia affected 9 patients whose intravenous skin and equipment sterilization was performed with 1:750 benzalkonium chloride from a contaminated stock bottle.[10] *Pseudomonas* contaminated blood cultures from 79 patients, again because of infected benzalkonium solutions.[11] These 3 articles describing not only the failure of benzalkonium to sterilize but its being the source of infection were published in the same edition of *The Journal of the American Medical Association* with the intent of attracting the attention of physicians. The editor[12] tells the story of the disobedient mule, whose attention could be stimulated only by whacking it on the head with a two-by-four. The analogy was drawn that we physicians are the mules and that our attention can be drawn to the uselessness of quaternary ammonium compounds only with this massive condemnation. These compounds are good for scrubbing walls and furniture, not skin and medical instruments. But we relinquish our habits only slowly. Please change to another disinfectant—now, please.

pHisoHex

A proprietary germicidal cleaning agent, pHisoHex is widely used for preoperative skin preparation around the eye. It contains 80% sodium octylphenoxyethoxyethyl ether sulfonate, 3% hexachlorophene, and lanolin esters. Ophthalmologists should be aware that the first ingredient is extremely toxic to the cornea.

Two near tragedies have been reported af-
ter use of pHisoHex.[13] In each case the operated eye was being removed with the patient under general anesthesia, and the normal remaining eye was unknowingly contaminated with the cleaning solution, which remained on the eye during surgery. At the close of surgery the good eye was noted to be red with a hazy cornea despite the fact that it had been covered to prevent exposure damage. Inflammation was severe by the first postoperative day, most of the corneal epithelium was absent, the cornea was diffusely hazy, and striate keratopathy was marked. Two weeks postoperatively the eye showed marked superficial punctate staining, heavy folds of Descemet's membrane, pigment keratitic precipitates, and aqueous flare. Folds in Descemet's membrane and photophobia were still present 6 weeks postoperatively. By 8 months, healing was complete, with only minor residual scarring, and the patient was asymptomatic. Both cases had a very similar course, as described.

Experimental exposure of a rabbit eye for as short a time as 30 seconds causes superficial punctate staining that lasts for 24 hours.[13] Exposures of 1 or 2 minutes cause damage lasting for 2 weeks. Histologic examination shows changes in all layers of the cornea, including sloughing of the endothelium.

Clearly, prevention is the preferred treatment of pHisoHex keratitis. This germicide should not be allowed to enter the eye even briefly. Particularly if the patient is under general anesthesia, ocular contamination with pHisoHex must be avoided, since the unconscious patient cannot complain. No local anesthetic should be placed in the fellow eye of a conscious patient, since the burning sensation of accidentally instilled germicide is of protective importance. Thorough irrigation of the eye should follow cleansing of the skin with pHisoHex.

During surgery for retinal detachment, which particularly requires a clear cornea, accidental contamination of the eye with even slight amounts of pHisoHex is immediately evident. The cornea dries rapidly, losing its luster and transparency. Conceivably, at least an occasional postcataract surgery deep striate keratopathy may be pHiso-Hex induced.

pHisoHex is a good germicide, but it is quite destructive to the cornea, hence representing a potential tragedy ready to happen in a careless moment.

Povidone-iodine

Presently we use povidone-iodine for our ophthalmic preoperative preparations. It will kill all bacteria in less than a minute, spores more slowly. It does not burn the skin, even though left on underneath the bandages. The stained skin is virtually impossible to reinfect for at least an hour. The stain is water soluble and washes off easily, unlike the stain of tincture of iodine. In routine preparation before eye surgery, using half-strength povidone-iodine, bacteria could be recovered in only 12% of cases following the preparation.[8] The effectiveness of a preoperative preparation is related not only to the germicide chosen but also to the thoroughness of the scrub. I believe that the importance of a meticulous prep cannot be exaggerated. Intraocular infections still happen—I see them at least every month on referral. *Be sure* your surgical eye is thoroughly cleaned, with special attention to the lid margins, and seriously consider using povidone-iodine. (Do not allow it to come in contact with the eye full strength—it burns, even through a topical anesthetic, but does no significant tissue harm.)

PRESERVATIVE
Chlorobutanol

One of the most popular preservatives for eye drops is 0.5% chlorobutanol solution. Although primarily bacteriostatic, chlorobutanol is often bactericidal when exposure is prolonged for 24 hours or more. Growth of *Pseudomonas* and of *Staphylococcus aureus* in nutrient broth was invariably prevented by 0.5% chlorobutanol solution.[14] Both gram-positive and gram-negative bacteria as well as many species of fungi are inhibited by chlorobutanol.

Chlorobutanol is stable and resists destruction by autoclaving at pH of 6.0 or less, but more alkaline solutions are rapidly hydrolyzed by heat. Since sodium fluorescein solutions are more alkaline than this, heat sterilization of chlorobutanol-preserved fluorescein completely destroys the preservative.

Although eye drops containing 0.5% chlorobutanol as a preservative have been instilled several times daily for years without ill effect, such solutions may not be tolerated as a continuous bath. Diffuse epithelial damage of the cornea results from bathing the eyes for as long as 20 minutes with 0.4% chlorobutanol in isotonic saline solution. Use of chlorobutanol-preserved solutions for gonioscopy is inadvisable, since epithelial damage lasting for several hours may ensue after this prolonged chemical contact. Biochemical studies indicate that chlorobutanol inhibits oxygen utilization of the cornea and loosens epithelial adhesion.[15]

In practice, chlorobutanol, 0.5% solution, is an effective and nonirritating preservative. It has been used continuously in all collyria used or dispensed at the Massachusetts Eye and Ear Infirmary since 1926. Such solutions have been used during intraocular surgery without causing endothelial or other damage. No instance of sensitization has been recognized during these many years of extensive use. In a survey of 576 bottles of eye medications containing chlorobutanol as a preservative, only a single instance of contamination (the organisms were *Pseudomonas*) was detected. The pharmacologic activity of ophthalmic medications is not reduced by chlorobutanol.

STERILIZING AGENTS
Cresol

An apparently effective solution (Post's solution No. 4) for chemical sterilization of sharp instruments contains the following constituents:

Liquor cresolis compound	8 ml
Oil of lavender	2 ml
Thymol crystals	2 g
Ethyl alcohol	88 ml

The thymol and oil of lavender are primarily to disguise the unpleasant odor of the cresol. This solution is not corrosive to metal instruments and does not dull sharp edges. Surgical instruments experimentally contaminated by bacteria are invariably sterilized within 2 minutes of immersion in this solution and usually within 60 seconds. Even when the solution has been contaminated by 5% whole blood and when spore-forming organisms such as *Bacillus subtilis* are used, materials difficult to sterilize, such as gauze or string, become sterile within 4 minutes.[16]

More recent evaluation of such chemical sterilizing solutions indicates that they are completely unreliable against spores.[17] The differences in method of evaluation include use of *Bacillus subtilis* strains with a high spore count, selection of culture media particularly adapted to growth of spores, saving of all solutions to identify presence of spores washed off but not killed, and drying of a proteinaceous film of spores on the instruments before use of the sterilizing solution. With these more rigid methods, all instruments were found to remain contaminated after 30 minutes of soaking in Post's solution No. 4. In most instances, Post's solution itself contained viable spores after 30 minutes.

The current belief is that no chemical method will effectively sterilize instruments contaminated with spores, with the exception of ethylene oxide.

Ethylene oxide

The sharp instruments used in eye surgery tend to be dulled by autoclaving, which is the reason for the rather extensive use of sterilizing solutions (which inadequately sterilize spores). Ethylene oxide sterilization has been shown to be efficacious for autoclaving and yet not damage sharp edges, glass, or plastic. This gas, in a concentration of 10 g/l of space, will sterilize even resistant organisms and spores within a 2-hour period. The explosive properties of pure ethylene oxide are eliminated by mixing it with hydrocarbon gases. The gas is toxic and should be handled with reasonable care. The ethylene oxide gas sterilizer is standard equipment in many hospitals. A small portable sterilizer has been developed and is practicable for private ophthalmic use.[18]

METALLIC GERMICIDES

Preantibiotic treatment of surface infections has included application of a variety of metallic salts, dyes, and so forth. Most of these medications do, indeed, have bacteriostatic or bactericidal activity, but their use on the eye is limited by ocular tolerance. Topical use of most of these medications is now obsolete.

Not only are the antiseptic solutions used in ophthalmology prior to the introduction of antibiotics relatively ineffective germicides, but actually they greatly delay healing of corneal epithelial defects and in most instances may cause permanent corneal opacity.[19] Such drugs include mild silver protein, 10%; merbromin (Mercurochrome), 2%; zinc sulfate, 0.5%; benzalkonium chloride (Zephiran), 1:3000; acriflavine (Neutroflavine), 1:1000; nitromersol (Metaphen), 1:2500; thimerosal (Merthiolate), 1:2500; and mercuric oxycyanide, 1:5000.

Mercury is a not infrequent allergen.[20] The typical reaction is delayed, reaching a peak 1 to 2 days after application of the Merthiolate. The area of skin around the eye exposed to mercury (as by skin preparation or preserved drops) is locally affected with a weeping, swollen, reddened allergic dermatitis of very typical appearance. It is more painful than itching. Perhaps a week is required for the reaction to subside.

Copper

Copper has been used to destroy bacteria, fungi, viruses, and algae. Copper sulfate has been shown to inhibit fungus (*Cephalosporium*) growth in vitro in concentrations as dilute as 0.06%. Topical application every hour of 0.12% copper sulfate solution was tolerated by the human eye and was believed to be helpful in treatment of two patients who developed keratitis resulting from *Cephalosporium*, although 8 weeks of therapy was necessary for one of the patients.[21] Increased penetration of copper may be attained by iontophoresis.

Copper sulfate iontophoresis is reported to be an effective treatment for herpes simplex keratitis, whether epithelial or stromal.[15] The rationale for this treatment is that the copper ion, with its known antimicrobial effect, may be forced into cell membranes by an electromotive force. Cocaine, 5% solution, was instilled at 2-minute intervals over a 10-minute period to render cell membranes more permeable and for its anesthetic effect. An aqueous solution of copper sulfate, 0.125%, was placed in a corneal bath electrode and connected to the anode of a 45-volt B battery. One milliampere of current was passed for 2 minutes. After treatment, 0.25% scopolamine solution was instilled and an eye pad was applied.

All 20 patients had a burning sensation in the eye immediately after the treatment, which lasted for 4 to 5 hours. Because this was anticipated, codeine was given before treatment. The treatment caused conjunctival hyperemia, loss of epithelium surrounding the ulcer, stromal edema, and slight anterior chamber flare. The eye may appear slightly worse the day after iontophoresis. On the average, corneal staining disappeared 4 to 5 days after iontophoresis. All 20 eyes (9 with dendritic ulcers, 10 with stromal keratitis, and 1 with disciform keratitis) healed following iontophoresis, although one patient required three treatments during a 2-week period. No case recurred during the period of 21 months between the first treatment and publication of the paper.[22]

Copper is selectively stored in the liver and in the central nervous system. Presumably, this selective storage explains the damage to these two organs in Wilson's hepatolenticular degeneration.[23] Certainly systemic toxic effects will not follow any ocular use of copper.

Silver

The ability of silver ions, even in a dilution of 10^{-5}M, to kill microorganisms is the basis for their ophthalmic use. This lethal action is not selective for microorganisms but is a protein denaturation that indiscriminately destroys conjunctival and corneal epithelium as well as bacteria. Silver nitrate is well suited to destroy surface organisms. For this reason, it is an effective eye prophylactic against gon-

orrhea if it is used immediately after birth. However, the anti-infectious potency of silver nitrate is not lasting, and it is too toxic for repeated instillations. Furthermore, the chemical burn of corneal epithelium temporarily reduces ocular resistance and predisposes the eye to pyogenic infections.

Tissue chlorides precipitate insoluble (and therefore inactivated) silver chloride. This precipitation prevents deep tissue penetration of protein destruction by silver (provided the solution is not too concentrated). Simultaneously it shields subsurface infection from cure. Presumably, this is the reason why bacteria that cause surface conjunctival infection (for example, gonococci) are destroyed, and why deeper infections (for example, the virus of inclusion blennorrhea and established gonococcal infections) are not cured.

Ocular tolerance

A 1% silver nitrate solution is extremely irritating, as anyone brave enough to try a drop in his own eye will testify. However, it is not extremely destructive, and usually within several days after silver prophylaxis the average newborn eye has stopped discharging. If 2% silver nitrate solution is used, prompt irrigation with saline solution is advised to prevent excessive eye irritation. A 6% silver nitrate solution causes extensive scar formation, and 12% may cause total blindness in rabbits.[24] Tragic results may follow confusion of 10% silver protein solutions (Argyrol) with silver nitrate, 10% solutions of which may blind a child. A survey of 85 ophthalmologists disclosed 17 who had encountered blindness that had resulted from use of excessively strong solutions of silver nitrate.[25]

Silver nitrate applicator sticks have been used as tissue-cauterizing devices. For example, exuberant granulation tissue in an exenteration socket can be eradicated by application of a silver nitrate stick. One horror story recounts the fate of a 35-year-old housewife who had the base of an incised chalazion cauterized with a silver nitrate stick. The eye was then patched. When next seen, the cornea was densely opaque, concealing all detail of the underlying iris. Corneal transplantation and cataract extraction were required. The corneal button was heavily infiltrated with silver granules.[26] Use of a silver nitrate stick within the eyelids does not seem prudent.

A nurse used a silver nitrate stick for ocular prophylaxis of a newborn.[27] Despite a perfectly dreadful initial reaction of extensive surface necrosis, only slight corneal scarring remained after 1 year. As Murphy's law states, "If anything can go wrong, it will, and at the worst possible moment." Never relax your vigilance.

Credé prophylaxis

In 1881 the incidence of gonorrheal ophthalmia was reduced from 10% to 0.5% simply by the instillation of a 2% silver nitrate solution into each conjunctival sac immediately after delivery. Except that the concentration of silver nitrate has been reduced to 1%, the Credé method is still practiced generally today and is legally required in most of the United States. Without doubt, silver nitrate prophylaxis reduces the frequency of gonorrheal ophthalmia. However, it does not eliminate all cases of gonorrheal ophthalmia, does not protect against virus inclusion conjunctivitis, and is not suitable for treatment of deeply invading bacterial infections.

Gonorrhea is still sufficiently prevalent (and actually may be increasing) that some type of eye prophylaxis continues to be desirable. The various antibiotics and sulfonamide drugs, systemically administered or topically instilled, have repeatedly been proved to be effective in gonorrheal prophylaxis, actually more effective than silver nitrate.[25,28,29] These newer drugs are far less irritating and also protect against eye infections from common pyogenic organisms, which are prevalent after the use of silver.

In the past, to prevent venereal disease after sexual intercourse, various chemical germicides such as silver were instilled into the urethra. This practice has been rendered obsolete by antibiotics. I am surprised that ophthalmologists still condone a similar half-century-old practice on infant eyes.[30] Perhaps it

can continue because a newborn child is more defenseless than a healthy young adult male.

Antiviral effect

Silver nitrate as well as a large number of other chemicals was evaluated in treatment of experimental herpes simplex keratitis.[31] Silver nitrate, mercuric chloride, benzoquinone, and chloranil all inactivated herpes virus when used in in vitro concentrations as dilute as $10^{-5}M$. A rather surprising finding was virus inactivation by prednisolone in a $10^{-2}M$ concentration. Iodine is effective in a $10^{-3}M$ concentration.

Unfortunately none of the large number of chemicals studied was found to be therapeutically effective when applied topically to the infected cornea in the form of drops. Presumably, this limitation exists because the virus lies within the epithelial cells and a virucidal chemical concentration is destructive to the cornea. Use of 0.17% silver nitrate solution was said to reduce the number of dendritic figures in 10 of 21 rabbit eyes, but did not shorten their duration. These results were interpreted as being equivocal.

Antibacterial effect

Silver nitrate is extremely toxic to microorganisms. For example, a concentration of 1 μg of $AgNO_3$/ml of solution killed 98.3% of *Pseudomonas* in 5 minutes and 99.997% in 15 minutes.[32] The presence of chloride ions in tissue fluids greatly reduces the antibacterial effectiveness of silver because of precipitation of insoluble silver chloride. Nevertheless, the minimal inhibitory concentrations for *Pseudomonas* are in the range of 20 to 40 μg/ml of silver nitrate, even in the presence of 7 mg sodium chloride/ml. The antibacterial activity of the medium seems to be related to the total concentration of silver and not only to the silver ions present.

Tissue toxicity of silver ions may be estimated by the measurement of respiration of skin cells in tissue cultures. One milligram per milliliter (0.1%) of silver nitrate caused a 22% inhibition of respiration; 2.5 mg/ml, 39% inhibition; 5 mg/ml, 61% inhibition; and

10 mg/ml, 76% inhibition. The minimal amount of silver nitrate causing inhibition of respiration of skin in tissue culture was 25 times greater than the minimal concentration of silver nitrate that inhibited growth of *Pseudomonas aeruginosa*. Obviously there is a favorable therapeutic index for the topical use of silver as an antibacterial agent. The author has advocated the use of 0.5% silver nitrate solution applied as a moist compress to prevent infection in burns of the skin.

Argyrosis

Argyrosis is the well-known bluish gray discoloration caused by tissue deposits of silver.[33] Because tissue chlorides are almost exclusively confined to the intercellular areas, silver staining of tissue is selectively deposited outside the cells.[34] This discoloration is permanent; however, superficial skin, conjunctival, and corneal silver deposits can be removed by subcutaneous or subconjunctival injection of a freshly prepared solution of sodium thiosulfate and potassium ferricyanide. Solutions of 12% sodium thiosulfate and 0.5% potassium ferricyanide are more stable than are the mixture. When mixed in equal proportions, a 6% and 0.25% solution of the respective drugs results. It must be used within 30 minutes of preparation. Topical ocular instillation is said to be effective but to act much more slowly. Deeper silver deposits (as on Descemet's membrane) cannot be removed in this way.[15]

CONTACT LENS STERILIZATION

Having smooth surfaces, the traditional "hard" methyl methacrylate contact lens is rather easily sterilized, cleaned, and washed. Almost any detergent or germicide can be used, providing that it is thoroughly rinsed off before insertion into the eye.

The hydrophilic "soft" lenses are porous and retain microorganisms as well as chemicals. Heat sterilization is the accepted method; however, 3% hydrogen peroxide will sterilize soft lenses within 5 minutes, destroying *Pseudomonas*, *Candida*, and all other common microorganisms. Hydrogen peroxide is painful to the eye but does not cause

any significant damage. Soaking the soft lens in 2.5% sodium thiosulfate solution (harmless to the eye) for 15 minutes will inactivate the hydrogen peroxide, after which the lens may be rinsed and inserted.[35]

A substantial mythology has arisen that soft contact lenses may concentrate the preservatives from eye drops and thereby damage the eye. This, of course, cannot happen. To the extent that the lens binds the preservative, it is not released to affect the eye. Dire consequences do not result from preservative binding.[36]

ULTRAVIOLET LIGHT

The germicidal properties of ultraviolet light are well known and widely used for sterilization. Before the discovery of antibiotics, ultraviolet radiation was successfully employed in treatment of corneal ulcers caused by microorganisms. Resistance of viruses, fungi, and many bacteria to antibiotics and the development of new ultraviolet radiation sources suggest reevaluation of this old method of therapy.

Peak germicidal activity occurs at a wavelength of about 2650 Å (most effective wavelength against viruses and fungi as well as against bacteria). Nucleoprotein absorption of ultraviolet light has a similar peak, which suggests that the germicidal effect is a result of nucleoprotein destruction. For some unexplained reason, actinic keratitis is produced most effectively at a wavelength of 2880 Å.[37] Superimposition of the germicidal and keratitis-producing spectral curves (Fig. 18-1) indicates that at 2537 Å the germicidal effect is 85% of maximum, whereas the keratitis effect is only 20% of maximum.[38] The 2537 Å wavelength was chosen because it is the wavelength emitted by a low pressure mercury-vapor lamp.

Experimental studies with 2537 Å ultraviolet light indicates that a dosage of as much as 1250 microwatt sec/cm² can be tolerated by the human cornea in a single dose without causing permanent scarring. Rabbit experiments indicate that stromal vascularization and scarring follows 5,000,000 microwatt sec/cm². Corneal epithelial damage is moderate-

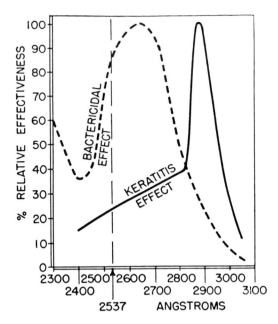

Fig. 18-1. Relative action spectra of bactericidal and keratitis-producing effects of ultraviolet light. (From Hudnell, A. B., and Chick, E. W.: Arch. Ophthalmol. **68:**304, 1962.)

ly severe following 800,000 microwatt sec/cm², but by 5 to 7 days after treatment, the cornea has returned to normal. In remarkable contrast to corneal resistance is bacterial susceptibility to this wavelength. Complete in vitro bacterial destruction requires only 2500 to 26,400 microwatt sec/cm². Fungus destruction requires 6600 to 330,000 microwatt sec/cm². Virus susceptibility is assumed to be in the same range as bacterial susceptibility. The human eye can tolerate without sequelae over three times the dose required to kill in vitro the most resistant microorganism tested.

Treatment appears to be quite simple, requiring only an accurately timed exposure of the cornea to the calibrated lamp, positioned 5 mm away. Apparently the energy output of these bulbs varies considerably (from 600 to 3000 microwatts/cm² at 5 minutes); hence each bulb requires individual calibration. Since the radiation intensity varies with the inverse square of the distance, accurate dosage requires precise positioning.

The discomfort of radiation keratitis can be

minimized by cycloplegics and patching and is said to be less severe than that of chemical cautery. Topical anesthesia is used prior to treatment. Mechanical removal of diseased epithelium or discharge presumably permits better ultraviolet penetration.

Hudnell and Chick[38] report treatment of only seven patients all having acute dendritic ulcers. One ulcer recurred but was successfully treated by repeat ultraviolet therapy. Unlike x-ray therapy, the ultraviolet effect is not cumulative. This presentation of ultraviolet treatment is most interesting, although it is not yet pragmatically established.

Exposure of a tonometer footplate to ultraviolet light within a special sterilizer holder destroyed all organisms within 15 minutes.[39] Challenge was by swabbing the footplate. This is not exactly the same as the in-use moist contact with the plunger, which moves up and down in the central cavity, shielded from ultraviolet light. Fortunately the applanation tonometer prism is an easily cleaned smooth surface.

REFERENCES

1. Thompson, R., Isaacs, M. L., and Khorazo, D.: A laboratory study of some antiseptics with reference to ocular application, Am. J. Ophthalmol. **20:**1087, 1937.
2. Theodore, F. H.: Newer concepts in treating external eye disease, Am. J. Ophthalmol. **40:** 744, 1955.
3. Glassman, H. N.: Surface-active agents and their application in bacteriology, Bacteriol. Rev. **12:**105, 1948.
4. Riegelman, S., Vaughan, D. G., and Okumoto, M.: Rate of sterilization as a factor in the selection of ophthalmic solutions, Arch. Ophthalmol. **54:**725, 1955.
5. Hok, R., Wachtel, J., and Havener, W. H.: Ultrasonic tonometer sterilization, Am. J. Ophthalmol. **58:**676, 1964.
6. Bell, R. P., and Johnson, L. V.: Cetydimethylbenzylammonium chloride—a new ophthalmic irrigation solution, Ohio State Med. J. **47:**231, 1951.
7. Lawrence, C. A.: Chemical preservatives for ophthalmic solutions, Am. J. Ophthalmol. **39:** 385, 1955.
8. Hale, L. M.: Povidone-iodine in ophthalmic surgery, Ophthalmic Surg. **1:**9, November-December, 1970.

9. Dixon, R. E., Kaslow, R. A., Mackel, D. C., Fulkerson, C. C., and Mallison, G. F.: Aqueous quaternary ammonium antiseptics and disinfectants, J.A.M.A. **236**:2415, November 22, 1976.

10. Frank, M. J., and Schaffner, W.: Contaminated aqueous benzalkonium chloride, J.A.M.A. **236**:2418, November 22, 1976.

11. Kaslow, R. A., Mackel, D. C., and Mallison, G. F.: Nosocomial pseudobacteremia, J.A.M.A. **236**:2407, November 22, 1976.

12. Hussey, H. H.: Benzalkonium chloride: failures as an antiseptic, J.A.M.A. **236**:2433, November 22, 1976.

13. Browning, C., and Lippas, J.: pHisoHex keratitis, Arch. Ophthalmol. **53**:817, 1955.

14. Murphy, J. T., Allen, H. F., and Mangiaracine, A. B.: Preparation, sterilization, and preservation of ophthalmic solution, Arch. Ophthalmol. **53**:63, 1955.

15. Grant, W. M.: Toxicology of the eye, Springfield, Ill., 1962, Charles C Thomas, Publisher.

16. Post, M. H., and Moor, W.: The sterilization of sharp instruments by chemical solutions, Am. J. Ophthalmol. **25**:579, 1942.

17. Riegelman, S., Vaughan, D. G., Jr., and Okumoto, M.: Evaluation of the sporicidal activity of Post's sterilizing solution, Arch. Ophthalmol. **53**:847, 1955.

18. Linn, J. G.: Use of gas sterilization for ophthalmic surgery, Arch. Ophthalmol. **62**:619, 1959.

19. Bellows, J. G.: Influence of local antiseptics on regeneration of corneal epithelium of rabbits, Arch. Ophthalmol. **36**:70, 1946.

20. Taub, S. J.: Delayed hypersensitivity to Merthiolate preservative, Eye Ear Nose Throat Mon. **49**:235, May 1970.

21. Byers, J. L., Holland, M. G., and Allen, J. H.: Cephalosporium keratitis, Am. J. Ophthalmol. **49**:267, 1960.

22. Brown, S. I., Holland, M. G., and Allen, J. H.: Treatment of herpes simplex keratitis with copper sulfate iontophoresis, Arch. Ophthalmol. **67**:453, 1962.

23. Gubler, C. J.: Copper metabolism in man, J.A.M.A. **161**:530, 1956.

24. Calvery, H. O., Lightbody, H. D., and Rones, B.: Effects of some silvery salts on the eye, Arch. Ophthalmol. **25**:839, 1941.

25. Wachter, H. E., and Pennoyer, M. M.: Prophylaxis in the eyes of newborn infants, Mo. Med. **53**:187, 1956.

26. Grayson, M., and Pieroni, D.: Severe silver nitrate injury to the eye, Am. J. Ophthalmol. **70**:227, 1970.

27. Hornblass, A.: Silver nitrate ocular damage in newborns, J.A.M.A. **231**:245, January 20, 1975.

28. Ormsby, H. L.: Ophthalmia neonatorum, Am. J. Ophthalmol. **39**:90, 1955.

29. Chapman, K. J.: A comparable study of Neo-Silvol and terramycin as prophylactic treatments in the eyes of the newborn, Ohio Med. J. **52**:591, 1956.

30. Berens, C.: Ophthalmia neonatorum prophylaxis, Am. J. Ophthalmol. **39**:87, 1955.

31. Sery, T. W., and Furgiuele, F. P.: The inactivation of herpes simplex virus by chemical agents, Am. J. Ophthalmol. **51**:42, 1961.

32. Ricketts, C. R.: Mechanism of prophylaxis by silver compounds against infection of burns, Br. Med. J. **1**:444, 1970.

33. Gutman, F. A., and Crosswell, H. H., Jr.: Argyrosis of the cornea without clinical conjunctival involvement, Am. J. Ophthalmol. **65**:183, 1968.

34. Collin, H. B.: Endothelial cell lined lymphatics in the vascularized rabbit cornea, Invest. Ophthalmol. **5**:337, 1966.

35. Gassett, A. R., Ramer, R. M., and Katzin, D.: Hydrogen peroxide sterilization of hydrophilic contact lenses, Arch. Ophthalmol. **93**:412, June 1975.

36. Mackeen, D. L.: The safety and efficacy of chemical disinfection with hydrophilic gel contact lenses, Contact Lens J. **8**:17, December 1974.

37. Cogan, D. G., and Kinsey, V. E.: Action spectrum of keratitis produced by ultraviolet radiation, Arch. Ophthalmol. **35**:670, 1946.

38. Hudnell, A. B., and Chick, E. W.: Corneal ultraviolet phototherapy, Arch. Ophthalmol. **68**:304, 1962.

39. Sherman, S. E.: Evaluation of an improved ultraviolet tonometer sterilizer, Am. J. Ophthalmol. **78**:329, August 1974.

19
IODIDE

When what to do one cannot decide
Then one prescribes iodide

The old German proverb just quoted indicates the status once enjoyed by iodide therapy. A wide variety of inflammatory and degenerative diseases, including those of the eye, were empirically treated with this drug.[1]

Of a series of 115 eyes with senile macular degeneration treated with oral administration of iodides (0.015 mg protiodide of mercury three times a day), 56 were reported to show improved visual acuity. However, 29 of these subsequently lost vision.[2] Contrary to the author's favorable interpretation, these statistics actually represent the expected spontaneous course of senile macular degeneration. In the discussion of heparin in Chapter 7, similar statistics are cited in a controlled study of senile macular degeneration.

Iodides were also considered to aid in the resorption of various pathologic deposits. Even today it is common to encounter patients who have been receiving iodide therapy for vitreous hemorrhages. Particularly when vitreous hemorrhage is caused by a retinal tear (and therefore occurs in an eye with considerable posterior vitreous separation), the blood may settle inferiorly very rapidly—sometimes within a few days. Such expected spontaneous rapid improvement can easily be misconstrued as "a dramatic cure" attributed to whatever therapy had been used. I have not personally observed any recognizable response to iodides with respect to clearing of vitreous hemorrhages, nor am I aware of any published data supporting such claims.

The physician prescribing systemic iodide should be aware that this drug can cause fever (as high as 104° F after 5 days of treatment with 3 ml of a saturated solution of potassium iodide in a daily dose). Skin eruptions, conjunctivitis, and coryza are other manifestations of iodide sensitivity.[3]

Treatment of herpetic keratitis

A strong solution of iodine (containing 7% iodine and 5% potassium iodide in alcoholic solution) was originally used in treatment of acute herpetic keratitis.[4] In the untreated control series (53 eyes) the average duration of conjunctival redness was 41 days, and the shortest period of corneal staining encountered in any eye was 10 days. In 97 eyes treated with iodine cautery the average duration of redness was 15 days, and in 85% corneal staining had disappeared by 10 days. Metaherpetic complications developed in 11 of the 53 control eyes and in 25 of the 97 treated eyes, a virtually equal incidence.

Topical instillation of a 5% potassium iodide solution alone was not helpful in treatment of dendritic ulcers. By contrast, epithelial curettement without chemical cautery definitely shortens the course of dendritic keratitis. Neither iodine cautery nor curettement benefits metaherpetic keratitis.

Because of the danger of permanent stromal scarring, the generous use of a strong solution of iodine has been abandoned in favor of the sparing use of a mild solution of iodine. The physician should avoid discoloration of Bowman's membrane, since such treatment causes irreversible, although superficial, corneal damage.

Specific antiviral therapy with topical idoxuridine and vidarabine has displaced chemical cauterization for herpetic keratitis to a second-choice position.

Potassium iodide, 1%, every 1 to 2 hours reduces the corneal reaction to fungal ulcers.[5] This benefit is believed to be a result of the potassium ion, which helps an injured cornea maintain its water pump system and glycolytic cycle. The iodide ion may not be helpful.

REFERENCES

1. Goodman, L., and Gilman, A.: The pharmacologic basis of therapeutics, ed. 4, New York, 1970, The Macmillan Co.
2. Laird, R. G.: Iodide therapy for senile macular degeneration, Am. J. Ophthalmol. **28:**287, 1945.
3. Steffen, G. E.: Iodide fever, J.A.M.A. **192:**571, 1965.
4. Gundersen, T.: Herpes corneae, Arch. Ophthalmol. **15:**225, 1936.
5. Newmark, E., Ellison, A. C., and Kaufman, H. E.: Pimaricin therapy of cephalosporium and fusarium keratitis, Am. J. Ophthalmol. **69:**458, 1970.

20
OSMOTIC AGENTS

Intraocular pressure may be reduced by use of osmotic agents, which increase the osmotic pressure of the plasma relative to that of aqueous and vitreous. Such osmotherapy is very effective for a brief period of time and is therefore useful as an emergency measure in the management of acute glaucoma. Osmotherapy has no role in the treatment of chronic glaucoma.

Maintenance of a plasma-aqueous osmotic gradient ideally requires use of a small molecule (greater osmotic effect per unit weight) that is nontoxic and has relatively poor ocular penetrance. Although it meets the first two requirements, sodium chloride diffuses into the aqueous rapidly and will not maintain the body fluids hypertonic with respect to the eye. Since they penetrate the eye poorly, sucrose and sorbitol will maintain an osmotic differential but cause renal damage and require very large doses (because of high molecular weight). Urea, mannitol, and glycerol will effectively reduce acutely elevated intraocular pressure and are clinically useful for this purpose.

UREA

A prompt and marked drop of intraocular pressure can be achieved in almost all cases of glaucoma by intravenous infusion of urea. If 30% urea solution is given at the rate of 90 to 120 drops/minute, the reduction in tension occurs within 30 to 45 minutes, with return to pretreatment pressure in 5 to 6 hours. The maximum effect is attained about 1 hour after urea infusion is begun.

Mechanism of action

The mechanism of action of urea is quite different from that of other antiglaucomatous medications, being entirely an osmotic phenomenon. Urea does not readily penetrate the barrier existing between blood and intraocular fluids. This poor penetration has been attributed to low lipoid solubility and high nitrogenous content. Being a small molecule, urea is able to exert a strong osmotic effect across a semipermeable membrane relatively impervious to its passage. The amount of lowering of intraocular and cerebrospinal fluid pressures is directly related to the increased osmotic pressure of the blood caused by intravenous urea and is accomplished by a withdrawal of intraocular water into the intraocular blood vessels.

The relationship between blood and aqueous urea levels has been studied after intravenous urea administration in human beings; the aqueous was obtained at the time of surgery, with simultaneous drawing of the blood sample.[1] In all patients the aqueous urea concentrations were always lower than the blood urea concentrations. Blood and aqueous urea levels at different time intervals after cessation of urea infusion are shown in Fig. 20-1. Naturally the blood levels were highest initially and dropped rapidly with renal excretion of the urea. Blood urea levels are essen-

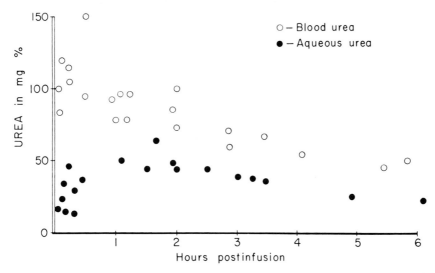

Fig. 20-1. Blood and aqueous urea values determined in human subjects immediately after intravenous administration of urea, 1 g/kg, given as a 30% solution at rate of 3 ml/minute. (Modified from Galin, M. A., Nano, H., and Davidson, R.: Arch. Ophthalmol. **65:**805, 1961.)

tially normal within 24 hours. Because of delay in passing the blood-aqueous barrier, aqueous urea levels are still quite low when the infusion is terminated and require 1 to 2 hours to reach their peak. By far the greatest concentration differential exists initially, with return to an essentially normal blood-to-aqueous ratio by 5 hours. Thus the known osmotic differential coincides exactly with the clinically observed pressure drop, which is greatest 30 to 45 minutes after the infusion is begun, and which relapses to pretreatment levels after 5 hours (provided the filtration angle is still closed).

The hypotensive effect of urea is produced not only by its effect on the aqueous humor but also by osmotic alteration of the vitreous body. The urea concentrations in blood, aqueous, and vitreous after a rapid (10 minutes) intravenous injection of 1 g urea/kg body weight (rabbits) are shown in Fig. 20-2[2]; the vitreous concentration of urea changes quite slowly and is proportionately below that of the blood for 4 to 5 hours. (The normal ratio of blood-to-aqueous-to-vitreous urea concentrations is 5:4:3.5.) The hypotensive effect of urea continues during this entire time, which is considerably longer

than the several hours during which the blood-to-aqueous ratio is altered.

Increased vitreous osmolality results within 1 hour after intravenous administration of osmotic agents (including urea, mannitol, and glycerin) to rabbits. This finding indicates vitreous dehydration. Inasmuch as the vitreous volume is much greater than any other part of the eye, it is probable that vitreous dehydration is the primary mechanism whereby hyperosmotic agents lower intraocular pressure.[3]

About 5 to 7 hours after injection the vitreous concentrations of urea become proportionately higher than the normal ratio with blood concentrations and remain elevated for many hours. During this time the blood-to-eye osmotic relationships may acctually tend to increase intraocular pressure.

The volume of the vitreous body changes after urea administration. Vitreous volume is least when its osmotic pressure is lower than the normal blood-to-vitreous ratio and greatest when its osmotic pressure is higher. The anterior chamber may deepen by as much as 0.2 mm after urea treatment, a result important in the treatment of angle-closure glaucoma.

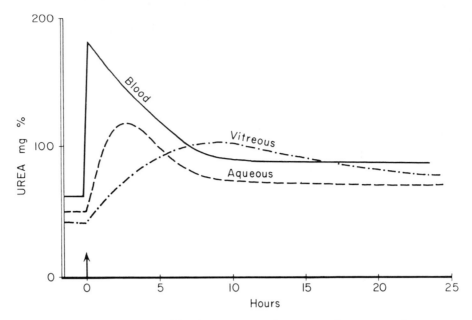

Fig. 20-2. Urea concentration in blood, aqueous, and vitreous after 1 g urea/kg given intravenously within 10 minutes. (Modified from Bleeker, G. M., Haeringen, N. J., and Glasius, E.: Am. J. Ophthalmol. **56:**561, 1963.)

A decrease in rabbit vitreous weight of 3% to 4% occurs subsequent to osmotherapy with urea, mannitol, or glycerol. This experimental study is compatible with the clinical observation that the vitreous volume can be reduced by osmotherapy.[4]

Measurements of the localization of radioactive carbon–labeled urea in the rabbit eye[5] are in agreement with the already cited biochemical determinations. Two hours after intravenous infusion of radioactive carbon–labeled urea, its aqueous concentration was only 36% of that in plasma. Autoradiographs of these eyes showed a relatively high concentration of labeled urea in the ciliary processes and the anterior surface of the iris. The therapeutic significance, if any, of this localization is not evident.

The possibility that "osmoreceptors" in the brain have some neural regulatory effect on intraocular pressure has been suggested by the observation that small intravenous doses of hyperosmotic agents will cause a small drop (2 or 3 mm Hg) in intraocular pressure in the normal eye but not in an eye with a transected optic nerve.[6-9]

Preparation and administration

For intravenous administration, a 30% solution of urea is used. This must be freshly prepared because stale solutions decompose to ammonia, which is toxic. The urea is dissolved in a 10% invert sugar solution to prevent hemolysis of erythrocytes. Dissolving of urea is an endothermic reaction; hence the solution becomes extremely cold during preparation. Although it may be well to warm the solution somewhat before intravenous injection, warming it to about 50° C will cause ammonia formation and should be avoided.

The dosage is 1 g urea/kg body weight. The usual rate of infusion is 90 to 120 drops/minute. Because of the marked diuretic effect, an indwelling catheter is required for anesthetized patients. Meperidine, 25 mg, and promethazine, 25 mg, may be given intravenously through the tubing immediately after the infusion is begun to prevent some of the unpleasant side effects that are commonly encountered.

Because extravasation of 30% urea solution will cause tissue necrosis and sloughing that

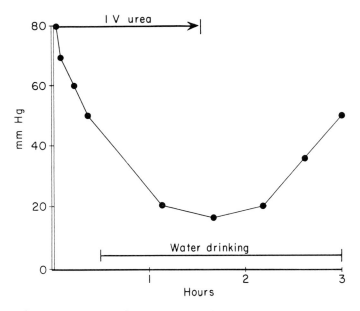

Fig. 20-3. Secondary rise of intraocular pressure resulting from drinking of water after control of glaucoma with intravenous administration of urea. (Modified from Hill, K., Whitney, J., and Trotter, R.: Arch. Ophthalmol. **65:**497, 1961.)

may be extremely destructive, the physician must be absolutely certain the needle is securely within the vein. The site of administration should be observed frequently to be certain the needle does not become accidentally dislodged. In one case, litigation proceedings were instituted when a slough of the back of a hand so severe as to expose a number of the extensor tendons resulted from extravasation of urea. Since wrist motion may cause the needle to pierce out of the small wrist veins, these vessels probably should not be used unless the larger veins of the forearm are completely unsuitable.

Drinking of water will nullify the hypotensive effect of urea, with a resultant secondary rise of intraocular pressure, as shown in Fig. 20-3.[10] Since the dehydration caused by urea characteristically causes thirst, the physician must caution the patient against drinking. Small amounts of cracked ice will relieve the sensation of thirst without causing hemodilution. Unless patients are specifically forbidden to drink, they will certainly do so, thereby blocking the effect of the urea.

When administered orally, urea is also effective in reducing intraocular pressure. A dosage of 1.5 g/kg will cause a substantial drop in pressure within 2 hours. As expected, intraocular pressure returns to pretreatment levels in about 7 hours. The response of a patient with congenital glaucoma is shown in Fig. 20-4.[11] In contrast to the resistance of congenital glaucoma to control by miotics, osmotic therapy is quite effective. Unfortunately oral urea therapy is not suitable for long-term control of glaucoma.

Although the drug is unpalatable, 20 patients were all able to take a single dose of urea administered as a 50% solution in cherry syrup on cracked ice; therefore this method is feasible for one-dose therapy, as in acute glaucoma.[11] However, the nausea of acute glaucoma will often interfere with oral medication. Surgeons preferring general anesthesia will need to use intravenous urea. The blood urea nitrogen does not return to normal for about 36 hours after urea dosage. Since the effect of urea depends on creating a blood-aqueous osmotic differential, repeat doses cannot be given often enough to

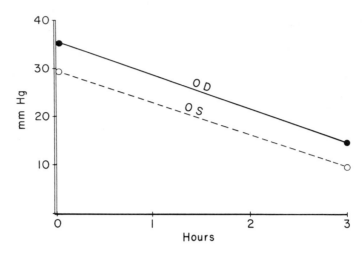

Fig. 20-4. Effect of oral administration of urea, 1.5 g/kg, on congenital glaucoma. (Modified from Galin, M. A., Aizawa, F., and McLean, J.: Arch. Ophthalmol. **62:**1099, 1959.)

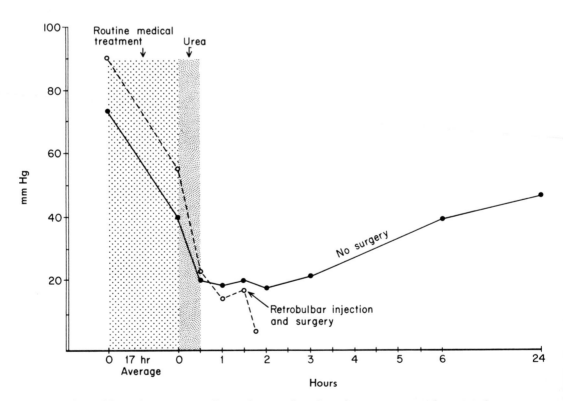

Fig. 20-5. Additive hypotensive effects of acetazolamide and miotics, urea infusion, and retrobulbar anesthesia with massage are illustrated in a series of 14 patients with acute glaucoma. Note that in patients not operated on pressure returned to preurea levels within 6 hours despite continuing miotic therapy. (Modified from Tarter, R. C., and Linn, J. G.: Am. J. Ophthalmol. **52:**323, 1961.)

maintain a prolonged, constant pressure control.

Use with other medications

The hypotensive effect of urea is additive to that of other types of antiglaucoma medications. Fig. 20-5 shows the drop of pressure produced in 14 patients with acute angle-closure glaucoma by the use of acetazolamide, pilocarpine or carbachol, eserine, and in some cases epinephrine.[12] This group of patients did not respond sufficiently to such therapy, although the average pressure drop was 35 mm Hg prior to administration of urea. Routine medical treatment was continued for an average of 17½ hours (3 to 24 hours) before urea was started. Within 30 minutes after administration of urea, all tensions dropped sharply to normal levels. Of particular interest is the still further reduction of pressure achieved by retrobulbar anesthetic injection and massage, which indicates that this must be the result of yet another mechanism of action.

In practice, miotics and carbonic anhydrase inhibitors are always used concomi-

tantly with urea in the management of acute glaucoma, and they almost always will control the pressure even after the osmotic effect is lost. For this reason, surgery is not scheduled to coincide with the 30- to 45-minute peak osmotic effect but is delayed, if pressure is controlled, for several days to permit the eye to recover from its inflamed condition (which predisposes to synechiae and vascular complications), to bring the patient to optimal physical condition (control of dehydration or other problems and performing of adequate physical and laboratory examinations), and because of the practical reason of scheduling convenience.

Indications

Primary acute glaucoma. The main ophthalmic use for urea is in the control of cases of narrow-angle acute glaucoma that have not responded to miotic and carbonic anhydrase inhibitor therapy. Because of the potential hazards inherent in urea treatment, these other medications should be used first. The use of urea is indicated by failure of the glaucoma to respond within a reasonable time.

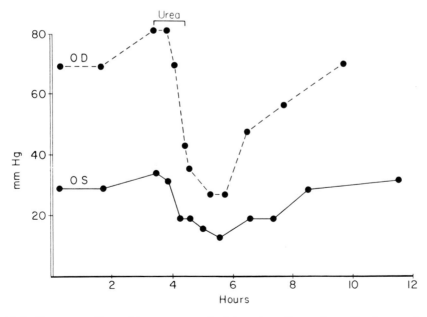

Fig. 20-6. Transient effect of intravenous administration of urea in angle-closure glaucoma with peripheral anterior synechiae. Within 8 hours, despite use of miotics, pressure was up again. (Modified from Davis, M., Duehr, P., and Javid, M.: Arch. Ophthalmol. **65:**526, 1961.)

A dramatic drop in pressure can confidently be expected within 30 minutes after osmotic therapy is begun. Even pressures that have been completely resistant to miotic and secretory inhibitor therapy will drop to low normal levels with urea.

Urea-induced hypotension is transient, with return to pretreatment pressures within 7 hours if the angle-closure defect is not relieved (Fig. 20-6).[13] Such a return to high tensions despite miotic therapy is proof that a filtering operation will be required. If the reduction of pressure produced by urea can be maintained by miotics, the angle is sufficiently open so that peripheral iridectomy will be adequate.

From the practical standpoint, the surgeon can assume that almost all acute primary glaucoma of only 1 or 2 days' duration will be controlled by miotics alone after the angle block is opened by the urea-induced vitreous shrinkage and deepening of the anterior chamber. (Angle opening may be confirmed by gonioscopy if desired.) Hence it is usually not necessary to perform iridectomy as an emergency procedure under adverse circumstances.

Glaucoma secondary to hyphema. The anterior chamber deepening effect of urea may open the trabecular block sufficiently to permit escape of some blood and may lower pressure enough to permit the intraocular musculature to respond to miotics and maintain better outflow. Presumably, because of such actions, urea may reduce the pressure accompanying an "eight-ball hemorrhage," not only transiently but also often permanently. Hence the surgeon should consider use of urea to be definitive treatment of glaucoma secondary to hyphema and not merely a means of dropping pressure at the time of surgery. Surgical evacuation of intraocular blood is an extremely hazardous procedure that may leave the eye much worse than before the operation. Surgery should be performed only after all medical measures, including urea, have failed to control pressure.

Repair of perforating injuries. If vitreous and/or uveal tissue bulge from a wounded eye, repair is difficult and will entail further loss of vital intraocular structure. Urea-induced softening of such an eye will prevent further vitreous loss during surgical manipulation and will enhance reposition of the iris and similar maneuvers such as re-formation of the anterior chamber. Urea-induced hypotension causes a quite dramatic falling together of previously gaping wound edges, with retraction within the eye of beads of protruding vitreous.

Removal of an intraocular foreign body or of a dislocated lens is almost invariably accompanied by vitreous loss. This may be minimized by the use of urea.

Glaucoma secondary to inflammation. Maintenance of an osmotic differential between plasma and aqueous is dependent on a functioning blood-aqueous barrier. Inflammation reduces the effectiveness of this barrier and permits aqueous electrolyte concentrations to approach those of the plasma. Theoretically, the pressure-reducing response to intravenous injection of urea should be diminished in the presence of ocular inflammation. The urea concentrations in blood, normal aqueous, and inflammatory aqueous have been studied in rabbits given a severe chemical iritis by injection of 0.1 normal sodium hydroxide.[14] As shown in Fig. 20-7, aqueous urea nitrogen concentrations are higher in the inflamed eye than in the normal eye. No intraocular pressures were reported in this experiment; however, it is implied that urea will be less effective in treating inflamed glaucomatous eyes. I consider this supposition to be more theoretical than an actual clinical problem, for if the blood-aqueous barrier were to be completely broken down and the plasma-aqueous osmotic differential were lost, the intraocular pressure would be subnormal, and no indication for urea therapy would exist.

However, it is clinically reported that if the blood-aqueous barrier is defective, as in secondary glaucoma, the blood-aqueous osmotic difference cannot be maintained for long and the intraocular pressure more rapidly returns to pretreatment levels[15] than in other types of glaucoma.

Retinal detachment surgery. The use of

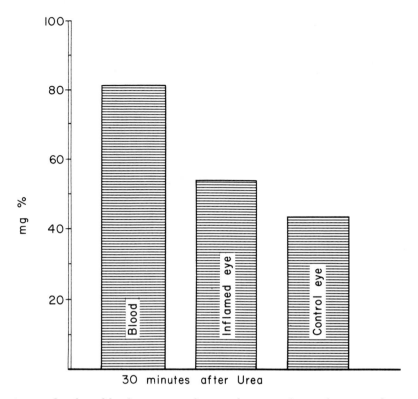

Fig. 20-7. Urea levels in blood, aqueous of eye with severe chemical iritis, and normal eye. (From Galin, M. A., and Davidson, R.: Arch. Ophthalmol. **68:**633, 1962.)

urea to decrease ocular volume has been suggested as an aid in retinal detachment surgery. If indicated, this would be particularly useful in volume-reducing procedures such as silicone implant, circling fascia, and scleral overlap. Inasmuch as most of my own practice is devoted to the care of retinal detachment patients, I feel qualified to state that a well-planned and executed procedure can be carried out without the nuisance of using urea or the danger of paracentesis. The type and extent of operation selected do not depend exclusively on the number or distribution of the retinal tears but must also take into account other factors, including the volume of removable subretinal fluid. Since undetached tears should be treated with cryotherapy or photocoagulation rather than with surgery, the problem of infolding the sclera in the absence of subretinal fluid does not exist. If optical obstacles (fixed small pupil) prevent photocoagulation, simple diathermy will effectively seal these flat tears,

but it is much more traumatic than photocoagulation or cryotherapy.

In the Custodis polyviol method of treating retinal detachment, an elastic substance is sutured firmly against the sclera at the diathermied site of the tear.[16] No subretinal fluid is released. Urea administered during this type of detachment procedure may soften the eye sufficiently to permit better indentation of the sclera.

Cataract extraction. Urea has been used prior to cataract extraction, but the results hardly seem to warrant the effort. In a series of 100 cases,[17] vitreous loss occurred four times, 10 patients complained of severe headache, and four patients became irrational and agitated, one to the extent of requiring postponement of surgery. A consistent softening of the eye was attained with use of urea, but similar softening is more safely induced by retrobulbar anesthesia with hyaluronidase followed by adequate massage.

If osmotic dehydration of the vitreous softens the eye before cataract surgery, what will happen when it rehydrates postoperatively? Apparently no clinically significant increase of pressure occurs, no doubt because aqueous outflow is sufficiently rapid to maintain normal pressures. Two cases of air block glaucoma have been reported to follow cataract extraction subsequent to oral administration of 150 ml of 50% glycerol.[18] In these cases the eye was so soft that a very large bubble of air was spontaneously aspirated and remained within the anterior chamber at the close of surgery. Acutely painful air pupillary block glaucoma occurred during the subsequent day.

Air pupillary block glaucoma may be prevented by avoiding a large air bubble in the anterior chamber. Medical treatment with osmotic agents and mydriatics will control pressure until the air is absorbed. Surgical removal of the air is not necessary.

Vitreocorneal contact. Osmotic removal of

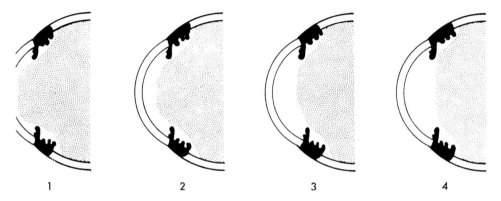

Fig. 20-8. Change of position of anterior vitreous face. **1,** Before administration of hypertonic urea solution. **2,** One hour after administration of hypertonic urea solution. **3,** Two hours after administration of hypertonic urea solution. **4,** Three hours after administration of hypertonic urea solution. (From Kornblueth, W., and Gombos, G.: Am. J. Ophthalmol. **54:**753, 1963.)

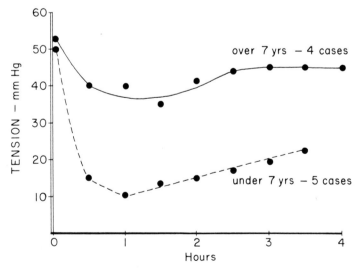

Fig. 20-9. Hypotensive action of urea in absolute glaucoma. Failure of pressure to respond to urea is encountered only in those eyes that have been blind for many years. (From Tarter, R. C., and Linn, J. G.: Am. J. Ophthalmol. **52:**323, 1961.)

fluid from the vitreous by means of hypertonic urea causes retraction of the vitreous body. The effect of urea on an aphakic eye with vitreous in the anterior chamber is illustrated in Fig. 20-8.[19] Within 3 hours the vitreous body had entirely retracted from the anterior chamber. Vitreocorneal contact may be treated by intravenous administration of urea followed by miotics to prevent return of vitreous to the anterior chamber.

Absolute glaucoma. The hypotensive effect of urea is absent only in eyes suffering from absolute glaucoma of many years' duration. (Fig. 20-9).[12] Presumably, such eyes have suffered extensive thrombosis and atrophy and have lost the extensive choroidal and retinal vascular bed across which the osmotic effect of urea is exerted. Obviously no significant benefit results from transient control of pressure in a blind eye, even if it is attained.

Sickle cell crisis. Urea will break the hydrophobic bonds that mediate sickling of red cells and will terminate an acute sickle cell crisis. A high concentration of urea is required—150 to 200 mg%—and is achieved by intravenous infusion continued until pain disappears. The induced diuresis is undesirable and must be compensated for by prompt and continuous hydration. Seventeen

patients experiencing acute sickle crisis were successfully treated by intravenous urea in sugar solution (the dextrose or glucose is necessary to prevent hemolysis).[20]

Complications

The complications of urea administration are shown in Fig. 20-10. All patients have rapid and massive diuresis that requires indwelling catheterization for about 3 hours. Serious distention of the bladder may occur in an anesthetized, noncatheterized patient during urea administration. Severe headache, probably caused by cerebral dehydration, affects 92% of patients, begins in 5 minutes, and may last as long as 45 minutes after the infusion. The headache of urea treatment results from reduced intracranial pressure and is quite similar to a lumbar puncture headache. It may be minimized by keeping the patient in bed without elevation of the head during urea administration and the subsequent 3 hours. Although drinking water will promptly stop this headache, it also stops the therapeutic osmotic effect of urea treatment. Meperidine helps both the headache and the arm pain that distress 84% of the patients. The arm pain stops as soon as the infusion is discontinued unless there is extrav-

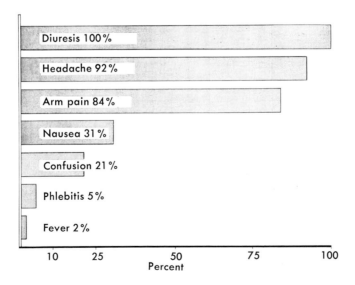

Fig. 20-10. Complications of urea administration. (Modified from Tarter, R. C., and Linn, J. G.: Am. J. Ophthalmol. **52:**323, 1961.)

asation of the solution into the tissues or thrombophlebitis develops (5%). Do not permit the urea solution to extravasate into the tissues, since this will cause extensive sloughing of skin and underlying tissue. One third of the patients are nauseated and vomit about 30 minutes after urea is started. Phenothiazine prophylaxis is helpful. Confusion and disorientation with hyperactivity affect 21% of patients and may be controlled with pentobarbital given intravenously. Fever is a rare complication (2%) and may last for several hours.

Death from subdural hematoma is a rare complication of urea-induced dehydration.[21] Stretching and possible rupture of bridging veins coursing between the sagittal sinus and the brain surface are postulated as the probable source of hemorrhage. Such subdural hemorrhages are reproducible in cats by urea administration. Urea dehydration may cause retraction of the brain as much as 0.5 cm from the skull. Prompt rehydration minimizes such complications. The one reported death occurred about 6 hours after urea infusion. Prior to death the patient was confused. Autopsy confirmed a fresh subdural hematoma accompanied by downward herniation of the brainstem.

Theoretically, the use of urea to reduce intraocular pressure prior to antiglaucoma surgery might decrease the frequency of intraocular hemorrhage. Because of the low incidence of such hemorrhage, valid statistics are difficult to assemble. A thought-provoking report describes the clinical course of a 54-year-old diabetic patient with pupillary block glaucoma after cataract extraction.[22] One hour after urea infusion his pressure had dropped from 50 to 9 mm Hg (Schiøtz), at which point the anterior chamber spontaneously filled with blood. Two weeks later the eye was enucleated because of continuing bleeding and pain. In a second patient an expulsive subchoroidal hemorrhage developed during surgery for acute narrow-angle glaucoma, even though the pressure had been reduced from 60 to 30 mm Hg by preoperative infusion of urea.

Obviously urea given preoperatively does

Table 20-1. Osmotic characteristics of urea and sucrose

	Molecular weight	*Milliosmols/70 g*
Urea	60.06	1165.5
Sucrose	342.30	204.52

not eliminate the risk of operative bleeding. Indeed, a sufficiently profound drop in pressure resulting from urea administration may in itself predispose to intraocular hemorrhage. Having observed these two hemorrhagic complications, the authors[22] advocate slower urea administration—up to 2½ hours —and state that side reactions are fewer and pressure reduction is adequate.

Osmotic stresses might be expected to manifest themselves across blood-eye barriers, possibly resulting in local tissue damage. Such tissue damage actually does occur if urea is given intra-arterially, thereby causing acute osmotic stress. In monkeys, intra-arterial urea causes widespread physical rupture of the ciliary epithelium and of the retinal pigment epithelium.[23,24] There is no evidence of clinically significant damage to these barrier structures when the urea is given intravenously.

Comparison with other osmotic agents

Because of its low molecular weight, urea is a considerably more effective osmotic agent than is sucrose, which has in the past been used similarly.[25] Osmotic effect is a function of the number of molecules, not of their molecular weight. As indicated in Table 20-1, a 70 g dose of urea will contain 1165.5 milliosmols, as compared to only 204.52 in 70 g of sucrose. It is evident that, weight-for-weight, urea has more than five times the osmotic effect of sucrose.

The data given in Fig. 20-11 clinically confirm the greater effectiveness of urea as an osmotic agent for the reduction of intraocular pressure.[26] The upper half of the figure shows the rate of drop in pressure after intravenous injection of 1 g urea/kg. The same glaucomatous patient was the subject for both of these

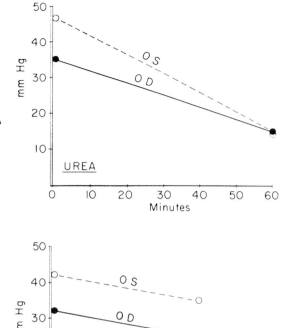

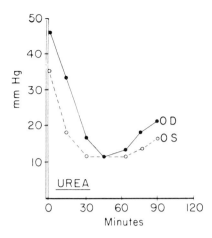

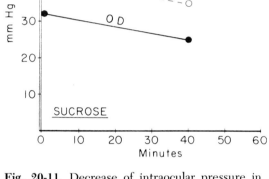

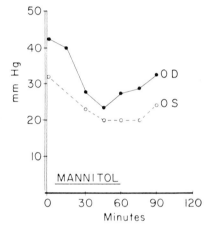

Fig. 20-11. Decrease of intraocular pressure in same glaucomatous patient after intravenous administration of 1 g/kg of urea, **A,** and of sucrose, **B.** Note the far greater drop of pressure produced by urea. (Modified from Galin, M. A., Aizawa, F., and McLean, J.: Arch. Ophthalmol. **63:**281, 1960.)

Fig. 20-12. Comparison of hypotensive effect of mannitol and urea when both are given in the same dose (1 g/kg). (From Galin, M. A., Davidson, R., and Pasmanik, S.: Am. J. Ophthalmol. **55:**244, 1963.)

studies. Urea caused a far more rapid drop than did sucrose.

Comparison of the osmotic effects of urea and mannitol in identical dosages of 1 g/kg demonstrates urea to have a more profound and more prolonged effect in the control of glaucoma (Fig. 20-12).[27] However, if the dosage of mannitol is increased to 2 or 3 g/kg (which is well tolerated by the patient), the same ocular hypotensive effect may be achieved as with a urea dosage of 1 g/kg.

Mannitol has fewer side effects than urea and deserves preferential use. The most

noteworthy advantage of mannitol is that its accidental extravasation into the tissues does not cause necrosis or any other serious consequence.

Glycerol is a convenient, effective, and relatively palatable osmotic medication given orally. Its use is certainly much easier than urea injection.

MANNITOL

Mannitol is more useful than urea as an intravenously administered osmotic agent for reducing intraocular pressure. The indications for mannitol use are the same as those already outlined for urea. The mannitol molecule is three times larger than that of urea, but it exerts a comparable osmotic effect, since mannitol is concentrated in the extracellular fluid compartments, which contain only one third of the total body water (urea diffuses more freely throughout the body water). As with urea, the mannitol-induced pressure-lowering effect coincides with the increase in serum osmotic pressure (Fig. 20-13).[28-30] This ocular hypotensive effect occurs in 30 to 60 minutes, depending on the rate of infusion, and lasts for about 6 hours. Because of vitreous dehydration, the anterior chamber deepens with intravenous infusion of mannitol as with urea.

Mannitol dosage is 2 g/kg of a 20% solution given intravenously during a 30-minute period. For a 50-kg adult, this would be 500 ml of a 20% solution. The rate of administration may vary from 20 to 45 minutes. Patients may not drink fluid during the period of osmotic dehydration or the therapeutic effect is lost. They must be specifically cautioned against drinking because mannitol dehydration causes thirst. Provision must be made for the marked diuresis that results. Since

mannitol is soluble only to a 15% concentration in cold water, the 20% preparation should be warmed prior to administration. This will eliminate the crystals that may be present in cold solutions.[29] Administration of the intravenous solution through a blood filter will also eliminate entry of crystals into the bloodstream.

Mannitol is stable in solution; therefore it can be heat sterilized and stored without the risk of deterioration. This avoids the bothersome preparation necessary with urea.

Its osmotic (and ocular hypotensive) effect depends not only on the amount given but also on the rate. The anesthesiologist gave one of my patients 40 ml of a 20% mannitol solution within about 2 minutes. The eye, previously very hard, suddenly became very soft. This solution, commercially available in ready-mixed vials,* is very convenient to use and can be administered rapidly, vial after vial, until the eye is titrated to the softness desired during the surgical procedure.

Since mannitol is not absorbed from the intestinal tract, it does not reduce intraocular pressure when given orally.

Mannitol is not metabolized to a significant degree; hence it may be used in diabetic patients without creating metabolic problems. Mannitol is the reduced form of mannose and does *not* give a positive Benedict reaction for urine sugar. Renal disease does not contraindicate mannitol infusion. Mannitol is less toxic than urea and hence has fewer side effects. Possibly one of the greatest advantages of mannitol over urea is freedom from tissue necrosis if the solution extravasates. Approximately 100 ml of a 20% mannitol solution extravasated in one reported case with no harmful effect except transient swelling.[30] Thrombophlebitis is less likely to occur with mannitol than with urea. Thrombosis and local irritation are not reported. The headaches of decreased intracranial pressure do occur and may be minimized by bed rest. The patient may have chills during mannitol infusion. An alarming but apparently not serious complication is angina-like chest

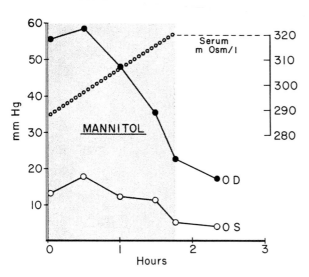

Fig. 20-13. Intraocular pressure-lowering effect of a 20% mannitol solution (2.2 g/kg) on acute angle-closure glaucoma that had not responded to pilocarpine and acetazolamide therapy. (Modified from Weiss, D. I., Shaffer, R. N., and Wise, B. L.: Arch. Ophthalmol. **68:**341, 1962.)

---

*Baxter Laboratories, Morton Grove, Ill.

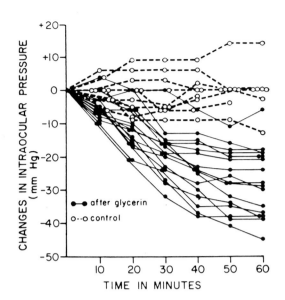

pain. This pain was sufficiently severe to cause delay of surgery in four patients of one series (the total number of patients in the series was not specified) but left no residual cardiac or pulmonary damage.[30] Whether the chest pain results from increased blood volume or from some specific irritant property of mannitol is undetermined.

An acute allergic reaction with unconsciousness occurred immediately after mannitol infusion in a patient severely allergic to penicillin, procaine, various buffering agents in ophthalmic drops, and a variety of other allergens. A subsequent skin test with mannitol was positive, producing a 3 cm flare.[31] Certainly such a response is extremely rare; nevertheless, I consider it worthy of comment to remind us that in such acute allergic reactions the emergency treatment is 0.1% epinephrine hydrochloride, 0.4 ml subcutaneously.

Fig. 20-14. Decrease of intraocular pressure resulting from oral administration of glycerol in doses from 1 to 1.5 g/kg given to glaucoma patients. Control patients had tonometric examinations at similar intervals but received no medication. (From Thomas, R.: Arch. Ophthalmol. **70:** 625, 1963.)

GLYCEROL (GLYCERIN)

Glycerol may be used as an osmotic agent to reduce intraocular pressure. It has the advantages of being effective when taken orally and of being nontoxic. The oral dosage is

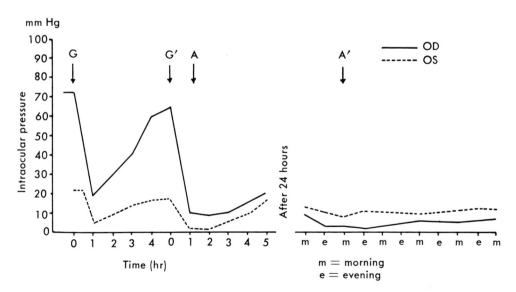

Fig. 20-15. Response of acute glaucomatous eye (solid line) and normal fellow eye (broken line) to oral administration of glycerol, 1.5 g/kg. Glycerol was given at G and again at G'. Acetazolamide (given at A and at A'), 250 mg, prevented the postglycerol pressure rise. (From Virno, M., and associates: Am. J. Ophthalmol. **55:**113, 1963.)

1 to 1.5 g/kg of a 50% glycerol solution dissolved in 0.9% saline solution. One milliliter of a 50% glycerol solution contains 0.62 g of glycerol. Addition of lemon or orange juice and refrigeration make it more palatable.

A drop in intraocular pressure usually begins within 10 minutes after oral administration of glycerol and is almost always quite marked by 30 minutes (Fig. 20-14). Pressure rises again to pretreatment levels in about 5 hours unless other medication (such as miotics or carbonic anhydrase inhibitors) is used. A second dose 5 hours after the first will again cause a pressure drop (Fig. 20-15).[32]

Because glycerol is the most easily used osmotic agent, it is most suitable for office use in the initial treatment of acute glau-

coma. However, its pressure-lowering effect is inferior to that of mannitol or urea (Fig. 20-16).[33] Because of uncertain absorption, the hypotensive response to glycerol is quite variable. Glycerol aqueous levels are appreciably higher in the inflamed eye than in the normal eye, indicating a decreased osmotic effect in treatment of an inflamed eye with acute glaucoma (Fig. 20-17).[33] If office administration of glycerol does not control pressure in a case of acute glaucoma, subsequent administration of mannitol in a hospital is indicated.

Ocular inflammation (induced by injection of 0.1 ml of 0.1M sodium hydroxide into the rabbit anterior chamber) does not significantly alter aqueous mannitol concentrations from those in the uninflamed eye (Fig. 20-

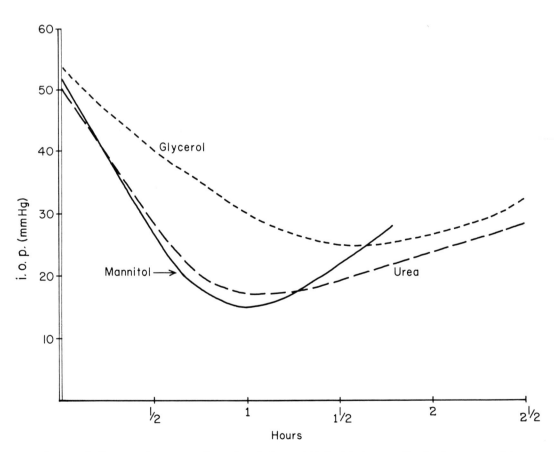

Fig. 20-16. Pressure-lowering effect of oral glycerol (1.5 ml/kg), urea (1 g/kg intravenously), and mannitol (3 g/kg intravenously). All drugs used in each of 30 glaucoma patients. (From Galin, M. A., Davidson, R., and Shachter, N.: Am. J. Ophthalmol. **62:**629, 1966.)

18).[33] For this reason, mannitol is believed to be a more effective osmotic agent than urea or glycerol in treatment of an inflamed eye with acute glaucoma.

Mechanism of action

Similar to other osmotic agents, glycerol works by increasing serum osmolarity to a higher level. This opposes the osmotic pull within the eye, which is responsible for maintenance of normal intraocular pressure.

In one series of cases the pressure-reducing effect of oral glycerol was transient and ineffective despite careful removal of the patients' water pitchers.[34] This failure was found to result from the ministrations of a humane young nurse who thoughtfully provided the suffering patients with coffee!

An ingenious experiment has demonstrated that patients with total aniridia are fully responsive to the hypotensive effect of glycerol osmotherapy.[35] This indicates that the iris surface, presenting more than 200 mm² of potentially dehydrating surface to the aqueous humor, is not essential for the clinical effect of hyperosmolar drugs. Actually the greatest surface for water transfer is behind the iris. The ciliary epithelium and retina-choroid surface provide an area of dehydrating interface seven times greater than the iris.

To determine whether osmotherapy reduces vitreous volume, the carefully dissected vitreous body of a pig eye was immersed in 50% glycerol for 15 minutes. The average weight loss in these experiments was

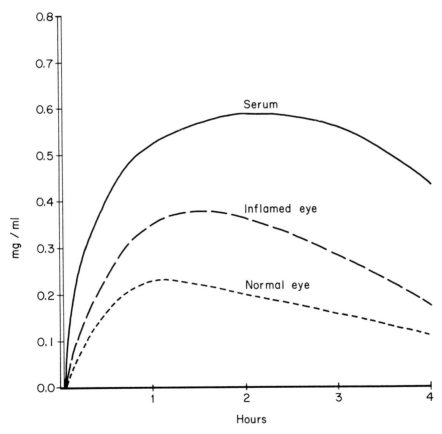

Fig. 20-17. Glycerol concentrations in serum and in aqueous of normal and inflamed rabbit eyes after oral glycerol, 2.4 g/kg. (From Galin, M. A., Davidson, R., and Shachter, N.: Am. J. Ophthalmol. **62:**629, 1966.)

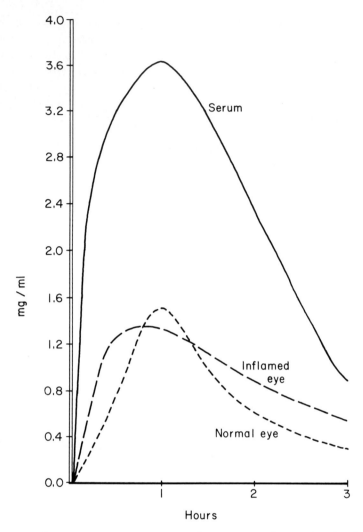

Fig. 20-18. Mannitol concentrations in serum and in aqueous of normal and inflamed rabbit eyes after intravenous dose of 3 g/kg of a 20% solution. (From Galin, M. A., Davidson, R., and Shachter, N.: Am. J. Ophthalmol. **62:**629, 1966.)

38.5%. A correspondingly marked visible decrease in vitreous volume accompanied the weight loss. This experimental finding confirms the clinical observations that osmotherapy does indeed reduce vitreous volume.[36]

Toxicity

Glycerol is a naturally occurring component of body fats, usually representing about 1% of body weight. It may be utilized as a carbohydrate and causes no harmful effect even when as much as 40% of the dietary calories are derived from glycerol.[37] Hyperglycemia and glycosuria can result from oral administration of glycerol.

Glycerol given orally is virtually free of side effects. It usually does not cause gastrointestinal upset or diuresis. Nausea is not uncommon. Accidental ingestion of 23 g/kg of glycerol was not fatal to a 2½-year-old child.[37] Approximately 2 g/kg has been given to human beings three times a day for 50 days without ill effect.

Headache resulting from decreased intracranial pressure is the chief annoying side

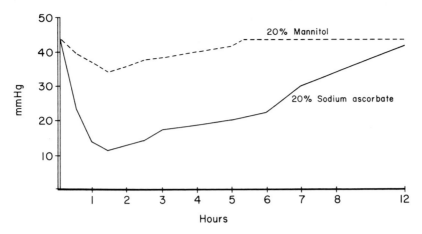

Fig. 20-19. Hypotensive effect of 20% sodium ascorbate, 1 g/kg intravenously, and of 20% mannitol, 1 g/kg intravenously, given to the same patient with congenital glaucoma on 2 consecutive days. (From Virno, M., and associates: Am. J. Ophthalmol. **62:**824, 1966.)

effect of glycerol given orally.[38] This type of headache results from treatment with any effective osmotic agent and is comparable to a lumbar puncture headache. It is relieved by lying down.

Dismissal of elderly patients immediately after oral glycerol administration is unwise. Not only does the intraocular pressure escape observation (and presumably glycerol would not be used in the absence of a serious pressure problem) but systemic problems may also arise. For example, an 82-year-old woman was permitted to go home after drinking 200 ml of 50% glycerol. On the bus she developed a convulsive seizure with disorientation. Medical evaluation indicated the basic problem was dehydration caused by osmotic diuresis. Her intraocular pressure, 60 mm before glycerol, dropped to 17 mm within an hour, at which time she left the office. As would be expected, pressure was again 60 mm when measured the next day.[39]

Hyperosmolar coma is a very serious complication of osmotherapy. It is essentially a severe dehydration of the patient, affecting the brain. The patient becomes confused and disoriented and may be misdiagnosed as having suffered an acute cerebrovascular accident. Patients with renal, cardiovascular, or diabetic disease are more susceptible, particularly if they are elderly and already somewhat dehydrated. Treatment is prompt hydration with hypotonic solutions, such as half-normal saline. More important is avoidance of excessive dehydration of unhealthy patients. A reported case was a 29-year-old diabetic man with renal failure and neovascular glaucoma. He received glycerol twice within 24 hours and acetazolamide, 250 mg, every 6 hours for four doses. Presumably fluids were restricted during this entire 24-hour period. Anorexia, vomiting, and increasing lethargy developed. He required 8 liters of hypotonic saline for rehydration.[40]

Given intravenously in dosages ranging from 0.25 to 2 g/kg, 30% glycerol in saline solution causes hematuria in both rabbit and man. The hematuria is caused by damage of the afferent glomerular arterioles, which undergo severe vasoconstriction for 30 to 40 minutes after glycerol administration. Subsequent reflex vasodilation lasting 5 to 8 hours is sufficiently severe to cause diffuse hemorrhage.[41]

The hemorrhagic effect of intravenous glycerol can be avoided by simultaneous administration of 20% sodium ascorbate buffered to pH 7.2 to 7.4 (with 30% glycerol in the same solution). Hematuria and/or histologically demonstrable renal damage do not result from simultaneous intravenous administration of this combined medication.

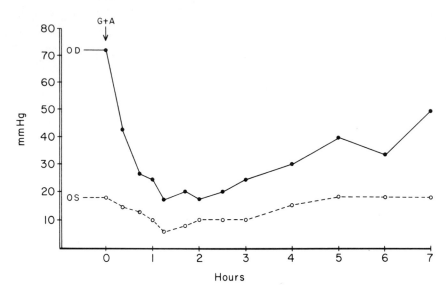

Fig. 20-20. Hypotensive effect of combined 20% sodium ascorbate (0.28 g/kg) and 30% glycerol (0.6 g/kg) given intravenously during 20 minutes in patient with acute congestive glaucoma of right eye. (From Virno, M., and associates: Am. J. Ophthalmol. **62:**824, 1966.)

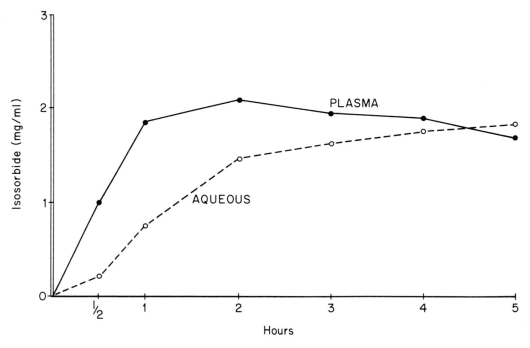

Fig. 20-21. Plasma and aqueous concentrations of isosorbide after oral administration of 2 g/kg in rabbits. (Modified from Becker, B., Kolker, A. E., and Krupin, T.: Arch. Ophthalmol. **78:**147, 1967.)

Not surprisingly, 20% sodium ascorbate, pH 7.2 to 7.4, 1 g/kg, is itself an effective osmotic agent, producing a maximum hypotensive effect within 70 minutes from the start of intravenous infusion (given over a 15- to 20-minute period). No untoward side effects were reported, except that fluctuations of blood pressure result if the pH values are higher or lower than the 7.2 to 7.4 range. The hypotensive effect of 20% sodium ascorbate is greater than that of 20% mannitol (Fig. 20-19).[41]

The combined effect of 30% glycerol and 20% sodium ascorbate is osmotically additive and produces a marked hypotensive effect in a dosage of 2 ml/kg given intravenously within 15 to 20 minutes (Fig. 20-20).[41] This combined medication has the advantage of high potency, low toxicity, small volume, and short administration time. At the time of this report it had been used in 16 glaucomatous patients with good results and no significant side effects. In rabbits the lethal intravenous dose of glycerol is 11 g/kg and that of sodium ascorbate is 6 g/kg.

Use in corneal clearing

The osmotic effect of glycerol has long been used by ophthalmologists to clear edematous corneas. This will remove fluid, thereby restoring transparency in conditions such as Fuchs' endothelial dystrophy and acute glaucoma. Osmotic clearing will not remove scar tissue, cellular infiltrations, blood vessels, deposits of calcium or fat, or any other material except excess water. Used as indicated, topical application of glycerol is most valuable in permitting the gonioscopic and ophthalmoscopic examinations vital to make the proper decisions regarding definitive treatment of the diseased eye.[42]

Since topical application of glycerol is painful, its use should be preceded by a local anesthetic such as tetracaine that will eliminate all discomfort. Concentrations ranging from 50% to pure anhydrous 100% glycerol are effective in clearing the cornea of edema within 1 or 2 minutes. Additional glycerol may be used as the gonioscopic lubricant to prolong the clearing effect. No corneal dam-

age results from glycerol application. In fact, glycerol dehydration is desirable before tonometry, since it collapses epithelial blebs, thereby preventing their mechanical rupture by the tonometer footplate.

Unfortunately osmotic dehydration is too transient to be of therapeutic value in diseases causing corneal edema. Measurements with the vapor-pressure osmometer indicate that after instillation of 0.2 ml of a 2.5% salt solution into the lower cul-de-sac, the tears bathing the eye are back to normal osmotic pressure (0.91 to 1.14 mm Hg average values) within only 90 seconds.[43] This explains why the treatment of edematous corneal conditions with hypertonic solutions is generally ineffectual.

Lens dehydration

Glycerol, 50%, has been used experimentally to dehydrate the lens by direct instillation into the anterior chamber of rabbits. No corneal, iris, or other damage resulted; however, the lens rapidly became dehydrated. The wrinkled capsule of the shrunken lens could easily be grasped by forceps, whereas previously it had been too tense. The authors[44] suggested glycerol dehydration as an aid in grasping the capsule of intumescent cataracts. Since the erysiphake or cryophake is quite effective, I doubt there is any real occasion for such use of glycerol. I myself would not consider using such a hypertonic solution within a human eye.

ISOSORBIDE (HYDRONOL)

Isosorbide is a hyperosmotic agent that can be given orally, as can glycerol. Isosorbide resembles mannitol in chemical structure. It is readily absorbed from the gastrointestinal tract and 95% of the dose is excreted unchanged in the urine. Isosorbide is not metabolized and provides no calories (in contrast to glycerol). It does enter the aqueous, but at a slower rate than plasma levels are attained; therefore it is effective in reducing intraocular pressure (Fig. 20-21).[45] The maximum hypotonic effect is achieved 1 hour after ingestion (Fig. 20-22).[45]

In comparison with glycerol, isosorbide

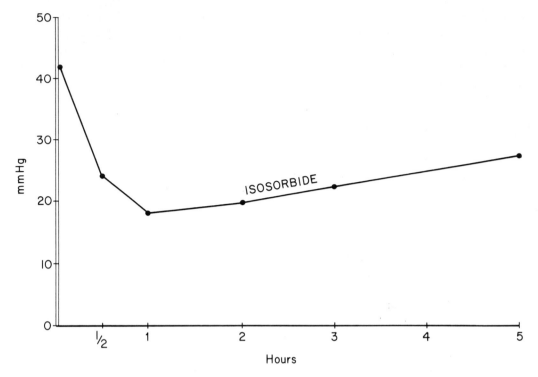

Fig. 20-22. Reduction of intraocular pressure after oral administration of isosorbide (2 g/kg) to patient with secondary glaucoma. (Modified from Becker, B., Kolker, A. E., and Krupin, T.: Arch. Ophthalmol. **78:**147, 1967.)

seems to cause less nausea and vomiting. Minimal nausea followed isosorbide administration in 2 of 10 patients. Four of these patients had previously been unable to tolerate glycerol treatment because of nausea and vomiting.

With suitable doses the fall of intraocular pressure following oral isosorbide is comparable to that after oral glycerol, intravenous urea, or mannitol. A dose of 1.5 to 2 g/kg of isosorbide (given in 50% solution) is comparable to 1 to 1.5 g/kg of glycerol.

Isosorbide causes the same general side effects as all other hyperosmotic agents (headache, dehydration, diuresis, urinary retention, and occasional disorientation). Cardiac or renal disease may contraindicate its use.[46-49]

ETHANOL

The hyperosmotic effect resulting from ethanol does not result from addition of osmotic molecules to the plasma but is medi-

ated by inhibition of the antidiuretic hormone, with resultant hypotonic diuresis. This loss of water increases the blood osmolality, resulting in an effective osmotic gradient across the blood-eye barrier. The associated intoxication is a sufficiently undesirable side effect so that this method of osmotherapy is rarely employed.[50]

DEXTROSE

A 50% dextrose solution is not currently advocated for use in osmotic hypotensive ocular therapy. It has been reported to destroy iris cysts when used to irrigate their cavity.[51] The technique was to fill a 1 ml syringe with a 50% dextrose solution in water and to attach it to a No. 26 needle through which the cyst contents had already been evacuated. The dextrose solution was washed into the cyst, aspirated four or five times, and finally withdrawn until the cyst was completely deflated. The cyst did not recur. The eye tolerated the procedure well, showing only a mild postoperative reaction for several weeks. I would consider the use of a 50% dextrose solution to be safer than the more caustic solutions such as iodine and trichloracetic acid that have been advocated for cyst destruction. Complete surgical excision of these postoperative or posttraumatic iris cysts is most difficult and more hazardous than their chemical or electrolytic destruction.

DISTILLED WATER

The surgeon should be absolutely certain that only isotonic solutions are used for intraocular irrigation. Permanent, dense corneal opacity follows the irrigation of rabbit anterior chambers with distilled water.[52] Moistening of the cornea with distilled water during ophthalmic surgery causes corneal edema. This is particularly distressing during surgery for retinal detachment.

I have seen at least three cases of permanent corneal opacity known to follow anterior chamber irrigation with distilled water during cataract extraction. An alarming diffuse corneal opacity develops within minutes of the irrigation, presumably caused by excessive hydration. Irreversible damage to the endothelium has presumably been sustained as soon as corneal hydration is obvious. Attempts to remedy the situation by irrigation with saline or some hypertonic solution are irrational, since this only causes additional mechanical damage. Electrolyte diffusion from the eye itself will restore the fluid in the anterior chamber to normal osmotic levels before the surgeon recognizes the problem and the nurse can substitute saline solution for the erroneously used distilled water. Subsequent biomicroscopy shows endothelial irregularity vaguely resembling endothelial dystrophy, diffuse stromal opacity, normal epithelium, and some degree of iris atrophy. Corneal transplantation was successfully performed in one case.

We do not permit distilled water in the eye surgical room.

The osmotic action of water is, of course, the basis for the well-known water-drinking provocative test for glaucoma. Plasma dilu-

tion results in hypersecretion of aqueous, the increased volume of which cannot be handled by an inadequate outflow mechanism.[53]

TOPICAL HYPERTONIC AGENTS

Elevated intraocular pressure cannot be reduced by topical application of hyperosmotic solutions; however, they do have limited usefulness in dehydration of the decompensated cornea. Reference has been made in the section on glycerol to use of this agent for temporary clearing of the edematous cornea associated with acute angle-closure glaucoma. Sodium chloride in 2% to 5% solution may be used in treatment of mild cases of stromal and epithelial edema caused by endothelial damage. Unfortunately, its effect is transient and only mild cases are helped.[54,55]

Used in combination with a bandage soft lens, 5% saline may be instilled four times daily, or more frequently. This is particularly helpful in the relief of pain from severe bullous keratopathy.[56] When used with a soft lens on damaged corneas, solutions should contain a preservative. Contrary to previous suspicions, preservatives do not concentrate in the soft lens and damage the cornea. Actually, preservatives are important to prevent contamination of the solutions to be used with the soft bandage lens.

REFERENCES

1. Galin, M. A., Nano, H., and Davidson, R.: Aqueous and blood urea nitrogen levels after intravenous urea administration, Arch. Ophthalmol. **65**:805, 1961.
2. Bleeker, G. M., Haeringen, N. J., and Glasius, E.: Osmotically induced protrusion of the ocular diaphragm, Am. J. Ophthalmol. **56:** 561, 1963.
3. Duncan, L. S., Hostetter, T., and Ellis, P. P.: Vitreous osmolality changes following administration of hyperosmotic agents, Invest. Ophthalmol. **8**:353, 1969.
4. Robbins, R., and Galin, M. A.: Effect of osmotic agents on the vitreous body, Arch. Ophthalmol. **82**:694, 1969.
5. Goren, S. B., and Newell, F.: The autoradio-

graphic localization of urea C-14 in the rabbit eye, Am. J. Ophthalmol. **54**:63, 1962.

6. Podos, S. M., Krupin, T., and Becker, B.: Effect of small-dose hyperosmotic injections on intraocular pressure of small animals and man when optic nerves are transected and intact, Am. J. Ophthalmol. **71**:989, 1971.

7. Krupin, T., Podos, S. M., Lehman, R. A. W., and Becker, B.: Effects of optic nerve transection on intraocular pressure in monkeys, Arch. Opththalmol. **84**:668, 1970.

8. Podos, S. M., Krupin, T., and Becker, B.: Mechanism of intraocular pressure response after optic nerve transection, Am. J. Ophthalmol. **72**:79, 1971.

9. Krupin, T., Podos, S. M., and Becker, B.: Effect of optic nerve transection on osmotic alterations of intraocular pressure, Am. J. Ophthalmol. **70**:214, 1970.

10. Hill, K., Whitney, J., and Trotter, R.: Intravenous hypertonic urea in the management of acute angle-closure glaucoma, Arch. Ophthalmol. **65**:497, 1961.

11. Galin, M. A., Aizawa, F., and McLean, J.: Oral urea as an osmotic ocular hypotensive agent, Arch. Ophthalmol. **62**:1099, 1959.

12. Tarter, R. C., and Linn, J. G.: A clinical study of the use of intravenous urea in glaucoma, Am. J. Ophthalmol. **52**:323, 1961.

13. Davis, M., Duehr, P., and Javid, M.: The clinical use of urea for reduction of intraocular pressure, Arch. Ophthalmol. **65**:526, 1961.

14. Galin, M. A., and Davidson, R.: Hypotensive effect of urea in inflammed and noninflamed eye, Arch. Ophthalmol. **68**:633, 1962.

15. Galin, M., Aizawa, F., and McLean, J.: Urea as an osmotic ocular hypotensive agent in glaucoma, Arch. Ophthalmol. **62**:347, 1959.

16. Galin, M. A., and Baras, I.: Intravenous urea in retinal detachment surgery, Arch. Ophthalmol. **65**:652, 1961.

17. Friedman, B., Bryon, H., and Turtz, A.: Urea in cataract extraction, Arch. Ophthalmol. **67**:421, 1962.

18. Jaffe, N. S., and Light, D. S.: The danger of air pupillary block glaucoma in cataract surgery with osmotic hypotonia, Arch. Ophthalmol. **76**:633, 1966.

19. Kornblueth, W., and Gombos, G.: The use of intravenous hypertonic urea in cataract extraction, Am. J. Ophthalmol. **54**:753, 1962.

20. Nalbandian, R. M., Shultz, G., Lusher, J. M., Anderson, J. W., and Henry, R. L.: Sickle cell crisis terminated by intravenous urea in

sugar solutions, Am. J. Med. Sci. **261**:309, 1971.

21. Marshall, S., and Hinman, F.: Subdural hematoma following administration of urea for diagnosis of hypertension, J.A.M.A. **182**:233, 1962.

22. Croll, L. J., and Aragones, J. V.: Observation on intravenous urea, Am. J. Ophthalmol. **55**:807, 1963.

23. Laties, A. M., and Rapoport, S.: The blood-ocular barriers under osmotic stress, Arch. Ophthalmol. **94**:1086, July 1976.

24. Shabo, A., Maxwell, D., and Kreiger, A.: Structural alterations in the ciliary process and blood-aqueous barrier of the monkey after systemic urea injections, Am. J. Ophthalmol. **81**:162, February 1976.

25. Dyar, E. W., and Matthew, W. B.: Use of sucrose preparatory to surgical treatment of glaucoma, Arch. Ophthalmol. **18**:57, 1937.

26. Galin, M. A., Aizawa, F., and McLean, J.: A comparison of intraocular pressure reduction following urea and sucrose administration, Arch. Ophthalmol. **63**:281, 1960.

27. Galin, M. A., Davidson, R., and Pasmanik, S.: An osmotic comparison of urea and mannitol, Am. J. Ophthalmol. **55**:244, 1963.

28. Weiss, D. I., Shaffer, R. N., and Wise, B. L.: Mannitol infusion to reduce intraocular pressure, Arch. Ophthalmol. **68**:341, 1962.

29. Adams, R. E., Kirschner, R. J., and Leopold, I. H.: Ocular hypotensive effect of intravenously administered mannitol, Arch. Ophthalmol. **69**:55, 1963.

30. Smith, E. W., and Drance, S. M.: Reduction of human intraocular pressure with intravenous mannitol, Arch. Ophthalmol. **68**:734, 1962.

31. Spaeth, G. L., Spaeth, E. B., Spaeth, P. G., and Lucier, A. C.: Anaphylactic reaction to mannitol, Arch. Ophthalmol. **78**:583, 1967.

32. Virno, M., Cantore, P., Bietti, C., and Bucci, M. G.: Oral glycerol in ophthalmology, Am. J. Ophthalmol. **55**:1133, 1963.

33. Galin, M. A., Davidson, R., and Shachter, N.: Ophthalmological use of osmotic therapy, Am. J. Ophthalmol. **62**:629, 1966.

34. Trevor-Roper, P. D.: Experience with the use of glycerol and other hypotensive agents in glaucoma, Eye Ear Nose Throat Mon. **44**:74, 1965.

35. Galin, M. A., Binkhorst, R. D., and Kwitko, M. L.: Ocular dehydration, Am. J. Ophthalmol. **66**:233, 1968.

36. Kapetansky, F. M., and Higbee, J. M.: Vitreous deturgescence, Eye Ear Nose Throat Mon. **48**:313, 1969.
37. Thomas, R.: Glycerin, Arch. Ophthalmol. **70**:625, 1963.
38. Drance, S. M.: Effect of oral glycerol on intraocular pressure in normal and glaucomatous eyes, Arch. Ophthalmol. **72**:491, 1964.
39. D'Alena, P., and Ferguson, W.: Adverse effects after glycerol orally and mannitol parenterally, Arch. Ophthalmol. **75**:201, 1966.
40. Oakley, D. E., and Ellis, P. P.: Glycerol and hyperosmolar nonketotic coma, Am. J. Ophthalmol. **81**:469, April 1976.
41. Virno, M., Bucci, M. G., Pecori 'Giraldi, J., and Cantore, G.: Intravenous glycerol–vitamin C (sodium salt) as osmotic agents to reduce intraocular pressure, Am. J. Ophthalmol. **62**:824, 1966.
42. Bietti, G. B., and Giraldi, J. P.: Topical osmotherapy of corneal edema, Ann. Ophthalmol. **1**:40, 1969.
43. Mastman, G., Baldes, E., and Henderson, J. W.: The total osmotic pressure of tears in normal and various pathologic conditions, Arch. Ophthalmol. **65**:509, 1961.
44. Vass, Z., and Katona, J.: The effect of glycerol on the eye lens of experimental animals, Acta Ophthalmol. **44**:843, 1966.
45. Becker, B., Kolker, A. E., and Krupin, T.: Isosorbide—an oral hyperosmotic agent, Arch. Ophthalmol. **78**:147, 1967.
46. Wisznia, K. I., Lazar, M., and Leopold, I. H.: Oral isosorbide and intraocular pressure, Am. J. Ophthalmol. **70**:630, 1970.
47. Mehra, K. S., and Singh, R.: Lowering of intraocular pressure by isosorbide, Arch. Ophthalmol. **86**:623, 1971.
48. Wood, T. O., Waltman, S. R., West, C., and Kaufman, H. E.: Effect of isosorbide on intraocular pressure after penetrating keratoplasty, Am. J. Ophthalmol. **75**:221, 1973.
49. Mehra, K. S., Singh, R., Char, J. N., and Rajyashree, K.: Lowering of intraocular tension, Arch. Ophthalmol. **85**:167, 1971.
50. Kolker, A. E.: Hyperosmotic agents in glaucoma, Invest. Ophthalmol. **9**:418, June 1970.
51. Esposito, A. C.: Treatment of a traumatic implanation cyst of the iris, Am. J. Ophthalmol. **41**:115, 1956.
52. Binder, R. F., Gerras, T., Milthaler, C., and Wahl, S. C.: Experimental intraocular hemolysis, Am. J. Ophthalmol. **58**:946, 1964.
53. Armaly, M. F.: Water-drinking test, Arch. Ophthalmol. **83**:169, 1970.
54. Marisi, A., and Aquavella, J. V.: Hypertonic saline solution in corneal edema, Ann. Ophthalmol. **7**:229, February 1975.
55. Green, K., and Downs, S.: Reduction of corneal thickness with hypertonic solutions, Am. J. Ophthalmol. **75**:507, March 1973.
56. Aquavella, J. V.: Chronic corneal edema, Am. J. Ophthalmol. **76**:201, August 1973.

21
OXYGEN

Oxygen therapy is better known to ophthalmologists for its toxic effect on the eye than for any possible beneficial effects. Excessive concentrations of oxygen damage the eyes of both infants and adults, although the adult retina is much more resistant to damage.

EFFECT ON PREMATURE INFANT

Kinsey's study of retrolental fibroplasia and the use of oxygen established beyond doubt the causative role of oxygen in damaging the eyes of premature infants.[1] Oxygen in high concentrations has the remarkable capability of selectively obliterating growing retinal vessels in immature animals.[2] For practical purposes, there is no concentration of oxygen in excess of that in air that is not associated with some additional risk of developing the retinopathy of prematurity. (This condition is rarely seen in very small infants who received no oxygen.) The length of time the infant is in an oxygen-enriched atmosphere is the important factor in causing retinal damage. As short an exposure as 11 hours was found to cause some degree of retinal scarring. Survival of the premature infant is not jeopardized by withholding supplemental oxygen, except when it is necessary for respiratory abnormalities.

When the use of oxygen has been necessary, it should be terminated as soon as possible, without any tapering off. Gradual withdrawal from oxygen, instead of minimizing ocular toxicity, provides the added amount of oxygen that may suffice to make an initially nontoxic dose damaging.[3]

Knowledge of the etiology of retrolental fibroplasia will not prevent this disease unless the knowledge is applied. One eastern clinic has encountered 10 cases of severe retrolental eye damage in children born since 1958.[4] Excess oxygen must be used with great care in the management of premature infants.

EFFECT ON ADULT

Severe ocular and general toxic effects result from prolonged exposure to 90% to 100% oxygen at atmospheric pressure. More than half of adult dogs maintained at such oxygen levels developed bilateral retinal detachment within 2 to 3 days.[5] Removal from oxygen caused spontaneous reattachment. Other changes included ciliary cysts, iritis with hyphema, and edema of the cornea and conjunctiva. Continuous oxygen exposure for 3 days was fatal to all of 10 adult dogs so exposed and to six of nine dogs removed to normal atmospheric oxygen for 1 to 2 hours daily.

During these experiments, promazine was used as a tranquilizer to facilitate handling the dogs. Subsequent experiments revealed this sedative to have significant retinotoxicity in combination with oxygen. The toxic effect of oxygen on the retina was greatly increased by simultaneous administration of phenothiazine or chloroquine.[6] Concurrent exposure to 98% oxygen and daily intramuscular injection of 50 mg of promazine caused extensive retinal detachment in 27 of 37 dogs within 4 days, whereas oxygen alone caused only localized detachments in 2 of 10 dogs. Apparently, additive inhibition of vital enzymes results from simultaneous use of high concentrations of oxygen and retinotoxic drugs such as the phenothiazine tranquilizers.

The mechanism of this oxygen-induced retinal detachment is not established; however, the probability of choriocapillaris damage has been suggested.[7] The rods and cones of rabbits selectively degenerate when exposed to high oxygen concentration.[8] In rabbits, death of the visual cells occurs after 5 days in 60% oxygen or after 2 days in 90% oxygen. In man, breathing pure oxygen causes marked vasoconstriction of retinal arteries and veins. Since serious eye damage can regularly be produced in experimental animals by 90% to 100% oxygen, such high levels should not be administered to human beings for prolonged periods of time.

A 32-year-old man was unable to breathe because of myasthenia gravis. Respiration was maintained with an iron lung, and 80% oxygen was administered for about 150 days. At the end of this period the patient complained of rapid, almost complete loss of vision occurring within a 2-day span. The reti-

nal arterioles were severely constricted and sheathed. The visual loss was permanent, one eye seeing hand movements and the other totally blind.[9]

HYPERBARIC OXYGEN

Under hyperbaric conditions, oxygen is even more toxic. ERG recordings during exposure of rabbits to 100% oxygen under pressures as high as 7 atmospheres indicated more rapid loss of retinal function with greater pressures (Fig. 21-1).[10] The b wave was extinguished after less than 1 hour of exposure to 100% oxygen under 6 atmospheres of pressure.

Breathing pure oxygen under 3 atmospheres of pressure caused a 10% decrease in the diameter of retinal arterioles (photographic documentation) in healthy young men.[11] During this oxygen exposure, the blood P_{CO_2} was not significantly altered; hence the vasoconstriction is oxygen induced and is unrelated to CO_2 changes.

As might be expected, the toxic effects of hyperbaric oxygen are manifested earlier in diseased eyes. For example, a patient with old inactive retrobulbar neuritis exposed to 100% oxygen at 2 atmospheres of pressure developed an almost complete loss of the visual field of the affected eye within 2 hours.

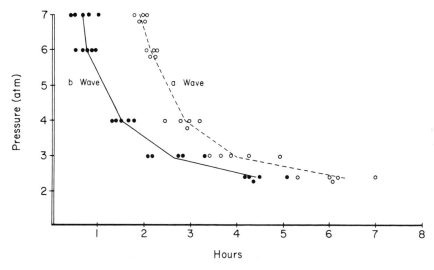

Fig. 21-1. Survival times of a and b waves of ERG under hyperbaric conditions. (From Bridges, W. Z.: Arch. Ophthalmol. **75:**812, 1966.)

The normal eye was unaffected. It was several weeks before the field loss completely cleared again.[12] Since a diseased eye may have reduced oxygen tolerance, hyperbaric oxygen exposure should not be used indiscriminately in the management of various circulatory disorders. Actually, no lasting visual improvement has been reported in the treatment of a variety of degenerative diseases with hyperbaric oxygen.

Visual field constriction also occurs with anoxia.[13]

Corneal vascularization (rabbit) after alkali burns was not inhibited by 100% oxygen under 2 atmospheres pressure.[14] The animals could not survive this hyperbaric oxygen for longer than an hour at a time, alternated with an hour of normal room air. No evidence indicates that increased tissue oxygen has any effect in retarding corneal neovascularization.[15]

Exposure to 3 atmospheres pressure under 100% oxygen caused guinea pigs to die within 7 to 16 hours. Not only retinal cellular damage but also extensive destruction of the nuclei of the corneal endothelium and the lens epithelium occurred.[16]

THERAPY

Oxygen has been suggested for emergency treatment of occlusion of the central retinal artery. A mixture of 95% oxygen and 5% carbon dioxide is supposed to supply additional oxygen for diffusion to the retina from the choroid. The purpose of the carbon dioxide is to induce vasodilation. The toxicity of oxygen in this concentration will of necessity limit treatment to short periods of time. However, the nature of retinal arteriolar occlusion is such that retinal death rapidly occurs; hence, unless function is restored promptly, prolonged further treatment is futile.

Experimental treatment of laser-induced retinal arteriolar occlusions in adult cats and monkeys showed that breathing 100% oxygen at atmospheric pressure gave little or no protection to the ischemic inner retinal layers.[17]

Inhalation of 100% oxygen at 3 atmospheres of pressure was not of benefit in the management of two cases of branch retinal arteriolar occlusion and one case of central retinal artery occlusion.[18] The distance from the choriocapillaris to the inner retinal layers is too far for effective oxygen diffusion, other essential nutrients are not supplied, or the accumulation of toxic metabolites is responsible for the death of the retina.

Hyperbaric oxygen (3 atmospheres) renders relatively anoxic cancer cells significantly more vulnerable to radiation therapy.[19] Quite possibly, radiation response of melanoma and retinoblastoma may be enhanced by hyperbaric oxygen radiotherapy.

REFERENCES

1. Kinsey, V. E.: Retrolental fibroplasia, Arch. Ophthalmol. **56**:481, 1956.
2. Ashton, N.: Oxygen and the growth and development of retinal vessels, Am. J. Ophthalmol. **62**:412, 1966.
3. Patz, A., and Eastham, A. B.: Oxygen studies in retrolental fibroplasia, Arch. Ophthalmol. **57**:724, 1957.
4. Zacharias, L.: Retrolental fibroplasia, Sight Sav. Rev. **24**:17, 1964.
5. Beehler, C. C., Newton, N. L., Culver, J. F., and Tredici, T. J.: Retinal detachment in adult dogs resulting from oxygen toxicity, Arch. Ophthalmol. **71**:665, 1964.
6. Beehler, C. C., and Roberts, W.: Experimental retinal detachments, Arch. Ophthalmol. **79**:759, 1968.
7. Yanoff, M., Miller, W. W., and Waldhausen, J. A.: Oxygen poisoning of the eyes, Arch. Ophthalmol. **84**:627, 1970.
8. Noell, W. K.: Metabolic injuries of visual cell, Am. J. Ophthalmol. **40**:60, 1955.
9. Kobayashi, T., and Murakami, S.: Blindness of an adult caused by oxygen, J.A.M.A. **219**:741, 1972.
10. Bridges, W. Z.: Electroretinographic manifestations of hyperbaric oxygen, Arch. Ophthalmol. **75**:812, 1966.
11. Anderson, B., Jr., Saltzman, H., and Frayser, R.: Changes in arterial pCO_2 and retinal vessel size with oxygen breathing, Invest. Ophthalmol. **6**:416, 1967.
12. Nichols, C. W., Lambertsen, C. J., and Clark, J. M.: Transient unilateral loss of vision associated with oxygen at high pressure, Arch. Ophthalmol. **81**:548, 1969.

13. Wolf, E., and Nadroski, A. S.: Extent of the visual field, Arch. Ophthalmol. **86**:637, 1971.

14. Lazar, M., Lieberman, T. W., and Leopold, I. H.: Hyperbaric oxygenation and corneal neovascularization in the rabbit, Am. J. Ophthalmol. **66**:107, 1968.

15. Kaiser, R. J., and Klopp, D. W.: Hyperbaric air and corneal vascularization, Ann. Ophthalmol. **5**:44, 1973.

16. Nichols, C. W., Yanoff, M., Hall, D. A., and Lambertsen, C. J.: Histologic alterations pro-duced in the eye by oxygen at high pressure, Arch. Ophthalmol. **87**:417, 1972.

17. Flower, R. W., and Patz, A.: The effect of hyperbaric oxygenation on retinal ischemia, Invest. Ophthalmol. **10**:605, 1971.

18. Anderson, B. Jr., Saltzman, H. A., and Heyman, A.: The effects of hyperbaric oxygenation on retinal arterial occlusion, Arch. Ophthalmol. **73**:315, 1965.

19. Wildermuth, O.: The case for hyperbaric oxygen radiotherapy, J.A.M.A. **191**:986, 1965.

22
QUININE

Quinine is of ophthalmologic interest because of its limited usefulness in the treatment of myokymia and because of its characteristic ocular toxicity.

TREATMENT OF MYOKYMIA

The refractory period of skeletal muscle is increased by quinine and the motor end plate becomes less sensitive. These changes are responsible for the curare-like effect of quinine. Persistent and annoying twitching of the orbicularis muscle may be relieved by oral administration of quinine.[1] The customary dosage is 0.32 g, which may be repeated several times daily. (As much as 2 g/day is used in therapy of malaria.)

This curariform effect has also been used as a provocative test for myasthenia gravis, which is made worse by quinine. In general, provocative tests for myasthenia are dangerous and give no more information than do the much safer therapeutic tests—neostigmine (Prostigmin) or edrophonium (Tensilon).

TOXICITY

Eight grams is the approximate fatal oral dose of quinine for an adult. In lesser doses it may cause assorted toxic symptoms. Eye involvement includes blurred vision, disturbed color vision, constricted visual fields, scotomas, and blindness. Individuals vary widely in their susceptibility to the toxic effects of quinine.

The typical onset of quinine amblyopia, as described in seven patients, is often quite sudden. Vision is dim, or light perception may be completely absent. A dose of approximately 4 g caused total blindness within 4 hours in one of these patients, an adult. Smaller doses may be toxic to children. Characteristically, vision is partially recovered, but marked optic atrophy and retinal arteriolar constriction persist. Arteriolar attenuation does not occur for about 10 days—at the onset of blindness the retinal vessels are dilated. At about 2 weeks the appearance of quinine poisoning is very similar to that of bilateral acute occlusion of the central retinal artery, with retinal edema and a cherry red macula.

Two cases of congenital blindness were reported in which the eye findings were typical of quinine amblyopia. During pregnancy both mothers had taken enough quinine to induce tinnitus. An intrauterine toxic effect of quinine was postulated to have produced this result.[2] In view of more recent knowledge as to the teratogenic effect of drugs, the possibility of quinine poisoning of the fetus seems quite likely.

Vasodilator therapy has been advised for quinine amblyopia on the assumption that the characteristic severe vasoconstriction is the cause of visual loss. Actually, in acute quinine poisoning, severe field constriction and visual loss may occur rapidly (for example, within 2 days during which 5.4 g of quinine sulfate was taken), while the ophthalmoscopic appearance is entirely normal.[3] In this reported case, optic atrophy and arteriolar attenuation were first recognizable 2 weeks after loss of vision.

Quinine amblyopia is considered to be a toxic effect that acts directly on the ganglion cells. Edema of this layer of the retina simulates occlusion of the central retinal artery, another aspect of this disorder that suggests a vascular mechanism. However, vasodilator therapy gives only equivocal results (difficult to evaluate because of the tendency to spontaneous partial recovery) and is not rational if the primary toxic effect is directly on the ganglion cells.

In another case of acute quinine amblyopia, the patient received immediate intravenous therapy with ACTH, thiamine, vitamin B_{12}, and tolazoline.[4] The threadlike arterioles were ophthalmoscopically unchanged by therapy during the 7-month course of observation; in fact, they gradually grew thinner. Vision improved from complete absence of light perception to 20/20 within 24 hours, but visual fields were constricted to the central 20 degrees and during the subsequent 7 months further decreased to the central 10 degrees. Vasodilator therapy with nicotinic acid, thiamine, and vitamin B_{12} was used for months without effect. A total of 0.8 g of quinine and 1.4 g of quinidine had been taken in 4 days for therapy of peripheral vascular disease. This isolated case seems to indicate that vasodilators and ACTH are ineffective against quinine arteriolar constriction. No other therapy is known to benefit quinine amblyopia. Fortunately spontaneous partial recovery commonly occurs.

Chronic quinine poisoning can be produced in dogs. This experimental poisoning causes progressive attenuation of the retinal vessels with subsequent pallor of the optic disc and blindness.[5]

Quinidine may also cause toxic amblyopia comparable to that of quinine.[6]

Iris abnormalities after quinine poisoning include a dilated irregular pupil with poor light reaction. Slit-lamp retroillumination shows marked patchy loss of the pigment epithelium of the posterior iris. In severe cases the anterior iris structure becomes atrophic, with loss of the normal stromal pattern. Quinine-induced damage to the iris arteries has been postulated as a possible cause of this iris atrophy.[7]

REFERENCES

1. Givner, I., and Jaffe, N. S.: Myokymia of the eyelids, Am. J. Ophthalmol. **32:**51, 1949.
2. Richardson, S.: The toxic effect of quinine on the eye, South. Med. J. **29:**1156, 1936.
3. Bard, L. A., and Gills, J. P.: Quinine amblyopia, Arch. Ophthalmol. **72:**328, 1964.
4. Lincoff, M.: Quinine amblyopia, Arch. Ophthalmol. **53:**382, 1955.
5. Catcott, E. J.: Ophthalmoscopy in canine practice, J. Am. Vet. Med. Assoc. **121:**35, 1952.
6. Monninger, R., and Platt, D.: Toxic amblyopia due to quinidine, Am. J. Ophthalmol. **43:**107, 1957.
7. Knox, D. L., Palmer, C. A. L., and English, F.: Iris atrophy after quinine amblyopia, Arch. Ophthalmol. **76:**359, 1966.

23
RADIOACTIVE PHOSPHORUS

Sodium radiophosphate (^{32}P) emits only beta particles. This radiation is rapidly dissipated within tissues, being entirely extinguished at a depth of 8 mm. Phosphorus (either stable or radioactive) is concentrated in rapidly proliferating tissues such as bone marrow, lymph nodes, liver, spleen, sites of recent injury, and certain neoplasms. ^{32}P has been advocated as an aid in the diagnosis of malignant melanoma, but it is not selectively concentrated in retinoblastomas.

During the first 4 minutes after intravenous injection, ^{32}P radioactivity is almost exclusively confined to the blood. Within the next 15 minutes, appreciable amounts of ^{32}P have already escaped through the capillary walls. At 1 hour, Geiger counting measures the considerable radioactivity still present within the blood as well as that of local tissue. Hence vascular areas (such as a site of inflammation) give abnormally high counts at 1 hour. From 24 to 48 hours are required for ^{32}P to reach an equilibrium in nucleoprotein. The nucleoprotein-bound portion of the ^{32}P is that which is related to tissue growth or neoplastic activity. For these reasons, counts made a day or more after injection are of greater value in differential diagnosis than counts made at 1 hour.[1]

Repeated counts in rabbits with experimental melanoma indicated that the increased percentage uptake of ^{32}P characteristic of melanoma was approximately the same at 2, 5, or 9 days following dosage. Hence, there is no advantage in waiting more than 2 days after ^{32}P administration before applying the counting probe.[2]

The distribution of radioactivity within the eye is not at all uniform. The following measurements (counts/second/gram of tissue) were recorded 45 hours after intravenous injection of ^{32}P: extraocular muscle, 180; choroid and retina, 86; ciliary body, 72; cornea, 27; lens capsule and cortex, 16; aqueous, 6; sclera, 2; vitreous, 1; and lens nucleus, 0.9. If the counting tube is held over a rectus muscle, the count is increased by as much as 70% above that obtained from an area between the muscles. Since an increase of 30% is considered suggestive of a melanoma, the importance of counting in corresponding areas in the control and suspect eyes is apparent.

Inflammations of the eye may increase the count to as much as 300% of the measurements in the control eye. In an experimental series using rabbits, surgery of the superior rectus muscle increased radioactivity by 80% on the third postoperative day.[3] The ^{32}P test is unreliable for as long as 6 weeks after surgery or injury. Even the trauma of gonioscopy will alter the ^{32}P uptake. Retinoblastomas do not show a significant uptake of ^{32}P. Serous retinal detachments, cysts, and other avascular lesions do not selectively concentrate ^{32}P. Hemorrhages and inflammatory masses do give higher counts, especially soon after injection.

470

^{32}P tests were performed on 66 eyes following a variety of ocular surgical procedures.[4] Positive tests (a 30% increase being considered positive) occurred in 56% of the eyes measured at 6 weeks, in 63% at 8 weeks, and in 18% at 10 weeks. If a 100% increase was required to designate a test as positive, 6% of the eyes were positive at 6 weeks and none at longer intervals. Since the experience of Solomon and associates[4] with melanomas indicated that a melanoma always gave more than a 100% increase in radioactivity, they advocated that a ^{32}P test for neoplasm be performed 8 weeks after surgery if the criterion for a positive neoplasm test was a 100% increase.

The technique of the ^{32}P test requires the usual precautions in handling radioactive material. The intravenous dose of 500 microcuries is selected because it is reasonably safe and because it provides enough radioactivity to count within a practical length of time. Calculation of this dose depends on the 14.3 day half-life of ^{32}P. At the end of 1 hour, 1-minute counts are made in the area of the lesion, seeking the site of highest radioactivity. Four to six 1-minute counts are made at this site of greatest activity, and an average count is calculated. The control count may be from a corresponding area in the other eye, from some neutral part of the body, or from some other arbitrary standard. In a series of 488 cases the control count was the average count from the 3, 6, 9, and 12 o'clock positions of the fellow eye.[5]

Using the criterion of a 30% increase over control measurements at 24 hours as indicating a positive test for melanoma, 123 of these 488 eyes were diagnosed as containing a melanoma. Of these, 13 were false positive tests. In addition, there were eight false negative tests. In this series of melanomas the ^{32}P test was 86% accurate in diagnosis. It should be pointed out that even this degree of accuracy is dependent on the ability of the ophthalmologist to screen out cases of recent injury that would be likely to record as false positive tests. Diagnosis of posterior lesions is particularly unreliable, since the position of the probe is uncertain and variable. Tilting the probe or holding its tip a few millimeters from the counting site introduces considerable error into the test.

Performance of the ^{32}P test in evaluation of a tumor located in the posterior part of the eye requires that the area of the tumor be precisely located on the sclera by indirect ophthalmoscopy at surgery and that the scleral location be marked, just as a retinal hole is localized. The Geiger counter is then positioned precisely on the sclera, exactly at the site of the tumor. Faulty technique will give unreliable readings far less than the 30% increase of diagnostic significance. Hemangiomas do not give a positive ^{32}P test.[6]

Since the radioactive uptake correlates with the rate of formation of new nuclei, one might expect the ^{32}P test to correlate quantitatively with the degree of malignancy. Indeed, in a study of 29 eyes, the higher counts were found in epithelioid and mixed melanomas and the lower counts were associated with spindle cell tumors. Unfortunately, there was such a wide variance of values that clinically accurate predictions of cell type could not be made from the ^{32}P test.[7]

The advocates of the ^{32}P test specify that it is not intended to replace clinical judgment, interpretation, and experience. Although pathologic reports suggest that as high as 20% of eyes enucleated as melanomas are erroneously diagnosed, it is my conviction that most such errors are committed by physicians relatively inexperienced in the diagnosis of melanoma. During the past 10 years I recall only a single instance of erroneous enucleation among the hundreds of eyes seen in consultation by the active members of our staff. This eye contained a choroidal hemangioma rather than a melanoma. We do not consider the ^{32}P test worth its expense and bother.

The ^{32}P test may not be without hazard. The amount of systemic radiation from this test is 20 to 30 rads to liver-spleen-bone marrow. This is approximately one third the dose of ^{32}P used to treat polycythemia vera. Repeated ^{32}P testing would, of course, increase the dosage. The incidence of acute leukemia in ^{32}P-treated polycythemia is 11%, as compared with less than 1% in the nonradiated group. Evidently the radiation hazard is not negligible.[8]

Orbital and cerebral scanning following the injection of radioisotopes such as technetium-99 pertechnetate may be helpful in measurement of orbital blood flow,[9] in quantitation of tear secretion,[10] and in detecting neoplasms.[11,12]

REFERENCES

1. Bettman, J. W., and Fellows, V.: Radioactive phosphorus as a diagnostic aid in ophthalmology, Arch. Ophthalmol. **51**:171, 1954.
2. Ruiz, R. S., and Pernoud, J. M.: Time and dose for optimum radioactive phosphorus uptake measurement in rabbit uveal melanoma, Am. J. Ophthalmol. **82**:218, August 1976.
3. Solomon, O. D., Moses, L., and Eigner, E. H.: Radioactive phosphorus uptake, Am. J. Ophthalmol. **55**:1238, 1963.
4. Solomon, O. D., Gans, J. A., and Levine, B.: Reliability of radioactive phosphorus uptake test after ocular surgery, Am. J. Ophthalmol. **70**:281, 1970.
5. Carmichael, P. L., and Leopold, I. H.: The radioactive phosphorus test in ophthalmology, Am. J. Ophthalmol. **49**:484, 1960.
6. Hagler, W. S., Jarrett, W. H., II, and Humphrey, W. T.: The radioactive phosphorus uptake test in diagnosis of uveal melanoma, Arch. Ophthalmol. **83**:548, 1970.
7. Char, D. H., Crawford, J. B., Irvine, A. R., Hogan, M. J., and Howes, E. L., Jr.: Correlation between degree of malignancy and the radioactive phosphorus uptake test in ocular melanomas, Am. J. Ophthalmol. **81**:71, January 1976.
8. Gaasterland, D. E.: Systemic radiation during the radioactive phosphorus uptake test, Am. J. Ophthalmol. **81**:691, May 1976.
9. Schachar, R. A., Weiter, J. J., Ernest, J. T., Stark, V., and Hoffer, P. B.: The measurement of relative blood flow to each orbit by dynamic isotope scanning using pertechnetate-99M, Am. J. Ophthalmol. **77**:223, February 1974.
10. O'Nan, W. W., Wirtschafter, J. D., and Preston, D. F.: Sodium pertechnetate Tc 99m in lacrimal secretion, Arch. Ophthalmol. **91**:187, March 1974.
11. Grove, A. S., Jr., and Kotner, L. M., Jr.: Radionuclide arteriography in ophthalmology, Arch. Ophthalmol. **89**:13, 1973.
12. Grove, A. S., Jr., and Kotner, L. M., Jr.: Orbital scanning with multiple radionuclides, Arch. Ophthalmol. **89**:301, 1973.

24
RADIOPAQUE CONTRAST MEDIA

Injection of radiopaque fluids is well suited for the study of obstructions to lacrimal drainage. Ethyl iodophenylundecylate (Pantopaque) is an excellent contrast medium for this purpose. It causes no damage to cornea, conjunctiva, canaliculi, or lacrimal sac. Even without anesthesia, this drug causes only a slight burning sensation. Its consistency is that of an oil of low viscosity; hence it injects freely with the usual lacrimal needle. Its contrast is sharp, thereby showing clearly the fine details of importance in dacryocystography.[1,2]

The technique of dacryocystography is comparable to that of lacrimal irrigation. Retained secretions and debris should be washed out with saline solution, and the lacrimal sac should then be expressed as completely as possible. The amount of radiopaque medium is determined by the ease of injection. Irrigation of the conjunctival sac will remove surplus contrast media that might otherwise cast confusing shadows. Posteroanterior and lateral x-ray films taken immediately after filling of the lacrimal sac will show clearly the size and extent of the lacrimal passages and will reveal the level of obstruction, abnormal fistulas, communication with sinuses, and other information.[3] Dacryocystography might be particularly useful when the obstruction is caused by fracture, since such injury may considerably disrupt the normal anatomy.

The physiologic function of an unobstructed lacrimal sac may also be studied by dacryocystography. The normal emptying time is 15 to 30 minutes, after which the contrast medium is no longer visible. Considerably prolonged emptying time is found in patients complaining of epiphora despite the fact that saline solution can be irrigated freely through the lacrimal passages into the nose.

Intubation of the canaliculus with an intravenous catheter placed 3 mm inside the punctum and taped to the cheek simplifies the procedure. Ultrafluid Lipiodol (viscosity 25 centipoise) is injected via the lower canaliculus, although the upper may also be used.[4,5]

ORBITAL CONTRAST STUDIES

The injection of oily or highly concentrated radiopaque contrast media is not a satisfactory method for evaluation of possible orbital neoplasms. Such radiopaque substances tend to be irritating, do not diffuse uniformly throughout the orbit, and are unsuitable for clinical use.

Iodopyracet (Diodrast), a water-soluble compound, contains 50% iodine; hence it tends to cause considerable tissue damage. In rabbits, injection of 35% iodopyracet solution (amount comparable to 5 ml in the human orbit) causes marked edema and exophthalmos and subsequent scleral necrosis.[6]

473

Larger volumes of injection cause severe orbital cellulitis and may result in scleral rupture. X-ray–detectable amounts of iodopyracet remain in the orbit for as long as 3 hours.

The irritating effect of iodopyracet may be greatly reduced by prior injection of hyaluronidase (50 TRU), which hastens disappearance of the dye from the orbit. Most of the iodopyracet disappears from the orbit within 15 minutes when preceded with hyaluronidase; hence films must be exposed rapidly after injection. This technique (1 ml of 3% procaine solution with 50 TRU of hyaluronidase, followed in 12 minutes by 5 ml of 35% iodopyracet solution) was used in 17 patients. Almost all suffered several hours of orbital and frontal pain and had considerable edema.[6] In five subsequently enucleated blind eyes there was no evidence of ocular necrosis or other damage from this injection. "Satisfactory" x-ray films were obtained in only 10 of the 17 eyes. In two cases, circumscribed filling defects were presumed to be neoplasms, but subsequent surgery showed no tumor to be present. Cadaver studies indicate that iodopyracet injections often were not evenly distributed through the orbit, thereby simulating tumors. In one patient, acute spasm of the central retinal artery developed immediately after iodopyracet injection, and vision was greatly reduced for 24 hours.

Orbitography with the use of 20% diatrizoate methylglucamine (Renografin) was reported as helpful in the evaluation of 20 patients suspected of having a space-occupying orbital lesion.[7] Two to four milliliters of this contrast medium (diluted with lidocaine to the proper concentration) is injected into the muscle cone before x-ray exposures are taken. No complications were reported with this technique.

Injection of opaque media permits verification of the accuracy of positioning of the retrobulbar needle and reveals some unexpected findings. Attempted orbitography with 5 ml of 30% Hypaque given by retrobulbar injection outlined the optic nerve perfectly, suggesting injection into the subdural space.[8] Ten minutes after injection, the radiopaque material had vanished from the orbit and was found to be in the lumbosacral subdural space!

REFERENCES

1. Milder, B., and Demorest, B. B.: Dacryocystography, Arch. Ophthalmol. **51:**180, 1954.
2. Milder, B.: Lacrimal fistula, Am. J. Ophthalmol. **39:**220, 1955.
3. Waldapfel, R.: Location of congenital dacryostenosis in children, Am. J. Ophthalmol. **37:**768, 1954.
4. Hurwitz, J. J., Welham, R. A. N., and Lloyd, G. A. S.: The role of intubation of macrodacryocystography in management of problems of the lacrimal system, Can. J. Ophthalmol. **10:**361, 1975.
5. Hurwitz, J. J., and Welham, R. A. N.: The role of dacryocystography in the management of congenital nasolacrimal duct obstruction, Can. J. Ophthalmol. **10:**346, 1975.
6. Manchester, P. T., Jr., and Bonmati, J.: Iodopyracet (Diodrast) injection for orbital tumors, Arch. Ophthalmol. **54:**591, 1955.
7. Beisner, D. H., and Sumerling, M. D.: Orbitography, Am. J. Ophthalmol. **68:**205, 1969.
8. Kaufer, G., and Augustin, G.: Orbitography, Am. J. Ophthalmol. **61:**795, 1966.

25
SECRETORY INHIBITORS

When the increased outflow of aqueous resulting from miotic therapy is insufficient to control glaucoma, the ophthalmologist usually resorts to medications that reduce aqueous secretion. These medications can be classified into four groups:

I. Carbonic anhydrase inhibitors
   A. Acetazolamide
   B. Methazolamide
   C. Dichlorphenamide
   D. Ethoxzolamide
II. Inhibitors of sodium-potassium–activated ATP
   A. Digitalis glycosides
   B. Ouabain
III. Sympathomimetic agents
   A. Levo-epinephrine
   B. Phenylephrine
IV. Monoamine oxidase inhibitors

Carbonic anhydrase inhibitors and inhibitors of sodium-potassium–activated adenosine triphosphatase (ATP) are considered in this chapter. The sympathomimetic agents were discussed in Chapter 12.

CARBONIC ANHYDRASE INHIBITORS
Acetazolamide (Diamox)

Acetazolamide is the most commonly used carbonic anhydrase inhibitor of value in the management of glaucoma.

Mechanism of action

Enzyme inhibition. The combination of carbon dioxide with water to form carbonic acid as well as the reversal of this process is catalyzed by carbonic anhydrase. Acetazolamide, a potent carbonic anhydrase inhibitor, blocks this process. Since the bicarbonate ion is the main osmotic constituent existing in rabbit aqueous in excess of plasma concentration, and since it is responsible for maintenance of intraocular pressure, acetazolamide would logically be expected to reduce intraocular pressure.[1] Unfortunately the chloride ion rather than the bicarbonate ion is believed to be primarily responsible for the osmotic maintenance of intraocular pressure in man. Hence the mechanism of action of acetazolamide in clinical use is not readily explained simply by a decreased bicarbonate secretion into the aqueous.

Demonstrable blocking of aqueous secretion occurs in the presence of acetazolamide concentrations as small as 10^{-6} M. This effect was demonstrated by photographic measurement of the rate of shrinkage of isolated rabbit ciliary processes.[2] The inhibitory effect of acetazolamide appeared only when the pH was 7.0 or below and not at pH 7.4 or higher (Fig. 25-1).

The finding that acetazolamide inhibits ciliary secretion only in an acid environment is compatible with the clinically recognized fact that ammonium chloride may enhance the effect of carbonic anhydrase inhibitors. The theoretical explanation of this phenomenon is that the secretory cells retain an acid excess as a result of producing an alkaline aqueous. Disposal of this acid residue is ac-

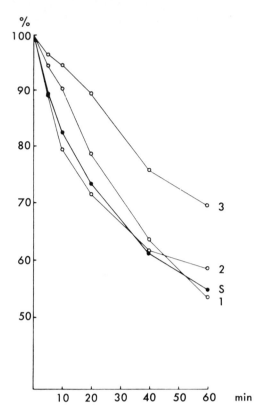

Fig. 25-1. Acetazolamide inhibition of ciliary process shrinkage. Vertical scale: percent of original size of ciliary process. Horizontal scale: time. *S*, Standard rate of decrease in size; *1* and *2*, rate of decrease with acetazolamide at pH 7.7 and 7.4, respectively; *3*, rate of decrease with acetazolamide at pH 7.0. (From Berggren, L.: Invest. Ophthalmol. 3:266, 1964.)

complished at least partially by the buffering effect of the carbonic anhydrase system. Obviously the more acid the environment, the more difficult the disposal of the acid residue. Hence secretion is hampered by the combination of an acid environment and the loss of carbonic anhydrase function.

Severe acidosis alone will lower intraocular pressure in human beings.[3] This is doubtless the cause of the mushy soft eye of diabetic coma.

The decrease of intraocular pressure resulting from acetazolamide correlates with the drop in blood pH resulting from metabolic acidosis.[4] A comparable drop of intraocular pressure results if the same amount of aci-

dosis is induced with calcium chloride or with ascorbic acid. These findings suggest that systemic acidosis is the mechanism of action whereby carbonic anhydrase inhibitors reduce intraocular pressure.

The response of rabbit eyes to acetazolamide is at least partially determined by diet. Animals on low salt intake respond poorly, whereas an increased salt intake causes a hypotensive response to acetazolamide.[5] Administration of the salt-retaining adrenal steroids increases the responsiveness of rabbits to the hypotensive effect of acetazolamide. Complete inhibition of the ciliary body carbonic anhydrase activity of the nonresponsive rabbit eye may cause no reduction of intraocular pressure.[6]

The rate of exchange of carbon dioxide between plasma and aqueous is almost incredibly rapid. Within less than 1 minute after intravenous injection of radioactive carbon–labeled bicarbonate, the concentration of labeled carbon dioxide in posterior chamber aqueous has already become 20% greater than the plasma concentration! (It is estimated that the half-life of carbon dioxide in the posterior chamber aqueous is less than 10 seconds.) In the acetazolamide-treated rabbit, 5 minutes elapse before the posterior chamber aqueous labeled carbon dioxide reaches a similar excess over plasma carbon dioxide. The anterior chamber aqueous does not reach its equilibrium with the plasma for about 15 minutes; this time lag accounts for the time lapse between intravenous administration of acetazolamide, its virtually instantaneous inhibition of ciliary body carbonic anhydrase, and a clinically recognizable drop of intraocular pressure.[7]

The molecular dimensions of carbonic acid and of the active end of carbonic anhydrase inhibitor molecules are virtually identical. This leads to the supposition that the carbonic anhydrase enzyme may have a shape complementary to these molecules (Fig. 25-2).[8] Obviously obstruction of the enzyme surface with the inhibitor would block its catalytic availability. The same active configuration exists in the molecules of the clinically useful carbonic anhydrase inhibitors—aceta-

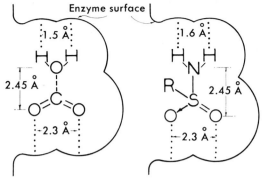

Enzyme surface

1.5 Å   1.6 Å

H O H   H N H

2.45 Å   R S   2.45 Å

O═C═O   O   O

2.3 Å   2.3 Å

Diagrammatic representation of enzyme substrate and enzyme inhibitor complexes

Fig. 25-2. Configuration of carbonic anhydrase enzyme (scalloped line) and the virtually identical dimensions of H_2CO_3 and the active end of the acetazolamide molecule. (From Becker, B.: Am. J. Ophthalmol. **47:**342, 1959.)

zolamide, methazolamide, and ethoxzolamide. A double active configuration exists in the dichlorphenamide molecule.

The relatively prolonged action of acetazolamide on the eye is best explained by the concept of a preferential affinity for certain tissues. Intravenous injection of radioactive sulfur–labeled acetazolamide into rabbits, with subsequent autoradiography of sections of the eye (frozen 2 hours after injection), shows a considerably higher concentration of acetazolamide to exist in the iris and ciliary processes than in other portions of the eye.[9] The drug is not distributed solely on the basis of random diffusion into body fluids. Although logical and long familiar to biochemists, the concept of specific chemical affinity of a drug for the physiologic structure on which it acts is sometimes overlooked by physicians.

These studies with radioactive acetazolamide also reveal that this drug is not metabolized within the eye. As a matter of fact, acetazolamide is not metabolized anywhere within the body and is excreted unchanged in the urine.

In dogs, adrenalectomy reduces the ocular hypotensive action of acetazolamide. Ocular instillation of beta adrenergic blocking agents will also reduce acetazolamide effect. These findings suggest that the adrenergic system is in some way related to the mechanism of action of acetazolamide.[10]

In a series of 25 control and 25 test patients the ocular hypertensive response to succinylcholine was completely abolished by 500 mg acetazolamide given intravenously 2 minutes before succinylcholine.[11] The mechanism of this effect, if confirmed, is entirely obscure to me.

In a group of four patients with elevated intraocular pressure uncontrolled by glaucoma surgery, miotics, and epinephrine, the administration of acetazolamide was found to cause immediate and continuing good control of pressure. The facility of outflow in these patients ranged from 0.03 to 0.10 before acetazolamide and increased to 0.20 to 0.45 on a dosage of 5 mg/kg four times a day (up to 1.5 g acetazolamide daily). Lesser doses did not control the glaucoma. All four patients were maintained for more than 3 years on acetazolamide alone. Since no toxic symptoms are reported, apparently this high dosage was satisfactorily tolerated. No reduction of the rate of aqueous flow was demonstrable in these patients. The authors[12] believe the usual mechanism of action of acetazolamide is inhibition of aqueous production, but improved outflow facility may also be an effect that is more prominent in a few patients. They briefly discuss the potential errors in tonographic assumptions.

Secretory inhibition. The most convincing evidence that acetazolamide acts by decreasing aqueous secretion is provided by tonography. Although substantial lowering of intraocular pressure follows treatment with acetazolamide, the facility of outflow does not change.[3]

In both human beings and rabbits, tonographic studies indicate 50% to 60% inhibition of aqueous flow by acetazolamide.[13,14] No further decrease in secretion occurs with even a tenfold increase in acetazolamide dosage. This suggests that the uncatalyzed hydration of carbon dioxide in the ciliary processes is sufficiently rapid to permit 40% of normal secretion in the absence of carbonic anhydrase.

Fluorophotometry may be used to determine the rate of disappearance of fluorescein from the anterior chamber of the normal human eye. In normal human subjects, 500 mg of acetazolamide will reduce the rate of fluorescein disappearance by 38%.[15] Thus fluorophotometry confirms the tonographic supposition that acetazolamide acts by decreasing the flow of aqueous.

In very large doses (100 mg/kg intravenously), acetazolamide is capable of inhibiting aqueous flow by as much as 75% in dogs.[16]

Since this decrease in secretion occurs even in rabbits that are "unresponsive" (that is, show no decrease in intraocular pressure), it has been postulated and demonstrated that these animals are able to maintain their pressure by a compensatory decrease to 40% of normal outflow. This may explain some cases of human failure to respond to acetazolamide. If the outflow mechanism is so damaged that it cannot carry off even half of the normal secretion, then carbonic anhydrase inhibitors will not be effective. Such cases are exemplified by extensive peripheral anterior synechiae, hemorrhagic glaucoma with vascular occlusion of the angle, and similar findings.

Another method of measuring aqueous flow, the fluorescein appearance time, also indicates that acetazolamide inhibits the rate of aqueous flow by slightly more than 50%.[17]

Unlike the mechanism of action of the miotics, the carbonic anhydrase inhibitors do not control glaucoma by improving facility of outflow; indeed, the reverse may occur. Although acetazolamide does not alter the coefficient of outflow in advanced glaucoma, an acetazolamide-induced decrease in outflow facility has been reported in normal eyes and in eyes with very early glaucoma.[18] Possibly this is a compensatory decrease to maintain intraocular pressure; at any rate it does not occur in most glaucoma patients—fortunately.

Prolonged acetazolamide therapy does not result in any maintained posttreatment improvement of outflow or decrease of aqueous secretion (Fig. 25-3).[19] After a mean duration

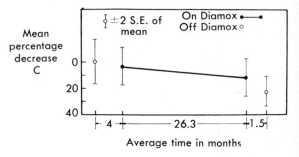

Fig. 25-3. Average decrease in outflow facility, C, during long-term acetazolamide (Diamox) therapy. (From deCarvalho, C. A., Cartaret, L., and Stone, H. H.: Arch. Ophthalmol. **59**:840, 1958.)

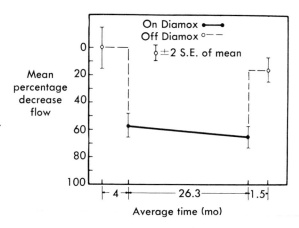

Fig. 25-4. Average acetazolamide-induced decrease in flow in 38 eyes with chronic simple glaucoma. (From deCarvalho, C. A., Cartaret, L., and Stone, H. H.: Arch. Ophthalmol. **59**:840, 1958.)

of therapy of 27 months, the coefficient of outflow of 38 eyes averaged 25% less than before therapy (Fig. 25-4). In this respect, secretory inhibition with carbonic anhydrase inhibitors differs from that achieved with levo-epinephrine, which improves outflow facility in a high proportion of patients. Incidentally, 59% of this series of patients required acetazolamide therapy after surgery had failed to control their tension.

Diuretic-hypotensive relationship. The hypotensive effect of acetazolamide is not a result of its diuretic action. No such response follows the use of other diuretics. Particular confusion has arisen because of the simi-

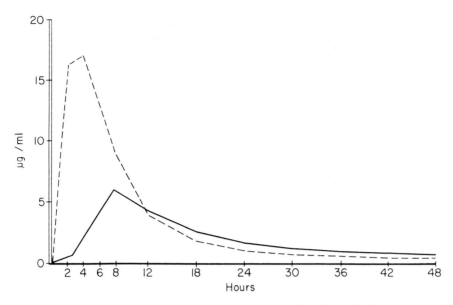

Fig. 25-5. Plasma levels of acetazolamide. Broken line: levels after oral administration of 500 mg of acetazolamide. Solid line: levels after administration of 500 mg of sustained-release acetazolamide. (Modified from Lederle Laboratories research data.)

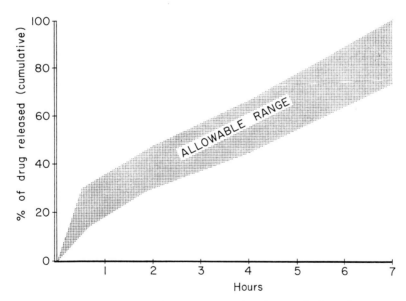

Fig. 25-6. Rate of release of coated form of acetazolamide. (Lederle Laboratories research data.)

larity of the brand names of two diuretics, acetazolamide (Diamox) and chlorothiazide (Diuril). Chlorothiazide, although a potent diuretic, has no effect on intraocular pressure. This has repeatedly been demon- strated, as, for instance, in 36 patients with chronic simple glaucoma that was controlled by acetazolamide but not by chlorothiazide.[20-23]

Acetazolamide will reduce intraocular

pressure in nephrectomized rabbits; hence its action cannot be mediated by diuresis or other renal mechanism.[3]

Hydrochlorothiazide (Esidrix), a very potent diuretic with a mechanism of action more closely related to mercurial diuretics than to carbonic anhydrase inhibition, has been evaluated in 45 normal and 37 glaucomatous patients.[24] The resulting drop of intraocular pressure was usually less than 3 mm Hg, an insignificant change. Diuretics that are not carbonic anhydrase inhibitors are not clinically useful in the treatment of glaucoma.

Absorption

Oral administration. Orally administered acetazolamide is rapidly absorbed; plasma levels of the drug reach near maximum levels by 2 hours (Fig. 25-5).[25] High plasma levels persist for 4 to 6 hours and then rapidly drop because of urinary excretion of acetazolamide.

The effect of acetazolamide may be prolonged by dispensing it in a coated granule form (Diamox Sequels). This sustained-release acetazolamide not only maintains more prolonged plasma levels and therapeutic effect but is also better tolerated because of the less severe side effects. The rate of release of acetazolamide from these coated granules is shown in Fig. 25-6.

Intravenous injection. The intravenous injection of acetazolamide, 50 mg/kg, in cats causes a decrease of intraocular pressure that is already recognizable 1 minute after injection.[26]

Intravenous administration is, of course, necessary if nausea and vomiting (as in acute glaucoma) prevent the patient from retaining the tablets given orally. The more prompt response to intravenous injection of acetazolamide is advantageous in treatment of acute glaucoma. However, if as long as an hour will elapse before the intravenous preparation can be obtained and administered, immediate administration of a capsule of uncoated acetazolamide is much easier and equally effective.

Local use. Local ocular use of acetazol-amide (topical, subconjunctival, or by iontophoresis) does not cause a drop of intraocular pressure, even though carbonic anhydrase inhibition is demonstrable in the iris and ciliary body. This suggests that an effect of acetazolamide on the blood plasma is necessary to reduce aqueous secretion.[3] Since red blood cells contain very high concentrations of carbonic anhydrase, elimination of the action of this enzyme from the highly vascular ciliary body apparently cannot occur without systemic administration of acetazolamide.

Intracameral injection of 0.1 ml of a 1% acetazolamide solution does not reduce intraocular pressure. Intracameral injection of a 10% solution causes acute pain and acute corneal edema that persist for a week or more.[27]

Hypotensive response

Dose-response relationships are relatively complex in the case of enzyme-inhibiting drugs. Specifically, acetazolamide causes only insignificant lowering of intraocular pressure until given in sufficient dosage to inhibit at least 98% of carbonic anhydrase activity. Furthermore, when two thirds of aqueous secretion is inhibited, the remaining one third is unaffected by virtually unlimited increase in the dosage of acetazolamide (Fig.

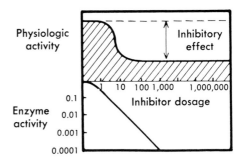

Fig. 25-7. Relationship of physiologic activity and enzyme activity to inhibitor dosage. The slightest measurable inhibitory effect is not noted until only 10% of enzyme activity remains. A tenfold increase in dosage reduces enzyme activity to 0.01% of normal and achieves maximum inhibitory effect. Further inhibition of physiologic activity does not occur, even if the dose is increased 1 million times! (From Friedenwald, J. S.: Am. J. Ophthalmol. **40:**139, 1955.)

25-7).[28] This is because the reaction CO_2 + H_2O = H_2CO_3 proceeds at a considerable velocity even in the complete absence of carbonic anhydrase.

The ocular hypotensive effect of acetazolamide parallels its plasma concentration (Fig. 25-8). The maximum effect of a single oral dose is attained within 2 hours and is maintained for 2 to 6 hours after administration. The effect of a single capsule of the sustained-release form of acetazolamide may extend over a 24-hour period.

"Excellent to good" response to sustained-release acetazolamide was achieved in 83% of 141 eyes with chronic simple glaucoma under treatment for periods ranging up to 30 months.[29] The average reduction of intraocular pressure was 9.2 mm Hg (range, 3 to 22 mm Hg). The greatest fall of pressure occurred in the patients with the highest initial pressures. Most of these patients received 500 mg of sustained-release acetazolamide every morning. A few required this dosage twice daily.

As would be expected, the occasional patient with hypersecretion glaucoma responds exceptionally well to carbonic anhydrase in-

hibitor therapy. A type of hypersecretion glaucoma follows paracentesis of the anterior chamber, and its response to acetazolamide is of interest.

As would be expected, use of acetazolamide after paracentesis of the anterior chamber does reduce the rate of re-formation of aqueous and delays restoration of the anterior chamber. Characteristically, after paracentesis the human eye exhibits a hypertensive response whereby the intraocular pressure rises to higher than normal for several hours. This hypertensive response is exaggerated in glaucomatous eyes. Acetazolamide not only delays restoration of intraocular pressure to preparacentesis levels but also reduces or eliminates the hypertensive response. (The physiologic significance of this is not yet established, but obviously it suggests that hypersecretion may be responsible for the excessively high pressure rebound.) Presumably, much the same type of aqueous response follows surgical or traumatic anterior chamber loss.[30] The effect of acetazolamide treatment of such cases is illustrated in Fig. 25-9. In this figure the solid line represents the levels of intraocular pres-

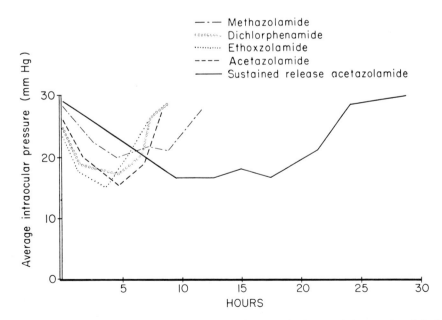

—·— Methazolamide
··········· Dichlorphenamide
·········· Ethoxzolamide
---- Acetazolamide
——— Sustained release acetazolamide

Fig. 25-8. Response of intraocular pressure to carbonic anhydrase inhibitors. (Modified from Garner, L. L., Carl, E. F., and Ferwerda, J. R.: Am. J. Ophthalmol. **55:**323, 1963.)

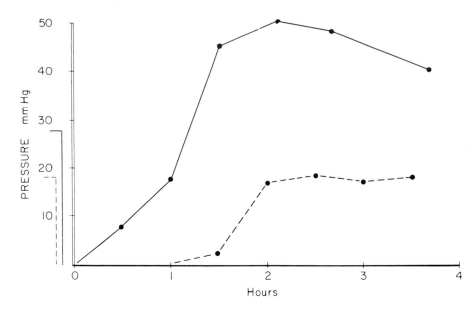

Fig. 25-9. Response of aqueous to anterior chamber loss. Solid line: hypertensive response to paracentesis of glaucomatous human eye. Broken line: delay in restoration of intraocular pressure in same eye after acetazolamide administration. (Modified from Kronfeld, P., and Freeman, H.: Am. J. Ophthalmol. **50:**1141, 1960.)

Table 25-1. Response of chronic simple glaucoma to therapeutic combinations*

Preparation	No. of eyes	No. of eyes controlled
Miotics alone	117	58 (49.6%)
Miotics + acetazolamide sustained-release capsules	89	58 (65.1%)
Miotics + levo-epinephrine	110	77 (70.0%)
Miotics + levo-epinephrine + acetazolamide sustained-release capsules	75	60 (80.0%)

*From Garner, L. L., Carl, E. F., and Ferwerda, J. R.: Acetozolamide in glaucoma, Exhibit, Sixty-Sixth Annual Convention, American Academy of Ophthalmology and Otolaryngology, 1961.

sure after paracentesis of a glaucomatous eye (initial pressure, 28 mm Hg). The broken line represents pressure when paracentesis was performed in the same eye after 2 days of administration of acetazolamide, 250 mg, three times a day (initial pressure, 19 mm Hg). Paracentesis was done with a No. 27 needle, great care being taken to form a beveled, leakproof wound. Note that acetazolamide caused about an hour's delay in restoration to previous pressure levels (which were attained, even so, within 2 hours), and that the marked hypertensive response shown before acetazolamide was eliminated with treatment.[30]

Therapeutic combinations

Only rarely is chronic glaucoma treated with acetazolamide alone. Ordinarily carbonic anhydrase inhibitors are added to miotic therapy when the latter has proved inadequate to control a difficult case of chronic simple glaucoma. Levo-epinephrine and carbonic anhydrase inhibitors have a similar mechanism of action, both decreasing aqueous secretion. In combination with miotic therapy, either levo-epinephrine or acetazolamide will increase the percentage of cases adequately controlled medically (Table 25-1).[31] Usually epinephrine is prescribed first because it has fewer side effects than acetazolamide, it also increases facility of outflow with long-term use, it minimizes the visual problems of extreme miosis, and it is less expensive. When both acetazolamide and epinephrine are used together with a miotic, their additive effect further improves glaucoma control.

Clinical use

Acute angle-closure glaucoma is routinely treated with intensive pilocarpine installation and oral or intravenous acetazolamide (depending on whether nausea and vomiting interfere with oral administration, and on the severity of attack and availability of the intravenous preparation). Osmotic hypotensive drugs may also be necessary.

Short-term glaucoma control. Acetazolamide has proved to be a valuable supplementary medication for short-term control of various types of acute primary and secondary glaucoma. Both narrow-angle and open-angle primary glaucomas respond nicely, as well as other types of glaucoma such as pigmentary, capsular exfoliation, infantile, and glaucoma secondary to uveitis. Patients with extensive peripheral anterior synechiae and marked impairment of outflow (for example, hemorrhagic glaucoma) respond very poorly. Of 406 eyes on short-term therapy (250 mg four times a day), 344 responded with a pressure drop of more than 10 mm Hg. However, of 17 glaucomatous eyes secondary to venous occlusion, only two responded to acetazolamide.[32,33]

Long-term glaucoma control. To evaluate the effect of long-term administration of acetazolamide, 50 patients with chronic simple glaucoma were selected for study, using the criteria that their glaucoma was previously uncontrolled by miotics alone and that initial therapy with acetazolamide (in addition to miotics) did control pressure.[34] The usual dose of acetazolamide was 250 mg every 6 hours or 500 mg of sustained-release acetazolamide every 12 hours. Of these patients, 62% were successfully controlled for more than 6 months. However, 26% of the patients were not successfully controlled because of intolerable side effects, usually gastrointes-

tinal. In only 12% of these patients was failure caused by inadequate control.

A similar study of 10 patients with secondary glaucoma resulted in failure to control 50% of patients, usually because of poor control of pressure in cases of severe outflow impairment. Even worse results followed attempted treatment of 10 cases of chronic narrow-angle glaucoma—80% failed.

In another study, 60% of 111 poorly controlled glaucoma patients were controlled with the addition of acetazolamide for 6 to 20 months.[32] The majority of patients (80%) receiving acetazolamide therapy have more or less annoying side effects. In addition, the cost of treatment is not inconsiderable ($148.90 year for 1 g/day in 1978).

In another report, satisfactory control was achieved in 12 of 20 patients treated for an average of 10½ months.[35]

These (and other) reports indicate that long-term use of acetazolamide should be considered when intensive topical medical therapy does not adequately control glaucoma. A considerable number of such patients will respond well to this treatment. There are, of course, patients in whom poor control or intolerance of medical treatment will ultimately lead to surgery (which is also not always successful).

Acetazolamide should not be used in inadequate dosage. Most patients with chronic simple glaucoma uncontrolled by miotics will require 250 to 500 mg every 4 to 6 hours. A single measurement of intraocular pressure is not necessarily representative of the 24-hour control and may be particularly misleading if the patient takes a single daily dose of acetazolamide several hours before the office visit.[36]

Ammonium chloride, in doses of 1 to 2 g every 6 hours, will potentiate the pressure-lowering effect of acetazolamide in some patients. Potassium chloride, 1 g three times a day, relieves side effects in some patients.[34]

Prevention of vitreous loss. Use of acetazolamide prior to intraocular surgery presumably decreases intraocular pressure and thereby reduces vitreous loss. Whether this is of any benefit when used in cataract surgery in addition to adequate preoperative local anesthesia and ocular massage is questionable. Quite often such routine preoperative medications may be prescribed indiscriminately, without regard for known pharmacologic effects; for example, one paper reports, "Acetazolamide was routinely prescribed the evening prior to surgery."[37] Obviously, unless surgery was performed at midnight, the hypotensive effect of this dose had long passed at the time of surgery.

In the repair of a lacerated eye or the removal of an intraocular foreign body, retrobulbar injection and ocular massage are usually contraindicated. In such cases, intraocular pressure may be reduced by intravenous acetazolamide. However, the intravenous osmotic agents (urea and mannitol) are much more effective.

Scleral buckling procedures. Use of acetazolamide prior to scleral surgery for retinal detachment has been suggested to soften the eye and permit a larger buckle. Since surgical planning should take into account the amount of subretinal fluid available for release, supplementary means of reducing pressure are rarely required. Intravenous injection of osmotic agents reduces ocular volume more rapidly and to a much greater extent than do secretory inhibitors.

Flat anterior chamber. Acetazolamide briefly enjoyed the reputation of restoring flat or shallow anterior chambers to normal after cataract or glaucoma surgery.[38-40] This effect has been variously attributed to a reduction of vitreous "edema," to improved healing of a leaky wound after reduced aqueous secretion, and to coincidence. Such a chamber-restoring effect is pharmacologically inexplicable and has not been substantiated by any controlled study. Pretreatment with acetazolamide *increases* the time required for re-formation of the anterior chamber in animals[41] and in man.[30]

Applanation tonometry after 85 consecutive uncomplicated cataract extractions showed that the average intraocular pressure had returned to normal preoperative levels within less than 24 hours (Fig. 25-10).[42] Obviously the popular belief in "postoperative hypotony" is erroneous, and excessively soft pressure must be interpreted to indicate a wound leak. These wound leaks, with consequent shallow chambers and choroidal detachments, may be avoided by careful surgery and especially by the use of multiple

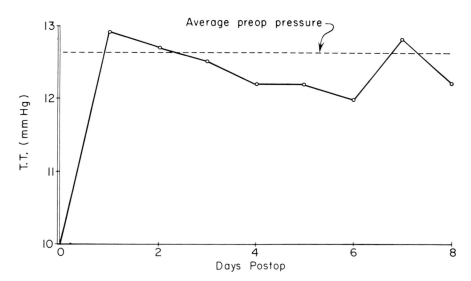

Fig. 25-10. Average applanation intraocular pressure measurements during first week following uncomplicated cataract extraction. Obviously average preoperative pressures are regained within first day after surgery. (Modified from Galin, M. A., Baras, I., and Perry, R.: Arch. Ophthalmol. **66:**80, 1961.)

corneoscleral sutures (five or more). There is no logical reason for the use of the various drugs that have been advocated for the treatment of flat chambers, since effective treatment requires sealing of the leak—a result that frequently occurs spontaneously but that is not promoted by medical management.

Hyphema. It has been postulated that reduced intraocular pressure postoperatively might reduce the incidence of the minor wound disruptions responsible for postoperative hyphema. The incidence of hyphema in 100 consecutive cataract patients given 250 mg of acetazolamide twice a day was 25%.[43] The preceding 120 patients, untreated, had only 17% hyphema. Similar results were cited in other unpublished series of cases.

Interestingly, late loss of the anterior chamber occurred in 6 of 130 acetazolamide-treated patients and in 6 of 150 untreated patients. This chamber loss despite routine use of acetazolamide certainly casts doubt on its therapeutic effectiveness in treatment of flat chamber. It seems clear to me that hyphema and chamber loss are complications of faulty surgical wound closure and may be avoided by better surgery, not by medical therapy with no rational basis.

Sickle cell retinopathy. Acetazolamide therapy will within 1 hour reduce by one half the proportion of sickle cells in sickle cell anemia.[44] Inactivation of carbonic anhydrase slows the reduction of hemoglobin to the abnormal rod form that alters erythrocyte contour. Long-term acetazolamide therapy arrests hemolysis and permits recovery from the anemia of sickle cell disease. Such therapy may have ocular value in those patients suffering from typical sickle cell retinopathy.

Pseudotumor cerebri. Carbonic anhydrase inhibitors, such as acetazolamide, reduce cerebrospinal fluid formation by 20% to 30%.[45] Diuretics, such as chlorothiazide, do not duplicate this effect of acetazolamide.

In treatment of pseudotumor cerebri, acetazolamide is used to titrate the symptoms. Dosage may vary from 500 mg sustained-release acetazolamide every other day to every 6 hours when necessary. Corticosteroid therapy is less effective than acetazol-amide. Osmotic agents such as glycerol are effective but last for only a few hours and cannot be used for extended periods of time.

If progressive visual field loss occurs despite medical therapy (as will happen in only a few cases), blindness may result. Surgical decompression of the optic nerve sheath should be performed in such cases. Decompression on one side may actually reduce the pressure on both optic nerves.[46]

Contraindications

The most important ocular contraindication to acetazolamide therapy is potential angle-closure glaucoma that the physician has elected to treat medically. Most eyes that have suffered an attack of acute angle-closure glaucoma would benefit from peripheral iridectomy, but for a variety of individual reasons, miotic therapy may be desirable for a shorter or longer period. If it is successful, miotic therapy may defer surgery for a considerable time without harm to the eye (unless an acute attack recurs). If miotic therapy inadequately opens the angle, peripheral anterior synechiae will progressively form, occlude portions of an angle, and cause a gradual pressure rise somewhat simulating open-angle glaucoma. Acetazolamide therapy is definitely contraindicated at this point; although it will reduce pressure temporarily, the false reassurance of tonometric control obscures the continuing destruction of the angle, which ultimately will preclude successful iridectomy and will force the surgeon to perform a considerably less satisfactory filtering operation.[47] (Do not misunderstand this contraindication. Acetazolamide may be of value in the short-term preoperative management of acute angle-closure glaucoma.)

Acetazolamide should not be used if the patient's pressure is adequately controlled by miotics. Its side effects are too severe to warrant such indiscriminate prescription.[36]

Surprisingly often a patient is treated with acetazolamide during the downhill course of severe unilateral glaucoma. Blindness ensues, the remaining eye is easily controlled with miotics alone, and yet the patient is continued on intensive acetazolamide therapy and is thereby uselessly subjected to expense and distressing side effects.

Because of its tendency to cause potassium loss, acetazolamide is contraindicated in Addison's disease and adrenal insufficiency. Patients with cirrhosis of the liver may become disoriented after acetazolamide therapy.

Side effects

Gastrointestinal upsets are the most frequent cause of acetazolamide intolerance severe enough to force discontinuance of treatment. Symptoms may range from vague abdominal discomfort and a peculiar metallic taste to severe nausea and diarrhea. Frequency of urination may be very annoying to some patients but usually decreases with time. Paresthesias commonly affect the hands and feet and the circumoral region. This numbness and tingling may be so severe as to interfere with dexterity. Drowsiness and malaise affect some patients.

These functional side effects are much less troublesome with the sustained-release form of acetazolamide. This form of carbonic anhydrase inhibitor has been well tolerated, being acceptable to 20 of a series of 23 new patients.[29] Of 42 patients who had been unable to tolerate carbonic anhydrase inhibitors, 36 could take sustained-release acetazolamide for many months. The annoying effect of nocturia could be avoided simply by giving the medication in the morning. The convenience of less frequent dosage is also noteworthy.

Potassium depletion may be responsible for the troublesome side effects of acetazolamide therapy and for resistance of the intraocular pressure to control by this form of treatment. Replacement therapy of 2 g of potassium chloride/day has been claimed to decrease the side effects and enhance the hypotensive action of acetazolamide.[48]

Does long-term acetazolamide treatment reduce body potassium? Does supplemental potassium enhance glaucoma control by the carbonic anhydrase inhibitors? Apparently the answer to both these questions is "No."

Fifteen patients with glaucoma receiving a daily dose of 500 to 750 mg acetazolamide for an average time of 2 years were studied to answer these questions.[49] In no patient was there any depletion of total body potassium. Apparently, if the patient receives a normal diet, long-term use of acetazolamide does not cause potassium depletion. This is in contrast to the characteristic potassium loss occurring in the first few weeks of treatment, a loss that is replaced spontaneously despite continuing therapy. In these 15 patients the average intraocular pressure was 19.25 mm Hg. After 2 weeks of supplemental potassium chloride therapy, the average intraocular pressure was 19.9 mm Hg, not a significant change and certainly not a drop in pressure.

The absence of measurable potassium depletion, the failure of supplemental potassium to reduce further the intraocular pressure, and the serious hazard of potassium-induced intestinal ulcerations all suggest that potassium treatment of glaucomatous patients is not indicated.

Hirsutism was reported to follow 16 months of acetazolamide, 125 mg/day, given to a 2½-year-old girl to control congenital glaucoma.[50] A heavy growth of long dark hair covered her back and lower legs. No endocrine abnormality was found and the hair disappeared within a year after the acetazolamide was discontinued. The mechanism was postulated to be acetazolamide stimulation of the adrenal glands.

Comparative tolerance

Patients differ in their tolerance of the various carbonic anhydrase inhibitors. All of these drugs cause similar side effects, but the severity may vary. The individual with acetazolamide intolerance may do well with another carbonic anhydrase inhibitor. Listed in order of increasing frequency of side effects, these drugs are as follows: sustained-release acetazolamide, dichlorphenamide, acetazolamide, methazolamide, and ethoxzolamide (Table 25-2).[31]

In another study, 10 glaucomatous patients were given acetazolamide (250 mg), ethoxzol-

Table 25-2. Comparative tolerance and efficacy of carbonic anhydrase inhibitors*

				Effect on intraocular pressure		
Drug	Dosage (mg)	Total treated	Total not tolerated	Onset (hr)	Maximum (hr)	Duration (hr)
Methazolamide	100 t.i.d.	44	24 (55%)	4	4-8	10-12
Dichlorphenamide	50 t.i.d.	74	27 (36%)	2	4	8
Ethoxzolamide	125 t.i.d.	20	13 (65%)	1½	3.5	7
Acetazolamide tablets	250 q.i.d.	93	44 (47%)	2	4	6-8
Acetazolamide sustained-release capsules	500 o.d.	83	9 (11%)	2	8-18	22-30

*From Garner, L. L., Carl, E. F., and Ferwerda, J. R.: Acetazolamide in glaucoma, Exhibit, Sixty-Sixth Annual Convention, American Academy of Ophthalmology and Otolaryngology, 1961.

amide (125 mg), and dichlorphenamide (50 mg), each for 10-day periods.[51] The purpose of this triple-blind study was to determine adequacy of intraocular pressure control and the relative incidence of systemic side effects. All drugs achieved essentially the same control. Side effects were greatest with dichlorphenamide and least with ethoxzolamide. Obviously these results differ from those cited in the preceding paragraph.

Toxicity

It is virtually impossible to kill an experimental animal with a single dose of acetazolamide. Dogs will survive intravenous administration of as much as 2000 mg/kg. However, 1000 mg/kg given intravenously daily for 3 days will result in death from potassium depletion.

Since acetazolamide is a sulfonamide derivative (but has no antibacterial action), it may cause the various toxic responses associated with other sulfonamides. These include agranulocytosis,[52] thrombocytopenia,[53] exfoliative dermatitis, hypersensitivity nephropathy,[54] renal calculi, and transient myopia.

The acetazolamide-induced predisposition to the formation of renal calculi results from the 60% to 90% reduction in urinary citrate after use of this drug. (Urinary citrate improves calcium solubility.) Since acetazolamide, methazolamide, and dichlorphenamide equally decrease urinary citrate, the problem of renal calculus formation cannot

be avoided by substituting another carbonic anhydrase inhibitor for acetazolamide.[55]

Acetazolamide-induced myopia. Uncommonly acetazolamide will cause rapidly developing transient myopia. The amount of this myopia in eight cases varied from 1.00 to 7.00 D.[56] Accommodative spasm is not the mechanism responsible for this myopia since it persists despite cycloplegia and does not change accommodative amplitudes. Presumably as in diabetes, an increase in the refractive power of the lens is responsible for this transient myopia. Since ingestion of as little as 500 mg of acetazolamide may cause this response, the affected patient must have some type of idiosyncrasy or heightened sensitivity to the medication.

Acetazolamide-induced myopia may develop within 8 hours of ingestion of the drug and requires several days to clear. Subsequent administration of acetazolamide may or may not cause a recurrence of myopia. The depth of the anterior chamber is unchanged during and after acetazolamide-induced myopia. (No change in anterior chamber depth occurs in normal patients who have taken acetazolamide.) Furthermore, reduction of anterior chamber depth from 3 to 0.5 mm would account for only about 3.00 D of myopia. After a report of two intensively studied cases and a pertinent theoretical discussion, the authors[57] concluded that the phenomenon was a "sensitivity reaction." I do not understand why such a drug sensitivity would not be consistently reproducible and prefer the classic explanation for diabetic myopia—changes in lens hydration. By this theory, inconstant myopic response to acetazolamide would be explained on the basis of electrolyte variations.

Transient myopia has been reported with other sulfonamide derivatives, including ethoxzolamide,[58,59] hydrochlorothiazide,[60] and others.[61]

Although high concentrations of carbonic anhydrase activity are demonstrable in the lens,[62] cataract formation has not been reported to follow prolonged treatment with acetazolamide.

Aplastic anemia. Fatal aplastic anemia occurred in a 69-year-old man receiving 116 g of acetazolamide over a period of 4½ months for treatment of glaucoma. This was believed to be a sulfonamide-induced hematopoietic suppression.[63]

In the evaluation of causes of drug-induced blood dyscrasias, acetazolamide was believed to account for 10 of 652 cases of agranulocytosis and for 3 of 266 cases of aplastic anemia. Glaucoma therapy resulted in the deaths from aplastic anemia of a 72-year-old man taking acetazolamide and a 71-year-old woman taking methazolamide.[64]

Teratogenicity. About one third of the offspring of rats given acetazolamide during early pregnancy have malformations of the forepaw usually characterized by absence of the fourth and fifth digits. The dosage required would be comparable to 0.5 to 1.5 g/day in humans. Mice and hamsters develop a comparable defect, but monkeys do not. No human cases have been reported, but ophthalmologists are cautioned against giving carbonic anhydrase inhibitors to women during the first trimester of pregnancy.[65]

Methazolamide (Neptazane)

Methazolamide is a carbonic anhydrase inhibitor chemically similar to acetazolamide. Its use in the control of glaucoma is comparable to that of acetazolamide.

Pharmacology

Since methazolamide more readily penetrates the blood-aqueous and blood-brain barriers (as much as 50 times higher concentration of methazolamide than acetazolamide can be attained in human cerebrospinal fluid) and because it is a more potent carbonic anhydrase inhibitor (in vitro red blood cell enzyme inhibition 60% greater than that with acetazolamide), it is more effective in lower dosage than is acetazolamide.[66] The suggested dosage is 50 to 100 mg two or three times daily, depending on the response of

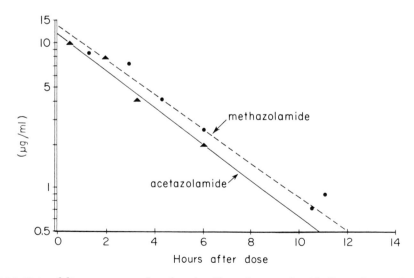

Fig. 25-11. Rate of disappearance of methazolamide and acetazolamide from plasma after intravenous dose of 5 mg/kg in dog. (From Lederle Laboratories research data.)

the individual patient. Almost complete carbonic anhydrase inhibition is attained by 5 mg/kg of methazolamide, and little additional therapeutic effect results from increasing the dose to as much as 100 mg/kg.

Both methazolamide and acetazolamide are stable, are absorbed from the intestinal tract within 2 hours, produce comparable plasma levels that are virtually gone in hours (Fig. 25-11), and are selectively concentrated in red cells (although methazolamide concentrations in red blood cells are double those of acetazolamide at 24 hours; 20% of the administered dose is retained in red blood cells as compared to 10%). Within 24 hours 90% of a dose of acetazolamide can be recovered from the urine, in contrast to 15% of methazolamide. About 50% of methazolamide is unaccounted for at 24 hours and is presumed to have been metabolized.

Toxicity

The toxicity of methazolamide is approximately 10 times greater than that of acetazolamide; however, this is of little clinical significance because of the wide margin of safety with both drugs. Dogs tolerate 100 mg of methazolamide/kg for 3 months, although it does cause acidosis and loss of sodium, potassium, and bicarbonate. The lethal intravenous dose of methazolamide is 500 mg/kg in the dog, death resulting from convulsions and central nervous system changes. Dogs have survived 2000 mg/kg of acetazolamide given intravenously. Much lower doses are required for therapeutic effect. Methazolamide was said not to interfere with urinary excretion of citrate and therefore to be less likely to cause renal calculi than is acetazolamide. However, calcium phosphate renal stones have been reported following methazolamide therapy.[67]

The side effects of acetazolamide and methazolamide differ. Acetazolamide is not tolerated because of nausea and vomiting, paresthesias, and diuresis. Methazolamide causes drowsiness, fatigue, malaise, and minimal gastrointestinal disturbance. Almost no diuresis results from 50 to 100 mg doses of methazolamide.

No ocular toxicity is evident with either medication. Comparable chemical changes in human aqueous are produced by the two drugs, including decreased chloride, decreased pH, decreased flow, and increased bicarbonate. Neither acetazolamide nor methazolamide will reduce intraocular pressure when applied topically, although both can be demonstrated to penetrate into the aqueous after local instillation.

Clinical use

The main indication for use of methazolamide appears to be chronic glaucoma inadequately controlled by acetazolamide (and miotics). In a series of 50 such patients, 14 (28%) were successfully controlled with methazolamide.[68] Success was defined as maintenance of pressure below 30 mm Hg, no progression of visual field loss, and tolerable side effects, extending for at least a 2-year period. Of 34 patients intolerant to acetazolamide, 12 (35%) could be maintained on methazolamide. Of 16 patients whose acetazolamide failure resulted from poor control, only two (13%) were satisfactorily controlled by methazolamide. About half of the patients with chronic simple glaucoma uncontrolled by miotics alone can be maintained at pressures below 24 mm Hg with the addition of carbonic anhydrase inhibitors. Acetazolamide, rather than methazolamide, is recommended as the carbonic anhydrase inhibitor of first choice in the management of glaucoma. This recommendation is based on the facts that methazolamide is not quite as effective as acetazolamide in controlling intraocular pressure and that its onset action is slightly slower (of possible importance in management of acute glaucoma).

Neither methazolamide nor acetazolamide should be used as a substitute for surgery in angle-closure glaucoma. Perhaps it is appropriate to comment that the management of all types of glaucoma requires accurate diagnosis, a reasonable amount of clinical experience, and appropriate routine testing, including perimetry, tonometry, gonioscopy, and ophthalmoscopy. It is not possible for a physician who has not devoted a considerable amount of time to eye work to manage glaucoma according to acceptable standards, and the advent of new drugs does not change this basic fact. However, the help of all physicians is necessary in the early diagnosis of glaucoma, which is the major preventable cause of blindness and will be found in 2% of patients over the age of 40 years.

Dichlorphenamide (Daranide)
Pharmacology

Dichlorphenamide contains within its molecule two configurations (sulfamyl group) resembling carbonic acid. Very probably this dual structure is the reason for its considerably greater carbonic anhydrase inhibitor potency and resulting smaller dosage. Only 50 mg of dichlorphenamide is the therapeutic equivalent of 250 mg of acetazolamide. The maintenance dosage is 25 to 100 mg three times a day. This must be adjusted to the needs of the individual patient.

Unlike the other carbonic anhydrase inhibitors, dichlorphenamide increases chloride excretion (in addition to increased sodium, potassium, and bicarbonate excretion). As a result, metabolic acidosis is less frequent and less marked after dichlorphenamide than after other carbonic anhydrase inhibitors. The decrease likelihood of acidosis causes pa-

tients usually to diurese even with frequently repeated doses. This is in contrast to acetazolamide, chronic administration of which usually does not maintain diuresis (an undesirable side effect in glaucoma therapy).

Dichlorphenamide is readily water soluble and is promptly absorbed after oral administration. Intraocular pressure drops within 30 minutes after dichlorphenamide ingestion, is at its lowest within 2 to 4 hours, and returns to normal in 6 to 12 hours. In a series of 30 normal and 20 glaucomatous eyes, a single oral dose of 200 mg of dichlorphenamide reduced aqueous humor formation by an average of 40%. Although the intraocular pressure was reduced by an average of 2.4 mm Hg in the normal eyes and 8.1 mm Hg in the glaucomatous eyes, the coefficient of outflow was unchanged in both groups.[69] The range of variation of individual response is shown in Fig. 25-12.

Clinical use

Dichlorphenamide, just as the other carbonic anhydrase inhibitors, is a supplement to standard miotic therapy of glaucoma and is not used alone except perhaps in the very rare case of hypersecretion glaucoma. Dichlorphenamide was effective in the treatment of patients who had previously re-

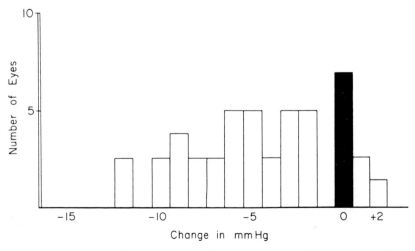

Fig. 25-12. Change in intraocular pressure in glaucomatous eyes 2 hours after oral administration of 100 mg of dichlorphenamide. (Modified from Gonzalez-Jiminez, E., and Leopold, I. H.: Arch. Ophthalmol. **60:**427, 1958.)

sponded well to acetazolamide. In addition, it was successful in the control of 10 of 17 patients who were not controlled by acetazolamide.[70] Some patients tolerate the side effects of dichlorphenamide better than those of acetazolamide; hence patients intolerant or refractory to the latter drug may benefit from a trial of dichlorphenamide.

The side effects of chronic use of dichlorphenamide are comparable to those of other carbonic anhydrase inhibitors. Hypokalemia may be avoided by simultaneous oral administration of potassium, which does not interfere with the antiglaucoma therapeutic effect. The ophthalmologist should not be annoyed by the glaucoma patient who seems depressed, confused, and querulous. These symptoms should indicate the possibility of toxicity from carbonic anhydrase inhibitor therapy and may require reduction in dosage or substitution of other methods of treatment. The presence of anorexia or nausea, paresthesias, dizziness, or ataxia and tremor confirms the diagnosis of toxicity. If these symptoms are drug induced, they should disappear when the medication is discontinued.

Ethoxzolamide (Cardrase)

The mechanism of action, therapeutic results, and side effects of ethoxzolamide are essentially the same as those for acetazolamide.

The intraocular pressure of normal and glaucomatous eyes is reduced by ethoxzolamide. The average dose used is 125 mg every 6 hours. After 125 mg, the intraocular pressure is reduced within 2 hours, the fall is maximal at 5 hours, and pressure has returned to normal in 12 hours. At the time of maximum effect this dosage reduces aqueous formation by 40%. Facility of outflow is unaffected. In a series of 36 glaucomatous eyes inadequately controlled by miotics, addition of ethoxzolamide caused an average drop in pressure of 43% (Fig. 25-13).[71]

Although the side effects of ethoxzolamide are similar to those of acetazolamide, patients who cannot tolerate acetazolamide may tolerate ethoxzolamide and vice versa.[72]

INHIBITORS OF SODIUM-POTASSIUM–ACTIVATED ATP
Digitalis glycosides

Just as carbonic anhydrase inhibitors reduce intraocular pressure, so also it has been possible to decrease aqueous flow by inhibiting sodium-potassium–activated adenosine triphosphatase.[73] This enzyme is necessary for aqueous formation in human beings and may be inhibited by the digitalis glycosides.

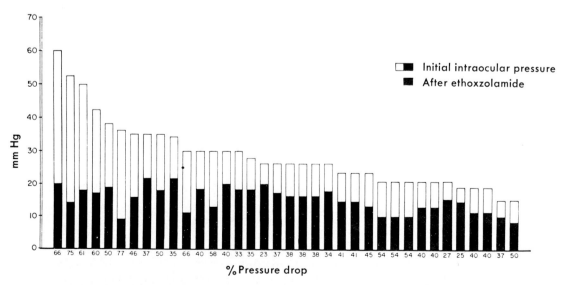

Fig. 25-13. Percentage drop of intraocular pressure in 36 miotic-treated eyes after ethoxzolamide treatment. (From Drance, S. M.: Arch. Ophthalmol. **62:**679, 1959.)

As shown in Fig. 25-14, treatment of a patient's congenital glaucoma with digoxin resulted in a marked drop of intraocular pressure. In the patients studied, digoxin suppressed aqueous formation by 45%, acetazolamide suppressed aqueous formation by 50%, and a combination of these two inhibitors reduced aqueous formation by 65%.

Selective concentration of digitoxin in the ciliary body has been demonstrated by use of radioactive tracer studies.[74] Presumably, this is related to the capability of this drug to alter aqueous secretion. By far the highest concentration of digitoxin was found in the retina. Demonstration of this high concentration of digitoxin within the retina is compatible with the belief (supported by electroretinography) that the visual phenomena of digitalis intoxication are caused by direct action on the retina rather than by cerebral effects of the drug.[75]

A single daily dose of digoxin is sufficient to maintain the secretory inhibition. The digitalizing dose is 0.03 mg/pound, and the maintenance dose is one half of this each day. For the average adult, 2 to 4 mg of digoxin is required for digitalization and about 0.5 mg/day for maintenance. As is well known, digitalis preparations are highly toxic and must be given with care. Toxic effects include diarrhea and abdominal discomfort, headache, disturbance in color vision, confusion, and cardiac arrhythmias such as extrasystoles and paroxysmal tachycardia.[76,77] Death may occur from ventricular fibrillation. Evaluation by electrocardiogram is desirable before use of these drugs. Administration of epinephrine should be avoided when a patient is digitalized.

Although a small additive effect is obtained from simultaneous use of acetazolamide and digoxin, combined medication is not recommended because of the frequency of unpleasant side effects. A drop in dosage of acetazolamide while digoxin is continued is reported to cause severe nausea and vomiting. Apparently, nausea is less likely to occur if digoxin is discontinued first.

Clinical use

It appears that digoxin might be useful in the management of glaucomatous patients who cannot tolerate acetazolamide and yet need inhibition of aqueous humor formation

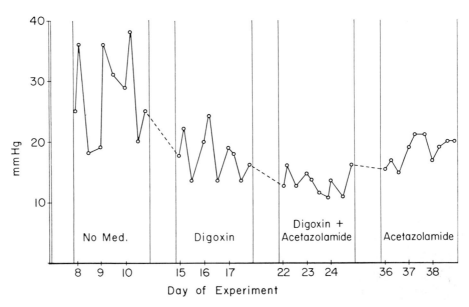

Fig. 25-14. Reduction of human intraocular pressure with digoxin is comparable to that achieved by acetazolamide. Note variations in pressure that are characteristic of glaucoma. (Modified from Simon, K., and Bonting, S. L.: Arch. Ophthalmol. **68:**227, 1962.)

to maintain adequate pressure control. Use of digoxin will be limited by its greater potential toxicity. Perhaps most of all, this discovery gives promise of an ever-increasing number of drugs that will alter the metabolism of the eye for a therapeutically useful purpose.

The stepwise progression of our knowledge is often interesting. Information that sodium-potassium phosphatase inhibitors inhibit aqueous secretion would naturally suggest histochemical investigation of the ciliary epithelium for the presence of this enzyme. Dense concentrations of phosphatase activity are found at the boundary between the pigmented and nonpigmented ciliary epithelium. Presumably, this is the site of the "sodium pump" that causes aqueous secretion.

Digitalization of 14 glaucomatous patients inadequately controlled by intensive standard treatment with miotics, carbonic anhydrase inhibitors, and epinephrine did not significantly reduce their intraocular pressures (Fig. 25-15).[78] Hence digitalization cannot be expected to improve the status of poorly controlled glaucomatous patients.

Topical ocular administration of 0.5% digi-

toxin ointment will lower human intraocular pressure but is not of practical value because it causes digitalis keratopathy. This keratopathy is characterized by diffuse epithelial edema and large folds in Descemet's membrane and is quite painful.[79]

Ouabain

As little as 0.5 μg of ouabain (another cardiac glycoside that is a strong inhibitor of sodium-potassium–activated adenosine triphosphatase), when injected intravitreally, will reduce the intraocular pressure of rabbits for as long as 2 weeks (Fig. 25-16).[80] For some unexplained reason, intravenous injection of as much as 250 μg/kg failed to alter intraocular pressure. In a dosage of 67 μg/kg of body weight, ouabain will reduce aqueous secretion by 40% in cats.[81] High concentrations of sodium-potassium–activated phosphatases are histochemically demonstrable in the ciliary epithelium and can be inhibited by intravitreal ouabain injection.[82]

The mechanism whereby cardiac glycosides cause corneal swelling has been studied by means of the reversible hydration caused by temperature drop.[83] Apparently, ouabain in a concentration of 10^{-4}M will cause a 50% inhibition of corneal deturgescence. These experiments suggest that the normal

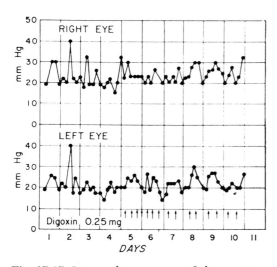

Fig. 25-15. Intraocular pressures of glaucomatous patient receiving intensive treatment with echothiophate, epinephrine, and acetazolamide before and after digitalization (started on the fifth day). (From Peczon, J. D.: Arch. Ophthalmol. **71**:500, 1964.)

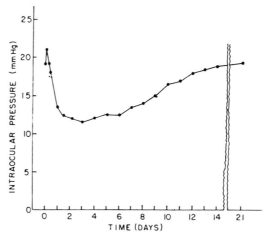

Fig. 25-16. Intraocular pressure drop after intravitreal injection of 0.5 μg of ouabain. (From Becker, B.: Invest. Ophthalmol. **2**:325, 1963.)

mechanism of corneal dehydration is an active sodium transfer from the cornea, primarily by the endothelium.

MONOAMINE OXIDASE INHIBITORS

Possibly monoamine oxidase inhibitors will prove useful as secretory inhibitors. Intravenous injection of nialamide, 50 mg/300 g body weight, caused a significant drop of intraocular pressure in 9 of 15 albino rabbits. Histochemical examination confirmed inhibition of ciliary body monoamine oxidase activity by the nialamide.[84]

REFERENCES

1. Becker, B.: Decrease in intraocular pressure in man by a carbonic anhydrase inhibitor, Diamox, Am. J. Ophthalmol. 37:13, 1954.
2. Berggren, L.: Direct observation of secretory pumping in vitro of the rabbit eye ciliary processes, Invest. Ophthalmol. 3:266, 1964.
3. Becker, B.: The mechanism of the fall in intraocular pressure induced by the carbonic anhydrase inhibitor, Diamox, Am. J. Ophthalmol. 39:177, 1955.
4. Bietti, G., Virno, M., Pecori-Giraldi, J., and Pellegrino, N.: Acetazolamide, metabolic acidosis, and intraocular pressure, Am. J. Ophthalmol. 80:360, September 1975.
5. Kinsey, V. E., Camacho, E., Cavanaugh, G. A., Constant, M., and McGinty, D. A.: Dependence of IOP—lowering effect of acetazolamide on salt, Arch. Ophthalmol. 53:680, 1955.
6. Green, H., Bocher, C. A., Calnan, A. F., and Leopold, I. H.: Carbonic anhydrase and the maintenance of intraocular tension, Arch. Ophthalmol. 53:463, 1955.
7. Kinsey, V. E., and Reddy, D. V. N.: Turnover of total carbon dioxide in the aqueous humor and the effect thereon of acetazolamide, Arch. Ophthalmol. 62:78, 1959.
8. Becker, B.: Carbonic anhydrase and the formation of aqueous humor, Am. J. Ophthalmol. 47:342, 1959.
9. Goren, S. B., Newell, F. W., and O'Toole, J. J.: The localization of Diamox-S^{35} in the rabbit eye, Am. J. Ophthalmol. 51:87, 1961.
10. Thomas, R. P., and Riley, M. W.: Acetazolamide and ocular tension, Am. J. Ophthalmol. 60:204, 1965.
11. Carballo, A. S.: Use of acetazolamide in an-

aesthesia for ophthalmic surgery, Can. J. Ophthalmol. 1:112, 1966.
12. Galin, M. A., and Harris, L.: Acetazolamide and outflow facility, Arch. Ophthalmol. 76:493, 1966.
13. Becker, B., and Constant, M. A.: Experimental tonography, Arch Ophthalmol. 54:321, 1955.
14. Becker, B.: The effect of acetazolamide on ascorbic acid turnover, Am. J. Ophthalmol. 41:522, 1956.
15. Bloom, J. N., Levene, R. Z., Thomas, G., and Kimura, R.: Fluorophotometry and the rate of aqueous flow in man. I. Instrumentation and normal values, Arch. Ophthalmol. 94:435, March 1976.
16. O'Rourke, J., Macri, F. J., and Berghoffer, B.: Studies in uveal physiology, Arch. Ophthalmol. 81:526, 1969.
17. Friedenwald, J. S.: Carbonic anhydrase inhibition and aqueous flow, Am. J. Ophthalmol 39:59, 1955.
18. Kronfeld, P. C.: Effects of acetazolamide on human aqueous dynamics, Arch. Ophthalmol. 68:442, 1962.
19. de Carvalho, C. A., Cartaret, L., and Stone, H. H.: Acetazolamide (Diamox) therapy in chronic glaucoma, Arch. Ophthalmol. 59:840, 1958.
20. Stepanik, J.: The effect of chlorothiazide (diuril, chlotride) on ocular tension in humans, Ophthalmologica 138:361, 1959.
21. Henry, M. M., and Lee, P.-F.: Clinical comparison of dichlorphenamide, chlorothiazide, and sulocarbilate with acetazolamide in control of glaucoma, Am. J. Ophthalmol. 47:199, 1959.
22. Schimek, R. A., Balian, J. V., Lepley, F. J., and Ottum, J. A.: Evaluation of dichlorphenamide as an ocular hypotensive agent, Arch. Ophthalmol. 60:1054, 1958.
23. Gonzales-Jiminez, E. R., and Leopold, I. H.: Chlorothiazide and ocular pressure, Arch. Ophthalmol. 60:70, 1958.
24. Fajardo, R. V., Hamilton, R., and Leopold, I. H.: The effect of hydrochlorothiazide (Esidrex) in intraocular pressure in man, Am. J. Ophthalmol. 49:1321, 1960.
25. Diamox and Diamox Sequels in glaucoma, Lederle Laboratories research data.
26. Macri, F., and Brown, J.: The constrictive action of acetazolamide on the iris arteries of the cat, Arch. Ophthalmol. 66:570, 1961.
27. Foss, R. H.: Local application of Diamox, Am. J. Ophthalmol. 39:336, 1955.

28. Friedenwald, J. S.: Current studies on acet-azolamide (Diamox) and aqueous humor flow, Am. J. Ophthalmol. **40:**139, 1955.

29. Garner, L. L., Carl, E. F., and Ferwerda, J. R.: Advantages of sustained-release therapy with acetazolamide in glaucoma, Am. J. Ophthalmol. **55:**323, 1963.

30. Kronfeld, P., and Freeman, H.: The effect of acetazolamide on the response to anterior chamber puncture in man, Am. J. Ophthalmol. **50:**1141, 1960.

31. Garner, L. L., Carl, E. F., and Ferwerda, J. R.: Acetazolamide in glaucoma, Exhibit, Sixty-Sixth Annual Convention, American Academy of Ophthalmology and Otolaryngology, 1961.

32. Leopold, I. H., and Carmichael, P. L.: Prolonged administration of Diamox in glaucoma, Trans. Am. Acad. Ophthalmol. **60:**210, 1956.

33. Leopold, I. H.: Experiences with Diamox in glaucoma, Am. J. Ophthalmol. **39:**885, 1955.

34. Becker, B., and Middleton, W. H.: Long-term acetazolamide (Diamox) administration in therapy of glaucomas, Arch. Ophthalmol. **54:**187, 1955.

35. Kupfer, C., Lawrence, C., and Linner, E.: Long-term administration of acetazolamide (Diamox) in the treatment of glaucoma, Am. J. Ophthalmol. **40:**673, 1955.

36. Becker, B.: Misuse of acetazolamide, Am. J. Ophthalmol. **43:**799, 1957.

37. Harley, R. D., and Mishler, J. E.: Acetylcholine in cataract surgery, Am. J. Ophthalmol. **54:**817, 1964.

38. Thorpe, H.: Acetazolamide (Diamox) in glaucoma surgery, Arch. Ophthalmol. **54:**221, 1955.

39. Morales, L. A.: Vitreous edema, Am. J. Ophthalmol. **39:**83, 1955.

40. Murphy, E. U.: Diamox in cataract wound healing, Am. J. Ophthalmol. **39:**86, 1955.

41. Leopold, I. H., Eisenberg, I. J., and Tasuna, J.: Experiences with acetazolamide (carbonic anhydrase inhibitor; Diamox) in glaucoma, Arch. Ophthalmol. **53:**150, 1955.

42. Galin, M. A., Baras, I., and Perry, R.: Intraocular pressure following cataract extraction, Arch. Ophthalmol. **66:**80, 1961.

43. Vail, D.: Diamox to prevent hyphema after cataract extraction, Am. J. Ophthalmol. **44:**637, 1957.

44. Hilkovitz, G.: Sickle cell disease: new method of treatment, Br. Med. J. **2:**266, 1957.

45. Kister, S.: Carbonic anhydrase inhibition VI. The effect of acetazolamide on cerebral spinal fluid flow, J. Pharmacol. Exp. Ther. **117:**402-405, 1956.

46. Lubow, M., and Kuhr, L.: Pseudotumor cerebri. In Glaser, J. S., editor: Neuro-ophthalmology, vol. IX, 1977, The C. V. Mosby Co.

47. Chandler, P. A.: Use and misuse of acetazolamide (Diamox) in the treatment of glaucoma, Arch. Ophthalmol. **57:**639, 1957.

48. Harrison, R.: Annual review—glaucoma, Arch. Ophthalmol. **70:**842, 1963.

49. Spaeth, G. L.: Potassium, acetazolamide, and intraocular pressure, Arch. Ophthalmol. **78:**578, 1967.

50. Weiss, I. S.: Hirsutism after chronic administration of acetazolamide, Am. J. Ophthalmol. **78:**327, August 1974.

51. Garrison, L., Roth, A., Rundle, H., and Christensen, R. E.: A clinical comparison of three carbonic anhydrase inhibitors, Trans. Pac. Coast Otoophthalmol. Soc. **51:**137, 1967.

52. Pearson, J. R., Binder, C. I., and Neber, J.: Agranulocytosis following Diamox therapy, J.A.M.A. **157:**339, 1955.

53. Reisner, E. H., Jr., and Morgan, M. C.: Thrombocytopenia following acetazolamide (Diamox) therapy, J.A.M.A. **160:**206, 1956.

54. Glushien, A. S., and Fisher, E. R.: Renal lesions of sulfonamide type after treatment with acetazolamide (Diamox) J.A.M.A. **160:**204, 1956.

55. Constant, M. A., and Becker, B.: The effect of carbonic anhydrase inhibitors on urinary excretion of citrate by humans, Am. J. Ophthalmol. **49:**929, 1960.

56. Muirhead, J., and Scheie, H.: Transient myopia after acetazolamide, Arch. Ophthalmol. **63:**315, 1960.

57. Galin, M. A., Baras, I., and Zweifach, P.: Diamox-induced myopia, Am. J. Ophthalmol. **54:**237, 1962.

58. Beasley, F. J.: Transient myopia—ethoxzolamide, Arch. Ophthalmol. **68:**490, 1962.

59. Halpern, A. E., and Kulvin, M. M.: Transient myopia, Am. J. Ophthalmol. **48:**534, 1959.

60. Beasley, F. J.: Transient myopia and retinal edema during hydrochlorothiazide (Hydrodiuril) therapy, Arch. Ophthalmol. **65:**212, 1961.

61. Michaelson, J. J.: Transient myopia due to hygroton, Am. J. Ophthalmol. **54:**1146, 1962.

62. Reich, T.: Anhydrase activity of bovine lenses, Am. J. Ophthalmol. **36:**500, 1953.

63. Lubeck, Marvin J.: Aplastic anemia following

acetazolamide therapy, Am. J. Ophthalmol. **69:**684, 1970.

64. Wisch, N., Fischbein, F. I., Siegel, R., Glass, J. L., and Leopold, I. H.: Aplastic anemia resulting from the use of carbonic anhydrase inhibitors, Am. J. Ophthalmol. **75:**130, 1973.

65. Maren, T. H.: Teratology and carbonic anhydrase inhibition, Arch. Ophthalmol. **85:**1, 1971.

66. Lederle Laboratories research data.

67. Shields, M. B., and Simmons, R. J.: Urinary calculus during methazolamide therapy, Am. J. Ophthalmol. **81:**622, May 1976.

68. Becker, B.: Use of methazolamide (Neptazane) in the therapy of glaucoma, Am. J. Ophthalmol. **49:**1307, 1960.

69. Gonzales-Jiminez, E., and Leopold, I. H.: Effect of dichlorphenamide on the intraocular pressure of humans, Arch. Ophthalmol. **60:**427, 1958.

70. Harris, J. E., Beaudreau, O., and Hoskinson, G.: Clinical and laboratory experiences with the carbonic anhydrase inhibitor, dichlorphenamide, Am. J. Ophthalmol. **45:**120, 1958.

71. Drance, S. M.: The effects of ethoxzolamide (Cardrase) on intraocular pressure, Arch. Ophthalmol. **62:**679, 1959.

72. Drance, S. M.: Ethoxzolamide (Cardrase) in the management of chronic simple glaucoma, Arch. Ophthalmol. **64:**433, 1960.

73. Simon, K., and Bonting, S. L.: Possible usefulness of cardiac glycosides in treatment of glaucoma, Arch. Ophthalmol. **68:**227, 1962.

74. Lufkin, M. W., Harrison, C. E., Jr., Henderson, J. W., and Ogle, K. N.: Ocular distribution of digoxin-^{3}H in the cat, Am. J. Ophthalmol. **64:**1134, 1967.

75. Lissner, W., Greenlee, J. E., Cameron, J. D., and Goren, S. B.: Localization of tritiated digoxin in the rat eye, Am. J. Ophthalmol. **72:**608, 1971.

76. Langdon, H. M., and Mulberger, R. D.: Visual disturbance after ingestion of digitalis, Am. J. Ophthalmol. **28:**639, 1945.

77. Wagener, H. P., Smith, H. L., and Nickeson, R.: Retrobulbar neuritis and complete heart block caused by digitalis poisoning, Arch. Ophthalmol. **36:**478, 1946.

78. Peczon, J. D.: Clinical evaluation of digitalization in glaucoma, Arch. Ophthalmol. **71:**500, 1964.

79. Smith, J. L., and Mickatavage, R. C.: The ocular effects of topical digitalis, Am. J. Ophthalmol. **56:**889, 1963.

80. Becker, B.: Ouabain and aqueous humor dynamics in the rabbit eye, Invest. Ophthalmol. **2:**325, 1963.

81. Oppelt, W. W., and White, E. D., Jr.: Effect of ouabain on aqueous humor formation rate in cats, Invest. Ophthalmol. **7:**328, 1968.

82. Shiose, Y., and Sears, M.: Localization and other aspects of the histochemistry of nucleoside phosphatases in the ciliary epithelium of albino rabbits, Invest. Ophthalmol. **4:**64, 1965.

83. Brown, S. I., and Hedbys, B. O.: The effect of ouabain on the hydration of the cornea, Invest. Ophthalmol. **4:**216, 1965.

84. Tarkkanen, A., and Mustakallio, A.: Inhibition of monoamine oxidase in the rabbit ciliary epithelium, Acta Ophthalmol. **44:**558, 1966.

26
TRICHLORACETIC ACID

Trichloracetic acid may be very useful as a cauterizing agent in ophthalmology. It is dispensed in crystalline form and must be kept in tightly closed bottles because it is so hygroscopic that it will dissolve completely in water adsorbed from the air. For use, several crystals are placed in a glass container, and a single tiny drop of water is added. Since a saturated solution is desired, an excessive amount of water should not be used. It is applied with a toothpick, around which is tightly wound a very small amount of cotton, twisted to a point. Adequate local anesthesia is obtained by appropriate drugs. The part of the eye to be treated is gently wiped dry. The toothpick applicator is dipped into the trichloracetic acid solution, the excess fluid is touched off on the edge of the container, and the acid is gently applied to the dried surface. Almost immediately the surface will turn a milky white color. Application is continued until the entire area to be treated has been covered, as indicated by the white color. Saline irrigation is advised to wash away any acid remaining on the surface.

Trichloracetic acid cautery may be used successfully for cautery of the dendritic figures of herpetic keratitis, for surface sterilization of infected ulcers, for removal of epithelium prior to placement of a conjunctival flap, and for closure of very small leaking wounds. I must confess to having been highly skeptical of the value of trichloracetic acid in closing wounds, but its use has been repeatedly demonstrated to my satisfaction. If by means

of fluorescein a tiny wound leak has been demonstrated to cause a shallow chamber after cataract extraction, a single application of trichloracetic acid may cause enough tissue swelling to close the leak. Similarly, very small leaks persisting after suture of irregular corneal lacerations may be sealed by such treatment.

The protein-denaturing effect of trichloracetic acid is rapidly expended, so that deeper layers of tissue are unaffected. The corneal epithelium may be safely removed without damaging Bowman's membrane. On one occasion I successfully treated an epithelial downgrowth of the trabeculum with trichloracetic acid, causing no more postoperative irritation than would have been expected from the mechanical trauma of surgery.

Trichloracetic acid cautery has been advocated for treatment of iris prolapse.[1] Repeated cautery of such a prolapse is said to cause adequate scar formation to cover the wound securely. This treatment was advocated before the quality of present-day needles greatly simplified the surgical repair of iris prolapse. I believe that in virtually all cases of iris prolapse the eye would be in better condition after iris excision or replacement and direct suturing of the wound than if cautery were used. Rarely, there may occur a tiny and nonprogressive iris prolapse of perhaps a millimeter's size with virtually no gaping of the wound. In such a case a trial of trichloracetic cautery may well be justified since it is certainly easier and probably less hazardous than surgical repair. Freezing with a cryoprobe will also eradicate filtering blebs and small iris prolapses and is probably safer and more effective than chemical or thermal cautery.

REFERENCE

1. Bettman, J. W., and Barkan, H.: Trichloracetic acid in the treatment of iris prolapse, Am. J. Ophthalmol. **20:**131, 1937.

27
VASODILATORS

The rationale for the use of vasodilators in the therapy of a variety of retinal disorders is the assumption that vascular spasm directly or secondarily affects the vessels in the neighborhood of these retinal lesions.[1] Included among these disorders are tobacco amblyopia, retrobulbar and optic neuritis, acute exudative chorioretinitis, central angiospastic retinopathy, and acute closure of the central retinal artery. Subcutaneous injection of 100 mg of sodium nitrite daily was reported to be helpful in such cases.

Presumably, vasodilator treatment of a variety of degenerative disorders (notably senile macular degeneration) is similarly based on the assumptions that decreased blood supply is the primary fault and that this is reversible by vasodilation.

RESPONSE OF CHOROIDAL VESSELS

Direct observation of the choroidal vessels (rabbit) through a plastic window inserted in the sclera showed that the systemic administration of vasodilating drugs caused pallor of the choroid and decreased speed of blood flow.[2] Presumably, this effect was a result of dilation of the vessels throughout the body, with resultant shunting of blood to areas other than the eye. When observed through the scleral window, choroidal vessels did not dilate in response to tolazoline (50 mg by retrobulbar injection or 75 mg intravenously), papaverine (0.5 g intravenously), or sodium nitrite (200 mg intravenously).[3]

In a somewhat similar experiment, observation of the choroidal vessels through dehydrated (and therefore translucent) sclera showed no vasodilation after administration of nicotinic acid (1 mg/kg) and sodium nitrite (2 mg/kg).[4]

Probably the best method now available for the study of intraocular blood volume is the use of radioactive phosphorus–labeled red cells.[5] By this method the radioactivity of the blood remains almost constant for more than 1½ hours. Since the beta particles of radioactive phosphorus penetrate only 3 to 8 mm of tissue, the measured radioactivity must originate from the eye itself and not from other parts of the head. Unfortunately this method cannot differentiate radioactivity emanating from the retina and that from the choroid. However, it is known that the choroid contains far more blood than the retina and is therefore responsible for most of the measured radioactivity.

One of the best vasodilators is 10% carbon dioxide, which almost immediately doubles the chorioretinal blood volume (Fig. 27-1). In marked contrast is the complete lack of blood volume change resulting from 90% oxygen (Fig. 27-2).

Extensive experimental studies in cats with radioactive phosphorus–labeled red blood cells have established beyond question that systemic administration of effective peripheral vasodilators *decreases* the intraocular blood volume.[6] Popular vasodilators such as hexamethonium chloride, isoxsuprine

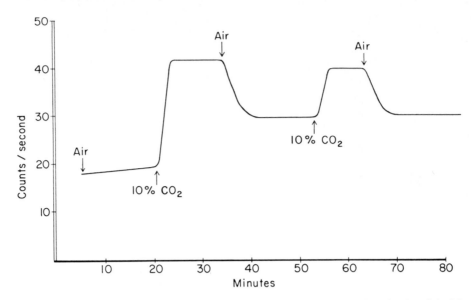

Fig. 27-1. Retinal and choroidal vasodilation produced by 10% carbon dioxide. (Modified from Bettman, J. W., and Fellows, V. G.: Am. J. Ophthalmol. **42:**161, 1956.)

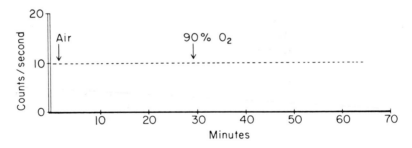

Fig. 27-2. Absence of change in retinal and choroidal blood volume during inhalation of 90% oxygen. (Modified from Bettman, J. W., and Fellows, V. G.: Am. J. Ophthalmol. **42:**161, 1956.)

(Vasodilan), methacholine (Mecholyl), nylidrin hydrochloride (Arlidin) (Fig. 27-3), and tolazoline (Priscoline) will cause within minutes of injection a decrease of intraocular blood volume as great as 30%. Nicotinic acid, one of the most popular vasodilators used by ophthalmologists, was given intravenously in 50 mg doses (considerably higher by weight than the human oral dose), but did not measurably alter intraocular blood volume. Intraocular blood volume was increased by vasoconstrictors, including epinephrine, norepinephrine (levarterenol) (Fig. 27-4), and nicotine, but these medications are not advocated for the treatment of ocular circulatory deficiencies.

Because the choroidal blood flow is actually decreased by systemically administered vasodilators, the use of such medications is contraindicated in those ocular disorders characterized by vascular occlusion or ischemia.[7]

RESPONSE OF RETINAL VESSELS

Therapy of "spasms" of the retinal circulation in various diseases presupposes that the retinal vessels to be treated are capable of spastic contraction. Experimentally, retinal

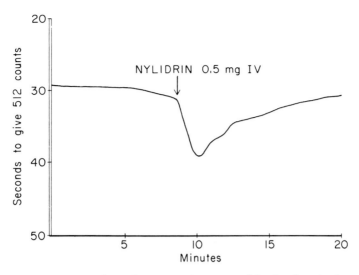

Fig. 27-3. Decrease in intraocular radioactivity (measuring blood volume) after intravenous administration of nylidrin. (Modified from Bettman, J. W., and Fellows, V. G.: Trans. Am. Acad. Ophthalmol. **66:**480, 1962.)

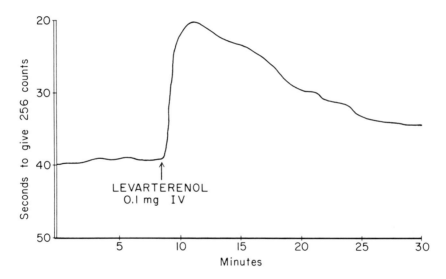

Fig. 27-4. Increase in intraocular radioactivity (measuring blood volume) after intravenous administration of levarterenol. (From Bettman, J. W., and Fellows, V. G.: Trans. Am. Acad. Ophthalmol. **66:**480, 1962.)

arteriolar constrictions can be induced by photocoagulation, electric stimulation, and direct mechanical trauma. Similar retinal arteriolar constriction can easily be induced in human beings during therapeutic photocoagulation. Venous constrictions cannot be induced by these methods.[8]

Arteriolar spasms initially affect the stimulated site and subsequently extend to involve adjacent sections of the vessel. Spasm does not extend to unstimulated vessels. (Note that these experiments were on cats, in which the retina is supplied with individual cilioretinal arterioles, unlike the human eye, which is usually nourished by a single central retinal artery. Possibly in the human eye a single lesion could cause the entire arteriolar tree to constrict.) Constriction may increase for up to 10 minutes after mechanical stimulation, but the vessel partially recovers within 30 minutes and is usually completely recovered by an hour.[8] Sectioning of the sympathetic and parasympathetic nerve supply did not alter the course of arteriolar constrictions.

The response of mechanically induced spasm of retinal arterioles to various medications has been evaluated by intravenous administration and by direct topical application to the exposed retinal arterioles. The most effective vasodilators were papaverine hydrochloride, tolazoline hydrochloride, and caffeine sodium benzoate.[9] Papaverine also relieved the arteriolar spasm when given intravenously. Inhalation of 90% oxygen and 10% carbon dioxide also reduced spasm. None of these drugs completely prevented or relieved the arteriolar spasm. Occasional vasodilation resulted from nicotinamide and phentolamine hydrochloride (Regitine). Because of the variable intensity of spasm, the results from these less effective drugs were difficult to evaluate. No vasodilating effect was recognizable after topical application of vasopressin (Pitressin), histamine, epinephrine, and neostigmine.

Documented by fundus photography, marked vasodilation of the retinal and choroidal vessels of the dog results from inhalation of 10% carbon dioxide.[10] Vessel size increased by as much as one third. Furthermore, the actual volume of cerebral blood flow is increased as much as 50% by inhalation of carbon dioxide.

Photography of human retinal vessels demonstrated that sublingual administration of 0.64 mg nitroglycerin to persons in a seated position caused a 6% and a 5% increase in the caliber of retinal arterioles and veins, respectively (seven subjects evaluated). However, retinal venous blood oxygen saturation was measured by a relative density photographic method and was found to drop from a normal of 60% saturation to 52% saturation during the nitroglycerin effect. This finding indicates that estimates of flow

changes in the retina should not be based on caliber changes of visible vessels, since this nitroglycerin vessel dilation actually reduced the flow rate of blood through the retina.[11] Use of the same technique to evaluate papaverine in a dosage of 64 mg intravenously resulted in no significant change in vessel caliber or venous oxygen saturation.

The retinal circulation time may be measured by densitometric measurement of fluorescein in serial fundus photographs and averages 4.7 seconds. Sublingual nitroglycerin, although it dilates retinal vessels, lengthens the circulation time by 40%, again indicating that measurements of vessel diameter may not correlate directly with flow rate of blood through the vessels.[12] By this method of measurement, oxygen-induced retinal arteriolar constriction was estimated to reduce the oxygen delivery rate by 50%. This response appears to protect the retina from the delivery of excessive oxygen.

The oxygen concentration of blood in the retinal vessels may be measured by comparison of the optical density of the vessels as photographed through red and green filters.[13] As measured by this technique, retinal arteriolar oxygen saturation when breathing atmospheric air is 55%. Breathing 100% oxygen increases retinal arteriolar oxygen saturation to 82% despite causing arteriolar attenuation. Breathing 90% oxygen and 10% carbon dioxide eliminates the arteriolar attenuation and increases oxygen saturation to 88%.

What clinical possibilities follow from these experiments? Effective vasodilating drugs might be beneficial in diseases causing acute constriction of the retinal arterioles. These drugs include papaverine, tolazoline, and inhalation of carbon dioxide and oxygen. It is doubtful that venous caliber is influenced by these medications, and chronic venous occlusive disease is unlikely to benefit from treatment with vasodilators.

SYSTEMIC EFFECTS

When given in moderately large clinical doses—for example, nicotinic acid, 100 mg three times a day after meals; nicotinyl alcohol (Roniacol), 50 mg three times a day after meals; tolazoline, 25 mg three times a day after meals; and nylidrin, 6 mg three times a day after meals—vasodilator drugs induce characteristic general responses.[14] The skin flushes and causes chilly sensations. The patient may feel as if the hair is rising on the back of the head. Lightheadedness and faintness may be disturbing. Heartburn and stomach discomfort are minimized by taking the medication after meals, but peptic ulceration is reported.

Use of drugs that materially lower blood pressure may be dangerous in patients with coronary insufficiency. Since tolazoline increases gastric secretion of hydrochloric acid, its use is contraindicated in patients predisposed to gastrointestinal peptic ulceration.

Very large doses of nicotinic acid (3000 to 6000 mg/day) will lower blood cholesterol but cause marked side effects, including flushing, itching, diarrhea, and vomiting. In one patient receiving 6000 mg/day for over a year, paracentral scotomas and reduced visual acuity (20/30) resulted but cleared within 3 days after nicotinic acid therapy was discontinued.[15] In such large doses, nicotinic acid will seriously impair diabetic control, causing hyperglycemia and ketosis despite increased insulin.[16] (The usual ophthalmologic prescription is for 150 to 300 mg of nicotinic acid/day.)

One should be willing to recognize that drugs may have actions other than the presumed mechanism. Niacin, in dosage of 3.0 g/day, can sustain over a 5-year period a 10% drop in serum cholesterol levels and a 26% drop of serum triglyceride levels. This dosage level was given to 1119 myocardial infarction patients in a controlled research protocol. As compared to the placebo group, niacin treatment did not reduce mortality. It did increase serum uric acid (and clinical gouty arthritis) and elevated serum glucose.[17] Of course, this has nothing to do with eyes, but it does illustrate that niacin does other things besides dilate vessels.

CLINICAL USE

Adequately controlled studies supporting the use of vasodilators for any ocular condi-

tion are hard to find. I am inclined to doubt that reduced blood flow that can be improved by vasodilator drugs is responsible for any purely ocular disease except embolic arteriolar occlusion. Experimental ocular data[9] and knowledge gained from the use of vasodilators in general medical disorders indicate that arteriolar spasms associated with direct irritation (as by an embolus) are benefited by vasodilators.

When vasodilators are used to increase ocular blood flow, the patient should be recumbent. Otherwise dependent pooling of blood in the dilated vessels of the systemic circulation will reduce rather than improve ocular blood flow. (Reduced cerebral blood flow in erect patients after excessive vasodilation may be readily evident—the patient faints.)

In fairness to the opposite point of view, a representative article strongly advocating vasodilator therapy of senile macular degeneration is cited. Of 203 patients with assorted macular degenerative conditions treated three times a day with nylidrin, 6 mg, only 16% suffered further visual loss when followed for periods of up to 13 years.[14] Fourteen percent showed improvement; the rest were unchanged. Unfortunately the study included no comparative control series of untreated cases. The clinical classification was sufficiently indefinite to preclude a reasonably reliable estimate as to the spontaneous course of the disorders. Hence I find it impossible to interpret the significance of these results.

SUMMARY

Although vasodilators applied directly to the retinal vessels (experimentally) do indeed relax induced retinal arteriolar "spasms," systemic administration of vasodilators demonstrably shunts blood away from the eye (when the patient is erect). Since vasodilators therefore ordinarily reduce rather than enhance ocular blood flow, and because little evidence exists that arteriolar constriction reversible by vasodilators causes any type (except embolic and hypertensive) of ocular pathology, I can see no reason (other than a placebo effect) for the use of vasodilators in the practice of ophthalmology. An exception to this might be the management of a fresh embolus to the retinal circulation.

Perhaps the clinician will have a more accurate concept of the tissue effects of vasodilators if the term "stagnator" is substituted, indicating that blood flow is slowed rather than enhanced by such drugs.

REFERENCES

1. Cordes, F. C.: The use of vasodilators in acute fundus disease, Am. J. Ophthalmol. **26:** 916, 1943.
2. Wudka, E., and Leopold, I. H.: Experimental studies of the choroidal vessels, Arch. Ophthalmol. **55:**857, 1956.
3. Paul, S. D., and Leopold, I. H.: The effect of vasodilating drugs on choroidal circulation, Am. J. Ophthalmol. **42:**899, 1956.
4. Stein, H. A., Wakim, K. G., and Rucker, C. W.: In vivo studies on the choroidal circulation of rabbits, Arch. Ophthalmol. **56:**726, 1956.
5. Bettman, J. W., and Fellows, V. G.: A technique for the determination of blood-volume changes, Am. J. Ophthalmol. **42:**161, 1956.
6. Bettman, J. W., and Fellows, V.: Effect of peripheral vasodilator and vasoconstrictor drugs on the intraocular (choroidal) blood volume, Trans. Am. Acad. Ophthalmol. **66:**480, 1962.
7. Friedman, E.: Choroidal blood flow, Arch. Ophthalmol. **83:**96, 1970.
8. Lende, R. A., and Ellis, P. P.: Induced spasm in the retinal arterioles of cats. I. Mechanisms and characteristics, Arch. Ophthalmol. **71:** 701, 1964.
9. Ellis, P. P., and Lende, R. A.: Induced spasm in the retinal arterioles of cats. II. Influences of physical factors and drugs, Arch. Ophthalmol. **71:**706, 1964.
10. Spalter, H. F., TenEick, R. E., and Nahas, G. G.: Effect of hypercapnia on retinal vessel size at constant intracranial pressure, Am. J. Ophthalmol. **57:**741, 1964.
11. Frayser, R., and Hickam, J. B.: Effect of vasodilator drugs on the retinal blood flow in man, Arch. Ophthalmol. **73:**640, 1965.
12. Hickam, J. B., and Frayser, R.: A photographic method for measuring the mean retinal circulation time using fluorescein, Invest. Ophthalmol. **4:**876, 1965.
13. Frayser, R., and Hickam, J. B.: Retinal vascular response to breathing increased carbon dioxide and oxygen concentrations, Invest. Ophthalmol. **3:**427, 1964.
14. Laws, H. W.: Peripheral vasodilators in the treatment of macular degenerative changes in the eye, Can. Med. Assoc. J. **91:**325, 1964.
15. Harris, J. L.: Toxic amblyopia, Am. J. Ophthalmol. **55:**133, 1963.
16. Janovsky, R. C.: Diabetogenic effects of nicotinic acid, Ohio Med. J. **64:**1139, 1968.
17. The coronary drug project research group: Clofibrate and niacin in coronary heart disease, J.A.M.A. **231:**360, January 27, 1975.

28
VISCOUS MEDICATIONS

Because of their viscosity and wetting characteristics, methylcellulose, polyvinyl alcohol, silicone fluids, and various polymers are of value to the ophthalmologist.

The wetting characteristics of various materials can be studied by measuring the contact angle of a drop of saline on the experimental surface. This measurement indicates the effectiveness of the preparation in causing wettability of the cornea or of a contact lens. This wetting angle measurement changes considerably with various additives, whether they be viscous agents, wetting agents, polymers, preservatives, stabilizers, or other chemicals. Hence the final properties of a preparation may be modified greatly by its formulation. The contact angle measurements of 12 popular ocular contact lens solutions varied from 51° to 20°.[1] For reference, bovine salivary mucin has a contact angle of 24°.

A significant factor in corneal integrity is the break-up time of the tear film. This may be increased by wetting agents (such as methylcellulose) but can be reduced by ointment vehicles.[2] Hydrophilic ointments are not, of course, effective wetting vehicles.

METHYLCELLULOSE

Methylcellulose is a viscous, transparent, nonirritating, water-soluble compound used in ophthalmology as a lubricant and as a vehicle that substantially prolongs the contact time of topically applied drugs. Methylcellulose is nearly inert chemically and is entirely compatible with the drugs commonly used in ophthalmology. It is stable and may be sterilized by boiling. Growth of microorganisms is not supported by methylcellulose.[3]

Toxicity

Methylcellulose is nonirritating to ocular tissue and may be used without fear of eye damage. Topical instillation of 1% solutions can be continued indefinitely without altering the appearance of the normal eye. The healing of experimental corneal epithelial wounds is not slowed by a 2% methycellulose solution.[4] Subconjunctival injection (in rabbits) of 0.1 ml of a 1% methylcellulose solution causes no irritation.[3]

The tolerance of the rabbit eye to 1.4% polyvinyl alcohol in isotonic saline solution and to 0.5% methycellulose in isotonic saline solution was studied by introducing 0.2 ml of each solution into the anterior chamber.[5] Mild to moderate conjunctival hyperemia was the result in 5 of 24 polyvinyl alcohol–treated eyes and in 28 of 36 methylcellulose eyes. Corneal edema occurred in eight of the methylcellulose–treated eyes, but in none of the polyvinyl alcohol–treated eyes.[5] This reaction has subsequently been shown to be caused by a 0.9% sodium chloride solution. When 0.1 ml of 0.5% methylcellulose in balanced salt solution (a mixture of electrolytes designed to approximate the composition of tissue fluids[6]) was injected into the anterior chamber, no irritation resulted other than would be expected from the trauma of the needle. After such injection, traces of methylcellulose are detectable in the aqueous for 3 days.[7]

Before demonstration that the 0.9% saline solution was responsible for the mild iridocyclitis, ophthalmologists were advised not to use methylcellulose solutions during intraocular surgery. However, there now appears to be no reason to fear that clinically useful concentrations of methylcellulose will affect the intraocular structures adversely.

Experimentally, glaucoma may be produced by filling the anterior chamber with 2.5% methylcellulose. This solution is too viscous to escape through the trabecular spaces and produces an acute rise in pressure.[8]

Preparation

The 4000 centipoise viscosity of methylcellulose is preferable for ophthalmic use. It is not readily dissolved in water; hence the following procedure is recommended. The methylcellulose fibers should be boiled for 20 to 30 minutes in half the desired volume of water. The suspension is then cooled to 5° to 10° C, and the remaining water is added. Methylcellulose is more soluble in cold water than in hot, but the resistance of the dry fibers to wetting is decreased by boiling. Concentrations of 0.5% to 2% are used in ophthalmology.

Clinical use

Methylcellulose, 0.5%, in a 0.9% sodium chloride solution makes excellent artificial tears. Lubrication with such a solution is helpful to patients with keratoconjunctivitis sicca, neuroparalytic keratopathy, or exposure keratopathy.

At least in theory, lacrimal substitutes (artificial tears) should correspond in chemical composition to the precorneal film. This precorneal film seems to be a most complex fluid sheet that resists evaporation, has excellent wetting characteristics, and is optically perfect. The film has both water and fat solubility characteristics. An hypothesis of the structure of the precorneal tear film suggests it is a thin sheet of water (and dissolved elements) lined both anteriorly and posteriorly by a monomolecular lipid layer.[9] One is led to speculate whether the ideal artificial tear might be some type of emulsion formulated to duplicate the lipid- and water-soluble, wetting, protective, and lubricating properties of the normal precorneal film. Clearly, such a simple substitute as normal saline solution is not an adequate tear replacement solution for therapeutic use.

Contact lenses may be moistened with methylcellulose solution. More viscous solutions (1%) are desirable for application of gonioscopic lenses, the three-mirror prism, and similar optical devices. The thick solution achieves a good contact with the cornea and is not readily lost during application.

In higher concentrations, methylcellulose becomes sufficiently viscous to be classified as an ointment. A 2.5% methylcellulose ointment may be used for gonioscopy and has the advantage of ensuring an optically tight fit with no tendency to leakage of coupling solution. A recommended formula is as follows:

Methylcellulose powder, 4000 centipoise	2.5 g
Methylparaben	0.023 g
Propylparaben	0.01 g
Sodium chloride	1.2 g
Distilled water as needed to	100 ml

If care is taken to prepare this ointment free of bubbles, it is optically perfectly clear. The preservatives maintain sterility and yet are nonirritating to the cornea.[10]

The abrasive effect of a tonometer on the cornea may be reduced by instillation of a 1% methylcellulose solution immediately prior to tonometry.[11] The methylcellulose may be incorporated in the anesthetic vehicle; however, this prolongs the anesthetic duration somewhat, which itself causes minor corneal damage. The viscosity of a 1% methylcellulose solution does not alter tonometer readings, but stronger solutions may slow plunger movement because of capillary attraction.

The incorporation of methylcellulose in ophthalmic solutions causes the medication to remain in contact with the cornea for a longer time and thereby enhances its effect.

The effect of a methylcellulose vehicle for a 2% pilocarpine concentration was compared with a 2% aqueous solution of pilocarpine in 17 patients with chronic simple glaucoma.[12] After 1 week without medication, these patients received 1 drop of aqueous pilocarpine in the right eye and 1 drop of methylcellulose pilocarpine in the left eye. The following week the solutions were placed in the opposite eyes. Pupil size was measured by photography before and 6 hours after medication. Tensions were taken 6 hours after medication. The average pupil diameter of all eyes and 2.6 mm after methylcellulose pilocarpine. Average intraocular pressure was 22.2 mm Hg after aqueous pilocarpine and 20.5 mm Hg after methylcellulose pilocarpine.

In an experimental study in which *Pseudomonas* organisms were injected into a rabbit cornea and followed by hourly instillations of neomycin in different vehicles, 76% of the infections were prevented by 1% neomycin in a methylcellulose vehicle, as compared to 44% in a polyvinyl alcohol vehicle and 38% in a polyvinylpyrrolidone vehicle. Presumably the results were caused by enhanced contact time with the methylcellulose vehicle.[13]

Actually, the contact time of topical medications with the eye is far shorter than one would imagine. Computerized microscintigraphy, using technetium 99m, will show the rate of loss of the labeled vehicle from a human eye. After 90 seconds, only 2.9% of radioactivity remains when using a saline vehicle. Only 4.3% remains with polyvinyl alcohol 1.4%. Only 8.8% remains with hydroxypropyl methylcellulose 0.5%.[14] Of course, 90 seconds later, a comparable percentage drop of the remaining material will again occur. Obviously, medication contact time is not very long.

POLYVINYL ALCOHOL

Polyvinyl alcohol, 1.4%, in water or isotonic saline solution, is another vehicle useful in prolonging the ocular contact of ophthalmic medications.[15] It is nontoxic, compatible with most ophthalmic medications and preservatives, and readily sterilized by autoclaving or filtering.

Studies of the regeneration of damaged corneal epithelium suggest that polyvinyl alcohol instillation only slightly retards regeneration of corneal epithelium. The variability of these experiments precluded a definite conclusion as to whether epithelial regeneration was more rapid with isotonic saline solution, methylcellulose, or polyvinyl alcohol. Actually all three types of drops were reported to slow healing of rabbit corneas slightly more than no treatment at all.

Polyvinyl alcohol is much less viscous than methylcellulose. A 1.4% solution has a viscosity of 4.4 centipoise in contrast to 50 centipoise for a 0.5% solution of methylcellulose.

Because it remains in the aqueous vehicle and does not penetrate the corneal epithelium, nickel chloride was selected as a test substance to determine ocular contact time after topical application in various solutions (0.5% methylcellulose, 1.4% polyvinyl alcohol, and isotonic saline solution). The time in minutes after application of a 0.5% nickel chloride solution was measured until nickel was no longer demonstrable on the conjunctiva by the dimethylgloxime test. In saline solution the nickel disappeared in 9 to 12 minutes; in methylcellulose, 10 to 13 minutes; and in polyvinyl alcohol, 11 to 13 minutes. Although contact time is prolonged by both methylcellulose and polyvinyl alcohol, their effect obviously lasts for only a very few minutes and is not comparable to the effect of a long-lasting ointment vehicle.

SILICONE FLUIDS

Lubrication of artificial eyes with silicone fluids has increased the comfort of wearing such a prosthesis and has improved prosthesis appearance. In a series of 35 patients, 28 reported socket irritation to be reduced by silicone use.[16] In addition, the silicone prevented discharge from crusting on the lids and the prosthesis. The glistening silicone film on the prosthesis surface also imparted a more lifelike appearance to the artificial eye.

The silicone used was Medical Fluid 360.* Viscosities of 100 and 350 centistokes were

---

*Dow Corning Corp., Midland, Mich.

used, with almost equal patient acceptance (slight preference for the thinner fluid, 100 centistokes). Frequency of use was variable, depending on the patient's comfort, but was usually three or four times daily.

Silicone usage did not decrease the volume of discharge or otherwise benefit socket infection. Although silicones are inert and do not support bacterial growth, they have no antibacterial properties.

Silicone eye drops of 100 centistokes of viscosity are preferable to the use of methylcellulose drops for the lubrication of artificial eyes if the lids do not close during sleep. Dry crusts of methylcellulose and mucus form on the prosthesis if the lids do not close and may be irritating to the lids. However, silicone drops have the disadvantage of making the prosthesis water repellent. Once used, the silicone drop must be continued daily, since tears will not properly moisten and lubricate the prosthesis thereafter.[17]

POLYMER DERIVATIVES

Reasoning that the most important component of the normal tear film is the mucus layer, and assuming that the mucus functions by adhering to the corneal epithelium and increasing its surface tension, an attempt has been made to duplicate the characteristics of mucus with a mixture of ethylene glycol polymers and polyvinylpyrrolidone. This preparation, Adapt,* also contains 0.5% hydroxyethyl cellulose, 0.004% thimerosal, and 0.1% EDTA. This "artificial mucus" was originally introduced as a contact lens wetting solution but was found to be comparably effective in wetting the dry cornea.[18,19] It binds persistently to solids and has a very high surface tension, thereby producing an easily wettable surface.[20]

---

*Burton, Parsons & Co., Inc., Washington, D.C.

REFERENCES

1. Lemp, M. A., and Szymanski, E. S.: Polymer adsorption at the ocular surface, Arch. Ophthalmol. **93**:134, February 1975.
2. Norn, M. S.: Topical fluorescein penetration, Am. J. Ophthalmol. **79**:335, February 1975.
3. Swan, K. C.: Use of methylcellulose in ophthalmology, Arch. Ophthalmol. **33**:378, 1945.
4. Alexander, C. M., and Newell, F. W.: The effect of various agents on corneal epithelization, Am. J. Ophthalmol. **48**:210, 1959.
5. Krishna, N., and Mitchell, B.: Polyvinyl alcohol as an ophthalmic vehicle, Am. J. Ophthalmol. **59**:860, 1965.
6. Merrill, D. L., Fleming, T. C., and Girard, L. J.: The effects of physiologic balanced salt solutions and normal saline on intraocular and extraocular tissues, Am. J. Ophthalmol. **49**: 895, 1960.
7. Fleming, T. C., Merrill, D. L., and Girard, L. J.: Studies of the irritating action of methylcellulose, Arch. Ophthalmol. **61**:865, 1959.
8. Virno, M., Bucci, M. G., Pecori-Giraldi, J., and Cantore, G.: Intravenous glycerol-vitamin C (sodium salt) as osmotic agents to reduce intraocular pressure, Am. J. Ophthalmol. **62**:824, 1966.
9. Ehlers, N.: The precorneal film, Acta Ophthalmol. **81** (supp.):1, 1965.
10. Miller, D., Aquino, M. V., and Fiore, A. S.: Gonioscopy ointment, Am. J. Ophthalmol. **67**:419, 1969.
11. Jervey, J. W.: Tonometry and the cornea, Arch. Ophthalmol. **56**:109, 1956.
12. Haas, J. S., and Merrill, D. L.: The effect of methylcellulose on responses to solutions of pilocarpine, Am. J. Ophthalmol. **54**:21, 1962.
13. Bach, F. C., Riddel, G., Miller, C., Martin, J. A., and Mullins, J. D.: The influence of vehicles on neomycin sulfate prevention of experimental ocular infection in rabbits, Am. J. Ophthalmol. **69**:659, 1970.
14. Trueblood, J. H., Rossomondo, R. M., Carlton, W. H., and Wilson, L. A.: Corneal contact times of ophthalmic vehicles, Arch. Ophthalmol. **93**:127, February 1975.
15. Krishna, N., and Brow, F.: Polyvinyl alcohol as an ophthalmic vehicle, Am. J. Ophthalmol. **57**:99, 1964.
16. Morgan, J. F., and Hill, J. C.: Silicone fluid as a lubricant for artificial eyes, Am. J. Ophthalmol. **58**:767, 1964.
17. Spivey, B. E., Allen, L., and Burns, C. A.: The Iowa enucleation implant, a 10-year evaluation of technique and results, Am. J. Ophthalmol. **67**:171, 1969.
18. Flanary, L. M., and Block, J. H.: Mucus substitutes for the dry-eyed contact lens wearer, J. Contact Lens Soc. Am. **4**:36, 1970.
19. Barsam, P. C., Sampson, W. G., and Feld-

man, G. L.: Treatment of the dry eye and related problems, Ann. Ophthalmol. 4:122, 1972.

20. Holly, F. J., and Lemp, M. A.: Surface chemistry of the tearfilm; implications for dry eye syndromes, contact lenses, and ophthalmic polymers, J. Contact Lens Soc. Am. 5:12, 1971.

29
VITAMINS

Deficiencies of vitamins are well known to cause typical ocular disorders. Night blindness and corneal xerosis result from vitamin A deficiency. Thiamine lack results in neurologic deficits, notably affecting the optic nerve. Scorbutic orbital hemorrhages may produce exophthalmos of sudden onset. Unless irreversible tissue changes have developed, vitamin therapy will restore function. No diseases other than the specific deficiency conditions are benefited by vitamins. Treatment with a large excess of vitamins is of no more benefit than the required amount. In-

deed, excessive doses of vitamins A, D, and K may be toxic. The recommended daily therapeutic doses are as follows: vitamin A, 25,000 units; thiamine, 2 mg; riboflavin, 2 mg; niacin, 20 mg; pyridoxine, 2 mg; cyanocobalamin (B_{12}), 1 μg; ascorbic acid, 100 mg; and vitamin D, 800 units.

Multivitamin preparations are now very extensively (and unnecessarily) used. The massive amounts of vitamins in many of these capsules are far greater than established therapeutic dosages and normal vitamin requirements. The widespread excessive use of

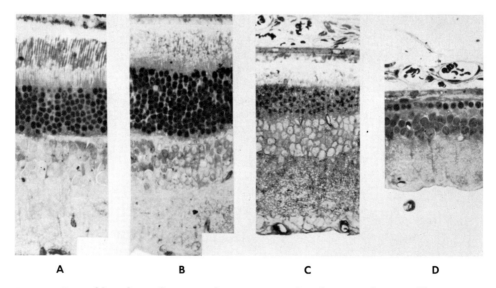

A B C D

Fig. 29-1. Retinal histology of rats raised on vitamin A–free diets supplemented by vitamin A acid. **A,** Control rats. **B,** Two-month deficiency. **C,** Six-month deficiency. **D,** Ten-month deficiency. (From Dowling, J.: Am. J. Ophthalmol. **50:**875, 1960.)

vitamins has fostered the erroneous conviction among laymen (and probably among some physicians) that extra vitamins increase resistance to disease, retard degenerative changes, and in general promote good health.

VITAMIN A
Effect of deficiency on the retina

A combination of the aldehyde derivative of vitamin A with visual protein (opsin) results in rhodopsin, the visual pigment of the rod visual system. A variety of isomers of vitamin A exist, but not all are capable of forming rhodopsin. Only the 7-*cis* isomer of vitamin A can join with opsin to form visual pigment. Rhodopsin bleaching releases the *trans* isomer of vitamin A, which is inactive and cannot be utilized to resynthesize rhodopsin. Enzymes within the eye catalyze the transformation of the inactive isomers to the 7-*cis* form.

In addition to rhodopsin, iodopsin (the cone visual pigment) is also synthesized from 7-*cis* vitamin A. This explains why both rod and cone vision deteriorate in vitamin A deficiency.

In the early stages of night blindness, treatment with vitamin A will cure the dysfunction within hours. Later, however, some degree of night blindness will remain for months despite high-dosage vitamin A. One explanation for this delayed recovery supposes that chronic deficiency causes loss of the protein opsin. Rhodopsin is not only a functional part of the visual cell but it is also an important structural part. About 40% of the dry weight of a frog rod is rhodopsin. Actual structural changes in the outer segments of the visual cells occur with long-standing vitamin A deficiency. These structural changes repair very slowly or not at all if destruction is sufficiently advanced.[1]

The functional and structural retinal damage caused by vitamin A deficiency has been clearly demonstrated in rats raised on a vitamin A–deficient diet supplemented by vitamin A acid.[2] Vitamin A acid prevents the symptoms of vitamin A deficiency in all tissues except the retina. The acid cannot be converted in vivo to either retinene or vitamin A, which are both necessary for rod and cone function. Vitamin A–deficient young rats die in about 2 months, at which time retinal deterioration is just beginning. Addition of vitamin A acid to their diet maintains the rats in good health indefinitely and yet permits retinal damage to develop as in untreated deficiency. In this way, the entire sequence of retinal destruction by vitamin A deficiency may be studied. Fig. 29-1 shows retinal sections from control and vitamin A–deficient rats (supplemented by vitamin A acid) after 2-, 6-, and 10-month deficiencies. The first histologic changes occur in the rod outer segments after about 2 months of deficiency. By 6 months the outer segments are almost completely gone, and fewer than half the cells of the outer nuclear layer remain. After 10 months the visual cells are entirely gone, but the inner layers of retina are relatively normal.

As might be expected, treatment with vitamin A will restore the damaged cells to health as long as they survive (even though they are not functional while deficient). When the visual cells have disappeared, no amount of treatment with vitamin A will restore vision. Recovery with treatment is shown in Fig. 29-2. Comparison with the control rat shows that the rat deficient for 6½ months has lost about half its visual cells. Sixteen days after this 6½-month deficiency is treated with vitamin A the surviving nuclei have regained their normal form and have regenerated outer segments. The tracings are ERG responses to graded light intensities. The deficient retina shows great loss of light sensitivity, which is markedly improved by treatment, but does not return completely to normal.

Because of the variability of preexisting liver stores of vitamin A, the degree of vitamin A dietary deficiency, species differences, and other conditions, the time required for the development and the cure of human vitamin A deficiency may be quite different from that for these rats. Nevertheless, these experimental findings supplement and are compatible with the clinical knowledge that the night

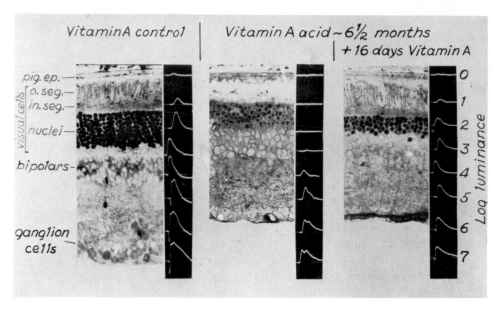

Fig. 29-2. Recovery of remaining visual cells after treatment of vitamin A deficiency of 6½ months' duration. (From Dowling, J.: Am. J. Ophthalmol. **50:**875, 1960.)

blindness of vitamin A deficiency is completely reversible in its early stages, but that vitamin A deficiency may cause permanent damage if it is prolonged and severe.

The emphasis placed on photochemical utilization of vitamin A leads us to imagine that vitamin A deficiency will cause solely rod and cone degeneration. This is not true, for this deficiency causes damage also to the retinal pigment epithelium and to all layers of the retina, including Mueller's glial cells. Actually, pigment cell changes precede those in the outer segments.[3] Whitish spots similar to those seen in retinitis punctata albescens and fundus albipunctata (disorders affecting the pigment epithelium) may appear in vitamin A deficiency and disappear with adequate treatment.

Vitamin A transport

The complexity of photochemical metabolism is well known to all visual scientists since Wald's Nobel Prize work. Even the transport of vitamin A is complex. It does not exist in plasma as a free vitamin but is firmly bound to a small specific protein known as retinol binding protein (RBP). By radioactive labeling, this RBP is found to have a specific affinity for the choroidal surface of the retinal pigment cells (not for the neuroreceptors themselves). The retinol then enters the pigment cell, which transfers it to the rod or cone.[4] Discovery of this specific binding mechanism of vitamin A transport identifies another way in which nutritional disorders may cause eye damage. (Refer to the section on xerophthalmia for discussion of the clinical importance of protein transport in malnutrition.)

An example of such a defect may exist in familial hypobetalipoproteinemia, a rare condition in which this lipid carrier molecule is deficient. Plasma vitamin A concentrations are often very low in hypobetalipoproteinemia. Atypical retinitis pigmentosa is a part of this syndrome, suggesting that perhaps this retinal disorder is a manifestation of vitamin A transport deficiency. Unfortunately for this supposition, water-soluble preparations of vitamin A do not prevent retinal degeneration in hypobetalipoproteinemia. Also, retinitis pigmentosa does not develop in vitamin A deficiency states.[5]

Optic nerve damage. Blindness in calves deficient in vitamin A has long been known.[6] The traditional mechanism of such blindness,

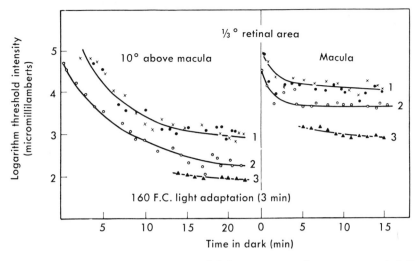

Fig. 29-3. Dark adaptation curves. *Curve 1:* solid dots represent chronic vitamin A deficiency; crosses indicate response after 8 days of vitamin A therapy. *Curve 2:* after 4 months of normal diet and high vitamin supplements. *Curve 3:* normal person. (From Steffens, L. F., and Sheard, C.: Am. J. Ophthalmol. **23:**1325, 1940.)

failure of rhodopsin synthesis and consequent neuroepithelial degeneration, is apparently only partially responsible for this optic atrophy. The vitamin A–deficient calves develop a long overgrowth of the skull that markedly narrows the optic foramen. Constriction of the optic nerve by the narrowed optic foramen ultimately results in ischemic necrosis of the nerve.

Use of electroretinography. Electroretinography is of considerable theoretical and some practical value in vitamin A deficiency. The ERG is rather abruptly extinguished when the vitamin A level of the blood falls to a level that causes the clinical manifestations of night blindness. This threshold is about 20 units of vitamin A/100 ml of plasma. The ERG may be completely extinguished even though the retina is still structurally normal and only functionally affected. At this stage the condition is still reversible by vitamin therapy. Electroretinography should be of help in differentiating malingering from organic diseases in a patient complaining of night blindness despite an ophthalmoscopically normal fundus. In contrast to nyctalopia, no direct relationship exists between vitamin A deficiency and xerosis. Further-

more, xerosis often does not respond well to treatment with vitamin A.[7]

Determination of plasma levels. The laboratory measurement of blood levels of vitamin A is a considerably more sensitive indicator of vitamin deficiency than is study of dark adaptation.[8] Furthermore, the vitamin A blood level is a specific and objective measurement in contrast to the nonspecific and subjective nature of dark adaptation studies. Normally, 100 ml of serum should contain from 75 to 150 units of vitamin A.

Dark adaptation. The visual response to intensive vitamin A treatment of chronic vitamin deficiency is shown in Fig. 29-3.[9] These dark adaptation curves were obtained from a patient after having been on a deficient diet for 9 months (curve 1, solid dots), after 8 days of high vitamin A therapy (curve 1, crosses), and after 4 months of high vitamin intake and normal diet (curve 2). Clearly the effect of severe vitamin A deficiency is only slowly and incompletely reversible by dietary replacement.

The normal rate of dark adaptation cannot be improved by supplemental vitamin A treatment of normal persons. The normal individual has a sufficient excess of vitamin A so that no visual abnormalities will result from a month of vitamin A dietary deficiency.[10]

Night blindness is, of course, not only a symptom of vitamin A deficiency but is also caused by numerous diseases of the eye, including glaucoma, optic neuritis, and others, as well as retinitis pigmentosa, the classic cause.[11]

Surface manifestations. Bitot's spots are popularly considered to be evidence of vitamin A deficiency. They are slightly refractile, silvery gray, often foamlike, frequently triangular surface deposits ordinarily situated near the temporal limbus. Conjunctival xerosis (keratinization) usually accompanies Bitot's spots. During a study of Ethiopian children, 891 vitamin A and carotene serum levels were measured—422 from schoolchildren with Bitot's spots and 469 from control children.[12] There was no significant difference in the vitamin A serum levels in the two groups. Furthermore, dark adaptation studies were normal in both groups of children. This study suggested that Bitot's spots were a sign of nonspecific nutritional deficiency but showed no correlation with vitamin A deficiency.

Faulty gastrointestinal absorption of vitamin A may cause the characteristic corneal changes of avitaminosis that respond readily to parenteral administration of vitamin A.[13]

Two cases of secondary bacterial corneal ulceration superimposed on xerotic corneas were encountered in chronic alcoholics with vitamin A deficiency. Conjunctival biopsy showed marked keratinization and complete absence of the conjunctival goblet cells. After 2 months of therapy with 25,000 units of vitamin A daily, the cornea and conjunctiva regained their normal lustrous appearance and a repeat biopsy showed a reappearance of the conjunctival goblet cells.[14]

Xerophthalmia (keratomalacia). Corneal damage resulting from vitamin A deficiency is considered to be a leading cause of bilateral blindness in preschool children living in poverty-stricken countries. Corneal destruction is invariably associated with severe generalized malnutrition.

El Salvador was identified as being the Central American country with the highest incidence of hypovitaminosis A. Because of this, a survey of 9508 children was made by house-to-house visiting of the rural and slum population. Only 3 children in the entire group were found to have bilateral corneal scarring believed most likely to be caused by vitamin A deficiency. No active cases were found. Statistical projections from this sample to the entire population suggest that there may be 43 new cases per year of bilateral corneal scarring caused by vitamin A deficiency in El Salvador.[15]

Nationwide distribution of vitamin A supplements twice a year to all children has been proposed as a method of prophylaxis against xerophthalmia. The method proposed is to assemble children between 1 and 5 years of age at distribution centers, where 200,000 units of vitamin A are placed into each child's mouth. Additional efforts are made to seek out absent children. Evaluation of the effectiveness of this program was attempted by study of the admissions to the principal pediatric hospital in El Salvador, an institution offering wide geographic coverage of the entire country. During the 12 months preceding the mass administration of vitamin A, 33 hospitalized children were diagnosed as having vitamin A deficiency corneal destruction. During the subsequent 12 months, 31 children were diagnosed.

It has been assumed, without proof, that mass distribution of vitamin A will prevent keratomalacia. Why did the program fail? One third of the affected patients were under the age of 1 year, which had not been expected because breast feeding (apparently abandoned) supplies vitamins. Another reason why prophylaxis was not advised for this group under 1 year of age is that 200,000 units of vitamin A commonly is toxic to the infant. Twelve percent of the affected patients were over 6 years of age. Hence half of the affected children were ineligible for the prophylactic program. Also, measles serologic studies suggested that only 80% of the target population was actually reached. (Measles vaccine and vitamin A were administered simultaneously.)

Actually, only half of the dose of 200,000 units is absorbed by normal children. Malnutrition interferes with both absorption and utilization of the vitamin. Finally, 2 children with monocular keratomalacia lost their second eye despite massive oral and parenteral vitamin A therapy.

Unfortunately, therefore, it must be concluded that prophylaxis with vitamin A alone is inadequate to prevent xerophthalmia in a population with many severely malnourished children.[16]

The age distribution of vitamin A deficiency corneal scarring as found in northern Haiti is shown in Fig. 29-4.[17] This identifies the first 3 years of life as being the time of greatest incidence, with relatively fewer cases occurring subsequently. Bilateral corneal involvement was present in 65% of these children. Although 5589 children were examined in Haiti and 17 cases of presumed xerophthalmia were identified, not a single Bitot's spot was encountered. Obviously, Bitot's spots are of no diagnostic value in malnourished children. Significant amounts of keratomalacia occur in the complete absence of Bitot's spots, which cannot be used as an index of the vitamin A status of the population.

The mortality of nonhospitalized malnourished children with keratomalacia is about 50%, which reduces the percentage of eye damage found in older, surviving children.[17]

Although a specific nutritional deficiency has been classically represented as being the cause of ulceration and perforation of the xerophthalmic cornea, this concept does not fully explain the sporadic incidence of the disease within large groups of malnourished children, the suddenness of corneal damage apparently unrelated to worsening nutrition, and the apparent resistance of some cases to massive vitamin treatment. During a 2-year period, 100 cases of hypovitaminosis A with xerophthalmia were seen in the Philippines.[18] Bacterial cultures of the eye demonstrated pathogenic bacteria in 86%. Of 29 cases with corneal ulceration and 22 additional cases with corneal perforation, all but 2 harbored pathogenic bacteria (such as *Pseudomonas aeruginosa*, *Diplococcus pneumoniae*, and *Staphylococcus aureus*). Whether because of reduced resistance in a malnourished child, poor hygiene, or some other cause, bacterial infection is the major cause of corneal ulceration or perforation in xerophthalmia. Clearly, the traditional treatment with vitamin A is insufficient—*antibiotics are necessary!*

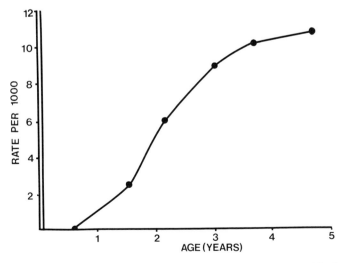

Fig. 29-4. Age-related prevalence of corneal abnormalities presumed caused by hypovitaminosis A. (Modified from Sommer, A., and associates: Am. J. Ophthalmol. **82:**439, September 1976.)

Keratomalacia can also occur in Boston, Massachusetts, and must be kept in mind when severely cachectic patients develop corneal damage.[19] The vitamin A protein transport system described on p. 512 is disrupted by inadequate dietary protein or by malabsorption states. Vitamin A serum levels do not correlate well with the occurrence of ocular disease. Apparently the vitamin breaks down or cannot be utilized in the absence of the specific retinol binding protein transport system, a fact not fully appreciated by clinicians.

Treatment consists of systemic vitamin A (50,000 units intramuscularly), oral vitamin A (25,000 units), topical vitamin A (25,000 units of vitamin A palmitate/ml, four times daily), protein supplement via stomach tube (if necessary), soft contact bandage lens, artificial tears, topical antibiotics, and 20% acetylcystine eye drops to decrease collagenase activity. Do not just give the patient vitamin capsules!

Teratogenicity. Extreme maternal deficiency of vitamin A in rats will result in severe eye defects of the offspring. These changes include abnormal retinal development such as coloboma and eversion, hypoplasia of the iris and anterior chamber, a faulty cornea and conjunctiva, and failure of lid fusion.[20]

Topical use

Topical corneal application of vitamin A in the treatment of assorted degenerative and inflammatory conditions is of doubtful value.[11] Epithelial regeneration of experimentally denuded animal corneas proceeds at the same rate whether treated with codliver oil or liquid petrolatum (provided the animals are not vitamin deficient).[21] The articles advocating such topical therapy date from long ago and are not very convincing.[22]

Toxicity

Vitamin A poisoning usually affects children receiving excessive vitamin dosage. Only rarely are adults affected. Manifestations of vitamin A toxicity do not appear until after many months of treatment. (Enormous single doses, for example, 350,000 units for an infant, may cause an acute rise in cerebrospinal fluid pressure.) Toxic manifestations include increased intracranial pressure with papilledema, very mild exophthalmos, conspicuous hair loss, rash and peeling of skin, widespread migratory arthritic pains, hypoprothrombinemia with bleeding, hepatomegaly and splenomegaly, hypomenorrhea, and generalized malaise.[23]

Severe retinal damage occurs in chronic vitamin A toxicity. The pigment cells are particularly damaged, showing infiltration with lipoid (vitamin A compounds?) as well as structural damage. The neuroepithelium is also damaged.[3]

Although they are uncommon, the central nervous system manifestations are the feature of vitamin A poisoning most likely to result in ophthalmologic consultation. The cause of the increased intracranial pressure is presumed to be hypersecretion of cerebrospinal fluid. Typical papilledema may be found with accompanying headaches. Extraocular muscle paresis and diplopia sometimes occur.

Because of liver storage, excessively high blood levels of vitamin A may persist for a month or more after the medication is discontinued. For this reason, symptoms are not relieved until 1 or 2 weeks after vitamin A is stopped and do not disappear completely for several months. Papilledema will not disappear for a month or more; this delayed response often causes the ophthalmologist to waver in the diagnosis and to become greatly concerned as to the possibility of brain tumor. However, the other typical symptoms and findings as well as the history of ingestion of several hundred thousand units of vitamin A daily for some months are sufficient to make a reliable diagnosis.

Carotenemia. Because conversion of carotene to vitamin A is not sufficiently rapid to accumulate toxic amounts of vitamin A, carotenemia is harmless. The syndrome of carotenemia usually develops after ingestion of large amounts of carotene-rich foods on the assumption that "carrots are good for your eyes." Carotenemia is recognizable by the typical yellow discoloration of the skin. Unlike jaundice, carotenemia does not cause ocular discoloration.[24]

THIAMINE (VITAMIN B₁)

Nutritional amblyopia as encountered in prisoners of war is not a result of vitamin A deficiency. Night blindness is infrequently encountered in such patients. Rather, they have central scotomas typical of the retrobulbar neuritis of thiamine deficiency, and general symptoms of beriberi are common. Dense central, paracentral, or centrocecal scotomas are characteristic of thiamine-deficiency amblyopia. On the average, about 11 months elapse between capture and onset of visual symptoms, suggesting that vitamin reserves may last for almost a year. About three fourths of a series of 22 patients with nutritional amblyopia had recognizable mild to marked temporal pallor of the optic nerves with vision of 20/100 or less.[25] In many patients the ERG showed reduced amplitude but in none was it completely extinguished.

Only one of these patients regained vision after high vitamin and protein therapy, which indicates that vision loss is caused by irreversible neural changes. The one patient who improved had 20/30 vision before treatment and was considered to have only very early thiamine deficiency.

Nutritional damage to the optic nerve of more than 6 months' duration is unlikely to improve in response to vitamin and dietary treatment.[26]

The inadequate diet associated with severe chronic alcoholism may cause marked impairment of central vision, with central or centrocecal scotomas (Fig. 29-5).[27] In the usual patient no ophthalmoscopic changes are visible. Thiamine treatment will often improve vision even though alcoholism continues. Ultimately visual loss becomes irreversible. At this stage, pathologic examination shows atrophy of the papillomacular bundle in the optic nerves, chiasm, and tracts.

In a series of 104 patients with isolated

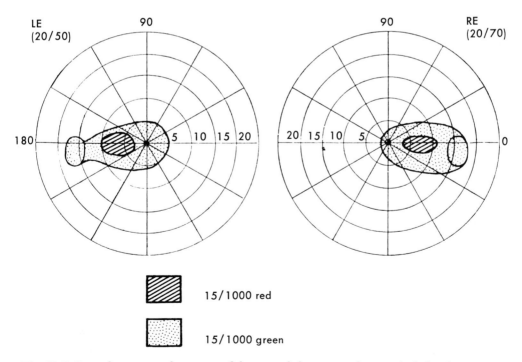

15/1000 red

15/1000 green

Fig. 29-5. Typical cecocentral scotoma of thiamine deficiency in chronic alcoholic. (From Victor, M., Mancall, E. L., and Dreyfus, P. M.: Arch. Ophthalmol. 64:1, 1960.)

abducens paralysis, only a single case was caused by vitamin deficiency in an alcoholic man. This paralysis recovered completely after 3 weeks of treatment with thiamine and nicotinic acid. Intensive vitamin B therapy was tried without benefit in four patients presumed to have diabetic neuropathy.[28]

Thiamine is not of value in treatment of toxic optic neuritis. As an example, two patients with visual field loss resulting from tryparsamide poisoning continued to lose field despite intensive thiamine treatment (30.1 mg/day by injection).[29]

RIBOFLAVIN (VITAMIN B₂)

A case of corneal disease caused by ariboflavinosis was diagnosed on the basis of deficient nutrition, low blood riboflavin, and characteristic corneal appearance.[30] Limbal vascularization uniformly surrounded the cornea and consisted of parallel vascular loops engorged with blood, extending 2 to 3 mm through the superficial stroma. Subepithelial opacities and scattered ulcers were present. Treatment with 15 mg of riboflavin/day resulted in collapse of the vessels within a month; only biomicroscopically visible ghost vessels remained.

Improvement of acne rosacea keratitis after riboflavin treatment has been reported[31] and denied.[32]

PYRIDOXINE (VITAMIN B₆)

Experimental deficiency of pyridoxine causes vascular congestion, hyperkeratosis, and hair loss of the eyelid margins. Corneal neovascularization occurs. The deficient animals have many other general symptoms, notably skin disorders and weight loss. In severe deficiency the ears become necrotic and fall off.

The similarity of these changes to the appearance of human angular blepharoconjunctivitis suggested study of pyridoxine levels in such patients. Normal control patients had 4 to 6 μg of pyridoxine/100 ml of urine. Values in patients with angular blepharoconjunctivitis were 1 to 2 μg/100 ml in five patients, 2 to 3 μg in seven patients, and 3 to 4 μg in six patients.[33] In only three of these 18 patients

with angular blepharoconjunctivitis were bacteria found to be responsible for the condition. Angular stomatitis, glossitis, and seborrheic dermatitis accompany angular blepharoconjunctivitis in human cases of pyridoxine deficiency—all of these symptoms may be cured by pyridoxine therapy.

Moraxella strains survive slightly longer in the conjunctival sac of pyridoxine-deficient guinea pigs than in normal animals. This increased bacterial survival time was found to be related to a decreased tear flow, inasmuch as it occurred only in animals with a decreased Schirmer test wetting of the filter paper strip. No metabolic cause for reduced resistance was demonstrable.[34]

CYANOCOBALAMIN (VITAMIN B₁₂)

Retrobulbar neuritis with typical central scotoma may be caused by pernicious anemia. This may be associated with the general symptoms of pernicious anemia or with the numbness and tingling of the extremities typical of subacute combined sclerosis (pernicious anemia neural changes) or may be an isolated symptom affecting one eye. Although folic acid stimulates hematopoiesis, it does not prevent the neurologic complications of pernicious anemia. Adequate treatment with vitamin B₁₂ can cure the retrobulbar neuritis of pernicious anemia.[35] Several months of treatment are required before disappearance of the scotoma.

Although cyanocobalamin is the commonly used form of vitamin B₁₂, hydroxocobalamin has been reported to be considerably more effective.[36] As little as 10 mg of hydroxocobalamin may maintain elevated vitamin B₁₂ levels for as long as a year. In contrast, comparable cyanocobalamin treatment may be effective for only a month.

Subnormal levels of vitamin B₁₂ were found in patients with tobacco amblyopia. The theory was advanced that tobacco amblyopia is a result of the failure to detoxify cyanide derived from tobacco smoke. Apparently, vitamin B₁₂ is necessary for this detoxification. The B₁₂ deficiency is apparently an independent factor unrelated to the tobacco smoking.[37]

A very similar neurologic syndrome is produced by deficiency of thiamine, nicotinic acid, and riboflavin and by tobacco amblyopia, drinking of Jamaican ginger, and Nigerian tropical amblyopia. Apparently the common mechanism of the latter three conditions is cyanide inhibition of cytochrome oxidase. In the Nigerian patients a cassava diet contains a glycoside metabolized to hydrocyanic acid. Diffuse neurologic malfunction characterizes this tropical amblyopia, impaired vision or blindness being present in 80% of cases. These patients were deficient in hydroxocobalamin, which detoxifies cyanide.[38]

B_{12} shots have been given indiscriminately for treatment of obscure neurologic or functional disorders, a use in which they can serve only as a placebo. Cyanocobalamin and hydroxocobalamin are effective only in conditions in which there is a vitamin B_{12} deficiency. Such deficiency occurs in patients who fail to absorb the vitamin. In pernicious anemia and gastrectomy patients this failure results from absence of gastric intrinsic factor, which must combine with the vitamin before it can be absorbed via the ileum. Loss of the ileum by surgery will also prevent absorption. Vitamin B_{12} deficiency also occurs in severe alcoholic liver disease (ingestion and storage failure) or in fish tapeworm (*Diphyllobothrium latum*) infestation (competition of parasite for the vitamin). The daily requirement is 0.1 μg, and perhaps 1500 μg is normally stored in the liver. Hence a 2- to 5-year supply may exist in a treated patient, who will not show signs of deficiency for some years after stopping therapy. Ultimately, however, a relapse will occur, with hematologic and neurologic damage. Hence, a patient with true vitamin B_{12} deficiency will require infrequent lifetime treatment.[39]

NIACIN (NICOTINAMIDE, NICOTINIC ACID)

A gradual decrease in vision in both eyes and measurable central scotomas without significant ophthalmoscopic evidence of abnormality of the disc or macula may be caused by pellagra.[40] Restoration of vision by vitamin treatment requires many weeks of therapy before maximum improvement is attained. If the vitamin deficiency has been sufficiently severe, the optic nerve is presumably irreversibly damaged, since visual recovery is incomplete. Since pellagrous polyneuritis is not benefited by niacin, but requires thiamine, pellagrous optic neuritis is probably really a manifestation of thiamine deficiency.

Nicotinamide is the coenzyme of the alcohol dehydrogenase system required to oxidize vitamin A to retinene, the first step in rhodopsin synthesis. Theoretically, a nicotinamide deficiency (as in pellagra) should cause night blindness, even in the presence of adequate amounts of vitamin A.

ASCORBIC ACID (VITAMIN C)

Hemorrhagic exophthalmos of sudden onset in children may be caused by scurvy.[41] Vitamin C treatment may result in disappearance of the exophthalmos in less than a week.

The routine prophylactic preoperative use of vitamins C (ascorbic acid) and K (menadione) does not decrease the frequency of postoperative anterior chamber hemorrhage.[42]

Despite Linus Pauling, there is no evidence that immense doses of vitamin C (1 g or more daily) will prevent or modify the common cold. Such doses may increase urinary oxalate excretion (possible hazard of calculus formation), may cause diarrhea, and mobilize calcium from the bones; hence excessive doses are not without possible toxicity.[43,44]

VITAMIN D

Excessive dosage of vitamin D may cause pathologic calcification of many areas of the body. Conjunctival and corneal opacities, typically a band-shaped keratopathy, appear in such patients.[45] Scleral calcification has also occurred, especially in patients with rheumatoid arthritis predisposed to scleral disease.[46] Abnormal calcification may also affect the renal parenchyma and cavities, blood vessels, joints, and meninges as well as other body structures.

Excessive vitamin D administration during

infancy has been recognized as the cause of "idiopathic" hypercalcemia. The more severe cases of this disorder cause osteosclerosis and are of interest to the ophthalmologist because of encroachment of the narrowed optic foramina on the optic nerves. Optic atrophy, possibly preceded by an appearance comparable to that of optic neuritis or papilledema, may result. The optic discs may be recognizably small, presumably because of arrested growth. Convergent strabismus, sometimes associated with abducens paresis, is reported. Systemic abnormalities include anorexia and vomiting, mental retardation, dwarfism, craniostenosis, and renal damage with hypertension.[47]

VITAMIN E

Vitamin E (alpha-tocopherol) has been advocated for treatment of a variety of ocular disorders, none of which seems to have benefited, Dosages ranging from 100 to 200 mg three times a day for 15 months in 12 patients with diabetic retinopathy did not improve these eyes.[48] Treatment of retinopathy of prematurity with vitamin E also failed.

VITAMIN K

Paradoxically, excessive amounts of vitamin K or its analogues will cause prothrombin deficiency and bleeding problems. Indiscriminate and excessive use of vitamin K is a common error in the management of bleeding unrelated to prothrombin deficiency. Hemorrhagic glaucoma, postoperative hyphema, spontaneous vitreous hemorrhage, and similar conditions are practically never a result of defective coagulation mechanisms. Treatment of such conditions with large doses (for example, 50 mg/day for several weeks) of vitamin K will not be of benefit and may actually induce hemorrhages.[49]

Before use of vitamin K, the patient's prothrombin time should be determined. Even if the patient does indeed have a prothrombin deficiency, vitamin K is commonly given in excessive dosage and over too prolonged a time. Hypoprothrombinemia caused by serious liver disease cannot be corrected by vitamin K therapy. If spontaneously low prothrombin levels do not improve within several days of vitamin K treatment, further vitamin K is more likely to cause harm than benefit.

REFERENCES

1. Wald, G.: The photoreceptor process in vision, Am. J. Ophthalmol. **40:**18, 1955.
2. Dowling, J.: Night blindness, dark adaptation, and the electroretinogram, Am. J. Ophthalmol. **50:**875, 1960.
3. Amemiya, T.: Vitamin A and the retina, Eye Ear Nose Throat Mon. **50:**50, September 1971.
4. Heller, J., and Bok, D.: A specific receptor for retinol binding protein as detected by the binding of human and bovine retinol binding protein to pigment epithelial cells, Am. J. Ophthalmol. **81:**93, January 1976.
5. Yee, R. D., Herbert, P. N., Bergsma, D. R., and Biemer, J. J.: Atypical retinitis pigmentosa in familial hypobetalipoproteinemia, Am. J. Ophthalmol. **82:**64, July 1976.
6. Hayes, K. C., Nielsen, S. W., and Eaton, H. D.: Pathogenesis of the optic nerve lesion in vitamin A–deficient calves, Arch. Ophthalmol. **80:**777, 1968.
7. Dhanda, R. P.: Electroretinography in night blindness and other vitamin A deficiencies, Arch. Ophthalmol. **54:**841, 1955.
8. Bodansky, O., Lewis, J. M., and Haig, C.: Comparative value of blood plasma vitamin A concentration and dark adaptation as a criterion of vitamin A deficiency, Science **94:**370, 1941.
9. Steffens, L. F., and Sheard, C.: Dark adaptation and dietary deficiency in vitamin A, Am. J. Ophthalmol. **23:**1325, 1940.
10. Isaacs, B. I., Jung, F. T., and Ivy, A. C.: Clinical studies of vitamin A deficiency, Arch. Ophthalmol. **24:**698, 1940.
11. Schmidtke, R. L.: Hypovitaminosis A in ophthalmology, Arch. Ophthalmol. **37:**653, 1947.
12. Paton, D., and McLaren, D. S.: Bitot spots, Am. J. Ophthalmol. **50:**658, 1960.
13. Goldberg, H. K., and Schlivek, K.: Necrosis of the cornea due to vitamin A deficiency, Arch. Ophthalmol. **25:**122, 1941.
14. Sullivan, W. R., McCulley, J. P., and Dohlman, C. H.: Return of goblet cells after vitamin A therapy in xerosis of the conjunctiva, Am. J. Ophthalmol. **75:**720, 1973.
15. Sommer, A., Quesada, J., Doty, M., and Faich, G.: Xerophthalmia and anterior-segment blindness among preschool-age children

in El Salvador, Am. J. Ophthalmol. **80**:1066, December 1975.

16. Sommer, A., Faich, G., and Quesada, J.: Mass distribution of vitamin A and the prevention of keratomalacia, Am. J. Ophthalmol. **80**:1073, December 1975.

17. Sommer, A., Toureau, S., Cornet, P., Midy, C., and Pettiss, S. T.: Xerophthalmia and anterior segment blindness, Am. J. Ophthalmol. **82**:439, September 1976.

18. Valenton, M., and Tan, R. V.: Secondary ocular bacterial infection in hypovitaminosis A xerophthalmia, Am. J. Ophthalmol. **80**:673, October 1975.

19. Baum, J. L., and Rao, G.: Keratomalacia in the cachectic hospitalized patient, Am. J. Ophthalmol. **82**:435, September 1976.

20. Warkany, J., and Schraffenberger, E.: Congenital malformations induced in rats by maternal vitamin A deficiency, Arch. Ophthalmol. **35**:150, 1946.

21. deRötth, A.: Local action of oils containing vitamin A, Arch. Ophthalmol. **24**:281, 1940.

22. de Grosz, S.: Local use of vitamin A preparations in ophthalmic practice, Arch. Ophthalmol. **22**:727, 1939.

23. Oliver, T. K., and Havener, W. H.: Eye manifestations of chronic vitamin A intoxication, Arch. Ophthalmol. **60**:19, 1958.

24. Abrahamson, I. A., Sr., and Abrahamson, I. A., Jr.: Hypercarotenemia, Arch. Ophthalmol. **68**:34, 1962.

25. King, J. H., and Passmore, J. W.: Nutritional amblyopia, Am. J. Ophthalmol. **39**:173, 1955.

26. Roberts, W. L., and Willcockson, T. H.: Postneuritic optic atrophy in repatriated prisoners of war, Am. J. Ophthalmol. **30**:165, 1947.

27. Victor, M., Mancall, E. L., and Dreyfus, P. M.: Deficiency amblyopia in the alcoholic patient, Arch. Ophthalmol. **64**:1, 1960.

28. Shrader, E., and Schlezinger, N.: Neuroophthalmologic evaluation of abducens nerve paralysis, Arch. Ophthalmol. **63**:108, 1960.

29. Leinfelder, P. J., and Stump, R. B.: Thiamine hydrochloride in the treatment of tryparsamide amblyopia, Arch. Ophthalmol. **26**:613, 1941.

30. Mann, I.: Ariboflavinosis, Am. J. Ophthalmol. **28**:243, 1945.

31. Johnson, L. V., and Eckardt, R. E.: Rosacea keratitis and conditions with vascularization of cornea treated with riboflavin, Arch. Ophthalmol. **23**:899, 1940.

32. Wise, G.: Ocular rosacea (not cured with riboflavin), Am. J. Ophthalmol. **26**:591, 1943.

33. Irinoda, K., and Mikami, H.: Angular blepharoconjunctivitis and pyridoxine (vitamin B_6 deficiency, Arch. Ophthalmol. **60**:303, 1958.

34. van Bijsterveld, O. P.: The survival of *Moraxella* on the conjunctiva in pyridoxine deficiency, Am. J. Ophthalmol. **74**:948, November 1972.

35. Ellis, P. P., and Hamilton, H.: Retrobulbar neuritis in pernicious anemia, Am. J. Ophthalmol. **48**:95, 1959.

36. Glass, G. B., Lee, D. H., Skeggs, H. R., and Stanley, J. L.: Hydroxocobalamin, J.A.M.A. **183**:425, 1963.

37. Foulds, W. S., Chisholm, I. A., Bronte-Stewart, J., and Wilson, T. M.: Vitamin B_{12} absorption in tobacco amblyopia, Br. J. Ophthalmol. **53**:393, 1969.

38. Osuntokun, B. O., and Osuntokun, O.: Tropical amblyopia in Nigerians, Am. J. Ophthalmol. **72**:708, 1971.

39. McCurdy, P. R.: "B_{12} shots" flip side, J.A.M.A. **231**:289, January 20, 1975.

40. Fine, M., and Lachman, G. S.: Retrobulbar neuritis in pellagra, Arch. Ophthalmol. **20**:708, 1937.

41. Dunnington, J. H.: Exophthalmos in infantile scurvy, Arch. Ophthalmol. **6**:731, 1931.

42. Kirby, D. B.: Advanced surgery of cataract, Philadelphia, 1955, J. B. Lippincott Co.

43. Dykes, M. H., and Meier, P.: Ascorbic acid and the common cold, evaluation of its efficacy and toxicity, J.A.M.A. **231**:1073, March 10, 1975.

44. Karlowski, T. R., Chalmers, T. C., Frenkel, L. D., Kapikian, A. Z., Lewis, T. L., and Lynch, J. M.: Ascorbic acid for the common cold, a prophylactic and therapeutic trial, J.A.M.A. **231**:1038, March 10, 1975.

45. Wagener, H. P.: The ocular manifestations of hypercalcemia, Am. J. Med. Sci. **231**:218, 1956.

46. Gartner, S., and Rubner, K.: Calcified scleral nodules in hypervitaminosis D, Am. J. Ophthalmol. **39**:658, 1955.

47. Harley, R. D., DiGeorge, A. M., Mabry, C. C., and Apt, L.: Idiopathic hypercalcemia of infancy: optic atrophy and other ocular changes, Trans. Am. Acad. Ophthalmol. Otolaryngol. **69**:977, 1965.

48. De Hoff, J. B., and Ozazewski, J.: Alpha-tocopherol to treat diabetic retinopathy, Am. J. Ophthalmol. **37**:581, 1954.

49. Smith, A. M., Jr., and Custer, R. P.: Toxicity of vitamin K, J.A.M.A. **173**:503, 1960.

30
LABEL WITH NAME OF DRUG

Addition of the five words in the title of this chapter to every prescription would benefit both patient and physician. The traditional secrecy as to content of a prescription is archaic, dangerous, and unwarranted. The following advantages accrue from labeled prescriptions.

1. If the patient is taking more than one medication, a change in instructions is less likely to cause confusion. ("Which bottles do I stop using?")

2. When one of multiple prescriptions is exhausted, it can be identified for refilling. ("I need more of the medicine in the round bottle.")

3. Several physicians caring for the same patient can more easily coordinate treatment. ("Why are you giving me Diamox for my eyes when the heart doctor uses it for my swollen ankles?")

4. A consultant or new physician need not change or discard perfectly adequate, but unknown, medications. This is a common and unnecessary expense to patients. Also, if a given medication has not been of benefit, this knowledge should prevent the new physician from prescribing the same type of drug again.

5. Medications to which there is a known allergy are less likely to be given without the patient's recognition. Because of the frequency and severity of drug allergies, the physician should inquire concerning allergy before prescribing medications with known allergic potential. Potent sensitizers such as horse serum and penicillin should certainly not be given before the history of possible allergy has been determined. When a drug-induced allergic response is observed, the physician should inform the patient as to the cause to enable him to avoid future trouble.

6. In case of emergency the nature of the patient's medications can more rapidly be determined. Such prompt identification is particularly urgent in accidental poisoning. Poisoning ranks as the fourth cause of accidental death in children.

One third of the 2240 calls to the University of Rochester Poison Control Center in 1962 concerned possible poisoning from misuse of medications.[1] Four fifths of all calls concerned children. The frequency of these incidents underscores the necessity for cautioning patients, "These drops, just as all other potent medications, should be kept out of reach of children."

An identification guide based on the physical characteristics of the various tablets and capsules has been published.[2] However, more than 5000 different kinds of tablets exist, and they are most confusing. Identification of unlabeled liquid medications is even more difficult; indeed, it is impossible.

7. If recurrence of disease calls for use of the same medication, the patient can, on your advice, safely and accurately resume treatment with the leftover tablets or drops.

8. Economy, in these days of high costs, is achieved for the various reasons just given.

9. Dispensing errors may be readily detected. (And they happen!)

In summary, a great deal of confusion could be avoided if prescriptions were clearly identified. Certainly, in matters as important as human health there is no room for uncertainty.[3]

REFERENCES

1. Misused medicine: 30% of 2,240 poison cases, Medical Tribune, p. 11, February 11, 1963.
2. Identification guide for solid dosage forms, J.A. M.A. **182:**1145, 1962.
3. Council on Drugs: To label or not to label, J.A. M.A. **194:**1311, 1965.

PART TWO

CURRENTLY EMPLOYED OPHTHALMIC THERAPY

This title has been selected with the express purpose of disavowing any conviction that the subsequent recommendations are the "right" therapy. The uncertainties of clinical responses are so enormous that diametrically opposed schools of thought commonly arise. For example, does pilocarpine or atropine benefit hyphema? In contrast to the tendency for a proposed national formulary to standardize medical usage into a rigid mold, I hope this section on current therapy will not be considered to represent the ultimate ideal therapy. It is the best I can do at the moment; nevertheless, I perceive clearly the numerous inconsistencies, conflicting recommendations, and uncertainties inherent in this material. Please recognize that many dogmatic assertions have been made to express various methods of treatment. Accept them with several grains of salt, consider the alternatives and the yet unpublished information available to you when you read these recommendations, and prescribe thoughtfully and responsibly.

Primum non nocere!

31
CATARACT*

The medical management of cataract will be discussed under the following categories:

Use of drops to postpone cataract extraction
Prevention of cataract
Treatment of lens trauma
Prevention of surgical infection
Preoperative sedation
Anesthesia
Dilating drops
Aids to hypotony
Irrigating solutions
Alpha-chymotrypsin
Miotics
Corticosteroids
Postoperative hyphema
Postoperative shallow chamber
Postoperative miotic iritis
Postoperative infection
Intraocular lenses
Postoperative glaucoma
Postoperative edema of posterior pole
Filamentary keratitis
Congenital cataract

USE OF DROPS TO POSTPONE CATARACT EXTRACTION

The patient with a moderately advanced nuclear cataract will frequently see more clearly when the pupil is dilated. Sight is not restored to normal, but mydriasis may cause enough improvement so that the patient is willing to instill drops regularly to enjoy this benefit. Mydriatic therapy is particularly ap-

*Reprinted in part from New Orleans Academy of Ophthalmology: Symposium on ocular pharmacology and therapeutics, St. Louis, 1970, The C. V. Mosby Co.

plicable to patients unable or unwilling to have cataract surgery because of age, general health, one-eyed status, etc. Whether sufficient benefit is derived to justify mydriatic therapy can only be determined by trial in the individual patient.

Because glare is the usual reason requiring cataract extraction and because glare is increased by dilation of the pupil, most patients do not benefit sufficiently from mydriasis to postpone surgery.

Phenylephrine, cyclopentolate, or any other effective drug may be used, depending on the physician's choice. The greater tendency for a parasympatholytic drug to elevate the intraocular pressure of an eye predisposed to glaucoma should be considered in making this choice. Since most patients with cataract have lost useful accommodation, the cycloplegic effect of a parasympatholytic drug is not usually a problem. The precaution of checking intraocular pressure of the dilated eye is indicated with greater frequency than if no drops were used.

Sometimes a patient with cataract prefers to have a small pupil. This is likely to be true during the early stages of a cataract when irregularities within the lens cause distortion or doubling of the image. Topical guanethidine, 10% three or four times daily, has been reported to abolish monocular diplopia in 18 of 19 cases of early cataract ("double-focus" lens). Monocular diplopia is believed to be caused by a refractive index difference within the lens substance. The second image may be

527

abolished by miosis, use of a pinhole, or by blocking part of the pupil with a card. Although effective in eliminating diplopia, pilocarpine induces troublesome accommodative myopia in younger patients. Topical guanethidine does not alter accommodation but does cause a cosmetically displeasing Horner syndrome of obvious ptosis on the treated side. Because of cosmetic reasons or the inconvenience of regular use of drops, only five of the previously cited 19 patients continued treatment rather than experience diplopia.[1]

Glaucomatous patients with cataract particularly object to the decreased vision caused by miotic therapy. Use of sympathomimetic drugs alone or in combination with the miotic, as necessary to control pressure, is often helpful in improving vision in such patients.

Dionin is the time-honored drop reputed to arrest cataract growth. I periodically encounter patients who have been using Dionin for many years (prescribed elsewhere). Despite use of the drop, their cataracts have progressed to require surgery. Discussion with some of the older ophthalmologists who have used Dionin indicates to me that they usually consider this to have solely a placebo effect, reassuring patients that they are not neglecting their eyes and tiding them over the awkward period when the cataract handicap is not yet sufficient to justify surgery. I do not remember meeting anyone who was personally convinced of the unquestionable value of Dionin, nor have I encountered any significant positive research findings on this subject. The notoriously unpredictable rate of progression of cataracts would seriously complicate evaluation of a cataract-inhibiting drug.

PREVENTION OF CATARACT

Although we know of no way to slow the progress of senile cataract, correction of metabolic abnormalities is known to arrest the development of certain types of cataract. Galactose cataract, diabetic cataract, and hypoparathyroid cataract are the classic examples of preventable or reversible metabolic cataracts.

Galactose cataract

The reversibility of early galactose cataracts is demonstrable in 1-month-old rats maintained on a cataractogenic galactose diet.[2] Withdrawal of the galactose diet prior to the seventh or eighth day frequently results in clearing of the lens vacuoles. After 12 to 18 days the lens opacities are dense and irreversible. Obviously these time factors are not applicable to the human infant with galactosemia, but the clearing of these early rat lens opacities is compatible with clinical reports that sufficiently early diagnosis and treatment of galactosemia will prevent cataract formation or reverse early stages of cataract.

Experimental galactose cataract begins with a reduction of the number of lens epithelial cells entering mitosis.[3] This reduction of epithelial mitoses may occur as soon as 5 days after the administration of large amounts of galactose or is of slower onset with less galactose. Removal of galactose from the diet permits the mitotic cycle to return to normal within a month's time. Thereafter new cortex is again normal and transparent; however, the zonular cataract laid down during the period of abnormal mitosis persists as an opaque layer. The clinical implication of this finding is that galactosemia cataracts are "reversible" in that their continued formation may be stopped with proper diet. Furthermore, new zones of opacity must indicate transitory periods of galactosemia. Such new opacities may be a highly sensitive guide to the adequacy of dietary galactose restrictions.

The conversion of galactose to glucose requires at least three specific enzymes. Deficiency of galactose-1-phosphate uridyl transferase is responsible for the classic galactosemia syndrome, which is associated with cataract, galactosuria, hepatosplenomegaly, mental retardation, nutritional deficiency, and death. Deficiency of another enzyme, galactokinase, does not cause these multiple systemic manifestations but may cause congenital cataracts that have been described as zonular, Y-sutural, central, posterior cortical, or embryonal. Galactosuria may be absent; hence a normal urine sugar test does not exclude the diagnosis of galactokinase deficiency, which can only be made by assay of red blood cells for the enzyme galactokinase.

Galactokinase deficiency is an autosomal recessive trait. Two homozygous persons were reported as having cataract surgery in childhood.[4] Heterozygotes showed scattered small lens opacities not recognizably different from those commonly encountered in the general population. If familial galactokinase deficiency can be recognized early, removal of dietary galactose will not only prevent progression of cataract but may result in improved visual acuity despite the presence of some permanent lens opacities.

Identical twins with galactokinase deficiency were found to have bilateral zonular cataracts at 4 months of age. A galactose-free diet arrested the progress of the cataracts, but they did not regress.[5] It was suggested that the metabolic deficiency must be detected and proper diet instituted by 1 month of life if cataract is to be prevented.

A fetus in the fifth month, aborted because of amniocentesis-diagnosed galactosemia, was found to have extensive vacuolation and degeneration of the lens epithelium and the lens fibers. Such changes were not present in metabolically normal fetuses. This finding indicates that the onset of galactose cataract may occur even before birth, resulting from fetal inability to metabolize transplacental galactose. No doubt the variations in the severity and type of enzyme deficiency result in different ages of onset of cataract. Biochemically, galactose easily enters the lens and is metabolized to dulcitol, which does not readily escape through the lens capsule and is not metabolized. The osmotic excess of dulcitol within the lens causes lens damage by hydration.[6]

Diabetic cataract

The classic "endocrine" type of cataract, consisting of innumerable tiny opacities of the superficial cortex, is known to develop during periods of severe diabetic acidosis. Clearly, diabetic acidosis is primarily of concern because it threatens life; however, good diabetic control will also prevent this type of acutely developing metabolic cataract.

Although diabetic cataracts are ordinarily irreversible, a case has been reported in which a 54-year-old diabetic patient developed blurred vision in the left eye only. When seen 2 days after the onset, he had extensive feathery posterior subcapsular opacities OS, with vision of counting fingers at 10 feet. His poorly controlled diabetes was treated and within 1 week the feathery opacities disappeared and vision improved to 20/40.[7] The biochemical mechanism of such reversible cataract formation is that during hyperglycemia sugars such as glucose or galactose penetrate rapidly into the aqueous humor and then into the lens. The glucose within the lens is metabolized to sorbitol, which cannot readily diffuse from the lens and accumulates in osmotic excess. The consequence is entry of water into the lens, causing variations in refractive index and opacity of the posterior subcapsular region. The acute diabetic cataract is not caused by lens protein or cellular damage and as a result is potentially reversible with prompt control of the hyperglycemia. The sorbitol within the lens is further metabolized to fructose, which is able to diffuse from the lens, thereby restoring normal osmotic relationships. Judging from this one case, acute lens opacity associated with poor diabetic control indicates prompt control of the hyperglycemia.

Hypoglycemic cataract

The metabolism of both the central nervous system and the lens is based on glucose, suggesting that hypoglycemia could cause permanent damage to both brain and lens. Thirteen cases of infantile cataract and mental retardation associated with hypoglycemia (either neonatal, ketotic, or idiopathic) have been reported.[8] These were typical lamellar cataracts. In two patients the cataracts progressed to complete maturity. In two children the eyes were recorded as being normal before the attack of hypoglycemia. Presumably, early detection and treatment of the hypoglycemia would prevent or minimize the cataract.

Hypoparathyroid cataract

Similarly, early recognition of hypoparathyroidism and appropriate medical replacement therapy will correct hypocalcemia and prevent cataract formation.

Absence of calcium significantly alters lens permeability in vitro by reducing potassium concentration to 65% of normal, doubling penetration of sucrose and mannitol, and tripling sodium penetration.[9] These changes are not cited as being necessarily causative of cataract, but they do indicate the considerable metabolic changes induced in the lens by hypocalcemia.

Toxic cataract

The possibility of poisoning, as by *p*-dichlorobenzene, should be considered in young patients with a relatively sudden onset of cataract. This chemical is commonly used as a moth repellant. Jaundice, weight loss, and weakness are characteristic of chronic *p*-dichlorobenzene poisoning. Onset of cortical cataract is delayed for many months after the start of chronic poisoning and may begin long after *p*-dichlorobenzene exposure stops. Although there is no specific therapy for toxic cataract, recognition of the cause and removal of the poison may arrest or slow cataractous change.[10]

Iatrogenic cataracts may result from a variety of medications. Dinitrophenol (a weight reducer) and MER 29 (effective in decreasing cholesterol levels) are well-known historical examples of medications capable of causing cataract in susceptible individuals. Although these medications are obsolete, currently acceptable medical therapy includes two groups of drugs recognized to be cataractogenic. These are the corticosteroids and the "irreversible" cholinesterase inhibitors.

Although the literature contains conflicting reports as to the cataractogenic potential of corticosteroid treatment, the general consensus is that sufficiently high doses given over a prolonged period do cause posterior subcapsular cataract. For example, 60% of 58 rheumatoid arthritis patients receiving intramuscular triamcinolone acetonide therapy were found to have posterior subcapsular opacities.[11] A period of 6 to 9 months of therapy elapsed before onset of cataract. One third of the patients who had received from 500 to 1000 mg of triamcinolone showed cataract. Lens opacities affected all patients who had received more than 2000 mg of this corticosteroid. Cataract surgery was necessary in 14 eyes of 8 patients in this series of 58.

The physician must also be alert to the possible development of posterior subcapsular cataract during long-term use of topical corticosteroids. For example, two young patients developed cataracts after 7 and 11 months of topical corticosteroid therapy following penetrating keratoplasty. Apparently such cataracts do not progress if the corticosteroid therapy is discontinued promptly.[12]

The evidence that indicates that strong anticholinesterase drugs have cataractogenic potential has been summarized in Chapter 12.

Sodium cyanate, 30 mg/kg, once daily, will inhibit red blood cell sickling, thereby reducing hemolysis and sickle cell crises. A patient is reported in whom bilateral small posterior subcapsular cataracts developed after 6 months of cyanate therapy. Two months after therapy was stopped the cataracts disappeared. Following another treatment period they reappeared, only to disappear again when treatment was stopped. A second patient on cyanate developed small posterior subcapsular cataracts that reduced vision to 20/25 and did not disappear 6 months after therapy was stopped.[13]

As is true throughout medicine, the anticipated benefits from these potent medications must be balanced against the possible hazards of their use.

DEHYDRATION CATARACT

A reversible loss of lens transparency can be produced experimentally by preventing closure of the eye. If long continued, this will result in anterior subcapsular cataract. A human counterpart of this condition follows paralysis of cranial nerve VII. Of 29 patients with operated acoustic neuroma resulting in seventh nerve paralysis, 5 developed unexplained anterior subcapsular cataract.[14] One required cataract extraction; the others retained 20/30 vision. The onset of these dehydration cataracts was 1 to 6 years after the development of paralysis of eyelid closure. In these 5 patients other cataractogenic factors (such as corticosteroid therapy, iritis, or corneal perforation) were absent. Development of an anterior subcapsular cataract under circumstances of poor lid closure apparently indicates additional attention to maintaining corneal moisture.

TREATMENT OF LENS TRAUMA

Glaucoma associated with a subluxated or dislocated lens has commonly been considered primarily a surgical problem. Actually, medical management is more likely to be successful. Posttraumatic glaucoma is usually caused by contusion angle deformity, which is not improved by extraction of a dislocated lens, but which may spontaneously regress or be controlled by conventional antiglaucomatous medications. An excellent analysis of the clinical course of 166 cases of dislocated lenses indicated that surgical complications were numerous and serious and clearly suggested the advantages of conservative medical management.[15] For example, vitreous loss occurred in 41% of these lens extractions, and blindness resulted in one third of the cases with vitreous loss. Lens extraction improved vision in only 13 of 41 eyes with lens dislocation caused by injury. Finally, the eye was found to tolerate an intact dislocated lens very well (a conclusion with which I am in complete agreement).

When the lens is subluxated, pupil-block glaucoma may become worse with miotics and be improved by mydriatics.[16] The mechanism of response is lessening of the contact between the lens and the dilated iris. Cycloplegic drugs may also tighten the zonular fibers and pull the lens backward. Vitreous block of the pupil will also be relieved by mydriasis.

Although surgical removal of a dislocated lens is a hazardous procedure and is *not* routinely indicated, if such an operation is necessary, preoperative softening of the eye by medical methods is important. Use of carbonic anhydrase inhibitors and oral or intravenous hypertonic solutions is of value.

The perennial miosis or mydriasis question is again encountered in the case of very tiny perforations of the anterior lens capsule. Some authors recommend miotic therapy with the intent of encouraging posterior synechiae that are supposed to seal the wound. However, posterior synechiae are undesirable because vessels may extend from synechiae to form a dense fibrovascular membrane. Use of atropine was reported in two cases of intralenticular small foreign bodies.[17] In both cases, spontaneous closure of the capsular wound occurred, without progression of the localized cataractous changes, and both eyes regained 20/20 phakic vision. I believe cycloplegic therapy of such cases to be more logical than use of miotics.

PREVENTION OF SURGICAL INFECTION

Twenty-two cases of bacterial endophthalmitis were reported to follow 20,000 cataract operations.[18] The rate of infection was 12 times greater in eyes receiving no topical antibiotics (4 of 660; 0.6%) than in antibiotic-treated eyes (12 of 19,340; 0.06%). Antibiotic treatment was started at the time of hospitalization and consisted of hourly drops for five instillations and ointment at night. Antibiotic ointment was also instilled at the end of the operation.

Selection of antibiotic was based on the assumption that about one half of the infections are caused by *Staphylococcus aureus* and about one fourth by *Pseudomonas*. Combinations of antibiotics were usually prescribed (for example, chloramphenicol and sulfacetamide; neomycin, polymyxin B, and erythromycin).[19]

Since several days may be required to eradicate bacteria from the lids, home use of antibiotics for a few days prior to cataract surgery seems rational.

Although 122 surgeons operated on these 20,000 cases, four surgeons had two or more infections (9 of the 22 infections). The same staphylococcal strain that destroyed two eyes was recovered from the surgeon's nose.

Clearly the operating room personnel can be the source of operative infection, despite antibiotics, and must observe the rules of sterile technique.

The patient origin of many postoperative intraocular infections has been well established. For this reason we carefully exclude from surgery patients with clinically recognizably infection such as chronic dacryocystitis or marginal blepharitis. Patients are *not* immune to their own microorganisms.

Bacterial cultures taken from the lower conjunctival sac after complete surgical scrubbing and draping of the patient immediately before surgery begins will startle the surgeon. In 81 of 100 such cases, positive cultures were obtained.[20] In seven cases the organism recovered was *Staphylococcus aureus;* in two cases it was *Pseudomonas.* Three of these 100 patients had used topical antibiotics for 2 days preoperatively—none of these three demonstrated bacterial growth.

Our own laboratory has confirmed the high frequency of contamination of the eye surface immediately before surgery. I attribute this finding to the uniformly poor quality of preoperative preparation carried out by beginning residents assigned to this lowly but vital duty. Invariably they will pay little attention to the lid margins, even though these structures border the operative field and are notorious harbors for germs. Mucous strands remaining within the cul-de-sac, especially beneath the upper lid or in the inner canthus, are mute testimony to incomplete irrigation. Center-out scrub technique is not used; commonly the contaminated sponge from the upper periphery will be returned to touch the lower lid margin, for instance. Rarely one observes that the final sponge is used to dry the contaminated opposite eye before it is used for a last pat on the eye to be operated on! Grossly visible contaminated material adherent to the base of the eyelashes is regularly present at the close of the eye preparation.

Fortunately the eye is somehow able to survive all this contamination. However, I refuse to tolerate such preparation of my cataract patients and recommend that new residents be observed closely as they scrub the eye preoperatively. The resident must be instructed that the lid margins are best cleaned by vigorous scrubbing with applicator sticks. Hold the lid everted by pressure on the brow or cheek and scrub horizontally along the lid margin and lash bases. Do not introduce the contaminated swab into the conjunctival sac.

Despite such vigorous scrubbing with Betadine, generous rinsing with saline solution, painting with 2% tincture of iodine, and rinsing with 70% ethyl alcohol, cultures of the draped eyelid immediately before surgery were positive in 24 of 100 patients.[21] Conjunctival cultures were positive in 12 of the 100 patients. In one of those patients, *Staphylococcus albus* was recovered from an aqueous sample taken immediately after surgery.

In a small series of cataract patients whom I personally prepared with Argyrol stain and Betadine scrub, preoperative cultures of the draped surface of the eye showed not a single microorganism to be present. In contrast, cultures of the resident preparations uniformly grew dozens if not hundreds of organisms! You must get the garbage off the lid margin, or else you will sooner or later be unpleasantly surprised with a case of endophthalmitis a day or two following surgery.

Confirmation that patients are commonly the source of their own infection originates from the correlation of preoperative conjunctival culture findings with postoperative endophthalmitis. For example, 2508 cataract extractions (no prophylactic antibiotics) were followed by 11 cases of endophthalmitis.[22] In all of these infections the responsible organism, *Staphylococcus aureus*, had been present in the preoperative cultures. Only six cases of endophthalmitis were encountered during the subsequent 7662 cataract extractions performed in the same institution. The decrease in frequency of infection was attributed to instillation of antibiotic ointment (type determined by surgeon) five times during the day preceding surgery.

Subdivision of these patients into various groups further substantiates the assumption that infections commonly originate from the patient's own microflora. In 2263 cases (of the 7662), *Staphylococcus aureus* was not present in preoperative conjunctival cultures, and none of these patients developed endophthalmitis. In 567 cases, *Staphylococcus aureus* and other pathogenic microorganisms were identified in preoperative culture; therefore surgery was postponed until antibiotic therapy had sterilized the conjunctival sac, and again no endophthalmitis occurred in these cases.

The surgeon should be aware that after local antibiotic treatment is discontinued, the same pathogen will commonly return to the eye within 24 hours. Other sites on the patient's body surface harbor the organism, thereby permitting its speedy return.

The ophthalmologist must decide whether preoperative cultures are practical in the routine. In most general hospitals the administrative problems and cost discourage routine cultures. Clearly, however, the information gained from this large series of cultures proves the wisdom of eradicating through antibiotic use any recognizable surface infection before cataract extraction is performed.

Quantitative counts of the number of organisms reveal that in the average patient a cotton swab rubbed on the conjunctiva and lid margin will pick up tens of thousands of microorganisms.[23] A repeat culture on these same patients 2 or 3 days after cataract extraction (no antibiotics used) showed in most cases a substantial increase in microorganisms, often numbering in the hundreds of thousands per swab. The bandaged human eye is an excellent incubator for bacterial growth, as is clinically recognizable from the generous amount of discharge accumulating overnight under an eye bandage. Fortunately a properly closed incision is invulnerable to invasion by such surface bacteria.

Subconjunctival injection of 100,000 units of crystalline penicillin G and 66 mg of streptomycin in 0.2 ml of normal saline solution given at the conclusion of intraocular surgery will reduce the incidence of postoperative endophthalmitis. In an 18-month study, alternate patients received antibiotics (480) or were untreated (494 cases), except that penicillin was not given to patients with a history of sensitivity. Seven of the untreated patients developed serious postoperative infections, as compared to only one antibiotic-treated patient. After this study, all patients received routine antibiotic therapy. Of 1480 consecutive intraocular operations for which the patients received routine antibiotics, only two eyes developed postoperative infections. These two infections were caused by *Proteus vulgaris* and *Pseudomonas aeruginosa*. Both organisms were resistant to penicillin and streptomycin.[24] Should infection occur after such prophylactic therapy, the organism should be presumed to be resistant to the prophylactic drugs. Immediate treatment with an antibiotic such as colistimethate should begin when the diagnosis of endophthalmitis is made.

No postoperative infection occurred in a series of 1212 consecutive cases of cataract extraction.[25] This freedom from infection was attributed to the use of 200,000 units of penicillin combined with either 20,000 units of streptomycin or 20 mg of colistimethate (Coly-Mycin). This antibiotic combination was injected beneath the inferior conjunctiva at the close of surgery. Penicillin was used in every case, even in 52 patients who reported a penicillin sensitivity. Two of these patients developed hives and four developed allergic blepharitis, but in no case did eye damage result. The author points out that *Proteus vulgaris* is resistant to colistimethate and that *Pseudomonas* is resistant to streptomycin. Fungi and viruses are, of course, not inhibited by these antibiotics.

Although use of a repository type of vehicle would seem to be a rational way to prolong the therapeutic effect of subconjunctivally injected penicillin, effective intraocular antibiotic concentrations may not result after such injections. Table 31-1 shows the aqueous concentrations attained at the specified times after subconjunctival injection of 100 mg each of potassium penicillin G, procaine penicillin G, and benzathine penicillin G.[26]

Note that the peak concentrations of 6000 μg/ml are enormously in excess of the 0.1

Table 31-1. Aqueous concentrations in micrograms per milliliter*

Hours after injection	Potassium penicillin G	Procaine penicillin G	Benzathine penicillin G
1	6000	Trace	0.0024
2	6000	24	0.0024
4	360	24	0.0024
6	60	24	0.0010
8	6	24	0.0010
24	0	Trace	Trace
48	0	0	Trace
72	0	0	Trace
96	0	0	Trace

*Modified from Records, R. E.: Arch. Ophthalmol. **78:** 380, 1967.

μg/ml concentration required to inhibit the growth of most penicillin-susceptible microorganisms. These enormous concentrations achieved by subconjunctival injection of potassium penicillin G last for hours and would seem preferable to the much lower but somewhat more prolonged levels achieved by use of procaine penicillin G. Effective antibacterial aqueous titers of penicillin were never attained after injection of the benzathine penicillin G. Because subconjunctival injection of potassium penicillin G is well tolerated, such injection of 200,000 units of this antibiotic may be a very useful form of ocular therapy.

The antibiotic chosen for subconjunctival injection varies with the surgeon. A currently popular choice is gentamicin, 20 mg in 0.5 ml of saline solution. Gentamicin has a wide spectrum of activity but may cause considerable redness and irritation for several days.

Although prophylactic subconjunctival antibiotics have traditionally been given at the end of cataract surgery, a more rational time of injection is just before surgery. Such timing permits antibiotic action during the dangerous period when the eye is open and makes the antibiotic immediately available for penetration into the eye as soon as the blood-aqueous barrier is broken down by the incision.

I instill Neosporin ointment at the close of surgery because such a combination of antibiotics has a wide spectrum, including *Pseudomonas*, and because it does not cause the conjunctival hyperemia and chemosis that may persist at the antibiotic injection site for days.

PREOPERATIVE SEDATION

On the day of this writing I visited another surgeon during performance of a cataract operation. The initial sedation of the patient appeared good—he was relaxed, tranquil, unconcerned, and joked about golfing. Retrobulbar anesthesia was uneventfully given and well tolerated. Shortly after the corneoscleral incision was performed, the iris began to prolapse, although the eye had been very soft. A minute later the patient raised one hand, then the other, breaking free from the restraining drapes. His head jerked and turned. He complained in a garbled and confused manner about nausea and the covers on his nose and mouth. For perhaps 5 minutes the surgeon endured one of the most dreaded experiences—an uncontrollable patient with a wide open cataract incision. During this time the patient's blood pressure was 80 systolic (normal, 140), with a very weak pulse.

What happened to cause this? The surgeon said the patient was "just scared." The patient only vaguely remembered that something unusual had occurred. An anesthesiologist described the incident when he knew nothing about it except the premedication.

What was the premedication and why was the reaction predictable? The patient, a robust elderly man, had received two different tranquilizer drugs in addition to a barbiturate and a narcotic. The combined effect of these medications is to produce hypotension. Relaxing from his initial apprehension after the operation had started, slightly anoxic from the drapes covering his mouth and nose, and hypotensive from premedication, the patient with average cerebral arteriosclerosis inevitably becomes disoriented from cerebral anoxia.

The use of these various combinations of tranquilizers, sedatives, and narcotics has become popular, doubtless because the patient is usually quiet and does not bother the surgeon. Episodes of disorientation from cerebral anoxia, as just described, frequently occur and are attributed to "anesthetic reaction," "bad patient," or "inadequate sedation." The surgeon who encounters such hypoxic reactions should recognize they represent oversedation with synergistic drugs and should reduce the premedication accordingly.

The treatment for acute cerebral anoxia is, of course, administration of oxygen. This can be given by a tube slipped under the drapes near the patient's mouth. In this instance, oxygen resulted in the prompt cure of the patient's disorientation.

I continue to use simply a barbiturate-narcotic combination, that is, 100 mg pentobarbital and 75 mg meperidine, for the average adult. Addition of the various tranquilizers to this premedication is too unpredictable for consistent safety.

ANESTHESIA

Advocates of general or of local anesthesia continue to do battle in the literature. Discussion of this question with specialists in anesthesiology is thought provoking. Without exception, every anesthesiologist with whom I have discussed this matter has unequivocally stated a strong preference for local anesthesia for cataract surgery or any other short operation that can be performed equally well with the patient under local anesthesia. After performing a large number of retinal detachment operations with the patient under general anesthesia, I am quite familiar with the high incidence of postoperative aches and pains, nausea and vomiting, and malaise and weakness after general anesthesia. The surgeon who marches triumphantly from the room at the completion of surgery will not see the patient cough, heave, and retch during recovery; nevertheless, this commonly occurs.

Should general anesthesia be necessary for cataract surgery, as in the case of a deaf or mentally unstable patient, I believe the same retrobulbar anesthetic injection and lid block should be given as for surgery to be done with the patient under purely local anesthe-

sia. This will effectively block squeezing and eye movement should the anesthesia inadvertently become light, which is not a rare occurrence during routine anesthesia. Also, retrobulbar anesthesia followed by massage is perhaps the most important method of achieving hypotony.

Since the techniques of local anesthesia are well known to all ophthalmologists, a detailed description of how to enter the muscle cone or to perform an Atkinson akinesia is superfluous. The advantages of a large volume of retrobulbar injection are, however, less well known and deserve comment. The usual orbit will accept a 5 to 6 ml retrobulbar injection of 1% lidocaine with epinephrine and 150 TRU of hyaluronidase. After 5 minutes of massage, such a large volume will diffuse throughout the orbital tissues, resulting in a block of all extraocular muscles except the superior oblique. Sub-Tenon's diffusion will elevate Tenon's capsule from the sclera, aiding preparation of the conjunctival flap. Placement of the superior rectus traction suture is completely painless. Hypotony is profound. Incidentally, a 1% concentration of lidocaine is optimal for local anesthesia. A 2% solution does not increase anesthetic effectiveness and doubles the amount of toxic drug. Not more than 0.5 g of lidocaine should be given to a patient at one time. This is 50 ml of a 1% solution or 25 ml of a 2% solution.

The advent of more complex techniques of cataract surgery (phacoemulsification, intraocular lens implantation) has resulted in greater stress on the surgeon. Many surgeons deem it appropriate to devote their full attention to the operation, without distraction from the patient. With this rationale, they choose either general anesthesia or local standby anesthesia. In either instance the presence of the anesthesiologist permits a more precise titration of the medications to match the physical and emotional condition of the patient with safety. If an individual surgeon thinks that a better operation can be delivered in this way, the surgeon is probably correct and should utilize the services of an anesthesiologist. On the other hand, if this costs $100 more per case, such management of next year's 400,000 cataract extractions would cost the nation $40,000,000. Is this cost-effective? I do not think that we can afford it.

DILATING DROPS

The choice of drops for preoperative pupil dilation is a matter of wide individual variation. Most surgeons prefer cataract extraction through a widely dilated pupil. If desired, maximum dilation can best be achieved by a combination of parasympatholytic and sympathomimetic drugs, for example, 1% atropine and 10% phenylephrine. Should the pupil constrict during surgery, a valuable drug is 0.1% epinephrine, which can be instilled directly into the anterior chamber at this time. Within minutes, maximum dilation will result.

The phacoemulsifiers have shown that endothelial damage is a cumulative phenomenon. Mechanical trauma, toxicity from the irrigating solution, preservatives or osmotic stresses from intraocular instillation of solutions such as epinephrine, prolonged surgery, as well as genetic vulnerability, all contribute to the final total damage that may result in corneal decompensation. Do not add to this stress total by instilling anything unnecessary into the anterior chamber.

I personally prefer cataract extraction through a widely dilated pupil but agree that this is certainly not essential. In some types of lens delivery (for example, erysiphake or cryoextraction assisted by an iris spatula), adequate opening of the pupil may be achieved by mechanical stretching. Peripheral iridectomy is easier if the pupil is not excessively dilated. Repositing the iris and protection of the vitreous face may be simplified by a relatively small pupil.

Constriction of the pupil during surgery, despite atropinization, is caused by liberation of histamine or prostaglandins from the injured tissues. Histamine, of course, acts directly on the constrictor iridis musculature and is an effective miotic even in the presence of complete blockage of the parasympathomimetic innervation. Should the surgeon wish to prevent traumatic miosis from

occurring during surgery, he may administer an effective systemic antihistaminic drug preoperatively. For example, promethazine, 25 mg given 2 hours before surgery, maintained a well-dilated pupil in 12 of 14 cataract extractions as contrasted to 8 of 13 control eyes.[27]

Long-continued miotic therapy may result in a fibrotic pupil that will not dilate in response to any medications. This may be true even though the miotic has been discontinued for days or weeks before surgery. (The miotic should be discontinued before surgery to avoid postoperative miotic iridocyclitis, even if the pupil does not dilate.) Forcible delivery of the cataract through such a small pupil will tear and stretch the iris, leaving a flaccid and distorted pupil. The solution to this problem is mechanical, not medical. Perform sphincterotomies at the 4:30 and 7:30 positions or cut radially from a 12:00 peripheral iridectomy to the pupil.

AIDS TO HYPOTONY

The easiest, safest, fully effective method of achieving hypotony before cataract extraction is massage after retrobulbar anesthesia. This technique requires nothing more than the routine adequate retrobulbar anesthesia followed by up to 5 minutes of intermittent massage. Profound softness of the eye can be achieved by this method, providing the outflow mechanism is reasonably normal. No toxic side effects or disadvantages exist other than would occur from the retrobulbar injection given for purposes of anesthesia alone.

Whether induced by massage or by osmotherapy, hypotony is perpetuated by surgical opening of the anterior chamber. This precludes any "rebound" of vitreous pressure such as has been feared by some authors.[28] The rate of fluid loss from the vitreous body is proportional to the hydrostatic pressure gradient across a semipermeable membrane. The pressure gradient is 3 mm Hg, the pressure remaining within the vitreous cavity after opening the anterior chamber. Water and small-molecule electrolytes leave the vitreous body of the open rabbit eye at a rate of 5 mg/minute. In a 20-minute period (perhaps the duration of an open eye during cataract surgery) the weight of the rabbit vitreous will decrease by 100 mg.[29]

Secretory inhibitors and osmotic agents are often used to reduce intraocular pressure preoperatively. Such medications may be useful in preparation of the glaucomatous eye for surgery but seem to have more drawbacks than benefits when used as a routine management for normotensive eyes.

Acetazolamide is commonly used preoperatively with the intent of softening the eye. Although there can be no doubt that secretory inhibition does somewhat reduce the intraocular pressure of a normal eye, mushy softness comparable to that attainable by postanesthetic massage does not result. Nevertheless, many authors have recommended preoperative acetazolamide and cite excellent operative results.

Does 250 mg acetazolamide given the evening before cataract extraction actually benefit the surgeon? Or is such medication a manifestation of pharmacologic ignorance? Acetazolamide-induced hypotony lasts not more than 8 hours after a given dose of drug. Unless a surgeon plans to operate at midnight, the evening dose of uncoated acetazolamide must be considered as nothing more than a waste of the nurse's time.

Osmotic hypotensive agents such as glycerol or mannitol produce mushy soft hypotony even in glaucomatous eyes and are of genuine value in such cases. Again, however, the surgeon must recognize the short duration of osmotic hypotension, perhaps 2 to 4 hours. Oral glycerol the night before cataract extraction serves no useful purpose.

The numerous undesirable side effects of osmotic medications must be considered in the decision as to whether they will help or hinder a given cataract operation. Diuresis, for example, regularly occurs. A nice little old lady who has to void in the middle of the cataract extraction but is too embarrassed to say so is really in a predicament. Perhaps she can be excused for shifting about on the table a bit, but nevertheless this movement is still quite unwelcome to the surgeon.

"Palatable and well tolerated" as glycerol

is said to be, nausea and vomiting commonly occur after ingestion of an adequate dose. I doubt the wisdom of administering glycerol before cataract surgery. Uncontrollable vomiting during cataract extraction should occur only in the surgeon's bad dreams and not at the operating table.

Thirty patients were given 50% glycerol, 1.2 g/kg, orally before cataract surgery and compared with 30 patients receiving 50% isosorbide, 2.0 g/kg.[30] Before use of the glycerol, antiemetics, such as Compazine, 10 mg intramuscularly, or Tigan, 250 mg orally, were administered. No antiemetic was given with the isosorbide. Five glycerol patients were nauseated, one vomited, and one had a headache. No isosorbide-treated patients were nauseated, but two had diarrhea. Both drugs lowered the average intraocular pressure from 17 to 12 mm Hg 1 hour later.

Urea has the distressing ability to cause extensive sloughing of tissue should it extravasate. Some years ago I saw a lady who had extravasated urea from an intravenous site in the back of her hand. The entire dorsal part of her hand had sloughed, completely exposing all the extensor tendons. The severity of these local reactions to urea has resulted in the general use of mannitol as our osmotic agent of choice.

Cerebral dehydration results from all effective osmotic agents and is not unique to any one drug. Confusion and disorientation may ensue. Cerebrovascular accidents have been reported in association with osmotherapy. The dehydrating effects of osmotic drugs are immediately reversible simply by giving the patient water to drink. Of course, the therapeutic dehydrating effect is also dissipated immediately if the patient drinks. This is a practical consideration, since osmotherapy makes the patient compulsively thirsty and he will certainly drink unless it is specifically prohibited. Incidentally, an excessively thirsty patient also tends to complain and move during surgery.

From this recital of complications it is evident that I do not endorse osmotherapy as a routine step in cataract surgery, but reserve it as an aid in the rare patient who must be operated on during an episode of uncontrolled glaucoma. An example of such a problem would be glaucoma secondary to a swollen injured lens. Effective osmotherapy would consist of 1 to 2 g of mannitol/kg of body weight given intravenously about 30 minutes before maximum softness of the eye is desired.

Contrary to popular belief, devastating complications do not necessarily follow cataract extraction from a hard eye. In 16 cases of acute phacolytic glaucoma unresponsive to acetazolamide and pilocarpine, cataract extraction was undertaken despite pressures of 40 to 60 mm Schiøtz measured at surgery. In no case was there hemorrhage, vitreous loss, or other serious complications. In fact, the vitreous volume seemed reduced, the anterior vitreous face being deeply concave in all cases, with spontaneous entry of air into the anterior chamber.[31]

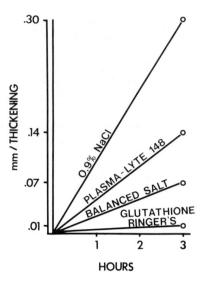

Fig. 31-1. Increase in corneal thickness following perfusion with designated solution. (Modified from Edelhauser, F., and associates: Am. J. Ophthalmol. **81:**473, 1976.)

IRRIGATING SOLUTIONS

In theory, the ideal irrigating solution for the anterior chamber would contain in proper concentration all the ions normally found in the aqueous humor. In practice, anterior chamber irrigation should be performed sparingly with minimal amounts of solution. Under such conditions, ionic equilibration rapidly occurs across the damaged blood-aqueous barrier.

A clinical comparison of the effect of irrigation with physiologic saline solution or balanced salt solution was made on 50 consecutive cataract extractions. Recognizable corneal haze persisted 4.1 days after saline solution and 3.5 days after balanced salt solution. Statistical evaluation indicated these variations were within chance limits, the standard deviation being 2 days. The incidence of striate keratitis was equal in the two series of cases.[32] Hence the common practice of limited irrigation with physiologic saline solution seems acceptable.

The rate of increase of thickness of the excised rabbit cornea and the appearance of the endothelium (both scanning and transmission electron microscopy) were studied for various solutions.[33] As shown in Fig. 31-1, 3 hours of perfusion with 0.9% sodium chloride resulted in a corneal thickness increase of 0.3 mm. This was reduced to 0.14 mm with Plasma-lyte 148 (the standard phacoemulsification solution), 0.11 with lactated Ringer's solution, 0.07 with balanced salt solution, and 0.01 with glutathione-bicarbonate Ringer's solution. The amount of endothelial damage demonstrated by microscopy correlated directly with the amount of corneal swelling.

After only 4 hours of perfusion with Plasma-lyte 148, the endothelium was severely disrupted and extensively vacuolated.[33] In contrast, after 7 days of incubation in McCarey-Kaufman (M-K) medium, human cornea endothelium appeared normal to electron microscopic examination.[34] Furthermore, 26 of 28 human corneas stored for up to 7 days in M-K medium remained clear after transplantation, indicating adequate endothelial survival. Even after 12 days of storage in M-K medium, rabbit corneas are suitable for penetrating keratoplasty.[35]

Trypan-blue staining identifies dead cells. After 4 days of storage of excised cat corneas in M-K medium, less than 5% of the endothelial cells stained with trypan blue.[36]

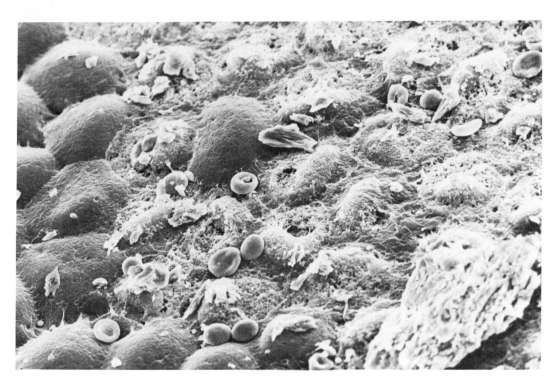

Fig. 31-2. Cat endothelium after phacoemulsification. (From Binder, P. S., and associates: Am. J. Ophthalmol. **82:**48, July 1976.)

Specular microscopic studies also confirm the superior viability of endothelial cells in glutathione-bicarbonate Ringer's solution as compared to the other irrigating media.[37]

The devastation that can be produced by irrigation with 500 ml of Plasma-lyte 148 and phacoemulsification is best demonstrated by a scanning electron microscope photograph such as shown in Fig. 31-2.[38] Irrigation alone, without use of ultrasound, causes severe damage.

Large volumes (125 to 850 ml) of irrigating solution are also used during vitrectomy. That this is toxic to the eye is demonstrable by measurement of corneal thickness. In aphakic patients undergoing vitrectomy for proliferative diabetic retinopathy, an increase of corneal thickness of 0.14 to 0.19 mm occurred when the irrigating solution was lactated Ringer's. In contrast, only 0.04 mm of increased thickness occurred with use of glutathione-bicarbonate Ringer's solution.[39]

The lens damage associated with vitrec-tomy is also attributable to the toxicity of irrigating solutions. Incubation of excised monkey lenses in glutathione-bicarbonate Ringer's solution maintained clarity in all lenses for 24 hours (some stayed clear as long as 96 hours). In contrast, all lenses were cataractous after 24 hours in Ringer's or Ringer's lactate.[40]

Unawareness of the destructive effect of anterior chamber irrigation with distilled water seems widespread. Generous irrigation with this hypotonic fluid will immediately destroy the corneal endothelium. Loss of corneal transparency develops during the surgical procedure and identifies this serious error—but too late. Postoperatively, the cornea is diffusely and uniformly edematous (in contrast to the localized edema of mechanical trauma or vitreocorneal contact).

I have followed two such cases in which distilled water is known to have been used and have seen other damaged eyes in which this diagnosis has seemed probable. Endothelial destruction by distilled water is irreversible. None of these severely damaged eyes has recovered spontaneously. Corneal transplantation was successfully performed in one of these cases.

ALPHA-CHYMOTRYPSIN

Doubt as to the zonulytic capability of alpha-chymotrypsin has long since been dispelled. Whether this enzyme is used in any particular operation now depends on the surgeon's decision as to whether the potential advantages of zonulysis outweigh the possible toxic effects of the drug.

Wound disruption and loss of the anterior chamber are slightly more common after use of alpha-chymotrypsin. Although these problems in wound healing were originally attributed to some type of enzymatic effect on the incision, they are now known to result from disruption of the wound by a transient enzyme-induced glaucoma. In a consecutive series of 100 cataract extractions performed without zonulysis, 4% had complications attributable to wound healing.[41] In 100 comparable cases operated on with zonulysis (2 to 4 ml of a 1:5000 solution), 11% had wound healing complications. Furthermore, all 11 of these wound complications occurred in patients in whom enzyme-induced glaucoma had been demonstrated. Other authors have also reported this threefold increase of incisional complications after enzyme use.[42] There is general agreement that use of multiple corneoscleral sutures is an effective method of preventing wound disruption, whether resulting from enzyme-induced glaucoma or another cause.

Enzyme-induced glaucoma characteristically appears from 2 to 5 days after surgery and usually spontaneously disappears in about 2 weeks. It is accompanied by a decrease in the facility of outflow (Fig. 4-9).[41] A deep anterior chamber and open angle differentiate enzyme-induced glaucoma from pupil-block glaucoma. Enzyme-induced glaucoma may or may not respond to 4% pilocarpine therapy, which should be initiated if high pressures are recognized. Although trabecular inflammation has been

suggested as a possible cause, corticosteroid therapy is not of benefit.

Alpha-chymotrypsin–induced glaucoma is dose related in that its frequency and severity increase with use of a larger volume of enzyme solution. Fig. 4-10 charts the highest (not average) pressure encountered in groups of 20 cataract extractions performed with the given volume of 1:5000 alpha-chymotrypsin.[43] Obviously the use of greater volumes causes very substantial pressure increases. Even the smallest volume used (0.25 ml) caused 55% of cases to develop postoperative pressures of 24 mm Hg or higher. Use of 1.5 ml increased this to 70%. The cataract surgeon is advised to use the smallest dose of alpha-chymotrypsin necessary to produce satisfactory zonulysis. Be reminded that 2 to 4 ml of 1:5000 alpha-chymotrypsin was routinely used when this form of postoperative glaucoma was discovered.[43]

As little as 0.2 ml of 1:5000 alpha-chymotrypsin and certainly not more than 0.5 ml will usually suffice to produce zonulysis. Indeed a 1:10,000 dilution is adequate. Obviously, differences in zonular strength will be anticipated in young and old patients and appropriate dosage adjustments may be made. Should undue zonular resistance be encountered after the first enzyme instillation, there is no reason why the enzyme irrigation cannot be repeated.

A disputed clinical point concerns the need to irrigate the anterior chamber to remove alpha-chymotrypsin after it has been allowed 2 minutes of action.[44] Such irrigation has been advocated to reduce potential toxic effects to the interior of the eye. However, it seems likely that spontaneous enzyme inactivation occurs, provided only small amounts have been introduced into the eye.

The enzyme-inhibiting property of human aqueous humor was evaluated by 15-minute incubation of equal volumes of 1:5000 alpha-chymotrypsin and of human secondary aqueous. Inhibitory activity measured in this way destroyed from 5% to 67% of the alpha-chymotrypsin potency (aqueous samples studied from 10 eyes). No enzyme activity could be detected in secondary aqueous obtained from five eyes in which alpha-chymotrypsin had been used for cataract extraction (0.4 ml of a 1:5000 solution, allowed to stand for 2 minutes). Judging from these findings, there seems to be no need to irrigate away or to neutralize the enzyme following its use for cataract extraction.[45]

However, irrigation probably removes much of the zonular and pigmentary debris that has been shown to be responsible for "enzyme" glaucoma; hence I do advocate such irrigation.

Primary human aqueous has also been shown to inactivate alpha-chymotrypsin.[46]

No correlation exists between preoperative intraocular pressure and susceptibility to enzyme-induced glaucoma. Hence, if indicated, the use of alpha-chymotrypsin need not be avoided during cataract extraction in patients with glaucoma. In a series of 15 patients with bilateral cataract and intraocular pressure ranging from 21 to 29 mm Hg in each eye, enzymatic zonulysis was used in the right eye but not in the left. In only two eyes in which zonulysis was used was there a transient 6 mm elevation above the pressure of the control eye.[47]

Of a control series of 200 cataract extractions performed without use of alpha-chymotrypsin, postoperative glaucoma (not detected prior to surgery) was found in six patients within 8 weeks after surgery. Three such cases of glaucoma occurred in the treatment series of 200 operations performed with 0.75 to 1 ml of a 1:5000 solution of Chymar.[48] Such a late onset of glaucoma is not characteristic of enzyme-induced glaucoma and does not represent a delayed type of enzyme damage (obviously, since it occurred in even greater frequency in patients not receiving enzyme).

Perhaps the greatest contraindication to enzymatic zonulysis is the youth of the patient. Lens-vitreous adhesions are usually very firm in patients under 20 years of age. Since such adhesions are not dissolved by alpha-chymotrypsin, intracapsular removal of the young lens is commonly accompanied by extensive vitreous loss. Irreparable retinal detachment often results. Enzymatic

zonulysis is not recommended for extraction of congenital, developmental, or traumatic cataracts in infants and children.[49]

The older patient usually has such fragile zonules that their dissolution is unnecessary. Over the age of 60 years, intracapsular extraction presents little difficulty, particularly since cryoextraction has become popular. Little reason exists for routine use of enzyme in the old eye.

The possibility of "intracapsular" removal of an extensive secondary cataract with the aid of zonulysis should be considered. Good results were reported in 16 eyes so treated.[50] I have personally found the results of this technique to be most encouraging.

MIOTICS

Immediately after cataract extractions some surgeons advise the use of a miotic. Miosis is stated to protect the vitreous face and to help prevent iris incarceration. Acetylcholine, pilocarpine, and carbachol have been recommended to achieve postoperative miosis. When these drugs are introduced directly into the anterior chamber, very dilute concentrations give an excellent pharmacologic response. For instance, 0.01% carbachol reduced pupil size from an average of 6 to 3 mm within 2 minutes after cataract extraction in human eyes.[51] Although maximum carbachol miosis lasts less than 2 hours, some pupillary constriction is recognizable for as long as 6 hours after medication.

Pilocarpine has long been used to achieve postoperative miosis and is, of course, effective. The standard 1% solution may be dropped on the cornea at any stage of the operation after delivery of the lens. Pilocarpine will give prolonged and good miosis, but it has the disadvantage of increasing postoperative pain.

Eserine or any indirectly acting parasympathomimetic drug acts by inhibiting destruction of acetylcholine. Since no acetylcholine is produced at the nerve terminals during the period of retrobulbar anesthesia, eserine will not cause miosis during surgery and cannot be used for this purpose.

Reliable preparations of 1% acetylcholine

are now available and have become relatively popular. To achieve miosis, this solution may be irrigated into the anterior chamber immediately after lens delivery.[52] Pupil constriction is prompt but lasts for only a few minutes. This provides the advantages of miosis during surgery but avoids postanesthetic discomfort.

I am skeptical of the value of miotics after cataract extraction. Proper surgical re-formation of the anterior chamber with saline solution will hold back the vitreous quite as well as does the iris. To my knowledge, no one fears to dilate an aphakic eye lest the vitreous face rupture or prolapse through the pupil. I have recognized no relationship between pupil size and ease of repositing the iris after cataract extraction.

The insertion and positioning of an iris-supported intraocular lens may be helped by miosis.

CORTICOSTEROIDS

The routine postoperative use of corticosteroids has become increasingly popular and is vigorously supported by its advocates, who cite the "obvious" benefits. Presumably the eye looks better and heals better. For example, the repository form of methylprednisolone acetate (Depo-Medrol) was injected beneath Tenon's capsule at the close of surgery in 200 consecutive cataract extractions.[53] The complications in this series of cases were compared with the frequency of complications reported in the literature. Although the validity of such comparisons appears doubtful, the authors concluded that corticosteroid therapy reduced the incidence of wound-healing problems such as flat and shallow anterior chambers, iris prolapse, uveitis, infection, and glaucoma. Only the frequency of filtering blebs (6% versus 1.4%) was greater in the corticosteroid-treated series.

In another series of 200 cataract patients a double-blind study was used to evaluate the effect of dexamethasone (Decadron), 0.1% drops instilled three times daily for 3 weeks postoperatively, as compared with placebo drops.[54] The amount of reaction in the various parts of the eye was recorded as well as intraocular pressure, complications, and the impression of the surgeons as to which drop they believed was being used. The postoperative courses of the treated and untreated groups were identical except that six corticosteroid-treated eyes developed filtering bleb, but none of the control group did so. The surgeons' attempts to guess which patients were receiving corticosteroid gave results no better than a chance guess. Perhaps the most interesting finding was that 27 patients had sufficient anterior chamber inflammatory response so that their physician removed them from the study and instituted therapy with known dexamethasone. Of these 27 patients, 13 had been receiving dexamethasone in the study and 14 were given control drops. This indicates that corticosteroid therapy does not significantly alter the course of postoperative traumatic iritis. The authors concluded that the superior results of modern cataract surgery are a result of technical advances (such as fine sutures). Postoperative corticosteroid therapy became popular during the same period of time and received undeserved credit for the appearance of the eyes. I am in complete agreement with this conclusion, never use routine postoperative corticosteroids, and attribute the comfort of the eyes to the use of 10-0 nylon sutures.

POSTOPERATIVE HYPHEMA

Minor amounts of blood clot adherent to the iris at the close of cataract surgery do not contribute to development of postoperative hyphema, spontaneously disappear before the first dressing, and require no attention or concern. Serious technical errors damaging the ciliary body or venous collector channels may produce immediate or early postoperative extensive hemorrhage. Most postoperative hyphemas arise from disruption of the wound edges before healing is secure but after capillary ingrowth has developed. The time of highest incidence of such hyphemas is toward the end of the first postoperative week.

Although much has been written concerning medical therapy of postoperative hyphema, these measures are not demonstrably effective. In contrast, appropriate surgical techniques can virtually eliminate the problem.

Systemic causes

Although patients suffering from blood dyscrasias, anticoagulant poisoning, or vitamin deficiencies would certainly be predisposed to postoperative hypema, such systemic conditions are not a significant cause of clinical bleeding after eye surgery. For instance, deficiency of vitamins C or K was not found to be a cause of postoperative hemorrhage in 96 patients with hyphema after cataract surgery.[55]

Use of vitamin K as a preoperative routine to prevent intraocular bleeding is unwarranted. Prothrombin levels were found to be normal in all but 1 of 133 cases of postcataract intraocular hemorrhage.[56] Subsequently, vitamin K therapy restored this one patient's prothrombin time to normal, and cataract extraction was performed on the other eye, which also developed a severe hemorrhage.

I have the undocumented clinical belief that heavy ethanol consumption predisposes to hyphema following cataract extraction. This possibility occurred to me during performance of retinal detachment surgery under general anesthesia induced by intravenous ethanol and morphine (an experimental anesthetic technique). From the standpoint of an eye surgeon, this is a totally unsatisfactory anesthetic because the eyes become grossly congested (so does the skin) with blood within a maximally dilated capillary bed. Everything bleeds! Subsequent to this experience, I have had four hyphemas in my own postcataract patients. Three of these patients were moderately heavy drinkers, charitably describable as socially functional alcoholics. Since realizing the probability of a relationship between ethanol and postoperative hyphema, I have instructed such patients to refrain from drinking for 2 weeks after surgery. Fortunately, I've had no more hyphemas—but who knows what that proves?

Estrogen therapy

As an example of the type of favorable report concerning medical therapy of postoperative hyphema, estrogens are said to decrease bleeding by increasing the amount of acid polysaccharide surrounding capillary walls. In a study of 223 cataract extractions,[57] half the patients received 20 mg of estrogen intravenously about 15 minutes preoperatively, followed by a 2.4 mg tablet (Premarin) four times a day for 7 days. The other half received placebo injection and tablets. Six hyphemas occurred in the 111 estrogen-treated patients (5.4%), and of these, five were quite small. Of the 112 placebo patients, 21 (18.8%) had hemorrhages, only three of which were small. Total hyphema filled the anterior chamber in three placebo cases, and one eye was blinded by hemorrhage. The explanation for this incredible 18% incidence of hyphema is not apparent but presumably is related to surgical technique.

Most studies of estrogen antihemorrhagic therapy are not so encouraging. For instance, postoperative hyphema developed in exactly 13% of 100 cataract extractions treated with a comparable dose of conjugated estrogens and also in 13% of 100 similar patients on placebo treatment.[58] These hyphemas did not differ in severity in the two groups.

Surgical techniques

Evidence that prevention of hyphema after cataract surgery is more a matter of surgical technique than of medical management is provided by many clinical studies correlating incision and suture techniques with the incidence of postoperative bleeding. For example, in a comparative study of 300 cases in which operation was performed before the development of modern corneoscleral sutures, when the incision was closed by superficial sutures, the incidence of hyphema was 15%.[59] In contrast, the use of a Stallard-type suture with a firm bite in the cornea and sclera reduced the incidence of postcataract hyphema to 6.6%.

Since the advent of the high-quality needles and sutures that permit easy and accurate placement of seven or more corne-oscleral sutures, wound disruptions causing significant anterior chamber hemorrhage are, fortunately, very rare. After a well-sutured cataract extraction, the incidence of complications such as hyphema or flat chamber is not increased by immediate reasonable activity, providing the eye is shielded against direct injury.[60] Medications do not achieve this result; good surgery does.

POSTOPERATIVE SHALLOW CHAMBER

Medical therapy of flat or shallow anterior chambers after cataract extraction is a curious mixture of frustrated optimism. Miotics, mydriatics, acetazolamide, restricted activity, and a variety of other treatments have all been used, sometimes with dramatic success. The unpredictable and often self-limited course of these shallow chambers suggests that coincidence is responsible for many of the claimed therapeutic responses.

Etiology

A truly rational therapeutic approach requires accurate understanding of the causes of shallow chamber after cataract extraction. Actually, at least two major types of postoperative shallow chamber exist—delayed re-formation of the chamber (early) and delayed loss of the chamber (late).[61]

The cause of postoperative shallow or flat chambers occurring within the first few days after surgery is almost certainly aqueous leakage through an area of faulty wound closure. Often the Seidel fluorescein test will disclose such a leak. In the most pronounced cases a green rivulet may be seen flowing through the layer of orange fluorescein. In other instances a diffuse color change from orange to green occurs very rapidly, indicating aqueous leakage. Convincing proof of this mechanism is offered by a series of 50 cataract extractions in which the eye was closed with two sutures as compared with 50 eyes closed with five corneoscleral sutures. All were done with the same technique other than for the number of sutures and by the same ophthalmologist.[62] The striking dif-

Table 31-2. Comparison of two techniques of cataract extractions (50 cases each)*

	Two sutures	Five sutures
Flat chamber	6	0
Shallow chamber	4	0
Iris incarceration or prolapse	7	1
Hyphema	4	1
Average final astigmatism	1.78 D	0.74 D

*From New Orleans Academy of Ophthalmology: Symposium on ocular pharmacology and therapeutics, St. Louis, 1970, The C. V. Mosby Co.

ferences encountered are recorded in Table 31-2.

Early shallow chamber

The medical management of early postoperative shallow chamber requires identification of the site of the wound leak by use of fluorescein. A generous amount of fluorescein enhances the visibility of the leak. A very small leak can be sealed by cautery with trichloracetic acid. The area around the leak should be touched with an acid-saturated toothpick tightly wrapped with only a thin layer of cotton fibers. If effective, the acid cautery will seal the leak immediately and the chamber will be reformed by the next day. Be warned not to substitute trichloracetic acid for the proper resuturing of a ruptured wound. An early fault in closure large enough to disclose a visible iris prolapse will gradually increase in size, and proper suturing should not be delayed by the foredoomed ineffectual use of trichloracetic acid.

Very small corneal perforations or incisional gaps may be closed by application of the surgical adhesive M-heptyl-2-cyanoacrylate.[63] This adhesive polymerizes instantaneously as soon as it contacts any fluid containing ions (such as tissue fluid or tears). The cyanoacrylate plug adheres to the tissue for at least several days, permitting the corneal tissue to grow together behind it. Minor tissue irritation accompanies the presence of this adhesive, but it is insufficient to damage the eye. The procedure is very simple, requiring only application of the adhesive to the clean surface of the edges of the corneal perforation. Local patching with surgical adhesives is the treatment of choice for small corneal perforations, replacing entirely the more complex surgical procedures such as keratoplasty.

Ophthalmic surgeons who frequently encounter early flat or shallow chamber problems must face the unpleasant truth that their technique is faulty. Five to seven properly placed corneal sutures will virtually eliminate the leaky wounds that cause soft eyes with flat chambers (and subsequent aphakic glaucoma). Convincing proof of the value of multiple sutures is provided by a consecutive series of 355 cataract extractions closed by five to seven sutures, complicated by not one single flat chamber. In contrast, the incidence of flat chamber was 9.1% in a series of 155 consecutive extractions performed by the same man but closed by only two sutures.[64]

In a later publication the same ophthalmologist reported a series of 702 consecutive cataract extractions without a single flat chamber.[65] This success was attributed to use of five to seven corneoscleral sutures.

Late shallow chamber

"Late" loss of the anterior chamber does not begin until perhaps 4 days after cataract extraction and may appear as long as 3 weeks postoperatively. In a series of 200 cataract extractions, "early" shallow chamber was entirely eliminated by careful wound closure, and yet 14 cases of late shallow chamber developed.[66] A possible external leak was demonstrable in only one of these eyes, although in five others a filtering bleb was transiently observed. Each of the 14 eyes showed evidence of obstruction of aqueous flow through the pupil. The concept was proposed that pupillary block is a major cause for late postoperative shallow chamber.

Medical therapy effective in breaking this pupillary block deepened the anterior chamber within 30 to 90 minutes in all of these 14 eyes. None required surgery such as posterior sclerotomy or air injection into the anterior chamber. Note that the moderate mydriasis of atropine alone is insufficient to break this pupillary block. The pupil *must* be maximally dilated by repeated instillation of 10% phenylephrine combined with a parasympatholytic drug such as atropine or cyclopentolate.

In one patient the shallow chamber recurred four times during a 10-day period. Invariably, however, the chamber re-formed promptly with extreme mydriasis. After the fourth dilation the chamber remained deep.

Miosis has been suggested for treatment of shallow chamber, but it usually fails or even worsens the condition. Infrequently a miotic may open a clogged iridectomy, thereby breaking the pupil block.

The aqueous appearance time of intravenous fluorescein (which enters the eye from ciliary processes) has been used to demonstrate an increased physiologic pupil block in aphakic eyes with vitreous prolapse into the anterior chamber.[67] In such eyes the appearance time of fluorescein in the anterior chamber averaged 1.7 minutes, almost three times the period required in eyes with a flat vitreous face behind the pupil (0.6 minute). These studies confirm the existence in some aphakic eyes of a physiologic pupil block that could worsen by inflammatory adhesions or benefit from wide dilation.

Fluorescein penetration into the aphakic vitreous of eyes with shallow or flat anterior chambers took 4 to 8 minutes in eight eyes with normal or elevated intraocular pressure. Vitreous fluorescein penetration in three eyes with flat chamber, massive choroidal detachment, and marked hypotony was said to be much slower (time unspecified). Inhibition of aqueous secretion was suggested as an explanation of this poor fluorescein entry into soft aphakic eyes with flat chambers.

Choroidal detachment

The choroidal detachment often found in eyes with shallow chamber appears to be a secondary phenomenon related to hypotony. Perhaps the most convincing argument against causation of shallow chamber by choroidal detachment is found in retinal detachment surgery. Small and sometimes large choroidal detachments are often found in eyes softened by release of subretinal fluid. Whether phakic or aphakic, these eyes never develop shallow chambers. (Massive posterior hemorrhages can cause a shallow chamber, but these eyes are hard.) Once established, a large choroidal (and ciliary body) transudative detachment is said to inhibit aqueous secretion,[68] accounting for continued softness of the eye.

Any evaluation of the response of medications of the intraocular tension of the postoperative cataract eye must take into account the expected normal course. Fig. 31-3 shows the average intraocular pressures in a series of 50 postoperative cataract patients.[69] After the first week, the average tensions were below 10 mm Hg. Clearly, therefore, low pressures in the range of 5 to 10 mm Hg cannot be considered abnormal postoperatively and do not in themselves require treatment.

Choroidal detachment is a unique fluid collection that disobeys Starling's law (requiring free fluid to enter the capillary bed) because it occurs in a position away from the capillary bed; hence it is not exposed to capillary pull. No matter how soft an eye, subretinal transudation does not occur because of the proximity of the choriocapillaris. A

high proportion of very soft eyes—whether due to surgery for glaucoma, cataract, or retinal detachment or to injury—will develop choroidal detachment. Such a choroidal detachment will spontaneously disappear whenever the intraocular pressure rises sufficiently high to force the fluid out of the eye, either transsclerally or into the large choroidal vessels. The fluid of a choroidal detachment is not effectively exposed to the capillary osmotic pull of mannitol, to the hyposecretory effect of acetazolamide, or to the outflow increase of pilocarpine. Fortunately, since we have no effective treatment anyway, choroidal detachment is a benign condition in itself, requiring no particular concern.

Vitreous block

Statistics from a "pupil block" advocate are thought provoking.[70] Of 3000 cataract extractions, only eight required surgery for postoperative shallow chamber associated with hypotony. All other shallow chambers (5% of nonbasal and 2% of basal iridectomies) responded to medical treatment alone! In these eight cases, posterior synechiae (resulting from inflammation) prevented medical dilation of the pupil. In all eight cases the an-

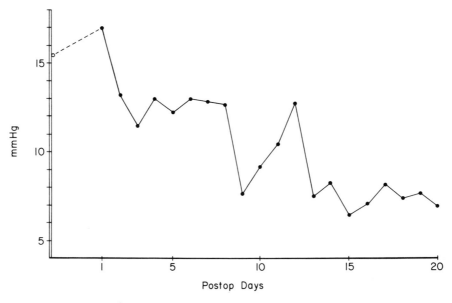

Fig. 31-3. Mean intraocular pressures in 50 eyes after cataract surgery. (Modified from Gormaz, A.: Am. J. Ophthalmol. **53:**832, 1962.)

terior chamber was restored by surgical iridectomy alone, without resorting to air injections, sclerotomy for drainage of suprachoroidal fluid, intentional rupture of the vitreous face, or resuturing of the limbal cataract incision. This suggests that the success after air injection may simply be because of the unknowing rupture of the pupillary block.

In a later publication the concept of "pupillary block" was widened to "vitreous block."[70] Vitreous block can occur with either peripheral or sector iridectomy and can exist with hypotony or glaucoma. Gonioscopy of 2000 aphakic eyes disclosed that 25% of the sector iridectomies and 33% of the peripheral iridectomies did not extend to within 1 mm of the root of the iris. Vitreous block was relatively frequent when the iris opening extended only halfway from the pupil to the root of the iris, but was seldom present with truly basal iridectomies. Hence the problem of the postoperative shallow chamber may be avoided not only by secure wound closure but also by an adequate iridectomy (either sector or peripheral) extending to within 1 mm of the iris root.[71]

The most precise explanation of why mydriasis reversibly alleviates glaucoma caused by continuing pupil block by an intact vitreous face is offered by measurements of the resistance to flow through the hyaloid membrane.[72] The C value/mm^2 of vitreous face is about 0.04. The resistance to aqueous flow through intact vitreous plugging a pupil will therefore increase rapidly with miosis, inversely to the square of the radius of the pupil. This explains why mydriasis will permit a pressure drop, although the vitreous face still appears in contact with the dilated pupil throughout its circumference. (Of course, this explanation is unnecessary if the dilated pupil is seen to separate completely from the vitreous face, thereby allowing unobstructed flow of aqueous.)

Secretory-inhibitor therapy

An attempt to evaluate the effect of acetazolamide on postcataract shallow anterior chamber utilized the hospital records of 150 cases compiled during the preceding decade.[73] Acetazolamide had been used in 55

of these episodes of flat or shallow chamber (dosage was apparently variable, probably 250 mg three or four times daily). If treatment was started within 48 hours, 79% of the chambers were re-formed within 2 additional days, as contrasted to only 45% of the control group. On the basis of these statistics, the paper concludes that acetazolamide is a valuable medication. Presumably the drug acts by reducing outflow pressure during the time required for a leaking wound to heal.

It is only fair to point out certain weaknesses in this study that may invalidate the conclusion. Evaluation of a case solely on the basis of old hospital records often leaves much to be desired; to quote from the paper, "It was therefore impossible at times to determine from old records the exact duration of the anterior chamber." The selection of the cases for treatment was not on the basis of predetermined random criteria and may have been influenced by factors that would distort the outcome. For instance, 23% of the nonacetazolamide-treated cases required surgical repair. Has this group of most severely leaking wounds been selectively placed into the untreated category, thereby altering the statistics? Consideration only of the total duration of the shallow chamber indicated that recovery occurred within 8 days in 92% of all (recalculated from total figures) untreated and 96% of treated eyes—hardly an imposing difference. Finally, the composition of one of the control groups appears to have been tampered with. Supposedly it is composed of eyes with absence of anterior chambers *for 48 hours.* With this requirement, 22 untreated cases that spontaneously re-formed within 2 days were discarded from consideration—hardly fair! Recalculation, including these cases, gives percentages that are virtually identical for the treated or untreated eyes. Hence this paper really indicates that acetazolamide treatment does not significantly alter the course of postcataract flat or shallow chamber.

Osmotic therapy

Pupillary-block shallow chamber glaucoma after cataract extraction may be successfully treated by systemic use of osmotic agents such as glycerol or mannitol, thereby avoiding surgical iridectomy. Medical treatment alone was effective in both of a series of two cases.[74] Severe vitreous adherence to the cornea was relieved by osmotic therapy alone in only one of five cases; the other four required posterior sclerotomy and air injection. The mechanism of action of osmotic agents in these two types of postcataract complications is, of course, shrinkage of the vitreous volume to free the vitreous from contact with pupil or cornea. I have had only one occasion to try glycerol therapy for pupil-block glaucoma. The patient vomited and the pressure was not relieved. Performance of a generous prophylactic iridectomy at the time of cataract extraction will virtually eliminate the complication of pupil-block shallow chamber glaucoma.

Osmotic-mydriatic therapy

Ten patients with shallow or flat anterior chamber after cataract extraction were treated with both 50% glycerol (1 ml/pound body weight, orally) and dilation (1% cyclopentolate and 10% phenylephrine, 1 drop of each every 10 minutes for four times). In every eye the anterior chamber was demonstrably deeper within 2 hours. In four cases a single treatment caused permanent deepening of the anterior chamber. A second treatment cured three additional eyes. Three and four treatments were required for one eye each. Only a single eye failed to respond permanently to four treatments and was operated on using air injection. Nausea was experienced by five patients. Two had severe headaches and one vomited.[75]

The rationale of this treatment is osmotic shrinkage of the vitreous body and release of iris-vitreous contact that might block aqueous flow into the anterior chamber. This osmotic-mydriatic method is recommended as a safe and effective way of treating the postoperative shallow or flat anterior chamber occurring in a soft eye.

Results of medical therapy of flat chamber

Of 8533 cataract extractions, 7.6% were complicated by postoperative flat anterior chamber.[76] These eyes were treated by a variety of medical regimens, including mydriatics, miotics, osmotic agents, and acetazolamide. Subsequent to such medications and/or pressure dressings, the anterior chamber re-formed in 78% of eyes. This author[77] specified that this re-formation may well have occurred spontaneously and regardless of the medical therapy chosen. The statistical information does not permit inferences as to the relative value of the different types of medical therapy. My purpose in citing these articles is to indicate that at least four out of five flat chambers will recover without surgery.

Soft contact lens for early flat chamber

An incisional leak large enough to cause continuing early flat or shallow anterior chamber can be occluded by covering it with a hydrophilic contact lens.[78] This method is apparently more effective than a pressure bandage external to the eyelids. Covering with a soft lens should be used only in cases selected because of small size of the gap, good alignment of the edges, and absence of prolapsed uveal tissue.

Epithelial downgrowth etiology of shallow chamber

Fistulization of an epithelial downgrowth may occur as late as 8 months or more (personal observation) after intraocular surgery.[79] This complication may be recognized by the shallow anterior chamber, choroidal detachment, intraocular infection, hypotony, or decreased visual acuity.

No medical therapy is effective for this cause of shallow chamber. Radiation or surgical treatment may benefit selected cases.

POSTOPERATIVE MIOTIC IRITIS

I particularly wish to call attention to a little appreciated but not uncommon cause of inflammation after cataract extraction. The permeability of the blood-aqueous barrier is increased during the period of effect of miotic therapy. This miotic-induced breakdown of the barrier is of considerable clinical significance because it results in extensive inflammatory changes after intraocular surgery on glaucoma patients.

Miotic iritis is relatively insidious in that the affected eye does not seem to be overly irritable. Nevertheless, posterior synechiae become gradually more extensive, a delicate connective tissue membrane creeps across the vitreous face, scattered pigment deposits appear over the vitreous face, and the pupil becomes firmly bound down, distorted, and unresponsive to dilation. Reduction in visual acuity corresponds to the density of the membrane and pigment covering the vitreous face.

Prevention of postoperative miotic iritis requires that the miotic be discontinued sufficiently long before surgery so that its action may be completely dissipated. In the case of pilocarpine this requires about 2 days, whereas the longer acting miotics such as isoflurophate may require 3 weeks. Since one hesitates to omit treatment of glaucoma for weeks, a practical expedient might be to change from a strong miotic to pilocarpine a month before surgery and then to discontinue the pilocarpine at least 2 days before cataract extraction.

Postoperatively, the glaucomatous patient should be watched more closely than most patients. If tolerated, cycloplegia is desirable to help prevent miotic iritis. Pressure control should be achieved by the use as necessary of secretory inhibitors such as acetazolamide and of sympathomimetic drugs such as epinephrine. The danger period for postoperative miotic iritis extends as long as a month after surgery. Miotic use should be avoided altogether or certainly held to a minimum during this period.

POSTOPERATIVE INFECTION

Perhaps the most dreaded postcataract complication is intraocular infection. The number of such infections in the United States has been estimated to approximate 800 to 1000 per year.[80]

The first problem confronting the ophthalmologist in the management of postoperative infection is differential diagnosis. Knowing the urgency of early diagnosis, the surgeon is realistically concerned by inflammatory reactions that might represent beginning endophthalmitis. A premature diagnosis of infection, leading to vigorous therapeutic overresponse, is very common and cannot really be condemned.

Undue pain, excessive redness and swelling, corneal edema, aqueous flare and cells, indistinct iris markings, debris on the vitreous face, and a poor red reflex are the usual findings suggesting postoperative endophthalmitis. Essentially identical findings may exist in eyes subjected to undue surgical trauma, irritated by retained foreign debris (powder or lint), irrigated by improper solutions, poisoned by preservatives and germicides retained on instruments, allergic to gut sutures, responding to retained lens material, suffering from anterior uveitis (whatever that is), or responding to a true infection by viruses or bacteria of such low virulence that spontaneous cure will result.[81-83] These conditions, to be considered in the differential diagnosis of endophthalmitis, will tend toward spontaneous recovery, may benefit from corticosteroid therapy, and will usually not be harmed (or helped) by antibiotics unless given by destructive routes or in excessive dosage.

From the practical standpoint, these relatively minor causes of concern far outnumber cases of truly dangerous infection. Most of the red and painful eyes viewed with alarm by the residents do not represent instances of infection and do not warrant potentially hazardous diagnostic and therapeutic measures.

More severe cases of aseptic iritis also occur and may cause fairly severe engorgement of iris vessels, transudation of fibrin into the anterior chamber, and even a small hypopyon.[84] Differentiation between such a severe case and a case of true infectious endophthalmitis may be virtually impossible, especially when the condition is first seen. The time of onset may be helpful, since a traumatic or toxic response will usually be evident at the first dressing in 24 hours, whereas the usual incubation period for a bacterial infection is 48 hours or longer. I believe that the most certain sign of bacterial endophthalmitis, in distinction from aseptic iritis, is a gray opacification of the cornea. Such corneal opacification does not occur in iritis but is typical of established endophthalmitis.

If the condition is caused by iritis, intensive cycloplegic and mydriatic therapy will usually promptly reduce the abnormal permeability of the iris vessels, with recognizable lessening of the severity of the inflammation. Warm compresses are helpful. Such management may be preferable initially if the cornea is transparent and the hypopyon is absent. However, you must watch the eye very closely, perhaps every 4 to 6 hours, to detect worsening of the condition despite cycloplegic therapy, which would occur if the diagnosis was really an infection. Many physicians advocate prompt corticosteroid usage also. Although this will help to clear iritis, corticosteroids will reduce resistance to infectious agents. If there is serious consideration of the possibility of infection, I advocate withholding corticosteroids until the response to cycloplegics, occurring within a day or two, proves the diagnosis to be iritis. Fortunately, in most cases, several days of observation and conservative treatment will result in disappearance of the problem.

The value of surface cultures of the limbal wound edge in deciding whether the diagnosis is endophthalmitis is virtually nil. In a series of 50 uncomplicated postoperative cataract patients, 36% of cultures of the conjunctival incision showed bacterial growth. I am surprised that almost all did not show growth; however, the reason is probably that routine topical antibiotic therapy was continued postoperatively in these cases.[85]

The diagnostic value of anterior chamber paracentesis in postoperative endophthalmitis has been evaluated in a retrospective study of 22 years of records from the Proctor Foundation.[80] During this period, 14 aqueous specimens from eyes with postoperative endophthalmitis were submitted to the laboratory. Of these 14 specimens, five produced positive cultures (three *Staphylococcus aureus*, one paracolon bacillus, and one *Bacillus subtilis*). Smears of these five specimens showed polymorphonuclear leukocytes in each instance. Four of the 14 specimens showed a mononuclear cell response, presumably indicating a diagnosis of postoperative uveitis. The authors believe that the information to be gained from the procedure far outweighs its risks and cite another study of 103 patients on whom paracentesis was performed after the diagnosis of uveitis was made, resulting in only five anterior chamber hemorrhages, all of which cleared.

While accurate identification of the sensitivity of a microorganism is undeniably desirable, the practical aspects of paracentesis deserve some consideration. Is paracentesis warranted before the infection is so severe as to be undeniable? At that stage of severity, will the eye survive long enough for sensitivity determinations to be helpful? In how many instances will the culture-guided therapy differ from "shotgun" therapy with systemic penicillin or chloramphenicol and topical administration of gentamicin or Neosporin? Is paracentesis of an inflamed eye with a 3-day-old cataract incision really as safe as a diagnostic tap for uveitis? Do five positive cultures in 22 years establish the value of paracentesis? Clearly, each individual eye will require careful, intelligent, and difficult decisions.

If the working diagnosis of bacterial endophthalmitis is made, token therapy with antibiotic drops is inappropriate. Prompt and intensive antibacterial therapy is necessary. My choice is chloramphenicol, 2 g initially, followed by 1 g every 3 hours. Chloramphenicol solubility characteristics permit ready intraocular penetration. Also, it has a reasonably wide antibacterial spectrum (does not include *Pseudomonas*).

Another regimen[86] advises oxacillin, 2 g every 4 hours, given as a 15- to 30-minute intravenous infusion. (Oxacillin is effective against penicillinase-producing staphylococci). Simultaneously, gentamicin is given intravenously in dosage of 5 mg/kg/day divided into three doses. In this dose level nephrotoxicity and ototoxicity will be produced in 2% to 3% of patients—these are truly devastating complications! Also, 80 mg of prednisone is given daily by mouth. In addition, 100 mg oxacillin, 40 mg gentamicin, and 4 mg dexamethasone are given by retrobulbar injection. Also, corticosteroids, oxacillin, gentamicin, and atropine are applied as topical eye drops.

The intraocular penetration of penicillin derivatives is enhanced by high serum levels, such as are achieved by intravenous injection over a 15-minute period. Such rapid injection achieves much better aqueous levels than result from continuous slow infusion.

The preceding suggestions for antibiotic therapy of endophthalmitis are, of course, arbitrary and should be superseded by definitive therapy if a microorganism can be isolated.

The use of corticosteroids in treatment of endophthalmitis is controversial. It seems completely irrational and contraindicated to me.

The treatment of fungus endophthalmitis is rarely successful. A single sub-Tenon's injection of 5 mg of amphotericin B is reported to have cured two cases of postcataract fungus infection with restoration of 20/20 vision in both eyes! Unfortunately, there was no laboratory identification of any microorganisms.[87]

INTRAOCULAR LENSES

Iris-supported lenses may become displaced if the pupil is dilated widely, hence cycloplegics and mydriatics should be avoided or used with caution in cases without secure bonding of the lens to the iris by sutures or synechiae. Eyes containing intraocular lenses are susceptible to iridocyclitis and often are treated with topical corticosteroids for prolonged periods.

The increased hazard of infection resulting from implantation of foreign bodies is generally recognized and has been specifically documented for intraocular lenses. For example, an epidemic resulting in loss of 12 eyes was reported as being caused by contaminated lens solutions.[88] Corticosteroid therapy of such cases only hastens corneal perforation and loss of the eye.[89]

That the lens itself may be toxic is suggested by tissue culture studies in which cytotoxicity to the lens loops was demonstrated.[90]

POSTOPERATIVE GLAUCOMA

A considerable variety of causes may result in glaucoma after cataract extraction. Obviously the glaucoma may be unrelated to the surgery. Ordinary chronic simple glaucoma, undetected before surgery or developing sometime subsequent to surgery, is undoubtedly the most common such cause. This may be treated with epinephrine and acetazolamide shortly after surgery; subsequently, standard miotic therapy with long-acting parasympathomimetic drugs is appropriate. A variant of this is corticosteroid glaucoma, in which a genetically predisposed individual temporarily manifests glaucoma during corticosteroid treatment for postoperative inflammation. Treat as for ordinary glaucoma and discontinue corticosteroids.

Enzyme-induced glaucoma has already been discussed in Chapter 4. Pupil-block glaucoma has been discussed in the shallow chamber section of this chapter.

Two types of transient open-angle deep chamber glaucoma after intracapsular cataract extraction have been described.[91] One type, caused by partial angle closure by redundant peripheral iris, responds to miotic therapy and is made worse by cycloplegia. The second type, caused by inflammatory changes of the angle, responds to corticosteroids. Early treatment of both types may reverse the abnormality and prevent development of permanent glaucoma. The differentiation of these two types of glaucoma requires gonioscopy, which is reasonably safe postoperatively if multiple sutures have been used. Unless a pupil-block etiology (which should cause a shallow chamber glaucoma and which is treated by dilating the pupil) is suspected, postoperative deep chamber glaucoma should receive a trial of miotic therapy. Commonly such miotic therapy may be discontinued after a month or so without recurrence of the glaucoma.

Another, fortunately rare, cause of glaucoma after cataract extraction is nonexpulsive choroidal hemorrhage. This condition differs from choroidal detachment in that the anterior chamber is deep rather than shallow and the pressure is elevated rather than soft. In both conditions a large dark choroidal mass is visible. Choroidal hemorrhage glaucoma can be treated with osmotic agents such as intravenous mannitol. Several courses of mannitol may be required before the hemorrhage stops and pressure remains normal. Mydriatic or miotic therapy does not benefit glaucoma resulting from choroidal hemorrhage.[92] Markedly elevated pressures should not be permitted to continue in the recently operated eye, since there is appreciable hazard of spontaneous wound rupture with subsequent loss of the eye. Release of the choroidal hemorrhage through a posterior sclerotomy is not without hazard but should seriously be considered if osmotherapy does not control the pressure.

POSTOPERATIVE EDEMA OF POSTERIOR POLE

Persistent edema of the macula, disc, or posterior retina occurs in 1% to 2% of eyes after cataract extraction.[93] This condition may vary in severity from slight edema to frank serous retinal detachment (without hole) and may be mistaken for papilledema or optic neuritis. It may occur any time after cataract surgery, even as long as 6 months postoperatively. Uncorrectibly reduced vision is the presenting complaint. Fluorescein photography suggests this condition is caused by intraretinal leakage of serous exudate from the retinal capillaries.[94]

Detailed examination of 25 such eyes indicated that the edema was localized in areas of the posterior pole to which a detached vitreous body was still adherent. Spontaneous partial or complete release of the vitreoretinal traction may result in disappearance of the edema and return of good acuity; this happened in four of nine eyes followed up for more than 3 months. Vision did not improve during this period in the other five eyes, in which the vitreoretinal adhesions persisted. In view of the demonstrated etiology of vitreoretinal traction (and also from empirical trial), we must doubt the value of medical therapy (steroids, vasodilators, iodides, and anticoagulants) of posterior pole edema after cataract extraction. Recovery depends on spontaneous release of traction and is not enhanced by medications.

Prednisone treatment, 20 to 40 mg/day, of 17 of 18 patients with macular edema after cataract extraction was followed by 20/30 vision or better in 83% of the patients.[95] The average duration of treatment was 5½ weeks. The single untreated patient also achieved 20/30 vision. The data presented in this report, devoid of control material, do not permit conclusions as to whether the course of macular edema was influenced by systemic corticosteroid therapy.

Recall that topical epinephrine may cause posterior pole edema in aphakic patients. Treatment is to discontinue epinephrine use. Be particularly alert to any visual complaints during the first 3 months after cataract extraction. Not yet corrected with glasses and unaware of what they should really be seeing, patients are particularly vulnerable to serious disease at this time of their convalescence. Failure to detect the early stages of epinephrine maculopathy in the newly postoperative aphakic patient with glaucoma may lead to permanent macular damage.

FILAMENTARY KERATITIS

Development of filamentary keratitis after cataract extraction may be treated by mechanical removal of the filaments followed by application of lubricants, such as methylcellulose. Doubtful additional benefit accrues to use of 0.5% silver nitrate solution to moisten the applicators used for removal. Soft contact lenses may relieve irritation.[96]

CONGENITAL CATARACT

Since the principal cause for loss of an eye after congenital cataract surgery is pupillary block leading to intractable glaucoma, and also because of the high incidence of persistent postoperative inflammation with secondary membranes, *prolonged* atropinization is important.[97] Atropine should be continued for as long as 3 or 4 months after the eye appears entirely white and even though there appears to be no need for continuing cycloplegia.

REFERENCES

1. Hales, R. H.: Monocular diplopia: its characteristics and response to guanethidine, Am. J. Ophthalmol. **63**:459, 1967.
2. Lerman, S.: Pathogenetic factors in experimental galactose cataract, Arch. Ophthalmol. **65**:334, 1961.
3. Cotlier, E.: The mitotic cycle of the lens epithelium, Arch. Ophthalmol. **68**:801, 1962.
4. Levy, N. S., Krill, A. E., and Beutler, E.: Galactokinase deficiency and cataracts, Am. J. Ophthalmol. **74**:41, 1972.
5. Oberman, A. E., Wilson, W. A., Frasier, D., Donnell, G. N., and Bergren, W. R.: Galactokinase-deficiency cataracts in identical twins, Am. J. Ophthalmol. **74**:887, November 1972.
6. Vannas, A., Hogan, M. J., Golbus, M. S., and Wood, I.: Lens changes in a galactosemic fetus, Am. J. Ophthalmol. **80**:726, October 1975.
7. Epstein, D. L.: Reversible unilateral lens opacities in a diabetic patient, Arch. Ophthalmol. **94**:461, March 1976.
8. Merin, S., and Crawford, J. S.: Hypoglycemia and infantile cataract, Arch Ophthalmol. **86**:495, 1971.
9. Thoft, R. A., and Kinoshita, J. H.: The effect of calcium on rat lens permeability, Invest. Ophthalmol. **4**:122, 1965.
10. Berliner, M. I.: Cataract following the inhalation of paradichlorobenzene vapor, Arch. Ophthalmol. **22**:1023, 1939.
11. Spencer, R. W., and Andelman, S. Y.: Steroid cataracts, Arch. Ophthalmol. **74**:38, 1965.
12. Wood, T. O., Waltman, S. R., and Kaufman, H. E.: Steroid cataracts following penetrating keratoplasty, Ann. Ophthalmol. **3**:496, 1971.
13. Nicholson, D. H., Harkness, D. R., Benson, W. E., and Peterson, C. M.: Cyanate-induced cataracts in patients with sickle-cell hemoglobinopathies, Arch. Ophthalmol. **94**:927, June 1976.
14. Goren, S. B.: Cataract associated with long-term facial paralysis, Am. J. Ophthalmol. **80**:300, August 1975.
15. Jarrett, W. H.: Dislocation of the lens, Arch. Ophthalmol. **78**:289, 1967.
16. Chandler, P. A.: Choice of treatment in dislocation of the lens, Arch. Ophthalmol. **71**:765, 1964.
17. Galin, M. A., Taylor, A., and McLean, J.: Intralenticular foreign bodies, Arch. Ophthalmol. **66**:830, 1961.
18. Allen, H. F., and Mangiaracine, A. B.: Bacterial endophthalmitis after cataract extraction, Arch. Ophthalmol. **72**:454, 1964.
19. Allen, H. F., and Mangiaracine, A. B.: Bacterial endophthalmitis after cataract extraction. II. Incidence in 36,000 consecutive operations with special reference to preoperative topical antibiotics, Trans. Am. Acad. Ophthalmol. Otolaryngol. **77**:OP-583, September-October 1973.
20. Chalkley, T. H. F.: Sepsis and intraocular surgery, Am. J. Ophthalmol. **56**:142, 1963.
21. Constantaras, A. A., Metzger, W. I., and Frenkel, M.: Sterility of the aqueous humor following cataract surgery, Am. J. Ophthalmol. **74**:49, 1972.
22. Locatcher-Khorazo, D., and Gutierrez, E.: Eye infections following cataract extraction: with special reference to the role of Staphylococcus aureus, Am. J. Ophthalmol. **41**:981, 1956.
23. Burns, R. P., and Oden, M.: Antibiotic prophylaxis in cataract surgery, Am. J. Ophthalmol. **74**:615, 1972.
24. Kolker, A. E., Freeman, M. I., and Pettit, T. H.: Prophylactic antibiotics and postoperative endophthalmitis, Am. J. Ophthalmol. **63**:434, 1967.
25. Cassady, J. R.: Prophylactic subconjunctival antibiotics following cataract extraction, Am. J. Ophthalmol. **64**:1081, 1967.
26. Records, R. E.: Subconjunctival injection of the repository penicillins, Arch. Ophthalmol. **78**:380, 1967.
27. File, T. M.: Studies on the use of antihistamines in cataract surgery, Am. J. Ophthalmol. **51**:1240, 1961.
28. Schimek, R. A., Cooksey, J. C., Landreneau, M., and Steigner, J. B.: The recovery phase after ocular hypotension induced by compression, Arch. Ophthalmol. **85**:288, 1971.
29. Brubaker, R. F., and Riley, F. C., Jr.: Vitreous body volume reduction in the rabbit, Arch. Ophthalmol. **87**:438, 1972.
30. Krupin, T., Kolker, A. E., and Becker, B.: A comparison of isosorbide and glycerol for cataract surgery, Am. J. Ophthalmol. **69**:737, 1970.

31. Lazar, M., Bracha, R., and Nemet, P.: Cataract extraction during acute attack of phacolytic glaucoma, Trans. Am. Acad. Ophthalmol. Otolaryngol. **81**:OP-183, January-February 1976.

32. Struve, C. A., Gage, T. D., Bishop, D. W., and Rock, R. L.: Saline versus balanced salt solution in intraocular surgery: a double-blind study, Am. J. Ophthalmol. **51**:159, 1961.

33. Edelhauser, H. F., Van Horn, D. L., Schultz, R. O., and Hyndiuk, R. A.: Comparative toxicity of intraocular irrigating solutions on the corneal endothelium, Am. J. Ophthalmol. **81**:473, April 1976.

34. Bigar, F., Kaufman, H. E., McCarey, B. E., and Binder, P. S.: Improved corneal storage for penetrating keratoplasties in man, Am. J. Ophthalmol. **79**:115, January 1975.

35. Breslin, C., Sherrard, E. S., and Rice, N. S. C.: McCarey-Kaufman technique of corneal storage before penetrating keratoplasties in rabbits, Arch. Ophthalmol. **94**:1976, November 1976.

36. Van Horn, D. L., Schultz, R. O., and De-Bruin, J.: Endothelial survival in corneal tissue stored in M-K medium, Am. J. Ophthalmol. **80**:642, October 1975.

37. Edelhauser, H. F., Van Horn, D. L., Hyndiuk, R. A., and Schultz, R. O.: Intraocular irrigating solutions, Arch. Ophthalmol. **93**:648, August 1975.

38. Binder, P. S., Sternberg, H., Wickham, M. G., and Worthen, D. M.: Corneal endothelial damage associated with phacoemulsification, Am. J. Ophthalmol. **82**:48, July 1976.

39. Waltman, S. R., Carroll, D., Schimmelpfennig, W., and Okun, E.: Intraocular irrigating solutions for clinical vitrectomy, Ophthalmic Surg. **6**:90, Winter 1975.

40. Christiansen, J. M., Kollarits, C. R., Fukui, H., Fishman, M. L., Michels, R. G., and Mikuni, I.: Intraocular irrigating solutions and lens clarity, Am. J. Ophthalmol. **82**:594, October 1976.

41. Kirsch, R. E.: Further studies on glaucoma following cataract extraction associated with the use of alpha-chymotrypsin, Trans. Am. Acad. Ophthalmol. Otolaryngol. **69**:1011, 1965.

42. Galin, M. A., Barasch, K. R., and Harris, L.: Enzymatic zonulolysis and intraocular pressure, Am. J. Ophthalmol. **61**:690, 1966.

43. Kirsch, R. E.: Dose-relationship of alpha-chymotrypsin in production of glaucoma after cataract extraction, Arch. Ophthalmol. **75**:774, 1966.

44. Bedrossian, R. H.: Irrigation after chymotrypsin? Arch. Ophthalmol. **74**:882, 1965.

45. Bedrossian, R. H., and Weimar, V.: Inhibitory effect of aqueous humor on alpha-chymotrypsin, Trans. Am. Acad. Ophthalmol. Otolaryngol. **67**:822, 1963.

46. Scheie, H. G., Yanoff, M., and Tsou, K. C.: Inhibition of α-chymotrypsin by aqueous humor, Arch. Ophthalmol. **73**:399, 1965.

47. Gombos, G. M., and Oliver, M.: Cataract extraction with enzymatic zonulolysis in glaucomatous eyes, Am. J. Ophthalmol. **64**:68, 1967.

48. Koke, M. P.: Alpha-chymotrypsin combined with penicillin in cataract extraction, Am. J. Ophthalmol. **63**:1706, 1967.

49. Girard, L. J., Neeley, W., and Sampson, W.: The use of alpha-chymotrypsin in infants and children, Am. J. Ophthalmol. **54**:95, 1962.

50. Mendelblatt, F. I.: Enzymatic zonulolysis, Am. J. Ophthalmol. **59**:1106, 1965.

51. Beasley, H., Borgmann, A. R., McDonald, T. O., and Belluscio, P. R.: Carbachol in cataract surgery, Arch. Ophthalmol. **80**:39, 1968.

52. Schimek, R. A.: Intraocular instillation of acetylcholine in anterior segment operations, Eye Ear Nose Throat Dig. **28**:63, 1966.

53. Buxton, J. N., Smith, D. E., and Brownstein, S.: Cataract extraction and subconjunctival repository corticosteroids, Ann. Ophthalmol. **3**:1376, 1971.

54. Burde, R. M., and Waltman, S. R.: Topical corticosteroids after cataract surgery, Ann. Ophthalmol. **4**:290, 1972.

55. DeVoe, G.: Hemorrhage after cataract extraction, Arch. Ophthalmol. **28**:1069, 1942.

56. Owens, W., and Hughes, W.: Intraocular hemorrhage in cataract extraction, Arch. Ophthalmol. **37**:561, 1947.

57. Swan, J.: Estrogens in cataract surgery, Am. J. Ophthalmol. **55**:1142, 1963.

58. Watt, R. H.: Conjugated estrogens in cataract surgery: a negative report, Am. J. Ophthalmol. **57**:426, 1964.

59. Lee, O. S.: Corneoscleral suture in operations for cataract, Arch. Ophthalmol. **37**:591, 1947.

60. Beard, C.: Overhospitalization—"The Medicare syndrome," Arch. Ophthalmol. **77**:577, 1967.

61. Weisel, J., and Swan, K. C.: Mydriatic treatment of shallow chamber after cataract extraction, Arch. Ophthalmol. **58**:126, 1957.

62. Taylor, D. M.: Optimum wound closure in cataract surgery, Am. J. Ophthalmol. **48:** 660, 1959.

63. Webster, R. G., Slansky, H. H., Refojo, M. F., Boruchoff, S. A., and Dohlman, C. H.: The use of adhesive for the closure of corneal perforations, Arch. Ophthalmol. **80:**705, 1968.

64. Taylor, D.: Prevention of flat chamber in cataract surgery, Am. J. Ophthalmol. **53:** 93, 1962.

65. Taylor, D. M.: Is the flat anterior chamber syndrome necessary? Arch. Ophthalmol. **74:** 161, 1965.

66. Weisel, J., and Swan, K.: Mydriatic treatment of shallow chamber after cataract extraction, Arch. Ophthalmol. **58:**126, 1957.

67. Portney, G.: Fluorescein studies in the aphakic eye, Am. J. Ophthalmol. **63:**934, 1967.

68. Chandler, P., and Maumenee, A. E.: A major cause of hypotony, Trans. Am. Acad. Ophthalmol. Otolaryngol. **65:**563, 1961.

69. Gormaz, A.: Ocular tension after cataract surgery, Am. J. Ophthalmol. **53:**832, 1962.

70. Swan, K. C.: Relationship of basal iridectomy to shallow chamber following cataract extraction, Arch. Ophthalmol. **69:**191, 1963.

71. Haik, H., and Larson, D. W.: Flat chambers after cataract extraction, South. Med. J. **58:** 342, 1965.

72. Grant, W. M.: Experimental aqueous perfusion in enucleated human eyes, Arch. Ophthalmol. **69:**783, 1963.

73. Fine, L.: Acetazolamide in the treatment of postoperative absent anterior chamber, Arch. Ophthalmol. **73:**19, 1965.

74. Jaffe, N. S., and Light, D. S.: Treatment of postoperative cataract complications by osmotic agents, Arch. Ophthalmol. **75:**370, 1966.

75. Leone, C. R., Jr., and Callahan, A.: Restoration of the anterior chamber with glycerol 50% and mydriasis, Am. J. Ophthalmol. **63:**1686, 1967.

76. Cotlier, E.: Aphakic flat anterior chamber. I. Incidence among 8,533 cataract extractions, Arch. Ophthalmol. **87:**119, 1972.

77. Cotlier, E.: Aphakic flat anterior chamber. II. Effect of spontaneous reformation and medical therapy, Arch. Ophthalmol. **87:**124, 1972.

78. Gasset, A. R., and Bellows, R. T.: Hydrophilic contact lenses in the treatment of shallow or flat chambers, Ann. Ophthalmol. **6:** 996, October 1974.

79. Chee, P. H. Y.: Epithelial downgrowth, Arch. Ophthalmol. **78:**492, 1967.

80. Allansmith, M. R., Skaggs, C., and Kimura, S. J.: Anterior chamber paracentesis, Arch. Ophthalmol. **84:**745, 1970.

81. Chishti, M., and Henkind, P.: Spontaneous rupture of anterior lens capsule (phacoanaphylactic endophthalmitis), Am. J. Ophthalmol. **69:**264, 1970.

82. Francois, J.: Glaucoma and uveitis after congenital cataract surgery, Ann. Ophthalmol. **3:**131, 1971.

83. Wilson, W. A.: Uveitis—immediate and delayed—complicating cataract surgery, Ann. Ophthalmol. **3:**949, 1971.

84. Allen, H. F., and Grove, A. S., Jr.: Early acute aseptic iritis after cataract extraction, Trans. Am. Acad. Ophthalmol. Otolaryngol. **81:**OP-145, January-February 1976.

85. Abelson, M. B., and Allansmith, M. R.: Normal conjunctival wound edge flora of patients undergoing uncomplicated cataract extraction, Am. J. Ophthalmol. **76:**561, October 1973.

86. Baum, J. L., and Rao, G.: Treatment of postcataract bacterial endophthalmitis with periocular and systemic antibiotics and corticosteroids, Trans. Am. Acad. Ophthalmol. Otolaryngol. **81:**OP-151, January 1976.

87. Allen, H. F.: Amphotericin B and exogenous mycotic endophthalmitis after cataract extraction, Arch. Ophthalmol. **88:**640, December 1972.

88. O'Day, D. M.: Fungal endophthalmitis caused by *Paecilomyces lilacinus* after intraocular lens implantation, Am. J. Ophthalmol. **83:**130, January 1977.

89. Mosier, M. A., Lusk, B., Pettit, T. H., Howard, D. H., and Rhodes, J.: Fungal endophthalmitis following intraocular lens implantation, Am. J. Ophthalmol. **83:**1, January 1977.

90. Galin, M. A., Chowchuvech, E., and Galin, A.: Tissue culture methods for testing the toxicity of ocular plastic materials, Am. J. Ophthalmol. **79:**665, April 1965.

91. Gorin, G.: Deep-chamber glaucoma following cataract extraction, Am. J. Ophthalmol. **55:**279, 1963.

92. Oberman, A. E.: Nonexpulsive choroidal hemorrhage, Am. J. Ophthalmol. **63:**1800, 1967.

93. Tolentino, F. I., and Schepens, C. L.: Edema of posterior pole after cataract extraction, Arch. Ophthalmol. **74:**781, 1965.

94. Gass, J. D. M., and Norton, E. W.: Cystoid

macular edema and papilledema following cataract extraction, Arch. Ophthalmol. **76:** 646, 1966.

95. Gehring, J. R.: Macular edema following cataract extraction, Arch. Ophthalmol. **80:** 626, 1968.

96. Dodds, H. T., and Laibson, P. R.: Filamentary keratitis following cataract extraction, Arch Ophthalmol. **88:**609, December 1972.

97. Chandler, P. A.: Surgery of congenital cataract, Trans. Am. Acad. Ophthalmol. Otolaryngol. **72:**341, 1968.

32
EXTERNAL DISEASES

LIDS
Common infections

Being located on the surface of the body, the lids are exposed to all types of environmental contamination. *Staphylococcus*, however, is the microorganism most capable of invading the lid structures and causing infection. In 1946 culture of 350 eyes with blepharitis showed the presence of *Staphylococcus* in 130 eyelids.[1] *Pityrosporum ovale* (seborrheic dermatitis or dandruff organism) was present in 100 cases. In 102 cases, both *Staphylococcus* and *Pityrosporum* were present. These findings, as well as the therapeutic responses, could be reproduced today.

Topical application of sulfonamide ointment, shampoos of scalp and greasy facial skin, and vigorous mechanical cleaning of the lid margins were reasonably effective in correcting blepharitis in conscientious patients. A very high proportion of patients apparently did not follow instructions, since they showed more improvement when treated in the clinic daily than when supposedly using the same treatment themselves. Prolonged treatment simply was not carried out reliably, resulting in persistence or recurrence of the blepharitis.

In addition to problems of cooperation and reinfection, diagnostic uncertainties such as the presence of allergic blepharitis or resistant organisms interfere with the percentage of success obtained. For example, in a small series of 15 cases a 10% solution of sulfacet-amide applied four times daily, 3 drops each time, corrected lid inflammatory symptoms in only 8 patients, even though a bacteriologic "cure" had been demonstrated by culture.[2] Another 15 patients (double-blind controls) were treated similarly with sulfacet-amide drops combined with a 0.2% solution of prednisolone—of these, all 15 became asymptomatic and did so more rapidly than the first group. Symptoms were controlled in 3 to 4 days with combined sulfa-corticosteroid therapy, in comparison with 6 to 8 days with the sulfa alone. No details were given as to the subsequent course of the blepharitis, but the condition was said to have been "rendered asymptomatic" rather than "cured." Presumably this means the expected relapses did in fact occur.

Another source for reinfection of the lid is contaminated eye cosmetics. Samples of used mascara and eye shadow obtained from 233 women were cultured, producing a growth of fungi in 12% of the samples and a growth of bacteria (mostly *Staphylococcus*) in 43%.[3] The clinical significance of this is illustrated by one patient with staphylococcal blepharitis so severe as to cause loss of eyelashes. To cover the cosmetic blemish, she used a generous coating of heavily contaminated cosmetic, thereby perpetuating the initial problem. Another potential hazard is presented by the woman who arrives in the operating room with a heavy layer of germ-laden cosmetics painted on the eye to be operated. The authors advocated discontinuance of cosmetic use at least 1 week prior to surgery.

Because of the great frequency of chronic marginal blepharitis, the crusting and irritation typical of this disorder are frequently present in patients whose primary complaint is another ocular problem. Having suffered from the blepharitis for a long time, the patient has either grown accustomed to its presence or despairs of a cure and fails to mention this complaint. This opportunity for treatment should not be overlooked by the ophthalmologist because of the patient's lack of complaint. Invariably I have found such patients appreciative of the antibiotic prescription and instructions about proper hygiene of the lids.

Selenium sulfide

Although troublesome to use, sulfur has long been known empirically to benefit seborrheic dermatosis. Selenium sulfide (Selsun), similar to sulfur in its physical and chemical properties, has also been found to have an antiseborrheic value.

In a concentration of 2.5%, selenium sulfide has been found to be nontoxic when properly applied. After a soap shampoo, 10 ml of selenium sulfide suspension is vigorously massaged into the scalp and left for 5 minutes. Then the hair is thoroughly washed several times to remove all traces of selenium. This selenium treatment must be repeated weekly to maintain control of seborrheic scalp disorders. Of 140 patients so treated for 2 years, 89% maintained good control of their seborrheic problems.[4]

Toxicity. The patient must be aware that selenium is highly poisonous and can easily be absorbed orally in toxic quantities. Hands and fingernails must be adequately rinsed after use to prevent contamination of food. The drug must be kept out of reach of children. Gastrointestinal and respiratory symptoms are prominent in animals suffering from selenium poisoning.

Selenium should not be applied to skin ulcers or lacerations, since absorption occurs through such wounds. About one third of patients using selenium sulfide shampoos develop excessive oiliness of hair and scalp. This can be partially controlled by tincture of green soap shampoos. Selenium use causes an orange discoloration in about one fifth of patients with gray hair. Keratoconjunctivitis results from the irritant action of a 2.5% concentration of selenium sulfide if it is permitted to enter the eyes. Skin sensitivity to the detergent vehicle has been reported.

Clinical use. Although the treatment of scalp seborrhea has been advocated as an adjunct to the management of marginal blepharitis, no correlation was found between the severity of scalp and lid involvement in 59 patients.[5] The marginal blepharitis in these patients was treated by direct application to the lid margins of a 0.5% selenium sulfide jelly. As a control, some of these eyelids were treated with ammoniated mercury ointment. After 4 weeks of treatment, 79% of the selenium-treated lids were classified as being cured as compared to 90% of the ammoniated mercury–treated lids. This difference was not statistically significant; however, it is obvious that selenium sulfide is not a more effective method of treatment of seborrheic blepharitis than a variety of other common medications, including antibiotics after careful cleaning with warm compresses.

Relapse of seborrheic blepharitis is common when treatment is discontinued.[6]

Less common infections

A nasty case of dermatophytosis (ringworm) affected the eyelids of a 4-year-old boy.[7] (This infection is self-limiting and heals spontaneously after 10 to 12 weeks.) Of interest is that improvement was attributed to the use of warm milk packs, another illustration of the fact that success will accompany the use of any treatment if it is only started at the right time.

The typical vesicular eruption of herpes simplex skin infections will respond to topical application of IDU ointment.[8] Secondary infection may change the presenting appearance to a dark, crusted ulceration somewhat

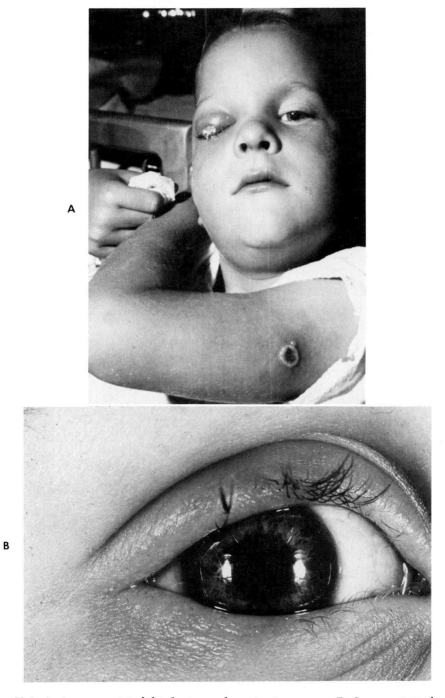

Fig. 32-1. A, Acute vaccinia lid infection and vaccination source. **B,** Same patient showing typical loss of eyelashes after healing of vaccinia ulcer. (From Gould, E., and Havener, W. H.: Am. J. Ophthalmol. **56:**830, 1963.)

comparable in appearance to a herpes zoster crusted ulcer.

Vaccinia is a classic cause of lid infections that are in some instances sufficiently severe to cause permanent loss of eyelashes (Fig. 32-1).[9]

Hyperkeratotic (rough-surfaced) viral warts of the eyelid may be treated by painting with a 0.7% solution of cantharidin in collodion.[10] Of 27 such warts, 13 were cured with a single application and 9 with repeated applications (at 8- to 10-day intervals). Because cantharidin is irritating to the cornea, it should not be used on lesions in contact with the cornea.

Allergy

The ocular manifestations of hay fever and similar common allergic states are best treated by general management of the disease (for example, desensitization, avoidance of allergens, and antihistaminic drugs). Prolonged local use of strong corticosteroid preparations should be avoided because of the possibility of developing glaucoma and cataract.

Baffling cases of conjunctival, lid, and corneal irritation may be caused by the use of cosmetics, germicidal soaps, perfumes, aftershave lotions, dyes, hair dressings, detergents, etc.[11] Itching, tearing, redness, and swelling may be caused by such irritation. The most effective therapy is avoidance of all such substances.

Allergy to ophthalmic drugs is quite common. Unsightly depigmentation of the eyelids occurred in four black patients using eserine ointment.[12] Merthiolate (mercury) allergy following preoperative skin decontamination causes a characteristic weeping, itching area, spotted with small white pustules. The thickened, dry, cracked skin of atropine allergy is similar in appearance to that of neomycin allergy. Proparacaine and cyclopentolate cause acute superficial punctate breakdown of the corneal epithelium. Pilocarpine allergy causes a follicular thickening of the lower cul-de-sac. In all instances

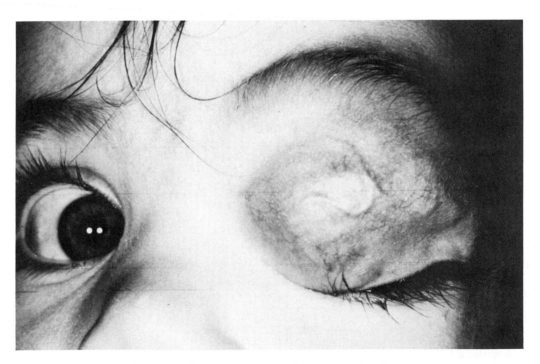

Fig. 32-2. Hemangioma of eyelid at 6 months of age.

the offending drug should be discontinued. Attempts to continue the medication, together with corticosteroid treatment for the allergy, are generally unsatisfactory.

Faulty lid position

Bell's palsy apparently does not respond to corticosteroids, vitamin B_{12}, nicotinic acid, or surgical decompression.[13]

Adequate corneal protection, depending on the severity of the eyelid fault, may be achieved by lubricant drops or ointments, by various types of tarsorrhaphy, or by application of protective covers such as a layer of clear plastic wrap (Saran) taped to cover the eye.[14]

Congenital eversion of the eyelids is particularly likely to occur in persons with Down's syndrome.[15] Although the horizontally elongated and relaxed lid responsible for this eversion may be treated surgically, spontaneous repositioning of the lids will occur after several months of conservative medical therapy with lubricant and antibiotic ointment and protection with clear plastic wrap.

Hemangioma

Cavernous hemangiomas in children are often treated with radiation, freezing, sclerosing injections, or corticosteroids. The results from such management are often more disfiguring than the hemangioma itself. Actually, the natural course of a congenital cavernous hemangioma is spontaneous disappearance. Such a dramatic disappearance is shown in Figs. 32-2 (appearance at 6 months of age) and 32-3 (appearance at 10 years of age).[16] This child received *no* treatment whatsoever to cause this improvement.

CONJUNCTIVA
Infection

We have been taught that the tears and the conjunctiva are sterile. Apparently this sterility is variable, being influenced by climate and environment as well as by host resistance. For example, conjunctival staphylococci were found in 34% of "normal" eyes in England, 60% of eyes in India, and 95% of eyes in Egypt.[17]

A population of southwestern American Indians receiving prolonged antibiotic (tetracycline and erythromycin) therapy for trachoma provided an opportunity to study the effect of such medication on the usual bacterial flora. Before treatment, 83% of the eyes showed *Staphylococcus*. After 6 weeks of treatment the recovery of *Staphylococcus* dropped to about 50%. This moderate decrease in the isolation of bacteria was purchased at the price of a 30-fold increase in the number of strains resistant to erythromycin.

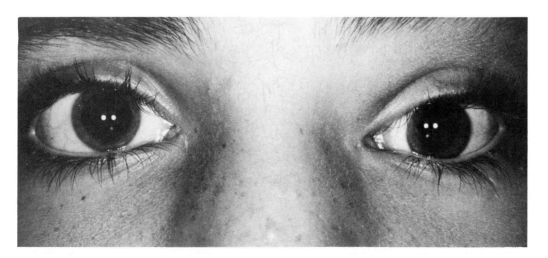

Fig. 32-3. Same patient at 10 years of age. Hemangioma has spontaneously disappeared.

The disadvantages in terms of development of resistant bacterial strains must be seriously considered in any long-term antibiotic regimen.[18]

Oculogenital infections

A surprisingly large number of eye infections originate in one way or another in the genital tract.[19] These include inclusion conjunctivitis (ophthalmia neonatorum, obstetrician's conjunctivitis, TRIC disease, *Chlamydia* infection), *Candida albicans* infection, gonorrhea, syphilis, lymphogranuloma venereum, *Trichomonas*, *Lactobacillus*, and *Mycoplasma* infection, pubic louse infestation, and even herpes simplex. Quite probably some of the common surface bacterial infections also have genital reservoirs.

We fail to perceive the epidemiologic relationships of many of these infections. For example, Reiter's syndrome, characterized by eye inflammation (conjunctivitis, iridocyclitis, or keratoconjunctivitis), arthritis, and urethritis, is unquestionably a venereal disease.[20,21] *Chlamydia* was isolated from 12 of 23 patients with Reiter's syndrome; was demonstrated in a married couple, both of whom had iritis[22]; and is characteristic of inclusion conjunctivitis (TRIC diseases).[23]

The therapeutic implications of the oculogenital nature of the diseases are that the patient must be treated for a systemic infection (not simply a local eye problem requiring topical therapy) and that the epidemiologic aspects of transmission of infection to and reinfection from a partner must be considered in achieving a lasting cure.

Following an epidemic of 602 cases of *Shigella* dysentery aboard a warship, nine patients developed a typical Reiter's syndrome with conjunctivitis, urethritis, and arthritis.[24] The conjunctivitis developed about 3 weeks after infection (usually 1 or 2 weeks after recovery from the dysentery), lasted less than 1 week, and disappeared without residual symptoms. Topical and systemic antibiotics and corticosteroids did not alter the spontaneous course of the disease. That author felt certain that no venereal transmission was involved. The inferences to be drawn from this article are that triads of symptoms may well have more than one etiology and that physicians should not be too arbitrary in their suspicions.

Reiter's syndrome may follow chlamydial infection or dysentery or be of unknown cause. About 90% of patients with Reiter's syndrome have the HLA-27 antigen, which occurs in only 4% to 8% of the normal population. This antigen is common in other arthritic syndromes and also in patients with anterior uveitis. Apparently this represents a genetic susceptibility that may be initiated by infection, to become spontaneously recurrent thereafter. Reiter's syndrome, even if associated with demonstrable *Chlamydia*, is nonresponsive to tetracycline treatment. Nonspecific treatment of the iritis includes use of corticosteroids, cycloplegics, butazolidine, and salicylates.

An excellent review[25] of the laboratory and clinical characteristics of *Chlamydia* infections also summarizes the accepted treatment. Neonatal inclusion blennorrhea responds to sulfonamide, tetracycline, or erythromycin given topically four times daily for at least 3 weeks. Such topical treatment will reduce the severity of ocular disease in adults, but is not curative. Adults require full dosage of oral tetracyclines for at least 3 weeks. Since this is sexually transmitted, the partners of the patient must also be treated, otherwise reinfection will occur.

Trachoma is treated with 3 to 5 weeks of oral tetracyclines, sulfonamides, or erythromycin. Penicillin and chloramphenicol inhibit the virus in vitro but are not very effective clinically. Trachoma organisms are resistant to streptomycin, vancomycin, gentamicin, neomycin, polymyxin B, and bacitracin. Topical tetracycline twice daily for 6 to 10 weeks is an alternate method of therapy. Reinfection from home contacts characteristically occurs. Little benefit results from treating a schoolchild but not his infected family.

Superior limbic keratoconjunctivitis

Superior limbic keratoconjunctivitis, a condition of unknown etiology, responds poorly to local corticosteroids or antibiotics. Swabbing the upper palpebral conjunctiva with a cotton applicator moistened with a 0.5% solution of silver nitrate was reported to be successful therapy in all of a series of 14 patients.[26] This condition is identified by its localization in the superior palpebral and bulbar conjunctiva and in the superior limbus and cornea. Punctate staining and filaments are common. Although polymorphonuclear neutrophilic leukocytes are characteristically found on conjunctival scrapings, a culture search for viral, fungal, or specific bacterial etiology has not been conclusive.[27,28]

Of a series of 10 cases of superior limbic keratoconjunctivitis,[29] five patients suffered from thyrotoxicosis. It was suggested that the condition was an immune reaction, although it is nonresponsive to topical corticosteroid therapy (and also to IDU).

Vernal conjunctivitis

Vernal conjunctivitis is a relatively benign, although annoying disease usually presumed to be of allergic origin. It is characteristically a disease of the young; 80% of a series of 400 patients were under 15 years of age. Diagnosis is easily made from the typical flattened papillary hypertrophy, most marked on the upper border of the superior tarsal conjunctiva. Itching and photophobia are the most prominent symptoms, the latter being particularly prominent in cases with corneal involvement. Seasonal variations with remission during the winter are common; however, severe cases (11% of the aforementioned 400 patients) may persist virtually unchanged throughout the entire year. The duration of the disease varies greatly, from several weeks to three decades, the average being about 4 years.

Medical evaluation of the patient with vernal conjunctivitis does not ordinarily provide information of therapeutic benefit. Two thirds of these patients have chronic ear, nose, or throat pathology, most commonly chronic vasomotor rhinitis. Half of the patients have positive skin tests to bacterial or fungus antigens, but only a few patients show positive skin tests to pollen or foodstuffs.

Specific desensitization is of little therapeutic value. Only 11% of the series of 400 patients cited previously gave a history of other allergic conditions. A familial incidence was present in 28%, and in 15 cases there were more than two patients with vernal conjunctivitis in the same family. Of 50 conjunctival cultures, 49 showed bacterial growth; however, these were mostly nonpathogenic organisms, presumably secondary invaders. No fungi were found in 30 cultures. Since 72% of the 400 patients were male, endocrinologic factors were suspected; however, clinical endocrinologic studies were nonproductive.

A possible explanation of the mechanism of vernal conjunctivitis arises from the discovery that tears contain immunoglobulin E, the immunoglobulin component capable of mediating atopic hypersensitivity.[30] Of 15 normal subjects, only one had high tear levels of this immunoglobulin. In contrast, high tear levels of immunoglobulin E were found in all of five patients with vernal conjunctivitis and in two of four patients with ragweed conjunctivitis. It is apparent that the presence of elevated amounts of immunoglobulin E in tears provides an acceptable explanation for immune phenomena localized to the eye. Immunoglobulin-containing plasma cells are demonstrable in the conjunctival cobblestone excrescences of vernal conjunctivitis.[31]

Although topical corticosteroid therapy gives symptomatic relief, the duration of the disease and the treatment is so long that the hazard of glaucoma and cataract is an unacceptable risk. Actually, equally prompt and effective symptomatic relief may be obtained from sympathomimetic drugs, such as 0.12% phenylephrine. The popular ocular decongestants such as Murine and Visine contain a sympathomimetic active ingredient and do, in fact, relieve the redness and itching of allergic conjunctivitis.

Iatrogenic conjunctivitis

"Overtreatment conjunctivitis" is a reaction to antibiotics or other medications prescribed for the treatment of acute or chronic conjunctivitis.[32] Ocular irritation continues even after the bacteria are eradicated and is relieved only when medication is stopped. Because of the frequency of overtreatment conjunctivitis, cases of chronic conjunctivitis that fail to respond to prolonged treatment may deserve a trial of several days without any medication at all.

This condition is initially a toxic process, but a continuum of transition forms shades indistinguishably into overt and obvious allergy to medications.

Erythema multiforme exudativum (Stevens-Johnson syndrome)

Stevens-Johnson syndrome is generally considered to be an allergic reaction manifested in patients predisposed to allergy to a great variety of medications, including among others sulfonamides, barbiturates, salicylates, codeine, bromides, iodides, phenylbutazone, phenytoin, thiouracil, coal tar derivatives, and food additives in margarine and chocolate.[33] In the natural course of the disease an upper respiratory infection appears 7 to 10 days before the skin and mucous membrane manifestations. Quite naturally the respiratory symptoms will be treated using one or more of the above-mentioned drugs, which then is blamed for the onset of the full-blown syndrome several days later. One brave investigator prescribed the same sulfonamide for tonsillitis occurring 3 months after Stevens-Johnson syndrome—no abnormal reaction resulted. Such a drug challenge is generally considered imprudent and strongly advised against.[34]

Viral, rickettsial, or *Mycoplasma* organisms have been incriminated in Stevens-Johnson syndrome. Some authorities believe that as many as one third of the cases can be attributed to herpes simplex virus.

It is customary to treat the acute ocular involvement of Stevens-Johnson syndrome with topical corticosteroids; however, these cases are so infrequent and variable in severity that a truly accurate evaluation of the effect of such therapy is most difficult. In any study of this problem the patients should receive corticosteroid therapy of the worse eye only, the other eye serving as a control.

In a series of 13 cases of Stevens-Johnson ocular disease, *Staphylococcus aureus* superinfection was reported[35] to be "common." Appropriate antibiotics should be used to treat such secondary bacterial infections. Anterior uveitis is also a component of the Stevens-Johnson syndrome and should be treated with atropine or other cycloplegic drugs. Leaving the pseudomembranes intact has been advocated, in the belief that the resulting raw surface was likely to promote scarring. (I would suppose toxic substances within the pseudomembrane might also cause scarring. The preferred management of these pseudomembranes is not established.)

Patients should be evaluated with Schirmer's test after recovery. Eyes that are dry or irritated are likely to develop severe corneal complications. Lubrication with tear substitutes and ointments may minimize these corneal problems.

The protective effect of therapeutic soft contact lenses may be of great value in the management of these mucus- and tear-deficient eyes.[36] The generalization that no medications can be used because they are retained in the lens and gradually released is, of course, illogical. If a medication is desirable, its prolonged delivery by a soft lens would also be desirable, if not to be sought after.

Ocular cicatricial pemphigoid

Chronic cicatricial conjunctivitis (ocular pemphigoid) continues to be a disease of unknown etiology that is unresponsive to treatment.[37] Although corticosteroid therapy is generally advised, the complications resulting from prolonged use can be so serious as to contraindicate such treatment. Of five patients with chronic cicatricial conjunctivitis treated with corticosteroids, three developed glaucoma, two developed cataract, and one had a herpetic infection.

Since no definitive treatment exists for this condition, only symptomatic management is possible. Epilation of the lashes is most important to prevent corneal damage from trichiasis.[38] Lubricating drops or ointments help to protect the cornea against dryness. Scleral contact lenses will hold open the conjunctival fornices, minimizing subconjunctival shrinkage and symblepharon formation, and will also increase comfort and corneal clarity. Well-fitted soft lenses probably are the treatment of choice for advanced ocular pemphigoid. Surgical plastic procedures with mucous membrane grafts are usually disappointing.

In a 56-year-old woman with typical ocular cicatricial pemphigoid, immunofluorescent antibodies conjugated with the basement membrane of the conjunctiva.[39] Despite this evidence of an immune mechanism, the condition did not respond to subconjunctival injections of triamcinolone. Perhaps the cicatricial stage of the disease is no longer responsive to corticosteroids.

In another study[40] 3 of 10 patients with ocular cicatricial pemphigoid showed immunoglobulin deposition on the conjunctival basement membranes.

Two patients developed unilateral ocular cicatricial pemphigoid following use of echothiophate iodide *only* in the affected eye for 6 and for 9 years. Immunoglobulin staining of the conjunctival basement membrane was present in only one of the 2 eyes.[41] The etiologic implications of this drug-induced immunologic response are not yet clearly explained.

Ligneous conjunctivitis

Ligneous conjunctivitis, a chronic pseudomembranous conjunctivitis with associated unusually hard induration of the eyelids, has its onset in early childhood and is usually bilateral. As would be expected in such a condition, many types of microorganisms can be cultured from the moist, warm surface membrane. Particular significance has been attached to repeated isolation of adenoviruses and of *Streptococcus* (well-known inducers of pseudomembrane formation). Although only about 50 cases of this rare condition have been reported, a familial occurrence has been noted seven times. This suggests a genetic deficiency, perhaps a faulty immune mechanism, permitting continuing infection and re-formation of the pseudomembrane.

Topical therapy with antibiotics, corticosteroids, hyaluronidase, and alpha-chymotrypsin has not been effective. Some benefit was reported with systemic corticosteroids in one case.[42,43]

On the theory that the mucopolysaccharide constituent of the ligneous membranes could be dissolved by enzymatic action, 8 patients from Turkey were treated with topical drops of hyaluronidase, 175 units/ml, and alpha-chymotrypsin 1:5000, instilled hourly for 3 months, then six times daily for a year. Five patients recovered completely and one was greatly improved.[44] All of these patients seemed to be unusually vulnerable to infection—7 had bronchopneumonia, which was fatal in one case. The illustrations show absolutely dreadful white membranes growing across the conjunctival surfaces. One child lost both eyes to infection.

Conjunctival malignancy

The typical firm, elevated cancer presents no problem in diagnosis. When first seen, patients with conjunctival neoplasms may have diffuse, nonspecific ocular signs, with superimposed secondary infection. There is no question that microorganisms will be found on the irregular surface of a neoplasm, but their presence should not be allowed to confirm the diagnosis of "chronic persistent bacterial conjunctivitis resistant to antibiotics." The correct diagnosis may be made by biopsy or by cytologic examination of scrapings from the surface of the lesion. Scrapings are easier to obtain but require a more experienced pathologist. Suspicion of malignancy in a persistent "infection" is the key to diagnosis.[45,46]

Self-inflicted conjunctivitis

Various chemical and mechanical methods of inducing ocular irritation are available to the malingering individual and limited only by the imagination. Their detection is aided by the atypical appearance of the lesion and its resistance to therapy. The main reason for misdiagnosis is failure to think of the possibility. Also, an ophthalmologist finds it hard to comprehend that anyone would willingly damage anything so important as his own eye.

A folk remedy, the placing of flax seed into the conjunctival cul-de-sac, is believed by some patients to correct minor eye ailments. Typical inferior corneal abrasions and secondary infections complicate use of this "therapeutic" foreign body.[47]

CORNEA
Physiology

The cornea is a remarkable structure with many unique characteristics of significance in medical therapy. Modern experimental techniques continue to contribute to our understanding of the physiologic mechanisms involved in ion transport across the cornea. These phenomena are, of course, also of fundamental importance in the intracorneal and intraocular penetration of topically applied medications.

The corneal epithelium is the principal barrier to the passage of ions. Having a lipoid concentration 100 times that of the stroma, the epithelium is 40,000 times more resistant to the diffusion of sodium than would be an equal thickness of physiologic saline solution.[48] An electric potential of up to 40 mv (stromal side positive) exists across the intact epithelium and presumably has some effect on ion transfer.

Similarly, the lipoid-containing endothelium is 1900 times more resistant to passage of sodium or bromide ions than is an equal thickness of saline solution. However, it must not be concluded that epithelium and endothelium are completely impermeable to ions. In fact, in rabbits one half of the sodium in the corneal stroma exchanges with the sodium in the aqueous humor *every 14 minutes.* Ion movement across epithelium and endothelium may be via the intercellular spaces. Transfer through these spaces is shown in Fig. 32-4, which is an electron photomicrograph of rabbit corneal endothelium 3 hours after a suspension of thorium dioxide was placed in the aqueous. The aqueous suspension of particles is seen at the top of the pho-

tomicrograph, many particles are deposited on the endothelial surface, the intercellular spaces are densely filled with thorium particles, and numerous particles diffuse into Descemet's membrane. (Actually, thorium dioxide particles may be traced into Descemet's membrane within 30 minutes, but this photomicrograph was selected because the dense accumulation of the thorium is more readily visible.)

In contrast, fat-soluble substances pass readily through the epithelium and endothelium, presumably because the cell membranes have a high lipoid content and are therefore lipoid permeable.

The corneal stroma is composed primarily of collagen fibrils supporting a ground substance permeable to water-soluble ions. Diffusion through the stroma is slowed somewhat by its viscosity and varies with the molecular size of the ions. Ions with a molecular weight of up to 500,000 can diffuse through the corneal stroma. Sodium ions (6 Å diameter) diffuse twice as slowly through the stroma as they would in saline solution. Hemoglobin molecules (70 Å diameter) diffuse 10 times more slowly in stroma than in saline solution. (The erythrocyte cell membrane and Descemet's endothelium are the layers that prevent hemoglobin from entering the corneal stroma as a complication of hyphema.) Interestingly, ion diffusion through the stroma proceeds equally in anteroposterior or radial directions. This corresponds with the electrical resistance, which is the same in all directions through the stroma and is about 2.5 times greater than the resistance of aqueous humor. Evidently the collagen layers, oriented parallel to the corneal surface, do not impede ion transfer as they do vascular ingrowth (which is characteristically maintained at the same depth across the cornea).

For the purposes of medicinal penetration, the cornea may be considered to be a fat-water-fat sandwich. Substances such as the alkaloids, which can associate and dissociate to become alternately lipoid and water soluble, will penetrate the cornea most easily (see Fig. 2-1).

Ion penetration at the limbus differs great-

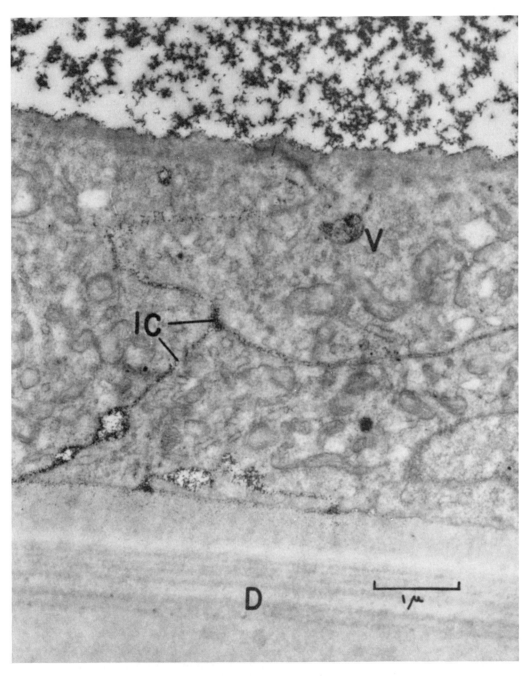

Fig. 32-4. Electron photomicrograph of rabbit endothelium 3 hours after contact with thorium dioxide suspension (suspension on aqueous side at top of photomicrograph). Intercellular spaces, *IC*, are filled with thorium particles that are also diffusing into Descemet's membrane, *D*. (From Donn, A.: Invest. Ophthalmol. 1:170, 1962.)

ly from that of the cornea proper, for here no selective membranes limit diffusion. In the limbal area (total extent, 0.2 cm²), solutes and water move freely in response to concentration and osmotic gradients. Although the limbal area is only one seventh that of the corneal surface, it transmits one fifth as much sodium exchange as does the entire rest of the cornea. Presumably, therefore, ionized medications can also selectively penetrate intraocularly via the limbus.

Although ions may diffuse from the limbus into the stroma (as previously described for intrastromal diffusion), there is no evidence for any flow of fluid from the limbus to the stroma. Spots of fluorescein placed in the peripheral stroma show no overall drift centrally. We must conclude, therefore, that systemic medications can reach the cornea only by diffusion (from limbus or aqueous).

Therapeutically, the corneal permeability may be greatly altered by cationic detergents such as benzalkonium chloride. A 1:10,000 concentration of benzalkonium increases corneal permeability to fluorescein 20-fold.[49] Electron microscopy suggests that this detergent-induced increase in corneal permeability occurs because of a widening of the intercellular spaces of the epithelium. Increasing the benzalkonium concentration to 1:1000 causes punctate epithelial defects and loosening of the adhesion between epithelium and stroma. Hence incorporation of benzalkonium chloride in a medication will increase intracorneal and transcorneal penetration. The toxic effects of preservative and detergent additives to a medication may be enhanced when a soft lens is being worn.

Of course, epithelial disease also enhances ion entry into the cornea. Antibiotics, for example, gain ready access to the corneal stroma in the presence of a bacterial ulcer. Increased intraocular pressure splits the superficial and basal cells of the epithelium (bedewing) and loosens the intercellular junctions. A pressure of 65 mm Hg for 1 hour increased the corneal permeability to fluorescein sixfold.[49]

Other valuable properties of the epithelium include great resistance to infection, resistance to water loss by evaporation, transparency, capability of attracting and maintaining the tear film, and an extraordinary rate of growth. Not only does this growth replace the epithelium itself but it also contributes heavily to the prompt healing of stromal wounds.[50]

As determined by studies with colchicine (which arrests mitosis in metaphase), 14% of the corneal epithelial cells are replaced daily.[51] At this rate, 100% of the cells should be replaced every 7 days.

Tritium-labeled thymidine is incorporated into cellular deoxyribonucleic acid only during the premitotic stage of cell division, and it remains there for the life of the cell. Autoradiographic studies of human corneas labeled by this method indicate that the turnover time of human corneal epithelium is, indeed, about 1 week.[52] The practical implication of this fact is that any epithelial defect continuing for as long as 1 week cannot be attributed to a single insult but must be caused by some type of persistent pathology, either continuing activity of the primary disease or some type of secondary factor (drying, for instance) that reduces cellular multiplication and migration.

The single cell layer of Descemet's endothelium is primarily responsible for preventing corneal decompensation. The endothelium is 1900 times more resistant to passage of an electrolyte ion than is an equal thickness of saline solution. This barrier helps to maintain the relative aqueous hypertonicity that dehydrates the cornea and that causes normal intraocular pressure. Failure of the endothelial function, whether resulting from dystrophy, injury, vitreocorneal contact, or some other cause, leads to bullous keratopathy.[53]

Supplementing a defective transendothelial osmotic pull with a transepithelial osmotic pull can be accomplished by topical application of hypertonic medications. The effectiveness of such medications is primarily determined by the duration of corneal contact and hence is influenced more by the vehicle than by the osmotic agent. For example, the reduction of corneal thickness

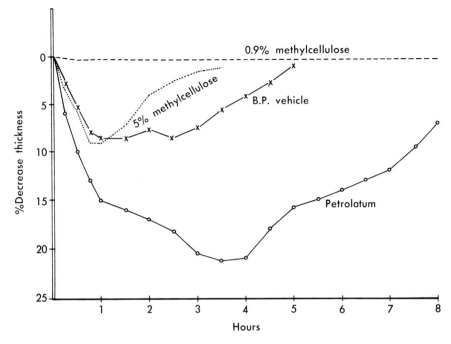

Fig. 32-5. Percent decrease in corneal thickness resulting from application of 5% sodium chloride in four different vehicles to edematous human corneas. (Data from Luxenberg, M. N., and Green, K.: Am. J. Ophthalmol. **71:**847, 1971.)

achieved in edematous human corneas by topical application of a 5% concentration of sodium chloride in various vehicles is illustrated in Fig. 32-5.[54] If the vehicle achieved poor duration of contact (0.9% methylcellulose), almost no dehydrating effect occurred. With long duration of contact resulting from a lanolin-petrolatum ointment vehicle, a decrease of as much as 20% in thickness was achieved, with the effect lasting up to 8 hours. Vehicles of 5% methylcellulose or a commercial polymer (an EKG-SOL prepared by Burton, Parsons and Co., Inc.) achieved intermediate dehydration, as illustrated. Let me repeat—the osmotic agent in all instances was 5% sodium chloride—the vehicle was changed, not the osmotic agent.[55]

Wound healing

The elusive goal of accelerated wound healing is perennially sought after. In general, we accept that the normal rate of tissue healing cannot be improved on, providing that nutritional deficiency and toxic factors such as infection and edema are avoided.

Because of the gingival collagen hyperplasia resulting from phenytoin, its effect on corneal wound healing was investigated. In rabbits the mean tensile strength of a central corneal incision was found to be 182 g/5 mm length of wound at the end of 1 week. At the end of the same 1-week period the tensile strength was 324 g in rabbits receiving 50 mg of oral phenytoin daily for 2 days preoperatively and twice weekly postoperatively. The increased strength of the phenytoin-treated wound persisted during the month following surgery (2-week values were treated, 279, and control, 214; 3-week values were 409 and 355, respectively; and 4-week values were 522 and 437, respectively).[56]

Reports praising the efficacy of autohemotherapy in the treatment of various diseases continue to appear and to be greeted with polite skepticism. In a controlled experiment involving the use of blood in the treatment of corneal abrasions, a 4 mm wide corneal abrasion was made in each eye of 12 rabbits.[57] The corneas were then covered by suturing the nictitating membrane to the temporal conjunctiva. Three drops of the rabbit's own blood were then placed between the cornea and the nictitating membrane on the right eye. In all 12 rabbits the right cornea healed more rapidly than the control left cornea. Treatment of more than 500 human corneal abrasions with antibiotic solution, homatropine, a few drops of the patient's own blood, and a 24-hour pressure bandage was reported by this investigator. The blood is squeezed from the patient's finger directly into the eye. Details of a series of 25 clinical corneal abrasions involving from about 10% to 50% of the corneal area treated with this method are also reported by this author (no controls). Seventeen were healed within 1 day, seven during the second day, and the remaining one by the third day. The reason for the effectiveness of this treatment is not known, but it was suggested it may be because of the blood content of amino acids, adenosine triphosphate, fibrin, thrombin, or other substances. Perhaps structural support by fibrin could be invoked. Certainly use of the patient's own blood is less expensive and more convenient than commercial preparations of these substances.

In other experimental situations the benefit of a method of therapy is obviously related to avoidance of tissue damage. For example, dimethylsulfoxide prevents destruction of the endothelial cells during carefully controlled cryopreservation.[58]

Infection

Of 115 central corneal ulcers, 41% were found to be staphylococcal.[59] A degenerative precursor such as neurotrophic keratitis, exposure keratopathy, or chronic glaucomatous edema was present in 28% of these eyes. Only 10% of the patients had a history of trauma. Surprisingly, no cultures at all were taken in half of these patients, who had corneal ulcers sufficiently severe to warrant hospitalization. Perhaps this is the main message from this series of patients—that the causative organisms of corneal ulcers are so diverse that their identification and specific therapy require culture studies.

The management of bacterial corneal ulcers is no different from any other antibiotic treatment of infection. The only unique feature is the ease with which disastrous consequences such as scarring and perforation can result from an infection no larger than a medium-sized facial acne lesion.

Even after the death of many microorganisms, toxic products may be liberated to cause corneal damage. Such toxins are characteristic of fungi and staphylococci and have also been demonstrated for pneumococci.[60] Traditional management recommends specific antibiotic therapy and assumes that the eye will dispose of the toxins. The role of corticosteroids in treatment of infections is controversial. Some ophthalmologists advocate corticosteroid therapy to reduce the inflammatory component of the infection; others (including myself) condemn reduction of resistance as enhancing growth of the microorganisms.

An advocate of high-dosage corticosteroid treatment reports 75 patients with central stromal keratitis treated hourly with topical 1% prednisolone (6:00 A.M. to 10:00 P.M., 17 drops/day) for 3 weeks or more.[61] In addition to the corticosteroid therapy, specific topical antiviral, antibacterial, or antifungal treatment was advocated. The duration and severity of keratitis was supposedly lessened in 74 of the 75 cases (no controls). This intensive corticosteroid therapy was advocated whether the etiology was viral, fungal, or bacterial. The rationale for corticosteroid therapy of infections having these diverse etiologies was suppression of leukocytic invasion of the cornea. Corneal stromal breakdown is presumed to be a lytic effect of the polymorphonuclear leukocytes; it may be prevented by corticosteroids. The specific purpose of corticosteroid therapy for corneal infection was said to be preservation of the corneal stromal structure. Infectious epithelial damage alone does not require corticosteroid therapy; in fact, corticosteroid treatment may itself promote epithelial breakdown (as well as immunologic incompetence).

The great probability of iatrogenic spread of epidemic conjunctivitis requires reemphasis. In a Canadian epidemic, 8 cases were traced to tonometry performed subsequent to examination of the original patient.[62] This infection was caused by adenovirus type 19. Wash your hands and clean your equipment!

Allergy

Measurement of immunoglobulins in the various parts of the human eye showed by far the highest concentrations to be in the cornea, which contained up to half the serum concentration of these immune proteins. Almost as much immunoglobulin was found in the conjunctiva and a somewhat smaller amount in the choroid. Far lower concentrations existed in all other portions of the eye.[63] Similarly, high corneal concentrations of immunoglobulin occur in the rabbit eye.[64,65] Presence of immunoglobulins in these surface tissues undoubtedly enhances resistance but also allows allergic responses to develop.

Allergic corneal infiltration can be completely suppressed by corticosteroid therapy. As an example, the corneal hypersensitivity reaction to injected bovine albumin in rabbit corneas was blocked by subconjunctival injection of dexamethasone 21-phosphate (Decadron injectable), 0.2 ml (4 mg/ml) every other day.[66] Corticosteroid therapy was not effective in experimental eyes that had already been permitted to develop extensive neovascularization and did not prevent cellular infiltration and corneal edema in such cases.

The most dramatic immunologic response of the cornea is transplant rejection. A common form of this is lymphocytic destruction of the transplanted endothelium, which can be seen with the biomicroscope as a rapidly (several days) progressing endothelial rejection line composed of masses of lymphocytes on the posterior corneal surface. Prompt and vigorous corticosteroid therapy,

both systemic (100 mg prednisone daily) and topical (hourly prednisolone), may reverse the immunologic rejection process and salvage a clear graft.[67]

Scanning electron microscope study of corneal graft rejection in rabbits shows that the endothelial destruction is caused by lymphocyte attack on the donor cells. Topically applied corticosteroids cause a cytolytic effect on the lymphocytes, which can be seen to rupture, disintegrate, and finally disappear altogether from the treated cornea. The scanning electron microscope has demonstrated that corneal homograft destruction is mediated by sensitized lymphocytes and that their most vulnerable target is the donor endothelium. This technique has also demonstrated the importance of the lymphocyte cytolytic effect of corticosteroids as the mechanism whereby immunosuppression is achieved.[68]

However, intensive corticosteroid therapy of corneal transplant patients is not without drawbacks. Healing of experimental corneal wounds is significantly retarded by topical instillation of 1% prednisolone every hour for 14 hours each day. Epithelial healing is slowed; after 24 hours, 19% of the area of a standard abrasion was unhealed in prednisolone-treated eyes, in contrast to a 4% unhealed area in control eyes (average of 20 eyes). Although statistically significant, this slowing of epithelial healing is transient and clinically unimportant.

Similar treatment of stromal wounds showed a substantial decrease of tensile strength. After 11 days the treated corneas ruptured with a 19-g pull, as contrasted with a 54-g pull necessary to rupture untreated fellow eyes. This considerable difference persisted after 18 days, rupture occurring with 117 g in treated eyes and 211 g in untreated fellow eyes. After 18 days rabbit controls treated with only saline solution ruptured with 382 g. In rabbits receiving steroid in one eye enough systemic steroid absorption occurred from the treated eye to retard healing of the supposedly "untreated" fellow eye control. (One drop of a 1% solution of prednisolone fourteen times daily equals 7 mg of corticosteroid. In these rabbits this dosage was comparable on a weight basis to 200 mg prednisolone/day in an adult human.)

If no corticosteroid was used during the first 10 postoperative days, subsequent treatment for 8 days did not significantly retard healing. From the practical clinical standpoint, this suggests that corticosteroid therapy should not be used during the first 10 days postoperatively, but that subsequent use will not impair healing of corneal stroma.[69]

An interesting story illustrates how easily even the wisest clinicians can misinterpret their observations. Heteroplastic transplantation of animal corneas to man was the first approach to the surgical correction of corneal scarring. Since these efforts were unsuccessful, von Hippel in 1877 tried a homotransplant. Unfortunately this patient lost his eye from panophthalmitis—a worse result than had followed heterotransplants. Because of the influence of von Hippel, homotransplants were considered to be contraindicated for more than a decade.[70]

In 3 cases of Mooren's indolent ulcer of the cornea, fluorescent techniques demonstrated abnormal immunoglobulins in the conjunctiva. This suggests the possibility that the progressive and relentless erosion of Mooren's ulcer is an autoimmune phenomenon.[71]

Phlyctenular keratoconjunctivitis is apparently caused by some type of immunologic response to microorganisms, including tuberculosis, *Candida albicans*,[72] and *Staphylococcus aureus*.[73] Although corticosteroid therapy might seem rational, the staphylococcal phlyctenule perforated the cornea subsequent to corticosteroid therapy.

Trauma
Alkali burns

A unique corneal response to trauma is the elaboration of collagenase by the injured epithelial cell.[74-77] Although this response was first recognized in alkali burns, it also occurs in a variety of other injuries, including herpes simplex infection and dehydration. The significant corneal response to the collagenase is stromal dissolution—the "melting" of the cornea, as is seen in alkali burns, herpetic ulcers, and dellen.[78,79]

Collagenase production has been demonstrated in cultures of corneal epithelial cells obtained from 10 cases of corneal diseases associated with acute or chronic corneal ulceration (pemphigus, Stevens-Johnson syndrome, radiation keratitis, rosacea, metaherpes, alkali burn, and rheumatoid keratitis). No collagenase activity was demonstrable in 16 epithelial cell cultures obtained from normal corneas or diseased corneas without ulceration (bullous keratopathy, interstitial keratitis, old corneal scars, and dystrophy).[80]

Electron microscopy showed that at the edge of alkali burns the basal cells of the epithelium increased in number and sent cytoplasmic processes into the stroma. These processes contained vesicles, suggesting a secretory capability. The stromal collagen fibers near these epithelial cell processes were frayed and disintegrated and became continuous with an amorphous mass of debris. Such abnormalities were not present in the nonulcerated cornea. These anatomic findings are compatible with the hypothesis that modified epithelial cells may secrete substances responsible for collagen destruction.[81]

Even 3 months after a severe alkali burn (rabbit eye), electron microscopy shows exposed collagen fibrils of stroma at the base of the ulcer and an incomplete layer of grossly damaged and undermined epithelium.[82]

The damage of an alkali burn is not confined to the epithelium but may extend to involve the entire anterior segment of the eye. The endothelium, for example, may suffer only localized destruction from a small alkali burn, and it responds by regeneration. Following severe burns, however, the entire endothelium is destroyed and is replaced by a fibroblastic retrocorneal membrane.[83] Such a membrane, of course, is incapable of maintaining corneal dehydration and can be presumed to exist behind every densely scarred burned cornea.

Within 2 minutes (probably within seconds) of application of 0.1 ml 2N sodium hydroxide to the rabbit cornea, the pH of the aqueous was 12. (The NaOH solution had a pH of 13.) Continuous flushing of the eye with saline reduced the pH only to 10 even after 2 hours of irrigation. In contrast, paracentesis and irrigation of the anterior chamber with buffered solution promptly reduced the pH to 9, with drop thereafter to 8, within 30 minutes. The authors advocated paracentesis of the anterior chamber and irrigation with buffered solution as emergency treatment even several hours after severe alkali burns.[84] However, no information was given as to whether the clinical course of the severe alkali burn is improved by such a paracentesis and irrigation.

The effects of severe alkali burns on intraocular pressure have obvious anatomic explanations. In moderately severe burns the outflow channels are damaged and chronic glaucoma develops. In more destructive burns the ciliary processes are destroyed, resulting in hypotony or even phthisis.[85] Another manifestation of aqueous secretory damage from alkali burns is marked reduction in aqueous and stromal glucose levels.[86]

Following severe alkali burns, there occur three separate types of glaucoma.[87] The first rise in pressure is transient, appearing within 1 minute and lasting for less than 10 minutes. It is a result of collagen shrinkage. The second rise reaches a maximum at 1 hour, then gradually falls to normal in about 3 hours. It is caused by prostaglandin release and can be opposed by prostaglandin inhibitors such as polyphloretin or beta adrenergic drugs (phenylephrine). The long-term and clinically significant post-burn glaucoma is caused by mechanical blockage of the filtration angle and is treated as appropriate for such a secondary glaucoma.

Treatment. In the immediate management of chemical burns of the eye there is no substitute for prompt, copious irrigation with ordinary water. The time lost in searching for an antidote more than nullifies any possible benefit to be gained through specific neutralization. Studies conducted to compare the relative effectiveness of a phosphate buffer and distilled water indicate that there is no difference in the healing rate and final condition of chemically burned corneas adequately irrigated with these two fluids.[88] These were well-controlled studies of standard rat cornea burns produced by hydrochloric acid, nitric acid, and sodium hydroxide.

Specific neutralization of alkali burns of the cornea with neutral ammonium tartrate has been advocated but seems without merit. In a controlled study of 107 rabbits, irrigation of sodium hydroxide corneal burns with neutral ammonium tartrate (0.35N) was of no value whatsoever.[89]

Following severe alkali burns, irrigation should be continued for at least a half hour. The pH level of the cornea has usually returned to normal by then. If desired, the use of pH indicator paper can be used to confirm the absence of excess alkalinity. Long-continued irrigation (for many hours) probably causes more irritation than benefit.[90]

Be sure to remove any particles of alkaline material that may be adherent to the conjunctiva. Eversion of the upper lid and careful inspection of both upper and lower cul-de-sacs is important.

Since the denuded corneal stroma is vulnerable to infection, antibiotic therapy is appropriate, as is the use of lubricant solutions and ointments if the burn has compromised the conjunctival and lacrimal secretory apparatus. Symblepharon develops rapidly and may be minimized by separating the apposed conjunctival surfaces, although this will not prevent late contraction of a scarred cul-de-sac. Iritis is always present and should be treated with cycloplegics. Watch for glaucoma, which may be caused by trabecular damage or a swollen cataract.

Prevention of stromal loss and corneal perforation may be achieved with the use of collagenase inhibitors.[91-93] Rabbit experiments indicate that burns of only part of the cornea rarely perforate, but that burns of the total cornea and surrounding conjunctiva always perforate if untreated. Hence it was concluded that partial corneal burns in humans would do well simply with topical antibiotics and cycloplegics; this was the case in 11 partial burns, all of which healed uneventfully. Total corneal and surrounding scleral burns of 25 human eyes were treated with 0.2M cysteine (collagenase inhibitor), 2 drops six times daily, beginning on the seventh day after injury. All but one of these eyes healed, and that one perforated during a 2-week period after emergency cataract extraction when cysteine was not used. Seven comparably burned eyes were treated with antibiotic and cycloplegic alone. Five of these seven eyes perforated.[94]

Healing of the alkali-burned cornea is complete when the epithelium *completely* covers the corneal surface. The absence of even a small area of epithelium identifies an area of potential ulceration. Healing of these eyes is extremely slow, taking as long as 9 months.[95]

Corneal collagenase is dependent on the presence of calcium for its activation. Chelation of calcium by EDTA, 0.2M, will inhibit collagenase (20 corneal ulcers healed with EDTA therapy of 35 patients),[96] but this inhibition is reversible by the addition of more calcium. Cysteine irreversibly inhibits collagenase, presumably by attaching to the enzyme molecule.[95] However, the ability of burned tissue to produce new collagenase is not impaired; hence regular and continuing use of cysteine is necessary until the epithelium is completely healed.[97]

Although cysteine is effective in inhibiting collagenase, it is unstable and relatively difficult to obtain. Acetylcysteine is readily available in most pharmacies as a 20% preparation (Mucomyst), is stable in solution for 96 hours, and is well tolerated by the human eye. Treatment with acetylcysteine six times daily was effective in preventing perforation of experimental alkali burns in rabbits. Argyrol 10% was also found to be helpful[98]—whether this was because of inactivation of protein enzymes or bacterial inhibition was not established.

Application of another collagenase inhibitor, penicillamine in a 0.15M solution, 1 drop four times a day, was found to be at least as effective as cysteine in preventing ulceration of alkali-burned human corneas.[99] The solution is stable for 7 days, as compared to 2 days for cysteine. The formula for the penicillamine solution was as follows:

Penicillamine hydrochloride	417 mg
Sodium hydroxide, 2N	1.1 ml
Distilled water to	15 ml

The sodium hydroxide is added to achieve a pH of 6.5

Corticosteroids augment the lytic action of collagenase, causing up to 12 times as much lysis in vitro. However, this potentiating effect of corticosteroids may be reversed by simultaneous use of collagenase inhibitors.[100] Be careful about using corticosteroids in treatment of alkali burns—they will melt the cornea.

Study of the characteristics of alkali burns in 200 rabbits indicated that spontaneous perforation occurred in 28% of untreated eyes with burns of the cornea only, in contrast to 90% of eyes with both corneal and scleral burns. Viability and continuing integrity of the alkali-burned cornea were closely related to the extent of neovascularization. Apparently, fibroblasts accompany the advance of neovascularization and help to protect the cornea from perforation. Twenty eyes were treated with 1% prednisolone three times daily following corneoscleral burns. Such corticosteroid treatment prevented neovascularization and return of living cells to the cornea and resulted in perforation of all eyes! This study suggested that neovascularization of alkali-burned eyes is a favorable prognostic development and should not be hindered, as by corticosteroid therapy.[101]

Destruction of the conjunctiva and lacrimal ducts results in a severe dry eye after healing of the acute effects of an alkali burn. Adequate replacement of moisture may be an impossible task.

To avoid misunderstanding, alkali burn does not refer only to corneal damage induced by sodium hydroxide or lye. Ammonia burns from refrigerants or fertilizers are exceptionally severe alkali burns.[102-104] A less obvious alkali burn results from fireworks such as sparklers or flares. These burns are not only thermal but are also intensely alkaline because of the magnesium in the fireworks.[103]*

Acid burns

In contrast to the dreadful injuries produced by alkali, acid burns of the eye are almost benign. In a case of generalized sulfuric acid burn so severe as to cause death in 5 days, the pathologic examination of the eyes showed severe damage to the lid skin, the conjunctiva, the epithelium of the cornea, and the stroma. Descemet's endothelium was partially intact and the deeper structures (iris, lens, and trabeculum) were entirely normal.[105]

Tear gas injury

The active incredient of tear gas weapons (Mace, etc.), chloracetophenone, is an irreversible inhibitor of sulfhydryl enzymes. In higher concentrations it denatures tissue proteins. Severe lacrimation and disability result from small amounts of this irritant dispersed in an aerosol spray. Close-range (3 to 6 feet) discharge of tear gas weapons can cause permanent corneal damage. This is particularly likely to occur when the chemical is delivered by an explosive cartridge.[106,107]

The therapy given in the reported cases consisted of topical corticosteroids, antibiotics, and cycloplegics. No specific antidote was discussed or advised.

The sulfhydryl group is one of the chemical radicals essential to growth and survival of tissues. Its use (as Hydrosulphosol) has been advocated in treatment of chemical burns of the eye.[108,109] Benefit from such use of sulfhydryl would be unexpected, since it is well known that provision of excess amounts of enzymes, vitamins, and similar substances does not promote growth or healing. Indeed, controlled animal experiments confirm the failure of sulfhydryl treatment to alter the rate of healing of corneal injuries.[110-115]

The only exception to the ineffectiveness of sulfhydryl treatment of corneal burns is in the management of tear gas burns. Many of

*For an excellent review of alkali burns, see reference 104.

these lacrimating gases (for example, iodoacetate) act by inhibiting sulfhydryl enzymes. Prompt sulfhydryl replacement is of considerable therapeutic value, in one experimental instance curing an eye in 4 days as contrasted to the control, which was still not healed after 14 days.[110] Although data as to the time of application are not available, general biochemical information suggests that greatest benefit would result from sulfhydryl treatment within minutes of the tear gas burn. From the practical standpoint, it is doubtful that sulfhydryl medication (glutathione and Hydrosulphosol) would be available soon enough after an iodoacetate burn to be of much therapeutic value.

Dimercaptopropanol (BAL) is not of value in treatment of tear gas burns. Its sulfhydryl groups are not available for tissue utilization but rather act as a most efficient competitor for toxic heavy metal ions such as arsenic, which are thereby removed from their tissue sulfhydryl linkages.

In summary, sulfhydryl therapy is rational only in a few rather unusual types of chemical burns in which there is an actual deficiency of sulfhydryl ions because of action of a specific inhibitor—and here only if promptly available.

Another mechanism of action of sulfhydryl-containing medications is inhibition of collagenase. Possibly this accounted for some of the therapeutic results reported in the earlier literature.

Glaucoma medications

Bullous keratopathy in several patients improved on withdrawal of medication used for glaucoma. Following this observation, the commonly used miotics were placed in epithelial tissue cultures, using 1:1000 dilutions of commercially available miotics. Cytotoxic changes such as vacuolation and granularity were conspicuous.[116]

An atypical paracentral band keratopathy was recognized in 18 patients receiving long-term glaucoma therapy.[117] None of the diseases commonly responsible for band keratopathy were present in these eyes. Treatment was by denuding the epithelium under topical anesthesia and dripping on 0.02M EDTA over a 15-minute period. In all cases in which the opacity was completely removed, no recurrence occurred despite continued miotic treatment. If a portion of the cornea was not included in the EDTA treatment, this area tended to develop further calcification.

Band keratopathy

Apparently simple mechanical scraping of the area of superficial calcification with a scalpel will remove band keratopathy as effectively as dissolving it with EDTA.[118]

Proprietary medications

Various shampoos, skin creams, decongestant drugs, aerosol preparations, etc. can cause mild toxic keratopathy.[119] The main significance of these problems is that our awareness of the possibility of such drug-induced corneal irritation may lead to detection and elimination of the cause of the patient's discomfort.

On an empirical basis, IDU has been recommended for treatment of aerosol keratitis. In a series of 84 cases of aerosol keratitis, treatment with lubricants, corticosteroids, and various lytic enzymes was ineffective, but relief was obtained with several drops of IDU instilled three or four times daily. The rationale for this is unexplained. Possibly IDU promotes cellular desquamation and thereby hastens release of the irritant spray particles embedded within the epithelium.[120]

Rust rings

Corneal "rust rings" surrounding imbedded corneal foreign bodies will themselves cause a chronic inflammatory reaction that may last for some weeks. For this reason, such rust rings should be curetted cleanly from the cornea, preferably with biomicroscopic observation. Following thorough removal of the brown discoloration, antibiotic and cycloplegic (if necessary) therapy is used as after the removal of an ordinary foreign body. Chemical identification of the "rust

ring" showed the presence of iron in 13 of 14 such rings.[121] Nineteen of twenty foreign bodies removed from corneas with rust rings were identified as iron. Of 20 foreign bodies without surrounding rust rings, only six were iron. It is clearly established that rust rings truly represent iron discoloration of the cornea, and apparently the characteristic chronic irritation is a toxic effect of the iron.

Topical use of deferoxamine (10% ointment) was suggested in management of corneal rust from multiple small iron particles (as might result from explosion of iron filings). The drug does not penetrate the intact corneal epithelium very well and hence is not very effective after epithelial healing has occurred. Topical deferoxamine therapy for 4 or 5 days immediately following injury was reported to remove residual rust staining in human eyes.[122]

Mechanical protection

In cases of temporary corneal exposure such as Bell's palsy, endocrine exophthalmos, and lid trauma, effective corneal protection may be obtained by taping a square of plastic food wrap (Saran Wrap) over the eye. An antibiotic ointment may be desirable if an infectious component is present.[123,124]

"Bandage" contact lenses

The protective effect of soft contact lenses has now been established for conditions such as bullous keratopathy.[125,126] The effect of 5% sodium chloride drops in reducing chronic epithelial edema is enhanced by retention within the contact lens.[127] The severe dry eye syndromes[128,129] and chronic herpetic ulcers[130] also respond to soft lens protection. Soft lenses may also be used to enhance the delivery of medication.[131]

The carrying case[132] or the wetting solutions and soft lenses themselves[133] may be the source of *Pseudomonas* contamination, which can lead to severe corneal scarring.[134] Continuous wearing of soft contact lenses can result in extensive corneal vascularization, the progression of which has been demonstrated by fluorescein angiography.[135] Wetting solutions show considerable variability and may themselves cause irritation; this is particularly true of solutions containing cationic detergents, which have been found to vary in pH and to be particularly irritating in acidic batches.[136]

Assorted keratopathies

The following material is a disorganized potpourri of suggestions from the literature concerning the treatment of a variety of corneal conditions.

Neuroparalytic keratitis

Neuroparalytic keratitis is probably caused by at least two separate factors, dryness of the eye and metabolic disturbances ("trophic" changes). Two groups of patients with fifth nerve paralysis were studied; they differed only in regard to whether the lacrimal innervation was interrupted by the neurosurgical procedure.[137] Initially, Schirmer's test measurements showed a marked decrease in tearing of all patients. After some months the Schirmer measurements returned to normal in those patients with intact greater superficial petrosal nerves. Lacrimal secretion was permanently impaired in patients with secretory nerve section; however, obliteration of the punctae via electrocoagulation improved the Schirmer readings and gave symptomatic relief in several cases. Neuroparalytic keratitis was more severe in the patients with greater tear deficiency but occurred to some extent in all patients with corneal anesthesia. Whether this is a result of metabolic "trophic" disturbance or unrecognized minor trauma is not clear. Nevertheless, the importance of maintaining adequate lubrication of eyes predisposed to neuroparalytic keratitis is certain. Use four times daily of methylcellulose, 2.5%, and topical antibiotics was quite effective in the management of one series of patients.[138]

Dellen

Dellen are small saucerlike excavations at the edge of the cornea adjacent to paralimbal elevations (for example, swelling following strabismus surgery). This corneal change is caused by dehydration and thinning of the cornea. Treatment is rehydration of the cornea, which may be achieved by patching the eye, frequent use of lubricating drops, or eliminating the paralimbal elevation (as by corticosteroid therapy of an allergic elevation).[139]

The lesion occurs 1 to 3 weeks postoperatively and heals spontaneously within a few days to 1 month. Neither corticosteroids nor antibiotics hasten healing. The most important point in therapy is to avoid overtreatment, since iodine cautery (for the misdiagnosis of virus keratitis) simply prolongs the defect.[140]

Filamentary keratitis

The possibility that some cases of filamentary keratitis are caused by viral infection is suggested by the cure of two such patients by 1 week of IDU therapy. One of these cases had been thought to be of allergic origin; the other followed cataract extraction.[141] An alternate explanation for this therapeutic result might be the inhibition of whatever epithelial activity is responsible for filament formation.

Topical acetylcysteine therapy four times daily was said to produce more uniform wetting and to benefit keratitis sicca.[142] Of course, artificial tears are the standard recommendation.[143]

Microcystic dystrophy

Should recurrent corneal erosions occur in this mild epithelial defect, hyperosmotic therapy, as with sodium chloride, is advised.[144]

Recurrent corneal erosion

Although our knowledge of the pathology of recurrent corneal erosion has been advanced by electron microscopic demonstration of absence of the basement membrane in areas of recurrent erosion, no new treatments are available.[145] Recommended management of stubbornly recurrent erosions includes mild cauterization of the involved area with 2% iodine followed by mechanical removal of the loose epithelium with a knife blade. Bedtime instillation of hypertonic ointment has been suggested in the belief that edema of the diseased site may thereby be avoided.

Because it seriously and deeply damages the cornea, use of a strong iodine solution (7%) is definitely contraindicated in the treatment of any corneal problem.[146]

Scleromalacia perforans

The value of corticosteroid treatment of scleromalacia perforans is questionable. An attempt was made to evaluate cortisone therapy in a series of 43 cases.[147] The author did not present statistical data, but offered general observations: "The initial response to steroid therapy was usually satisfactory but this success was short-lived, for after a varying period of time (six months to four years) the affected eye had to be enucleated. The development of necrogranulomatous scleritis is characterized by exacerbations and remissions and it is therefore difficult to be certain whether the initial beneficial effects are due to the cortisone. It is equally difficult to assess the long term effects of cortisone.[147]

There is general agreement that the red eye of the patient with severe rheumatoid arthritis becomes more comfortable with topical corticosteroid use, but the probability of enhanced scleral loss is suspected by many clinicians.

Wegener's granulomatosis

Necrotizing scleritis and ring ulcers of the cornea may accompany Wegener's syndrome.[148] Systemic use of cyclophosphamide and prednisone was beneficial in one case, causing dramatic improvement of the scleral damage. Subconjunctival injection of heparin had been of no value.[149] Heparin injections have been advocated in the treatment of peripheral corneal lesions on the supposition that they represent ischemic damage. Of 28 peripheral lesions so treated, 26 were said to have improved (no controls).[150] Since the corneal nutrition derives primarily from the aqueous, the basis for the assumption of ischemic damage is unclear.

Rosacea keratitis

The intravenous use of riboflavin (1 mg/day) is reported to cure promptly rosacea keratitis, superficial marginal keratitis, and catarrhal ulcers.[151] This article suggests "overwork and irregular lunching" as the cause of such corneal ulcers and does not cite convincing evidence of therapeutic response. Based on such articles, vitamin therapy of corneal ulcers is sporadically used, but seems to be a nonspecific and ineffectual treatment.

Intensive riboflavin therapy (as much as 10 mg/day intravenously for 2 weeks, followed by 20 mg/day orally for 1 month) failed to cure any of 21 cases of rosacea keratitis.[152] Secondary staphylococcal infection was present in most of these patients, was mainly responsible for the corneal scarring, and was controlled with topical sulfonamides.

Burdock burr ophthalmia

A chronic keratoconjunctivitis of sudden onset, completely unresponsive to medication, may be caused by mechanical irritation by a foreign body. Such an etiology should be particularly suspected if the corneal lesions are linear, as would be expected if abrasions were produced by a sharp object in the upper lid. The common burdock burr is a classic cause of such a keratoconjunctivitis that is often undiagnosed because of the extremely small size of the bristle. The burdock plant also contains chemical irritants.

Only with the biomicroscope can one see the hair-thin bristle embedded in the center of a reddened area in the upper tarsus and hidden beneath a covering of mucus. Mechanical extraction, quite difficult because the shaft is barbed, immediately cures the condition.[153,154]

Chlorpromazine keratopathy

Very high doses of chlorpromazine (2000 mg/day) produced characteristic corneal epithelial changes in 19 of 30 schizophrenic patients. The entire exposed corneal epithelium developed a faint white diffuse opacification. Gray or brown lines, sufficiently distinct to be barely perceptible grossly, formed in the epithelium. No patient lost more than one Snellen line of visual acuity. Although greatly improved, the epithelial keratopathy was still faintly visible in all cases 2 months after chlorpromazine was discontinued. Epithelial keratopathy occurs only in patients receiving a high daily dosage, in contrast to the lens and deep corneal changes seen only after a high total dose (500 to 1000 g).[155]

Keratoconus

The acute corneal edema associated with rupture of Descemet's membrane in keratoconus (acute keratoconus) typically clears as soon as the defect is covered by regenerating endothelium.[156] Depending on the size of the lesion, this regeneration usually occurs within 1 month. Although pressure dressings and carbonic anhydrase inhibitors have been advised, their value seems unproved and their use without clear rationale. Any treatment started about 1 month after onset of the acute keratoconus will be followed promptly by a "cure," which is simply the spontaneous course of the disease.

REFERENCES

1. Thygeson, P.: Etiology and treatment of blepharitis, Arch. Ophthalmol. **36:**445, 1946.
2. Aragones, J. V.: The treatment of blepharitis: a controlled double blind study of combination therapy, Ann. Ophthalmol. **5:**49, 1973.
3. Wilson, L. A., Kuehne, J. W., Hall, S. W., and Ahearn, D. G.: Microbial contamination in ocular cosmetics, Am. J. Ophthalmol. **71:**1298, 1971.
4. Bereston, E. S.: Use of selenium sulfide shampoo in seborrheic dermatitis, J.A.M.A. **156:**1246, 1954.
5. Wong, A. S., Fasanella, R. M., Haley, L. D., Marshall, C. L., and Krehl, W. A.: Selenium (Selsun) in the treatment of marginal blepharitis, Arch. Ophthalmol. **55:**246, 1956.
6. Lavyel, A.: Selsunef ointment to treat squamous blepharitis, Am. J. Ophthalmol. **49:**820, 1960.
7. Ostler, H. B., Okumoto, M., and Halde, C.: Dermatophytosis affecting the periorbital region, Am. J. Ophthalmol. **72:**934, 1971.
8. Nauheim, J. S., and Sussman, W.: Herpes simplex of the lids and adjacent areas. Trans. Am. Acad. Ophthalmol. Otolaryngol. **75:**1236, 1971.
9. Gould, E., and Havener, W. H.: Vaccinia lid infection, Am. J. Ophthalmol. **56:**830, 1963.
10. Bock, R. H.: Treatment of palpebral warts with cantharon, Am. J. Ophthalmol. **60:**529, 1965.
11. Irvine, S. R.: Missed diagnoses, Arch. Ophthalmol. **71:**291, 1964.
12. Jacklin, H. N.: Depigmentation of the eyelids in eserine allergy, Am. J. Ophthalmol. **59:**89, 1965.
13. Adour, K. K., and Swanson, P. J., Jr.: Facial paralysis in 403 consecutive patients, Trans. Am. Acad. Ophthalmol. Otolaryngol. **75:**1284, 1971.
14. Levine, R. E., House, W. F., and Hitselberger, W. E.: Ocular complications of seventh nerve paralysis and management with the palpebral spring, Am. J. Ophthalmol. **73:**219, 1972.
15. Stern, E. N., Campbell, C. H., and Faulkner, H. W.: Conservative management of congenital eversion of the eyelids, Am. J. Ophthalmol. **75:**319, 1973.
16. Magnuson, R. H.: Untreated hemangioma, Arch. Ophthalmol. **94:**685, April 1976.
17. Tomar, V. P. S., Sharma, O. P., and Joshi, K.: Bacterial and fungal flora of normal conjunctiva, Ann. Ophthalmol. **3:**669, 1971.
18. Olson, C. L.: Bacterial flora of the conjunctiva and lid margin, Arch. Ophthalmol. **82:**197, 1969.
19. Thygeson, P.: Historical review of oculogenital disease, Am. J. Ophthalmol. **71:**975, 1971.
20. Mills, R. P., and Kalina, R. E.: Reiter's keratitis, Arch. Ophthalmol. **87:**447, 1972.
21. Ostler, H. B., Dawson, C. R., Schachter, J., and Engleman, E. P.: Reiter's syndrome, Am. J. Ophthalmol. **71:**986, 1971.
22. Dawson, C. R., Schachter, J., Ostler, H. B., Gilbert, R. M., Smith, D. E., and Engleman, E. P.: Inclusion conjunctivitis and Reiter's syndrome in a married couple, Arch. Ophthalmol. **83:**300, 1970.
23. Schachter, J.: Complement-fixing antibodies to Bedsonia in Reiter's syndrome, TRIC agent infection, and control groups, Am. J. Ophthalmol. **71:**857, 1971.
24. Noer, H. R.: An "experimental" epidemic of Reiter's syndrome, J.A.M.A. **197:**693, 1966.
25. Dawson, C. R.: Lids, conjunctiva, and lacrimal apparatus, Arch. Ophthalmol. **93:**854, September 1975.
26. Corwin, M. T.: Superior limbic keratoconjunctivitis, Am. J. Ophthalmol. **66:**338, 1968.
27. Theodore, F. H.: Further observations on superior limbic keratoconjunctivitis, Trans.

Am. Acad. Ophthalmol. Otolaryngol. **71:** 341, 1967.

28. Theodore, F. H., and Ferry, A. P.: Superior limbic keratoconjunctivitis, Arch. Ophthalmol. **84:**481, 1970.

29. Cher, I.: Superior limbic keratoconjunctivitis, Arch. Ophthalmol. **82:**580, 1969.

30. Brauninger, G. E., and Centifano, Y. M.: Immunoglobulin E in human tears, Am. J. Ophthalmol. **72:**558, 1971.

31. Allansmith, M. R., Hahn, G. S., and Simon, M. A.: Tissue, tear, and serum IgE concentrations in vernal conjunctivitis, Am. J. Ophthalmol. **81:**506, April 1976.

32. Thygeson, P., and Kimura, S. J.: Chronic conjunctivitis, Trans. Am. Acad. Ophthalmol. Otolaryngol. **67:**494, 1963.

33. Greenberg, L. M., Mauriello, D. A., Cinotti, A. A., and Buxton, J. N.: Erythema multiforme exudativum (Stevens-Johnson syndrome) following sodium diphenylhydantoin therapy, Ann. Ophthalmol. **3:**137, 1971.

34. Coursin, D. B.: Stevens-Johnson syndrome—nonspecific parasensitivity reaction? J.A.M.A. **198:**113, 1966.

35. Howard, G. M.: The Stevens-Johnson syndrome, Am. J. Ophthalmol. **55:**893, 1963.

36. Gasset, A., and Kaufman, H.: Soft lenses in therapy, Am. J. Ophthalmol. **69:**252, 1970.

37. Chalkley, T. H. F.: Chronic cicatricial conjunctivitis, Am. J. Ophthalmol. **67:**526, 1969.

38. Bedell, A. J.: Ocular pemphigus, Am. J. Ophthalmol. **60:**99, 1965.

39. Herron, B. E.: Immunologic aspects of cicatricial pemphigoid, Am. J. Ophthalmol. **79:** 271, February 1975.

40. Furey, N., West, C., Andrews, T., Paul, P. D., and Bean, S. F.: Immunofluorescent studies of ocular cicatricial pemphigoid, Am. J. Ophthalmol. **80:**825, November 1975.

41. Patten, J. T., Cavanagh, H. D., and Allansmith, M. R.: Induced ocular pseudopemphigoid, Am. J. Ophthalmol. **82:**272, August 1976.

42. Chambers, J. D., Blodi, F. C., Golden, B., and McKee, A. P.: Ligneous conjunctivitis, Trans. Am. Acad. Ophthalmol. Otolaryngol. **73:**996, 1969.

43. Kanai, A., and Polack, F. M.: Histologic and electron microscope studies of ligneous conjunctivitis, Am. J. Ophthalmol. **72:**909, 1971.

44. Firat, T.: Ligneous conjunctivitis, Am. J. Ophthalmol. **78:**679, October 1974.

45. Thygeson, P.: Observations on conjunctival neoplasms masquerading as chronic conjunctivitis or keratitis, Trans. Am. Acad. Ophthalmol. Otolaryngol. **73::**969, 1969.

46. Dykstra, P. C., and Dykstra, B. A.: The cytologic diagnosis of carcinoma and related lesions of the ocular conjunctiva and cornea, Trans. Am. Acad. Ophthalmol. Otolaryngol. **73:**979, 1969.

47. Humphrey, W. T.: Flaxseeds in ophthalmic folk medicine, Am. J. Ophthalmol. **70:**287, 1970.

48. Donn, A.: The movement of ions and water across the cornea, Invest. Ophthalmol. **1:** 170, 1962.

49. Green, K., and Tonjum, A.: Influence of various agents on corneal permeability, Am. J. Ophthalmol. **72:**897, 1971.

50. Dohlman, C. H.: The function of the corneal epithelium in health and disease, Invest. Ophthalmol. **10:**383, 1971.

51. Bertalanffy, F. D., and Lau, C.: Arch. Ophthalmol. **68:**546, 1962.

52. Hanna, C., Bicknell, D. S., and O'Brien, J. E.: Cell turnover in the adult human eye, Arch. Ophthalmol. **65:**695, 1961.

53. Irvine, A. R., Jr.: The role of the endothelium in bullous keratopathy, Arch. Ophthalmol. **56:**338, 1956.

54. Luxenberg, M. N., and Green, K.: Reduction of corneal edema with topical hypertonic agents, Am. J. Ophthalmol. **71:**847, 1971.

55. Green, K., and Downs, S.: Reduction of corneal thickness with hypertonic solutions, Am. J. Ophthalmol. **75:**507, 1973.

56. Kolbert, G. S.: Oral diphenylhydantoin in corneal wound healing in the rabbit, Am. J. Ophthalmol. **66:**736, 1968.

57. Christenberry, K. W.: Treatment of corneal abrasion with topical whole blood, Arch. Ophthalmol. **63:**948, 1960.

58. Polack, F. M., Bernier, G., and Slappey, T. E.: Incorporation of radioactive sulphate by corneal stroma during cryopreservation, Am. J. Ophthalmol. **72:**906, 1971.

59. Brightbill, F. S.: Central corneal ulcers, Ann. Ophthalmol. **4:**331, 1972.

60. Johnson, M. K., and Allen, J. H.: Ocular toxin of the pneumococcus, Am. J. Ophthalmol. **72:**175, 1971.

61. Aronson, S. B., and Moore, T. E., Jr.: Corticosteroid therapy in central stromal keratitis, Am. J. Ophthalmol. **67:**873, 1969.

62. Jackson, W. B., Davis, P. L., Groh, V., and

Champlin, R.: Adenovirus type 19 keratoconjunctivitis in Canada, Can. J. Ophthalmol. **10**:326, 1975.

63. Allansmith, M. R., Whitney, C. R., McClellan, B. H., and Newman, L. P.: Immunoglobulins in the human eye, Arch. Ophthalmol. **89**:36, 1973.

64. Allansmith, M., Newman, L., and Whitney, C.: The distribution of immunoglobulin in the rabbit eye, Arch. Ophthalmol. **86**:60, 1971.

65. Allansmith, M., Newman, L. P., and Hutchison, D. S.: Immunoglobulin G in the rabbit cornea, Arch. Ophthalmol. **82**:229, 1969.

66. Olson, C. L.: Subconjunctival steroids and corneal hypersensitivity, Arch. Ophthalmol. **75**:651, 1966.

67. Levenson, J. E., and Brightbill, F. S.: Endothelial rejection in human transplants, Arch. Ophthalmol. **89**:489, 1973.

68. Polack, F. M.: Lymphocyte destruction during corneal homograft reaction, Arch. Ophthalmol. **89**:413, 1973.

69. Aquavella, J. V., Gasset, A. R., and Dohlman, C. H.: Corticosteroids in corneal wound healing, Am. J. Ophthalmol. **58**:621, 1964.

70. Leigh, A. G.: Corneal transplantation, Oxford, 1966, Blackwell Scientific Publications.

71. Brown, S. I., Mondino, B. J., and Rabin, B. S.: Autoimmune phenomenon in Mooren's ulcer, Am. J. Ophthalmol. **82**:835, December 1976.

72. Wong, V. G., and Kirkpatrick, C. H.: Immune reconstitution in keratoconjunctivitis and superficial candidiasis, Arch. Ophthalmol. **92**:335, October 1974.

73. Ostler, H. B.: Corneal perforation in nontuberculous (Staphylococcal) phlyctenular keratoconjunctivitis, Am. J. Ophthalmol. **79**:446, March 1976.

74. Brown, S. I., and Weller, C. A.: Cell origin of collagenase in normal and wounded corneas, Arch. Ophthalmol. **83**:74, 1970.

75. Pfister, R. R., McCulley, J. P., Friend, J., and Dohlman, C. H.: Collagenase activity of intact corneal epithelium in peripheral alkali burns, Arch. Ophthalmol. **86**:308, 1971.

76. Brown, S. I., and Hook, C. W.: Isolation of stromal collagenase in corneal inflammation, Am. J. Ophthalmol. **72**:1139, 1971.

77. Brown, S. I., Weller, C. A., and Wassermann, H. E.: Collagenolytic activity of alkali-burned corneas, Arch. Ophthalmol. **81**:370, 1969.

78. Gnadinger, M. C., Itoi, M., Slansky, H. H., and Dohlman, C. H.: The role of collagenase in the alkali-burned cornea, Am. J. Ophthalmol. **68**:478, 1969.

79. Brown, S. I., Weller, C. A., and Akiya, S.: Pathogenesis of ulcers of the alkali-burned cornea, Arch. Ophthalmol. **83**:205, 1970.

80. Slansky, H. H., Gnadinger, M. C., Itoi, M., and Dohlman, C. H.: Collagenase in corneal ulcerations, Arch. Ophthalmol. **82**:108, 1969.

81. Matsuda, H., and Smelser, G. K.: Epithelium and stroma in alkali-burned corneas, Arch. Ophthalmol. **89**:396, 1973.

82. Henriquez, A. S., Pihlaja, D. J., and Dohlman, C. H.: Surface ultrastructure in alkali-burned rabbit corneas, Am. J. Ophthalmol. **81**:324, March 1976.

83. Matsuda, H., and Smelser, G. K.: Endothelial cells in alkali-burned corneas, Arch. Ophthalmol. **89**:402, 1973.

84. Paterson, C. A., Pfister, R. R., and Levinson, R. A.: Aqueous humor pH changes after experimental alkali burns, Am. J. Ophthalmol. **79**:414, March 1975.

85. Stein, M. R., Naidoff, M. A., and Dawson, C.: Intraocular pressure response to experimental alkali burns, Am. J. Ophthalmol. **75**:99, 1973.

86. Pfister, R. R., Friend, J., and Dohlman, C. H.: The anterior segments of rabbits after alkali burns, Arch. Ophthalmol. **86**:189, 1971.

87. Paterson, C. A., and Pfister, R. R.: Intraocular pressure changes after alkali burns, Arch. Ophthalmol. **91**:211, March 1974.

88. Bahn, G. C., Sonnier, E., and Allen, J. H.: Therapeutic studies in experimental chemical injury of the cornea, Am. J. Ophthalmol. **49**:1331, 1960.

89. Geeraets, W. J., Aaron, S. D., and Guerry, D., III: Alkali burns of the cornea and neutral ammonium tartrate, Va. Med. Mon. **91**:493, 1964.

90. Girard, L. J., Alford, W. E., Feldman, G. I., and Williams, B.: Severe alkali burns, Trans. Am. Acad. Ophthalmol. Otolaryngol. **74**:788, 1970.

91. Brown, S. I., and Weller, C. A.: Collagenase inhibitors in prevention of ulcers of alkali-burned cornea, Arch. Ophthalmol. **83**:352, 1970.

92. Brown, S. I.: Treatment of the alkali-burned cornea, Sight Sav. Rev. **41**:83, 1971.

93. Brown, S. I., Akiya, S., and Weller, C. A.: Prevention of the ulcers of the alkali-burned cornea, Arch. Ophthalmol. **82**:95, 1969.

94. Brown, S. I., Tragakis, M. P., and Pearce, D. B.: Treatment of the alkali-burned cornea, Am. J. Ophthalmol. **74:**316, 1972.

95. Brown, S. I., and Hook, C. W.: Treatment of corneal destruction with collagenase inhibitors, Trans. Am. Acad. Ophthalmol. Otolaryngol. **75:**1199, 1971.

96. Slansky, H. H., Dohlman, C. H., and Berman, M.: Prevention of corneal ulcers, Trans. Am. Acad. Ophthalmol. Otolaryngol. **75:**1208, 1971.

97. Anderson, R. E., Kuns, M. D., and Dresden, M. H.: Collagenase activity in the alkali-burned cornea, Ann. Ophthalmol. **3:**619, 1971.

98. Evans, R. M., McCrary, J. A., III, and Christensen, G.: Mucomyst (acetylcysteine) in the treatment of corneal alkali burns, Ann. Ophthalmol. **4:**320, 1972.

99. Francois, J., Cambie, E., Feher, J., and Van den Eeckhour, E.: Collagenase inhibitors (penicillamine), Ann. Ophthalmol. **5:**391, 1973.

100. Brown, S. I., and Weller, C. A.: The pathogenesis and treatment of collagenase-induced diseases of the cornea, Trans. Am. Acad. Ophthalmol. Otolaryngol. **74:**375, 1970.

101. Brown, S. I., Wassermann, H. E., and Dunn, M. W.: Alkali burns of the cornea, Arch. Ophthalmol. **82:**91, 1969.

102. Helmers, S., Top, F. H., Sr., and Knapp, L. W., Jr.: Ammonia and eye injuries in agriculture, Sight Sav. Rev. **41:**9, 1971.

103. Harris, L. S., Cohn, K., and Galin, M. A.: Alkali injury from fireworks, Ann. Ophthalmol. **3:**849, 1971.

104. Lemp, M. A.: Cornea and sclera, Arch. Ophthalmol. **92:**158, August 1974.

105. Schultz, G., Henkind, P., and Gross, E. M.: Acid burns of the eye, Am. J. Ophthalmol. **66:**654, 1968.

106. Thatcher, D. B., Blaugh, S. M., Hyndiuk, R. A., and Watzke, R. C.: Ocular effects of chemical Mace in the rabbit, Ophthalmol. Dig. **33:**29, 1971.

107. Laibson, P. R., and Oconor, J.: Explosive tear gas injuries of the eye, Trans. Am. Acad. Ophthalmol. Otolaryngol. **74:**811, 1970.

108. Cruthirds, A. E.: Importance of sulfhydryl in treatment of corneal and x-ray burns, Am. J. Surg. **72:**500, 1946.

109. Kuhn, H. S.: The use of hydrosulphosol in the treatment of chemical and/or thermal burns of the eyes, Trans. Am. Acad. Ophthalmol. **52:**157, 1948.

110. Harley, R. D.: An experimental study on the evaluation of hydrosulphosol in the treatment of ocular injuries due to chemical burns, Am. J. Ophthalmol. **35:**1653, 1952.

111. Havener, W. H., Falls, H. F., and McGee, H. B.: Experimental hydrosulphosol therapy of thermal and chemical ocular burns in rabbits, Eye Ear Nose Throat Mon. **32:**201, 1953.

112. Rocknem, R. E.: Evaluation of wounds of the rabbit cornea treated with calsulfhydryl (Hydrosulphosol), Arch. Ophthalmol. **50:**696, 1953.

113. Horwich, H., and Turtz, A.: Experimental evaluation of hydrosulphosol, Am. J. Ophthalmol. **37:**239, 1954.

114. Marr, W. G., Wood, R., and Grieves, M.: Further studies on the effect of agents on regeneration of corneal epithelium, Am. J. Ophthalmol. **37:**544, 1954.

115. Bahn, G., and Allen, J.: Calsulfhydryl in chemical injury of cornea, Arch. Ophthalmol. **54:**22, 1955.

116. Krejci, L., and Harrison, R.: Antiglaucoma drug effects on corneal epithelium, Arch. Ophthalmol. **84:**766, 1970.

117. Kennedy, R. E., Roca, P. D., and Landers, P. H.: Atypical band keratopathy in glaucomatous patients, Am. J. Ophthalmol. **72:**917, 1971.

118. Wood, T. O., and Walker, G. G.: Treatment of band keratopathy, Am. J. Ophthalmol. **80:**553, 1975.

119. Dahl, A. A., and Grant, W. M.: Unusual keratitis from a household remedy, Am. J. Ophthalmol. **68:**858, 1969.

120. MacLean, A. L.: Aerosol keratitis, Am. J. Ophthalmol. **63:**1709, 1967.

121. Zuckerman, B., and Lieberman, T.: Corneal rust ring, Arch. Ophthalmol. **63:**254, 1960.

122. Harris, L. S., Galin, M. A., and Mittag, T. W.: Corneal rust stain removal, Am. J. Ophthalmol. **71:**854, 1971.

123. MacCarthy, C. F., and Hollenhorst, R. W.: Protective moist-chamber eye dressing, Am. J. Ophthalmol. **71:**1333, 1971.

124. Golden, S.: Thin plastic shield for prevention of exposure keratitis, Am. J. Ophthalmol. **55:**384, 1963.

125. Leibowitz, H. M., and Rosenthal, P.: Hydrophilic contact lenses in corneal disease, Arch. Ophthalmol. **85:**283, 1971.

126. Gasset, A. R., and Kaufman, H. E.: Bandage lenses in the treatment of bullous keratopathy, Am. J. Ophthalmol. **72:**376, 1971.

127. Takahashi, G. H., and Leibowitz, H. M.:

Hydrophilic contact lenses in corneal disease, Arch. Ophthalmol. **86:**133, 1971.

128. Gasset, A. R., and Kaufman, H. E.: Hydrophilic lens therapy of severe keratoconjunctivitis sicca and conjunctival scarring, Am. J. Ophthalmol. **71:**1185, 1971.

130. Kaufman, H. E., Uotila, M. H., Gasset, A. R., Wood, T. O., and Ellison, E. D.: The medical use of soft contact lenses, Trans. Am. Acad. Ophthalmol. Otolaryngol. **75:** 361, 1971.

130. Leibowitz, H. M., and Rosenthal, P.: Hydrophilic contact lenses in corneal disease, Arch. Ophthalmol. **85:**163, 1971.

131. Aquavella, J. V., Jackson, G. K., and Guy, L. F.: Therapeutic effects of bionite lenses: mechanisms of action, Ann. Ophthalmol. **3:** 1341, 1971.

132. Winkler, C. H., Jr., and Dixon, J. M.: Bacteriology of the eye, Arch. Ophthalmol. **72:** 817, 1964.

133. Milauskas, A. T.: Pseudomonas aeruginosa contamination of hydrophilic contact lenses and solutions, Trans. Am. Acad. Ophthalmol. Otolaryngol. **76:**511, 1972.

134. Golden, B., Fingerman, L. H., and Allen, H. F.: Pseudomonas corneal ulcers in contact lens wearers, Arch. Ophthalmol. **85:**543, 1971.

135. Dixon, W. S., and Bron, A. J.: Fluorescein angiographic demonstration of corneal vascularization in contact lens wearers, Am. J. Ophthalmol. **75:**1010, 1973.

136. Sussman, J. D., and Friedman, M.: Irritation of rabbit eye caused by contact-lens wetting solutions, Am. J. Ophthalmol. **68:**703, 1969.

137. deHaas, E. B.: Desiccation of cornea and conjunctiva after sensory denervation, Arch. Ophthalmol. **67:**439, 1962.

138. Weinstock, F. J.: Treatment of neurotrophic keratitis, Am. J. Ophthalmol. **67:**150, 1969.

139. Baum, J. L., Mishima, S., and Boruchoff, S. A.: On the nature of dellen, Arch. Ophthalmol. **79:**657, 1968.

140. Nauheim, J. S.: Marginal keratitis and corneal ulceration after surgery on the extraocular muscles, Arch. Ophthalmol. **67:**708, 1962.

141. Thomas, C. I., Purnell, E. W., and Rosenthal, M. S.: Treatment of herpetic keratitis with IDU and corticosteroids, Am. J. Ophthalmol. **60:**204, 1965.

142. Messner, K., and Leibowitz, H. M.: Acetylcysteine treatment of keratitis sicca, Arch. Ophthalmol. **86:**357, 1971.

143. Donaldson, D. D.: Corneal degeneration, Ann. Ophthalmol. **5:**561, 1973.

144. Trobe, J., and Laibson, P. R.: Dystrophic changes in the anterior cornea, Arch. Ophthalmol. **87:**378, 1972.

145. Goldman, J. N., Dohlman, C. H., and Kravitt, B. A.: The basement membrane of the human cornea in recurrent epithelial erosion syndrome, Trans. Am. Acad. Ophthalmol. Otolaryngol. **73:**471, 1969.

146. Hood, C. I., Gasset, A. R., Ellison, E. D., and Kaufman, H. E.: The corneal reaction to selected chemical agents in the rabbit and squirrel monkey, Am. J. Ophthalmol. **71:** 1009, 1971.

147. Sevel, D.: Necrogranulomatous scleritis, clinical and histologic features, Am. J. Ophthalmol. **64:**1125, 1967.

148. Ferry, A. P., and Leopold, I. H.: Marginal (ring) corneal ulcer as presenting manifestation of Wegener's granuloma, Trans. Am. Acad. Ophthalmol. Otolaryngol. **74:**1276, 1970.

149. Brubaker, R., Font, R. L., and Shepherd, E. M.: Granulomatous sclerouveitis, Arch. Ophthalmol. **86:**517, 1971.

150. Aronson, S. B., Elliott, J. H., Moore, Thomas E., Jr., and O'Day, D. M.: Pathogenetic approach to therapy of peripheral corneal inflammatory disease, Am. J. Ophthalmol. **70:** 65, 1970.

151. Conners, C. A., Eckardt, R. E., and Johnson, L. V.: Riboflavin for rosacea keratitis, marginal corneal ulcers, and catarrhal corneal infiltrates, Arch. Ophthalmol. **29:**956, 1943.

152. Wise, G.: Ocular rosacea, Am. J. Ophthalmol. **26:**591, 1943.

153. Havener, W. H., Falls, H. F., and McReynolds, W. U.: Burdock burr ophthalmia, Arch. Ophthalmol. **53:**260, 1955.

154. Breed, F. B., and Kuwabara, T.: Burdock ophthalmia, Arch. Ophthalmol. **75:**16, 1966.

155. Johnson, A. W., and Buffaloe, W. J.: Chlorpromazine epithelial keratopathy, Arch. Ophthalmol. **76:**664, 1966.

156. Wolter, J. R., and Henderson, J. W.: Ruptures of Descemet's membrane in keratoconus, Am. J. Ophthalmol. **63:**1689, 1967.

33
EXTRAOCULAR MUSCLES

ACCOMMODATIVE ESOTROPIA

The ratio between accommodation and accommodative convergence can be dramatically changed by topical use of anticholinesterase drugs or cycloplegics. These medications alter the myoneural junctions of the ciliary musculature so as to require less or more innervation to produce a given amount of accommodation. Because comparable amounts of innervation are sent to the ciliary muscles and the medial recti during the act of focusing on a near object and because medial rectus innervation is unaffected by topical autonomic medications, the ratio of accommodation to accommodative convergence must change with these medications. Weak cycloplegics increase the convergence associated with a given amount of accommodation and theoretically might benefit convergence insufficiency. Anticholinesterase drugs reduce the amount of convergence associated with a given amount of accom-

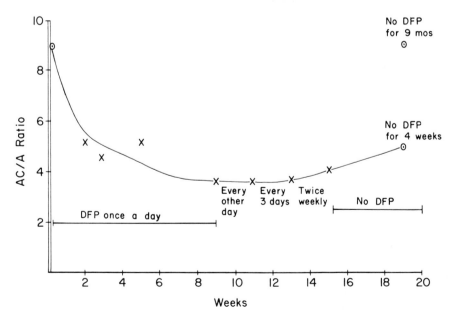

Fig. 33-1. Decrease in AC/A ratio during DFP therapy and subsequent return to previous values. (Modified from Sloan, L., Sears, M., and Jablonski, M.: Arch. Ophthalmol. **63:**283, 1960.)

584

modation and are well known to benefit convergence excess. Although the ratio of accommodative convergence to accommodation is changed by autonomic medications, the total strength of accommodative convergence itself is not altered. Fusional convergence is *not* affected by autonomic drugs.[1]

Although the effectiveness of anticholinesterase therapy of accommodative strabismus may be determined empirically on a clinical trial-and-error basis, determination of the AC/A ratio may permit quite accurate prediction of the therapeutic response.[2] The amount of therapeutic response to anticholinesterase treatment is substantially greater in patients with a high AC/A ratio and relatively small in those with a low AC/A ratio.

The effect of anticholinesterase drugs on muscle balance appears to be considerably more complex than simply causing increased tonus of the ciliary muscle. Continuous administration of a low concentration of diisopropyl flurophosphate (DFP) almost always reduces the AC/A ratio (Fig. 33-1).[3] Only patients with an initially very low AC/A ratio fail to respond in this fashion. As illustrated, the change in AC/A ratio requires at least 3 weeks before the maximal is attained. Reduction in frequency of administration after the first 3 weeks is desirable because it greatly decreases the incidence of cyst formation and yet maintains therapeutic effect. The effects of therapy persist for many weeks after DFP is discontinued.

A brief review of the method and theory of AC/A measurement is appropriate. Perhaps the most accurate yet simple method consists of fixation at a constant near distance (33 cm) while wearing full correction for any refractive error. Changes in accommodation

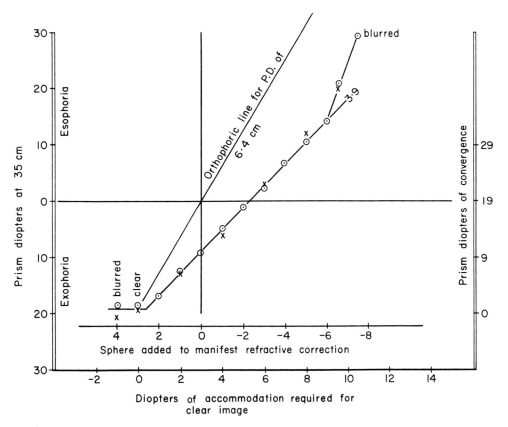

Fig. 33-2. Normal AC/A graph. (Modified from Sloan, L., Sears, M., and Jablonski, M.: Arch. Ophthalmol. **63**:283, 1960.)

are induced by adding minus or plus spheres. This method measures *accommodative* convergence only, since stimuli for fusional convergence are eliminated, and tonic and proximal vergence stimuli are constant. The plotting of data from a normal subject is shown in Fig. 33-2. Although the double labeling of the ordinate and abscissa may at first seem confusing, this diagram is easily understood when one recognizes that one ordinate and abscissa is numbered in terms of near fixation (33 cm), whereas the other is numbered in terms of distance fixation. The scale "prism diopters at 33 cm" has its zero point at the amount of convergence theoretically required for fixation at 33 cm (discussed later, along with the "orthophoric line"). The scale "prism diopters of convergence" has its zero at distance fixation, where the eyes should theoretically be parallel. "Diopters of accommodation required for clear image" has its zero at distance fixation, where the emmetropic eye should require no accommodation. "Sphere added to manifest refraction correction" has its zero at 3.00 D on the distance accommodation scale, since 3.00 D of accommodation is theoretically required to focus at 33 cm.

The "orthophoric line" represents the amount of convergence per unit of accommodation that will maintain the eyes perfectly converged on the fixation point at all distances. This is a simple linear relationship. The prism diopters of convergence required to fixate at a given distance may be determined by multiplying the meter angles of convergence by the interpupillary distance measured in *centimeters*. Fig. 33-3 (meter angle–prism diopter conversion drawing) shows this calculation, assuming an interpupillary distance of 6 cm. Since by definition meter angles of convergence and diopters of accommodation are always numerically equal for a given distance, 6 prism diopters of convergence is theoretically required for each diopter of accommodation exerted by an individual with a 6 cm interpupillary distance. This slope (AC/A = 6/1; AC/A ratio of 6) is the "orthophoric line" (different for each interpupillary distance).

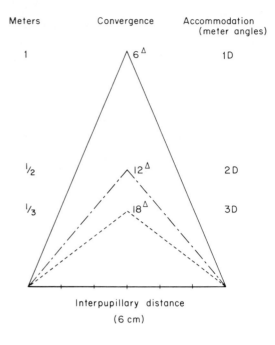

Convergence = Meter angles X P.D.

Fig. 33-3. Meter-angle value of convergence is equal to reciprocal of distance in meters (and therefore is also equal to diopters of accommodation required by an emmetrope at this distance).

The AC/A ratio is quite constant for each individual and does not necessarily bear any relationship to the amount of convergence that would be required to maintain the eyes straight (an adjustment made, if possible, by *fusional* convergence). Repeated tests indicate that the AC/A ratio of a given individual does not spontaneously change by more than ±0.5. Hypothetical AC/A graphs may be constructed (Fig. 33-4) to show the varying slopes that may be encountered and their significance. Clinical data indicate that normal persons without ocular symptoms practically always have AC/A ratios less than 6; the usual normal range is between 2 and 5. This is in accord with the common finding that normal persons, essentially emmetropic for distance, almost always have an exophoria for near.

The AC/A slope is not altered by the presence of basic phoria resulting from tonic vergence factors. Fig. 33-5 shows the effect of a

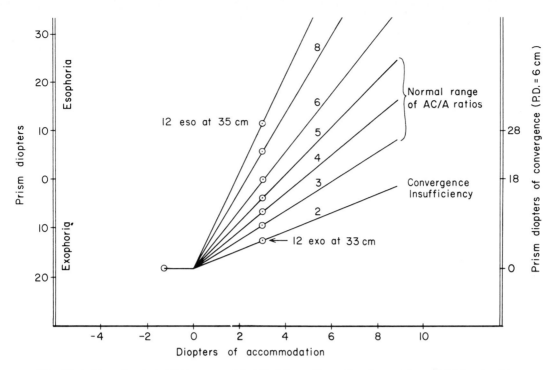

Fig. 33-4. Hypothetical AC/A ratios. (Modified from Sloan, L., Sears, M., and Jablonski, M.: Arch. Ophthalmol. **63:**283, 1960.)

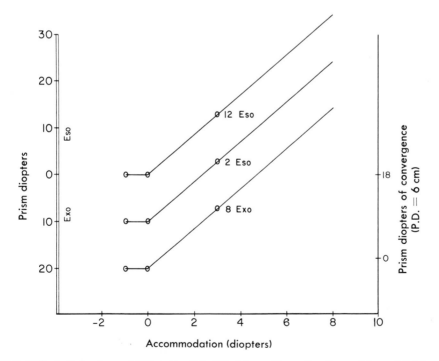

Fig. 33-5. Effect of phoria on AC/A ratio. (Modified from Sloan, L., Sears, M., and Jablonski, M.: Arch. Ophthalmol. **63:**283, 1960.)

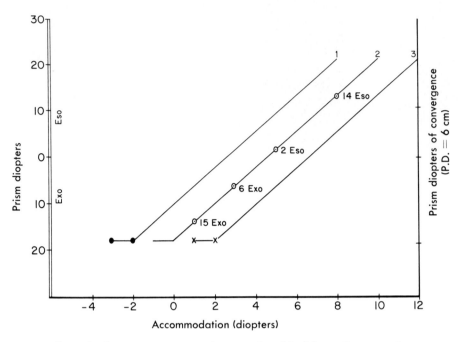

Fig. 33-6. Effect of refractive error on AC/A ratio. (Modified from Sloan, L., Sears, M., and Jablonski, M.: Arch. Ophthalmol. **63:**283, 1960.)

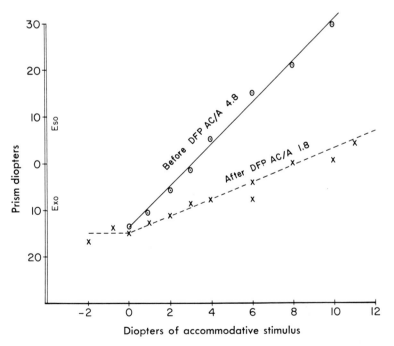

Fig. 33-7. Decrease in AC/A ratio after 21 weeks of DFP therapy. (Modified from Sloan, L., Sears, M., and Jablonski, M.: Arch. Ophthalmol. **63:**283, 1960.)

phoria, which is to shift the line in the direction of exodeviation or esodeviation, whichever it may be. The inclination of the slope (the AC/A ratio) does not, however, change. Similarly, uncorrected refractive error or lens-induced dioptric changes do not change the AC/A ratio. As shown in Fig. 33-6, spherical changes of accommodation simply shift the position horizontally. Although it is not directly relevant to the present pharmacologic discussion, note that the position of the AC/A line on the graph will indicate the existence of a phoria or an uncorrected refractive error.

The AC/A ratio obviously affects binocular relationships and may, if abnormal, cause or contribute to strabismus. Reduction of the ratio, which can usually be achieved with prolonged DFP therapy (Fig. 33-7), helps to restore normal binocular function in selected patients. Fortunately it is clinically possible to identify easily the majority of patients who will be helped by DFP. They consist of the group usually classified as exhibiting accommodative esotropia. These patients develop first intermittent and then constant esotropia, which is worse with near accommodative attention and with fatigue, which appears at age 2 to 4 years, and which is ordinarily associated with hyperopia of 2.00 D or more.

Most patients with accommodative esotropia can see clearly at distance by wearing their full hyperopic correction *and* using DFP. This is incompatible with the not uncommon oversimplification that suggests that DFP works simply by causing "peripheral accommodation." Were this the case, full hyperopic spectacle correction would never be tolerated. Clearly, the effect of DFP in strabismus is to reduce the amount of accommodative convergence required per diopter of accommodation and not to correct the hyperopia. Infrequently DFP will decrease the manifest hyperopia—such patients will not see clearly at distance through their full atropine correction and will require a weaker prescription—or perhaps their vision will remain straight with no glasses at all. This refractive change is transient, and the eye reverts to its original hyperopia when DFP is stopped.

The effect of short-term use of strong concentrations of anticholinesterase drugs is quite different from that of long-term usage. A marked spasm of accommodation develops, without necessarily producing any immediate decrease in the AC/A ratio. Fig. 33-8 shows the effect of a single dose of 0.1% DFP. In this case the accommodative spasm caused an 8.00 D hyperopic shift of the AC/A line, but there was no significant change in its slope. Perhaps this can be interpreted to indicate that the brain must have time to adapt to the new accommodative situation before it is able to respond with decreased convergence innervation.

Just as the AC/A ratio is increased by topically applied cycloplegic drugs, so also an increase would be expected after systemic administration of such drugs. Fig. 33-9 shows the increased AC/A ratio caused by orphenadrine citrate, 150 mg/day.[4] (Orphenadrine is an antimuscarinic drug used to treat muscle spasm in Parkinson's disease.) Tested in young adults, this drug caused an average increase of 2.6 prism diopters per diopter of accommodation and reduced accommodative amplitude by an average of 4.20 D (40% of original accommodation). Why such drugs cause reading difficulty in prepresbyopic patients is obvious.

Echothiophate iodide (Phospholine) was used in a series of 28 patients with accommodative esotropia greater for near than at distance (abnormally high AC/A ratio).[5] Concentration of the drug was 0.125% or 0.0625%. Instillation was at bedtime, once daily. During the course of treatment the concentration and frequency of echothiophate was reduced, depending on the therapeutic response.

Twenty of the 28 patients were restored to binocular vision at near by use of echothiophate. Analysis of the eight failures showed no significant difference from the successfully treated cases in refractive error, binocular status, or other reason that would be correlated with the failure. Bifocals had been worn by 17 patients before anticholinesterase

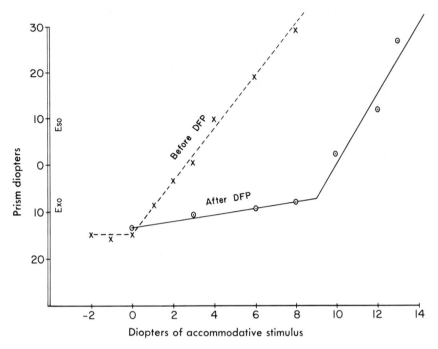

Fig. 33-8. Effect of single instillation of 0.1% DFP on AC/A relationship. (Modified from Sloan, L., Sears, M., and Jablonski, M.: Arch. Ophthalmol. **63:**283, 1960.)

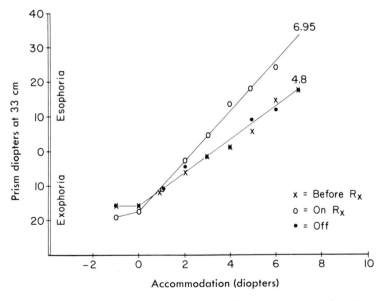

Fig. 33-9. Typical convergence/accommodation graph illustrating a normal AC/A ratio of 4.8, increase to 6.9 while on systemic orphenadrine, and subsequent return to normal. (Modified from Pemberton, J. W., and Brown, D. J.: Arch. Ophthalmol. **68:**348, 1962.)

therapy. All bifocals were discontinued, and in every case near binocularity was maintained or improved by echothiophate. The duration of successful treatment varied from 6 to 19 months in this series, indicating the continuing therapeutic effectiveness of long-term anticholinesterase therapy. Double-blind evaluation of an inert drop showed no therapeutic response in eight patients, indicating that echothiophate does not act as a placebo.

The complications of prolonged use of echothiophate are the same as those of other strong miotics. Half of these patients (51%) developed pupillary margin cysts within 1 to 6 months. The cysts regressed with decreasing frequency or strength of treatment, which was continued in all cases regardless of the appearance of these small lesions. That the incidence of iris cysts is primarily related to strength and frequency rather than to the type of anticholinesterase is indicated by comparison of this 51% incidence with echothiophate to a study reporting 23% cysts with echothiophate and 54% with DFP.[6] Obviously the incidence of cysts produced by any of these drugs will depend on the intensity of administration. No clinical data establish a different therapeutic/toxic ratio for the various "irreversible" cholinesterase inhibitors used in the treatment of accommodative esotropia.

Blurred vision was noted by one third of these patients. Refractions done in 14 patients showed a miotic-induced myopia of less than 0.50 D in nine patients and 0.50 to 1.00 D in the other five patients. Naturally those patients with the greater myopia noticed more subjective visual blurring. In most cases this induced myopia was transient, even though miotic treatment continued. Seven patients noted aching brows. Lid twitching annoyed two patients. These problems subsided as the patients became accustomed to treatment.

Another use for anticholinesterase therapy is suggested by the favorable response of two other patients (20 and 25 years of age) with accommodative insufficiency. Whereas both patients had previously required bi-

focals for comfort in near reading, under miotic treatment they could read well without glasses. The details given concerning these two patients do not permit exclusion of the diagnosis of a possible functional disorder responding to the placebo effect of glasses or drops. Nevertheless, use of echothiophate for accommodative insufficiency is theoretically rational.

Daily instillation of 1 drop of 0.06% echothiophate iodide for the treatment of esotropia in a group of 21 children resulted in a fall of blood cholinesterase to values ranging from 27% to 87% of pretreatment levels (mean drop to 48%). Return to normal values did not occur until several weeks after medication was discontinued. None of these children had systemic symptoms attributable to the medication. During a 5-year period the authors observed four children with abdominal cramping and diarrhea that were severe enough to require hospitalization of two with serious consideration of exploratory surgery.[7]

Prolonged respiratory paralysis may follow administration of succinylcholine (as a muscle relaxant during general anesthesia) to patients in whom cholinesterase has been reduced by medications or exposure to insecticides. Ophthalmologists should advise patients (or their parents) receiving echothiophate that this agent will modify the choice of drugs used during surgery. Patients should understand their responsibility to inform the physician that they are receiving echothiophate, so that any anesthetic can be given safely. Of course, this precaution also applies to eye surgery! Succinylcholine should not be used in patients who have received echothiophate within 6 weeks preceding surgery.

Use of 2.5% phenylephrine at the same time as the echothiophate (both drugs may be prescribed in the same solution) will prevent formation of iris cysts.[8]

Do not forget that miotic therapy may be used after strabismus surgery should an accommodative element persist.

Although the term "miotic therapy" is often used, only the cholinesterase inhibitors are useful in modifying the AC/A ratio and in clinical therapy of accommodative strabismus. Direct-acting parasympathomimetic drugs such as pilocarpine produce an accommodative spasm and persistent myopia (or decreased hyperopia). The increased depth of focus resulting from a small pupil is not the cause of the therapeutic benefit from anticholinesterase treatment of strabismus.[9]

Postoperative reactions

Catgut allergy must be considered in the differential diagnosis of conditions causing redness of the eye postoperatively. This characteristically causes itching, conjunctival hyperemia and chemosis, and lid edema. Proof that this reaction is caused by catgut allergy was obtained by burying a piece of plain catgut intradermally in the patient's forearm after strabismus surgery in 219 children.[10] Study of an additional 169 patients who underwent strabismus surgery further established the excellent correlation between this type of ocular reaction and a positive local response to the intradermal catgut.[11]

Catgut allergy may cause an immediate response (within 24 to 48 hours) or may be delayed until approximately 1 week after surgery. The time of onset depends on whether the patient has previously been sensitized to sheep collagen (catgut). Of 144 patients who had no previous surgery, none had an immediate response. Of these 144 patients, approximately one fourth had a delayed response. Of 25 patients previously operated on, more than one third developed immediate catgut allergy. Subsequent development of additional cases of delayed allergy brought the total incidence of catgut allergy to approximately one half of the children previously operated on.

Analysis of this data further indicates that chromic catgut is somewhat less likely to cause allergy than is plain catgut. The surgical cases reported in these studies were grouped in various categories; however, the figures of 27% allergy to plain gut and 19% to chromic catgut may be cited as being proportionately representative. These particular figures are the incidence of delayed allergy in children not previously operated on.

From the therapeutic standpoint, diagnosis of catgut allergy is important because, as expected, corticosteroid therapy does reduce the intensity and duration of the eye reaction. Furthermore, recognition of the allergic nature of this redness prevents the misdiagnosis of postoperative infection and the unnecessary use of antibiotics. The potential helpfulness of the catgut skin test in differential diagnosis is suggested by the fact that, of the total 388 patients reported in these two papers, only five had eye reactions not accompanied by a positive skin test. Three of these reactions were recognized as wound infections; two were caused by very extensive surgery. The routine placement of a short section of catgut suture in the forearm skin postoperatively is therefore suggested as a diagnostic aid, which will be expected to indicate presence of catgut allergy in almost one third of patients.

Systemic medications

Some day it may be possible to administer drugs that selectively inhibit or enhance convergence or divergence. Such effects are produced by alcohol, anesthesia, and anoxia, but not in clinically useful circumstances. An antimalarial drug, plasmocid, has been demonstrated to have selective neurotoxic effects, especially affecting the oculomotor nuclei.[12] Unfortunately other cerebral functions are also affected, and selective vergence modification is not achieved.

LATENT NYSTAGMUS

The amplitude, velocity, and frequency of the abnormal eye movements in latent nystagmus are reported to be demonstrably reduced by cycloplegia induced by 1% cyclopentolate.[13] Such treatment of affected children may result in improved visual acuity. Perhaps the mechanism of action is the increase in light entering the eye (latent nystagmus may be induced by neutral density filters as well as by covering one eye).

Six of ten cases of latent nystagmus were improved by cycloplegia,[14] three were unchanged, and one was worsened. Modification of latent nystagmus by cycloplegia may be of some value in the treatment of amblyopia (15% of a series of strabismus patients were reported to have latent nystagmus that markedly reduced monocular acuity with the amblyopic eye). For instance, one patient had 20/70 acuity of the amblyopic eye, which improved to 20/30 when the latent nystagmus was reduced by cycloplegia. (From the practical standpoint, I wonder whether loss of near vision from the cycloplegia would not more than counter improved distant acuity achieved by the use of cyclopentolate. If the same effect could be achieved by mydriasis alone, perhaps phenylephrine would be preferable.)

PTOSIS

Ptosis caused by Horner's syndrome may be temporarily relieved (for several hours) by the topical ocular administration of 1:1000 epinephrine.[15] Apparently the sensitized smooth muscle of Müller, lying just beneath the superior conjunctiva, is effectively reached by such topical therapy.

Phenylephrine is also effective in cosmetic treatment of mild ptosis. The effect may be varied by using the drug in different concentrations or time intervals. When 10% phenyl-

ephrine is instilled for mydriatic ophthalmoscopy, a normal lid will retract perceptibly. Postoperative cataract or retinal detachment patients often complain of ptosis on their first office visit. If my secretary has instilled phenylephrine to aid fundus examination, the ptosis will usually have miraculously disappeared by the time we discuss the condition, a circumstance quite reassuring to the patient.

A phenylephrine test may be used to predict the effectiveness of ptosis surgery.[16] If the lid elevates to a cosmetically acceptable level within 15 minutes after instillation of several drops of 10% phenylephrine, a surgical procedure consisting of resection and advancement of Müller's muscle is likely to accomplish the desired result.

The rate and amount of mydriatic response of postganglionic Horner's syndrome is illustrated in Fig. 33-10.[17] This represents the response to 0.05% epinephrine bitartrate applied to both corneas at 0, 5, and 10 minutes. Obviously the clinical observation of such a positive epinephrine diagnostic test could be made any time from 20 to at least 45 minutes after epinephrine instillation. The clinician should be aware that a de-

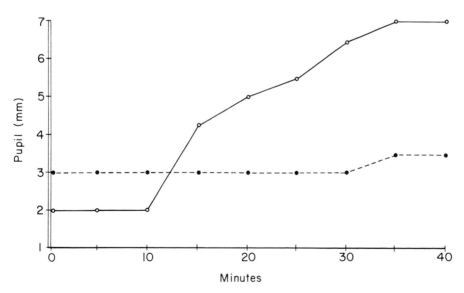

Fig. 33-10. Response of normal (solid) and Horner's (circle) pupil to 0.05% epinephrine. (Modified from Langham, M. E., and Weinstein, G. W.: Arch. Ophthalmol. **78:**462, 1967.)

nervation site proximal to the superior cervical ganglion (preganglionic) will result in minimal adrenergic sensitization. The clinical appearance of ptosis, miosis, and anhidrosis is identical, whether caused by a preganglionic or a postganglionic lesion. Either lesion will interrupt sympathetic impulses; however, only the postganglionic lesion will fail to dilate in response to an indirect-acting sympathomimetic drug (cocaine, hydroxyamphetamine [Paredrine]).

Ptosis may be caused by reserpine, presumably by a mechanism of norepinephrine depletion. Indeed, a mouse ptosis assay is used in measurement of reserpine activity. Drugs such as chlorpromazine (an alpha sympatholytic compound) augment reserpine-induced ptosis. Conversely, antihistaminic drugs (for example, tripelennamine) oppose reserpine activity by their adrenergic reinforcing effects.[18]

MYASTHENIA GRAVIS

The characteristic change in myasthenic involvement of muscles is accelerated tiring. This is easily demonstrated in extraocular muscles when the patient attempts to maintain gaze in the field of action of the involved muscle. Visible fatigue will develop within 15 seconds to 2 minutes, in contrast to normal muscles, which can maintain gaze for many minutes without tiring.[19] Histologically demonstrable necrosis, infiltration with inflammatory cells, and atrophy are commonly found in myasthenic muscles. This characteristic myopathy is not uniformly distributed, and it is well known that one or several extraocular muscles may be selectively involved in myasthenia. Becoming refractory to anticholinesterase therapy probably is caused by these histologic changes in muscle, which represent a later stage of the disease than the initial physiologic block of function.

Edrophonium (Tensilon) is a valuable drug in testing for the presence of myasthenia but has too short an action to be of therapeutic value (see Chapter 12).

The general medical treatment of myasthenia gravis consists of neostigmine and pyridostigmine, given in dosage titrated to the needs of the individual patient. Overdosage may cause a paradoxical increase in the severity of the disease manifestations. The edrophonium test is helpful in determining whether the problem is insufficient or excessive therapy, since the inadequately treated patient will improve with edrophonium and the excessively treated patient will not improve or may even worsen.

Patients with even minimal bulbar involvement can rapidly develop desperate respiratory or swallowing problems, precipitated by a minor respiratory infection. Because of this, an ophthalmologist is well advised to delegate the primary care of myasthenic patients to a neurologist or internist.

Perhaps 75% of myasthenic patients respond well to corticosteroid therapy in combination with the parasympathomimetic drugs. Alternate-day, large-dose prednisone treatment is one method of treatment.[20]

Another regimen is to give 10 to 20 mg of prednisone every 6 hours. On such a schedule, 11 of 22 myasthenic patients with ocular symptoms improved to a normal level of function.[21]

Ptosis and diplopia persisting after adequate systemic treatment of myasthenia gravis may benefit from local anticholinesterase therapy.[22] A recommended treatment plan starts with 0.25% eserine ointment instilled into the cul-de-sac of both eyes each morning for 2 weeks. Should no benefit ensue, dosage may be increased to three times daily for the following 2 weeks. If there is still no response, 0.025% DFP ointment should be started every evening, and 2 weeks later, 0.1% DFP should be started. The myasthenic patient is quite sensitive to the effect of DFP and, peculiarly, may react to an overdose as if it were curare. Any improvement followed by a relapse should suggest the possibility of overdosage. The patient should be maintained on the smallest effective amount of medication. Of 10 patients treated in this way, five were reported to have subjective and objective improvement in their ocular myasthenic signs and symptoms.

The initial symptoms of myasthenia gravis

often occur in the extraocular muscles, and in the late stages of this disease almost all patients suffer from extraocular muscle weakness. Both diagnostic and therapeutic reasons exist, therefore, for the use of topically effective medications. In a series of seven patients with myasthenia gravis, ptosis was relieved in five and diplopia in two by use of topical anticholinesterase drugs.[23] Neostigmine, 5%, or demecarium bromide (Humorsol), 0.1%, was used. Individual responses differ, and the drug of choice and frequency of instillation must be adapted to each patient. Use of drops may be selectively timed to enhance the effect of systemic medication as necessary. Drops may simply be instilled into the cul-de-sac, or more prolonged effect may be secured through the aid of a small cotton pack temporarily placed in the lower conjunctiva. Improvement of muscle functions is also demonstrable electromyographically. Although not all myasthenic patients show marked improvement, it is evident that in at least some patients a safe and rapid diagnostic test can be carried out by the ocular instillation of anticholinesterase agents. Echothiophate iodide is reported to be ineffective when applied locally, possibly because of poor penetration. Atropine-like drugs are antidotal to cholinergic toxic effects without impairing the myasthenic therapeutic effect.

The twitching of the orbicularis muscle sometimes complained of by glaucomatous patients after use of the strong anticholinergic drugs is further evidence of the penetration of topically applied drugs into adjacent muscular structures.

THYROID OPHTHALMOPATHY

Diagnostic uncertainty may arise when unilateral exophthalmos or extraocular muscle malfunction is not associated with obvious general physical signs of thyroid disease. If present, the characteristic lid retraction of thyroid disorder is virtually pathognomonic. Occasionally, however, the diagnosis of thyroid ophthalmopathy cannot be confirmed by physical examination. Such patients are usually euthyroid, hence the basal metabolic rate will be normal.

Because thyroid ophthalmopathy is a disorder of the hypothalamic-pituitary-thyroid system, special tests of the hormones involved in this function are the most sensitive diagnostic approach. The hypothalamus produces thyrotropin-releasing hormone (TRH), which stimulates the pituitary to produce thyroid-stimulating hormone (TSH), which in turn stimulates the thyroid to produce thyroxin. Thyroxin and triiodothyronine exert a feedback inhibition on the pituitary, causing decreased formation of TSH. The characteristic feature of the Graves disease is that the thyroid becomes autonomous, functioning independently of TSH. Simultaneously, the pituitary becomes unresponsive to TRH.

The most rapid test to confirm the diagnosis of thyroid ophthalmopathy is the TRH test. Intravenous injection of 500 μg of TRH causes the TSH level to increase three to five times over the basal level within 30 minutes in normal subjects. In disease of the hypothalamic-pituitary-thyroid system, the TSH level is not changed by TRH (Fig. 33-11).[24] The TRH test requires 60 minutes of

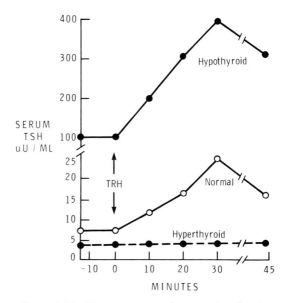

Fig. 33-11. Responses to thyrotropic-releasing hormone. (From Hyman, B. N., and Johnson, P. C.: Trans. Am. Acad. Ophthalmol. Otolaryngol. **79:**528, 1975.)

the patient's time and can be reported within 1 day. It is not affected by previous iodine intake. No toxic responses occur.[24]

The other test commonly used to evaluate the pituitary-thyroid relationships is Werner's triiodothyronine suppression test. This is performed by giving 75 to 150 μg of triiodothyronine daily for 8 days. This will cause at least a 50% decrease of ^{131}I uptake in normal subjects, whereas patients with Graves' disease do not show such a suppression of iodine uptake. Recent exposure to iodine invalidates this test. This dosage of triiodothyronine may cause symptoms of thyrotoxicity in many patients.

Unfortunately, there is relatively little that can be done for thyroid ophthalmopathy. High doses of systemic corticosteroids reduce acute cellular infiltration and orbital congestion.[25] Radiation (1500R) may reduce lymphocytic infiltration and is suggested as an alternative to surgical decompression for optic neuropathy.[26] Extraocular muscle function is not improved by radiation. Lubricants are helpful if corneal exposure threatens.

PAINFUL OPHTHALMOPLEGIA

Inflammations in the area of the superior orbital fissure may cause transitory paralysis of the nerves transmitted through the fissure.[27] Retro-orbital pain and limitation of extraocular movements are the characteristic manifestations. This syndrome (Tolosa-Hunt) apparently may be caused by a number of inflammatory etiologies; since syphilis may be a causative factor, serologic evaluation is in order.

Treatment with systemic corticosteroids is recommended. In one patient, prednisone in a dosage of 60 mg daily resulted in an improvement in symptoms within 2 days and full relief within 2 weeks.

REFERENCES

1. Parks, M.: Etiologic and compensatory factors of comitant horizontal deviations in children. In Haik, G. M., editor: Strabismus, St. Louis, 1962, The C. V. Mosby Co.
2. Chin, N. B., and Breinin, G. M.: Ratio of accommodative convergence to accommodation, Arch. Ophthalmol. 77:752, 1967.
3. Sloan, L., Sears, M., and Jablonski, M.: Convergence accommodation relationships, Arch. Ophthalmol. 63:283, 1960.
4. Pemberton, J. W., and Brown, D. J.: Accommodative convergence, Arch. Ophthalmol. 68:348, 1962.
5. Hill, K., and Stromberg, A.: Echothiophate iodide in the management of esotropia, Am. J. Ophthalmol. 53:488, 1962.
6. Miller, J. E.: A comparison of miotics in accommodative esotropia, Am. J. Ophthalmol. 49:1350, 1960.
7. Ellis, P. P., and Esterdahl, M.: Echothiophate iodide therapy in children, Arch. Ophthalmol. 77:598, 1967.
8. Simmons, R.: Personal communication, 1968.
9. Breinin, G. M.: Accommodative strabismus and the AC/A ratio, Am. J. Ophthalmol. 71:303, 1971.
10. Apt, L., Costenbader, F., Parks, M., and Albert, D.: Catgut allergy in eye muscle surgery. I. Correlation of eye reaction and skin test using plain catgut, Arch. Ophthalmol. 63:30, 1960.
11. Apt, L., Costenbader, F., Parks, M., and Albert, D.: Catgut allergy in eye muscle surgery. II. Correlation and comparison of eye reaction and skin test after the use of plain and chromicized catgut, Arch. Ophthalmol. 65:474, 1961.
12. Lyle, D., and Schmidt, I. G.: The selective effect of drugs upon nuclei of the oculogyric system, Am. J. Ophthalmol. 54:706, 1962.
13. Windsor, C. E.: Modification of latent nystagmus, Arch. Ophthalmol. 80:352, 1968.
14. Windsor, C. E., Burian, H. M., and Milojevic, B.: Modification of latent nystagmus, Arch. Ophthalmol. 80:657, 1968.
15. Hubert, L.: Diagnostic significance of epinephrine instilled into conjunctival sacs, Arch. Ophthalmol. 17:1076, 1937.
16. Putterman, A. M.: Jaw-winking blepharoptosis treated by the Fasanella-Servat procedure, Am. J. Ophthalmol. 75:1016, 1973.
17. Langham, M. E., and Weinstein, G. W.: Horner's syndrome, Arch. Ophthalmol. 78:462, 1967.
18. Aceto, M. D., and Harris, L.: Effect of various agents on reserpine-induced blepharoptosis, Toxicol. Appl. Pharmacol. 7:329, 1965.
19. Sears, M. L., Walsh, F. B., and Teasdall, R. D.: The electromyogram from ocular muscles in myasthenia gravis, Arch. Ophthalmol. 63:791, 1960.
20. Smith, J. L.: Therapy for ocular myasthe-

nia gravis, Trans. Am. Acad. Ophthalmol. Otolaryngol. **78**:OP-795, September-October 1974.

21. Cape, C. A.: Ocular response to corticotropin in myasthenia gravis, Arch. Ophthalmol. **90**:292, October 1973.

22. Giles, C. L., and Westerberg, M. R.: Clinical evaluation of local ocular anticholinesterase agents in myasthenia gravis, Am. J. Ophthalmol. **52**:331, 1961.

23. Leopold, I. H., Hedges, T. R., Montana, J., Krishna, N., and Beckett, S.: Local administration of anticholinesterase agents in ocular myasthenia gravis, Arch. Ophthalmol. **63**:544, 1960.

24. Hyman, B. N., and Johnson, P. C.: Thyro-

tropin-releasing hormone (a test to diagnose Graves' ophthalmopathy), Trans. Am. Acad. Ophthalmol. Otolaryngol. **79**:OP-524, May-June 1975.

25. Cohen, J. S.: Optic neuropathy of Graves disease, hyperthyroidism, and ocular myasthenia gravis, Arch. Ophthalmol. **90**:131, August 1973.

26. Ravin, J. G., Sisson, J. C., and Knapp, W. T.: Orbital radiation for the ocular changes of Graves' disease, Am. J. Ophthalmol. **79**:285, February 1975.

27. Milstein, B. A., and Morretin, L.: Report of a case of sphenoid fissure syndrome studied by orbital venography, Am. J. Ophthalmol. **72**:600, 1971.

34
GLAUCOMA

For purposes of therapy, glaucoma must be subdivided into chronic simple, acute, and secondary types. Use of the tonometer alone does not provide enough information to diagnose or to follow a case of glaucoma. The perimeter and tangent screen, slit-lamp microscope, ophthalmoscope, and visual acuity chart are absolutely essential. Gonioscopy often provides vitally important information. The techniques of electronic tonography, applanation tonometry, and provocative testing may be desirable in certain cases. No substitute exists for knowledge gained through practical experience (as in a residency or preceptee program). Manipulation of the instruments, interpretation of the findings, differential diagnosis, the response expected from the available drugs and combinations,[1] and the indications for surgery must be mastered by physicians before they can competently manage a case of glaucoma. In short, glaucoma is a specialist's disease. The general physician has an irreplaceable and vital role in case finding but is rarely equipped to manage glaucoma.

Instrumentation techniques and their interpretation are beyond the scope of this volume, and the following discussion assumes that proper clinical diagnosis and differentiation of the types of glaucoma have been made.

PRIMARY OPEN-ANGLE GLAUCOMA

The objective of therapy is to maintain throughout the patient's lifetime a normal visual acuity and visual field, if at all possible. This should be accomplished with as little inconvenience and discomfort as feasible and with maximum safety. It is presently accepted that a patient whose open-angle glaucoma is adequately controlled medically is *not* a candidate for surgery. This recommendation is made because of the complications arising from surgery, both early (0.5% loss of eyes) and late (40% frequency of development of cataract,[2,3] infection of filtering bleb, failure to control glaucoma, increase in severity of glaucoma, multiple nonspecific symptoms, and other complications). Surgery is clearly indicated when the anticipated course of a glaucoma refractory to medical management leads to future blindness.

Great emphasis has rightly been placed on tonometry as a guide to therapy. Opinions as to the top level of pressure that can be tolerated vary from 20 to 30 mm Hg or even higher. Maintenance of pressure below 20 mm Hg is definitely established as optimal and will prevent progression of glaucomatous damage more effectively than will less rigid pressure control. Continuing pressures above 40 mm Hg will almost invariably lead to blindness. It must be admitted that some eyes can withstand such pressures for 10 or even 15 years. Thereafter the patient contributes to the statistics that 12% of blindness is caused by glaucoma. Pressures between 20 and 30 mm Hg are borderline in that the physician is not really happy with them and will make further medical efforts to reduce the pressure. However, surgery, or even medication, may not be justified by a pressure of 30 mm Hg without other indications.

The concept of physiologic ocular hypertension is currently popular; it advocates that medical therapy not be instituted solely in response to the presence of elevated intraocular pressure. The patient should be observed for the appearance of some objective sign such as increased disc cupping (requires careful photographic documentation of the disc status) or early field changes (requires static, not kinetic, perimetry). Apparently there is no urgency in starting therapy, particularly since we now know (through corticosteroid provocative testing) that one third of the population carries a recessive gene for glaucoma. The time of starting therapy is also affected by the age of the patient (how great the life expectancy is; greater vulnerability of the disc over 70 years of age), family history of destructively severe glaucoma, presence of cataract, and other indi-

vidualized factors.[4,5] For example, low blood pressure and anemia may predispose to the circulatory vulnerability of the optic nerve. Diabetes of a severity requiring treatment is statistically associated with glaucomatous nerve damage. A vertically oval cup with a cup/disc (C/D) ratio greater than 0.5 or a 0.2 asymmetry with larger cup in the eye with higher pressure arouses concern.[6]

Currently, the therapeutic goals in glaucoma appear to be normalization of pressure and outflow measurements and prevention of field loss. Perhaps at some future time the susceptibility of the individual eye will also be evaluated and will afford the most reliable information as to what level of control (whether medical or surgical) is required to prevent further loss of function. Many clinicians have speculated as to a close relationship between ophthalmic artery pressure and susceptibility to glaucomatous damage.

A 3 mm white perimetric target may be rendered invisible by externally applied ocular pressure. Interestingly, the Bjerrum sco-

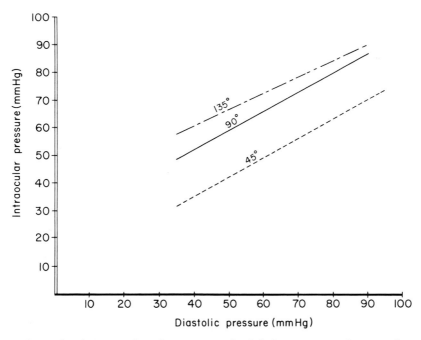

Fig. 34-1. Relationship between diastolic pressure of ophthalmic artery and intraocular pressure required to obliterate a 3/1000 white target in various parts of the upper Bjerrum scotoma area in glaucomatous eyes. (Modified from Vanderburg, D., and Drance, S. M.: Am. J. Ophthalmol. **62:**1049, 1966.)

toma area of the visual field is most suscepti-ble to this pressure-induced loss of function, and vulnerability increases as the blind spot is approached. As shown in Fig. 34-1, there is a consistent relationship between diastolic pressure of the ophthalmic artery and the externally induced ocular pressure required to obliterate the 3/1000 white target.[7] I would anticipate that tomorrow's clinicians will attempt to maintain intraocular pressure below some proportion of the diastolic oph-thalmic artery pressure that has empirically been found to prevent further functional loss.

The normal fluorescence of the optic disc is reduced in glaucomatous optic atrophy and in about half of the patients with glau-coma that has not yet caused atrophy.[8] This finding suggests an element of permanent interference with the blood supply of the optic disc in such cases. Since fluorescence

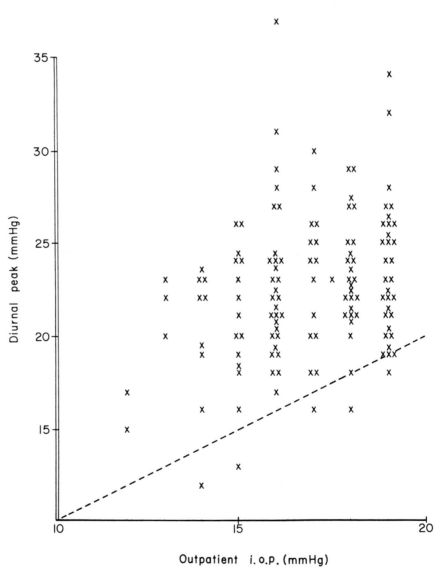

Fig. 34-2. In all but 11 (on or below dotted line) of 132 well-controlled cases of chronic simple glaucoma, peak of diurnal pressure curve was higher than that of outpatient pressure mea-surement. (Modified from Drance, S. M.: Arch. Ophthalmol. **70:**302, 1963.)

and ophthalmoscopically observed disc color are not necessarily correlated findings, the fluorescein test may have some clinical prognostic value in glaucoma.

Diagnosis
Tonometry

Tonometry performed four times a year is not, of course, proof that pressure control is maintained during the intervals. The diurnal curve of pressure, which is exaggerated in glaucomatous patients, reaches peaks in the early morning or late afternoon (variable in different patients), and damaging elevations of pressure may exist within a few hours before or after a normal tonometer reading.

For this reason, tonometry, although a reliable guide to uncontrolled pressure, will not by itself establish the existence of adequate control.

Unfortunately, marked diurnal variations of intraocular pressure continue to occur in patients with treated chronic simple glaucoma. In fact, in a series of 132 such patients under excellent control (outpatient pressures of 19 mm Hg or less), all but 11 patients were found to have higher pressures at some time during the diurnal curve (Fig. 34-2).[9] These diurnal variations are not correlated with coefficient of outflow values; hence they cannot be predicted by tonography (Fig. 34-3).[9] From a practical stand-

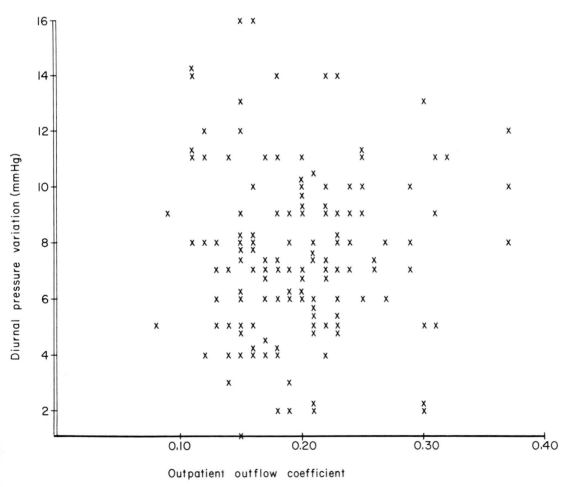

Fig. 34-3. Scattergram showing lack of correlation between coefficient of outflow and diurnal pressure variations. (Modified from Drance, S. M.: Arch. Ophthalmol. **70**:302, 1963.)

point, these data lead to the conclusion that the intraocular pressure should be measured at frequent intervals day and night (for example, 6 A.M., 9 A.M., 11:30 A.M., 1:30 P.M., 5 P.M., and 10 P.M.) when an apparently well-controlled glaucomatous eye is losing visual field. Medical therapy theoretically should be increased to eliminate these peak elevations of the diurnal curve.

In a series of 1280 eyes measured by applanation and Schiøtz tonometry the applanation pressure was higher by at least 5 mm Hg in 19% of the eyes.[10] In 4% of the eyes the applanation pressure was 9 mm Hg or more higher than the Schiøtz measurement. These differences are of sufficient magnitude and frequency to encourage the exclusive use of the applanation instrument by ophthalmologists. However, use of the 1948 scale for the Schiøtz tonometer gives values that are usually within 2 mm Hg of the applanation values.[11] Larger discrepancies are recognized to exist after surgery. Be aware that an inadequate amount of fluorescein will give falsely low applanation values.[12]

Neither the Schiøtz nor the Goldmann applanation tonometers give reliable readings on eyes with scarred or edematous corneas. The Mackay-Marg electronic applanation tonometer has been found in such difficult eyes to give readings closely comparable to simultaneous manometric pressure readings.[13]

Since decrease in scleral rigidity subsequent to the use of miotics could mislead ophthalmologists into believing that they had attained control of the glaucoma, the effect of drugs on scleral rigidity has been evaluated.[14] Decreased scleral rigidity occurred in only 6 of 62 patients treated with echothiophate iodide or demecarium bromide and was not consistently present in these six. Error as to the degree of glaucoma control is therefore unlikely to result from changed scleral rigidity. (Pilocarpine, phenylephrine, and cyclopentolate were found not to alter the scleral rigidity of normal eyes.)

Tonography before and after performance of a water drinking provocative test in a series of 41 glaucomatous patients showed no significant change in outflow facility or ocular rigidity.[15] This indicates that the mechanism of elevation of pressure results from an increased aqueous secretion. The increased aqueous secretion results from hemodilution of a magnitude of about 8 milliosmols after rapid drinking of 1 liter of water by a dehydrated patient. The period of maximum rise of intraocular pressure during a water drinking test occurs much sooner than is usually believed. The maximum rise occurred at 10 minutes in 78% of 159 normal eyes and 52% of 250 glaucomatous eyes. The highest pressure occurred at 30 minutes or later in only 4% of normal and 10% of glaucomatous eyes.[16] Hence the most important tonometric measurement is taken 10 minutes after the test. A rise of 9 (applanation) or 7 (Schiøtz) mm Hg is considered diagnostic of glaucoma.

Elevation of intraocular pressure following drinking of water is caused by a reduction of the osmotic pressure of the blood and the consequent more rapid entry of water into the relatively more hypertonic aqueous chamber. Restriction of fluid intake in the clinical management of glaucoma is almost entirely irrational. A water-drinking test is positive when patients have been dehydrated by many hours of abstinence from fluid, *and* when they drink far more water than is comfortable within 5 minutes, *and* when no electrolytes are simultaneously ingested. Drinking of normal amounts of fluid, at a reasonable rate, accompanied by food, not preceded by many hours of abstinence, does not materially alter blood osmotic pressure or intraocular pressure in normal or glaucomatous patients. Freely translated, if your glaucoma patient eats pretzels, drinking beer will not elevate the intraocular pressure.

Drinking of 1 liter of water by an average-sized adult human reduces the blood osmotic pressure by perhaps 8 milliosmoles. Fig. 34-4[17] illustrates levels of intraocular pressure in dogs following fluid administration resulting in no osmotic change (bottom curve), approximately 8 milliosmoles reduction in blood osmotic pressure (middle curve), and

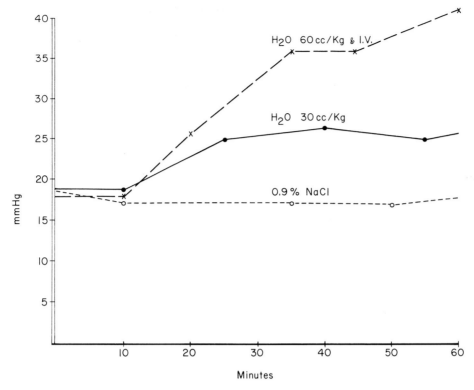

Fig. 34-4. Idealized composite drawing representing dog intraocular pressure changes. The lowest curve shows that the intraocular pressure remains unchanged with intravenous infusion of isotonic saline. The intermediate curve shows a small rise in pressure caused by ingestion of a moderate volume of water. The upper curve represents marked increase of intraocular pressure caused by oral and intravenous administration of large amounts of water. (Data from Galin, M. A., and associates: Am. J. Ophthalmol. **51**:601, April 1961.)

approximately 20 milliosmoles reduction (top curve). In this study a direct relationship between reduced blood osmolality and increased intraocular pressure was well demonstrated. The volume of fluid administered to the dog is not primarily responsible for the elevated intraocular pressure, as evidenced by the failure of normal saline to alter blood osmotic pressure or intraocular pressure. Naturally, however, larger amounts of water or hypotonic fluid will cause a greater dilution of the blood and a greater increase of intraocular pressure.

Tonography

Measurement of the facility of outflow by tonography is theoretically preferable to simple tonometry. Normalization of the facil-

ity of outflow (0.15 μ1/min/mm Hg or greater) predictably ensures maintenance of visual field in a high proportion of cases. Unfortunately, single tonographies are subject to error, they are more expensive than tonometry, and they may cause annoying visual blurring, sometimes lasting for hours afterward.

The usefulness of tonography in the management of glaucoma is evident from a study of 72 eyes in which pressure never exceeded 25 mm IIg during periods of 1 to 6 years.[18] As seen in the lower part of Table 34-1, these eyes were divided into those with pressures above 20 mm Hg and those with pressures below 21 mm Hg. Correlation of field loss with these pressure groupings was meaningless, with actually 41% field loss in the lower

Table 34-1. Correlation of visual field loss to C value and pressure control*

Average C	Number observed	Number field loss	% Field loss
0-0.12	30	13	43
0.13-0.17	20	9	45
0.18 and above	22	1	4
Total	72	23	
Pressure range			
Above 20	38	9	23
Below 21	34	14	41

*From Roberts, R. W.: Trans. Am. Acad. Ophthalmol. Otolaryngol. **65:**163, 1961.

Table 34-2. Prognostic significance of tonographic values in 250 glaucomatous eyes followed up for 3 years*

	Successful control
P_0 < 22	66%
C > 0.17	84%
P_0/C < 100	91%

*From Roberts, R. W.: Trans. Am. Acad. Ophthalmol. Otolaryngol. **65:**163, 1961.

pressure group and only 23% field loss in the higher pressure group. In contrast to the failure of correlation between pressure readings and field loss, tonographic readings were closely correlated with field changes. Of 50 eyes with tonographic readings of 0.17 or less, 44% lost field, but only 1 of 22 eyes with a C value of 0.18 or above lost field. We are forced to the conclusion that accurate tonography, if available, is of great value in ascertaining the adequacy of glaucoma control.

Further proof of the value of tonography is provided by data on 250 eyes studied for 3 years.[18] Table 34-2 indicates that 66% of the eyes with pressure of less than 22 mm Hg lost no field during this 3-year period. If C values were greater than 0.17, 84% lost no field. If P_0/C values were 100 or less, 91% lost no field.

Nevertheless, we are treating the eye and its response to glaucoma, not the tonographic record. As a specific example, the decision to operate for open-angle glaucoma is not made on the basis of tonographic values but rather on the demonstration of progressive ocular damage despite medical therapy.[19]

Following the discovery of tonography and the development of reliable instruments, its clinical use was widespread. At the present time, there has been a tendency to rely more on individual tonometric measurements inasmuch as these are expedient determinations of the effectiveness of therapy. Also, the concept of ocular hypertension, as a status of the

eye without field loss, has increased our interest in quantitative static perimetry. Perimetry is now considered to be a more important guide to the adequacy of medical therapy than is tonography. From the practical standpoint, the patient can afford only so much care, and perimetry alone is more cost effective than tonography and perimetry.

Perimetry

A cumulative record of eye damage is obtained through visual field measurement. Fields should be done routinely every 3 to 4 months in patients with chronic simple glaucoma. Tangent screen examination is considerably more sensitive than perimetry, although Rönne's nasal step is better demonstrated in many respects by the latter. Goldmann projection perimetry is superior to the older methods of tangent screen and arc perimetry. Static perimetric profiles obtained with the Goldmann instrument will demonstrate field defects completely unsuspected by the older kinetic methods.

Evidence of visual field loss caused by glaucoma indicates that the previous methods of control have been inadequate and that more intensive medical therapy is required. Field loss combined with borderline or high tension, not controllable medically, suggests the need for surgery. Progressive field loss may *not* be a result of glaucoma even though the defects are characteristic of glaucoma. The most common source of confusion is a slowly developing senile cataract. Cataracts cause concentric constriction of the visual field and will intensify any previously existing defect such as a Seidel scotoma. Decreasing acuity and field in a glaucomatous patient with *well-controlled* pressures are not infrequently found to be caused by a cataract.

Arcuate scotomas terminating sharply at the midline may be misinterpreted as incomplete Bjerrum scotomas. Actually, such field defects are virtually pathognomonic of chiasmal lesions. A case is reported in which 6 years of increasingly vigorous miotic therapy by 3 military ophthalmologists did not prevent slow progression of the perimetric defect to a complete temporal hemianopia with an early temporal field loss in the other eye. A 3½ cm chromophobe adenoma was removed surgically.[20] When one follows large numbers of patients in a clinic, it is dangerously easy to accept uncritically the old working diagnosis and to continue the previous treatment or mechanically and thoughtlessly to increase the dosage as the status of the patient deteriorates. It is even harder to realize that your own working diagnosis is wrong!

Miosis will cause an increase of field defects over that recorded through a larger pupil. Field constriction resulting from miosis may give the false impression of progressive glaucomatous atrophy and may lead to unnecessary therapeutic procedures if unrecognized.[21] Another symptom of miosis is accentuation of vitreous floaters. This optical phenomenon casts more discrete and annoying shadows on the retina, causes complaints from the new user of miotic drugs, and causes unwarranted concern in the ophthalmologist who has heard of an association between miotic use and retinal detachment.

Suggestive evidence that retinal detachment in glaucomatous patients is not caused by the use of miotics is the finding that in nine detachment patients with severe glaucoma, seven had retinal lesions before the use of any medical treatment for glaucoma.[22] Retinal detachment and glaucoma may occur together in eyes predisposed to both by age, disease, or genetic predisposition (for example, Marfan's syndrome). I am completely convinced that the use of miotic therapy before the detachment is purely coincidental.

Inasmuch as my ophthalmic subspecialty is retinal detachment and I have operated as many as 500 cases in a single year, my opinion on this particular subject is not without experience. Miotic therapy should not be used during the first few weeks after detachment surgery because it accentuates formation of posterior synechiae in the inflamed eye. When the reaction to surgical trauma has quieted, miotic therapy may be resumed as necessary.

Sudden development of subnormal pressure in an eye previously suffering from poorly controlled glaucoma is not a cause for rejoicing. Rather, this hypotony heralds the onset of a retinal detachment.

Visual acuity

Visual acuity is recorded on each visit because it is an easily measured and sensitive indication of ocular health. Decreasing acuity is a danger signal requiring complete reevaluation of the status of the given eye, for it may indicate development of other diseases as well as glaucomatous loss. A relatively sudden decrease in acuity is more likely to be caused by another disease than by glaucoma. Visual acuity checks are a very poor way of following the course of glaucoma. Since glaucomatous field loss is initially midperipheral, central acuity is not affected until very late.

Ophthalmoscopy

Ophthalmoscopic study of glaucoma is of value only with respect to the disc. The appearance of the optic nerve in glaucoma is closely correlated with its function. An almost normal nerve is incompatible with near blindness resulting from glaucoma. Typical "cupping" is an easily observed and unequivocal danger signal. Often it is impossible to differentiate physiologic cupping from early glaucomatous atrophy. The value of serial ophthalmoscopic examinations is severely limited by the examiner's inability to recall the exact details of a disc for an hour, let alone for 3 months. Recording of a simple drawing of two concentric circles, the outer circle representing the disc margins and the inner circle indicating the extent of the phys-

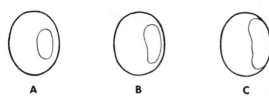

Fig. 34-5. Simple method of drawing extent of physiologic or glaucomatous cup within disc for purposes of serial recording. **A,** Physiologic cup. **B,** Borderline appearance. **C,** Definite glaucomatous cup.

iologic or pathologic cupping, is a rapid and helpful method of following a case of glaucoma (Fig. 34-5). Notation of the cup/disc ratio is appropriate. Vertical elongation of the "physiologic" cup strongly suggests the presence of glaucomatous damage.

Therapeutic miosis interferes with visualization of the fundus, with the exception of the optic nerve, which can usually be seen if their patients holds their eyes still. Dilatation of the pupil for careful fundus examination should be done routinely every several years or at any time for evaluating symptoms that would ordinarily indicate ophthalmoscopy. Eyes with *known open-angle* glaucoma can be dilated with impunity with sympathomimetic mydriatics. Often the decreased aqueous secretion resulting from these drugs will reduce intraocular pressure rather than raise it. Before the patient leaves the office, the pupils should again be constricted *without fail* if there is a gonioscopically narrow angle.

Reluctance to dilate the pupils of patients with chronic open-angle glaucoma for periodic fundus examination appears unjustified. The eyes of a series of 69 consecutive patients with miotic-treated open-angle glaucoma were dilated by use of 1% cyclopentolate, 2 drops every 15 minutes for three times.[23] Less than half of these patients responded with a pressure elevation greater than 6 mm Hg. The average pressure elevation in the responding patients averaged about 8 mm Hg. Obviously such pressure elevations are not hazardous and do not constitute a contraindication to properly dilating eyes of open-angle glaucoma patients for examination of

the fundus. Periodic observation of the optic nerve is necessary to identify possible progression of glaucomatous damage. Furthermore, 6% of the patients with retinal detachment have glaucoma.[24] Of course, narrow-angle eyes may develop acute glaucoma when dilated.

A pressure-elevation response to a cycloplegic drug marks an eye as strongly suspect for open-angle glaucoma. A 6 mm or greater increase of intraocular pressure after cycloplegia occurs in 23% of patients with known open-angle glaucoma but in only 2% of apparently normal patients.[25] This pressure rise begins 30 to 60 minutes after cycloplegic instillation, reaches a maximum in 90 to 120 minutes, and returns to normal 4 to 6 hours after the use of cyclopentolate. The use of 4% pilocarpine will reverse the pressure rise.

This pressure elevation is related to the effectiveness of cycloplegia and results from the use of cyclopentolate, homatropine, atropine, and scopolamine. Pressure elevation in open-angle glaucoma does not occur after use of sympathomimetic dilating drops such as phenylephrine or eucatropine or with weak cycloplegics such as 0.2% cyclopentolate or 0.5% tropicamide.

The changes in the coefficient of outflow produced by the use of 10% phenylephrine or 1% cyclopentolate in miotic-treated open-angle glaucoma patients are given in Table 34-3.[26] In this study, 3 drops of the phenylephrine or of the cyclopentolate were instilled 1 hour before tonography. This represents a use of these drugs in a manner comparable to their use for routine dilatation of pupils in office practice. As seen in the table, cyclopentolate caused a decrease in the coefficient of outflow in each case (and, as expected, a rise in intraocular pressure). In contrast, phenylephrine caused an increase in the coefficient of outflow in all eyes except the three that are underlined. It is noteworthy that the three eyes showing a decreased coefficient of outflow with phenylephrine all had a most precipitous drop in coefficient of outflow with cyclopentolate. One is tempted to assume that these eyes did not suffer from purely open-angle glaucoma but under con-

Table 34-3. Phenylephrine- and cyclopentolate-induced changes in coefficient of outflow of miotic-treated eyes with gonioscopically open angles while miotic*

Patient		Miotic regimen	Miotic regimen with 10% phenylephrine added	Miotic regimen with 1% cyclopentolate added
M. P.	OD	0.25	0.28	0.15
	OS	0.19	0.21	0.13
J. D.	OD	0.25	0.38	0.13
	OS	0.32	0.20	0.06
L. A.	OD	0.21	0.50	0.12
	OS	0.15	0.45	0.12
B. L.	OD	0.14	0.17	0.06
R. P.	OD	0.20	0.22	0.07
	OS	0.30	0.28	0.16
E. R.	OD	0.18	0.33	0.15
	OS	0.22	0.34	0.13
A. J.	OD	0.18	0.24	0.16
	OS	0.22	0.17	0.03
M. B.	OD	0.20	0.20	0.13
	OS	0.27		0.14
E. J.	OD	0.13	0.20	0.04
	OS	0.12	0.08	0.02

*Modified from Schimek, R. A., and Lieberman, W. J.: Am. J. Ophthalmol. **51:**781, 1961.

Table 34-4. Effect of 10% phenylephrine on demecarium-treated open-angle glaucoma (mean values of 16 patients)*

	Applanation pressure (mm Hg)	Outflow facility (C)	Pupillary size (mm)
Before demecarium bromide	29.8	0.09	3.2
After demecarium bromide	17.6	0.22	1.6
After demecarium bromide and phenylephrine, 10%	15.8	0.22	4.1

*From Kolker, A. E., and Hetherington, J., Jr.: Becker-Shaffer's diagnosis and therapy of the glaucomas, ed. 4, St. Louis, 1976, The C. V. Mosby Co.

ditions of mydriasis had developed angle-closure glaucoma. At the time of topography all pupils measured 5 to 6 mm in diameter, despite the preceding use of 0.5% to 4% pilocarpine, echothiophate, or demecarium.

The clinical implications of this study are clear-cut and practical. Use of phenylephrine (or other sympathomimetic mydriatics) is a safe and effective way of dilating the eyes of patients under miotic therapy for primary open-angle glaucoma. Such dilatation probably should be done routinely every 2 years or so and is mandatory for proper evaluation of any symptom compatible with the development of some other intraocular condition (for example, unexplained visual loss). Cyclopentolate (or other parasympathomimetic cycloplegics) should not be used for this purpose. (Dilatation of the eye with narrow-angle glaucoma is potentially hazardous even with phenylephrine, most particularly if the pressure is borderline or elevated even before dilatation.)

On the other hand, if part of the purpose

of examination is a routine tonometric screening for the presence of glaucoma, a higher proportion of glaucomas will be detected if the tonometry is done after cyclopentolate dilatation. This actually is somewhat of a provocative test, which may often elevate borderline pressures to diagnostic levels. Should phenylephrine be used for mydriasis before tonometry, the resultant drop in intraocular pressure will often produce a falsely normal tonometric reading. If an ophthalmologist prefers the use of sympathomimetic mydriatics, the tonometry should be performed before the pupil is dilated.

In cataract patients on miotic treatment for open-angle glaucoma, 10% phenylephrine hydrochloride may be used to improve vision if cataract is present without increasing intraocular pressure (Table 34-4).[27]

Gonioscopy

Gonioscopy is an essential part of the initial evaluation and classification of a glaucomatous patient. Because continuing growth of the lens may cause a previously open angle to close partially, it is appropriate to repeat gonioscopy every 5 years or so or when a critical decision is being made, such as the type of operation to be performed. Gonioscopic demonstration of an open angle reassures the physician that sympathomimetic mydriatics and the "irreversible" miotics may safely be used and is therefore of obvious importance to medical management. The most critical decision in gonioscopy is whether or not the angle is capable of closing.

Therapy

Medical therapy of chronic simple glaucoma customarily begins with a miotic, usually 1% pilocarpine, prescribed two or three times daily. Patients must be acquainted with the serious nature of the disease and the importance of faithful medication for the rest of their life. They must also be reassured that the burning and blurring from the drops will diminish with time. The first appointment following treatment should be scheduled in 1 or 2 weeks to evaluate the effect of treatment, to reemphasize the importance of faithful adherence to instructions, and to answer any questions that may have arisen. The frequency of appointments thereafter depends on the patient's response to treatment. A discouraging outlook should not be offered patients with early glaucoma; rather, they should be reassured that proper medical therapy will more than likely control the pressure and thereby protect their sight.

When confronted with the question of whether a given case of ocular hypertension (?) should be treated in the absence of field defect, a trial of miotic therapy of one eye only may be valuable. A substantial drop of pressure in only the treated eye confirms the actual effect of the medication, in contrast to the possibility that a drop in both eyes (if both were treated) might simply represent a diurnal variation.

The experienced clinician is aware that the presence of a great deal of melanin will reduce the ocular response to pilocarpine and epinephrine as well as to cycloplegics and mydriatics.[28] Hence darkly pigmented individuals are particularly likely to experience poor glaucoma control and require especially alert observation.

Failure to control the disease with 1% pilocarpine, three times a day, may be met by increasing the percentage up to 4% and the frequency up to five times daily. The use of 0.25% eserine ointment at night has been popular in hard-to-control cases, but it is preferable to add epinephrine in a search for a combination that will better control pressure.

Careful tonographic study of three glaucoma patients suggested that a maximum antihypertensive effect was achieved by either 4% pilocarpine or 1% physostigmine. Combined use of these two drugs in these concentrations did not produce an additive or enhanced pressure-lowering effect. The duration of therapeutic effect, rapidity of onset, and comfort of this drug combination were not evaluated, but were speculated to be possible benefits of the combined medication and require further investigation. This study did not support the simultaneous clinical use of pilocarpine and physostigmine in treatment of chronic simple glaucoma.[29]

Likewise, the simultaneous use of 4% pilocarpine and of 0.125% echothiophate does not result in more effective glaucoma control than does use of echothiophate alone.[30] Such a combination is irrational, inconvenient, wastefully expensive, and contraindicated.

The types of antiglaucoma medications available can be grouped as follows:
1. Miotics
   a. Short acting
   b. "Irreversible" cholinesterase inhibitors
2. Carbonic anhydrase inhibitors
3. Sympathomimetic mydriatics

Failure to control open-angle glaucoma with a medication from one of these groups suggests the addition of a drug from *another* group rather than substitution or addition from the same group. Changes within a group are not made for therapeutic reasons but because of intolerance of a given medication. For instance, carbachol is an excellent substitute miotic to use in the event of pilocarpine allergy but is not likely to control glaucoma uncontrollable by pilocarpine.[31] Similarly, Neptazane may not cause gastric distress in a given patient but will probably not control pressure any better than does Diamox.

The most rational approach to glaucoma therapy in difficult cases is to use combinations of medications from different groups. For example, if pilocarpine does not completely control a case, addition of acetazolamide or levo-epinephrine (or both, if necessary) is far more logical than addition or substitution of carbachol as the miotic. The "irreversible" miotics may control glaucoma more effectively than pilocarpine and have the advantage of infrequent instillation; however, their side effects are more intense.

The problem of decreased acuity resulting from miosis in a patient with cataract may be alleviated with sympathomimetic mydriatics. Discomfort from isoflurophate is least when it is instilled at bedtime. Gastric upsets from acetazolamide may be diminished by taking the tablets after meals. Danger of contamination and inconvenience is minimized by the commercially available plastic "squeeze" dropper bottles.

Abnormalities of the trabecular meshwork are accepted as the cause of chronic open-angle glaucoma. These abnormalities include pigment deposition, sclerosis and granularity of the trabecular collagen, and swelling and proliferation of the trabecular endothelium.[32] The trabecular meshwork of a glaucoma patient may be considered as a progressively less permeable filter. The rate of loss of permeability is extremely slow and varies in different patients. Considerable outflow reserve exists; therefore these aging changes do not cause elevated pressures in most eyes. Possibly specific endothelial changes may be responsible for glaucoma or may themselves be caused by increased pressure—a vicious cycle. Fortunately, decrease in aqueous production may occur and partially compensate for lost outflow facility.

From a therapeutic viewpoint, progressive deterioration of the trabecular meshwork explains nicely the need for gradually increasing treatment. No evidence suggests that miotics primarily reverse structural abnormalities or slow degenerative changes. Rather, they increase outflow by stretching more widely open the defective filtration apparatus. Loss of responsiveness to miotics is not usually to be interpreted as development of drug resistance, but as a progression of trabecular damage to the degree that a given miotic regimen can no longer adequately open the filtration spaces (Fig. 34-6). According to this concept, early use of miotic therapy, use of high drug concentrations, greater frequency of instillation, or selection of more potent miotics need not be avoided on the basis of "using up the effectiveness" of the given medication. Therapy in excess of that required to maintain normal intraocular pressure is objectionable, of course, because of cost, inconvenience, and side effects.

Occasional cases suggest that apparently an eye can develop resistance to the effect of pilocarpine and, after pilocarpine is discontinued for a suitable interval, may regain responsiveness to this drug. For this reason, medications such as pilocarpine should be

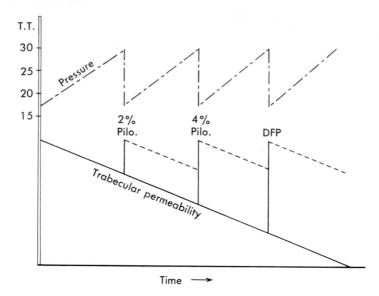

Fig. 34-6. Schematic representation of relationship between intraocular pressure and trabecular permeability as affected by miotic therapy. Trabecular permeability of a glaucomatous eye gradually decreases with time. This permeability may be increased a certain amount with 2% pilocarpine, more by 4% pilocarpine, and still more by DFP. As trabecular meshwork becomes less permeable with time, progressively stronger miotic therapy is required to maintain normal intraocular pressure. Ultimately not even the strongest miotic therapy may be effective, but it is assumed that this time is not hastened by previous treatment.

discontinued when they are no longer effective and replaced by another miotic. Sometimes resistance will develop to the "stronger" miotic, after which pilocarpine may again be effective.[33]

Since the stronger miotics are more effective in the control of glaucoma, one might logically propose their use as the first medication given a new glaucoma patient. Echothiophate, 0.125%, was tried in 29 patients with the result that 10 patients either stopped using the drug or did not return.[34] Apparently the side effects are too severe to be tolerated by these new patients, who have not yet been indoctrinated with the importance of glaucoma treatment.

Our glaucoma expert* reports a tendency for ophthalmologists to fear the use of the "irreversible" miotics, no doubt because of their well-publicized toxicity. However, the hazards of surgery or of nerve damage from inadequate pressure control are more serious

than the complications of strong miotic therapy. When glaucoma is no longer controlled by 4% pilocarpine four times daily combined with 1% epinephrine twice daily, a change to 0.06% echothiophate once daily is appropriate. Progressive increase to a dosage of 0.125% echothiophate twice daily is made as necessary. Dose-response studies indicate that a greater concentration or frequency of use of echothiophate is unlikely to improve the control of the glaucoma and therefore should be avoided.

In general, the smallest effective amount of any medication or combination of drugs should be sought. For example, 0.5% epinephrine once daily may be a very effective addition to the patient escaping control with 1% pilocarpine three times daily.

Incidentally, the usefulness of epinephrine in treatment of chronic simple glaucoma is not newly discovered but has been recognized for many years.[35] However, the advent of stable and comfortable preparations has made its wide use feasible.

---

*Kapetansky, F.: Personal communication, 1965.

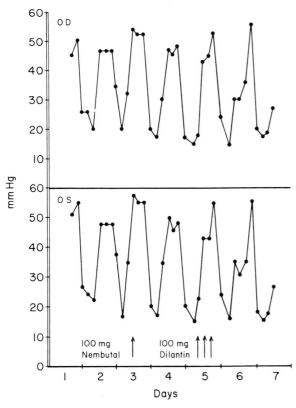

Fig. 34-7. Marked spontaneous diurnal variations of pressure in patient with chronic open-angle glaucoma. It is evident that Nembutal and Dilantin have not altered intraocular pressure, although this would seem to be the case if the observer were unaware of control measurements before and after drug administration. (Modified from Peczon, J. D., and Grant, W. M.: Arch. Ophthalmol. **72:** 178, 1964.)

General recommendations

Because of the vague clinical impression that glaucoma is worse in tense and worried individuals (may it be that patients with severe glaucoma are justifiably and realistically tense and worried?), general admonitions have been given to avoid excitement and stimulants and to relax, perhaps with the aid of sedatives. Do sedatives lower intraocular pressure and stimulants elevate pressure? A critical review of the literature, supported by careful measurement of diurnal tension curves of hospitalized patients with open-angle glaucoma, indicates that clinically significant changes of intraocular pressure do not follow use of stimulants or sedatives (including meperidine, chlorpromazine, promethazine, reserpine, meprobamate, mephenesin, methamphetamine, methylphenidate, pentobarbital, promidone, dextroamphetamine, and caffeine).[36] Use of these drugs may cause transient, but unsustained pressure changes, even on repeated administration. In evaluating the effects of such drugs on glaucoma, the ophthalmologist must be aware of the great diurnal changes that may spontaneously occur and be falsely interpreted as drug effect (Fig. 34-7).[36]

For some obscure reason, ophthalmologists occasionally further distress the unfortunate glaucomatous patient by unreasonable and unnecessary restrictions on general activity and use of the eyes. Reading, for example, may be forbidden or sharply curtailed. As a matter of fact, accommodation, far from being harmful, actually reduces intraocular pressure! The mechanism of this pressure drop is an increase of the coefficient of outflow during accommodation.[37] Careful study of 10 human subjects has established that within 3 to 4 minutes after accommodation, the intraocular pressure drops as much as 3 to 8 mm Hg (Fig. 34-8).[38] This pressure drop is directly related to accommodation and is not an artifact of repeated measurement.

The effect of drugs on the outflow of these accommodating eyes was pharmacologically predictable. Enhancing the effect of the physiologically produced acetylcholine, 0.25% eserine increased C values as high as 0.50. Treatment with 2% pilocarpine did not further increase the outflow beyond the effect produced by accommodation alone. In contrast, 1% cyclopentolate blocked the accommodation response and lowered the C value to an average of 0.20.[39]

In all of 19 subjects (including three with chronic simple glaucoma), exercise caused a drop of intraocular pressure.[40] Clearly, exercise should not be prohibited in patients with glaucoma.

Treadmill work performed to fatigue caused a drop of intraocular pressure averaging 33% and lasting from 10 minutes to over 3½ hours.[41] Serum osmolarity increases after

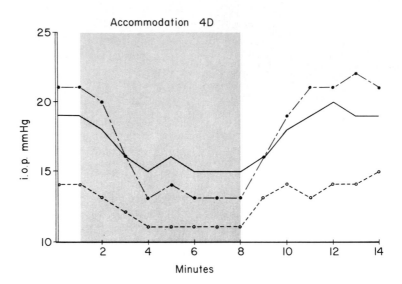

Fig. 34-8. Effect of accommodation on intraocular pressure. The three lines represent successive applanation tonometry readings of separate subjects. Pressures were recorded at 1-minute intervals. Shaded area represents the duration of accommodation. Note definite drop in pressure with accommodation and prompt return on relaxation. (Modified from Armaly, M. F., and Rubin, M. L.: Arch. Ophthalmol. **65:**415, 1961.)

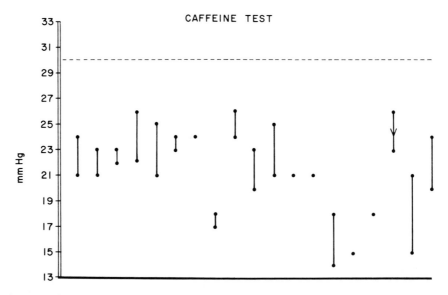

Fig. 34-9. Each vertical line represents increase of intraocular pressure of a single glaucomatous eye during 1 hour after drinking two cups of strong black coffee. (Arrow indicates drop of tension.) (Modified from Bloomfield, S., and Kellerman, L.: Am. J. Ophthalmol. **30:**869, 1947.)

exercise and is at least partly responsible for this decrease in intraocular pressure. However, a comparable increase in serum osmolarity achieved by giving small doses of oral glycerol did not cause as great an intraocular pressure drop. This finding indicates that other mechanisms also contribute to exercise-induced hypotension.[42]

Response to coffee

The drinking of coffee is often prohibited to patients with glaucoma. What happens to the intraocular pressure of patients with chronic simple glaucoma during the hour after ingestion of two cups of strong black coffee? Fig. 34-9 shows the maximum pressure rise in 19 glaucomatous eyes measured every 15 minutes for 1 hour after two cups of coffee.[43] Although a transitory rise was recorded for most of these eyes, in only a single instance did the increase exceed 6 mm Hg (Schiøtz). Incidentally, this evaluation did *not* exclude the hemodiluting effect of drinking two cups of fluid alone, which is half the volume used in a water drinking test. It seems unlikely that an occasional cup of coffee will be harmful to any but the most poorly controlled glaucoma patient—and such a patient is in trouble even without coffee.

In a series of 172 glaucomatous eyes the caffeine test (0.4 g caffeine in 150 ml water) caused a raise of intraocular pressure of 6 mm or more in only 15% of patients.[44] The effect of the water was greater than that of the caffeine.

Response to ethanol

Ethanol intake is not harmful to glaucomatous patients. Indeed, 50 ml of alcohol (contained in whisky or beer) caused a transitory decrease of intraocular pressure in 32 of 33 eyes of normal and glaucomatous subjects.[45] The intraocular pressure drop begins during the first hour and returns to normal after 4 or 5 hours. In general, the patients with higher pressures showed greater pressure drops, which averaged 9 mm Hg in the glaucoma patients. Facility of outflow was not increased. An osmotic mechanism of action seems likely and is apparently mediated through inhibition of the antidiuretic hormone.

Response to nicotine

A rise of intraocular pressure greater than 5 mm Hg occurred immediately after smoking a cigarette in 37% of 70 patients with untreated primary glaucoma but in only 11% of 70 nonglaucomatous persons. This pressure rise was transient, returning to baseline within 30 minutes.[46]

Response to marijuana

Smoking of 2 g of marijuana in a study of 21 adults disclosed an average intraocular pressure drop of 24% (varying from +4% to −45%) 1 hour afterward. Hyperemia of the conjunctival vessels was a consistent response, reaching a peak at 30 to 60 minutes after smoking. Very marked reduction of tear secretion occurred, with the wetting of a Schirmer test strip decreasing from 35 to 5 mm or less. This drying is sufficient so that contact lens wearers have lens tolerance difficulties during and after marijuana use. Even the lacrimation experienced while chopping onions is blocked. Pupillary dilation does not occur; in fact, slight constriction occurs in darkness. There is no change in the pupillary light response, Snellen visual acuity, refractive error, phoria, color vision, stereoscopic perception, or visual fields.[47]

Effect of systemic drugs

Since topical administration of anticholinergic (atropine-like) drugs is known to increase intraocular pressure in patients with chronic simple glaucoma, systemic administration of such medications has often been assumed to have a similar ocular hypertensive effect. If this assumption is correct, glaucoma patients should not use antispasmodic drugs for gastrointestinal problems, antihistaminics, antiparkinsonism drugs, psychotropic medications, or preanesthetic medications to control pulmonary secretions. In actual fact, most such medications will be used by physicians who are unaware the patient has glaucoma. Does this harm the patient?

To determine the effect of anticholinergic

medications, 29 patients with chronic open-angle glaucoma were given 0.6 mg of atropine sulfate orally, and this same dose was repeated 4 hours later (Fig. 34-10). Intraocular pressures were measured hourly by the Goldmann applanation instrument for 8 hours after the initial dose of atropine. This study demonstrated conclusively that therapeutic oral doses of atropine have no significant effect on the intraocular pressure of patients with chronic open-angle glaucoma. Even more impressive is the fact that these patients were *not* on miotic therapy at the time of the experiment.

Use of a proprietary cold remedy containing 0.2 mg of belladonna alkaloids, given twice daily for 4 days, caused no changes in applanation pressures in 27 normal volunteers and 37 patients with glaucoma (including 18 patients with "narrow" angles).[48]

Anticholinergic medication such as would be used for peptic ulcer (propantheline, 15 mg every 6 hours) was administered to 47 patients with open-angle glaucoma and seven

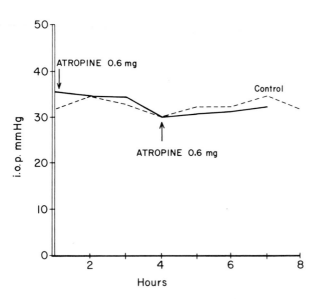

Fig. 34-10. Representative intraocular pressures in eye with chronic open-angle glaucoma, untreated (dotted line) and after two doses of atropine, 0.6 mg, given orally 4 hours apart (solid line). (Modified from Lazenby, G. W., Reed, J. W., and Grant, W. M.: Arch. Ophthalmol. **80:** 443, 1968.)

patients with narrow-angle glaucoma.[49] In the open-angle group only five eyes showed pressure increases greater than 4 mm Hg. These pressure increases occurred only when the patient was not using the glaucoma medication and were promptly controlled by 1% pilocarpine. Three of the untreated narrow-angle eyes responded to propantheline with a 15 mm Hg pressure elevation, which was readily controlled with 1% pilocarpine. It is apparent that the standard warnings against the use of such anticholinergic drugs in glaucoma patients are futile—only the unknown, untreated glaucoma patient is likely to respond with elevated pressure and such patients are, by definition, unidentified. These studies support our traditional advice that the treated glaucoma patient may safely receive any anticholinergic systemic drug indicated for the treatment of a general medical disorder.

In an unusually severe anticholinergic challenge, atropine sulfate, 0.6 mg, was given three times a day for 1 week to 21 patients with open-angle glaucoma.[50] In an attempt to predict which patients might respond with atropine-induced pressure elevation, the patients were categorized with respect to their response to topical 1% cyclopentolate (pressure rise greater or less than 5 mm Hg). Those eyes that did not respond with pressure elevation following cyclopentolate likewise did not show elevated pressures following a week of atropine. Nine of the 21 patients experienced a cyclopentolate-induced pressure rise of 5 mm Hg or more. Of these patients, the mean pressure before atropine was 24; after atropine it was 28. One patient with a C value of 0.08 and a P_o of 20 changed with 1 week of atropine to a C of 0.06 and a P_o of 34. Evidently occasionally a patient with severe glaucoma under borderline control will respond adversely to a systemically administered anticholinergic medication in very large dosage. A pressure-elevation response to anticholinergic medication is more closely related to impaired outflow facility than to the intraocular pressure level measured before the test.[51]

Hormones administered for fertility control (norethynodrel with mestranol [Enovid]) apparently reduce intraocular pressure. This medication (5 mg/day) was given for 2 weeks to 12 patients with open-angle glaucoma (in addition to their regular antiglaucoma therapy). The average intraocular pressure of the treated patients was 4 mm Hg lower than the average pressure of 10 control patients. (Pretreatment pressures were the same in both groups.) This difference was said to be statistically significant.[52,53] The mechanism of action of this hormone-induced pressure drop is apparently an increase in the facility of outflow.[54,55]

The nitrate vasodilators (nitroglycerin, amyl nitrite, and pentaerythritol tetranitrate) do not increase intraocular pressure in normal or glaucomatous patients.[56] Hence their use is not contraindicated in glaucomatous patients despite occasional comments to the contrary.

Systemically administered vasodilating drugs such as nitrites, nylidrin, tolazoline, aminophylline, and nicotinic acid do not cause intraocular pressure elevations in either open- or narrow-angle glaucoma.[57]

Motivation

In the management of a chronic disease such as glaucoma, physicians must recognize the differences between their cultural background and that of the patient. They assume that the patient's desire for health will override any other considerations. In many culture groups and in numerous individuals, recognition of long-range goals is poor. Such patients will be unable to evaluate present inconvenience as being preferable to prevention of a nebulous future evil.[58] Freely translated, this important gobbledygook means that all your knowledge of glaucoma diagnosis and therapy really *does not help your patient whatsoever*—until you have effectively explained to their satisfaction the need for treatment, have outlined adequately their instructions, and have through subsequent examinations determined the extent of their cooperation.

Evaluation of a sample of 94 patients from a large glaucoma clinic revealed that only 7% had normal vision in both eyes. At least 50% of the patients at least once daily did not follow instructions regarding use of their medications. A majority of these patients did not know what glaucoma is and did not know what would happen if they did not use their drops. The most significant correlation between proper use of medication and a demonstrable characteristic of the patient was the patient's knowledge of the nature of the disease. There was no correlation between proper medication use and the following variables: age, sex, race, income, occupation, apparent intelligence, or fear of blindness. Patients with considerable sight loss were less likely to neglect their medications. Specifically, frightening patients by telling them that they will go blind is not a very effective way of achieving cooperation in self-medication. An understandable explanation of the nature of glaucoma, its consequences, and its treatment is apparently the best way to achieve proper patient motivation.[59]

The return rate for treated patients is higher than it is for those who were untreated.[60] This has practical implications for the patient with ocular hypertension (?) who is to be followed without therapy. Possibly a homeopathic dosage (for example, 0.5% pilocarpine at bedtime) has merit in improving follow-up of patients whose status concerns the physician. It should be clearly understood by physicians that there is no evidence that this medication benefits the optic nerve and that they are simply using an approach that improves follow-up. I would prefer the more honest and direct approach of identifying the presence of borderline pressures and emphasizing the importance of keeping subsequent appointments.

Prognosis

We seek recognizable features that will alert us as to the greater probability of the existence of glaucoma or that may indicate a greater risk of future visual field loss. For example, patients with Marfan's syndrome or Sturge-Weber encephalotrigeminal angiomatosis are well known to be predisposed to glaucoma.

Krukenberg's spindles have been generally accepted as being associated with pigmentary glaucoma and therefore representing an indication of increased risk. However, a study of 43 patients[61] initially selected because of the presence of Krukenberg's spindle without field loss indicates that there is very little risk of glaucoma associated with this status. Corticosteroid provocative testing of these patients showed 43% to have an intermediate pressure rise and 29% to have a high pressure response (normal population response expected to be 29% and 5%), indicating a substantial predisposition to glaucoma. Yet only two of these patients developed field loss over a follow-up average time of 5.8 years. Since most of the patients were referred to a glaucoma clinic because of suspicious cupping, ocular hypertension (?), or familial glaucoma, they may represent a population biased toward glaucoma; if so, an isolated Krukenberg's spindle may have an even more benign prognosis.

The height of intraocular pressure may be an excellent predictor of subsequent field loss. Of 31 patients with unilateral field loss, 13 fellow eyes had an initial pressure greater than 26; 18 had pressures below 26. Of those above 26, 62% developed field loss, in contrast to only 6% of those with lower pressures. If under therapy the pressure exceeded 24 mm Hg, 64% lost field during a 3- to 7-year period of follow-up. Only 10% field loss occurred if pressure was controlled below 24 mm.[62] Despite the speculations we hear about ocular hypertension and optic nerve resistance, there *is* a direct relationship between elevated intraocular pressure and glaucomatous nerve damage.

A search for prognostic factors related to field loss in homozygous (GG) corticosteroid responders indicated that response to epinephrine was such a predictor. If the intraocular pressure dropped 5 mm or more after 1 day of treatment with 2% epinephrine instilled topically twice daily, 50% of patients

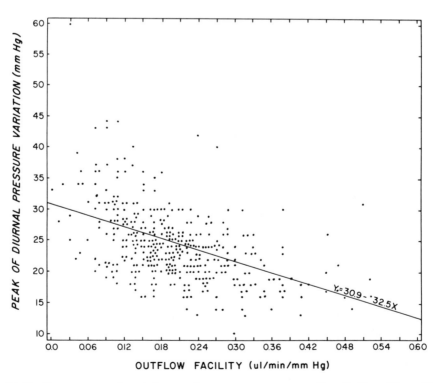

Fig. 34-11. Scattergram of peak intraocular pressure versus outflow facility. (From Phelps, C. D., and associates: Am. J. Ophthalmol. **77:**367, March 1974.)

developed field loss within 10 years. If the pressure dropped less than 5 mm in response to epinephrine, only 6.5% developed field loss. This response was unrelated to the original intraocular pressure, which was a less reliable predictor than the epinephrine response.[63] Although nontreatment of GG patients with pressures over 20 mm Hg is of obvious scientific value in a research institution, the consequences of this study cast doubt on the validity of following ocular hypertensive (?) persons. Of these 80 patients left untreated for 5 to 10 years, 25% developed field defects.

Another study determined the effect of unilateral epinephrine treatment in patients with symmetric ocular hypertension (?).[64] (I must confess that I do not really understand what "ocular hypertension" is. In this series the mean baseline intraocular pressure was 27.3 mm Hg and 32% of patients had a family history of glaucoma. Peaks of intraocular pressure greater than 30 mm Hg occurred in 74%. Is this "hypertension" or glaucoma?) At any rate, one eye of 19 such patients was treated with 1% or 2% epinephrine twice daily for 1 to 5 years. Field defects developed in 32% of the untreated eyes and in none of the treated eyes. (Since my grandfather went blind from glaucoma, if I ever develop a pressure of 27 mm Hg, I don't think I'll wait for a field defect before starting treatment!)

Once visual field damage has started, the damaged eye is more vulnerable to continuing loss than is the undamaged fellow eye, even though pressures are maintained the same. Of 11 patients with monocular field loss maintained at equal pressures, seven showed greater subsequent field loss in the already damaged eye.[65] Also, when one eye has developed field loss, the second eye has a 45% chance of developing field loss within 5 years. These facts suggest that the ophthalmologist should not uncritically withhold therapy of increased intraocular pressure simply because there is no field defect yet.

The predictive value of tonography has very little clinical value. Scattergram correlation of outflow facility versus peak diurnal pressure (presumed to be the most significant predictor of field loss) shows rather wide variations (Fig. 34-11).[66] In clinical usage the popularity of tonography has declined greatly during the past decade. Actually, the predictive value of the initial intraocular pressure is better than that of tonography!

The antigens HLA-B12 and HLA-B7 are more prevalent in primary open-angle glaucoma patients. The predictive value of these antigens in anticipating field loss was studied in 76 patients with GG response to corticosteroid testing and pressure over 20 mm Hg. This population of patients had been followed and studied in detail for 5 to 10 years. One of these antigens was present in 41% of the patients with field loss and neither was present in 5% of the patients with field loss. The presence or absence of these HLA antigens was a more valid predictor of field loss than any other known factors (including initial pressure, C/D ratio, and family history of glaucoma).[67] This suggests the possibility that there exists a histochemical basis for susceptibility to optic nerve damage by intraocular pressure.

The critical decision

Should therapy be started or not? Is it ocular hypertension, to be spared the ordeal of drops; or is it glaucoma, to be prevented from causing blindness? Our leading authorities differ as to early or late therapy.[68] Over the past 3 decades I have watched the pendulum swing back and forth; early surgery, late surgery; more intensive medication, early abandonment of medicine; early diagnosis, late diagnosis.

Obviously, the decision as to when a given eye is sufficiently threatened to justify treatment will depend on our perception as to the prognosis. Hence prognostic factors such as those we value from our past experience, or will accept in the future, will be the deciding factor as to when we start treatment. I tend to agree with Hans Goldmann,[69] who argues that we have failed in our responsibility to the patient if we wait and watch until the patient develops permanent field loss as we patiently observe. The risks of medication are relatively minor in comparison to field loss.

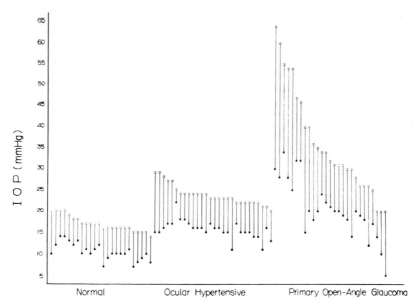

Fig. 34-12. Diurnal variations of intraocular pressure in 24 normal eyes, 28 eyes with ocular hypertension, and 27 eyes with primary open-angle glaucoma. Each vertical line represents the highest and lowest pressure recorded in that individual eye. (From Kitazawa, Y., and Horie, T.: Am. J. Ophthalmol. **79:**557, April 1975.)

However, surgery is another matter—to run the risks of an operation before field loss has occurred is not usually a very sensible course.

Of individuals with average pressures above 30 mm Hg, one fourth to one third will develop field loss.[68] This would seem unacceptably high to me if I were the patient, and I would want to be protected against this damage. Perhaps 10% of patients with pressures above 25 mm Hg will develop field loss. If the treatment was excessively burdensome, I would be less certain about tolerating unpleasant drops at a pressure of 25 mm Hg. If I could manage with once daily epinephrine, that would seem worthwhile. (Half of my maternal ancestors lost their sight because of glaucoma.)

The upper limit of normal intraocular pressure cannot be defined exactly because many eyes have a physiologic reserve that permits them to tolerate an abnormally high pressure without damage. Conversely, a few vulnerable eyes may continue to lose field with a pressure well below 20 mm Hg. A study of

20,000 eyes[70] indicated that the upper statistical limit of normal is about 25 mm Hg and that a very high probability of future optic nerve damage was associated with repeated pressures above 25 mm Hg.

The overlapping of the pressures of normal and glaucomatous patients, with the intervening group of ocular hypertensive persons, is particularly well illustrated when the wide range of diurnal pressure elevation is also considered (Fig. 34-12).[71]

"LOW PRESSURE" GLAUCOMA

The "low pressure" glaucoma syndrome may be characterized as showing typical glaucomatous field defects in association with excavated atrophy of the disc. The angles are open. The condition differs from the usual glaucoma in that the intraocular pressure is never found to be elevated. A group of 45 such patients was selected on the basis of no recorded pressure being above 24 mm Hg.[72] Of those tested, two thirds had a low pressure response to provocative corticosteroid testing. This is the same frequency distribution found in the general population and strongly suggests that low pressure glaucoma is an entirely different disease than genetic open-angle glaucoma. However, in eight patients, one eye was classified as low pressure glaucoma and the fellow eye met pressure criteria permitting the diagnosis of open-angle glaucoma. Obviously it is difficult to diagnose two different diseases in the same patient.

Seventeen of the patients had unilateral disease. Of these, 11 had an identifiable vascular lesion on the affected side. Of the 45 patients, 13 had experienced a severe hemodynamic crisis (gastrointestinal hemorrhage or cardiac arrest, for example). Seventeen patients had low blood pressures. A group of control patients did not show these two changes in comparable frequency. Eleven of the 45 patients were noted to have transient linear hemorrhages near the disc, suggesting vascular insufficiency of the optic nerve head. Only six patients showed radiologic calcification of the internal carotids.

The authors concluded that low pressure glaucoma is an ischemic atrophy of the optic disc. It may result from many interacting factors, all of which oppose or promote disc perfusion. This study included no observations of the response of low pressure glaucoma to traditional glaucoma therapy, but left the impression that such therapy was not usually relevant.

NARROW-ANGLE GLAUCOMA

Recognition of a narrow or closed angle is by gonioscopic observation. There is, however, a very close correlation between gonioscopy and a properly directed examination with the unaided biomicroscope. The slit beam is directed perpendicularly on the cornea just at the limbal junction. The viewing angle is positioned 60 degrees to the corneal side of the illumination. This permits a good view of the optical section of the cornea and periphery of the anterior chamber. The corneal thickness serves as the reference unit. If the depth of the peripheral anterior chamber is half the corneal thickness or greater, the angle is incapable of closure. If the chamber

is less than one fourth the corneal thickness, the angle is dangerously narrowed. A chamber depth between one fourth and one half the corneal thickness requires gonioscopy for more precise classification.[73]

The functional capability of an anatomically suspicious angle may be evaluated by a variety of provocative tests. The relative value of such tests was determined in a series of 19 eyes with very narrow angles.[74] A positive test was defined as a pressure elevation of 8 mm Hg or greater. The phenylephrine test (2 drops of 10% solution, repeated in 5 minutes; pressure measured at 90 minutes) was positive in 11% of patients. The cyclopentolate test (2 drops of 1% solution, repeated in 5 minutes; pressure measured at 90 minutes) was positive in 16% of patients. Dark room testing (light-tight occlusion for 1 hour) was positive in 53% of patients. Prone provocative testing (face down for 1 hour) was positive in 58% of patients. No method of testing precipitated any uncontrollable attacks of acute glaucoma. In one patient the dark room test caused a 42 mm Hg elevation of pressure, in contrast to a 5 mm Hg drop when the same eye was dilated with cyclopentolate.

The reason for emphasizing recognition of a narrow angle is that peripheral iridectomy corrects the condition if performed before the development of peripheral anterior synechiae. Serious consequences may follow prolonged medical treatment of eyes with asymptomatic chronic glaucoma and very narrow angles. Pressure control is difficult and variable despite use of all forms of medical therapy, and peripheral synechiae gradually develop.[75] These problems can be avoided by periodic evaluation of the angle, which may narrow with time.

In the management of acute angle-closure glaucoma, just as in open-angle glaucoma, intraocular pressure may be reduced by three entirely distinct medical methods: improvement of facility of aqueous outflow, reduction of ocular volume by use of osmotic agents, and reduction of aqueous formation. In practice, miotics and osmotic agents are both used in the initial treatment of a patient with acute glaucoma. Secretory inhibitors are useless if pressures are very high and are contraindicated in chronic management of patients with borderline pressure control.

Because of the rapidity with which very high pressure destroys the optic nerve, treatment of acute glaucoma, although qualitatively similar to management of chronic glaucoma, is much more urgent. Pilocarpine, 2%, is commonly instilled every 5 minutes for four times, then every 3 hours. Since the edematous cornea of acute glaucoma facilitates passage of medications, maximum miotic effect is certainly attained by this frequency of instillation. Commonly the frantic physician and the aides flood the eye repeatedly with large amounts of miotic for hours. It is doubtful that any benefit is obtained from such excessive and uncritical use of miotics, which also carries the risk of systemic toxicity. In one such reported case the unfortunate patient received 2 drops of 3% pilocarpine in each eye every 5 minutes. After 1 hour and 15 minutes of this intensive treatment the patient suffered cardiovascular collapse (blood pressure 60/30) so severe as to require consideration of myocardial infarction in the differential diagnosis.[76]

The "irreversible" cholinesterase inhibitors such as isoflurophate are contraindicated in acute glaucoma because they increase vascular congestion and may further close the angle. Furthermore, they cause postoperative inflammation ("miotic" iritis).

The "normal" fellow eye must always be treated with miotics also. Neglect of this simple precaution may confront the embarrassed young ophthalmologist with the problem of bilateral acute glaucoma. Pilocarpine, 2%, three times a day, is usually sufficient for short-term prophylactic therapy of the fellow eye. Again it must be stressed that isoflurophate and related drugs are contraindicated by narrow angles even if the pressure is initially normal. Epinephrine and other sympathomimetic drugs may occlude a narrow angle.

The dilated pupil of acute glaucoma may be completely resistant to miotic therapy. Unlike the dilated pupil produced by mydriatic or cycloplegic drugs, which may be overcome by frequent instillation of concentrated miotics, the paralyzed pupil of acute glaucoma may fail to respond to any amount of miotics. Above a critical pressure level (about 60 mm Hg) the sphincter muscle is paralyzed and nonresponsive.[77-79] Miotics instilled during this nonresponsive state are absorbed by the iris and will cause subsequent constriction if pressure later drops below the critical level. If a miotic-treated dog eye is cannulated so that intraocular pressure may be controlled simply by varying the height of a fluid reservoir connected to the eye, the pupil size may be changed at will simply by changing the pressure above or below the critical level that paralyzes the sphincter. Because miotic effect may be attained subsequent to pressure control, pilocarpine therapy is rational even in the presence of the highest pressures, since it anticipates pressure control by other types of medication. As previously mentioned, prolonged, excessive use of miotics does not increase the likelihood of constricting the pupil, is potentially quite toxic, and is irrational.

If angle-closure glaucoma is secondary to forward displacement of the lens (as may rarely occur spontaneously or following trauma), miotic therapy may worsen the glaucoma by increasing pupillary block. In unilateral cases, presence of a wide open angle in the fellow eye is an important clue to the lens-displacement mechanism in the affected eye. Mydriatic therapy will temporarily control this type of secondary angle-closure glaucoma, but iridectomy or cataract extraction is the definitive treatment.[80]

Reduction of ocular volume by osmotic agents, the second medical method, is accomplished with intravenous urea[81] or mannitol. These agents produce the most marked reduction of intraocular pressure possible with medical methods. Creating an osmotic gradient from intraocular fluids to the vascular bed, these agents act completely independently of the normal ocular outflow and inflow system. For this reason, the hypotonic effect of osmotic agents occurs despite the presence of complete and unrelieved acute angle closure and even if pilocarpine and acetazolamide therapy have failed. Osmotherapy will fail if the patient is allowed to drink hypotonic fluids such as water or coffee.

Since osmotic agents do not directly open the angle (although they often deepen the anterior chamber because of fluid withdrawal from the posterior eye), miotics should be used simultaneously. Because of simplicity and comfort, oral glycerol is used first in management of acute glaucoma. Intravenous mannitol is started if pressure has not fallen within several hours—by which time the patient will usually be in the hospital. In virtually all cases, pressure will be controlled within the hour.

The postosmotherapy pressure will help to determine whether iridectomy or filtering surgery is necessary. When pressure is controlled and the mannitol infusion is discontinued, 2% pilocarpine should be instilled every 3 or 4 hours. The pressure will remain normal if the filtration meshwork has been opened, indicating that simple iridectomy is the treatment of choice. If the pressure rises to abnormal levels within 1 or 2 days despite miotic treatment, control of the glaucoma will require filtering surgery. If the angle has been blocked by extensive peripheral anterior synechiae, the very high pressures of an attack of acute glaucoma may recur as soon as 5 hours after the first mannitol infusion. Fortunately this second pressure rise will be controlled by another intravenous administration of mannitol, which should be scheduled to start about 30 to 45 minutes before the time of operation. Since mannitol is rapidly excreted, the second infusion, by the time it is clinically recognized to be necessary, can again cause the plasma hypertonicity that effects the drop in eye pressure. Before the second dose of mannitol, if given only shortly after the first, the patient may be at least partially rehydrated, orally or intravenously. If an hour or more elapses after fluid administration to permit establishment of the rehydrated osmotic equilibraium between plasma and aqueous, the osmotic effect of the second dose of mannitol will be greater than if the patient were dehydrated.

Remember the indwelling catheter during surgery under general anesthesia, lest the osmotherapy result in a distended bladder.

Glycerol, 50%, is also useful in the management of acute glaucoma when applied directly to the eye. Topical glycerol does not reduce pressure, but it does clear edema from the cornea, thereby permitting a more accurate diagnosis. Secondary glaucoma (as associated with acute iridocyclitis, neovascularization of the iris and angle, bleeding melanoma, glaucomatocyclitic crisis, or hypermature cataract) may be confused with angle-closure glaucoma, especially if the cornea is cloudy. Since glycerol is painful, topical anesthesia (tetracaine, etc.) must precede its use. Several drops of 50% glycerol will cause remarkable clearing of a steamy cornea within minutes. The fundus is best viewed immediately after glycerol clearing and before miosis is attained. Knowledge of the health of the optic nerve and retina is essential to proper diagnosis and management.

Although in the recent past emergency surgery was the proper treatment for acute glaucoma, the more effective medical methods now available will control the acute rise of pressure and permit postponement of surgery for several days until the eye is less inflamed. After an acute attack of angle-closure glaucoma, the eye should almost always be operated. Reasonable exceptions should be made to this rule. If pressure can be *well controlled by miotics alone*, an elderly and infirm patient can often be spared the expense and trauma of surgery. This is particularly true if the angle closure was precipitated by mydriatic examination and had not spontaneously occurred previously. The best of surgeons encounter unforeseen and unpredictable complications.

The decision as to whether peripheral iridectomy or a filtering operation is to be done may be based (partially) on the adequacy of control by miotics alone following discontinuance of osmotherapy. Prompt relapse to high pressure indicates continuing, presumably permanent, angle closure that requires filtering surgery. Good pressure control by miotics alone occurs if the angle is functionally open; here peripheral iridectomy will prevent a recurrent attack and is the operation of choice. Gonioscopy and tonography may aid the surgical decision in borderline cases. Do *not* procrastinate and delay surgery if miotic treatment fails to give good pressure control, for such delay will rapidly destroy the angle function.

The third method of glaucoma control, reduction of aqueous formation by the use of acetazolamide or epinephrine, is not very useful in the management of acute glaucoma either before or after surgery. Since secretory inhibition is incomplete (decreasing aqueous formation by about 60%), elevated pressure will not be controlled by acetazolamide if the outflow mechanism is so severely damaged that it cannot handle even 40% of the normal rate. During an acute angle-closure attack the outflow is, of course, almost nil; hence the problem will usually not respond to acetazolamide. Through its mydriatic effect, epinephrine only worsens, if possible, the angle closure.

Acetazolamide is positively *not* to be used in the long-term control of angle-closure glaucoma, since this permits formation of extensive peripheral anterior synechiae. Once such adhesions have formed, the opportunity for cure by peripheral iridectomy is forever lost.

Reduction of aqueous inflow may also result from retrobulbar anesthesia. Unfortunately the excellent pressure-lowering effect obtained before cataract surgery through use of lidocaine, hyaluronidase, and massage usually does not occur after retrobulbar anesthesia of very hard eyes. Even though pressure is not thereby controlled, retrobulbar anesthesia (for example, 2 ml of 1% lidocaine) is a most valuable way to control pain and nausea. The almost instantaneous relief obtained in this way is most welcome to the patient. Caution should be observed in freeing uncooperative and unmanageable patients from pain—the false reassurance of comfort may cause them to refuse the further treatment urgently required for the control of pressure and the preservation of sight.[82]

The corticosteroid-induced pressure elevation typical of open-angle glaucoma is not regularly associated with narrow-angle glaucoma. None of 15 angle-closure glaucoma patients had a pressure elevation greater than 6 mm Hg following topical instillation of 0.1% betamethasone four times daily for 3 to 6 weeks.[83] This finding indicates that the therapeutic use of corticosteroids, if indicated for an inflammatory reaction following peripheral iridectomy, for instance, is not contraindicated by fear of inducing pressure elevation.

Dilation of the pupil may occasionally be necessary in an eye with a dangerously narrow angle. A technique of sector dilation with epinephrine may be useful in such a case. The eye is first anesthetized topically to prevent spreading of the epinephrine by tearing. The patient is to look steadily upward. A thin strip (1 × 5 mm) of filter paper is moistened at its tip with 1% or 2% epinephrine. This moist tip is inserted between the lower lid and the limbus at the 6 o'clock position and is allowed to remain for only 1 minute. Within a half hour, the lower part of the pupil will dilate several millimeters. This technique is said to be adequate to permit ophthalmoscopy, yet it does not result in elevation of intraocular pressure.[84]

SECONDARY GLAUCOMA

Accurate differential diagnosis between chronic simple glaucoma and secondary open-angle glaucoma is of therapeutic importance, since the former is almost always bilateral and lifelong, whereas the latter is often unilateral and may be temporary. Unnecessary treatment of a normal eye causes difficulty in seeing at night and reduced distance vision because of accommodative spasm. A past history of injury or uveitis should arouse suspicion that the glaucoma is secondary.

A multitude of secondary glaucomas exist. In most cases their management is comparable to that of primary glaucoma. In a few instances (traumatic angle damage and glaucomatocyclitic crisis), recognition of the cause may prevent unnecessary surgery.

Brief discussion of representative examples will illustrate the concepts of secondary glaucoma.

Postcontusion glaucoma

A cause-and-effect relationship is generally assumed to exist between a posteriorly dislocated lens after trauma and the postcontusion glaucoma. In accord with this assumption, lens extraction is frequently advised as treatment of the glaucoma. Pathologic study of 63 cases of glaucoma associated with traumatic posterior lens dislocation or subluxation has demonstrated the basis for this type of glaucoma and indicates that medical treatment may frequently be more appropriate than surgical treatment.[85] These cases were almost evenly divided into closed- (32) and open- (31) angle glaucoma. The angle closure was attributed to rubeosis iridis, vitreous block of the pupil, or organized hemorrhage. All but one of the open-angle cases showed the typical postcontusion angle deformity, consisting of posterior displacement of the iris root and deep tears into the ciliary body. These findings indicate that open-angle glaucoma associated with posterior lens displacement is primarily postcontusion glaucoma and is not directly caused by the abnormal lens position at all. "Hypersecretion" resulting from "irritation by the dislocated lens" has not been demonstrated; the glaucoma in these cases is caused by increased outflow resistance. Only 4 of the 31 open-angle cases showed any signs of lens-induced inflammation.

Obviously gonioscopy is most important in the evaluation of postcontusion glaucoma. If the angle is found to be open and abnormally widened, the principles of treatment should be the same as for chronic open-angle glaucoma. Extraction of the lens is indicated only if lens-induced uveitis or phacolytic glaucoma occur or for optical reasons. If the angle is closed, appropriate surgical correction is in order, and relief of glaucoma is more likely caused by iridectomy than by lens removal.

Postcontusion glaucoma is a result of a splitting of the ciliary body so that the circular muscle, iris root, and ciliary processes are displaced posteriorly, leaving the longitudinal muscle attached to the scleral spur.[86] (This is not a cyclodialysis.) Immediate damage to or subsequent deterioration of the trabecular meshwork results in a secondary open-angle glaucoma that is quite similar to chronic simple glaucoma in its response to therapy, both medical and surgical.

This type of glaucoma is diagnosed clinically by recognition of increased depth of the anterior chamber, posterior displacement of the iris root, and an unusually wide ciliary body.[87] A thin gray hyaline membrane may cover the injured angle.

The magnitude of ocular hypertensive response to 0.1% dexamethasone three times daily differs on a genetic basis.[88] Arbitrary classification of the hypertensive response as 0 to 5 mm, 6 to 14 mm, or greater was the basis of hypothetical designation as genotypes of low (P^L, P^L), intermediate (P^L, P^H), or higher pressure (P^H, P^H), respectively. Remarkably, this genetic model was validated in a study of 10 families (parents and offspring). Armaly[88] believes glaucoma transmission to be by polygenic inheritance. From the practical standpoint, this remarkable study indicates (as we already know) that the great majority of glaucoma patients (but not all) will develop a clinically significant pressure increase after prolonged topical use of potent corticosteroids.

Comparable study of traumatic angle recession glaucoma intended as a control disclosed the surprising fact that angle recession glaucoma is itself a manifestation of glaucomatous inheritance, occurring only in patients whose uninjured fellow eye (and also the injured eye) showed a dexamethasone hypertensive response greater than 5 mm Hg (consecutive series of 11 cases). This indicates the logical conclusion that secondary glaucoma is not exclusively dependent on the injury but also on the genetic status of the individual. Apparently we cannot assume that corticosteroids will not elevate the pressure of chronic secondary glaucoma—the reverse may commonly be true.

A study of 55 retired boxers identified nine

of 110 eyes (8.2%) as having contusion-angle deformity.[89] Despite an average duration of 33 years since the injury, none of these nine eyes had glaucoma. This casts doubt on the assumption that such an injury causes glaucoma. This common and probably false assumption arises from the usual method of presentation of clinical cases. A glaucoma-oriented physician encounters a unilateral glaucoma and finds a contusion-angle deformity. *Post hoc, ergo propter hoc.* (After this, therefore because of this.) Actually, the glaucoma is a genetically caused open-angle glaucoma, the onset of which may have been accelerated by the injury. Practically, the use of corticosteroids in such an eye will probably induce a glaucomatous response.

Further confirmation of the rarity of late glaucoma following contusion-angle deformity comes from a study of 50 patients with traumatic hyphema.[90] Of these 50, 33 had early glaucoma, but only four had elevated pressures 6 months later. After 10 years, 31 were still available for study. Of these, one eye had been enucleated for painful blindness, one had a pressure of 23 mm Hg, and one had a pressure of 32 mm Hg.

Glaucomatocyclitic crisis

The very uncommon syndrome known as a glaucomatocyclitic crisis is believed to represent a form of secondary glaucoma complicating mild anterior segment inflammation.[91] The most effective management is corticosteroid-mydriatic therapy exactly as would be used for a mild attack of iritis. Since glaucomatocyclitic crises are of short duration, lasting only for hours or at most a few days, the prolonged effect of atropine is undesirable, and the cycloplegics of choice are of the short-acting type. Corticosteroids alone, used topically every few hours, effectively shorten most attacks. Miotics are not helpful. The most common and also most serious error in management is surgical intervention. Not only do filtering operations not prevent future attacks, but they introduce the unnecessary hazard of intraocular surgery with its possible complications.

The diagnosis of glaucomatocyclitic crisis,

necessary to proper management, is made through awareness of the existence of this entity and because of the paradox of an acute attack of glaucoma in the presence of a gonioscopically open angle. Cells and flare are not marked during a crisis but may readily be observed with the slit lamp. Unfortunately cells and flare often are present during an attack of primary acute glaucoma and therefore are of no help in differential diagnosis. The history of previous, recurrent, self-limited attacks with an onset in relatively young adult life and without any optic nerve damage is compatible with the diagnosis of glaucomatocyclitic crisis. Although these crises usually affect only one eye, patients with binocular involvement have been reported.[92,93]

Tonography performed during a glaucomatocyclitic crisis shows a decreased coefficient of outflow of the aqueous.[94] During an attack, inflammatory signs are constantly present and include keratic precipitates, faint flare, and aqueous cells. Synechiae are not present. Since the duration of a glaucomatocyclitic crisis may be several months, failure to recognize the inflammatory features of this disease may result in erroneous diagnosis of unilateral chronic simple glaucoma in a young adult—which mysteriously disappears with time.

Topical corticosteroid therapy (every 2 hours the first day, reduced in frequency as pressure drops) will control the inflammation and reduce the pressure of a glaucomatocyclitic crisis within a few days. Relapse will occur if the corticosteroid is discontinued before the attack has run its course, which may last some weeks. The pressure of a glaucomatocyclitic crisis may also be controlled with pilocarpine, epinephrine, or carbonic anhydrase inhibitors[94]; however, the most fundamental and rational therapy would seem to be control of the inflammation with topical corticosteroids.

The nature of the glaucomatocyclitic syndrome has been challenged by a study of 11 patients with this diagnosis.[95] The gathering of these 11 cases required a 13-year period at the Washington University Glaucoma Center—a comment on the rarity of the condition. Critical evaluation of these cases showed many instances of elevated intraocular pressure of the affected and fellow eyes between crises, cupping and atrophy of the disc, bilateral visual field loss, and high responsiveness to corticosteroid testing. In short, a glaucomatocyclitic crisis may be only a variant of primary open-angle glaucoma and deserves long-term, careful evaluation of both eyes.

Although glaucomatocyclitic crises generally do not damage the optic nerve, occasional cases are sufficiently severe to do so. In two of five such cases, thermal sclerectomy was performed, with achievement of good filtration and control of pressure even during subsequent acute attacks.[96]

Because prostaglandin E causes elevation of intraocular pressure in animals, it was suspected as an explanation of glaucomatocyclitic crises.[97] Assay of PGE content of the aqueous humor in seven cases showed its concentration indeed to be increased. A correlation existed between higher levels of PGE and higher levels of intraocular pressure. In two cases PGE was assayed during an attack and also in remission. As expected, the PGE level was much higher during the attack (for example, 18.4 ng/ml during the attack and 3.2 ng/ml during remission in one case).

Indomethacin blocks the synthesis of PGE_2 from arachidonic acid and was given in dosage of 150 mg/day until the intraocular pressure was reduced to about 20 mm Hg. The average duration of treatment was 12 days. A dosage of 75 mg/day was found to be much less effective. Nausea resulted from the dosage of 150 mg/day. Fig. 34-13[97] compares the intraocular pressure in three cases treated with indomethacin with the response of the same eye during a previous attack

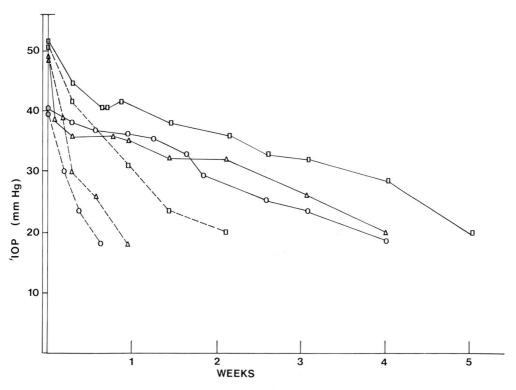

Fig. 34-13. Solid lines: response of glaucomatocyclitic crisis to acetazolamide, epinephrine, and dexamethasone. Interrupted lines: response of same eyes to indomethacin. The symbols (circle, triangle, square) designate the same eye. (From Masuda, K., and associates: Jpn. J. Ophthalmol. **19:**368, 1975.)

when treated with topical dexamethasone and epinephrine and 1000 mg of acetazolamide per day.

Polyphloretin phosphate is an antagonist of PGE_2. In three cases it was injected subconjunctivally in dosage of 3, 6, and 7.5 mg. This reduced intraocular pressure within an hour, more effectively with the larger doses (for example, 45 to 22 mm Hg within 1 hour with 6.0 mg). The effect of subconjunctival injection was transient and irritating, hence its clinical value is not yet established. Nevertheless, this confirms the significance of PGE in the etiology of glaucomatocyclitic crisis.[97]

Glaucoma with episcleritis

Two patients with long-standing rheumatoid arthritis had glaucoma with pressures of 45 and 50 mm Hg, associated with painless redness of the eyes. Traditional glaucoma therapy with pilocarpine, echothiophate, and epinephrine failed to control the pressure. One patient had faint flare and fine keratic precipitates; the other did not. The diagnosis of episcleritis was made and treatment was instituted with topical and systemic corticosteroids. Within a week the episcleritis had subsided and the pressures returned to normal.[98]

Under such circumstances the possibility of inflammatory glaucoma should be considered and a trial of corticosteroids instituted.

Glaucoma following interstitial keratitis

Patients who have had interstitial keratitis often suffer enough damage to the structures of the anterior chamber angle to predispose them to late development of chronic glaucoma. Such glaucoma was found in 17 of 88 cases of inactive interstitial keratitis[99] and is therefore of sufficient frequency to warrant routine tonometry in the periodic examinations of patients who have had interstitial keratitis. The onset of glaucoma occurred from 10 to 60 years after the acute interstitial keratitis (Fig. 34-14). Tonography shows marked reduction in the facility of outflow. The angles are gonioscopically open in this form of glaucoma. Treatment is by the usual medical means or, if necessary, by filtering surgery.

The glaucomas developing after syphilitic interstitial keratitis may either be open or closed angle in type. The open-angle cases are associated with inflammatory trabecular obstruction. The closed-angle cases are found in patients with reduced corneal diameter,

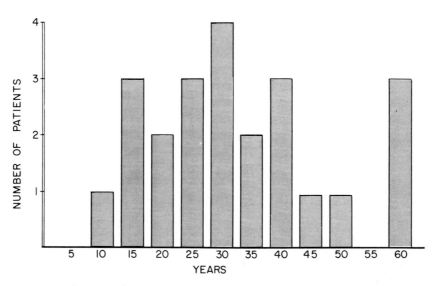

Fig. 34-14. Interval in years between active interstitial keratitis and onset of glaucoma. (Modified from Knox, D. L.: Arch. Ophthalmol. **66:**18, 1961.)

presumably caused by growth arrest by the disease.[100] Treatment is the same as for comparable cases of glaucoma uncomplicated by preexisting keratitis.

CONGENITAL GLAUCOMA

Treatment of congenital glaucoma must, of course, be based on accurate diagnosis. Tonometric measurements of the small eyes of infants through narrow palpebral apertures are difficult and subject to error. Furthermore, the pressure of newborn eyes may be slightly higher than the pressure in adults. The mean tension of 47 human infant eyes, measured with the infant under general anesthesia during the first day of life, was 22.2 mm Hg Schiøtz,[101,102] ranging from 16 to 29 mm Hg. The horizontal diameter of the newborn cornea is approximately 10 mm.

The diagnosis of congenital glaucoma should not be made on the basis of corneal opacity alone. The rare condition of congenital hereditary corneal dystrophy as well as other congenital faults may cause bilateral corneal opacities superficially similar to those of congenital glaucoma.[103] However, these nonglaucomatous conditions do not cause the typical enlargement of corneal diameter that is usually associated with marked corneal edema of glaucomatous origin. Furthermore,

the lacrimation, photophobia, and elevated intraocular pressure typical of glaucoma are not present in conditions such as congenital corneal dystrophy. Apparently it is not uncommon for goniotomy or other antiglaucoma surgery to be performed mistakenly in cases of congenital hereditary corneal dystrophy.

The structural changes responsible for congenital glaucoma are apparently resistant to miotic or mydriatic medical therapy. Pilocarpine, DFP, 10% phenylephrine, and atropine do not have any appreciable effect on the intraocular pressure or facility of outflow in patients with congenital glaucoma.[104]

The intraocular pressure of 181 eyes treated with miotics for infantile glaucoma is charted in Fig. 34-15.[105] The rarity of adequate medical control is obvious.

A trial of medical treatment for infantile glaucoma only allows time for further damage to the optic nerve. Surgery is the only treatment of value.[106]

Presumably medical therapy fails to control congenital glaucoma because of the structural anomaly of the angle. Normally the longitudinal fibers insert on the ciliary spur and through their contraction tend to open the trabecular spaces. Fig. 34-16 shows forward attachment of the ciliary fibers on the

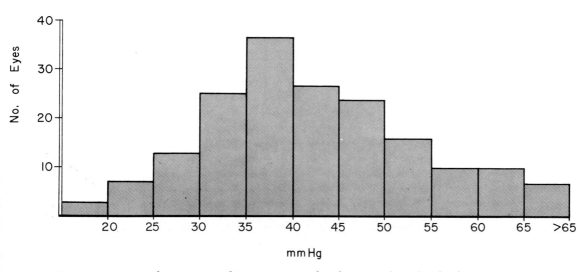

Fig. 34-15. Intraocular pressure of 181 eyes treated with miotics for infantile glaucoma. (Data from Haas, J.: Invest. Ophthalmol. 7:140, 1968.)

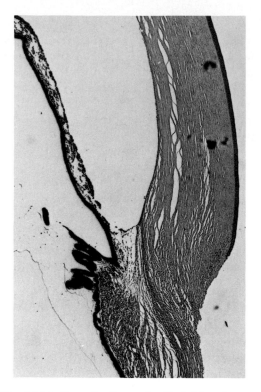

Fig. 34-16. Eye of a 5-month-old child with congenital glaucoma. Note abnormal forward attachment of ciliary fibers on trabeculum. (From Reeh, M. J.: Trans. Am. Acad. Ophthalmol. Otolaryngol. **65:**178, 1961.)

trabeculum in a 5-month-old eye with congenital glaucoma.[107] Pilocarpine-induced contraction of these abnormally inserted fibers cannot open the trabecular spaces.

Congenital glaucoma is not caused by absence of the canal of Schlemm, since jugular compression during gonioscopy readily causes visible filling of Schlemm's canal with blood.

Xanthogranuloma (nevoxanthoendothelioma) should be considered in the differential diagnosis of congenital glaucoma. The eye lesion consists of diffuse iris infiltration by large histiocytes that are shed into the aqueous and block the trabeculae with resultant glaucoma. Iris neovascularization frequently causes spontaneous intraocular hemorrhage. Diagnosis is made by the ocular appearance, by the skin lesions, and by biopsy of the iris

or skin. Medical therapy is of no avail, but x-ray treatment may be helpful.[108]

Another differential diagnosis to be considered is the battered child syndrome. A 9-week-old child with bilateral pressure of 60 mm Hg and enlarged hazy corneas was found also to have hyphema, iridodialysis, dislocated lenses, cataract, vitreous hemorrhage, and numerous cutaneous scars. His 17-year-old unmarried mother finally admitted to gross abuse of the child.[109] It is estimated that in 1966 there were at least 15,000 battered children in the United States, 30% of whom suffered permanent damage and 5% death.

GLAUCOMA REQUIRING SURGERY

This admittedly artificial category of glaucoma has been created to allow separate discussion of the medical aspects of glaucoma patients undergoing surgery.

Angle-closure glaucoma

Should iridectomy or filtering surgery be performed for acute glaucoma? Arbitrary recommendations based on duration of the acute attack are far less reliable than conclusions derived from therapeutic responses. For example, differentiation between appositional closure and synechial closure of a narrow-angle glaucoma may be made by gonioscopy after intravenous mannitol. The osmotic decrease in vitreous volume deepens the anterior chamber so that an initially occluded angle may open throughout its entire circumference. This finding will help the surgeon to decide between iridectomy and a filtering procedure.[110]

As another example, if good pressure control can be maintained by miotics alone after osmotic reduction of an attack of angle-closure glaucoma, iridectomy is obviously indicated. Several days' time may be required for evaluation of the effect of miotic therapy. During this period the inflammation of the acute attack will subside, leaving the eye more suitable for surgery.

After adequate peripheral iridectomy, eyes that have had angle-closure glaucoma may be dilated without fear of causing acute pressure elevation. Thirty-four such eyes were dilated with 10% phenylephrine instilled three times at 15-minute intervals— in no eye did dilation result in a pressure rise as great as 6 mm Hg. Similar use of 1% cyclopentolate caused a pressure rise greater than 6 mm Hg (average, 9.6 mm Hg) in seven of these 34 eyes, a response similar to that found in chronic simple glaucoma. All seven pressure-responding eyes had required medication for glaucoma control after iridectomy; hence these eyes appeared to have had both open- and closed-angle glaucoma.[111]

In 60 eyes following adequate iridectomy for angle-closure glaucoma, no angle closure followed use of 10% phenylephrine.[112] However, in another case the pigment layer was not included in the iridectomy, and phenylephrine, as expected, caused a severe acute attack of glaucoma.

Once daily 10% phenylephrine mydriasis after peripheral iridectomy has been advocated to prevent formation of posterior synechiae.[113] Such dilation does not ordinarily cause a pressure rise in cases of angle-closure glaucoma after iridectomy. In a series of over 300 such patients, acute angle-closure glaucoma was induced by phenylephrine dilation of two postiridectomy eyes. One was lost; the second was salvaged by miotic therapy. Both eyes had plateau-type irides, which permitted far peripheral closure despite a midperipheral iridectomy.

The importance of postoperative phenylephrine dilation to prevent posterior synechiae after iridectomy is indicated by the finding of 22 cases of immovable adherent pupil in a series of 100 peripheral iridectomies.[114] This troublesome complication is sufficiently frequent to require consideration in deciding postoperative medical management. A cycloplegic drug may also safely be used to dilate almost all eyes with normal pressure after iridectomy for angle-closure glaucoma. Of 65 such eyes dilated with 2% homatropine, only four developed pressure elevations greater than 8 mm Hg, and the average of these elevations was only 10 mm Hg.[114]

Should chronic pressure elevation persist after iridectomy in cases of primary angle-closure glaucoma, the strong miotics and epinephrine may be safely prescribed without fear of precipitating acute elevation of pressure.[115]

Tonography performed 2½ hours after instillation of 1% levo-epinephrine in a series of 39 glaucomatous eyes showed a more than 25% increase of facility of aqueous outflow in 23 eyes.[116] During this brief period a decrease in tension occurred in only nine of the eyes. (These 39 eyes were all cases of narrow-angle glaucoma in which peripheral iridectomy had been performed. Epinephrine was found to be useful in preventing postoperative synechiae, helped in control of residual pressure elevations, and was preferable to the use of parasympatholytic drugs.)

Occasionally a rather marked rise in pressure will follow an iridectomy done for narrow-angle glaucoma. In the belief that this is because of postoperative swelling of the iris and ciliary body, the use of miotics and 1% epinephrine bitartrate may be recommended.[117] The vasoconstrictor effect of epinephrine is supposed to reduce the uveal edema and vasodilatation, while its mydriatic effect is counteracted by the miotics.

Open-angle glaucoma

Medical therapy is accepted as the treatment of choice for open-angle glaucoma, except for the few unusually severe cases. Even when a case has entered the surgical category, however, the use or nonuse of medication may importantly influence its outcome.

The long-acting miotics (DFP, demecarium, and echothiophate) increase the postoperative inflammatory reaction and therefore should be discontinued at least 5 days before glaucoma surgery.[118] If control is reasonably adequate with pilocarpine, this short-acting miotic should be substituted some weeks before surgery.

Young ophthalmologists often feel uncertain about the use of atropine in the postoperative treatment of a glaucomatous eye after a filtering operation. If the operation is adequate, there is no possibility of precipitating glaucoma by cycloplegic dilation of the pupil. The purpose of atropine and corticosteroids at this time is to minimize iritis and scarring that might compromise the filtering procedure. Such treatment is unqualifiedly endorsed by experienced glaucoma surgeons.[119]

Drugs that inhibit aqueous secretion (for example, acetazolamide) should not be used immediately prior to filtering surgery or for several weeks thereafter. A free flow of aqueous is of great importance to maintenance of the filtering bleb. Blebs have been seen to flatten and disappear with acetazolamide therapy.[118]

Topical application of steroids four times a day after filtering antiglaucoma operations is advocated to minimize scarring of the operative site.[120] This seems to be a rational assumption, although I am not aware of any controlled study of the effectiveness of such treatment.

The expected hypertensive response of chronic simple glaucoma to corticosteroids may be beneficial after filtering surgery.[121] By temporarily blocking the normal outflow, corticosteroid therapy diverts the aqueous outflow into the surgical opening, thereby promoting its patency. Furthermore, the anti-inflammatory effect decreases scarring and postoperative reaction.

Prolonged corticosteroid medication may adversely affect the filtering blebs of glaucoma surgery. In one patient receiving prednisone (15 to 40 mg/day) for arteritis, leaks developed in the conjunctival surfaces of the blebs 2 months after surgery in one eye and 2½ years after surgery in the other eye.[122] No other leaks occurred after approximately 100 limboscleral trephinations done by the same technique over a 5-year period. Although this isolated bilateral case may have been caused by some reason other than prolonged steroid treatment, this possibility must be considered.

Leakage of the conjunctival suture line may cause a flat chamber after filtering surgery for glaucoma. If topical staining with fluorescein does not identify the site of the leak, injection of fluorescein solution into the anterior chamber via a knife-needle–beveled corneal incision will cause a recognizable flow of stained fluid from the area of faulty closure.[123]

A conjunctival leak following filtering glaucoma surgery may be sealed by application of cyanoacrylate tissue adhesive to the surface of the leak. Within 1 or 2 weeks the adhesive will fall off, but during this period the leak will most likely seal itself beneath the adhesive barrier.[124]

Following glaucoma surgery, an excessively filtering bleb may cause hypotony. Correction of this condition may be achieved by painting the bleb with trichloracetic acid or by destroying the epithelium with iodine and covering it with a fresh flap of conjunctiva.[125] A better way to deal with an undesired bleb is to freeze it. Within a month after cryotherapy, the frozen tissue shrinks markedly, often flattening completely. A similar technique will eradicate small iris prolapses.

Phacolytic glaucoma

Phacolytic glaucoma is an acute glaucoma resulting from blocking of an open trabecular meshwork by phagocytic cells entering the anterior chamber in response to liquefied lens material. Formerly, therapy was considered to be an emergency cataract extraction. The condition responds very well to osmotic and corticosteroid therapy, which should be used to obtain a quiet eye that can be scheduled for cataract extraction at a convenient time.

Malignant glaucoma

Malignant glaucoma is defined as a condition in which the aqueous flow becomes trapped within the vitreous cavity, displacing the iris and lens (if present) forward to collapse the anterior chamber. Malignant glaucoma may occur after surgery for glaucoma,[126] after cataract extraction, following the use of miotics,[127] or spontaneously.[128]

Approximately half of the cases of this dreaded complication after iridectomy or filtering surgery for narrow-angle glaucoma can be controlled by medical treatment. Intensive mydriatic-cycloplegic therapy with 1% to 4% atropine and 10% phenylephrine is required. Presumably the cycloplegia relaxes the ciliary muscle, tightens the zonular fibers, and thereby pulls the lens backward from its pupil-blocking position. This treatment is not useful in aphakic malignant glaucoma. Maximum mydriasis breaks the pupil block and permits the anterior chamber to reform. Although acetazolamide and osmotic agents may also be used to advantage, correction of the basic fault requires intensive cycloplegia. At least 4 days of intensive medical treatment is appropriate before deciding on surgery, because in most cases the anterior chamber re-forms only slowly after several days of treatment. Atropinization must be continued indefinitely, since malignant glaucoma will recur even months later, whenever atropine is stopped, and may not again be medically controllable. Pilocarpine or other miotics not only do not benefit malignant glaucoma, they actually make it worse.[129,130]

Since intravenous mannitol (20%, 2 g/kg) reduces vitreous volume and thereby deepens the anterior chamber, this type of osmotic therapy is suitable for treatment of malignant glaucoma.[131] Medical deepening of the anterior chamber with mannitol may break this malignant cycle; however, in two of the three reported cases, lens extraction was ultimately necessary to control the glaucoma.

REFERENCES

1. Grant, W. M.: Physiological and pharmacological influences upon intraocular pressure, Pharmacol. Rev. **7**:143, 1955.
2. Sugar, H. S.: Cataract and filtration surgery, Am. J. Ophthalmol. **69**:740, 1970.
3. Shaffer, R. N.: Cataract incidence, Am. J. Ophthalmol. **69**:368, 1970.
4. Sugar, H. S.: Principles of medical management in chronic open-angle glaucoma, Ann. Ophthalmol. **3**:579, 1971.
5. Armaly, M. F.: Interpretation of tonometry and ophthalmoscopy, Invest. Ophthalmol. **11**:75, 1972.
6. Hoskins, H. D., Jr.: The management of elevated intraocular pressure with normal optic discs and visual fields. II. An approach to early therapy, Surv. Ophthalmol. **21**: 479, May-June 1977.
7. Vanderburg, D., and Drance, S. M.: Studies of the effects of artificially raised intraocular pressure, Am. J. Ophthalmol. **62**: 1049, 1966.
8. Hayreh, S. S., and Walter, W. M.: Fluorescent fundus photography in glaucoma, Am. J. Ophthalmol. **63**:982, 1967.
9. Drance, S. M.: Diurnal variation of intraocular pressure in treated glaucoma, Arch. Ophthalmol. **70**:302, 1963.
10. Smith, J. L.: The incidence of Schiøtz-applanation disparity, Arch. Ophthalmol. **77**:305, 1967.
11. Johnson, C. C.: Goldmann tonometer, Arch. Ophthalmol. **78**:416, 1967.
12. Bucci, M. G.: Procedure for obtaining fluorescent semicircles in applanation tonometry, Am. J. Ophthalmol. **71**:1140, 1971.
13. Kaufman, H. E., Wind, C. A., and Waltman, S. R.: Validity of Mackay-Marg electronic applanation tonometer in patients with scarred irregular corneas, Am. J. Ophthalmol. **69**:1003, 1970.
14. Rosen, D. A., and Warman, A. G.: Observations on the clinical determination of scleral rigidity, Am. J. Ophthalmol. **54**:375, 1962.
15. Galin, M. A., Aizawa, F., and McLean, J. M.: The water provocative test in glaucomatous patients, Am. J. Ophthalmol. **52**:15, 1961.
16. Drance, S. M.: Studies with applanation water tests, Arch. Ophthalmol. **69**:39, 1963.
17. Galin, M. A., Aizawa, F., and Baras, I.: Studies on the mechanism of the water drinking test, Am. J. Ophthalmol. **51**:601, April 1961.
18. Roberts, R. W.: Tonography in the management of glaucoma, Trans. Am. Acad. Ophthalmol. Otolaryngol. **65**:163, 1961.
19. Podos, S. M., and Becker, B.: Tonography—current thoughts, Am. J. Ophthalmol. **75**: 733, 1973.
20. Trobe, J. D.: Chromophobe adenoma presenting with a hemianopic temporal arcuate scotoma, Am. J. Ophthalmol. **77**:388, March 1974.
21. Engel, S.: Influence of a constricted pupil on the field in glaucoma, Arch. Ophthalmol. **27**:1184, 1942.
22. Havener, W. H., and Podedworny, W.: Combined surgical procedure for retinal de-

tachment and uncontrolled glaucoma, Am. J. Ophthalmol. **58**:804, 1964.

23. Harris, L. S., and Galin, M. A.: Cycloplegic provocative testing, Arch. Ophthalmol. **81**:544, 1969.

24. Pemberton, J. W.: Schiøtz-applanation disparity following retinal detachment surgery, Arch. Ophthalmol. **81**:534, 1969.

25. Harris, L. S.: Cycloplegic-induced intraocular pressure elevations, Arch. Ophthalmol. **79**:242, 1968.

26. Schimek, R. A., and Lieberman, W. J.: The influence of Cyclogyl and Neo-Synephrine on tonographic studies of miotic control in open-angle glaucoma, Am. J. Ophthalmol. **51**:781, 1961.

27. Kolker, A. E., and Hetherington, J., Jr.: Becker-Shaffer's diagnosis and therapy of the glaucomas, ed. 4, St. Louis, 1976, The C. V. Mosby Co.

28. Melikian, H. E., Lieberman, T. W., and Leopold, I. H.: Ocular pigmentation and pressure and outflow responses to pilocarpine and epinephrine, Am. J. Ophthalmol. **72**:70, 1971.

29. Kronfeld, P. C.: The efficacy of combinations of ocular hypotensive drugs, Arch. Ophthalmol. **78**:140, 1967.

30. Kini, M. M., Dahl, A. A., Roberts, C. R., Lehwalder, L. W., and Grant, W. M.: Echothiophate, pilocarpine, and open-angle glaucoma, Arch. Ophthalmol. **89**:190, 1973.

31. Flindall, R. J., and Drance, S. M.: Dose response of intraocular pressures to single instillations of carbaminoylcholine chloride, Can. J. Ophthalmol. **1**:4, 1966.

32. Wolter, J. R.: Histopathology of the trabecular meshwork in glaucoma, Am. J. Ophthalmol. **49**:1089, 1960.

33. Becker, B.: Diagnosis and therapy of the glaucomas, St. Louis, 1961, The C. V. Mosby Co.

34. Levene, R. Z.: Initial glaucoma therapy with phospholine iodide, Am. J. Ophthalmol. **57**:429, 1964.

35. Wiener, M., and Alvis, B. Y.: The use of concentrated epinephrine preparations in glaucoma, iritis, and related conditions, Am. J. Ophthalmol. **20**:497, 1937.

36. Peczon, J. D., and Grant, W. M.: Sedatives, stimulants, and intraocular pressure in glaucoma, Arch. Ophthalmol. **72**:178, 1964.

37. Armaly, M. F., and Burian, H. M.: Changes in the tonogram during accommodation, Arch. Ophthalmol. **60**:60, 1958.

38. Armaly, M. F., and Rubin, M. L.: Accommodation and applanation tonometry, Arch. Ophthalmol. **65**:415, 1961.

39. Armaly, M. F., and Jepson, N. C.: Accommodation and the dynamics of the steady state intraocular pressure, Invest. Ophthalmol. **1**:480, 1962.

40. Lempert, P., Cooper, K., Culver, J. F., and Tredici, T. J.: The effect of exercise on intraocular pressure, Am. J. Ophthalmol. **63**:1673, 1967.

41. Lempert, P., Cooper, K. H., and Culver, J. F.: The effect of exercise on intraocular tension, Invest. Ophthalmol. **4**:243, 1965.

42. Stewart, R. H., LeBlanc, R., and Becker, B.: Effects of exercise on aqueous dynamics, Am. J. Ophthalmol. **69**:245, 1970.

43. Bloomfield, S., and Kellerman, L.: The relative value of several diagnostic tests for chronic simple glaucoma, Am. J. Ophthalmol. **30**:869, 1947.

44. Leydhecker, W.: Influence of coffee upon ocular tension, Am. J. Ophthalmol. **39**:700, 1955.

45. Peczon, J. D., and Grant, W. M.: Glaucoma, alcohol, and intraocular pressure, Arch. Ophthalmol. **73**:495, 1965.

46. Mehra, K. S., Roy, P. N., and Khare, B. B.: Tobacco smoking and glaucoma, Ann. Ophthalmol. **8**:462, April 1976.

47. Hepler, R. S., Frank, I. M., and Ungerleider, J. T.: Pupillary constriction after marijuana smoking, Am. J. Ophthalmol. **74**:1185, December 1972.

48. Mulberger, R. D.: Effect of a common cold product containing belladonna on intraocular pressure, Eye Ear Nose Throat Mon. **47**:61, 1968.

49. Hiatt, R. L., Fuller, I. B., Smith, L., Swartz, J., and Risser, C.: Systemically administered anticholinergic drugs and intraocular pressure, Arch. Ophthalmol. **84**:735, 1970.

50. Lazenby, G. W., Reed, J. W., and Grant, W. M.: Anticholinergic medication in open-angle glaucoma, Arch. Ophthalmol. **84**:719, 1970.

51. Harris, L. S., Galin, M. A., and Mittag, T. W.: Cycloplegic provocative testing after topical administration of steroids, Arch. Ophthalmol. **86**:13, 1971.

52. Meyer, E. J., Roberts, C. R., Leibowitz, H. M., McGowan, B., and Houle, R. E.: Influence of norethynodrel with mestranol on intraocular pressure in glaucoma, Arch. Ophthalmol. **75**:771, 1966.

53. Meyer, E. J., Leibowitz, H., Christman, E.

H., and Niffenegger, J. A.: Influence of nor-ethynodrel with mestranol on intraocular pressure in glaucoma, Arch. Ophthalmol. **75:**157, 1966.

54. Treister, G., and Mannor, S.: Intraocular pressure and outflow facility, Arch. Ophthalmol. **83:**311, 1970.

55. Lee, P., Donovan, R. H., and Mukai, N.: Effects of norethynodrel with mestranol on the rabbit eye, Arch. Ophthalmol. **81:**89, 1969.

56. Whitworth, C. G., and Grant, W. M.: Use of nitrate and nitrite vasodilators by glaucomatous patients, Arch. Ophthalmol. **71:**492, 1964.

57. Grant, W. M.: Ocular complications of drugs, J.A.M.A. **207:**2089, 1969.

58. Riffenburgh, R. S.: Glaucoma therapy, Arch. Ophthalmol. **75:**204, 1966.

59. Spaeth, G. L.: Visual loss in a glaucoma clinic, Invest. Ophthalmol. **9:**73, 1970.

60. Bigger, J. F.: A comparison of patient compliance in treated versus untreated ocular hypertension, Trans. Am. Acad. Ophthalmol. Otolaryngol. **81:**277, 1976.

61. Wilensky, J. T., Buerk, K. M., and Podos, S. M.: Krukenberg's spindles, Am. J. Ophthalmol. **79:**220, February 1975.

62. Kass, M. A., Kolker, A. E., and Becker, B.: Prognostic factors in glaucomatous visual field loss, Arch. Ophthalmol. **94:**1274, August 1976.

63. Becker, B., and Shin, D. H.: Response to topical epinephrine, Arch. Ophthalmol. **94:**2057, December 1976.

64. Shin, D. H., Kolker, A. E., Kass, M. A., Kaback, M., and Becker, B.: Long-term epinephrine therapy of ocular hypertension, Arch. Ophthalmol. **94:**2059, December 1976.

65. Harbin, T. S., Jr., Podos, S. M., Kolker, A. E., and Becker, B.: Visual field progression in open-angle glaucoma patients presenting with monocular field loss, Trans. Am. Acad. Ophthalmol. Otolaryngol. **81:** OP-253, March-April 1976.

66. Phelps, C. D., Woolson, R. F., Kolker, A. E., and Becker, B.: Diurnal variation in intraocular pressure, Am. J. Ophthalmol. **77:**367, March 1974.

67. Shin, D. H., and Becker, B.: The prognostic value of HLA-B12 and HLA-B7 antigens in patients with increased intraocular pressure, Am. J. Ophthalmol. **82:**871, December 1976.

68. Anderson, D. R.: The management of ele-vated intraocular pressure with normal optic discs and visual fields. I. Therapeutic approach based on high risk factors, Surv. Ophthalmol. **21:**479, May-June 1977.

69. Goldmann, H.: An analysis of some concepts concerning chronic simple glaucoma, Am. J. Ophthalmol. **80:**409, September 1975.

70. Leydhecker, W.: The intraocular pressure: clinical aspects, Ann. Ophthalmol. **8:**389, April 1976.

71. Kitazawa, Y., and Horie, T.: Diurnal variation of intraocular pressure in primary open-angle glaucoma, Am. J. Ophthalmol. **79:** 557, April 1975.

72. Drance, S. M., Sweeney, V. P., Morgan, R. W., and Feldman, F.: Studies of factors involved in the production of low tension glaucoma, Arch. Ophthalmol. **89:**457, 1973.

73. van Herick, W., Shaffer, R. N., and Schwartz, A.: Estimation of width of angle of anterior chamber, Am. J. Ophthalmol. **68:** 626, 1969.

74. Harris, L. S., and Galin, M. A.: Prone provocative testing for narrow angle glaucoma, Arch. Ophthalmol. **87:**493, 1972.

75. Pollack, I. P.: Chronic angle-closure glaucoma, Arch. Ophthalmol. **85:**676, 1971.

76. Greco, J. J., and Kelman, C. D.: Systemic pilocarpine toxicity in the treatment of angle closure glaucoma, Ann. Ophthalmol. **5:**57, 1973.

77. Tyner, G. S., and Scheie, H. G.: Mechanism of miotic-resistant pupil with increased intraocular pressure, Arch. Ophthalmol. **50:** 572, 1953.

78. Rutkowski, P. C., and Thompson, H. S.: Mydriasis and increased intraocular pressure, Arch. Ophthalmol. **87:**21, 1972.

79. Charles, S. T., and Hamasaki, D. I.: The effect of intraocular pressure on the pupil size, Arch. Ophthalmol. **83:**729, 1970.

80. Gorin, G.: Angle closure glaucoma induced by miotics, Am. J. Ophthalmol. **62:**1063, 1966.

81. Galin, M., Aizawa, F., and McLean, J.: Intravenous urea in the treatment of acute angle closure glaucoma, Am. J. Ophthalmol. **50:**379, 1960.

82. Icaza, M. J.: Medical treatment of acute glaucoma, Arch. Ophthalmol. **35:**361, 1946.

83. Kitazawa, Y.: Primary angle-closure glaucoma, Arch. Ophthalmol. **84:**724, 1970.

84. Bienfang, D. C.: Sector pupillary dilatation with an epinephrine strip, Am. J. Ophthalmol. **75:**883, 1973.

85. Rodman, H. I.: Chronic open-angle glaucoma associated with traumatic dislocation of the lens, Arch. Ophthalmol. **69**:445, 1963.

86. Alper, M. G.: Contusion angle deformity and glaucoma, Arch. Ophthalmol. **69**:455, 1963.

87. Pettit, T., and Keates, E. U.: Traumatic cleavage of the chamber angle, Arch. Ophthalmol. **69**:438, 1963.

88. Armaly, M. F.: Inheritance of dexamethasone hypertension and glaucoma, Arch. Ophthalmol. **77**:747, 1967.

89. Palmer, E., Lieberman, T. W., and Burns, S.: Contusion angle deformity in prizefighters, Arch. Ophthalmol. **94**:225, February 1976.

90. Kaufman, J. H., and Tolpin, D. W.: Glaucoma after traumatic angle recession, Am. J. Ophthalmol. **78**:648, October 1974.

91. Posner, A., and Schlossman, A.: Syndrome of unilateral attacks of glaucoma with cyclitic symptoms, Arch. Ophthalmol. **39**:517, 1948.

92. Levatin, P.: Glaucomatocyclitic crises occurring in both eyes, Am. J. Ophthalmol. **41**:1056, 1956.

93. Simpson, D. G.: Glaucomatocyclitic crises, Am. J. Ophthalmol. **50**:163, 1960.

94. Spivey, B. E., and Armaly, M. F.: Tonographic findings in glaucomatocyclitic crises, Am. J. Ophthalmol. **55**:47, 1963.

95. Kass, M. A., Becker, B., and Kolker, A. E.: Glaucomatocyclitic crisis and primary open-angle glaucoma, Am. J. Ophthalmol. **75**:668, 1973.

96. Hung, P. T., and Chang, J. M.: Treatment of glaucomatocyclitic crises, Am. J. Ophthalmol. **77**:169, February 1974.

97. Masuda, K., Izawa, Y., and Mishima, S.: Prostaglandins and glaucomatocyclitic crisis, Jpn. J. Ophthalmol. **19**:368, 1975.

98. Harbin, T. S., Jr., and Pollack, I. P.: Glaucoma in episcleritis, Arch. Ophthalmol. **93**:948, October 1975.

99. Knox, D. L.: Glaucoma following syphilitic interstitial keratitis, Arch. Ophthalmol. **66**:18, 1961.

100. Sugar, H. S.: Late glaucoma associated with inactive syphilitic interstitial keratitis, Am. J. Ophthalmol. **53**:602, 1962.

101. Kornblueth, W., Abrahamov, A., Aladjemoff, L., Magora, F., and Gombros, G.: Intraocular pressure in the newborn measured under general anesthesia, Arch. Ophthalmol. **67**:750, 1962.

102. Kornblueth, W., Aladjemoff, L., Magora, F., and Ben Dor, D.: Intraocular pressure in children measured under general anesthesia, Arch. Ophthalmol. **72**:489, 1964.

103. Keates, R. H., and Cvintal, T.: Congenital hereditary corneal dystrophy, Am. J. Ophthalmol. **60**:892, 1965.

104. Maumenee, E.: Further observations on the pathogenesis of congenital glaucoma, Am. J. Ophthalmol. **55**:1163, 1963.

105. Haas, J.: Principles and problems of therapy in congenital glaucoma, Invest. Ophthalmol. **7**:140, 1968.

106. Scheie, H. G.: Infantile glaucoma and juvenile glaucoma, Trans. Am. Acad. Ophthalmol. Otolaryngol. **67**:458, 1963.

107. Reeh, M. J.: Bilateral congenital glaucoma, Trans. Am. Acad. Ophthalmol. Otolaryngol. **65**:178, 1961.

108. Sanders, T. E.: Intraocular juvenile xanthogranuloma (nevoxanthogranuloma), Trans. Am. Acad. Ophthalmol. Soc. **58**:59, 1960.

109. Tseng, S. S., and Keys, M. P.: Battered child syndrome simulating congenital glaucoma, Arch. Ophthalmol. **94**:839, May 1976.

110. Weiss, D. I., Shaffer, R. N., and Wise, B. L.: Mannitol infusion to reduce intraocular pressure, Arch. Ophthalmol. **68**:341, 1962.

111. Harris, L. S., and Galin, M. A.: Cycloplegic provocative testing, Arch. Ophthalmol. **81**:356, 1969.

112. Lowe, R. F.: Primary angle closure glaucoma, Am. J. Ophthalmol. **60**:415, 1965.

113. Lowe, R. F.: Primary angle closure glaucoma, Am. J. Ophthalmol. **65**:552, 1968.

114. Godel, V., Stein, R., and Feiler-Ofry, V.: Angle-closure glaucoma, Am. J. Ophthalmol. **65**:555, 1968.

115. Forbes, M., and Becker, B.: Iridectomy in advanced angle closure glaucoma, Am. J. Ophthalmol. **57**:57, 1964.

116. Lowe, R. F.: Primary angle closure glaucoma, Am. J. Ophthalmol. **58**:581, 1964.

117. Chandler, P.: Angle closure glaucoma, Arch. Ophthalmol. **53**:305, 1955.

118. Shaffer, R. N.: Open-angle glaucoma, Trans. Am. Acad. Ophthalmol. Otolaryngol. **67**:467, 1963.

119. Iliff, C. E., and Haas, J. S.: Posterior lip sclerectomy, Am. J. Ophthalmol. **54**:608, 1962.

120. Scheie, H. G.: Filtering operations for glaucoma: a comparative study, Am. J. Ophthalmol. **53**:571, 1962.

121. Becker, B., and Hahn, K. A.: Topical corticosteroids and heredity in primary open-

angle glaucoma, Am. J. Ophthalmol. **57:** 543, 1964.

122. Sugar, H. S.: Clinical effect of corticosteroids on conjunctival filtering blebs, Am. J. Ophthalmol. **59:**854, 1965.

123. Friedman, B. B.: Flat anterior chamber, Am. J. Ophthalmol. **61:**912, 1966.

124. Grady, F. J., and Forbes, M.: Tissue adhesive for repair of conjunctival buttonhole in glaucoma surgery, Am. J. Ophthalmol. **68:** 656, 1969.

125. Sugar, H. S.: Treatment of hypotony following filtering surgery for glaucoma, Am. J. Ophthalmol. **71:**1023, 1971.

126. Balakrishnan, E., and Abraham, J. E.: Chandler's operation for malignant glaucoma, Arch. Ophthalmol. **82:**723, 1969.

127. Rieser, J. C., and Schwartz, B.: Mioticinduced malignant glaucoma, Arch. Ophthalmol. **87:**706, 1972.

128. Levene, R.: A new concept of malignant glaucoma, Arch. Ophthalmol. **87:**497, 1972.

129. Chandler, P. A., Simmons, R. J., and Grant, W. M.: Malignant glaucoma, Am. J. Ophthalmol. **66:**495, 1968.

130. Chandler, P. A., and Grant, W. M.: Mydriatic cycloplegic treatment in malignant glaucoma, Arch. Ophthalmol. **68:**353, 1962.

131. Weiss, D. I., Shaffer, R. N., and Harrington, D. O.: Treatment of malignant glaucoma with intravenous mannitol infusion, Arch. Ophthalmol. **69:**154, 1963.

35
INFECTION

For therapeutic purposes, organization of this subject matter according to the characteristics of the offending microorganism seems preferable to the usual arrangement based on ocular anatomy. Nevertheless, the behavior of the eye exposed to infection is our primary interest. A few general comments will precede description of the specific organisms.

GENERAL PRINCIPLES

The virulence and number of microorganisms are known to be parameters influencing the severity of an infection. Variations in host response are also significantly responsible for differences in the severity of an infection. The severity of 54 cases of blepharoconjunctivitis was found to correlate well with the serum immunoglobulin levels of the patients. The mean immunoglobulin (IgM) value for normal persons was 134 mg/100 ml; for patients with mild staphylococcal infection, 135 mg/100 ml; and for patients with severe disease, 95 mg/100 ml.[1] This demonstration of lowered host resistance explains the susceptibility of some individuals to recurrent severe blepharoconjunctivitis. Lacking innate antibacterial defenses, such patients will be more than usually dependent on antibiotic therapy repeated as often as required by recurrent blepharoconjunctivitis.

Indeed, ocular infections may be the first manifestation of a serious resistance-lowering systemic disease. For example, bilateral peripheral ring ulcers of the cornea heralded the onset of acute leukemia in a 53-year-old woman.[2] Ring ulcers have also been reported in association with the different collagen diseases and a variety of severe systemic infections; their occurrence should suggest the possibility of such serious systemic problems. As another example of reduced resistance, the frequent association of herpes zoster with blood dyscrasias is well known.

The importance of normal nasolacrimal function in defense against bacterial infections of the cornea and conjunctiva was experimentally demonstrated by diathermy occlusion of the rabbit lacrimal punctum.[3] Only the right lacrimal system was blocked; the left eyes served as a control. After complete healing, the existence of the punctum block was confirmed by a slit-lamp examination and the presence of epiphora. Uniform superficial corneal abrasions were made bilaterally, and each eye of 28 rabbits was inoculated with a drop of *Pseudomonas aeruginosa* broth culture. Corneal infection occurred in all 28 eyes with blocked puncta, but in only 1 of the 28 eyes with open lacrimal passages. From the clinical standpoint, interference with the normal cleaning flow of tears (as by patching of the eye) has an adverse effect on the healing of external ocular infections.

Patching of an eye promotes the growth of any microorganism that may happen to be in the conjunctival sac. All of 24 *Pseudomonas*-inoculated and patched rabbit eyes developed severe conjunctivitis.[4] In contrast, 20 of 24 similarly inoculated but unpatched eyes

636

showed no conjunctivitis at all after 48 hours. Clinical experience indicates that human eyes respond similarly—witness the frequent development of blepharoconjunctivitis in the patched but unoperated fellow eye in retinal detachment patients, for instance. Indeed, patching has been suggested as a means of increasing the severity of an obscure chronic lid infection to the point that the offending organisms can more easily be identified.

Without doubt an eye significantly infected by bacteria should not be patched unless effective antibiotics are simultaneously being used.

Attempts to prevent postoperative infection must consider the usual origin of ocular infections. Preoperative cultures were available in seven cases of postoperative infection.[5] In each instance the same organism found preoperatively (identified by phage typing) was responsible for the infection. This indicates that the patient is the usual source of postoperative eye infections. Hence special attention should be given to ensuring that lids, conjunctiva, and lacrimal apparatus are free of infection before intraocular surgery is performed. (This report originated from an institution using meticulous aseptic operative technique—obviously the operating room personnel can be the source of infection if they become careless.)

Although it is apparent that the microorganism causing an endophthalmitis is not necessarily the same as that recovered from the surface of the eye, such a similarity may exist. Separate cultures from lids and conjunctivas of each eye of 410 patients indicated that the presence of a given microorganism on one eye suggests strongly that it is present on the other eye.[6]

Since postoperative endophthalmitis commonly is caused by the patient's own microorganisms, a high correlation should exist between cultures of the conjunctival sac and the intraocular infection. Treatment of such infections should certainly include antibiotics capable of inhibiting organisms grown from conjunctival cultures. However, infections following penetrating wounds will commonly result from organisms on the foreign body, which are unlikely to be identified from surface cultures.

A variant of self-originating infection concerns the role of eye cosmetics in initiating and perpetuating minor or serious eye infections. Although eye cosmetics are sterile when purchased, repeated use often results in heavy contamination, as indicated in a study of 153 college students.[7] In a series of 22 women with chronic bacterial blepharitis, heavy contamination of their cosmetics with *Staphylococcus epidermidis* was uniformly present. A vicious cycle results, in which more contaminated mascara is applied to conceal the more severely infected lid. From the practical standpoint, use of eye makeup should be avoided before eye surgery.

UNDESIRABLE DRUGS

Probably through tradition, ophthalmologists tend to use streptomycin as part of a shotgun therapy of eye infections. For instance, treatment of five patients with postoperative endophthalmitis with methicillin (4 g/day), chloramphenicol (4 g/day), streptomycin (3 g/day), and prednisone (60 mg/day) was reported.[8] Such therapy is dangerously obsolete. Since the advent of streptomycin, a considerable number of less toxic antibiotics effective against gram-negative organisms have been developed. Chloramphenicol, the tetracyclines, and ampicillin are well-known examples. Streptomycin does not readily penetrate the blood-aqueous barrier and is therefore not nearly so effective as chloramphenicol against intraocular infections. Most strains of *Pseudomonas* are resistant to streptomycin. Most important, streptomycin causes irreversible vestibular nerve damage. It has been aptly stated that the current indications for streptomycin are limited to tularemia, tuberculosis, and the plague.

Corticosteroid therapy of acute ocular infections should also be questioned. Laboratory studies indicate that intraocular infections treated with adequate dosages of effective antibiotics may result in less scarring if corticosteroid therapy is also employed. In clinical practice the organism causing postoperative endophthalmitis is rarely known. (In none of the five cases cited in the previous paragraph was the causative organism reported.) The possibility of infection by a resistant bacterium, fungus, or virus is very real. Few facts in clinical therapy are more certain than that corticosteroids will reduce host resistance to microorganisms. I consider corticosteroid therapy of intraocular infection to be a very dangerous practice. Possibly the best indication for corticosteroid therapy of postoperative infections is the possibility of inaccurate diagnosis, the supposed "infection" really being a traumatic uveitis—which would, of course, respond to corticosteroid therapy.

Let us evaluate a study that concluded, "Retrobulbar corticosteroids in combination with effective antibiotic therapy effectively treated experimental bacterial endophthalmitis."[9] The experiment involved intravitreal injection of penicillin G–sensitive *Staphylococcus aureus* in 113 rabbits, subsequently treated with retrobulbar injection of 100 mg penicillin G, combined in some cases with 25 mg prednisolone or 4 mg dexamethasone, repeated daily for 10 days. At the end of 10 days the density of vitreous infiltrate was not significantly different between the antibiotic-corticosteroid and the antibiotic alone groups. However, at the end of 60 days, the fundus was visible in 64% of eyes treated with penicillin and corticosteroid, but in only 39% treated only with penicillin—a significant difference.

While this sounds good, the fine print reports that 14 corticosteroid-treated eyes *were eliminated from the study* because they developed corneal ulcers so severe as to preclude seeing the red reflex! *Only* corticosteroid-treated eyes developed such ulcers, indicating that this treatment has serious complications. The article cites only percentages instead of numbers of eyes, so accurate statistical correction for these 14 excluded eyes is not possible. However, only 59 animals (including controls) remained alive at 60 days. These 14 excluded eyes may have represented as many as 30% of the corticosteroid-treated eyes. Recalculation with this assumption indicates that 60% to 70% of the cortico-

steroid-treated eyes were so severely diseased as to preclude fundus visualization—essentially *the same* percentage as the eyes treated only with penicillin. It is hardly fair to sweep a 30% incidence of corneal ulcers under the rug just because you want to recommend corticosteroid use in treatment of infections.

SURGICAL INFECTIONS

Patients of retinal detachment surgeons seem to have more than their share of infections, a fact presumably related to the extensive procedures employed and to the use of implanted foreign materials.

Inflammatory changes after retinal detachment surgery may be caused by postoperative uveitis or by bacterial infection, a much more serious condition. Many surgeons use topical corticosteroid therapy routinely to suppress such postoperative inflammation. (I have personally avoided routine postoperative corticosteroid therapy because of concern about encouraging infection.) Corticosteroid therapy is useless and probably detrimental if the inflammation is caused by infection.

In a series of 231 scleral buckling procedures, eight cases of scleral abscess occurred.[10] Pain that becomes more severe on the fourth to ninth postoperative day is the most characteristic symptom. Proptosis, ecchymosis, prolapse of conjunctiva, and clouding of the vitreous confirm the diagnosis of scleral abscess. The causative organism can usually be cultured from the conjunctival sac. Intensive systemic use of antibiotics effective against the isolated organism will reduce the severity of reaction, but early removal of the implanted silicone buckling material is essential to maintain clear vitreous and a useful eye. Prompt recognition of the existence of infection and early implant removal is most important if endophthalmitis and destruction of the eye are to be avoided.

The chronic granulomas that occur (8% to 20% reported incidence) following placement of a hollow polyethylene circling tube do not respond to treatment with topical or systemic antibiotics and/or corticosteroids.[11,12] Surgical removal of the suture and flushing of the tube with antibiotic may clear the granuloma; however, usually the tube itself must be removed. Injection of chloramphenicol suspension into the tube at the time of surgery will prevent granuloma formation, which is a result of low-grade chronic infection of the dead space inside the tube. Actually, the use of tubes is now obsolete, having been superseded by solid silicone rods or by fascia lata.

The currently popular silicone sponge explants are prone to develop infection. This can be minimized by saturating the sponge with an antibiotic before insertion.

A 4% incidence of rejection of silicone material because of infection is fairly representative.[13] Interestingly, the preoperative preparation in this series consisted only of scrubbing and flushing the operative area with saline. Why a surgeon would not take advantage of the germicidal activity of preparation agents such as povidone-iodine (Betadine) is unclear to me.

Experimentally, the combination of infecting organisms, implanted silicone material, and scleral necrosis induced by diathermy was required to produce scleral abscess.[14] Substitution of cryotherapy for diathermy prevented experimental abscess formation. A mycotic abscess after silicone implantation required enucleation in one case.[15]

The most effective way to prevent late infection of implanted foreign circling material is to use donor human fascia lata for the implanted material. The technique is comparable to the use of any other circling material and has a number of advantages besides freedom from infection.* I have performed this procedure up to 500 times annually and have encountered late infection only in several cases. In each instance, exploration revealed the focus of infection to be at the site of a silk suture knot, while the fascial strip itself was free of infection.

---

*For a discussion of implantation technique, see Havener, W. H., and Gloeckner, S.: Atlas of diagnostic techniques and treatment of retinal detachment, St. Louis, 1967, The C. V. Mosby Co.

Corneal transplantation

Bacteriologic study of 240 donor eyes obtained for corneal transplantation showed 100% to be contaminated. The types of microflora were approximately comparable to those found in the living eye; however, the number of organisms was enormously greater in the dead eyes. *Pseudomonas* contamination affected 4% of the donor eyes.[16]

Various methods of attempted sterilization of donor eyes have been evaluated. Immersion in 1:5000 thimerosal (Merthiolate) for up to 45 minutes did not reduce the number of contaminating microorganisms. Sterilization of some eyes was achieved by 30-minute immersion in 1:1000 benzalkonium chloride, but this treatment caused the corneal stroma to become hazy. Exposure to 1:1000 benzalkonium together with ultrasonic agitation for 1 minute effectively sterilized the donor eyes but caused serious endothelial damage that rendered the cornea unsuitable for transplantation. Ethylene oxide gas sterilization for 2 hours was effective but also damaged the endothelium. Irrigation with Neosporin solution (polymyxin B, gramicidin, and neomycin), 0.5 ml for 2 minutes, resulted in sterile cultures from 16 of 22 eyes. Since treatment with Neosporin was the most effective method of destroying bacteria and because it did not damage the donor cornea, this method of caring for donor eyes has been recommended.[17]

Vitreous transplantation

Further proof of antibiotic penetration into normal eyes is provided by a study of the so-called antibacterial effect of human vitreous.[18,19] This phenomenon, found in vitreous from eye bank eyes, is caused by premortem antibiotic therapy in these patients or by antibiotics applied during postmortem storage.[20] No antibacterial effect was found in vitreous obtained from patients who had not received antibiotics. Penicillinase destroyed the antibacterial effect found in vitreous from four patients who had received penicillin. The effect of antibiotics used during eye bank storage was studied with the aid of a pair of eyes from the same patient. From one eye vitreous was immediately aspirated. The other eye was stored for several weeks in a contact with a solution containing 0.1% polymyxin B and 0.5% neomycin sulfate before aspiration and culture of vitreous. Sufficient antibiotic penetrated into the vitreous of the second eye to cause a marked antibacterial effect that was absent in the vitreous from the first eye. Storage of eye bank eyes in contact with antibiotics would seem to be of value.

Philosophically, the reasons why anyone would want to transplant a suspension of contaminated viscous debris into an eye escape me completely.

Tonometry

Tonometer sterilization is one of the most important ophthalmologic uses of bactericidal agents. Unfortunately the design of a Schiøtz tonometer is such that it is virtually impossible to sterilize by any practical means. Alcohol, ether, benzalkonium chloride (Zephiran), nitromersol (Metaphen), and many other similar sterilizing solutions not hazardous to the eye have been proved inadequate to destroy many types of virulent organisms and spores. Similarly, moist and dry heat and ultraviolet light are ineffective methods for tonometer sterilization. Covering the footplate of the tonometer with very thin, disposable sterile latex "Tonofilms" has been advocated as the only certain way to prevent spread of infection by the tonometer.[21]

Although the limitations of sterilizing solutions must be clearly recognized, clinical experience with the many thousands of pressure measurements that have been taken by conscientious ophthalmologists proves that infection is not a common problem if reasonable precautions are taken. Thorough periodic cleaning of the tonometer (at least once weekly, depending on frequency of use) and constant deep immersion of the footplate end in a solution such as 1:5000 benzalkonium chloride will eliminate a considerable number of microorganisms. Most important is avoidance of gross contamination of the tonometer by eyes red from infection or crusted with discharge. In addition to con-taminating the instrument, tonometry in such eyes predisposes them to self-infection of minor abrasions. Remember that sterilizing solutions tolerated by the eye will not dependably destroy viruses, bacteria, and fungi; therefore do not expect these solutions to compensate for failure to maintain the tonometer under clean conditions.

The applanation tonometer is not only more accurate, but it has a more sterilizable structure. The polished tip may simply be wiped with moist cotton. Experimental contamination with *Pseudomonas* was reliably removed by such simple wiping.[22] Viral contamination was also removed by simply wiping with moist cotton.[23] As a matter of fact, the transmission of adenovirus epidemic keratoconjunctivitis probably occurs more frequently via the contaminated hands of medical personnel than from infected instruments. Witness that the personnel themselves contract keratoconjunctivitis by touching their own eyes. *Wash your hands!*

ENDOPHTHALMITIS
Diagnostic technique

Faced with an apparent intraocular infection, the ophthalmologist must differentiate an aseptic inflammatory response from the presence of microorganisms. Although clinical criteria are helpful in preliminary differentiation, laboratory studies are more definitive and also permit identification of the specific organism and its sensitivity to antibiotics.

Unless specimen material is discharging through an incision or fistula leading to the interior of the infected eye, cultures of the surface of the eye or eyelids will not necessarily identify the same organism that exists within the eye. In the absence of faults of operating room technique, however, the microflora of the patient's own lids and lacrimal apparatus are the most likely source of endophthalmitis. Hence the responsible organism for a postoperative endophthalmitis might also exist on the eyelids.

The question of validity of intraocular specimens in diagnosing endophthalmitis was studied in rabbit eyes.[24] Staphylococci and *Pseudomonas* were inoculated into the anterior chamber. Of 17 eyes inoculated with *Staphylococcus albus*, 12 developed infection; from these 12, in nine cases the organism was identified by culture of aqueous obtained by paracentesis. In all the eyes developing infection resulting from *Staphylococcus aureus* or *Pseudomonas*, the organism was identified by paracentesis (Table 35-1).[24] Under the conditions of this study, therefore, the responsible organism could be identified in about 85% of cases of experimental endophthalmitis. This result suggests that there may be clinical cases (15%?) of endophthalmitis that would be mistakenly diagnosed as aseptic iritis on the basis of a negative culture. Still, an 85% correct yield suggests that paracentesis may be a valuable diagnostic technique.

In the clinical counterpart of the preceding study, intraocular cultures were obtained from 33 eyes diagnosed as endophthalmitis. Positive cultures were obtained from 14 eyes; of these, only three eyes retained useful vision. (*Staphylococcus epidermidis* was the organism recovered from all three salvaged eyes.) No growth was obtained from 14 eyes; of these, 13 eyes retained useful vision. In five eyes the isolation was considered questionable, since it was not present on more than one culture medium. The authors believed that sterile inflammation is present in most cases in which organisms cannot be recovered from paracentesis.

If diagnostic paracentesis is to be performed, it is probably better done in the operating room. Under these circumstances, the aspirated material is less likely to become contaminated. Also, facilities are available for dealing with unexpected contingencies. Of the above 33 eyes, "several" suffered dehiscence of a recent cataract incision or rupture of an infected filtering bleb. We have experienced rupture of a softened cornea during manipulation of an endophthalmitis about 1 week old. Obviously, paracentesis is not without inherent dangers and should not be done lightly, without adequate indications.

Analysis of 27 eyes with positive cultures indicated that the vitreous (if obtainable) was a more reliable sample than was the aqueous. Of these 27 eyes, there were 18 anterior chamber samples, of which 10 were positive. There were 20 vitreous samples, of which all 20 were positive (and seven concomitant aqueous samples were negative). Four dehiscent wound cultures were all positive.[25] In no instance was there a positive aqueous and a negative vitreous aspirate.

The technique used was razor blade limbal partial keratotomy (not quite entering the anterior chamber). Through this incision, a 25-gauge needle was introduced to obtain 0.1 to 0.2 ml of aqueous. Subsequently, a 22-gauge needle was passed through the same site to aspirate 0.2 to 0.3 ml of vitreous fluid.

Another method of obtaining vitreous samples is the use of a vitrectomy instrument.[26] This is aggressive management and should certainly be reserved for cases in which the diagnosis seems absolutely certain.

Therapy

Intravitreal instillation of antibiotics may be conveniently done immediately after these surgical diagnostic procedures. The tolerance of the eye for antibiotics introduced into the vitreous is very low. Only 0.1 to 0.2 mg of gentamicin is the maximum safe dose in the rabbit eye.[27] Larger amounts alter the ERG and cause cataract. Vision of 20/400 or

Table 35-1. Eyes inoculated with bacteria: comparison of clinical infection and positive isolation

Inoculum	No. of eyes	Clinical infection	Positive isolate*
Staphylococcus albus	17	12	9
Staphylococcus aureus	8	5	5
Pseudomonas fluorescens	9	5	5
Controls	15	0	0

From Tucker, D. N., and Forster, R. K.: Arch. Ophthalmol. **88**:647, December 1972. Copyright 1972, American Medical Association.

*Positive isolate only from group with clinical infection.

better was obtained in only six of 15 culture-positive eyes treated with intravitreal gentamicin, 0.1 mg, and cephaloridine, 0.25 mg. Five of these six effectively treated infections were caused by *Staphylococcus epidermidis*, the other, *Propionibacterium acnes*. Both of these are organisms of low virulence and would more likely have responded to conventional extraocular routes of antibiotic administration. The obvious question is whether the risk of intraocular antibiotic injection is justified, when contrasted to the effectiveness of parenteral or subconjunctival routes.

A higher dosage (0.4 mg) of gentamicin was injected intravitreally in five infected eyes.[28] The visual results were 20/50 *(Diplococcus pneumoniae)*, 20/300 *(Hemophilus influenzae)*, hand movements *(Proteus mirabilis)*, 20/400 *(Proteus morgani)*, and 20/40 *(Staphylococcus aureus)*. These eyes also were injected with 0.36 mg of dexamethasone.

Orbital cellulitis

The seriousness of this infection is indicated by the fact that 29% of 104 pediatric patients had bacteremia and four suffered meningitis. Paranasal sinusitis was present in 77 patients (84%). However, antibiotic management sufficed in all cases; no sinus surgery was performed. *Hemophilus influenzae* is a major cause of orbital cellulitis in children and requires fortified chocolate blood agar for its growth. Ampicillin (effective against *H. influenzae*) and methicillin (effective against penicillinase-producing staphylococci) were used in treatment of these cases.[29]

An unusual diagnostic characteristic of *Hemophilus* cellulitis is that it causes a blue-purple discoloration of the overlying skin, unlike the usual inflammatory redness.[30]

BACTERIA

On the basis of their ocular significance, the bacteria selected for discussion will include *Staphylococcus, Pseudomonas, Neisseria gonorrhoeae, Mycobacterium tuberculosis,* and *Clostridium.* Obviously a multitude of other organisms may infect the eye.

The microorganisms isolated from 2160 cases of suspected bacterial conjunctivitis (Los Angeles, 1962 to 1965) suggest the frequency with which various types of bacteria will be encountered in surface eye infections.[31] The commonest organism was *Staphylococcus* (47.8% coagulase negative; 14.7% coagulase positive). *Corynebacterium diphtheriae* was isolated in 13.4%; alpha hemolytic streptococcus, 8.6%; and *Pseudomonas,* 1.4%. Other organisms isolated were found with less than 1% frequency.

Representative antibiotic sensitivities of coagulase-positive staphylococci are reported

Table 35-2. Antibiotic sensitivity of coagulase-positive *Staphylococcus aureus* isolated from conjunctiva*

Antibiotic	Suie—1957 % sensitive of 115 cases	Nicholas—1965 % sensitive of 306 cases
Bacitracin	86.8	94
Chloramphenicol	72.6	96
Erythromycin	56.3	91
Neomycin	64.8	95
Novobiocin	—	97
Penicillin	62.6	65
Tetracycline	78.2	67

*Modified from Nicholas, J. P., and Goolden, E. B.: Arch. Ophthalmol. **75:**639, 1966.

Table 35-3. Antibiotic sensitivity of *Pseudomonas* species isolated from conjunctivae (31 isolates)*

Antibiotic	Number of isolates Sensitive	Resistant
Bacitracin	1	30
Chloramphenicol	8	23
Erythromycin	2	29
Neomycin	28	3
Novobiocin	0	31
Penicillin	0	31
Polymyxin B	30	1
Tetracycline	0	28

*From Nicholas, J. P., and Goolden, E. B.: Arch. Ophthalmol. **75:**639, 1966.

in Table 35-2.[31] Such data are of obvious value in guiding the arbitrary selection of antibiotics for use in treatment of minor surface infections of the eye.

The antibiotic sensitivities of *Pseudomonas* (Table 35-3) are quite different from those of *Staphylococcus.*

Conjunctival culture of 20 racetrack employees engaged in the handling of horses or stable maintenance confirmed the expectation that occupational exposure will increase the frequency of eye contamination.[32] Micrococci were isolated from all of these 40 eyes. Aerobic spore-forming bacilli were identified in seven eyes. Infection was not clinically evident in any of these eyes. The physician should be particularly alert to the danger of infection after injury or surgery of eyes of patients employed in a dirty environment.

Staphylococcus

Staphylococcus aureus is the potentially pathogenic microorganism most frequently found in and about the eye and was recovered in 33.6% of 6523 eye cultures.[33] Identification of a given strain of staphylococci is possible through bacteriophage typing, which consists of the determination of staphylococcal susceptibility to destruction by a given type of bacteriophage. In this study of 525 patients, 26 types of bacteriophage were used, and the following conclusions were drawn:

1. Only a single phage type of *Staphylococcus aureus* is generally present in an eye. This is true of infected or noninfected eyes.
2. An individual with one infected eye usually carries the same strain of *Staphylococcus* in the noninfected eye!
3. The same phage type of *Staphylococcus* found in the eye commonly exists in contiguous areas (nose, face, hands, ears).
4. An individual frequently carries the same strain of *Staphylococcus* for 6 months or more.
5. Elimination of staphylococci by antibiotics applied to the eye is usually temporary; reinfection presumably occurs from contiguous areas within a few days.
6. Family or hospital contacts are a source of infection and commonly carry the same staphylococcal strain as the patient.
7. In seven cases of postoperative eye infection, preoperative cultures were available, and in *every* case, the eye carried before operation the same phage type that was responsible for the infection. Furthermore, the same type was found also in the "uninfected" eye and in contiguous areas such as the nose.

Probably all people have *Staphylococcus aureus* on their eyelids from one fourth to one third of the time. It is not true that some people have staphylococci on their lids almost all the time whereas others almost never do. Because of the great variability of staphylococcal contamination, there is at least a 20% chance that *Staphylococcus aureus* will be present on the eyelids on the day of surgery, even if cultures were negative the day before.[34]

Culture of one nostril of 30 members of an ophthalmology staff permitted recovery of *Staphylococcus aureus* from 15 individuals.[35]

The infective potential of *Staphylococcus aureus* is well recognized clinically. This organism is responsible for about half of all cases of endophthalmitis occurring after cataract surgery. Experimental inoculation of the rabbit anterior chamber resulted in severe panophthalmitis when the inoculum contained 1000 to 3000 organisms of coagulase-positive *Staphylococcus aureus*. In contrast, 5 to 15 million organisms of *Staphylococcus pyogenes albus* were required to cause intraocular infection. Nevertheless, cases of *Staphylococcus pyogenes albus* endophthalmitis do occur following cataract surgery and the preoperative presence of this relatively benign organism cannot be ignored.[36]

The variable antibiotic resistance of staphylococcal strains is well known. Prediction of the most effective antibiotics for a given infection is not reliable without culture identification and sensitivity studies. Development of a penicillin (methicillin) resistant to the action of staphylococcal penicillinase has been invaluable in the management of staphylococcal infections. Of 8060 clinical staphylococcal isolates, 99% were sensitive to 6.25 μg/ml of methicillin.*

Staphylococcus epidermidis is typically described as being nonpathogenic. For example, preoperative cultures in 638 patients before retinal detachment surgery were reported as disclosing "contamination by pathogens" in 5%. The pathogens referred to were *Staphylococcus aureus, Proteus, Klebsiella,* and *Pseudomonas*. The presence of *Staphylococcus epidermidis* in 37% of cases was not included in the pathogenic classification. Yet, in this series, the silicone implant required removal because of infection in 4% of the cases, and half of these infections were caused by *Staphylococcus epidermidis*.[13]

Although *Staphylococcus epidermidis* is less virulent than the major pathogens, it is certainly capable of causing both extraocular and intraocular infections. Because of the great frequency with which it inhabits the body surface, *Staphylococcus epidermidis* may be a common cause of ocular infections.

Pseudomonas

Effective treatment of *Pseudomonas* infections requires recognition that these bacteria may persist in the eye for a long time despite therapy, that original infection or reactivation of infection may readily be produced by corticosteroid therapy, and that *Pseudomonas* infections commonly are contaminated with other bacteria (pneumococci or streptococci, for example) or viruses (such as herpes simplex).[37] Furthermore, *Pseudomonas* keratitis may be rapidly destructive.

Practical suggestions for treatment emphasize prompt diagnosis. The purulent exudate of a *Pseudomonas* ulcer fluoresces under a Woods' ultraviolet light. (The corneal ulcer itself does *not* fluoresce.) Long, thin, gram-negative bacteria may be recognized in the initial scrapings from the ulcer. Because of the variable growth characteristics, both liq-

uid (thioglycollate or broth) and solid culture media are recommended. The isolation of multiple varieties of microorganisms should be interpreted to mean infection by these multiple organisms and not culture contamination. *Pseudomonas pyocyanea* can inhibit growth of other microorganisms in the culture media.

Frequent topical applications of polymyxin B, colistin, or gentamicin will inhibit *Pseudomonas*. Almost all strains are highly sensitive to 6.25 μg/ml or less of these drugs. Subconjunctival injection of polymyxin B and colistin is severely irritating and of questionable additional value. Since polymyxin B is ineffective against gram-positive organisms and because mixed infections commonly occur, antibiotics effective against gram-positive organisms should also be used. Gentamicin is effective against both *Pseudomonas* and gram-positive organisms. Antibiotic instillation should be as frequent as every 30 minutes until the acute infection is controlled.

Case reports document severely destructive relapses of *Pseudomonas* infection as late as 2 months after control of the original ulcer. Most such eyes have been treated with corticosteroids in an attempt to reduce corneal scarring and vascularization. To my mind the concept of combined corticosteroid-antibiotic treatment of any infection is questionable, but in the case of *Pseudomonas* infection such management is positively contraindicated. The source of the reinfection after negative culture is not documented, but persistence of the germ on other body surfaces seems probable and has been well documented as a source of ocular reinfection by many other organisism. Do not use corticosteroids in the management of any stage of *Pseudomonas* keratitis, early or late.

Atropinization for associated iritis is appropriate.

Does *Pseudomonas* keratitis respond better to gentamicin, colistin, or polymyxin B? To answer this question, 0.05% solutions of each drug were instilled every 2 hours as treatment of experimental *Pseudomonas* keratitis in rabbits.[38] For practical purposes, the three drugs were equally effective.

---

* Data from Bristol package circular, 1968.

Carbenicillin, a semisynthetic penicillin derivative, is effective against *Pseudomonas*. Daily subconjunctival injection of 0.5 ml of a 20% solution of carbenicillin sterilized experimental *Pseudomonas* corneal ulcers (in rabbits) within 2 days. The use of a combination of gentamicin, 10 mg, and carbenicillin, 100 mg, was not significantly more or less effective than the use of either drug alone or of 5 mg of polymyxin B.[39]

The resistance of *Pseudomonas* to most antibiotics is well known. Of 400 clinically isolated strains of *Pseudomonas*, 88% were sensitive to colistin, 88% to polymyxin B, 55% to sulfacetamide, 19% to chloramphenicol, 10% to tetracycline, and 1% to penicillin.[40] Ophthalmologists find chloramphenicol most valuable because it penetrates the blood-aqueous barrier, but they must be aware that this drug is not likely to benefit *Pseudomonas* infections.

Gentamicin therapy of a *Pseudomonas*-infected rabbit cornea is not capable of controlling the infection and saving the cornea when treatment is begun after 24 hours of infection.[41]

A thought-provoking article indicates that the visual end result was essentially the same in *Pseudomonas* corneal ulcers whether or not they received specific antibiotic therapy.[42] Nine untreated patients from San Salvador were compared with nine California patients treated with colistin or polymyxin B. Vision of 20/400 or better was achieved by three San Salvador patients and by two California patients. One of each group required enucleation. In three San Salvador and six California patients the result was finger counting to light perception vision. Two San Salvador patients had no light perception.

A summary of reports from a number of investigators stated that 19 of 23 patients with *Pseudomonas* keratitis responded to topical application, 1 or 2 drops hourly, of a 0.1% solution of colistin. Visual results were not specified.[43]

Although keratoconjunctivitis is ordinarily considered to be a threat only to the eye, a premature infant has such poor resistance that conjunctival infection with a virulent organism may result in fatal systemic infection. Four fatal cases of *Pseudomonas aeruginosa* conjunctivitis in premature children[44] should alert us to the fact that conjunctivitis in the premature infant is potentially far more serious than in an adult. Identification by culture and prompt antibiotic treatment are indicated.

Flavobacterium meningosepticum is a gram-negative rod morphologically and culturally similar to *Pseudomonas*, but which differs in its antibiotic sensitivity. Isolation of a "*Pseudomonas* species" resistant to aminoglycosides and carbenicillin is sufficiently unique to question the accuracy of the identification. *Flavobacterium* may be sensitive to erythromycin, rifampin, and sulfonamides. The organism is discussed under the heading of *Pseudomonas* to emphasize the diagnostic difficulties that permit misidentification of microorganisms. In this particular case report,[45] *Flavobacterium* infection caused loss of an eye following corneal transplantation despite topical instillation of 1% prednisolone and hydrocortisone every 2 hours, daily sub-Tenon's injections of 4 mg of dexamethasone, and 80 mg of oral prednisone daily. I realize clinical mythology represents corticosteroid therapy as being capable of reducing the scarring of ocular infection. Still, the reports of lost eyes include the use of corticosteroids so frequently as to confirm the known facts that such treatment results in immunologic incompetence, thereby enhancing growth of microorganisms. For some reason, clinicians have difficulty comprehending that drugs can do harm to their own patients.

Neisseria gonorrhoeae

Gonorrheal keratoconjunctivitis is notorious for its ability to cause disabling permanent corneal scarring, particularly in the infant. Not quite 90 years ago, Credé reported the incidence of ophthalmia neonatorum to be 226 of 2266 newborns (10%). A single application of 2% silver nitrate reduced the disease incidence to 4 of 1160 infants (0.5%).

Although silver nitrate is unquestionably of benefit in reducing the frequency of gonorrheal ophthalmia, it has several disadvantages. As anyone brave enough to instill the drug into his own eye will testify, the pain is of disabling intensity. All patients develop a chemical conjunctivitis, which is commonly superinfected by staphylococci. Purulent bacterial conjunctivitis occurred in 17.5% of 1000 infants after silver nitrate prophylaxis.[46]

Perhaps the most serious potential objection to silver nitrate is the possibility of false reassurance to patient and physician. Gonococcal ophthalmia does occur despite silver nitrate prophylaxis. In fairness to silver nitrate, however, it is doubtful that a single instillation of any drug into the eyes of an infant actually exposed to infection will invariably prevent gonococcal ophthalmia.

Because prophylaxis is not always effective, reliance should be placed on observation of the baby's eyes during the postpartum period. Despite popular belief, the normal infant eye does not discharge (unless irritated by prophylaxis or infection, which is not normal). Antibiotic therapy is so reliable that not a single serious eye lesion resulted from any of 49 cases of gonorrheal ophthalmia neonatorum.[47] Hence, substituting observation for prophylaxis does not jeopardize the eye.

When the precaution of routine postpartum eye inspection is followed in the nursery, there is virtually no need for prophylaxis in good economic areas. Because of the high incidence in poor socioeconomic areas, routine postpartum eye inspection is most important in addition to and despite prophylaxis (Table 35-4).[47]

The value of prophylaxis in poor socioeconomic areas is clearly illustrated in Table 35-5.[47] At the end of 1956, mandatory prophylaxis was abolished in New York City. Nevertheless, customary medical practice continues to employ prophylaxis in most patients.

If prophylaxis is to be used, what is the best drug? Silver acetate is said to be as effective as silver nitrate, yet has the safety factor of insolubility beyond 1.2%. This prevents accidental use of excessively strong concentration.[48] Silver ions are bound and inactivated by the chlorides and protein in tear film, ocular discharge, and conjunctival surface. Permanent corneal scarring may be caused by accidental use of 10% silver nitrate.

The quaternary ammonium compounds are more effective germicides than is silver nitrate in the presence of serum and chlorides.[49] They are much less irritating to the eye, are good wetting agents and therefore penetrate well into the crevices of the cul-de-sac, and can also be used for cleaning the lids and face.[50] Sulfacetamide (10% ointment or 30% drops) has been advocated for the advantages of effectiveness, freedom from irritation, stability, and rarity of allergic reactions.[51,52]

Many authors have advocated the prophylactic use of antibiotics by local instillation or injection at birth. Being the first antibiotic,

Table 35-4. Effect of prophylaxis on prevalence of gonorrheal ophthalmia neonatorum in a poor socioeconomic group*

	Births	Cases	Rate/ 100,000
No prophylaxis	6,545	12	183
Silver nitrate, 1%	56,705	8	14
Various antibiotics	28,811	8	28
Penicillin (50,000 units/ml)	10,090	0	0

*Data from Greenberg, M.: Am. J. Public Health **51:** 836, 1961.

Table 35-5. Prevalence of gonorrheal ophthalmia neonatorum in New York City, 1956 to 1958*

	Births	Cases	Rate/ 100,000
Private patients only	78,189	0	0
Ward and private patients	292,190	21	7.2
Ward patients only	102,151	28	27.4

*Data from Greenberg, M.: Am. J. Public Health **51:** 836, 1961.

penicillin has received more than the usual share of praise.[53-58] Penicillin is extremely effective in the treatment of most strains of *Neisseria*, and it is nontoxic, tolerated very well, inexpensive, and easily administered. It has the disadvantage of having a considerable allergic potential.

Although in the past *Neisseria gonorrhoeae* has been uniformly susceptible to penicillin treatment, resistant strains have multiplied and as of 1962 accounted for as high as 20% of clinical infections. A severe case of penicillin-resistant gonorrheal conjunctivitis has been reported to respond well to ampicillin, 250 mg orally four times daily.[59]

Topical bacitracin has been used.[60]

The freedom of tetracycline-treated eyes from chemical inflammation and the stability of this group of drugs has been cited.[61]

The whole controversy over regulatory control of ophthalmia neonatorum prophylaxis seems quite anachronistic to me. If such regulations are really necessary, they should be changed to permit physicians to use a medication (for example, an antibiotic of their choice) effective against the gonococcus, instead of requiring exclusively silver nitrate. Ancient regulations of this sort hinder rather than help medical practice, unless they are rephrased to permit discretionary modification.[62]

Bound by tradition, a surprising number of public health personnel insist on putting silver nitrate on the conjunctiva. They would not consider silver nitrate swabbing of an infected throat or silver nitrate irrigation of a urethra, but they have failed to recognize that silver nitrate prophylaxis of the eye is equally outdated and barbaric.

Inclusion conjunctivitis must be considered in the differential diagnosis of ophthalmia neonatorum. The incubation period of this venereal disease is ordinarily about 1½ weeks, whereas the incubation period of gonococcal ophthalmia is less than 1 week. Inclusion conjunctivitis may also be transmitted in inadequately chlorinated swimming pools.[63,64]

Gonorrhea is among the most common diseases. In 1969, 495,000 cases were reported in the United States; in 1971, there were 625,000. Apparently only 10% to 20% of cases are reported, suggesting that we have millions of new cases each year. Throughout the world, 60 million new cases of gonorrhea are estimated to develop annually.[65] The adult eye is also susceptible to gonorrheal infection, and this diagnosis should be considered in any case of conjunctivitis characterized by excessively heavy purulent discharge. Whether occurring in infant or adult, gonorrheal conjunctivitis is a systemic disease and should be treated by systemic medication in addition to topical treatment. Eye drops should not be the only medication prescribed.

Before 1955 few gonococcal strains required more than 0.05 unit/ml of penicillin for inhibition in vitro. By 1965, 15% of strains were resistant to 0.5 unit/ml. Fortunately even the most resistant strains can be eradicated by sufficiently high doses of penicillin.[66] Current treatment recommendations for gonorrhea therefore specify much higher penicillin dosages than in the past. For example, probenecid, 1 g, should be given orally at least 30 minutes before penicillin injection to retard renal excretion of the antibiotic. A dose of 4,800,000 units of procaine penicillin G is then given, divided into two injection sites because of the volume required. This procaine penicillin G dosage will also abort incubating syphilis but will not treat established syphilis; hence appropriate examination and serologic testing for syphilis should be performed at the time of initial evaluation of the gonorrhea.

Alternate recommendations for gonorrheal treatment include 3.5 g of ampicillin and 1.0 g of probenecid given simultaneously at one time. A less desirable regimen because it cannot be accomplished under direct supervision at one time is tetracycline, 1.5 g initially, followed by 0.5 g four times daily to a total dose of 9 g.

Long-acting benzathine penicillin G and oral penicillin V are not advised.

A follow-up serologic test for syphilis is advisable after 3 months if these alternate methods are used, since only the 4,800,000 procaine penicillin G regimen is known to abort syphilis.

Mima polymorpha is a gram-negative intracellular diplococcus indistinguishable on smear from the gonococcus. It causes a hyperacute keratoconjunctivitis clinically comparable to that of gonorrhea. *Mima* organisms are so named because they mimic *Neisseria.* Both are venereal infections, capable of inhabiting urethral and conjunctival mucosa.

An 11-year-old Boston girl lost her eye from such an infection, which caused a corneal perforation.[67] Some details of this case are instructive. The patient was first seen with 20/40 vision and a 2-day history of severe conjunctivitis. She did not use the antibiotic drops given to her and returned 9 days later with the corneal perforation. Her father was reported to be under treatment for a "rash of the penis." She was hospitalized for corenal transplantation but never returned after discharge. The case history indicates that the patient's unreliability was largely responsible for loss of the eye. While there is often not very much we can do about patient unreliability, we should probably try harder to impress patients of the need for cooperation in instances of potentially destructive infection. Incidentally, tetracyclines are more effective than penicillin in *Mima* treatment.

The temptation to use penicillin and tetracycline simultaneously should be avoided because the combination is less effective than penicillin alone. Penicillin interferes with cell wall formation by inhibition of synthesis of mucopeptides. It is bacteriocidal but cannot act on nonmultiplying cells. Tetracyclines inhibit protein synthesis and prevent cell multiplication. Hence tetracyclines block the bacteriocidal effect of penicillin. This fact is demonstrable both in vivo and clinically. As an example, the fatality rate of pneumococcal meningitis was 30% in patients treated with penicillin alone but increased to 79% in patients treated with both penicillin and chlortetracycline. More is not necessarily better.[68]

Mycobacterium tuberculosis

The role of tuberculosis in causing ocular inflammation is uncertain. Although there is no doubt that tubercle bacilli have been found in eyes, the accuracy of etiologic diagnosis of uveitis has always been questionable. For example, the same clinician diagnosed a tuberculous etiology in 79% of cases of granulomatous uveitis in 1941, but only in 23% in 1954.[69] By 1958 the frequency of diagnosed tuberculous etiology had dropped to 4%. One cannot help but suspect that changing diagnostic criteria (which now include toxoplasmosis) are more responsible for these differences than are actual changes in disease prevalence.

Both the difficulty of making the diagnosis of tuberculous uveitis and the possible rewards of making such a diagnosis are substantiated in a careful study of the Middlebrook-Dubos hemagglutination test for tuberculosis.[70] This test was run on both serum and primary aqueous samples from 34 granulomatous iridocyclitis patients and 21 tuberculous rabbits. Data from additional uveitis patients on whom paracentesis was not done were also presented where appropriate.

An attempt was made to divide the uveitis patients according to tuberculous and nontuberculous etiology on the basis of skin tests, x-ray films, blood tests, and the isoniazid-streptomycin therapeutic test. The Middlebrook-Dubos titers on serum and aqueous were then compared for these two groups of tuberculous and nontuberculous patients. The serum titers were virtually identical (tuberculous, 77% positive; nontuberculous, 78% positive) for the two groups, thereby indicating that *serum* titers are of *no* value in the diagnosis of tuberculous iridocyclitis. *Aqueous* titers, however, did show a definite correlation with the clinical diagnosis of tuberculosis. Positive aqueous titers were found in 75% (three of four) tuberculous iridocyclitis patients and in only 15% (3 of 18) of nontuberculous patients. (Of the 34 patients, *serum* Middlebrook-Dubos tests were positive in 65% of patients, whereas the *aqueous* tests were positive in only 26%.) These data cast serious doubt on the value (if any) of systemic (skin or serum) tests for tuberculosis as customarily used to help diagnose the etiology of ocular disease. The tuberculin skin test is of value in uveitis diagnosis only if it is negative, in which case a tuberculous etiology is most unlikely. Although experimental tuberculous ocular infections may not produce a positive skin test, clinical ocular tuberculosis is not injected into the eye, but enters by hematogenous spread from infection existing elsewhere within the body and causing a positive skin test.

Response to the isoniazid-streptomycin therapeutic test correlated well with the *aqueous* Middlebrook-Dubos titers but insignificantly with the *serum* titers. Positive aqueous titers were found in 80% (four of five) of patients responding to isoniazid, but in only 19% (5 of 26) not responding to isoniazid. Obviously paracentesis and immunologic study of primary aqueous were reasonably successful in predicting the possibility of therapeutic response to isoniazid (of nine positive aqueous tests, four therapeutic responses; of 22 negative aqueous tests, only one therapeutic response). These studies indicate that antibodies are formed within the eye and do not simply leak through the blood-aqueous barrier. Further refinement of immunologic testing of aqueous humor may in the future permit more accurate diagnosis of the causes of uveitis.

The rabbit experiments confirmed the expectation that aqueous titers would be positive for tuberculosis by the Middlebrook-Dubos test. However, even after tuberculous iridocyclitis had existed for as long as a month, 3 of 12 rabbits had negative aqueous titers. During the first several weeks of horse serum–induced uveitis, several of the rabbits with systemic tuberculosis showed positive aqueous titers, presumably caused by antigen leakage from serum into the aqueous. These rabbit tests indicate that both false positive and false negative aqueous titers for tuberculosis can occur, although uncommonly. (In these paragraphs, "positive titer" has referred to any positive test, even if only in a 1:2 dilution.)

Statistically, the most important clinical feature of tuberculosis from the standpoint of the ophthalmologist is its tendency to reactivation by systemic corticosteroid treatment. In 1967 the Ohio State Medical Association endorsed a statement by the American Thoracic Society Committee on Chemoprophylaxis indicating that persons with a positive tuberculin test are in danger of reactivation of tuberculosis should they receive corticosteroid treatment. Recommended chemoprophylaxis for such individuals was isoniazid, 300 mg/day (10 mg/kg for children), to be given as a single daily dose for 12 months. Perhaps we should give more serious thought to the possible benefits and detriments of corticosteroid therapy before dispensing these potent drugs. A year of isoniazid treatment is not a small price to pay for a trial of corticosteroid therapy instituted for questionable indications. This therapeutic recommendation is still currently accepted medical practice.[71]

Tuberculin desensitization is currently believed to be of no value in the control of clinical tuberculosis.[72] Older studies suggested the benefit of tuberculin desensitization in rabbits[73] and patients.[74] However, the present infrequency of such treatment attests to its doubtful efficacy.

Local treatment of a tuberculous scleral ulcer is effective. Streptomycin sulfate was administered as an eye drop every 2 hours for 2 weeks, with no change in the appearance of the lesion. Subsequently, 75 mg of streptomycin sulfate was injected beneath the conjunctiva near the lesion every 3 days for seven times. Two months after treatment was started, the ulcer was completely healed. The diagnosis was established by biopsy and culture in a patient with extensive systemic tuberculous involvement.[75]

Mycobacterium fortuitum is an acid-fast bacillus rarely responsible for eye infection.[76] Four cases of *Mycobacterium fortuitum* keratitis are reported following corneal foreign body removal. All four cases were referred from the same physician and all had been treated with corticosteroids. The source must have been the same contaminated instrument. Incidentally, experimental infection cannot be produced in rabbits without reducing their resistance by corticosteroid treatment or some other means. The course of the infection was self-limited over a period of 5 months to a year, leaving a dense localized corneal scar. Treatment with rifampin, kanamycin, or streptomycin was not effective, nor are any other effective agents known.[77] Isoniazid is not effective.

Phlyctenular keratoconjunctivitis

The clinical association between phlyctenular keratoconjunctivitis and tuberculosis continues to be stressed by many authors. In an evaluation of 26 Eskimo children with phlyctenular keratoconjunctivitis, only one was found to have a negative tuberculin test.[78] Of 99 other children of the same age group, who had never had phlyctenular disease, 32 had negative tuberculin skin tests. Tubercle bacilli are not found in biopsy material from phlyctenules. Topical corticosteroid therapy is reported to clear phlyctenular inflammation within 1 or 2 days. If phlyctenulosis is caused by tuberculosis, and this seems likely in some cases, presumably the process is some type of allergic manifestation rather than a direct infection.

In the East-Central portion of the United States, phlyctenular keratoconjunctivitis is quite uncommon, and when seen does not incriminate the patient as a tuberculosis suspect. Presumably other types of bacterial sensitivity may also cause this lesion.

A series of 26 patients with phlyctenular keratoconjunctivitis showed dramatic response to the topical instillation of 2.5% cortisone acetate.[79] Drops were used hourly the first day, and four times a day thereafter. Although the duration of treatment was variable and not specifically stated, it appears to have been less than a week in most cases. There was a relapse in only three patients when cortisone was discontinued; all three responded promptly to retreatment.

Clostridium

Perforating wounds of the eye and orbit are no exception to the rule that tetanus must be feared from such an injury. Active immunization against tetanus should be universal. Human tetanus immune globulin is available for use in nonimmunized individuals occasionally encountered. Most strains of *Clostridium* are sensitive to the commonly used antibiotics. Adequate surgical cleaning of the wound with removal of contaminated foreign bodies is appropriate. Solid foreign bodies such as bullets or BB pellets may routinely be left embedded in soft tissue such as the orbit. In contrast, porous material such as wood is almost always poorly tolerated.[80,81]

Clostridium perfringens causes massive intraocular necrosis resulting from toxin formation, hence the eye will be destroyed despite antibiotic treatment. This is a devastating infection, destroying the eye within a day.[82]

Other bacteria

Virtually any microorganism can cause ocular infections. For example, *Serratia marcescens*, usually considered to be a nonpathogenic saprophyte, can cause eye infection not only in the diabetic patient[83] but also in the injured eye of an otherwise perfectly healthy person.[84] The clinical moral is that the only rational way to treat serious eye infections is by identification of the responsible microorganism and selection of an appropriate effective antibiotic.

Proteus infections of the eye are usually disastrous. The experimental treatment of *Proteus* corneal infections in rabbits consisted of twice daily subconjunctival injection of antibiotics for 3 days. The antibiotics used were gentamicin and tobramycin, and the dosage was 8 mg per injection. Gentamicin was more effective, reducing the average colony count to 56 after 3 days. For comparison, the average colony count was 240 for tobramycin and over 10,000 for the untreated controls.[85]

FUNGAL INFECTIONS

Fungus cultures were taken from both eyes of 158 normal persons twice (separated by a 1-week interval). About 7% of eyes were fungus positive (35 isolations). The majority of positive cultures were obtained from the eyelids and not from the conjunctival sac. Only six eyes were fungus positive on both cultures. Identical species of fungus were isolated in the environment of these persons. Environmental change resulted in prompt disappearance of these fungi from the patient's eyelids. Hence fungi on the healthy eyelids appear to originate from random external contamination, do not propagate, and are transient.[86]

In a study of 156 adults carried out in Little Rock, Arkansas, 25 patients (16%) were found to have fungi recoverable through conjunctival cultures.[87] Controls were run to exclude airborne contamination. None of these patients had been on local or systemic steroid therapy. This study establishes the fact that a large proportion of our population are asymptomatic ocular carriers of fungus infection. Just as a high proportion of postoperative bacterial intraocular infections are caused by organisms originating from the patient's own lids, conjunctiva, and lacrimal apparatus, so also it seems likely that fungus endophthalmitis may have a local origin.

Treatment of ocular fungus infection requires consideration of three separate items:

1. How does the ophthalmologist know the ocular disorder is caused by fungus infection?
2. What are the characteristics of the available fungistatic drugs?
3. What is the effect of other commonly used medications on fungus infection?

Diagnosis

Almost certainly, only a few ocular fungus infections will be recognized as such during the early stages. This diagnostic failure is explained by the difficulty of identifying fungus structures with commonly used isolation and staining methods, by the slow growth of fungi on culture media, and by the absence of pathognomonic characteristics with which to differentiate fungus infections from the vastly more common bacterial and virus infections.

Suspicion of corneal fungus infection usually arises when a corneal ulcer, usually of some weeks' duration, proves resistant to vigorous antibiotic therapy. A considerable number of the reported cases of corneal fungus infection have had hypopyon associated with the corneal infiltration and ulceration.[88] Suspicion should be aroused earlier if no pathogenic bacteria can be identified from an acute and severe corneal ulcer appearing to be infectious but not typical of herpes simplex. Although surface discharge may contain recognizable mycelia, scrapings of the ulcer are more certain to provide material of diagnostic value. The Gram technique will usually stain fungi (all are gram-positive). The methenamine-silver stain provides greater contrast and is superior to Gram and Giemsa stains for fungus identification. The potassium hydroxide wet mount is suitable only for gross examination of specimens containing abundant hyphae.[89] Not uncommonly smears may be reported as negative, although subsequent growth will appear on culture. *Repeated* smears and cultures are clearly indicated in the management of any serious and uncontrolled infectious corneal ulcer presumably caused by an unidentified microorganism.

Although Sabouraud agar is designed for fungus culture, it may be preserved with cyclohexamide, which inhibits growth of many of the fungi pathogenic to the eye. The ophthalmologist should specify use of agar that does not contain cyclohexamide. Also, fungi grow much better at room temperature (25° C) than in the incubator.[90]

Characteristics of keratomycosis

Certain clinical features are highly suggestive of keratomycosis. Historically, the injury occurs at least 5 days before severe inflammatory response and possibly as long as 3 weeks previously. (Bacterial infections ordinarily have a more prompt onset.) In all but one of 15 cases the injury was caused by vegetable matter.[91] The typical ocular reaction is extremely *severe*, often out of proportion to the superficial ulcer. Descemet's folds and hypopyon are common. *Branching lines* commonly radiate from the ulcer, in contrast to the necrotic margin of a bacterial ulcer. (Hyphae are usually identifiable well beyond the clinically obvious limits of a fungus corneal ulcer.) Rather firm, elevated areas may exist within the ulcer instead of the excavated, necrotic contour characteristic of bacterial infection. Whitish plaques may lie internal to the endothelium. A midperipheral white corneal ring comparable to that seen in allergic responses may develop surrounding the fungus antigen.

In the aforementioned series of 15 cases, routine culture on Sabouraud medium incubated at 37° C *never* resulted in the isolation of fungus! In contrast, incubation at 30° C on freshly prepared Sabouraud medium reliably produced fairly rapid fungus growth. The physician should remember that topical anesthetics contain antifungal preservatives. Before scrapings are taken, excess anesthetic should be rinsed out of the eye with saline solution. Immediate stain (Gram or Gridley fungus stain) of the scrapings on a slide will commonly demonstrate hyphae and permit a rapid diagnosis.

Fungus endophthalmitis may complicate intraocular surgery or penetrating injury, usually appearing at least a week and sometimes months after the injury. The infection develops more rapidly if the inoculum of organisms is large, or if it is placed near a vascular part of the eye. The eye becomes red and painful and usually develops a hypopyon, which may spontaneously disappear.[92] Localized grayish infiltrates appear within the vitreous and gradually become more extensive. Diagnosis is made by smear and culture of aspirated aqueous or vitreous.

Therapy

The effective fungistatic drugs that may be useful in treatment of ocular fungus infection are amphotericin B, pimaricin, and nystatin. These antibiotics are derived from *Streptomyces* cultures. The drugs do not penetrate the eye very well by any route other than direct intraocular injection, and they are highly toxic. Corneal fungus infections have been cured, both clinically and experimentally, by amphotericin B and/or nystatin.[93] Some weeks are required for the final healing of fungus corneal ulcers. This delay is caused by toxic substances that are quite damaging to the cornea even when applied as an extract of killed fungi. Corneal perforation may threaten if the keratitis has been severe— such eyes may be saved by lamellar keratoplasty. The visual results from such keratoplasty leave a great deal to be desired, but at least the eye is not totally lost through perforation. Therapy of intraocular fungus infections is quite unsatisfactory. Even though the fungus may be destroyed by heroic injections of nystatin and amphotericin B, intraocular scarring usually precludes useful vision.[94]

Amphotericin B

Amphotericin B is fungistatic against a wide variety of yeasts and fungi, including *Coccidioides, Histoplasma, Blastomyces,* and *Candida.*[95] It has no demonstrable effect against viruses, bacteria, or protozoa. Amphotericin B has a wider spectrum of activity than does nystatin and is more effective than stilbamidine. *Candida* strains resistant to amphotericin B can be developed in vitro and sometimes have an associated resistance to nystatin.

Amphotericin B is heat labile and light sensitive; therefore both the dry powder and the solutions should be refrigerated. Solutions should be prepared with 5% dextrose, since saline solution precipitates the drug. Amphotericin B is poorly absorbed from the gastrointestinal tract, so it is given intravenously in concentrations of 0.1 mg/ml. Renal excretion is slow, and demonstrable blood levels persist for 18 hours or more after a single intravenous dose. Amphotericin B cannot be identified in intraocular fluids after parenteral administration. Unpleasant and potentially dangerous side effects are almost inevitable at therapeutic dosage levels. Amphotericin B should be used only in hospitals under close clinical supervision for treatment of mycotic infections diagnosed by culture. The drug is too toxic for use in vague and undiagnosed conditions merely because a skin test for one of the fungi may be positive. Obviously this applies to most cases of uveitis. Quick cures should not be expected. Weeks or months of treatment may be necessary. (Amphotericin B is not fungicidal.) Treatment for less than a month may be followed by relapse. Dosage should be adjusted to minimize the toxic effects rather than increasing to high levels in the vain hope of obtaining a more prompt remission. Under no circumstances should the total daily dosage exceed 1.5 mg/kg of body weight. Therapy is initiated with a daily dose of 0.25 mg/kg, and gradually increased as tolerated.

Amphotericin B causes chills, fever, headaches, and anorexia. These symptoms may be helped by aspirin. Chemical thrombophlebitis is a hazard that may be minimized by reducing the rate of infusion or, if necessary, by using a solution more dilute than the usually recommended 0.1 mg/ml. Rapid intravenous injection sometimes causes death in rabbits. Renal damage must be guarded against by routine check of blood urea nitrogen levels and periodic kidney function tests if therapy is prolonged. For topical ocular use, a 0.3% solution of amphotericin B may be prepared in 5% glucose or distilled water.[96] Subconjunctival injection of 125 μg of amphotericin B is reasonably well tolerated but does not result in appreciable intraocular penetration. Intraocular injection is extremely toxic; however, 35 μg in a 0.05 ml volume may be tolerated by the eye. Use of amphotericin B in ointment form is not reported but would seem a rational way to prolong contact of the medication with a corneal ulcer and to reduce the frequency of instillation. Drops have been used as often as every 15 minutes but may be irritating and cause epithelial damage. In treatment of local fungal abscesses of the lids or orbit, 0.5 mg of amphotericin B may be injected directly into the infected site at weekly intervals.

Fig. 35-1[97] illustrates the degree of sensitivity exhibited by different fungi to amphotericin B.

Pimaricin

Pimaricin is an antifungal antibiotic that may be applied topically to the cornea as a 5% suspension every 2 hours. Such treatment may be clinically effective against *Aspergillus*, *Fusarium*, and *Cephalosporium* infections, for example. In vitro, *Aspergillus* growth is inhibited by 10 μg/ml of pimaricin.

Pimaricin is insoluble in water and will not penetrate into the cornea. Before use of pimaricin, necrotic surface tissue should be surgically removed—this provides diagnostic material in addition to enhancing the thera-

peutic effect. Subconjunctival injection is of no value whatsoever. The injected pimaricin simply remains as an insoluble mass.[98]

Fig. 35-2 indicates the sensitivity of fungi to pimaricin.[97] This is an effective drug and one of the least irritating to the eye. Unfortunately, it penetrates very poorly and is of no value except for corneal fungus infections, where it is usually the drug of choice.

Nystatin

Nystatin inhibits the growth of a wide variety of fungi, molds, and yeasts.[99] It has little

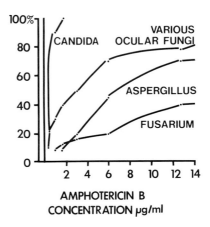

Fig. 35-1. Cumulative percent ocular fungi isolates sensitive to various concentrations of amphotericin B. (Modified from Jones, B. R.: Am. J. Ophthalmol. **79:**719, May 1975.)

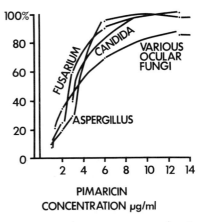

Fig. 35-2. Cumulative percent ocular fungi isolates sensitive to various concentrations of pimaricin. (Modified from Jones, B. R.: Am. J. Ophthalmol. **79:**719, May 1975.)

or no effect on other types of microorganisms. Despite the broad antifungal spectrum of nystatin, its therapeutic effect in systemic mycoses has been disappointing because toxicity prevents the administration of adequate quantities of the drug. Oral preparations are poorly absorbed. Intravenous injections cause chills and fever, and intramuscular injections cause local reactions. For practical purposes, therefore, nystatin is used topically and has been found clinically valuable in the treatment of surface fungus infections.

Nystatin is reasonably well tolerated by the eye as a topical ointment containing 100,000 units/g or by subconjunctival injection of 5000 units suspended in 0.5 ml saline solution. Neither method produces measurable intraocular concentrations of nystatin. Nystatin, 200 units, may be injected into the vitreous or aqueous chambers, but it causes hyperemia and leukocytic infiltration lasting several days to a week.[100] Vitreous assays show that nystatin levels sufficient to inhibit *Aspergillus* (6 to 12 units/ml) persist for only 24 hours after injection. Unfortunately a second intravitreal injection of 200 units of nystatin 36 hours after the first causes vitreous degeneration. Single intravitreal injections of 400 units of nystatin cause cloudiness of the vitreous persisting for at least a week.

Intravitreal injection of 1000 *Aspergillus* spores will destroy all untreated rabbit eyes. Eyes infected in this manner were treated by intravitreal injection of 200 units of nystatin.[100] Seven of eight eyes treated 24 hours after injection showed no fungus growth during observation periods of up to 7 weeks. Treatment 2 days or more after infection temporarily reduced the severity of infection but did not prevent destruction of the eyes. The intraocular injection of such toxic medications is not appropriate in clinical therapy.

Nystatin is very insoluble in water; only 300 to 600 units dissolve in 1 ml. As much as 200,000 units may be dissolved in 1 ml of the special diluent provided by Squibb. If the nystatin solution in diluent is placed into isotonic saline solution or water, a fine suspension results that may be used for topical ocular instillation. Refrigerated aqueous suspen-

sions retain 90% of original activity after storage for 2 weeks.

As shown in Fig. 35-3,[97] nystatin is a relatively ineffective drug against most fungi. This fact, combined with its poor solubility, limits its use to superficial keratomycosis caused by susceptible fungi. A 3% ointment is reasonably well tolerated.

Clotrimazole

As shown in Fig. 35-4,[97] clotrimazole is the drug of choice against *Aspergillus* infections.

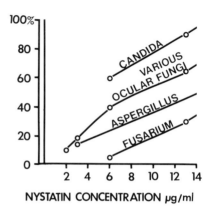

Fig. 35-3. Cumulative percent ocular fungi isolates sensitive to various concentrations of nystatin. (Modified from Jones, B. R.: Am. J. Ophthalmol. **79:**719, May 1975.)

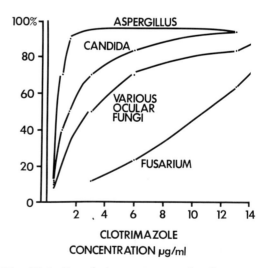

Fig. 35-4. Cumulative percent ocular fungi isolates sensitive to clotrimazole. (Modified from Jones, B. R.: Am. J. Ophthalmol. **79:**719, May 1975.)

It may be given orally in doses of 60 to 100 mg/kg/day. For keratomycosis, 1% clotrimazole in arachis oil may be instilled every 3 hours until clinical response is observed; thereafter administration should be four times a day for 2 to 3 months, as required by the duration of the infection.

Flucytosine

Flucytosine is the drug of choice for corneal and intraocular infections with *Candida* species (Fig. 35-5).[97] It is transformed to highly toxic 5-fluorouracil within susceptible fungi but is not metabolized in humans, hence is relatively nontoxic to man. Flucyto-

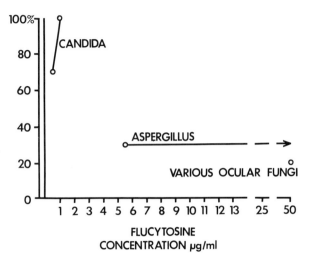

Fig. 35-5. Cumulative percent ocular fungi isolates sensitive to various concentrations of flucytosine. (Modified from Jones, B. R.: Am. J. Ophthalmol. **79:**719, May 1975.)

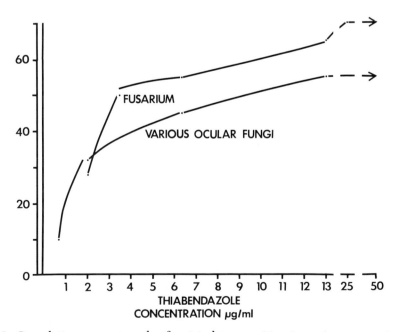

Fig. 35-6. Cumulative percent ocular fungi isolates sensitive to various concentrations of thiabendazole. (Modified from Jones, B. R.: Am. J. Ophthalmol. **79:**719, May 1975.)

sine is well absorbed orally and is given in dosage of 200 mg/kg/day. Solutions of 1.5% are nonirritating and may be given for keratomycosis, but they do not give satisfactory intraocular concentrations. Four months of oral therapy cured a case of *Candida albicans* endophthalmitis, with final vision of 20/20!

Thiabendazole

Thiabendazole is widely used in veterinary medicine and is effective against visceral larva migrans in dosage of 25 mg/kg/day. It has both antihelminthic and antifungal activity. A 4% suspension is tolerated by the eye on topical instillation. Thiabendazole is particularly useful against *Fusarium* species (Fig. 35-6).[97]

Miconazole and econazole are chemically related derivatives with improved antifungal activity, but they have poorer solubility and are more irritating on topical application.

Potassium iodide

The amount of corneal edema caused by intralamellar *Aspergillus* injections into rabbit corneas was measured by weighing a 7 mm trephine button removed from the central cornea.[101,102] The weight of normal corneal buttons averaged 19 mg; of untreated infected corneas, 43 mg; of pimaricin-treated corneas, 28 mg; and of pimaricin and potassium iodide–treated corneas, 22 mg. A 1% solution of potassium iodide was dropped on the cornea every 2 hours around the clock at the same time as pimaricin was applied.

The potassium may reduce corneal edema by supporting glycolysis and phosphorylation metabolic activity. According to this thesis, the effect of potassium iodide is to prevent corneal damage from secondary edema. No antifungal effect was demonstrable. Sodium iodide was ineffective. A 2% concentration of potassium iodide was too strong and interfered with healing. Oral potassium iodide was of no value. This study does not support the popular notion that iodides may be effective antifungal agents in concentrations not destructive to tissue.

Surgical adjunct therapy

Medical therapy of keratomycosis with nystatin or amphotericin B is irritating to the eye and may require weeks or months of treatment. Keratoplasty is not effective, since the pathogen extends far beyond the visible ulcer and cannot be effectively removed. For some reason, a thin Gundersen conjunctival flap covering the entire cornea gives dramatic relief of symptoms and arrests the disease. Superficial keratectomy with removal of as much damaged tissue as possible is performed in the region of the ulcer before positioning of the flap. (The keratectomy tissue is also valuable for diagnosis.) Apparently the flap does more than just hide the lesion; it actually cures it and is the treatment of choice.[91] The antifungal antibiotics penetrate tissue very poorly and their use is usually discontinued after placement of a conjunctival flap.

The role of vitrectomy in diagnosis and treatment of fungal endophthalmitis is not yet clearly defined. Although the operation itself is probably the most dangerous ophthalmic surgical procedure, it does provide an excellent approach to diagnosis. For example, the white fluff-balls in the vitreous in *Candida* endophthalmitis have been removed by vitrectomy and are found to consist of masses of fungal hyphae and necrotic inflammatory cells.[103] Because of the availability of a variety of antifungal medications and the differing sensitivities of fungi to these drugs, it is as important to obtain sensitivity studies in cases of fungal infection as in bacterial infection.

Furthermore, removal of dense intraocular inflammatory membranes may prevent pupil block glaucoma and traction detachment of the retina. Do not uncritically undertake diagnostic and therapeutic vitrectomy, however, for it is unnecessary in a mild infection and represents simply a two-stage enucleation in severely damaged eyes.

Effect of other medications
Antibiotics

Although it is commonly stated that antibiotics themselves enhance the growth of fungi, examination of the evidence on which this statement seems to be based is not convincing. Observation of luxuriant fungus growth on media containing streptomycin led to evaluation of the fungus-stimulating properties of this antibiotic.[104] Without doubt, in proportion to the increasing concentration of streptomycin, growth was stimulated in experiments in vitro with *Sporotrichum, Coccidioides, Histoplasma, Trichophyton,* and other fungi. Fungus activation in vivo by streptomycin has not been demonstrated. Saslaw[105] believed that the streptomycin molecule enhanced growth by providing nutrients that may not be present in an artificial medium but would be present in vivo.

Intrastromal corneal inoculation with *Candida* was performed in 11 young rabbits.[106] Terramycin, 1%, was added to the inoculum in the right eyes; left eyes were untreated infected controls. Corneal perforation was the result in eight treated eyes and one control eye. Although on first glance this eight-to-one statistic appears to indicate fungus potentiation by antibiotics, and has frequently been referred to as providing such proof, this is not necessarily the case. Intralamellar injection of tetracyclines is irritating and may, by this nonclinical method of application, have caused enough damage to the thin corneas of these young rabbits to account for the higher incidence of perforation. Furthermore, experiments with other types of fungi (including *Aspergillus*) in adult rabbits, treated with Aureomycin, showed no increased growth because of the presence of an antibiotic. These experiments,[106] characterized as "exploratory," certainly do not establish a contraindication to the clinical use of antibiotics in ocular therapy.

Intraperitoneal injection of 2 mg of Aureomycin in 17 mice and of 320 million *Candida* cells into 17 other mice resulted in no deaths.[107] However, when these doses of Aureomycin and *Candida* were combined and injected simultaneously, 16 of 17 mice died of *Candida* infection. In variations of this experiment, injection of Aureomycin 24 hours before the *Candida* caused the death of four of nine mice. However, when Aureomycin was given 8 or 24 hours after *Candida,* only one of 20 mice died. This experiment indicates that locally injected Aureomycin interferes for at least a day with normal defense mechanisms. Whether Aureomycin is a biologic activator of fungus infections or damages resistance under some conditions as a nonspecific irritant cannot be determined from the plan of this experiment.

The action of antibiotics in the eye should not be confused with that in the gastrointestinal tract, where destruction of inhibitory bacteria by antibiotics may permit a secondary overgrowth of fungi. Since no bacteria are normally present within the eye, antibiotic therapy cannot facilitate intraocular fungus growth by removal of inhibitory bacteria.

I believe that the concept of antibiotic potentiation of ocular fungus infection has not been clearly established. In view of the uncertainty of this concept, the diagnostic difficulty in distinguishing between bacterial and fungal ocular infection, the much commoner incidence of bacterial infection, and the ease with which bacterial superinfection of corneal defects can occur, withholding antibiotic therapy because of the possible presence of fungus infection is not statistically in the best interest of the patient.

Corticosteroids

Quite a different situation exists in regard to corticosteroid therapy, which is clearly established as a factor in promoting ocular fungus infection. Experimental work on ocular fungus infection, quite difficult before the advent of corticosteroids, is now routinely aided by corticosteroid treatment of the animals.[108] The facilitation of ocular *Candida* infection produced by a single injection of 60 μg of prednisolone will last for at least 2 weeks. The incidence of fungus culture from human eyes is increased from 18% to 67% by 3 weeks or more of topical corticosteroid therapy. The incidence of corticosteroid treatment of human eyes developing fungus infections is so high as to assume some diagnostic significance.[109]

Furthermore, *it is not clear that any benefits accrue from the use of corticosteroids in the treatment of corneal abrasions, purulent corneal ulcers, perforating wounds of the eye, or purulent endophthalmitis. Corticosteroid therapy is strongly contraindicated in the management of such ocular conditions.*

The literature presents conflicting opinions regarding the treatment of keratomycosis. On one side there is the belief that deep corneal abscesses exhibit an inflammatory response that can be benefited by corticosteroids. A single case report describes improvement of an *Aspergillus* corneal ulcer with topical prednisolone.[110] The report suggests that the improvement may have coincided with the withdrawal of amphotericin B therapy, to which the patient was highly intolerant. Also, keratoplasty became necessary after 10 days of corticosteroid therapy and fungus hyphae were found to extend through Descemet's membrane. Temporary and misleading improvement of bacterial keratitis is a well-recognized and characteristic response—a comparable response of keratomycosis would be expected. Finally, the concept of "covering" corticosteroid therapy with antifungal drugs is difficult to understand, since the antifungal drugs do not penetrate tissue well, whereas fungi and corticosteroids may do so.

Another recommendation for the management of deep keratomycosis is the mechanical removal of as much damaged surface tissue as possible, thereby exposing the deeper fungi to antifungal drug effect. Many authors have emphasized the frequency with which corticosteroid treatment of relatively minor injuries precedes keratomycosis.[111]

The majority opinion continues to be that fungus contamination responds adversely to corticosteroid therapy. A case of *Curvularia lunata* keratomycosis followed prolonged self-treatment with hydrocortisone.[112] Subconjunctival prednisolone enhanced the severity of experimental *Candida albicans* keratomycosis in rabbits.[113] Devastating sporotrichosis endophthalmitis destroyed an eye treated with systemic prednisone, 60 mg/day, and subconjunctival betamethasone, 6 mg.[114]

A 49-year-old woman with pars planitis died of *Nocardia* brain abscess 2½ months after starting prednisone (initial dose, 80 mg/day).[115] The author also cited another fatality from disseminated cytomegalovirus infection following prednisone therapy of a renal transplant. Systemic corticosteroid therapy is stated to be a predisposing factor to orbital and cerebral phycomycosis.[116]

Nocardia asteroides keratitis followed topical corticosteroid treatment of a corneal abrasion. The organism isolated from this patient was inoculated intralamellarly into six rabbit corneas and resulted in minor scars. Six similarly inoculated corneas were treated with dexamethasone, 0.1% four times daily for 3 weeks—these treated corneas developed large granulomatous lesions, which in two animals extended into the anterior chamber.[117]

Aspergillus niger contamination of the rabbit conjunctiva spontaneously disappears if untreated. Twice daily treatment with 0.2% hydrocortisone drops doubled the number of colonies cultured at 2 days.[118] In fact, exacerbation of corneal or intraocular infection following corticosteroid therapy has been cited as a diagnostic feature of mycotic infection.[119]

Cycloplegics

Atropinization is indicated in the treatment of most fungus infections of the eye. The benefits of atropine are the same as for any other cause of iridocyclitis.

Specific organisms
Candida albicans

Candida albicans was the most common cause of keratomycosis in Wisconsin, being the etiologic agent in four of seven cases.[120] This fungus can superinfect other corneal diseases, and two of these cases occurred in association with herpetic ulceration, one in exposure keratopathy.

This fungus can cause chronic and recurrent conjunctivitis, as occurred in one of our nurses who also had a candidal vulvitis. Thus fungi should be added to the list of causes of oculogenital infections.

Endophthalmitis caused by *Candida* may occur following intravenous contamination; for example, exchange transfusion in infancy,[121] mainline use of heroin or other substances by drug addicts,[122] or intravenous hyperalimentation.[123] Prolonged intravenous catheterization is prone to result in infection.

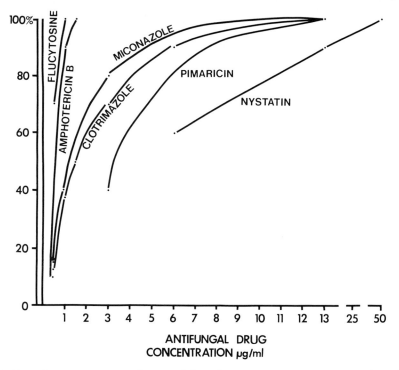

Fig. 35-7. Cumulative percent ocular *Candida* isolates sensitive to various antifungal drugs. (Modified from Jones, B. R.: Am. J. Ophthalmol. **79:**719, May 1975.)

Immunosuppression and generally reduced resistance predisposes to disseminated fungal infection, as may occur following organ transplants or chemotherapy for neoplasm.[124] Such endophthalmitis is not an isolated ocular problem but is part of a life-threatening systemic disease.

Candida endophthalmitis may also complicate cataract extraction.[125] Most such eyes are lost to enucleation or blindness, but in one case the eye regained 20/30 vision after eight sub-Tenon's injections of 500 to 750 μg of amphotericin B given every other day.

Fortunately, *Candida* is one of the most sensitive fungi to therapeutic medications. Fig. 35-7[97] depicts the cumulative percent of sensitivity to various antifungal drugs of *Candida* isolates from ocular infections. Flucytosine and amphotericin B are highly effective and are the drugs of first choice.

Aspergillus

This fairly common mold rarely causes ocular infection. It is relatively nonresponsive to treatment, and *Aspergillus* endophthal-

mitis usually destroys the eye. Immunosuppressive regimens, as following renal transplantation, predispose to such infections.[126]

Extraocular *Aspergillus* abscesses may present as slowly enlarging lumps of the lid or orbit. Diagnosis is made by biopsy excision, but removal of the infectious material is usually incomplete and the lesion tends to recur. Local injection of the recurrent mass with 0.5 mg of amphotericin B at 1- to 2-week intervals will destroy the organism without danger of systemic toxicity.[127]

Clotrimazole is the most effective drug against *Aspergillus* (Fig. 35-8).[97]

Fusarium solanae

The most common cause of keratomycosis in Florida is *Fusarium solanae*.[128] Pimaricin is the drug of choice for *Fusarium* keratomycosis (Fig. 35-9).[97]

Summary

The diagnosis of fungus infection should be strongly suspected in any case of purulent corneal ulcer from which pathogenic

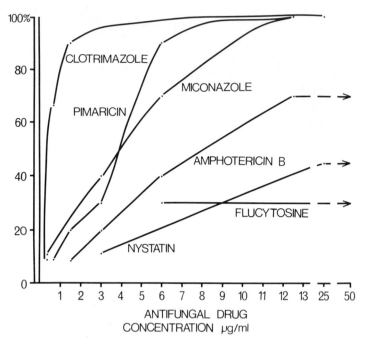

Fig. 35-8. Cumulative percent ocular *Aspergillus* isolates sensitive to various antifungal drugs. (Modified from Jones, B. R.: Am. J. Ophthalmol. **79**:719, May 1975.)

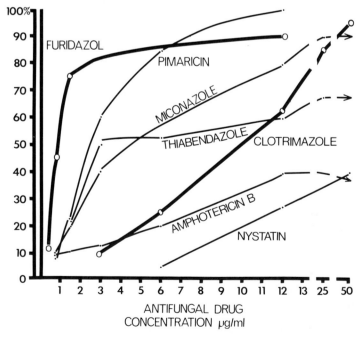

Fig. 35-9. Cumulative percent *Fusarium* isolates sensitive to various antifungal compounds. (Modified from Jones, B. R.: Am. J. Ophthalmol. **79**:719, May 1975.)

bacteria are not readily isolated, and appropriate microbiologic studies should be performed.

Amphotericin B, pimaricin, and nystatin therapy are of clinically and experimentally demonstrated value in the management of fungus-induced ulcers of the cornea.

The known value of antibiotics against bacterial infection should not be discarded in the case of a corneal ulcer of uncertain cause because the concept of antibiotic potentiation of fungus growth is not clearly established.

Corticosteroids unquestionably enhance fungus growth in vivo and are of no benefit to injured or infected eyes anyway. Hence corticosteroid therapy of injured or infected eyes is definitely contraindicated.

HISTOPLASMOSIS

"Presumed histoplasmic" choroiditis accounts for approximately 20% of the uveitis cases seen in midwestern eye clinics but is less common in other parts of the United States. The typical appearance of presumed histoplasmic choroiditis consists of disseminated atrophic peripheral foci less than one-half disc diameter in size, circumpapillary scarring, and clear vitreous. A characteristic dark, hemorrhagic, destructive lesion may develop at the macula.[129-131]

Experimentally, ocular lesions can be produced by local or systemic injection of *Histoplasma*. The preference of this organism for the choroid is indicated by the fact that intravitreal injection results in choroidal growth of *Histoplasma*—not retinal growth, as would be expected.[132-134]

Of 34 patients suspected of having histoplasmic chorioretinitis, 50% were nonreactive to the *Histoplasma* complement fixation test. Of 39 patients having suspected histoplasmic chorioretinitis, 88% were negative to the *Histoplasma* collodion agglutination test.[135] Apparently the correlation between the results of *Histoplasma* skin testing and serologic testing is very poor.[136]

The reader should be aware that the designation of "presumed histoplasmic" choroiditis is a working hypothesis and not an established fact.

Therapy

Amphotericin B, to a total dose of at least 25 mg/kg over 4 weeks, will dramatically improve the prognosis of severe systemic histoplasmosis. With such treatment, only 23% of 194 treated patients died, in contrast to 83% of 115 untreated patients.[137]

Treatment of 20 patients with presumed histoplasmic chorioretinitis with amphotericin B and corticosteroids failed to influence the course of the disease in 16 of these 20 patients, and three of the four favorable reactions showed only minimal improvement of acuity. Apparently, amphotericin B treatment of typical macular disease associated with a positive histoplasmin skin test is not justified.[138] Besides being ineffectual, this treatment is dangerous and unpleasant.

A case has been reported in which systemic corticosteroid therapy of systemic histoplasmosis was followed by worsening of the general condition, leading eventually to death.[139]

The treatment of presumed histoplasmic choroiditis is discouraging.[140] Moving from endemic areas seems of no value. Histoplasmin desensitization, amphotericin B, antihistaminics, or 6-mercaptopurine medication produced no better results than those found in a control group. Corticosteroid therapy (systemic or by sub-Tenon's injection) may reduce the severity of retinal scarring (undocumented clinical impression), but usually must be continued for 2 years before quiescence of a macular lesion. Immediate self-medication by corticosteroids is said to abort recurrent attacks of macular inflammation within hours or days. Knowing the tendency for an apprehensive patient to misinterpret symptoms as indicating a recurrent retinal detachment (which is not present), I would expect many patients to credit (inaccurately) immediate medication with the cure of a "recurrence."

Paramacular photocoagulation was used in 32 eyes with central presumed histoplasmic choroiditis, with retention of 20/50 or better vision in almost one third of the treated eyes.[140] However, comparable final acuity resulted in the same proportion of untreated eyes.

This rather dismal therapeutic response is compatible with the clinical supposition that no organisms are present in the destructive macular lesion. The break in the lamina vitrea is supposed to permit vascular invasion from the dense posterior choriocapillaris into the subpigment epithelium space. Connective tissue proliferation and contraction result in the typical deep hemorrhages. Such a lesion, very similar to senile disciform macular degeneration, would not be expected to respond to presently known methods of therapy.

Recent pathologic studies at The Ohio State University have revealed substantial lymphocytic infiltration of the choroid in fundus lesions that appeared ophthalmoscopically to be old, inactive scars. Intensive serial study of these eyes has permitted repeated discovery of organisms identical in morphologic characteristics to *Histoplasma capsulatum* in at least four separate eyes. We believe that the continuing presence of small numbers of living organisms, surrounded by a mass of sensitized lymphocytes, represents the specific lesion of clinical histoplasmosis. Defects in the lamina vitrea, subpigment epithelial neovascularization, and contraction of scar tissue are nonspecific secondary changes.[141]

During the 12 years preceding 1975, 540 cases of presumed histoplasmic choroiditis were seen at The Ohio State University. Controlled therapeutic evaluations were not performed, but the clinical impression has been that a combination of systemic corticosteroid therapy and photocoagulation (when permitted by location at least 0.25 DD from the fovea) gives the best results. At one time meticulously followed desensitization was considered to be effective (but again, this was an uncontrolled clinical impression).[142]

PARASITES
Trichinosis

The early diagnosis of trichinosis by its typical signs, including weakness and swelling of the extraocular muscles and subconjunctival hemorrhage, is of greater impor-

tance since the development of effective anthelminthic therapy. Thiabendazole (Mintezol) will kill not only the adult worms in the gastrointestinal tract but also the larval forms in the muscles. This drug is effective in a therapeutic dose of 50 mg/kg (compared to an LD_{50} dose of 3500 mg/kg). Dramatic and prompt clinical cure of a patient was reported with thiabendazole, 500 mg, every 12 hours for 7 days.[143]

In 1954, 21 million cases of human trichinosis were estimated to exist in North America. The flocculation test for trichinosis is said to be reliable. Muscle biopsy may be unreliable, showing parasites in only seven of 16 proved cases. The history of raw pork ingestion several days before diarrhea and abdominal pain, followed by diffuse myalgia and generalized weakness, is most helpful. Eosinophilia and fever are present. The larvae encyst only in striated muscle but may invade any part of the body, including the retina and cerebrospinal fluid.

In two patients with acute trichinosis, biopsy study of the deltoid muscle showed active larvae after 6 and 9 days of thiabendazole in a dosage of 50 mg/kg/day. Nausea, vomiting, and dermatitis occurred in four patients receiving thiabendazole. However, the patients' fever subsided and they felt subjectively improved within several days after treatment was begun. Clearly, thiabendazole is not a panacea for the treatment of trichinosis.[144]

Nematode endophthalmitis

The life cycle of *Toxocara canis*, probably the commonest intraocular parasite in North America, is incomplete in the human host. The worm leaves the intestine for other tissues, including the eye, and dies without returning to the intestine. Since piperazine and other antihelminthic drugs are effective only against parasites within the intestine, no benefit results from such treatment of ocular involvement with visceral larva migrans.[145]

Systemic corticosteroid therapy may decrease the ocular allergic reaction to the live organism and to the decomposition products of the dead nematode. Following the active stage, the ocular toxocaral lesion may remain unchanged in appearance for years and does not, of course, require treatment after the inflammatory response has subsided.

Thiabendazole treatment may be of benefit in this condition.

Onchocerciasis

Although we see this disease only in returned missionaries, onchocerciasis is a major cause of blindness in Africa.[146] In endemic areas, 25% to 40% of the population over the age of 40 years are blind as a result of infestation with this parasite.

The ocular destruction is caused by direct invasion by myriads of microfilariae. These organisms are 250 μ long and about 7 μ in diameter, are motile, and can be recognized in aqueous and vitreous by biomicroscopy. On death, the microfilariae release antigenic substances, causing focal inflammation.[147]

Oral diethylcarbamazine citrate (Hetrazan) will destroy microfilariae but is not effective against the encysted subcutaneous and intramuscular adult worms that produce the microfilariae. Consequently, continuing therapy is required. Topical 5% diethylcarbamazine instilled four times daily will eliminate the microfilariae from the anterior chamber within 48 hours.[148] No exacerbation of ocular inflammation has resulted from this therapy. The study of 10 blind eyes did not report the response of the posterior segment ocular inflammation to the topical diethylcarbamazine. Adequate penetration of topically applied medication to the choroid would be unexpected. Whether or not retrobulbar injection of the drug would be of any value was not reported and is probably not a particularly important question, since the oral medication is effective.

Phthiriasis palpebrarum

Crab louse infection of the eyelashes is readily recognized by slit-lamp identification of the louse grasping the base of the hair or the oval nits glued to the hair shaft. Treatment is fairly simple. Thorough shampooing of lashes, hair, and pubis, treatment of family members, and laundering of the bedding will eradicate the pest. If preferred, insecticides may be applied to the bedclothes.[149]

Suffocation of the louse by generous application of any greasy ointment to the lids may suffice if the lids alone are involved. Use of isoflurophate ointment on the lid margins has been suggested because of the relation of this drug to the potent anticholinesterase insecticides. Incapacitating ciliary spasms make the use of isoflurophate unpleasant, however.

Demodex folliculorum

Demodex folliculorum is an eight-legged, thick-bodied mite about 300 μ long. Growth from egg to adult requires 2 weeks. The mite can easily be demonstrated beneath the microscope in peanut oil preparations and was found by quick examination in 40% of 500 consecutive patients seen in a New York office practice.[150]

In Denmark a very thorough study demonstrated *Demodex* in virtually everyone over the age of 50 years and in at least 20% of children. The frequency of isolation depended on the extent of evaluation. Norn[151] estimated the *Demodex* population on the average middle-aged person to be at least 1000 organisms. Their greatest concentration is found in the follicles of the nasal skin— every other examined follicle harbored a *Demodex*. Every tenth eyelash follicle contained a *Demodex* demonstrable by epilating the lash. The oily parts of the face, forehead, and eyebrows were the main habitat. *Demodex* were rarely found on the body, arms, pubis, or axilla. Apparently the organism is adapted to live in oily sebaceous material. It can travel across the skin at a rate of about 1 cm/hour.

Fortunately infestation with this mite seems to be asymptomatic because eradication is difficult, if not impossible. *Demodex* is killed by ether, alcohol, sulfur ointment, and organophosphate cholinesterase inhibitors. Presumably an effective regimen would include vigorous and frequent facial scrubbing with alcohol, thorough mechanical scrubbing of the lid margins, epilation of loose lashes, and application of sulfacetamide ointment to the lid margins.

Electron microscopy shows *Demodex* specimens to be covered with various types of bacteria.[152] Presumably the mites may act as mechanical vectors in the spread of infection.

SPIROCHETES

In 1957 the U.S. Public Health Service estimated that 26,000 persons were blinded by syphilis—approximately 8% of all blindness.[153] Maintenance of these syphilitic blind cost 12½ million dollars and their estimated lifetime lost income totaled 76 million dollars.

Of 730 cases of syphilitic blindness, optic atrophy accounted for 494; interstitial keratitis, 76; chorioretinitis, 29; and iridocyclitis, 14.[154]

Reported cases of new syphilis in the United States have increased from 6399 in 1956 to 22,969 in 1964.[155] By some statistical legerdemain, this figure was extrapolated to a probable estimate of 120,000 cases in 1964, mostly unreported. Even cursory reading of current newspapers suggests that the changing habits of today's young population will increase this figure rapidly. Inevitably, these patients will arrive at our offices.

Diagnosis

Syphilis should be particularly suspected as a possible cause of six ocular manifestations.[156] These are (1) any pupillary abnormality not otherwise readily explained, (2) optic atrophy, (3) fundus changes suggesting retinitis pigmentosa (including bilateral cases), (4) chronic uveitis, (5) dislocated lenses (except Marfan's syndrome), and (6) chronic keratitis with deep vascularization. A high incidence of psychoneurotic or psychotic mental symptoms is observed in patients with late syphilis. Because of the significant frequency of false negative serologic reactions, patients strongly suspected as having syphilitic ocular changes should be studied with the specific treponemal tests (*Treponema pallidum* immobilization [TPI] and fluorescent treponemal antibody absorption). A negative standard serologic test does *not* rule out syphilis as a cause of these ocular changes.

The treponemal immobilization test should *not* be done on any patient receiving an antibiotic with antitreponemal activity. So long as such antibiotic persists in the serum, it will affect the test. The TPI test may remain positive for the rest of the patient's life, despite therapy, and should *not* be used to assess the results of treatment. Since it is quite expensive, the TPI test should *not* be ordered until the routine serologic examinations (which usually suffice for diagnosis) have been performed. The two indications for specific treponemal antigen testing are (1) detection of the biologic false positive reaction and (2) detection of seronegative syphilis.

Many physicians erroneously assume that negative serologic tests (Kahn, VDRL, etc.) exclude the possibility of syphilis from the differential diagnosis of an eye inflammation. Actually, a false negative serology is not uncommon in patients with ocular syphilis and neurosyphilis.[157] Of 718 sera positive to the FTA-ABS test, 39% were false negative with the VDRL test.[158] Inadequate antibiotic treatment of syphilis is particularly likely to produce the patient who is false negative by the standard serologic tests but who is correctly diagnosed with the TPI method.

An even more accurate test than the TPI is the fluorescent treponemal antibody-absorption (FTA-ABS) test for syphilis.[159] Although this is presently considered to be the ultimate test, it is not completely infallible since in repeated testing of borderline positive sera, 17% of originally positive sera cannot be reconfirmed as positive by the same test. Antibodies to related treponematoses such as yaws or pinta will also cause the FTA-ABS test to be positive. The FTA-ABS test is not affected by antibiotic therapy as is the TPI.

We tend to assume that "borderline" reports on serologic tests are probably of no significance. In fact, such a report identifies the real possibility that syphilis is present. Of 105 neuro-ophthalmologic patients with borderline FTA-ABS tests, 15% had "syphilitic" pupils, 29% had optic atrophy, and 9.5% had optic neuritis.[160]

Application of the FTA-ABS test to ophthalmology, particularly when used to study specimens of aqueous humor, has established the presence of spirochetes in a number of chronic eye infections suspected but not previously proved to be syphilitic.[161-167] Pitfalls of this rather demanding technique include a variety of artifact *"Treponema."*[168]

Optic atrophy

Although syphilis is a relatively uncommon etiology of optic neuritis, this is a blinding disease that can be effectively treated during its early stages. Hence serologic testing should without fail be part of the evaluation of every patient with optic neuritis. Direct spirochetal invasion of the optic nerve has been demonstrated to be the cause of luetic optic atrophy. Any ophthalmologist who has seen the numerous cases of syphilitic secondary optic atrophy in the blind wards of a veterans' hospital will not doubt the potential of this disease to cause optic neuritis with consequent primary optic atrophy.

The response of acute syphilitic optic neuritis to penicillin is rapid. A typical case of 2 weeks' duration in a 20-year-old female was treated with 600,000 units of procaine penicillin daily for 10 days.[169] Within 8 days after treatment was started, vision had improved from 20/40 to 20/20 and a field defect so large as to be almost hemianopic had nearly completely disappeared. Vision was still normal 2 years later.

Traditionally, temporal arteritis has been classified as a collagen disease, leading to the therapeutic implication that corticosteroid therapy is appropriate for this disorder. Reevaluation of our thinking is required by the unequivocal demonstration of *Treponema pallidum* in sections of the temporal artery and aspirated aqueous samples from an 83-year-old man with bilateral acute blindness from typical temporal arteritis.[170] The authors also found reactive FTA-ABS tests in four of 10 patients with biopsy-proved temporal arteritis.

Unfortunately intensive treatment with penicillin, corticosteroids, and anticoagulants did not restore sight to this patient. When ischemic necrosis has destroyed the optic nerve, any therapy is too late. However, detection of the syphilitic infection and its treatment might reasonably be expected to prevent subsequent vascular or neurologic disease elsewhere—perhaps in the other eye in a case of monocular blindness resulting from syphilitic temporal arteritis. (This is an unproved hypothesis, but the importance of the treatment of syphilis cannot be questioned.) From the practical standpoint, the diagnosis of temporal arteritis indicates the performance of serologic tests for syphilis.

Interstitial keratitis

To evaluate the effect of therapy on a given disease, one must first have an accurate picture of the natural course of that disease. Very few cases of active interstitial keratitis resulting from congenital syphilis are now seen in the United States, and the ophthalmologist whose experience is limited to recognition of a few old, typically scarred corneas will erroneously conclude that this is the usual outcome of interstitial keratitis.

A very good article presents detailed information on 128 Finnish patients with interstitial keratitis caused by congenital syphilis.[171] Keratitis developed between 4 and 12 years of age in 59% and between 13 and 22 years of age in 31%. Other typical stigmata of congenital syphilis were present in 90% of these patients. The commonest of these stigmata were the peg-shaped and notched Hutchinson's incisor teeth, which were found in 57% of all cases. Only three siblings of the 128 affected patients had interstitial keratitis, although these families averaged four children each. Serologic and clinical study identified only 20% of the children of syphilitic parents as having congenital syphilis. Wassermann or Kahn tests were positive in only 44% of patients. Only one patient showed the clinical manifestations of neurosyphilis and only two of 40 had spinal fluid changes.

The most functional statistic of final visual acuity is the vision of the patient's better eye. Of the better eyes, 31% saw 20/20 or better; 39%, 20/40; 22%, 20/80; 6%, 20/200; 2%, counts fingers; and 1% blind. If involvement of the second eye occurred, it appeared within 1 year in 93% of cases and in more than 5 years in only 4% of the bilateral cases. Of 88 treated patients, 80% were bilateral; of 32 untreated, 87% were bilateral.

Ten percent of patients with interstitial keratitis had strabismus. Myopia was present in 33% (normal incidence, 7%), and the cases of over 6.00 D were related to an early age of onset of the keratitis. Stromal scars were present in 95%, and deep blood vessels in 84%. Forty percent had iris atrophy, and 13 of 17 patients had goniosynechiae. Only 12% had syphilitic chorioretinitis.

Although the onset of syphilitic interstitial keratitis is usually considered to be in early infancy, this is not true. Fig. 35-10 shows the age of onset of ocular inflammation in a large series of cases recorded in the Johns Hopkins Hospital.[172]

The death blow has been dealt to the theory of an allergic etiology of syphilitic interstitial keratitis by the development of the fluorescent antibody stain for *Treponema pallidum*. This technique is far more sensitive than the older silver nitrate stains and

dark-field method. The classic study of experimental ocular syphilis in 1921 failed to demonstrate ocular spirochetes.[173] With the fluorescent antibody stain, *Treponema pallidum* has been demonstrated in both the aqueous and vitreous from a rabbit with luetic iritis and keratitis 23 months after subcutaneous inoculation with the organism.[174]

The persistent nature of syphilitic intraocular infection is proved by the histologic demonstration of many spirochetes within a blind, painful eye enucleated 42 years after the onset of acute interstitial keratitis.[175] A special silver nitrate stain was necessary. This patient showed the classic serologic pattern of late syphilis, seronegative to the usual tests but reactive to specific treponemal tests. However, of 20 cases of clinically diagnosed late syphilitic interstitial keratitis, the FTA-ABS test was reactive in only 35%.[176]

Therapy

Current recommendations for the treatment of syphilis with penicillin are as follows. Primary, secondary, latent, and early congenital (2 to 10 years of age) syphilis may be treated with a total of 6 million units. Procaine penicillin in oil with aluminum mono-

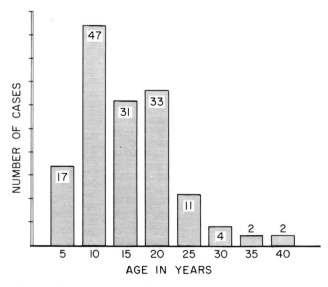

Fig. 35-10. Age of onset of acute interstitial keratitis. (Modified from Knox, D. L.: Arch. Ophthalmol. **66:**18, 1961.)

stearate, 1 million units/injection, may be given, at intervals of 2 to 7 days, to this total. Neurosyphilis, cardiovascular syphilis, and treatment failures should receive 7.2 million units. Some authors advise higher doses in problem cases.

Actually, the amount of treatment needed to eradicate spirochetes (if possible at all?) is unknown, since the recommended treatment may fail to eradicate spirochetes from the cerebrospinal fluid.[177] This is possibly because penicillin may not enter the cerebrospinal fluid in adequate concentrations to destroy the spirochetes.[178]

Penicillin-sensitive patients may be treated with erythromycin or a tetracycline, 3 g daily, for 10 days for primary syphilis and 15 days for neurosyphilis.

A quantitative decrease in the serologic test usually appears within 6 months after adequate treatment. Complete serologic nonreactivity may not occur as long as 2 years after treatment. Approximately half of the patients with late syphilis will *never* become nonreactive. Treatment solely to obtain a negative serology is expensive and cannot be justified medically. The purpose of therapy of neurosyphilis is to heal active lesions and to prevent further progress of the disease.

A repeat course of adequate treatment is indicated for the development of a progression of symptoms (for example, visual field loss) that can be attributed to syphilis relapse or reinfection. Failure of the spinal fluid to revert to normal (less than five cells) within 1 to 2 years after treatment indicates continuing neurosyphilitic activity, which should be treated.

Ocular therapy

In noninflamed human eyes the usual dose of penicillin G (600,000 to 1,200,000 units) yields barely assayable levels of aqueous humor activity. Not only does the blood-eye barrier block the entry of penicillin, but whatever antibiotic enters the eye is washed out by the aqueous flow and is selectively transported out of the eye by the ciliary body. Renal and ciliary body transport of penicillin is blocked by probenecid, which therefore has a dual mechanism for enhancing intraocular concentrations of penicillin.

To achieve measurable intraocular penicillin levels, probenecid, 0.5 g orally every 6 hours, was advised together with injections of 2,500,000 units of penicillin G or 1.5 g of ampicillin orally. Therapy of this magnitude resulted in aqueous levels approximating 1 μg/ml at 2 hours and 0.2 μg/ml at 5 hours. Without probenecid, no aqueous levels of penicillin were attainable at 2 hours.[179]

Although such intensive penicillin treatment (continued for 10 days or more) of treponemal uveitis usually resulted in a remission of clinical activity, more than half of the treated patients had a spontaneous recurrence of anterior uveitis. Treponemes were frequently demonstrated in the aqueous humor during these recurrences. *Treponema pallidum* divides at a rate of perhaps once every 30 hours. Inability to maintain adequate levels of penicillin constantly for such long periods of time may account for the incomplete destruction of the microorganisms.

What are the therapeutic implications of the finding of intraocular treponemes? Of a group of 36 patients with various ocular manifestations of syphilis, 12 were found to have the characteristic treponema in their aqueous humor.[180] (In four of these patients, both the VDRL and FTA-ABS serologic tests were negative, and in three additional patients the tests were only weakly reactive.) A treatment regimen of 1.5 g oral ampicillin and 0.5 g probenecid orally four times daily for 10 days was completed by only seven of these 12 patients (six cases of active uveitis and one of optic atrophy). (In four of these patients the VDRL and FTA-ABS tests were negative and in two additional patients the tests were only weakly reactive.) Of these six patients with treated uveitis, three improved clinically, and follow-up aqueous humor examinations did not reveal treponemes during 6 months of posttreatment observation. Two patients improved but relapsed into recurrent uveitis 2 and 4 months after treatment, at which time treponemes were again found in the aqueous. One patient continued to have active uveitis and demonstrable treponemes despite treatment.

Although many reports substantiate the recovery of spirochetes from aqueous humor in syphilitic eyes, treatment adequate to eradicate the intraocular infection is yet to be determined. For example, treatment and retreatment with penicillin in dosages up to 7.2 million units has failed to eradicate the intraocular spirochetes.[181] Even 9.2 million units of penicillin did not eliminate spirochetes from the aqueous humor of a 23-year-old woman with papillitis and chronic anterior uveitis.[182]

Retesting with the FTA-ABS test showed that of 67 patients supposedly adequately treated at least 13 years previously for late syphilis, 98% were still seropositive.[183] The clinician must recognize that there is no known method for eradicating the treponeme from man in the late stages of syphilis.[184]

The suggestion has been made that ocular tissues may provide a poor environment for spirochetal multiplication. Relatively dormant intraocular organisms would be immune to penicillin, since its action is to interfere with the synthesis of the cell wall mucopeptide, a process important only to growing spirochetes.[185] Another explanation for persistent intraocular organisms cites the poor intraocular penetration of antibiotics.

The reader will recognize a large number of clinical problems that will always remain unsolved in the management of a given case of possible syphilitic uveitis. Is the etiology syphilitic despite a negative (or positive) serology? Does adequate medication penetrate the eye? Is the patient faithful in taking medication? Did syphilitic reinfection occur after completion of antibiotic treatment? If the uveitis gradually subsides, is this because of antibiotic therapy, simultaneous use of corticosteroids, or spontaneous improvement? Scientifically acceptable answers to these questions are difficult to achieve.

Private physicians tend to have a perspective focused mostly on their own personal patients' disease to the relative exclusion of the public health aspects of this disease.

Such a view is entirely unacceptable in the management of syphilis. The damage caused by this eradicable disease will never be eliminated except by preventive public health measure, including the reporting and epidemiologic follow-up of all cases of syphilis. Knowledge of the rate of spread of syphilis indicates that treatment of 30% of all new cases before they can be transmitted to others will eradicate the disease in 8 years. As of 1965, however, 1 million active cases in the United States were estimated to require treatment. This represents a 225% increase over 1957. Unless treated, about one fourth of these infected individuals will develop the crippling late manifestations of the disease.[186]

TOXOPLASMOSIS

Multiple publications document the complex nature of ocular toxoplasmosis, which is now considered to be a frequent cause of posterior uveitis.[187-212]

Diagnosis

Correlation of the ophthalmoscopic picture of uveitis with its presumed etiology suggests that such classification may indeed be possible.[213] In 97% of patients with focal exudative retinochoroiditis with vitreous opacities, the toxoplasmin skin test and Sabin dye tests were found to be positive. In contrast, the toxoplasmin skin tests were positive in only 24% of patients with other types of uveitis. This finding strongly suggests that toxoplasmosis is a common, if not the usual, cause of focal exudative retinochoroiditis.

Transplacental toxoplasma infection of the retina is an unequivocally proved cause of congenital retinochoroiditis, optic neuritis, and encephalitis. For example, in eight autopsied cases of human congenital toxoplasmosis, all eyes showed microphthalmos and severe retinal necrosis.[214] The choroid was never involved except as a secondary change resulting from adjacent retinal infection. Retinal detachment and necrosis, as well as marked swelling of the optic disc, were described.

Coats' disease appears clinically compatible with the assumption that a chronic low-grade infection exists within the retina and perhaps also the choroid. That *Toxoplasma* infection is capable of causing the picture of Coats' disease is indicated by the typical case of a 17-year-old girl in whom *Toxoplasma* organisms were found in sections of the choroid and ciliary body and were isolated by mouse inoculation of ocular material obtained at enucleation.[215]

Unfortunately the ophthalmoscopic appearance of an individual case of posterior uveitis does not permit certain etiologic diagnosis. Until direct biopsy identification of the causative organism is possible, accurate specific diagnosis and therapy are impossible. A pertinent case report describes an acute uveitis diagnosed as caused by toxoplasmosis because of positive skin and blood tests.[216] Six months later the enucleated eye was found to have been destroyed by *Candida albicans*—a completely unsuspected endogenous fungus infection.

Prognosis

Attempts to define and predict the course of a given attack of toxoplasmic choroiditis (for purposes of evaluating therapeutic effect) cannot be successful because of the great spontaneous variations in the course of this disease.[217] Although the average duration of an active episode of toxoplasmic retinochoroiditis was 4.2 months, the duration varied from 1 week to 2 years in this series of 63 patients. Many episodes of toxoplasmic retinochoroiditis are self-limited, short, and benign. Any type of treatment of such mild attacks could be misinterpreted as being of impressive value. Such observations may be responsible for the popular but unproved assumption that prompt diagnosis and early treatment will shorten the course and severity of the disease. This carefully documented publication was of superior quality, containing excellent details and thoughtful evaluation, yet the authors have themselves emphasized that such retrospective studies of treatment response have little value. Essential parameters such as the duration of the symptoms before treatment, the length of the treatment regimens, and details as to drug changes are almost impossible to extract from old records even though detailed. Valid conclusions as to the effects of therapy in diseases such as uveitis will require carefully planned prospective evaluations designed to minimize the effect of spontaneous variations by matching significant numbers of comparable patients receiving well-defined treatment regimens. Variations in the origin of the patients preclude comparison with other published data. The aforementioned series of patients, for example, originated through referral to a renowned uveitis center; hence they would be weighted with unusually severe cases.

Different strains of *Toxoplasma* vary greatly in their virulence, as studied in tissue culture and by animal inoculation.[218] These variations in virulence, combined with differences in host resistance, apparently account for the unpredictable behavior of human intraocular infection presumably of toxoplasmic etiology. Because of these multiple variables, the clinical evaluation of uveitis therapy is understandably difficult.

Therapeutic response

Vision-threatening uveitis presumed to be of toxoplasmic origin may be treated by pyrimethamine and sulfonamides, usually accompanied by systemic corticosteroids. Such treatment of 90 patients suggested that improvement could usually be recognized after 2 weeks of therapy, with circumscribed inactive scarring achieved by 2 to 3 months.[219] In some cases, active inflammation continued for several more months. No control patients were available for comparison. The risks of such treatment require capable medical supervision, since the side effects are severe and unpleasant.

In another series of 84 patients, 43% were free of active uveitis after pyrimethamine and sulfonamide therapy.[220] Unfortunately no information is given as to the duration of treatment required to achieve this response. The inadequacy of existing clinical studies of the effectiveness of pyrimethamine therapy is generally acknowledged.[221]

A realistic evaluation of pyrimethamine and sulfonamide therapy of human uveitis presumed to be of toxoplasmic etiology concludes that it is "disappointing." Such treatment of 18 cases resulted in probable benefit to only four.[222]

Possible complications of corticosteroid therapy also require clinical consideration. During corticosteroid therapy a patient (42 years of age) developed a perforation of a diverticulum of the descending colon and died of peritonitis despite surgery and antibiotic therapy.[223] This patient had a negative *Toxoplasma* skin test and a negative dye test at 1:16. The dye test was positive only with undiluted serum. The eye lesions were refractory to large doses of topical and systemic corticosteroids. The postmortem examination of the eyes showed the foci of active retinochoroiditis to contain *Toxoplasma* cysts.

Experimental therapy

Corticosteroid treatment of *Toxoplasma*-infected animals causes a marked decrease in retinal and choroidal inflammation and destruction. Nineteen rabbits were infected by intravitreal injection.[224] Five rabbits were treated with 50 mg hydrocortisone injected subcutaneously two times a day; six were treated with 25 mg two times a day. The nine untreated controls all suffered diffuse and severe retinal and choroidal destruction. Ten of the 11 treated rabbits developed only focal chorioretinal lesions, much less severe than the untreated cases.

Unfortunately all 11 treated rabbits died (of the infection!) within 2 weeks, although all untreated animals survived until sacrifice. Since similar hydrocortisone treatment of rabbits with chronic toxoplasmosis did not cause reactivation of the disease or death, it seems that only acute infections are potentiated by corticosteroids. Concurrent therapy with pyrimethamine, sulfonamides, and corticosteroids was suggested as good clinical management for chorioretinitis presumed of toxoplasmic etiology; however, this suggestion was not based on experimental proof of its efficacy. This fatal corticosteroid-in-duced dissemination of toxoplasmosis is thought provoking.

Pyrimethamine and sulfonamide treatment did not protect guinea pigs against experimental ocular infection with toxoplasmosis.[225] However, guinea pigs metabolize these medications quite rapidly.[226]

Attempts were made to reactivate healed toxoplasmic retinochoroiditis (rabbit) by trauma, systemic epinephrine, and systemic corticosteroids.[227] None of these provocative methods resulted in clinical relapse.

Immunologic factors significantly affect the multiplication and encystment of *Toxoplasma gondii*. The organisms were grown in tissue culture (rabbit corneal endothelial cells). Addition of rabbit immune serum and complement factors resulted within 3 days in the formation of large numbers of toxoplasma cysts. Within 5 days cellular destruction was conspicuously less marked in the immunologically treated cultures than in the controls.[228] One can only speculate as to whether active or passive hyperimmunization would be of benefit to the patient, or whether induced encystment would protect the organisms against antibiotic therapy.

In a patient with polymyositis and a Sabin-Feldman dye titer of 1:32,000, repeated muscle biopsies failed to disclose any organisms.[229] Clindamycin, 300 mg every 6 hours for a month, resulted in a drop of the titer to 1:8000 and improvement in clinical symptoms.

Cryotherapy

The inflammations of all of a series of seven patients having presumed *Toxoplasma* retinochoroiditis treated with cryotherapy became inactive more rapidly than would have been anticipated without freezing.[230] These were quite severe inflammations, and yet they quieted within a few weeks after cryotherapy.

Photocoagulation

After prophylactic photocoagulation of 24 patients with inactive "*Toxoplasma*" lesions that had previously recurred at least once, no recurrences developed in the treated areas during follow-up periods of up to 3 years' duration.[231] In two patients, recurrences developed at untreated edges in the macular region. Because of the unpredictable timing of recurrences, evaluation of such prophylactic therapy is not really possible.

VIRUS INFECTIONS

The virus infections of ocular significance include adenovirus infections, cat-scratch disease, herpes simplex, herpes zoster, inclusion conjunctivitis, molluscum contagiosum, rubella, trachoma, and vaccinia. Although we are accustomed to dismiss treatment of virus diseases as being nonexistent, this is not really true. The following discussions will outline briefly some pertinent clinical features of these diseases and will cite therapeutic recommendations that appear representative of the literature to date.

Adenovirus infections

More than 30 antigenically different varieties of adenovirus have been isolated from man. Many of these may affect the conjunctiva, causing mild or severe conjunctivitis of short or prolonged duration, with or without corneal involvement. In some instances the eye findings are only a minor part of a highly infectious acute illness known as pharyngoconjunctival fever.

The laboratory confirmation of the clinical diagnosis of adenovirus infection requires the isolation of the virus in tissue culture or the demonstration of rising antibody titers. In a group of volunteers inoculated with type 3 adenovirus, vain attempts were made to find a more rapid diagnostic method. Fluorescent antibody techniques and various stains for conjunctival cytology did not give useful results.[232]

Two patients with adenovirus conjunctivitis caused by types 2 and 3 were treated by topical idoxuridine without response.[233]

Epidemic keratoconjunctivitis

As yet, there is no specific therapy for the epidemic keratoconjunctivitis caused by type 8 adenovirus. During an epidemic, 102 cases were studied at the Wills Eye Hospital.[234]

The empirically recommended treatment for these patients consisted of local antibiotics, corticosteroids, and cycloplegics. The authors specifically noted the absence of superinfection with bacteria, fungi, or other viruses. The need for, or the benefit from, antibiotic therapy is therefore not established. However, preventive antibiotic treatment during the period of epithelial staining (second and third week of the disease) does not seem unreasonable.

Local corticosteroid drops relieved discomfort during the acute stages of keratoconjunctivitis. The presence of anterior uveitis was considered to be another indication for corticosteroid treatment. Neither shortening nor prolongation of the disease was noted as a result of corticosteroid therapy.

Presumably cycloplegia was recommended for the usual indications of photophobia, discomfort, and aqueous flare or cells.

Prevention of the spread of infection is an important part of the management of epidemic keratoconjunctivitis. Although tonometry is usually condemned as the method of iatrogenic spread of the disease, the majority of patients infected in the hospital never had tonometry. Hand-to-eye transmission was considered proved by the appearance of the disease in patients of physicians themselves suffering from the initial stages of the infection. Use of a sterile cotton-tipped applicator for lid examination in the cornea service eliminated spread, even though all cases were referred to this area. In the cornea service it was the rule never to touch the patient's eyelids with the fingers during examination. Another control measure was the elimination of infected physicians and nurses from patient-care responsibility during the signs and symptoms of the acute stage of disease.

Recognition of epidemic keratoconjunctivitis in time to prevent the spread of infection is almost impossible in a sporadic case. For this reason, routine cleanliness (handwashing and general precautions to protect the patient from contamination) is essential in our medical practice.[235-237] The most frequent initial symptoms of epidemic keratoconjunctivitis are foreign body sensation, redness of the eye, and tearing. Only half the patients have tender preauricular nodes. Fever, malaise, and upper respiratory tract infections are rarely evident. The disease begins with the rather nonspecific conjunctival phase, characterized by hyperemia and edema of the bulbar and particularly the tarsal conjunctiva and by follicular hypertrophy. The characteristic corneal phase does not appear until about 11 days after onset of symptoms and begins with myriads of pinpoint epithelial-staining foci, involving the entire corneal area. The typical rounded subepithelial infiltrates traditionally used for diagnosis of epidemic conjunctivitis are recognized on an average of 20 days after symptoms begin. These infiltrates vary from 0.2 to 1.5 mm in size and last for weeks or months. Corneal sensitivity is not reduced in epidemic conjunctivitis, whereas this commonly occurs in herpes simplex or herpes zoster.

Viral typing studies have disclosed that epidemic keratoconjunctivitis is not characteristic of only type 8 adenovirus, but may also be caused by types 2, 4, 7, 9, 10, 14, 16, 19, and 29.[238] Symblepharon, uveitis, and hemorrhagic conjunctivitis may be components of the infection. The severity of the keratitis correlates somewhat with the antibody titers, low titers being associated with more severe keratitis.[239] Because positive viral isolations are difficult to obtain after the first week of illness, serologic tests were the most successful method of identification.

In a unique epidemic of 87 patients with epidemic keratoconjunctivitis, multiple etiologic agents were simultaneously present. Type 8 adenovirus was responsible for 47 cases; type 19 for 23; type 3 for two; type 7A for one; and herpes simplex for one. The virus responsible in the remaining cases was not identifiable. Contrary to the presumption that clinically apparent differences would be found between types 8 and 19, there was a spectrum of severity within the cases caused by each type, and clinical distinction was impossible. In both groups there were cases of conjunctivitis with no evidence of kera-

titis. Of special interest was the prospective study of 10 teachers at a school suffering an epidemic. Within 3 days of exposure, two teachers yielded positive cultures of adenovirus type 19. One of these developed conjunctivitis and increased serologic titer 26 days later. The other developed an increasing titer but never exhibited ocular disease. Obviously, the host response to adenoviruses varies widely.[240]

Superficial punctate keratitis

The diagnosis of superficial punctate keratitis is important because the symptoms respond well to corticosteroid therapy. Superficial punctate keratitis is a bilateral chronic corneal inflammation lasting from months to years, with remissions and exacerbations. The typical lesion is a microscopically small fluorescein-staining defect of the superficial epithelium. These defects are distributed throughout the corneal surface, may number 20 or more, and are responsible for the characteristic slight blurring of vision and ocular burning, irritation, and redness. They ultimately heal without scarring. Antibiotic or sulfonamide therapy is not helpful. IDU therapy is not helpful—in fact, it causes an increase in the size of the subepithelial opacities.[241] The etiology is unknown; however, a virus is suspected (adenovirus?). In a series of 29 cases, epidemiologic study failed to detect contact of the patients with other infected individuals, and no causative organism was recovered by routine culture, tissue culture inoculation, or rabbit corneal inoculation.[242] Except for one patient, all 29 of these patients experienced prompt symptomatic relief with topical corticosteroid treatment. The corticosteroid effect is suppressive rather than curative, since the epithelial lesions returned whenever corticosteroids were discontinued. The overall duration of the disease does not seem to be prolonged by symptomatic treatment with corticosteroids, nor does this cause exacerbations or scarring.

Cat-scratch disease

The oculoglandular syndrome of Parinaud may follow a cat scratch, but this classic syndrome was found in only six of 152 cases of cat-scratch disease.[243] Retrospective evaluation showed that of 40 patients treated with antibiotics, 20 had not improved after 1 week and 20 had possibly improved. Of 49 untreated patients, 34 improved and 15 had not improved after 1 week. Nearly all commonly used antibiotics were used; in particular, tetracycline was used. Several patients received three different antibiotics consecutively or simultaneously without benefit. Corticosteroid treatment was not helpful. Aspiration of suppurating nodes was suggested for symptomatic relief.

Since the oculoglandular syndrome of cat-scratch disease spontaneously improves, the effect of antibiotic treatment is difficult to evaluate. Although this is a virus disease, it has been suggested (without a controlled study) that chlortetracycline, 200 mg four times a day, may hasten recovery.[244]

Herpes simplex

Antibodies to this troublesome virus are present in over 90% of adults, although fortunately the great majority of these individuals have no significant disease manifestations.[245]

Acute ocular herpes simplex

Experimental ocular infection with herpes simplex virus inoculated by instilling a drop of virus suspension on the uninjured nonimmune rabbit eye reveals prompt virus growth in all layers of the cornea.[246] Virus could be recovered from the various lacrimal and conjunctival glands as early as 10 hours after inoculation. Only after 18 hours was virus recoverable from the cornea. After 2 days most of the corneas showed superficial staining and virus was recoverable in all cultures of corneal epithelium and stroma. Higher concentrations of virus were recoverable on the third and fourth day, at which time dendritic figures appeared. By the fifth day, corneal edema and iritis appeared in most animals, and virus was recoverable from all corneal layers, including the endothelium. Corneal edema could be correlated with endothelial virus infection. Clearly, the

old concept that herpes is solely an epithelial infection is an unsubstantiated myth despite the fact that chemical cautery "cures" dendritic keratitis.

Experiments studying the persistence of herpes simplex virus in the corneal epithelium of rabbits showed that the virus could be recovered from 100% of untreated eyes 5 days after infection, from 62% after 10 days, and from no eyes after 15 days.[247] Disappearance of detectable virus preceded spontaneous healing of the corneal ulcers. In contrast, when subconjunctival methyl prednisolone, 20 mg, or topical hydrocortisone, 0.5% three times a day, were used in treatment of the infected rabbits, virus could still be recovered on the fifteenth day in 71% (10 of 14) of the eyes. This is in agreement with many other studies that indicate that corticosteroids inhibit the ability to destroy virus.

In this same study, complete removal of all the corneal epithelium by curettage was performed on 24 eyes from which virus could still be recovered and on 35 eyes without recoverable virus. Recurrent dendritic keratitis occurred in 75% of the former group, but in only 3% of the latter. In rabbits, therefore, curettage seems to have no effect on the clinical course of corneal herpetic infection, recurrences being frequent if the virus was present at the time of treatment. No chemical sterilization was used in this experiment.

Is the rate of subsequent recurrence of human herpetic keratitis favorably or unfavorably affected by treatment of the active disease with the various methods of therapy? This question was evaluated in a study of 159 patients followed for a minimum of 2 years after an attack of herpetic keratitis. The recurrence rate after the first attack of dendritic keratitis was 26% of patients. During the 2 years following a second (or more) attack of herpetic keratitis, the recurrence rate was 43%. No statistically significant differences in recurrence rates were found in patients who had been treated with iodine cauterization, IDU, or corticosteroids.[248]

The physician tends to think in terms of therapeutic eradication of the germ causing a given infection. Apparently "cure" of herpes simplex corneal infection represents some type of inactivation or latency during which the virus nevertheless persists. Study of 50 rabbits with herpes simplex eye infections permitted virus recovery during 112 separate episodes up to 3 years (the length of the study) after the initial infection.[249] No recognizable clinical infection was present during 72% of these episodes of culture-proved virus presence. When the rabbit eye is infected with herpes simplex virus, a chronic inapparent infection probably persists during the lifetime of the animal and may be activated by various factors, including topical epinephrine.

Intramuscular injection of 0.5 ml of 1:500 epinephrine in oil for 3 consecutive days effectively reactivated herpetic keratitis in 12 of 22 attempts.[250] In one rabbit, four herpetic recurrences were reactivated over a 6-month period. The reactivating effect of epinephrine may offer a clue as to why herpetic recurrences are related to periods of stress.

Chronic persistence of herpes simplex virus in the human ocular adnexae can be demonstrated by staining with fluorescein-labeled antibody. This technique revealed virus antigen in sections of conjunctiva and lacrimal glands in three of four patients with active corneal herpes and in four of seven patients with clinically inactive disease.[251] Recurrent keratitis can easily be explained on the basis of reinfection from these extraocular sources. After "cure" of human herpetic keratitis, virus cannot be isolated from the cornea, and there is no evidence indicating that virus remains latent within corneal tissue of normal appearance.[252]

Another answer to the question of the location of herpes virus between attacks was provided by the sacrifice of rabbits 4 to 9 months after the original infection. Virus cultures were made of conjunctiva, nictitating membrane, lacrimal gland, cornea, iris, preganglionic trigeminal nerve, trigeminal ganglion, and central trigeminal nucleus. All these tissues were virus negative except the trigeminal ganglion. Nineteen of 26 ganglia (73%) were virus positive. This finding suggests that the trigeminal ganglia are the reservoirs of herpes simplex virus between attacks of clinical disease.[253]

Herpetic conjunctivitis

Herpes simplex may also cause acute or recurrent conjunctivitis unassociated with corneal disease.[254] Recognition of this etiology will permit prescription of IDU therapy.

Zoster dendrite

Superficial dendritic patterns resembling herpes simplex may occur in herpes zoster. The clinical distinction is of significance because corticosteroid therapy benefits the zoster lesions and harms the simplex lesions. The zoster pathology is a thickening of the epithelial cells, which appear to form an elevated gray plaque that stains only slightly with fluorescein. In contrast, simplex causes an ulcerated dendritic figure, with loss of epithelium in a trough-like contour that stains brightly. The zoster dendrite clears in 7 to 72 days (average 30 days).[255, 256]

Idoxuridine (IDU) therapy

Herpes simplex virus can be isolated from about 65% of active epithelial lesions. If IDU has been given within the 48 hours preceding culture, the chance of isolating the virus is reduced to about 8%, despite continuing presence of epithelial activity.[257]

To maintain effective action of IDU, 0.5% ointment must be applied five times daily (including bedtime application). Recognizable improvement of a dendritic ulcer should occur within 5 days in two thirds of the patients. (An inactive "ghost" pattern may persist for several weeks at the ulcer site and should not be misinterpreted as treatment failure.) Mechanical removal of the infected epithelium may be appropriate if response to IDU is not evident within 5 days.

Do not discontinue IDU if improvement is noted at 5 days. Rather, continue treatment for a total of 2 weeks. The reason for this is that all virus is *not* destroyed by treatment. Indeed, a rebound increase in virus titer occurs at the end of 1 week in rabbits.

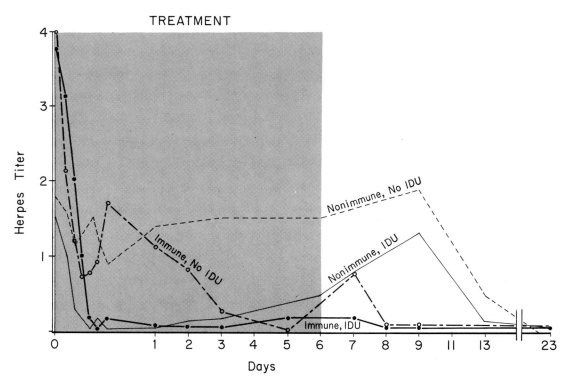

TREATMENT

Fig. 35-11. Herpes virus titer in experimental immune (heavy lines) and nonimmune (thin lines) rabbits and with (solid lines) and without (dotted lines) IDU treatment. Note increase in titer at 1 week, despite treatment. (Modified from Hughes, W. F.: Am. J. Ophthalmol. **67:**313, 1969.)

This 1-week rebound occurs in all animals, whether IDU-treated, untreated, immune to herpes, or nonimmune. However, the least virus rebound occurs in immune, IDU-treated animals (Fig. 35-11).[258]

Although IDU treatment may be discontinued after 2 weeks in the management of dendritic ulcers, more prolonged therapy may be required in the treatment of chronic herpetic keratitis. In such cases, overtreatment must be avoided, since drug-induced corneal changes may be misinterpreted as evidence of continuing herpetic activity. Superficial punctate erosions will occur in 10% to 20% of patients using IDU for periods of several months. Although IDU inhibits stromal regeneration experimentally and can contribute to delayed corneal healing clinically, this is not considered to be a common complication. Chronic inflammatory conjunctival thickening rarely occurs as a specific allergic response to IDU. Strains of virus resistant to IDU may be encountered.[259]

Corticosteroid response

Local corticosteroid treatment of acute herpetic keratitis is contraindicated. Experimentally, such management can produce all types of complicated herpetic lesions of the cornea. These include disciform keratitis, chronic ulceration, secondary bacterial invasion, uveitis, and corneal perforation.[260] The literature and practicing ophthalmologists seem to be in almost unanimous agreement with these conclusions.

Corticosteroid treatment of experimental herpetic keratitis induced by topical instillation of virus on rabbit corneas increased the time during which positive cultures could be obtained from 2 weeks in the control to as long as 3 weeks. Medrysone, 1%, and dexamethasone, 0.1%, were instilled four times daily for 10 days. Both corticosteroids enhanced virus recovery. In the natural course of rabbit herpes, encephalitic death is not uncommon. Such deaths occurred in six of the 15 control animals, nine of the 15 dexamethasone-treated animals, and 10 of the 15 medrysone-treated animals.[261]

Systemic corticosteroid therapy has also been considered to be responsible for the general spread of herpes simplex infection in man.[262]

Topical dexamethasone, 0.1%, applied four times daily for 10 days did not reactivate herpetic keratitis in rabbit eyes that had spontaneously recovered from virus infection 5 months to a year before the corticosteroid challenge. In these same eyes, virus could be recovered in culture following challenge with topical epinephrine, 2%, five times daily for 1 week.[263] A similar experiment showed no reactivation following 10 days of dexamethasone treatment of rabbit herpetic keratitis that had been allowed to heal for 2 months.[264]

Local cauterization

Prior to the development of specific antiviral drugs, herpes simplex corneal infections were treated, mostly ineffectually, by a wide variety of medications.[265] The most widely used treatment was chemical cauterization of the diseased corneal epithelium. Cautery is advised only in superficial epithelial disease, since it seems only to irritate and further scar the cornea when the stroma is involved. No one cauterizing agent seems superior to another, since their effectiveness is dependent on the destruction and removal of the infected cells. Iodine, trichloracetic acid, ether, silver nitrate, and various other caustics have been used as well as thermal cautery.[266]

Selection of drugs that are virucidal in vitro for use in the removal of corneal epithelium infected with herpes simplex has seemed rational therapy. Furthermore, such therapy is empirically successful—it works! Logically, cultures from corneas scrubbed with virucidal drugs such as iodine, silver nitrate, or ether should be found thereafter to be free of virus. Experimentally, this is not true, since herpes simplex virus was cultured from 13 of 32 infected rabbit corneas subsequent to epithelial removal with iodine, ether, or silver nitrate.[267] Apparently, complete destruction of infected cells is often not achieved, and virus persists, although it may be asymptomatic.

After epithelial removal with physiologic saline solution, virus could be recovered in eight of 13 eyes, a slightly higher rate of recovery than with the virucidal agents, but not a statistically significant difference. These findings suggest that in vitro virucidal activity is unrelated to the effectiveness of treatment of dendritic keratitis by epithelial removal. If extracellular virucidal properties are unimportant, then the primary clinical objective should be the removal of the infected tissue with as little trauma and scarring as possible.

In these experiments, vigorous use of iodine caused severe stromal scarring, induced vascularization, and retarded epithelial healing for more than 3 days in all eyes. (It is quite possible that excessive use of iodine may cause human corneal scarring and may prolong recovery time. This is particularly true in the delicate and thin corneas of infants.)

A precaution taken to evaluate possible contamination is of clinical interest. Twenty corneas in the right eye of rabbits were infected with herpes simplex. The following day the left corneas were extensively scarified. Three days later both eyes were cultured. Although virus was recovered from 19 of 20 inoculated corneas, not one of the scarified eyes contained virus. This finding is certainly consistent with the clinical experience that infection is not readily spread to the other eye. However, patients with simplex infection should certainly be cautioned against rubbing their eyes in such a manner as to abrade infected material into the cornea of the good eye.

Chemical cautery of dendritic ulcers with 0.5% zinc sulfate solution has been advocated as an effective alternate to IDU therapy.[268] The zinc solution is applied to the ulcer with a cotton applicator for 1 minute and 40 seconds, during which time the loose epithelium surrounding the ulcer is rubbed off. Treatment for longer than 2 minutes may cause permanent nebular corneal scarring and should be avoided. In a series of 40 dendritic ulcers, 50% were epithelized in 24 hours and 90% in 3 days after zinc treatment. Results such as this may be obtained with any form of effective chemical cautery.

Comparison between IDU and simple mechanical debridement of the epithelium with a dry cotton applicator (no chemical cautery) indicates that debridement may have significant advantages. This study was done in Tunisia, a country with very few trained ophthalmologists.[269] The average healing time with IDU treatment of epithelial ulcers was 13 days, as compared to 5 days for debridement. Fewer office visits and less professional time was required for debridement. The prolonged patient cooperation required for IDU therapy is unnecessary with debridement.

One third of the herpetic keratitis in Tunisia was found to be complicated by deep stromal damage, usually consequent to corticosteroid therapy initiated by poorly trained personnel. Apparently red eyes are routinely treated with antibiotics and corticosteroids, with little knowledge of differential diagnosis or therapeutic complications.

Enzyme therapy

Enzymatic debridement of dendritic corneal ulcers with chymotrypsin is reported to accelerate their healing.[270] A freshly prepared solution of lyophilized chymotrypsin in saline solution (10,000 to 30,000 units/ml) is instilled hourly or may be used in an eyecup to bathe the eye for 5 to 10 minutes. The solution is stable for only 4 days. It may cause a burning sensation and redness of the lids in some patients. In addition, antibiotic ointment is prescribed for night use with the intention of preventing secondary infection.[271]

Fifty-four patients with fresh dendritic ulcers treated with chymotrypsin were reported to all be symptomatically improved within 48 hours. Only 2 days of treatment cured 39 patients. In the remaining 15 patients the ulcers healed in 3 to 13 days. A faint, ground-glass appearance at the site of the ulcer persisted for a few weeks and then gradually disappeared. No permanent scarring was produced in any patient. Theoretically, only nonviable tissue is eliminated, and this permits healthy epithelium to regenerate rapidly. Eight cases of metaherpetic keratitis did not clear with chymotrypsin. Before prescribing this treatment, read on!

Trypsin, 50,000 units/ml, was used to treat eight infected rabbit corneas by means of 5-minute corneal baths. Purulent conjunctivitis and iritis and stromal destruction resulted, with corneal perforation in six of the eight eyes. Despite this treatment. herpes simplex virus was recovered from all eight eyes. Alpha-chymotrypsin, 1:5000, was similarly used and caused only minimal corneal damage, but it also failed to sterilize any eye.[267]

In another experiment, commercial trypsin and chymotrypsin preparations were instilled for 6 days on rabbit eyes infected with herpes simplex.[272] Corneal damage was much more severe in the treated eyes. These enzymes appear to remove the fibrin and necrotic protein, thereby exposing fresh tissue to the further advance of the virus.

I myself have performed corneal transplantation for a corneal perforation caused by topical drops of alpha-chymotrypsin. The patient had a 7-year history of herpetic keratitis with nine recurrences of metaherpetic activity. Within a few days of enzyme treatment (prescribed elsewhere) the patient noted dramatic improvement of vision (presumably because of dissolution of the opaque stroma). Shortly thereafter the cornea ruptured spontaneously. The central cornea was entirely absent except for Descemet's membrane, which had perforated (Fig. 35-13).

Antibiotics

The use of antibiotics to prevent secondary bacterial infection of herpetic corneal ulcers is as rational as antibiotic use for any other cause of epithelial damage. One occasionally hears the claim that virus ulcers are immune to bacterial infection. The falsity of this claim is documented by a report of proved pneumococcal hypopyon ulcer developing suddenly on a dendritic ulcer.[273] Actually, seven such superimposed infections were encountered in 99 cases of herpes simplex keratitis. The majority of these were caused by fungus infection, which was ascribed to corticosteroid therapy.

None of the antibiotics antagonize the herpes virus itself.[274-276] Reports suggestive of herpetic inhibition apparently document only the natural course of the disease, with spontaneous quiescence.

Vaccination

Repeated smallpox vaccination has been recommended as treatment for recurrent herpes simplex infections but has no rational basis. The two viruses are antigenically unrelated and no evidence exists to prove benefit from such treatment.[265]

Cryotherapy

The usefulness of cryotherapy in the treatment of herpes simplex was evaluated in experimental infections of the rabbit corneal epithelium.[277] The cryostylet at $-20°$ F was applied for 7 seconds on the second, fourth,

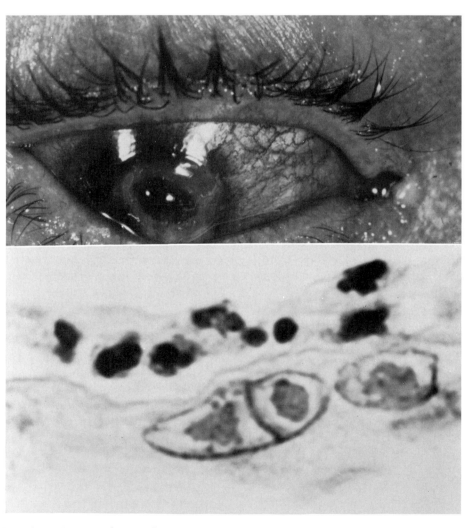

Fig. 35-12. Section of excised corneal button obtained at time of transplantation showing herpes virus inclusion bodies. (From Havener, W. H., and Stambaugh, N.: Am. J. Ophthalmol. **54:**756, 1962.)

and sixth day after herpes inoculation, causing recognizable stromal freezing. For comparison, 0.5% IDU ointment was applied three times daily, starting on the third day after inoculation. The results (Fig. 35-12) indicate that freezing has no significant effect on the course of herpes simplex keratitis.[227-279]

An interesting exchange of correspondence reviews the possible mechanisms of effect, if any, of cryotherapy for herpetic keratitis.[280] The final conclusion seemed to be that cryotherapy might be a means of destroying affected cells, somewhat akin to chemical cautery.

Occasionally papers report dramatic cures from cryotherapy, however.[281] For example, in patients treated for epithelial herpetic keratitis by cryotherapy, only one of 38 failed to heal in comparison to six failures in 27 patients treated with IDU. Also, the lesions undergoing cryotherapy healed in an average of 3.4 days as compared to 11 days for IDU.[282]

Photodynamic inactivation

Combination of herpes simplex virus with dyes such as neutral red, proflavine, or toluidine blue apparently renders the virus sensitive to disruption by light. Blue light is most effective. Conditions such as temperature, pH, duration of dye exposure, and duration of light exposure are critical.

Although this treatment has some effect in vitro, its clinical value is trivial compared with that of idoxuridine and it is not recommended for clinical use.[283-285]

Hormones

Hormonal suppression of the menstrual cycle was successfully used in the treatment of a case of herpes simplex keratitis that recurred at the start of five successive cycles despite IDU therapy.[286]

Contact lenses

Should dendritic keratitis occur in a patient wearing contact lenses, the use of the lenses should be promptly discontinued. Instillation of virus into six rabbit eyes fitted with contact lenses resulted in severe keratitis with scarring and vascularization of five corneas.[287] In contrast, mild keratitis without scarring developed in only two of the six fellow eyes (which served as controls without contact lenses). Wearing of the lenses 3 months after the infection subsided did not reactivate the healed keratitis.

Gamma globulin

Chronic postherpetic keratitis induced by corticosteroid treatment of herpes simplex–infected rabbits was significantly improved by one to three subconjunctival injections of 0.5 ml of human or rabbit gamma globulin. Gamma globulin injection was followed by improvement in 22 of 28 eyes, in contrast to worsening of 21 of 24 untreated controls.[288] Extensive corneal vascularization and associated iritis responded most favorably to the gamma globulin, whereas deep stromal opacities cleared only slowly. Since virus could not be recovered from these chronic lesions and because gamma globulin treatment during the stage of acute viral infection was unsuccessful, the mechanism of action was considered to be other than antiviral. Secondary bacterial infection was demonstrated in several of the chronically inflamed corneas; hence it is possible the gamma globulin acted by virtue of its antibacterial effect.

Five of six patients with chronic herpetic keratitis were reported to show improvement after subconjunctival injection of 0.3 ml gamma globulin.

BCG

Nonspecific resistance induced by BCG (*Mycobacterium bovis*) inoculations did not enhance the resistance of rabbits to herpes simplex corneal inoculations, as measured by clinical appearance or virus titer.[289]

Chronic herpetic keratitis

Chronic stromal herpetic keratitis apparently can be separated into a number of components, each of which requires a different therapeutic approach. These include (1) continuing virus infection, (2) a hypersensitive response, (3) a mechanical or neurotrophic ulceration, (4) iridocyclitis, and (5) secondary bacterial infection. Treatment for these different problems is by (1) IDU, (2) corticosteroids, (3) corneal protection, (4) cycloplegics, and (5) antibiotics.[290] Each of these treatments is specific for only the corresponding component, and will *not* benefit the others. Obviously combined therapy is usually necessary.

IDU treatment (0.5% ointment three times a day) of stromal keratitis must be continued for long periods (usually several months). The criterion of cure is complete absence of biomicroscopically visible corneal edema. Relapse will occur if even the slightest possible edema remains when therapy is discontinued. The majority of cases of stromal keratitis will not benefit from IDU alone, but also require treatment with corticosteroids and adequate mechanical protection. With combined treatment, 65 of 73 cases responded well.[290] Long-term IDU therapy is safe and does prevent recurrence of corneal herpes.

Corticosteroid treatment is advised three or four times daily by topical instillation of a drop or ointment. The theoretical rationale for this is a stromal hypersensitivity response to the virus infection. Empirically, combined treatment with corticosteroids and IDU is very effective against stromal herpes. Corticosteroid therapy alone, without IDU, is very likely to result in recurrent active virus keratitis; hence it should be avoided. The unprotected raw surface of a corneal ulcer is readily infected by secondary invaders, especially when the normal corneal resistance is reduced by chronic corticosteroid therapy. (IDU does not protect against bacterial infection.) For this reason, concurrent antibiotic treatment is important.[291]

Pathophysiology of chronic herpetic keratitis

Planning a rational treatment of chronic keratitis after herpes simplex infection requires knowledge of whether the lesion is caused by persistent virus or is some type of "allergic" or "trophic" phenomenon. Ordinarily cases of metaherpetic keratitis are said not to harbor virus. This "absence" of virus

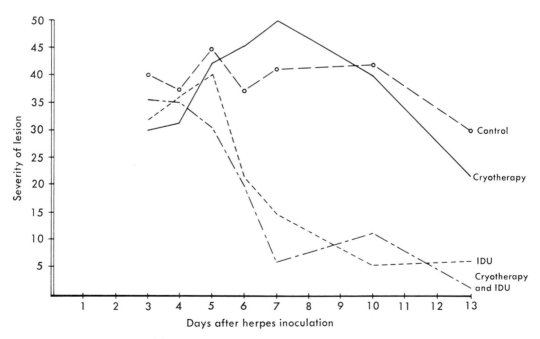

Fig. 35-13. Response of herpetic keratitis to cryotherapy. (Modified from Corwin, M. E., Copeland, R. L., and Birnbaum, S.: Am. J. Ophthalmol. **63:**399, 1967.)

may well be because of the proper reluctance of the physician to biopsy an adequate amount of tissue from the center of an already weakened cornea. Fig. 35-13 shows virus inclusion bodies found in a corneal button obtained at the time of corneal transplantation in a man who had herpes simplex 7 years prior to surgery (and nine recurrences).[292] I believe this finding strongly supports my conviction that the virus continues to be present in chronic herpetic keratitis, and that this is not an "allergic" phenomenon.

Comparable cases of herpes simplex virus isolation from the corneal stroma and deep retrocorneal scar tissue, by both electron microscopy and virus culture, have been reported,[293] and it is now generally accepted that living virus is harbored within the stromal keratocytes in chronic herpetic infection.[294] Even in stromal tissue from which virus cannot be cultured, immunofluorescent techniques reveal viral antigens still to be present.[295]

Stromal virus localization of experimental herpetic keratitis has been demonstrated by fluorescent antibody techniques and by electron microphotography.[296,297]

The concept that herpetic stromal keratitis is an immunologic phenomenon unrelated to the presence of active virus particles has been further challenged by the discovery by electron microscopy of virus particles in deep stromal cells from five of 19 specimens obtained from patients with chronic herpetic keratitis.[298] Each of these five patients had received corticosteroid drops. The herpes virus, unlike bacteria, does not produce destructive enzymes or toxins and presumably induces corneal inflammation by acting as an antigenic stimulus. Although corticosteroid therapy may reduce the inflammatory component of this antigenic response, it also suppresses host defenses and permits deeper penetration and proliferation of the virus, allowing more corneal destruction to take place. Hence corticosteroids should be used sparingly and together with IDU when stromal involvement exists.

Isolation of the herpes simplex virus from aqueous samples of patients with acute uveitis also supports the belief that active infection rather than an allergic response causes herpetic inflammation.[299]

Herpes simplex virus particles have been demonstrated by electron microscopy in iris tissue obtained at the time of surgery for secondary glaucoma in a patient with herpetic keratitis and uveitis. This finding establishes the fact that at least in this case the etiology of the uveitis was direct invasion of the iris by the microorganism and not some type of allergic response. In this patient, inflammation and pain could be controlled only with heavy corticosteroid therapy; however, despite this treatment (because of it?) the infection progressed to extensive corneal damage, uncontrollable glaucoma, cataract, iris atrophy, and scleritis.[300]

The persistent and recurrent oval corneal ulcers that develop after herpes simplex keratitis do not contain demonstrable virus and do not respond to IDU therapy. These ulcers may be comparable to the recurrent ulcerations that follow trauma. Indeed, the trauma of a complete corneal scrub with iodine may result in a 33% incidence of such sterile metaherpetic ulcers, as compared to 17% of patients treated with mechanical, nonchemical removal of infected epithelium.[301] The best treatment for such recurrent trophic ulcers is the use of adequate lubricant and protective ointments.

Endothelial damage appears to be responsible for at least part of the stromal edema associated with chronic herpetic keratitis.[302] Since this edema is often reversible by corticosteroid therapy, a component of hypersensitivity is also postulated.

Perhaps the best explanation for the corneal ulceration occurring in chronic herpetic keratitis is the development of collagenolytic activity by the chronically infected epithelial cells. Marked collagenolytic activity in vitro was demonstrable in 19 of 20 epithelial samples obtained from rabbit corneal viral ulcers but in only two of 14 normal control samples.[303] Apparently this collagenolytic effect is comparable to that known to follow alkali burns of the cornea.

Following penetrating keratoplasty for

herpetic damage, intensive and prolonged corticosteroid therapy is of value in controlling recurrent inflammation. Dexamethasone 0.1% is instilled six times daily for a month, then continued at a low level with careful observation to detect recurrent inflammation.[304]

An excellent review of herpes simplex is found in the September 1976 issue of *Survey of Ophthalmology* (Vol. 21).

Herpes zoster

Zoster virus can be recovered from the vesicles of the skin eruption, from blood, and from spinal fluid. With an immunofluorescent technique, zoster virus was demonstrated in 15 of 17 corneal scrapings taken during the first 8 days of the disease. After 10 days, all corneal scrapings were negative. Six conjunctival scrapings were also positive. In one case, disciform keratitis and iridocyclitis developed 8 months after the original infection. Corneal epithelial scrapings at that time showed virus fluorescence.[305] These findings leave no doubt but that the initial corneal lesions are caused by the presence of virus and are not some type of neurotrophic phenomenon.

Evaluation of the effect of cortisone on ophthalmic herpes zoster was the objective of a study of 70 patients.[306] Local treatment with cortisone, atropine, and chloramphenicol was started immediately on hospitalization of 45 patients, whereas 25 patients received only atropine and chloramphenicol. Allocation of the patients to the two groups was determined by chance factors related to hospital space assignments and disregarded eye symptoms. On admission and after 2 weeks of treatment special note was made of ocular findings, including observation of corneal infiltrates, corneal ulceration, aqueous flare, keratic precipitates, posterior synechiae, and increased intraocular pressure. Of most interest was the determination whether each of the above findings had worsened, remained unchanged, improved, or become cured within the 2-week period. Worsening of these findings occurred at five times the frequency in the noncortisone pa-

tients as compared to those treated with cortisone (dosage not specified). Cure was recorded in nine instances in the cortisone-treated group, as compared to none of the controls.

At the end of the 14-day study period, 13 of the 25 control patients had pronounced iridocyclitis and required corticosteroid therapy, which was started at that time. Because this later use of cortisone eliminated most of the control group, evaluation of the incidence of late sequelae was impossible. Only 25 of the 70 patients did not have some type of residual damage. The most frequent residual problem, postherpetic neuralgia, affected 28 of the 70 patients.

The importance of antibiotic therapy together with cortisone was stressed to counteract the lowered resistance caused by cortisone. Such antibiotic treatment is particularly vital in the presence of corneal ulceration. Since this precaution was observed in each case (chloramphenicol therapy), no adverse side effects to the use of cortisone were noted in any patient.

In a double-blind study of dermatologic herpes zoster, triamcinolone, 16 mg three times daily, was given for 7 days, followed by 8 mg three times daily for 7 days, followed by 8 mg twice daily for 7 days. There were 19 control and 15 triamcinolone-treated patients. The healing time of the skin lesions (2 to 4 weeks) was unchanged by corticosteroid treatment. Postherpetic neuralgia (defined as pain lasting more than 8 weeks) occurred in three (30%) of the triamcinolone-treated patients over 60 years old and in 15 (73%) of the control patients over 60 years old. During the first 2 weeks of the disease, no triamcinolone effect on the pain was noted. The triamcinolone did not cause increased severity of zoster in any patient.[307]

None of the existing antibiotics has any inhibiting action on the herpes zoster virus[308] and will not prevent any complications other than secondary bacterial infection. However, since secondary infection of the skin lesions is invariably present, thorough cleaning with the aid of hot packs and mechanical debridement of crusts, followed by local application of antibiotic ointment, should be recommended and will greatly reduce scarring. Similar prophylactic antibiotic treatment of corneal ulcerations is most important, as previously noted.

No very effective treatment exists for chronic postherpetic neuralgia.[309] Thiamine, nicotinic acid, tincture of belladonna, phenobarbital, cortisone, vitamin B_{12}, ascorbic acid, chlorpromazine, diathermy heat, and x-ray therapy were of no benefit in virtually all of a series of 35 patients. Analgesic blocking of the affected areas with intradermal procaine was the most valuable treatment, although in some cases avulsion of portions of the trigeminal nerve was necessary.

Do not forget that herpes zoster commonly affects patients with a generalized malignancy such as a lymphoma.[310] The patient should be evaluated for such an underlying condition.

Ophthalmic zoster in a 7-year-old child was associated with undetectable immunoglobulin A. Immunoglobulin deficiency is commonly found in patients with Hodgkin's disease and chronic lymphatic leukemia and may account for the greater frequency of zoster seen in these disorders.[311]

The diagnostic importance of iris atrophy was stressed in a study of 520 cases of ophthalmic herpes zoster.[312] Approximately 50% of these patients develop iritis and 25% have iris atrophy. Fluorescein angiography discloses marked vascular atrophy corresponding to the areas of pigment and mesodermal atrophy, suggesting a mechanism of ischemia following inflammatory vasculitis. Without statistics, it was stated that corticosteroid therapy greatly reduced the severity of the vasculitis, thereby preventing iris atrophy and secondary glaucoma. Since herpes simplex does not produce ischemic iritis, its appearance (recognized by transillumination through the areas of pigment loss) permits recognition of the zoster etiology and indicates intensive use of topical corticosteroids. A mechanism of infection was postulated in which the virus replicates in the trigeminal ganglion, migrates down the nerve axons, and produces the typical vascular damage in

iris and skin. The reader would conclude that topical corticosteroid therapy should also help the skin lesion if it benefits the iritis, but dermatologic use of corticosteroid was not mentioned.

Molluscum contagiosum

A persistent keratoconjunctivitis results from exposure of the eye to debris originating from a molluscum nodule on the lid margin.[313] Excision of the nodule results in prompt remission of symptoms. If for some reason surgical removal seems unwise, thermal or chemical cautery may be substituted and will be effective if the lesion is adequately destroyed.

Rubella

Prevention of the congenital rubella syndrome is the objective of vaccination with attenuated rubella virus and of administration of gamma globulin. A critical distinction must be recognized between these two medications as to time of use.

The rubella vaccine is a noncontagious living organism that induces viremia for 2 to 6 weeks and causes effective immunity. Rubella vaccine is *not* to be used in pregnant females or in women who may become pregnant, because it may be transmitted transplacentally and cause fetal damage (although this did not occur in 23 infants delivered of mothers vaccinated during their pregnancy[314]). The intended candidates for rubella vaccination are primarily kindergarten and elementary school pupils. The various contraindications of reduced resistance, other virus diseases or vaccinations, allergy, and the like should be observed.[315-317] By age 15 years, 80% of schoolchildren are already immune by virtue of having contracted rubella through natural contact.[318]

Human immune globulin contains rubella antibodies and may be given to rubella-susceptible pregnant women after exposure to the disease. The reliability of this preventive measure is doubtful.

In a small series of 33 passively immunized and 37 control children (dosage of 0.12 to 0.2 ml of gamma globulin/pound of body weight), the attack rate of rubella was 83% in the immunized group and 92% in the control group. A series of 31 infants suffered from proved congenital rubella syndrome despite attempted prophylaxis with gamma globulin.[319]

During a rubella epidemic in an institution for retarded children, clinical disease or a rise in rubella titer occurred in 16 of 21 residents who did not receive gamma globulin prophylaxis. Immune globulin, 0.5 ml/kg, was given to 22 patients who did not manifest rubella within a week after prophylaxis. Of these 22, 18 developed clinical disease or a rise in titer. Obviously this attempt at rubella prophylaxis was entirely unsuccessful.[320] A summary of eight other controlled studies reports that perhaps 70% protection against rubella has been attained, with a range from 0% to 87%.

Therapeutic abortion is another method of preventing the congenital rubella syndrome. Apparently extensive malformations occur in 25% of children born after a first trimester maternal infection.[321] More detailed study shows that lesser handicaps affect up to 90% of first trimester–infected children. Only seven of 24 children infected during the second trimester were entirely normal.[322] Rubella virus was recovered from nine of 10 fetuses obtained by therapeutic abortion after maternal rubella.[323] Serologic testing for maternal antibodies to rubella is now possible and is, of course, invaluable in establishing that a given mother is already immune to the disease; hence she need not consider therapeutic abortion because of an unidentified febrile illness during a rubella epidemic.

The continuing presence of demonstrable rubella virus in newborns with the typical rubella syndrome (cataract, deafness, congenital heart disease, as well as growth retardation, hepatosplenomegaly, and encephalomyelitis) not only confirms the etiology of this syndrome but also has some practical significance. These infants are capable of transmitting rubella infection and should be avoided by pregnant women in the first trimester (namely, the nursing personnel). Of 31 babies with the complete rubella syndrome, 61% harbored recoverable rubella virus.[324] In one case, virus was still recoverable from the cerebrospinal fluid of a 6-month-old child (initial maternal infection during early pregnancy). Four of five apparently normal infants born to mothers with first trimester rubella were deaf but without other apparent anomalies; hence all offspring of first trimester rubella-infected mothers should be observed carefully for deafness. Infant deafness is easily overlooked but is of considerable educational significance and should be suspected in all patients with ocular findings compatible with rubella.

Inclusion conjunctivitis (chlamydia)

The term "TRIC" (trachoma and inclusion conjunctivitis) agent has been applied to the almost indistinguishable viruses that cause trachoma and inclusion conjunctivitis. Despite the similarity of the viruses, the diseases are differentiated by the typical corneal scarring of trachoma. In contrast, inclusion conjunctivitis causes only minimal corneal damage, although severe follicular conjunctivitis may occur.

Micropannus (limited to the peripheral cornea) and minimal conjunctival scarring were found in six of nine children who had suffered neonatal inclusion conjunctivitis at the time of follow-up examination 7 months to 11 years later. In one 7-year-old patient, fluorescent antibody testing demonstrated persistent typical TRIC inclusion bodies.[325]

Inclusion conjunctivitis is an oculogenital disease, affecting the conjunctiva, the urethral and prostatic epithelium, and the cervical and rectal epithelium. The virus may persist for years in these sites, which represent potential sources for ocular reinfection. Fluorescent antibody studies are positive for TRIC agents in over half of male urethral and female cervical scrapings obtained from individuals having follicular conjunctivitis or from their sexual contacts.[326]

The clinical characteristics of inclusion conjunctivitis were nicely outlined in a study of 84 human volunteers.[327] From the therapeutic standpoint, topical tetracycline ointment did not reduce the number of positive conjunctival immunofluorescent smears, not did it modify the clinical course of the disease. Oral sulfisoxazole (Gantrisin) in a dosage of 2 to 3 g/day for 2 weeks would successfully terminate the infection. A few patients suffered relapses as long as several months later and required a second course of sulfisoxazole. Several volunteers developed iridocyclitis that responded to cycloplegic and topical corticosteroid treatment.

For some reason, inclusion conjunctivitis of the newborn is supposed to respond to topical sulfonamide therapy, whereas adult infections require a systemic drug.

Diagnosis of neonatal inclusion conjunctivitis most likely identifies a situation in which all members of the family should be treated. Treatment of the child before the twelfth day of life will completely prevent ocular scarring, which was found in nine of 12 patients either untreated or not treated until after 13 days of age. Topical chloramphenicol or tetracycline is effective. Five of 10 mothers and two of five fathers had positive complement fixation titers immediately after the birth of the affected child. Of 14 examined parents, two had active follicular keratoconjunctivitis, four mothers had pelvic inflammatory disease so severe as to require hospitalization, and two fathers had suffered from Reiter's syndrome of severe arthritis and conjunctivitis. Systemic tetracycline therapy is effective against *Chlamydia* infections.[328] I doubt that it would occur to most ophthalmologists to wonder where the infective agent of neonatal conjunctivitis came from or to do anything about it. The purpose of such a provocative challenge to you should be evident.

Trachoma

American ophthalmologists are almost unable to comprehend that 400 million people are afflicted with trachoma and that this disease is the world's leading cause of blindness. Our inexperience with trachoma is because of the obvious fact that the spread of this disease can be controlled by good personal hygiene and cleanliness. In addition, the trachoma virus is antibiotic susceptible.

The organism has limited antigenicity and does not induce effective immunity; hence vaccination against trachoma has not achieved more than partial success.[329] The limited antigenic resistance that can be demonstrated correlates with the presence of a secretory IgA immunologic agent from the conjunctiva. Serum antibodies do not seem to be important in preventing trachoma reinfection or modifying its severity.[330]

In virus cultures, trachoma growth is inhibited by penicillin, tetracyclines, chloramphenicol, sulfonamides, and nitrofurazone (Furacin). Streptomycin is ineffective.[331]

Unfortunately the trachoma virus is more resistant to antibiotics than are the common susceptible bacteria; therefore prolonged clinical treatment is required for cure. For example, 3 to 6 weeks of topical (three times daily) or systemic (tetracycline or sulfonamide) treatment are required to achieve an 80% cure rate.[332]

Study of Indian children at a boarding school showed a trachoma prevalence of 17%. The rate of infection of children free of trachoma was 14% during their summer vacation at home. Because of this high rate of new infection, at 1 year after treatment the treated group of children had approximately the same prevalence of active trachoma as did the untreated control group.[332] Existence of trachoma in a child may be considered synonymous with trachoma in other members of his family. As long as hygiene is poor, only one member of such a group cannot be cured of trachoma, since he will promptly become reinfected.

A Russian ophthalmologist has made a very sensible recommendation for the mass treatment of trachoma. Treat the entire population, *family by family*, thereby greatly decreasing the reinfection rate.[333] No doubt there are also sound group psychotherapeutic aspects to participation by the entire family in purification rites.

The two classic signs of childhood trachoma are prominent follicles of the upper tarsus, visible only on lid eversion (Fig. 35-14),[334] and early pannus. Biomicroscopy is necessary to detect the early extension of limbal

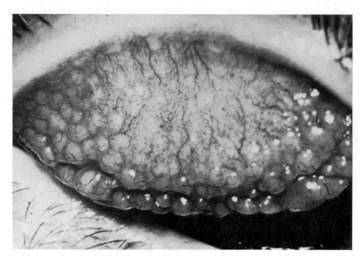

Fig. 35-14. Acute follicular stage of trachoma. (From Thygeson, P., and Dawson, C. R.: Arch. Ophthalmol. **75**:3, 1966.)

vascular loops on the cornea, which is most characteristic of trachoma and is only rarely present in other types of keratoconjunctivitis.

The severity of the clinical manifestations of trachoma varies widely within a population of patients. In Haiti there is a high prevalence of trachoma, but very few cases result in visual handicap. Of 43 Haitians, 23 were diagnosed clinically as having typical active trachoma, eight had atypical follicles, 10 had conjunctivitis, one had old corneal vascularization, and one was an anemic 5-year-old child with ocular findings. Chlamydial serum antibodies were sought and found in all these patients (except five with active trachoma who were not tested for some reason).[335]

The value of simple hygienic measures in the management of trachoma should not be forgotten. In a study of Saudi Arabian children the severity of trachoma was found to be definitely worse in those living in crowded and primitive conditions in an oasis as compared to similar children living in a townsite. Apparently reinfection and secondary infection are responsible for this difference.[336]

The frustrating experiences of epidemiologists could never be illustrated better than by a small group of 500 Arizona Indians. During a 4-year period of annual surveys and treatment the adult incidence of trachoma dropped from 12% to 2%. But the mission schoolchildren continued to have a 12% prevalence! The reason was that the school washroom continued to have only one cloth for communal hand and face drying.[337,338]

One year after paper towels were required, the prevalence of trachoma in the schoolchildren dropped to 5%.[339] An interesting correlation was attempted between television watching and trachoma. One third of the Indians did not watch any television, whereas one third watched more than 20 hours/week. No correlation existed between television watching and trachoma.

After this 5-year effort of surveying for trachoma, the authors concluded that the effort of single-disease screening was not warranted by the results and recommended that the annual trachoma survey should be replaced by routine eye examinations as part of the general medical care of the population. We tend to become enamored by our own little corner of the body and forget that general hygiene and care is sometimes more appropriate. Still, the authors did manage to reduce the overall prevalence of trachoma from 12% to 3% within 5 years.

Trachoma can be cured by three or four injections of repository preparations of long-

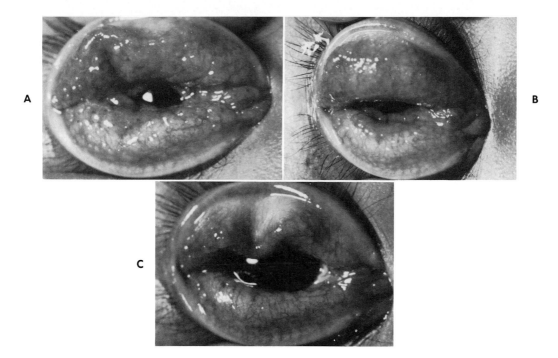

Fig. 35-15. **A,** Clinical picture of acute trachoma. **B,** Same eye 3 weeks after sulfonamide injection. **C,** Condition 8 weeks after treatment. (From Mitsui, Y., and associates: Am. J. Ophthalmol. **55:**782, 1963.)

acting sulfonamides administered at intervals of 1 to 2 weeks. This method of treatment is preferable in underdeveloped areas where the patients will not reliably take topical antibiotics or oral sulfonamides for the prolonged period necessary to cure the trachoma.

Repository acetyl sulfamethoxypyridazine (Kynex) was given to schoolchildren (weighing about 40 kg) in a dosage of 2.5 g/injection.[340] This preparation is a 250 mg/ml suspension; therefore it required a 10 ml volume of injection, which was given intragluteally. No other treatment was used

The results of treatment are shown in Fig. 35-15, which illustrates almost complete clearing of the conjunctiva within 2 months.[340] Clinical cure does not result until some time after the eradication of the virus. Treatment may therefore be stopped before the conjunctiva returns to a normal appearance. In cases from which inclusion bodies could be demonstrated, these had disappeared by the third day after injection. In experimental trachoma in human volunteers,

definite clinical improvement was evident in 1 week. Response in chronic trachoma patients was slower, requiring 2 to 3 weeks. No relapses were encountered during a 5-month period of observation. Several trachoma-like ocular inflammations resistant to therapy were encountered; these were thought not to be of trachomatous etiology.

The blood levels attained by intramuscular injection of acetyl sulfamethoxypyridazine are shown in Fig. 35-16.[340] Each arrow represents an injection of 2.5 g of medication.

Side reactions to the injections included definite pain at the injection site in all patients. Fever of 100° F lasting several days occurred in one third of the patients. Headache and loss of appetite were present for several days in one third of the patients. Urinalyses were normal. The known toxic effects of sulfonamides must be considered before advising such therapy.

A 70% cure rate of trachoma in Indian villages was achieved by the ingenious method of incorporating antibiotics in the black eye

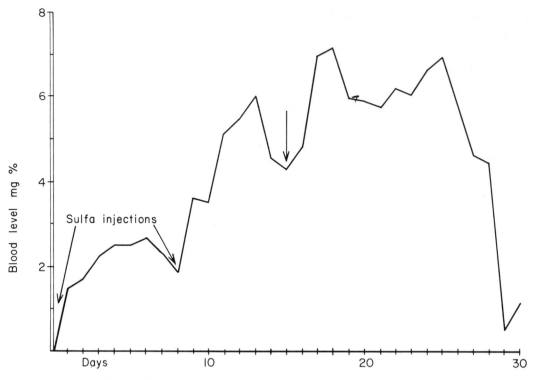

Fig. 35-16. Sulfonamide blood levels after intramuscular injection of Kynex. (Modified from Mitsui, Y., and associates: Am. J. Ophthalmol. **55:**782, 1963.)

cosmetics popularly used in the community. No particular medical instructions by professional personnel were required, since the natives simply applied the medication to the lid margins in the same way they were accustomed to use the cosmetic.[341] In fact, these patients were actually unaware that the cosmetic contained an antibiotic! Obviously vanity is a stronger motivation than desire for health.

Among Navajo Indians the sex ratio of trachoma is seven girls to one boy. This is attributable to the common use of contaminated eye cosmetics. In this group, 1 g of triple sulfonamide four times daily for 3 weeks achieved an 87% cure rate of trachoma.[342]

Some of the variables in trachoma treatment were illustrated in a Tunisian study.[343,344] Chlortetracycline 1%, erythromycin 1%, tetracycline 1%, rifampicin 1%, and boric acid 5% were compared to a no treatment control group. All medications were given in school twice daily 6 days per week for 10 weeks. The severity of the clinical disease, the recovery of *Chlamydia* by immunofluorescent stain, and the number of bacteria present were greatly decreased by all of the antibiotics, none of which showed significant superiority. The boric acid and control groups varied considerably resulting from the seasonal changes of prevalence of bacterial infection. Because of the occasional toxic reactions to systemic antibiotics, topical treatment for trachoma has been found to achieve greater acceptance within the treated population. Nevertheless, the economic and administrative burden of 10-week topical antibiotic treatment of all the affected population is beyond the medical capability of poverty-striken countries.

The student interested in trachoma may wish to read the 631-page *Symposium on Trachoma and Allied Diseases* published by the *American Journal of Ophthalmology*.[345] The therapeutic implications of this symposium may be summarized briefly as follows:

TRIC agents are curable by antibiotics. Sulfonamides, tetracyclines, erythromycin, and penicillin have all been used successfully in the treatment of these diseases. Apparently the antibiotic susceptibility of various strains of TRIC agents may differ considerably, just as is true for bacteria. However, sufficiently high concentrations of an antibiotic for an adequately prolonged period of time (which may be several months) will eradicate TRIC infections. Clinically, these facts mean that mass treatment of large groups of infected individuals will frequently be unsuccessful in a substantial percentage of cases. (Failures may be because of reinfection or patient unfaithfulness in treatment as well as because of resistant strains.) However, individual cases of TRIC infection such as might rarely be seen in practice in the United States can certainly be cured by adequate systemic and topical antibiotic therapy.

Sporadic cases of trachoma occur in the United States and may be unrecognized because of lack of suspicion. Trachoma should be suspected in any chronic conjunctivitis lasting more than 2 months, especially if follicles or papillae are present or if vascular pannus appears on the upper cornea. Giemsa smears will show inclusion bodies. Corticosteroid therapy will not only aggravate the disease but will also activate a latent case. Used for diagnostic purposes, topical corticosteroids will increase the percentage of positive Giemsa smears.[346]

Vaccinia

The epidemiology of ocular vaccinia was described in a series of 348 cases detected by follow-up of requests for vaccinia immune globulin. Of these eye infections, 70% occurred in association with a primary vaccination and 19% were acquired from another vaccinated individual. No underlying cause for infection (such as eczema or immunologic deficiency) was present in 95%. Of all patients, 58% were under 4 years of age. Only 2% of the lid vaccinia patients had residual scarring or loss of eyelashes. Only 22 patients had corneal involvement and of these only four had residual corneal scarring. None of the corneal scars were extensive.[347]

The reason for the punctate shape of the superficial keratitis induced by vaccinia virus is suggested by electron microscopy. Apparently the infection arises from a single infected cell. The release of virus particles when this cell dies results in a centrifugal spread of virus. All cells at a given distance from the center of the lesion tend to break down simultaneously, resulting in the typical circular pit.[348]

Clinical reports

In one case of vaccinia keratitis in a 2-year-old patient, marked improvement after 48 hours of IDU therapy was reported.[349] Three cases of eyelid vaccinia treated with vaccinia immune globulin (0.3 ml/pound) were reported to have cleared within 1 week.[350] Secondary bacterial infection was prominent in these cases and responded well to the use of warm compresses and topical antibiotics.

Systemic antibiotics have also been reported to benefit eyelid vaccinia, presumably by clearing secondary infection.[351,352] Staphylococci and pneumococci were isolated from the infected lids.

Experimental therapy

Experimental evaluation of therapy for vaccinial keratitis produced negative results. Groups of rabbits were treated with systemic and topical vaccinia immune globulin, with topical IDU, and with both medications together. No significant differences in the clinical course were noted between the control animals and any of those under the various treatment methods. Virus recovery from the infected corneas was possible during the first week in all animals, and all were free of recoverable virus after 10 days. The IDU that failed to sterilize the eye was confirmed to be active by demonstrating its ability to inhibit vaccinia virus in monkey kidney tissue culture.[353]

Although the duration of vaccinia keratitis was unchanged, its severity seemed less in the IDU-treated rabbits, suggesting the desirability of topical IDU therapy. Topical vaccinia immune globulin was of no benefit.

A single systemic dose of vaccinia immune globulin in the rabbits did not produce any unusual corneal response, but when systemic dosage was repeated daily for five doses, a large corneal scar persisting for more than a month resulted. Comparable persistent stromal clouding had been noted in four human patients treated with immune globulin. A corneal antigen-antibody reaction was postulated as the cause, since topical corticosteroid therapy (started *after* virus eradication) cleared the opacity.

Inoculation of vaccinia virus into the conjunctival sac of previously vaccinated rabbits caused conjunctivitis lasting 6 to 8 days. Comparable infection in nonimmune rabbits lasted 10 to 12 days.[354]

If interferon inducers (polyinosinic-polycytidilic acid) are given simultaneously with a vaccinia virus vaccine, the level of serum antibody after 1 month may be 20 times greater than without the poly I:C. Poly I:C apparently acts as a very effective adjuvant.[355]

REFERENCES

1. Bettman, J. W., Jr., and Aronson, S. B.: Host response in infectious ocular disease, Arch. Ophthalmol. **82:**30, 1969.
2. Wood, W. J., and Nicholson, D. H.: Corneal ring ulcer as the presenting manifestation of acute monocytic leukemia, Am. J. Ophthalmol. **76:**69, July 1973.
3. Primbs, G., Sand, B., and Straatsma, B.: Observations on experimental corneal ulcers, Arch. Ophthalmol. **66:**564, 1961.
4. McCulloch, J. C.: Origin and pathogenicity of Pseudomonas pyocyanea in conjunctival sac, Arch. Ophthalmol. **29:**924, 1943.
5. Locatcher-Khorazo, D., Sullivan, N., and Gutierrez, E.: Staphylococcus aureus isolated from normal and infected eyes, Arch. Ophthalmol. **77:**370, 1967.
6. Allansmith, M. R., Ostler, H. B., and Butterworth, M.: Concomitance of bacteria in various areas of the eye, Arch. Ophthalmol. **82:**37, 1969.
7. Wilson, L. A., Julian, A. J., and Ahearn, D. G.: The survival and growth of microorganisms in mascara during use, Am. J. Ophthalmol. **79:**596, April 1975.
8. Pincus, J., Deiter, P., and Sears, M. L.: Experiences with five cases of postoperative endophthalmitis, Am. J. Ophthalmol. **59:**403, 1963.
9. Baum, J. L., Barza, M., Lugar, J., and Onigman, P.: The effect of corticosteroids in the treatment of experimental bacterial endophthalmitis, Am. J. Ophthalmol. **80:**513, September 1975.
10. Lincoff, H. A., McLean, J. M., and Nano, H.: Scleral abscess, Arch. Ophthalmol. **74:**641, 1965.
11. Lincoff, H. A.: Intractable granuloma as a complication of polyethylene tube buckling procedures, Arch. Ophthalmol. **64:**201, 1960.
12. Everett, W. G., and Scott, D. C.: Chronic granuloma following scleral buckling procedures, Trans. Am. Acad. Ophthalmol. Otolaryngol. **66:**614, 1962.
13. Ulrich, R. A., and Burton, T. C.: Infections following scleral buckling procedures, Arch. Ophthalmol. **92:**213, September 1974.
14. Langston, R., Lincoff, H., and McLean, J. M.: Scleral abscess, Arch. Ophthalmol. **74:**665, 1965.
15. Milauskas, A. T., and Duke, J. R.: Mycotic scleral abscess, Am. J. Ophthalmol. **63:**951, 1967.
16. Polack, F. M., Locatcher-Khorazo, D., and Gutierrez, E.: Bacteriologic study of "donor" eyes, Arch. Ophthalmol. **78:**219, 1967.
17. Rollins, H. J., Jr., and Stocker, F. W.: Bacterial flora and preoperative treatment of donor corneas, Am. J. Ophthalmol. **59:**247, 1965.
18. Reed, H., and Platts, S.: The self-sterilizing properties of the vitreous, Am. J. Ophthalmol. **53:**501, 1962.
19. Zehetbauer, G., and Roberts, S. R.: Antibacterial effects in the vitreous, Am. J. Ophthalmol. **54:**797, 1962.
20. Hill, K.: The nature of the antibacterial effect of human vitreous, Trans. Am. Acad. Ophthalmol. Otolaryngol. **64:**298, 1960.
21. Wood, R.: Prevention of infection during tonometry, Arch. Ophthalmol. **68:**202, 1962.
22. Corboy, J. M., and Borchardt, K. A.: Mechanical sterilization of the applanation tonometer. I. Bacterial study, Am. J. Ophthalmol. **71:**889, 1971.
23. Corboy, J. M., Goucher, C. R., and Parnes, C. A.: Mechanical sterilization of the applan-

ation tonometer. II. Viral study, Am. J. Ophthalmol. **71**:891, 1971.

24. Tucker, D. N., and Forster, R. K.: Experimental bacterial endophthalmitis, Arch. Ophthalmol. **88**:647, December 1972.
25. Forster, R. K.: Endophthalmitis: diagnostic cultures and visual results, Arch. Ophthalmol. **92**:387, November 1974.
26. Abel, R., Jr.: Diagnostic and therapeutic vitrectomy for endophthalmitis, Ann. Ophthalmol. **8**:37, January 1976.
27. Forster, R. K., Zachary, I. G., Cottingham, A. J., Jr., and Norton, E. W. D.: Further observations on the diagnosis, cause, and treatment of endophthalmitis, Am. J. Ophthalmol. **81**:52, January 1976.
28. Peyman, G. A., Vastine, D. W., Crouch, E. R., and Herbst, R. W., Jr.: Clinical use of intravitreal antibiotics to treat bacterial endophthalmitis, Trans. Am. Acad. Ophthalmol. Otolaryngol. **78**:OP-862, November-December 1974.
29. Watters, E. C., Wallar, P. H., Hiles, D. A., and Michaels, R. H.: Acute orbital cellulitis, Arch. Ophthalmol. **94**:785, May 1976.
30. Londer, L., and Nelson, D. L.: Orbital cellulitis due to *Haemophilus influenzae*, Arch. Ophthalmol. **91**:89, February 1974.
31. Nicholas, J. P., and Goolden, E. B.: Bacteriologic culture results in conjunctivitis, Arch. Ophthalmol. **75**:639, 1966.
32. van Bijsterveld, O. P., and Richards, R. D.: Bacillus infections of the cornea, Arch. Ophthalmol. **74**:91, 1965.
33. Locatcher-Khorazo, D.: Bacteriophage types of Staphylococcus aureus, Arch. Ophthalmol. **63**:781, 1960.
34. Allansmith, M. R., Anderson, R. P., and Butterworth, M.: The meaning of preoperative cultures in ophthalmology, Trans. Am. Acad. Ophthalmol. Otolaryngol. **73**:683, 1969.
35. Lorentzen, S. E.: The nasal bacterial flora of the staff of an ophthalmic unit, Acta Ophthalmol. **45**:251, 1967.
36. Valenton, M. J., Brubaker, R. F., and Allen, H. F.: Staphylococcus epidermidis (albus) endophthalmitis, Arch. Ophthalmol. **89**:94, 1973.
37. Burns, R. P.: Pseudomonas aeruginosa keratitis: mixed infections of the eye, Am. J. Ophthalmol. **67**:257, 1969.
38. Furgiuele, F. P.: Treatment of Pseudomonas infection of the rabbit cornea, Am. J. Ophthalmol. **66**:276, 1968.

39. Bohigian, G., Okumoto, M., and Valenton, M.: Experimental Pseudomonas keratitis, Arch. Ophthalmol. **86**:432, 1971.
40. Hessburg, P. C., Truant, J. P., and Penn, W. P.: Treatment of Pseudomonas keratitis in rabbits, Am. J. Ophthalmol. **61**:49, 1966.
41. Furgiuele, F. P., Kiesel, R., and Martyn, L.: Pseudomonas infections of the rabbit cornea, Am. J. Ophthalmol. **60**:818, 1965.
42. Bohigian, G. M., and Escapini, H.: Corneal ulcer due to Pseudomonas aeruginosa, Arch. Ophthalmol. **85**:405, 1971.
43. Lund, M. H.: Use of colistin sulfate ophthalmic solution in therapy of Pseudomonas ocular infections, Ann. Ophthalmol. **3**:855, 1971.
44. Burns, R., and Rhodes, D. H.: Pseudomonas eye infection as a cause of death in premature infants, Arch. Ophthalmol. **65**:517, 1961.
45. LeFrancois, M., and Baum, J. L.: *Flavobacterium* endophthalmitis following keratoplasty, Arch. Ophthalmol. **94**:1907, November 1976.
46. Solomons, E.: The incidence of ophthalmia neonatorum without prophylaxis, Am. J. Obstet. Gynecol. **78**:513, 1959.
47. Greenberg, M.: Ophthalmia neonatorum, Am. J. Public Health **51**:836, 1961.
48. Mayou, M. S.: Observation on ophthalmia neonatorum, Br. Med. J. **2**:973, 1931.
49. Kaivonen, M.: Comparative tests on the bactericidal effect of certain antiseptics and antibiotics, Acta Ophthalmol. **36**:546, 1958.
50. Kaivonen, M.: Prophylaxis of ophthalmia neonatorum, Acta Ophthalmol. **79**(suppl.): 9, 1965.
51. Bickel, J. E.: Sodium sulfacetimide for the prophylaxis of gonorrheal ophthalmia neonatorum, J. Pediatr. **37**:854, 1950.
52. Fraser, I. T.: Treatment of ophthalmia neonatorum with sulphonamidobenzylaminepropionate ('Sulfomyl'), Practitioner **177**:71, 1956.
53. Harris, S. T.: Penicillin vs. silver nitrate in ophthalmia neonatorum prophylaxis, Sight Sav. Rev. **27-28**:152, 1957-1958.
54. Davidson, H. H., Hill, J. H., and Eastman, N. J.: Penicillin in the prophylaxis of ophthalmia neonatorum, J.A.M.A. **145**:1052, 1951.
55. Franklin, H. C.: Prophylaxis against ophthalmia neonatorum, J.A.M.A. **134**:1230, 1947.
56. Margileth, A. M.: Comparison of ocular re-

actions using penicillin and bacitracin ointments in ophthalmia neonatorum prophylaxis, J. Pediatr. **51**:646, 1957.

57. Sorsby, A.: Ophthalmia neonatorum, Practitioner **181**:525, 1958.

58. Mellin, G. W.: Ophthalmia neonatorum: yesterday, today and tomorrow, Sight Sav. Rev. **31-32**:102, 1961-1962.

59. Spaeth, G. L.: Treatment of penicillin resistant gonococcal conjunctivitis with ampicillin, Am. J. Ophthalmol. **66**:427, 1968.

60. Posner, C., Anderson, G., and Prigot, A.: Observations on the prophylaxis of ophthalmia neonatorum in a municipal hospital. In Welch, H., and Martí-Ibáñez, F., editors: Antibiotics annual, 1958-1959, New York, 1959, Interscience Publishers, Inc., p. 134.

61. Mathieu, P. L.: Comparison study: silver nitrate and oxytetracycline in newborn eyes, Am. J. Dis. Child. **95**:609, 1958.

62. Pearson, H. E.: Failure of silver nitrate prophylaxis for gonococcal ophthalmia neonatorum, Am. J. Obstet. Gynecol. **73**:805, 1957.

63. Thygeson, P., and Stone, W., Jr.: Epidemiology of inclusion conjunctivitis, Arch. Ophthalmol. **27**:91, 1942.

64. Schachter, J., Rose, L., and Meyer, K. F.: The venereal nature of inclusion conjunctivitis, Am. J. Epidemiol. **85**:445, 1967.

65. Friendly, D. S.: Gonorrheal ophthalmia, Trans. Am. Acad. Ophthalmol. Otolaryngol. **74**:975, 1970.

66. Rudolph, A. H.: Control of gonorrhea, J.A.M.A. **220**:1587, 1972.

67. Ward, M., Olive, G. M., Jr., and Mangiaracine, A. B.: Corneal perforation and iris prolapse due to *Mima* polymorphea, Arch. Ophthalmol. **93**:239, March 1975.

68. Schechter, R. J.: Treatment of Mima polymorphia conjunctivitis, Arch. Ophthalmol. **94**:338, February 1976.

69. Hallett, J. W., Wolkowicz, M. I., Leopold, I. H., and Wijewski, E.: The Middlebrook-Dubos test in uveitis, Arch. Ophthalmol. **63**:1016, 1960.

70. Schlaegel, T. F., Jr., Arbogast, J. L., and Estela, L. A.: The value of the Middlebrook-Dubos hemagglutination test for tuberculosis, Am. J. Ophthalmol. **51**:627, 1961.

71. McConville, J. H., and Rapoport, M. I.: Tuberculosis management in the mid-1970s, J.A.M.A. **235**:172, January 12, 1976.

72. Stein, S. C., and Hetherington, H. W.:
Fifteen years' experience with the tuberculin test, J.A.M.A. **173**:129, 1960.

73. Woods, A. C., and Burky, E. L.: Experimental studies of ocular tuberculosis, Arch. Ophthalmol. **29**:369, 1943.

74. Woods, A. C.: Ocular tuberculosis, Arch. Ophthalmol. **18**:510, 1937.

75. Bloomfield, S. E., Mondino, B., and Gray, G. F.: Scleral tuberculosis, Arch. Ophthalmol. **94**:954, June 1976.

76. Kirber, M. W., Kirber, H. P., and Dubin, I. N.: Experimental intraocular infection with *Mycobacterium fortuitum*, Am. J. Ophthalmol. **77**:173, February 1974.

77. Lazar, M., Nemet, P., Bracha, R., and Campus, A.: *Mycobacterium fortuitum* keratitis, Am. J. Ophthalmol. **78**:530, September 1974.

78. Farson, C.: Phlyctenular keratoconjunctivitis at Point Barrow, Alaska, Am. J. Ophthalmol. **51**:585, 1961.

79. Thygeson, P., and Fritz, M. H.: Cortisone in the treatment of phlyctenular keratoconjunctivitis, Am. J. Ophthalmol. **34**:357, 1951.

80. Walsh, T. J.: Clostridial ocular infections, Br. J. Ophthalmol. **49**:472, 1965.

81. Tsutsui, J.: Tetanus infection of cornea, Am. J. Ophthalmol. **43**:772, 1957.

82. Frantz, J. F., Lemp, M. A., Font, R. L., Stone, R., and Eisner, E.: Acute endogenous panophthalmitis caused by *Clostridium perfringens*, Am. J. Ophthalmol. **78**:295, August 1974.

83. Salceda, S. R., Lapuz, J., and Vizconde, R.: Serratia marcescens endophthalmitis, Arch. Ophthalmol. **89**:163, 1973.

84. Lazachek, G. W., Boyle, G. L., Schwartz, A. L., and Leopold, I. H.: Serratia marcescens, an ocular pathogen, Arch. Ophthalmol. **86**:599, 1971.

85. Okumoto, M., Smolin, G., Belfort, R., Jr., Kim, H. B., and Siverio, C. E.: *Proteus* species isolated from human eyes, Am. J. Ophthalmol. **81**:495, April 1976.

86. Wilson, L. A., Ahearn, D. G., Jones, D. B., and Sexton, R. R.: Fungi from the normal outer eye, Am. J. Ophthalmol. **67**:52, 1969.

87. Hammeke, J. C., and Ellis, P. P.: Mycotic flora of the conjunctiva, Am. J. Ophthalmol. **49**:1174, 1960.

88. Ley, A., and Sanders, T. E.: Fungus keratitis, Arch. Ophthalmol. **56**:57, 1956.

89. Forster, R. K., Wirta, M. G., Solis, M.,

and Rebell, G.: Methenamine-silver–stained corneal scrapings in keratomycosis, Am. J. Ophthalmol. **82:**261, August 1976.

90. Forster, R. K., and Rebell, G.: The diagnosis and management of keratomycoses. I. Cause and diagnosis, Arch. Ophthalmol. **93:**975, October 1975.

91. Kaufman, H. E., and Wood, R. M.: Mycotic keratitis, Am. J. Ophthalmol. **59:**993, 1965.

92. Anderson, B., Roberts, S. S., Gonzalez, C., and Chick, E. W.: Mycotic ulcerative keratitis, Arch. Ophthalmol. **62:**169, 1959.

93. Barsky, D.: Keratomycosis, Arch. Ophthalmol. **61:**547, 1959.

94. Mangiaracine, A., and Sumner, L.: Fungus keratitis (Aspergillus fumigatus), Arch. Ophthalmol. **58:**695, 1957.

95. Theodore, F. H., Littman, M. L., and Almeda, E.: The diagnosis and management of fungus endophthalmitis following cataract extraction, Arch. Ophthalmol. **66:**168, 1961.

96. Council on Drugs: J.A.M.A. **171:**651, 1959.

97. Jones, B. R.: Principles in the management of oculomycosis, Am. J. Ophthalmol. **79:**719, May 1975.

98. Ellison, A. C., and Newmark, E.: Effects of subconjunctival pimaricin in experimental keratomycosis, Am. J. Ophthalmol. **75:**790, 1973.

99. Bailey, J. C., and Fulmer, J.: Aspergillosis of orbit, Am. J. Ophthalmol. **51:**671, 1961.

100. Fine, B., and Zimmerman, L.: Therapy of experimental intraocular Aspergillus infection, Arch. Ophthalmol. **64:**849, 1960.

101. Ellison, A. C., and Newmark, E.: Potassium iodide in mycotic keratitis, Am. J. Ophthalmol. **69:**126, 1970.

102. Ellison, A. C.: Editorial, Am. J. Ophthalmol. **70:**152, 1970.

103. Snip, R. C., and Michels, R. G.: Pars plana vitrectomy in the management of endogenous *Candida* endophthalmitis, Am. J. Ophthalmol. **82:**699, November 1976.

104. Campbell, C. C., and Saslaw, S.: Enhancement of growth of certain fungi by Streptomycin, Proc. Soc. Exp. Biol. Med. **70:**562, 1949.

105. Saslaw, S.: Personal communication, 1960.

106. Ley, A. P.: Experimental fungus infections of the cornea, Am. J. Ophthalmol. **42:**59, 1956.

107. Seligmann, E.: Virulence enhancing activities of Aureomycin on Candida albicans, Proc. Soc. Exp. Biol. Med. **79:**481, 1952.

108. Montana, J. A., and Sery, T. W.: Effect of fungistatic agents on corneal infections with Candida albicans, Arch. Ophthalmol. **60:**1, 1958.

109. Mitsui, Y., and Hanabusa, J.: Corneal infections after cortisone therapy, Br. J. Ophthalmol. **39:**244, 1955.

110. O'Day, D. M., Moore, T. E., Jr., and Aronson, S. B.: Deep fungal corneal abscess, Arch. Ophthalmol. **86:**414, 1971.

111. Polack, F. M., Kaufman, H. E., and Newmark, E.: Keratomycosis, Arch. Ophthalmol. **85:**410, 1971.

112. Wind, C. A., and Polack, F. M.: Keratomycosis due to Curvularia lunata, Arch. Ophthalmol. **84:**694, 1970.

113. Smolin, G., and Okumoto, M.: Potentiation of Candida albicans keratitis by antilymphocyte serum and corticosteroids, Am. J. Ophthalmol. **68:**675, 1969.

114. Levy, J. H.: Intraocular sporotrichosis, Arch. Ophthalmol. **85:**574, 1971.

115. Zimmerman, L. E.: Changing concepts concerning the pathogenesis of infectious diseases, Am. J. Ophthalmol. **69:**947, 1970.

116. Hale, L. M.: Orbital-cerebral phycomycosis, Arch. Ophthalmol. **86:**39, 1971.

117. Newmark, E., Polack, F. M., and Ellison, A. C.: Report of a case of Nocardia asteroides keratitis, Am. J. Ophthalmol. **72:**813, 1971.

118. White, J. H., and Cinotti, A. A.: Experimental fungal contamination of the conjunctiva, Eye Ear Nose Throat Mon. **50:**441, 1971.

119. Hollwich, F., and Dieckhues, B.: Keratomycosis, Ann. Ophthalmol. **2:**744, 1970.

120. Chin, G. N., Hyndiuk, R. A., Kwasny, G. P., and Schultz, R. O.: Keratomycosis in Wisconsin, Am. J. Ophthalmol. **79:**121, January 1975.

121. Michelson, P. E., Rupp, R., and Efthimiadis, B.: Endogenous *Candida* endophthalmitis leading to bilateral corneal perforation, Am. J. Ophthalmol. **80:**800, November 1975.

122. Vastine, D., Horsley, W., Guth, S. B., and Goldberg, M. F.: Endogenous *Candida* endophthalmitis associated with heroin use, Arch. Ophthalmol. **94:**1805, October 1976.

123. Dellon, A. L., Stark, W. J., and Chretien, P. B.: Spontaneous resolution of endogenous *Candida* endophthalmitis complicating intravenous hyperalimentation, Am. J. Ophthalmol. **79:**648, April 1975.

124. Greene, W. H., and Wiernik, P. H.: *Can-*

dida endophthalmitis: successful treatment in a patient with acute leukemia, Am. J. Ophthalmol. **74:**1100, December 1972.

125. Rosen, R., and Friedman, A. H.: Successfully treated postoperative *Candida parakrusei* endophthalmitis, Am. J. Ophthalmol. **76:**574, October 1973.

126. Naidoff, M. A., and Green, W. R.: Endogenous *Aspergillus* endophthalmitis occurring after kidney transplant, Am. J. Ophthalmol. **79:**502, March 1975.

127. Wolter, J. R.: Diagnosis and management of orbital aspergillosis, Ann. Ophthalmol. **8:** 17, January 1976.

128. Forster, R. K., and Rebell, G.: Animal model of *Fusarium solani* keratitis, Am. J. Ophthalmol. **79:**510, March 1975.

129. Schlaegel, T. F., Jr., Weber, J. C., Helveston, E., and Kenney, D.: Presumed histoplasmic choroiditis, Am. J. Ophthalmol. **63:**919, 1967.

130. Schlaegel, T. F., Jr., and Kenney, D.: Changes around the optic nervehead, Am. J. Ophthalmol. **62:**454, 1966.

131. Walma, D., Jr., and Schlaegel, T. F., Jr.: Presumed histoplasmic choroiditis, Am. J. Ophthalmol. **57:**107, 1964.

132. Smith, J. L., and Singer, J. A.: Experimental ocular histoplasmosis, Am. J. Ophthalmol. **58:**1021, 1964.

133. Smith, J. L., and Singer, J. A.: Experimental ocular histoplasmosis, Am. J. Ophthalmol. **58:**3, 1964.

134. Salfelder, K., Schwarz, J., and Akbarian, M.: Experimental ocular histoplasmosis in dogs, Am. J. Ophthalmol. **59:**290, 1965.

135. Suie, T., Rheins, M. S., and Makley, T. A., Jr.: Serologic studies of presumed histoplasmic choroiditis, Am. J. Ophthalmol. **60:** 1059, 1965.

136. Sommers, J. M., Singer, J. A., Taylor, W. H., and Smith, J. L.: Histoplasmosis, Am. J. Ophthalmol. **60:**469, 1965.

137. Furcolow, M.: Comparison of treated and untreated severe histoplasmosis, J.A.M.A. **183:**823, 1963.

138. Giles, C. L., and Falls, H. F.: Amphotericin B therapy in the treatment of presumed histoplasma chorioretinitis, Am. J. Ophthalmol. **66:**101, 1968.

139. Spaeth, G. L.: Absence of so-called histoplasma uveitis in 134 cases of proven histoplasmosis, Arch. Ophthalmol. **77:**41, 1967.

140. Schlaegel, T. F., Cofield, D. D., Clark, G.,

and Weber, J. C.: Photocoagulation and other therapy for histoplasmic choroiditis, Trans. Am. Acad. Ophthalmol. Otolaryngol. **72:**355, 1968.

141. Makley, T. A., Jr.: Personal communication.

142. Makley, T. A., Jr., Long, J. W., and Suie, T.: Therapy of chorioretinitis presumed to be caused by histoplasmosis, Int. Ophthalmol. Clin. **15:**181, Fall 1975.

143. Spaeth, G. L., Adams, R. E., and Soffe, A. M.: Treatment of trichinosis, Arch. Ophthalmol. **71:**359, 1964.

144. Kean, B. H., and Hoskins, D. W.: Treatment of trichinosis with thiabendazole, J.A.M.A. **190:**852, 1964.

145. Unsworth, A. C., Fox, J. C., Rosenthal, E., and Shelton, P. A.: Larval granulomatosis of the retina due to nematode, Am. J. Ophthalmol. **60:**127, 1965.

146. Scheie, H. G., Shannon, R. E., and Yanoff, M.: Onchocerciasis (ocular), Ann. Ophthalmol. **3:**697, 1971.

147. Cordero-Moreno, R.: Etiologic factors in tropical eye diseases, Am. J. Ophthalmol. **75:**349, 1973.

148. Ben-Sira, I., Aviel, E., Lazar, M., Lieberman, T. W., and Leopold, I. H.: Topical Hetrazan in the treatment of ocular onchocerciasis, Am. J. Ophthalmol. **70:**741, 1970.

149. Moses, L.: Phthiriasis palpebrarum, Am. J. Ophthalmol. **60:**530, 1965.

150. Jacobson, J. H.: Demodex folliculorum, infestation of the eyelids, Trans. Am. Acad. Ophthalmol. Otolaryngol. **75:**1242, 1971.

151. Norn, M. S.: The follicle mite (Demodex folliculorum), Eye Ear Nose Throat Mon. **51:**187, 1972.

152. English, F. P., Iwamoto, T., Darrell, R. W., and DeVoe, A. G.: The vector potential of Demodex folliculorum, Arch. Ophthalmol. **84:**83, 1970.

153. U. S. Public Health Service, Publication No. 341, 1957 revision.

154. Freeble, C.: Syphilis as cause of blindness, J.A.M.A. **146:**1500, 1951.

155. Olansky, S., and Norins, L. C.: Current serodiagnosis and treatment of syphilis, J.A.M.A. **198:**165, 1966.

156. Smith, J. L., Singer, J. A., Moore, M. B., Jr., and Yobs, A. R.: Seronegative ocular and neurosyphilis, Am. J. Ophthalmol. **59:** 753, 1965.

157. Smith, J. L.: The TPI test in ophthalmology, Am. J. Ophthalmol. **57:**973, 1964.

158. Harner, R. E., Smith, J. L., and Israel, C. W.: The FTA-ABS test in late syphilis, J.A.M.A. **203**:545, 1968.

159. Deacon, W. E., Lucas, J. B., and Price, E. V.: Fluorescent treponemal antibody absorption (FTA-ABS) test for syphilis, J.A.M.A. **198**:624, 1966.

160. Seeley, R. L., Sarkar, M., and Smith, J. L.: The borderline fluorescent treponemal, Arch. Ophthalmol. **87**:16, 1972.

161. Wells, J. A., and Smith, J. L.: The fluorescent antibody tissue stain in experimental ocular syphilis, Arch. Ophthalmol. **77**:530, 1967.

162. Smith, J. L., and Israel, C. W.: Treponemes in aqueous humor in late seronegative syphilis, Trans. Am. Acad. Ophthalmol. Otolaryngol. **72**:63, 1968.

163. Taylor, W. H., Smith, J. L., and Singer, J. A.: Experimental seronegative syphilis, Am. J. Ophthalmol. **60**:1093, 1965.

164. Smith, J. L., and Israel, C. W.: The presence of spirochetes in late seronegative syphilis, J.A.M.A. **199**:126, 1967.

165. Smith, J. L., and Taylor, W. H.: The FTA-ABS test in ocular and neurosyphilis, Am. J. Ophthalmol. **60**:653, 1965.

166. Smith, J. L., Israel, C. W., McCrary, J. A., and Harner, R. E.: Recovery of Treponema pallidum from aqueous humor removed at cataract surgery in man by passive transfer to rabbit testis, Am. J. Ophthalmol. **65**:242, 1968.

167. Mackey, D. M., Price, E. V., Knox, J. M., and Scotti, A.: Specificity of the FTA-ABS test for syphilis, J.A.M.A. **207**:1683, 1969.

168. Montenegro, E. N., Nicol, W. G., and Smith, J. L.: Treponemalike forms and artifacts, Am. J. Ophthalmol. **68**:197, 1969.

169. Lorentzen, S. E.: Syphilitic optic neuritis— a case report, Acta Ophthalmol. **45**:769, 1967.

170. Smith, J. L., Israel, C. W., and Harner, R. E.: Syphilitic temporal arteritis, Arch. Ophthalmol. **78**:284, 1967.

171. Oksala, A.: Interstitial keratitis and chorioretinitis, Acta Ophthalmol. **30**:437, 1952.

172. Knox, D. L.: Glaucoma following syphilitic interstitial keratitis, Arch. Ophthalmol. **66**:18, 1961.

173. Brown, W. H., and Pearce, L.: Experimental syphilis in the rabbit. VII. Affections of the eyes, J. Exp. Med. **34**:167, 1921.

174. Wells, J. A., and Smith, J. L.: The fluorescent antibody tissue stain for Treponema pallidum in the eye, Am. J. Ophthalmol. **63**:410, 1967.

175. Montenegro, E. N. R., Israel, C. W., Nicol, W. G., and Smith, J. L.: Histopathologic demonstration of spirochetes in the human eye, Am. J. Ophthalmol. **67**:335, 1969.

176. Smith, J. L.: Testing for congenital syphilis in interstitial keratitis, Am. J. Ophthalmol. **72**:816, 1971.

177. Tramont, E. C.: Persistence of *Treponema pallidum* following penicillin G therapy, J.A.M.A. **236**:2206, November 8, 1976.

178. Mohr, J. A., Griffiths, W., Jackson, R., Saadah, H., Bird, P., and Riddle, J.: Neurosyphilis and penicillin levels in cerebrospinal fluid, J.A.M.A. **236**:2208, November 8, 1976.

179. Goldman, J. N.: Clinical experience with ampicillin and probenecid in the management of treponeme-associated uveitis, Trans. Am. Acad. Ophthalmol. Otolaryngol. **74**:509, 1970.

180. Christman, E. H., Hamilton, R. W., Heaton, C. L., and Hoffmeyer, I. M.: Intraocular treponemes, Arch. Ophthalmol. **80**:303, 1968.

181. Goldman, J. N., and Girard, K. F.: Intraocular treponemes in treated congenital syphilis, Arch. Ophthalmol. **78**:47, 1967.

182. Smith, J. L., and Israel, C. W.: Spirochetes in the aqueous humor in seronegative ocular syphilis. Persistence after penicillin therapy, Arch. Ophthalmol. **77**:474, 1967.

183. Atwood, W. G., Miller, J. L., Stout, G. W., and Norins, L. C.: The TPI and FTA-ABS tests in treated late syphilis, J.A.M.A. **203**:549, 1968.

184. Smith, J. L.: Recent observations on the treatment of late ocular syphilis and neurosyphilis, Trans. Am. Acad. Ophthalmol. Otolaryngol. **73**:1113, 1969.

185. Ryan, S. J., Hardy, P. H., Hardy, J. M., and Oppenheimer, E. H.: Persistence of virulent treponema pallidum despite penicillin therapy in congenital syphilis, Am. J. Ophthalmol. **73**:258, 1972.

186. Brown, W. J.: Something sensible you can do about syphilis, Consultant, 1965, p. 46.

187. Cassady, J. V.: Toxoplasmic uveitis, Arch. Ophthalmol. **58**:259, 1957.

188. Crawford, J. B.: Toxoplasma retinochoroiditis, Arch. Ophthalmol. **76**:829, 1966.

189. Darrell, R. W., Pieper, S., Jr., Kurland, L.

T., and Jacobs, L.: Chorioretinopathy and toxoplasmosis, Arch. Ophthalmol. **71**:63, 1964.

190. Desmonts, G.: Definitive serological diagnosis of ocular toxoplasmosis, Arch. Ophthalmol. **76**:839, 1966.

191. Editorial: Am. J. Ophthalmol. **48**:112, 1959.

192. Fair, J. R.: Congenital toxoplasmosis (part V), Guildcraft **34**:27, 1960.

193. Fair, J. R.: Congenital toxoplasmosis (part IV), Am. J. Ophthalmol. **48**:813, 1959.

194. Fair, J. R.: Congenital toxoplasmosis (part III), Am. J. Ophthalmol. **48**:165, 1959.

195. Forbes, S. B.: Ocular toxoplasmosis, Am. J. Ophthalmol. **44**:41, 1957.

196. Frenkel, J. K., and Jacobs, L.: Ocular toxoplasmosis, Arch. Ophthalmol. **59**:260, 1958.

197. Frenkel, J. K.: Ocular lesions in hamsters, Am. J. Ophthalmol. **39**:203, 1955.

198. Hogan, M. J., Kimura, S. J., and O'Connor, R.: Ocular toxoplasmosis, Arch. Ophthalmol. **72**:592, 1964.

199. Hogan, M. J., Zweigart, P. A., and Lewis, A.: Recovery of Toxoplasma from a human eye, Arch. Ophthalmol. **60**:548, 1958.

200. Hogan, M. J.: Ocular toxoplasmosis, Arch. Ophthalmol. **55**:333, 1956.

201. Hogan, M. J.: Ocular toxoplasmosis, Arch. Ophthalmol. **53**:916, 1955.

202. Jacobs, L., Naquin, H., Hoover, R., and Woods, A. C.: A comparison of the toxoplasmin skin tests, the Sabin-Feldman dye tests, and complement fixation tests for toxoplasmosis in various forms of uveitis, Trans. Am. Acad. Ophthalmol. Otolaryngol. **60**:655, 1956.

203. Jones, T. C., Kean, B. H., and Kimball, A. C.: Toxoplasmic lymphadenitis, J.A.M.A. **192**:87, 1965.

204. Kean, B. H., Kimball, A. C., and Christenson, W. N.: An epidemic of acute toxoplasmosis, J.A.M.A. **208**:1002, 1969.

205. Kimura, S. J.: The uveal tract, Arch. Ophthalmol. **63**:571, 1960.

206. O'Connor, G. R.: Precipitating antibody to Toxoplasma, Am. J. Ophthalmol. **44**:75, 1957.

207. O'Connor, G. R.: Anti-toxoplasma precipitins in aqueous humor, Arch. Ophthalmol. **57**:52, 1957.

208. Park, H. K., and Neville, M. A.: Determination of antibodies to toxoplasma and old tuberculin in uveitis patients, Am. J. Ophthalmol. **56**:235, 1963.

209. Park, H. K.: Toxoplasma hemagglutination test, Arch. Ophthalmol. **65**:184, 1961.

210. Sabin, A. B.: Human toxoplasmosis, Am. J. Ophthalmol. **41**:600, 1956.

211. Woods, A. C., Jacobs, L., Wood, R. M., and Cook, M. K.: A study of the role of toxoplasmosis in adult chorioretinitis, Am. J. Ophthalmol. **37**:163, 1954.

212. Yukins, R. E., and Winter, F. C.: Ocular disease in congenital toxoplasmosis in nonidentical twins, Am. J. Ophthalmol. **62**:44, 1966.

213. Van Metre, T. E., Jr., Knox, D. L., and Maumenee, A. E.: The relationship between toxoplasmosis and focal exudative retinochoroiditis, Am. J. Ophthalmol. **58**:6, 1964.

214. Manschot, W. A., and Daamen, C. B. F.: Connatal ocular toxoplasmosis, Arch. Ophthalmol. **74**:48, 1965.

215. Frezzotti, R., Berengo, A., Guerra, R., and Cavallini, F.: Toxoplasmic Coats' retinitis, Am. J. Ophthalmol. **59**:1099, 1965.

216. Wolter, J. R.: Endogenous fungus endophthalmitis, Arch. Ophthalmol. **68**:337, 1962.

217. Friedmann, C. T., and Knox, D. L.: Variations in recurrent active toxoplasmic retinochoroiditis, Arch. Ophthalmol. **81**:481, 1969.

218. Hogan, M., Yoneda, C., and Zweigart, P.: Growth of Toxoplasma strains in tissue culture, Am. J. Ophthalmol. **51**:920, 1961.

219. Ghosh, M., Levy, P. M., and Leopold, I. H.: Therapy of toxoplasmosis uveitis, Am. J. Ophthalmol. **59**:55, 1965.

220. Kaufman, H. E.: Uveitis accompanied by a positive toxoplasma dye test, Arch. Ophthalmol. **63**:767, 1960.

221. Acers, T. E.: Toxoplasmic retinochoroiditis, Arch. Ophthalmol. **71**:605, 1964.

222. Hogan, M. J.: Ocular toxoplasmosis, Trans. Am. Acad. Ophthalmol. Otolaryngol. **62**:7, 1958.

223. Zscheile, F. P.: Recurrent toxoplasmic retinitis with weakly positive methylene blue dye test, Arch. Ophthalmol. **71**:645, 1964.

224. Kaufman, H.: The effect of corticosteroids on experimental ocular toxoplasmosis, Am. J. Ophthalmol. **50**:919, 1960.

225. Hogan, M. J., Zweigart, P. A., and Lewis, A.: Experimental ocular toxoplasmosis, Arch. Ophthalmol. **60**:448, 1958.

226. Cole, J. G., and Byron, H. M.: Evaluation of 100 eyes with traumatic hyphema: intravenous urea, Arch. Ophthalmol. **71**:35, 1964.

227. Nozik, R. A., and O'Connor, G. R.: Studies

on experimental ocular toxoplasmosis in the rabbit, Arch. Ophthalmol. **83**:788, 1970.

228. Shimada, K., O'Connor, R., and Yoneda, C.: Cyst formation by *Toxoplasma gondii* (RH strain) in vitro, Arch. Ophthalmol. **92**:496, December 1974.

229. Samuels, B. S., and Rietschel, R. L.: Polymyositis and toxoplasmosis, J.A.M.A. **235**:60, January 5, 1976.

230. Dobbie, J. G.: Cryotherapy in the management of toxoplasma retinochoroiditis, Trans. Am. Acad. Ophthalmol. Otolaryngol. **72**:364, 1968.

231. Spalter, H. F., Campbell, C. J., Noyori, K. S., Rittler, M. C., and Koester, C. J.: Prophylactic photocoagulation of recurrent toxoplasmic retinochoroiditis, Arch. Ophthalmol. **75**:21, 1966.

232. Ellison, E. D., Kaufman, H. E., and Little, J. M.: Comparison of methods for the laboratory diagnosis of ocular adenovirus type 3 infection, Invest. Ophthalmol. **8**:484, 1969.

233. Boniuk, M., Phillips, C. A., Hines, M. J., and Friedman, J. B.: Adenovirus infection of the conjunctiva and cornea, Trans. Am. Acad. Ophthalmol. Otolaryngol. **70**:1016, 1966.

234. Laibson, P. R., and Dupre-Strachan, S.: Community and hospital outbreak of epidemic keratoconjunctivitis, Arch. Ophthalmol. **80**:467, 1968.

235. Dawson, C. R., Hanna, L., and Togni, B.: Adenovirus type 8 infections in the United States, Arch. Ophthalmol. **87**:259, 1972.

236. Golden, B., McKee, A. P., and Coppel, S. P.: Epidemic keratoconjunctivitis; a new approach, Trans. Am. Acad. Ophthalmol. Otolaryngol. **75**:1216, 1971.

237. Dawson, C. R., Hanna, L., Wood, T. R., and Despain, R.: Adenovirus type 8 keratoconjunctivitis in the United States, Am. J. Ophthalmol. **69**:473, 1970.

238. Burns, R. P., and Potter, M. H.: Epidemic keratoconjunctivitis due to adenovirus type 19, Am. J. Ophthalmol. **81**:27, January 1976.

239. Knopf, H. L. S., and Hierholzer, J. C.: Clinical and immunologic responses in patients with viral keratoconjunctivitis, Am. J. Ophthalmol. **80**:661, October 1975.

240. O'Day, D. M., Guyer, B., Hierholzer, J. C., Rosing, K. J., and Schaffner, W.: Clinical and laboratory evaluation of epidemic keratoconjunctivitis due to adenovirus types 8

and 19, Am. J. Ophthalmol. **81**:207, February 1976.

241. Thygeson, P.: Clinical and laboratory observations on superficial punctate keratitis, Am. J. Ophthalmol. **61**:1344, 1966.

242. Thygeson, P.: Further observations on superficial punctate keratitis, Arch. Ophthalmol. **66**:34, 1961.

243. Carithers, H. A., Carithers, C. M., and Edwards, R. O., Jr.: Cat-scratch disease, J.A.M.A. **207**:312, 1969.

244. Alfano, J. E., and Perez, A.: Cat-scratch disease, Am. J. Ophthalmol. **55**:99, 1963.

245. Leopold, I. H., and Sery, T. W.: Epidemiology of herpes simplex keratitis, Invest. Ophthalmol. **2**:498, 1963.

246. Pavan-Langston, D., and Nesburn, A. B.: The chronology of primary herpes simplex infection of the eye and adnexal glands, Arch. Ophthalmol. **80**:258, 1968.

247. Kaufman, H. E., and Maloney, E.: Experimental herpes simplex keratitis, Arch. Ophthalmol. **66**:99, 1961.

248. Carroll, J. M., Martola, E.-L., Laibson, P. R., and Dohlman, C. H.: The recurrence of herpetic keratitis following idoxuridine therapy, Am. J. Ophthalmol. **63**:103, 1967.

249. Laibson, P. R., and Kibrick, S.: Recurrence of herpes simplex virus in rabbit eyes: results of a three-year study, Invest. Ophthalmol. **8**:346, 1969.

250. Laibson, P. R., and Kibrick, S.: Reactivation of herpetic keratitis in rabbit, Arch. Ophthalmol. **77**:244, 1967.

251. Kaufman, H. E., Brown, D. C., and Ellison, E. D.: Herpes virus in the lacrimal gland, conjunctiva and cornea of man—a chronic infection, Am. J. Ophthalmol. **65**:32, 1968.

252. Brown, D. C., and Kaufman, H. E.: Chronic herpes simplex infection of the ocular adnexa, Arch. Ophthalmol. **81**:837, 1969.

253. Nesburn, A. B., Cook, M. L., and Stevens, J. G.: Latent herpes simplex virus, Arch. Ophthalmol. **88**:412, 1972.

254. Brown, D. C., Nesburn, A. B., Nauheim, J. S., Pavan-Langston, D., and Kaufman, H. E.: Recurrent herpes simplex conjunctivitis, Arch. Ophthalmol. **79**:733, 1968.

255. Piebenga, L. W., and Laibson, P. R.: Dendritic lesions in herpes zoster ophthalmicus, Arch. Ophthalmol. **90**:268, October 1973.

256. Marsh, R. J., Fraunfelder, F. T., and McGill, J. I.: Herpetic corneal epithelial dis-

ease, Arch. Ophthalmol. **94**:1899, November 1976.

257. Coleman, V. R., Thygeson, P., Dawson, C. R., and Jawetz, E.: Isolation of virus from herpetic keratitis, Arch. Ophthalmol. **81**:22, 1969.

258. Hughes, W. F.: Treatment of herpes simplex keratitis, Am. J. Ophthalmol. **67**:313, 1969.

259. Oshima, K.: Herpes simplex mutant isolated from IDU-resistant herpetic keratitis, Jpn. J. Ophthalmol. **11**:115, 1961.

260. Kimura, S. J., Diaz-Bonnet, V., and Okumoto, M.: Herpes simplex keratitis, Invest. Ophthalmol. **1**:273, 1962.

261. Takahashi, G. H., Leibowitz, H. M., and Kibrick, S.: Topically applied steroids in active herpes simplex keratitis, Arch. Ophthalmol. **85**:350, 1971.

262. Howard, R. O.: Herpes simplex keratoconjunctivitis, Am. J. Ophthalmol. **62**:907, 1966.

263. Kibrick, S., Takahashi, G. H., Leibowitz, H. M., and Laibson, P. R.: Local corticosteroid therapy and reactivation of herpetic keratitis, Arch. Ophthalmol. **86**:694, 1971.

264. Easterbrook, M., Wilkie, J., Coleman, V., and Dawson, C. R.: The effect of topical corticosteroids on the susceptibility of immune animals to reinoculation with herpes simplex, Invest. Ophthalmol. **12**:181, 1973.

265. Howard, G. M., and Kaufman, H. E.: Herpes simplex keratitis, Arch. Ophthalmol. **67**:373, 1962.

266. Kronenberg, B.: Treatment of herpetic keratitis with ether, Arch. Ophthalmol. **26**:247, 1941.

267. Kaufman, H. E., and Howard, G. M.: Therapy of experimental herpes simplex keratitis, Invest. Ophthalmol. **1**:561, 1962.

268. de Roetth, A.: Treatment of herpetic keratitis, Am. J. Ophthalmol. **56**:729, 1963.

269. Whitcher, J. P., Dawson, C. R., Hoshiwara, I., Daghfous, T., Messadi, M., Triki, F., and Oh, J. O.: Herpes simplex keratitis in a developing country, Arch. Ophthalmol. **94**:587, April 1976.

270. Stow, M. N., and Jenkins, B. H.: The use of chymotrypsin in the treatment of dendritic keratitis, Arch. Ophthalmol. **66**:61, 1961.

271. Jenkins, B.: Chymotrypsin in the treatment of dendritic ulcers, South. Med. J. **56**:275, 1963.

272. Chung, S., and Wong, A.: Proteolytic enzyme treatment of herpes simplex lesions of the rabbit cornea, Am. J. Ophthalmol. **53**:75, 1962.

273. Hogan, M. J., Kimura, S. J., and Thygeson, P.: Pathology of herpes simplex kerato-iritis, Am. J. Ophthalmol. **57**:551, 1964.

274. Thygeson, P., and Hogan, M. J.: Aureomycin in the treatment of herpes simplex cornea, Am. J. Ophthalmol. **33**:958, 1950.

275. Geller, H. O., and Thygeson, P.: Aureomycin, chloromycetin, and terramycin in experimental herpes-simplex virus infections, Am. J. Ophthalmol. **34**:165, 1951.

276. MacKneson, R. G., and Ormsby, H. L.: The effect of the broad and medium spectrum antibiotics on the virus of herpes simplex, Am. J. Ophthalmol. **39**:689, 1955.

277. Corwin, M. E., Copeland, R. L., and Birnbaum, S.: Cryogenic therapy, Am. J. Ophthalmol. **63**:399, 1967.

278. Corwin, M. E., and Tanne, E.: Cryotherapy in experimental herpes simplex keratitis, Am. J. Ophthalmol. **70**:33, 1970.

279. D'Alena, P., Okumoto, M., and Crawford, B.: Cryotherapy of stromal herpes simplex keratitis in rabbits, Am. J. Ophthalmol. **72**:134, 1971.

280. Bellows, J. G., and Hughes, W. F.: Letters to the editor, Am. J. Ophthalmol. **68**:362, 1969.

281. Bellows, J. G.: Low temperature treatment of herpes simplex keratitis, Eye Ear Nose Throat Mon. **45**:67, 1966.

282. Fulhorst, H. W., Richards, A. B., Bowbyes, J., and Jones, B. R.: Cryotherapy of epithelial herpes simplex keratitis, Am. J. Ophthalmol. **73**:46, 1972.

283. Kaufman, H. E.: Photodynamic inactivation of herpes simplex keratitis, Arch. Ophthalmol. **92**:536, December 1974.

284. Lahav, M., Dueker, D., Bhatt, P. N., and Albert, D. M.: Photodynamic inactivation in experimental herpetic keratitis, Arch. Ophthalmol. **93**:207, March 1975.

285. Stanley, J. A., and Pinnolis, M.: Light intensity on the photodynamic inactivation of herpes simplex keratitis, Am. J. Ophthalmol. **81**:332, March 1976.

286. Deutsch, F. H.: Recurrent herpes simplex keratitis, Am. J. Ophthalmol. **61**:1527, 1966.

287. Lawaczeck, E. J. J., Francis, R. D., and Dixon, J. M.: The effect of corneal contact lenses, Am. J. Ophthalmol. **55**:943, 1963.

288. Hudnell, A. B., and Osterhout, S.: Gamma globulin in experimental herpes simplex keratitis, Invest. Ophthalmol. **3**:366, 1964.

289. Smolin, G., Okumoto, M., Meyer, R., and Belfort, R., Jr.: Effect of immunization with attenuated *Mycobacterium bovis* (BCG) on experimental herpetic keratitis, Can. J. Ophthalmol. **10**:385, 1975.

290. Thomas, C. I., Purnell, E. W., and Rosenthal, M. S.: Treatment of herpetic keratitis, Am. J. Ophthalmol. **60**:204, 1965.

291. Dohlman, C. H., and Zucker, B. B.: Long-term treatment with idoxuridine and steroids, Arch. Ophthalmol. **74**:172, 1965.

292. Havener, W. H., and Stambaugh, N.: Corneal perforation in keratitis, Am. J. Ophthalmol. **54**:756, 1962.

293. Collin, H. B., and Abelson, M. H.: Herpes simplex virus in human cornea, retrocorneal fibrous membrane, and vitreous, Arch. Ophthalmol. **94**:1726, October 1976.

294. Kaufman, H. E.: Herpetic stromal disease, Am. J. Ophthalmol. **80**:1092, December 1975.

295. Metcalf, J. F., and Kaufman, H. E.: Herpetic stromal keratitis—evidence for cell-mediated immunopathogenesis, Am. J. Ophthalmol. **82**:827, December 1976.

296. Tanaka, N., and Kimura, S. J.: Localization of herpes simplex antigen and virus, Arch. Ophthalmol. **78**:68, 1967.

297. Edelhauser, H. F., Schultz, R. O., and Van Horn, D. L.: Experimental herpes simplex keratitis, Am. J. Ophthalmol. **68**:458, 1969.

298. Dawson, C., Togni, B., and Moore, T., Jr.: Structural changes in chronic herpetic keratitis, Arch. Ophthalmol. **79**:740, 1968.

299. Pavan-Langston, D., and Brockhurst, R. J.: Herpes simplex panuveitis (a clinical report), Arch. Ophthalmol. **81**:783, 1969.

300. Witmer, R., and Iwamoto, T.: Electron microscope observation of herpes-like particles in the iris, Arch. Ophthalmol. **79**:331, 1968.

301. Kaufman, H. E.: Epithelial erosion syndrome: metaherpetic keratitis, Am. J. Ophthalmol. **57**:983, 1964.

302. Kaufman, H. E.: Disease of the corneal stroma after herpes simplex infection, Am. J. Ophthalmol. **63**:878, 1967.

303. McCulley, J. P., Slansky, H. H., Pavan-Langston, D., and Dohlman, C. H.: Collagenolytic activity in experimental herpes simplex keratitis, Arch. Ophthalmol. **84**:516, 1970.

304. Langston, R. H. S., Pavan-Langston, D., and Dohlman, C. H.: Penetrating keratoplasty for herpetic keratitis—prognostic and therapeutic determinants, Trans. Am. Acad. Ophthalmol. Otolaryngol. **79**:OP-577, July-August 1975.

305. Hayashi, K., Uchida, Y., and Ohshima, M.: Fluorescent antibody study of herpes zoster keratitis, Am. J. Ophthalmol. **75**:795, 1973.

306. Bergaust, B., and Westby, R. K.: Zoster ophthalmicus local treatment with cortisone, Acta Ophthalmol. **45**:787, 1967.

307. Eaglstein, W. H., Katz, R., and Brown, J. A.: The effects of early corticosteroid therapy on the skin eruption and pain of herpes zoster, J.A.M.A. **211**:1681, 1970.

308. Laws, H. W.: Herpes zoster ophthalmicus complicated by contralateral hemiplegia, Arch. Ophthalmol. **63**:273, 1960.

309. Blaricom, L. S., and Horrax, G.: Chronic postherpetic neuralgia, J.A.M.A. **161**:511, 1956.

310. Blodi, F. C.: Ophthalmic zoster in malignant disease, Am. J. Ophthalmol. **65**:686, 1968.

311. Kielar, R. A., Cunningham, G. C., and Gerson, K. L.: Occurrence of herpes zoster ophthalmicus in a child with absent immunoglobulin A and deficiency of delayed hypersensitivity, Am. J. Ophthalmol. **72**:555, 1971.

312. Marsh, R. J., Easty, D. L., and Jones, B. R.: Iritis and iris atrophy in herpes zoster ophthalmicus, Am. J. Ophthalmol. **78**:255, August 1974.

313. Julianelle, L. A., and James, W. M.: Molluscum contagiosum of the eye, its clinical course and transmissibility, and the cultivability of the virus, Am. J. Ophthalmol. **26**:565, 1943.

314. Communicable Disease Center report, Medical Tribune, Wednesday, May 26, 1971, p. 25.

315. Buynak, E. B., Hilleman, M. R., Weibel, R. E., and Stokes, J., Jr.: Live attenuated rubella virus vaccines prepared in duck embryo cell culture, J.A.M.A. **204**:195, 1968.

316. Detels, R., Kim, K. S. W., Gutman, L., and Grayston, J. T.: Live attenuated rubella virus vaccine given in an orphanage just prior to a rubella epidemic, J.A.M.A. **207**:709, 1969.

317. Grayston, J. T., Detels, R., Chen, K. P., Gutman, L., Kim, K. S. W., Gale, J. L., and Beasley, R. P.: Field trial of live attenuated rubella virus vaccine during an epidemic on Taiwan, J.A.M.A. **207**:1107, 1969.

318. Grand, M. G., Wyll, S. A., Gehlbach, S. H., Landrigan, P. J., Judelsohn, R. G., Zendel,

S. A., and Witte, J. J.: Clinical reactions following rubella vaccination, J.A.M.A. **220:** 1569, 1972.

319. Cooper, L. Z., and Krugman, S.: Clinical manifestations of postnatal and congenital rubella, Arch. Ophthalmol. **77:**434, 1967.

320. Doege, T. C., and Kim, K. S. W.: Studies of rubella and its prevention with immune globulin, J.A.M.A. **200:**584, 1967.

321. Grayston, J. T., Peng, J.-Y., and Lee, G. C. Y.: Congenital abnormalities following gestational rubella in Chinese, J.A.M.A. **202:** 1, 1967.

322. Hardy, J. B., McCracken, G. H., Jr., Gilkeson, M. R., and Sever, J. L.: Adverse fetal outcome following maternal rubella after the first trimester of pregnancy, J.A.M.A. **207:** 2414, 1969.

323. Rawls, W. E., Desmyter, J., and Melnick, J. L.: Serologic diagnosis and fetal involvement in maternal rubella, J.A.M.A. **203:** 627, 1968.

324. Phillips, C. A., Melnick, J. L., Yow, M. D., Bayatpour, M., and Burkhardt, M.: Persistence of virus in infants with congenital rubella and in normal infants with a history of maternal rubella, J.A.M.A. **193:**1027, 1965.

325. Forster, R. K., Dawson, C. R., and Schachter, J.: Late follow-up of patients with neonatal inclusion conjunctivitis, Am. J. Ophthalmol. **69:**467, 1970.

326. Schachter, J., Dawson, C. R., Balas, S., and Jones, P.: Evaluation of laboratory methods for detecting acute TRIC agent infection, Am. J. Ophthalmol. **70:**375, 1970.

327. Dawson, C., Wood, T. R., Rose, L., and Hanna, L.: Experimental inclusion conjunctivitis in man, Arch. Ophthalmol. **78:**341, 1967.

328. Mordhorst, C. H., and Dawson, C.: Sequelae of neonatal inclusion conjunctivitis and associated disease in parents, Am. J. Ophthalmol. **71:**861, 1971.

329. Bietti, G. B., Guerra, P., Vozza, R., Felici, A., Ghione, M., Buogo, A., Lolli, B., Salomons, H., and Kebreth, Y.: Results of large-scale vaccination against trachoma, Am. J. Ophthalmol. **61:**1010, 1966.

330. Fraser, C. E. O., McComb, D. E., Murray, E. S., and MacDonald, A. B.: Immunity to chlamydial infections of the eye, Arch. Ophthalmol. **93:**518, July 1975.

331. Grayston, J. T., Wang, S.-P., Woolridge, R. L., Yang, Y.-F., and Johnson, P. B.: Trachoma—studies of etiology, laboratory diagnosis and prevention, J.A.M.A. **172:**1577, 1960.

332. Foster, S. O., Powers, D. K., and Thygeson, P.: Trachoma therapy: a controlled study, Am. J. Ophthalmol. **61:**451, 1966.

333. Maichuk, Y. F.: Some aspects of rational trachoma therapy, Am. J. Ophthalmol. **74:** 694, 1972.

334. Thygeson, P., and Dawson, C. R.: Trachoma and follicular conjunctivitis in children, Arch. Ophthalmol. **75:**3, 1966.

335. Nichols, R. L., Lahav, M., Albert, D. M., and Whittum, J. A.: Trachoma in a rural Haitian community, Am. J. Ophthalmol. **81:** 76, January 1976.

336. Bobb, A. A., Jr., and Nichols, R. L.: Influence of environment on clinical trachoma in Saudi Arabia, Am. J. Ophthalmol. **67:** 235, 1969.

337. Portney, G. L., and Portney, S. B.: Epidemiology of trachoma in the San Xavier, Arch. Ophthalmol. **86:**260, 1971.

338. Portney, G. L., and Hoshiwara, I.: Prevalence of trachoma among southwestern American Indian tribe, Am. J. Ophthalmol. **70:**843, 1970.

339. Portney, G. L., and Portney, S. B.: Five-year perspective on trachoma in the San Xavier Papago Indian, Arch. Ophthalmol. **92:**211, September 1974.

340. Mitsui, Y., Konishi, K., Kinouchi, T., and Kajima, M.: Treatment of trachoma by intramuscular injection of a repository sulfonamide, Am. J. Ophthalmol. **55:**782, 1963.

341. Gupta, U. C., Parthasarathy, N. R., and Gupta, C. K.: Study of broad spectrum antibiotic Kajal in mass control of trachoma, Am. J. Ophthalmol. **65:**778, 1968.

342. Lawler, D. J., Biswell, R., Sharvelle, D. J., and Carreno, O. B.: Trachoma among the Navajo Indians, Arch. Ophthalmol. **83:**187, 1970.

343. Dawson, C. R., Daghfous, T., Messadi, M., Hoshiwara, I., Vastine, D. W., Yoneda, C., and Schacter, J.: Severe endemic trachoma in Tunisia, Arch. Ophthalmol. **92:**198, September 1974.

344. Dawson, C. R., Hoshiwara, I., Daghfous, T., Messadi, M., Vastine, D. W., and Schacter, J.: Topical tetracycline and rifampicin therapy of endemic trachoma in Tunisia, Am. J. Ophthalmol. **79:**803, May 1975.

345. Symposium on trachoma and allied diseases, Am. J. Ophthalmol. **63:**1027, 1967.

346. Carroll, W. W., and King, R. G., Jr.: Tra-

choma surfaces in Virginia, Clin. Trends **11:** 8, 1973.

347. Ruben, F. L., and Lane, J. M.: Ocular vaccinia, Arch. Ophthalmol. **84:**45, 1970.

348. Matas, B. R., Spencer, W. H., Hayes, T. L., and Dawson, C. R.: Morphology of experimental vaccinial superficial punctate keratitis—a scanning and transmission electron microscopic study, Invest. Ophthalmol. **10:** 348, 1971.

349. Jack, M. K., and Sorenson, R. W.: Vaccinial keratitis treated with IDU, Arch. Ophthalmol. **69:**730, 1963.

350. Moses, L.: Vaccinia palpebrarum, Am. J. Ophthalmol. **60:**331, 1965.

351. King, J. H., Jr., and Robie, W. A.: Primary vaccinia of the eyelids, Am. J. Ophthalmol. **34:**339, 1951.

352. Kline, O. R., Jr.: Roentgen therapy of ocular vaccinia, Am. J. Ophthalmol. **34:**342, 1951.

353. Fulginiti, V. A., Winograd, L. A., Jackson, M., and Ellis, P.: Therapy of experimental vacinal keratitis, Arch. Ophthalmol. **74:** 539, 1965.

354. Knopf, H. L. S., Blacklow, N. R., Glassman, M. I., Cline, W. L., and Wong, V. G.: Antibody in tears following intranasal vaccination with inactivated virus (part II), Invest. Ophthalmol. **10:**760, 1971.

355. Knopf, H. L. S., Blacklow, N. R., Glassman, M. I., Cline, W. L., and Wong, V. G.: Antibody in tears following intranasal vaccination with inactivated virus (part III), Invest. Ophthalmol. **10:**750, 1971.

36
HEMORRHAGE*

From the therapeutic standpoint, intraocular blood can be subdivided according to vitreous or anterior chamber location.

VITREOUS HEMORRHAGE

A variety of systemic disorders may cause vitreous hemorrhage. Some, such as blood dyscrasias or hypertension, may receive effective systemic treatment. Others, such as diabetic retinopathy, are presently untreatable. Almost always systemic causes of vitreous hemorrhages produce ophthalmoscopically recognizable retinopathy in the fellow eye, even though the primarily affected retina is hidden by vitreous blood.

Completely spontaneous vitreous hemorrhages unassociated with evidence of injury, retinopathy of systemic disease, or previous chronic ocular symptoms are almost certainly caused by vitreoretinal traction. Indirect ophthalmoscopy, periodically repeated until the vitreous clears sufficiently, is the best method of recognizing the site of origin of such hemorrhage. Posterior sites of origin rarely tear through the relatively thicker posterior retina, pose no hazard of retinal detachment, and require no limitation of activity. Equatorial or peripheral tears usually disrupt the entire thickness of the retina and commonly lead to retinal detachment. Since

prophylactic cryotherapy will prevent detachment, the opportunity for effective surgical cure should not be lost during a period of placebo treatment.

No medical treatment will hasten the clearing of vitreous hemorrhage. The proprietary medications (mostly containing some form of iodine, vitamin, or vasodilator) commonly advocated for such purpose do not modify the spontaneous course of vitreous hemorrhage. The structural integrity of the vitreous body is the most important factor in determining the duration of a vitreous hemorrhage. A healthy young vitreous may suspend decolorized blood for months, whereas extensive posterior vitreous separation may permit even a large hemorrhage to settle inferiorly within a few days. These clinically unpredictable variations account for dramatic "cures" falsely attributed to concurrent medications.

Although prescription of a placebo to reassure the patient with a vitreous hemorrhage may be occasionally appropriate, I myself never do this, but rather prefer to explain the condition to the patient. Certainly the physician should never believe that any medication is adequate management of vitreous hemorrhage. Rather, it is essential to establish the cause of the hemorrhage.

Experimental therapy

Because the intact red cell cannot escape from the vitreous cavity, hemolysis of the red

---

*Reprinted in part from New Orleans Academy of Ophthalmology: Symposium on ocular pharmacology and therapeutics, St. Louis, 1970, The C. V. Mosby Co.

cell is the rate-determining step for the removal of hemoglobin from the vitreous. Acceleration of red cell destruction by inflammatory cells occurred in immunologic uveitis, which doubled the rate of disappearance of radioactive chromium–labeled red cells from rabbit vitreous. Unfortunately the ocular damage resulting from inflammation precludes clinical use of such a method of therapy.[1]

In three patients with vitreous hemorrhage of over 2 years' duration, 0.5 ml of central vitreous was aspirated and replaced with 25,000 units of urokinase. Urokinase is a plasminogen activator, and the intent of this therapy was to lyse the fibrin clot, supposedly present in the vitreous for years. Improvement of vision was reported in two of the three patients.[2] I would interpret any improvement to be more likely a result of mechanical disruption of the vitreous framework than of the biologic activity of the drug.

The role of vitreous-destructive operations in the management of vitreous hemorrhage is yet to be determined. Severe and irreparable complications may result, and the duration of the few reported dramatic successes is not established.

TRAUMATIC HYPHEMA

Simple hyphema per se does not cause permanent visual disturbance. Loss of vision after traumatic bleeding into the anterior chamber is the result of associated ocular injuries, secondary glaucoma, bloodstaining of the cornea, or traumatic iritis.

To a very large extent, the severity of injury predetermines the final visual acuity of an injured eye. Macular damage, vitreous organization, cataract, retinal detachment, endophthalmitis, phthisis bulbi, secondary glaucoma, corneal scarring, or optic nerve injury may be associated with (but not caused by) a hyphema and preclude restoration of vision. Presence of such lesions will greatly alter the management of a given hyphema. Complete absence of light perception is a clinical sign worthy of note, for it permits clinicians to predict that, with only rare exceptions, vision cannot be restored, even though they are unable to see within the eye.

Management

In the treatment of hyphema the ophthalmologist may wish to achieve one or more of the following results:

1. Arrest of continuing bleeding
2. Prevention of recurrent bleeding
3. Elimination of blood from the anterior chamber
4. Control of secondary glaucoma
5. Prevention of corneal bloodstaining
6. Treatment of associated injuries, including traumatic iritis
7. Detection and care of late complications

The relative importance of these factors will vary greatly from patient to patient. Because of this variability, the approach to treatment of an injured eye must be individualized. Unfortunately many critical questions relevant to the management of hyphema are unanswerable. These factors have resulted in conflicting beliefs and recommendations concerning the optimal treatment of hyphema.

Arrest and prevention of bleeding

Information as to the origin of hyphema may be derived from surgical experience. All ophthalmologists know that the normal iris can be cut with no fear of hemorrhage. In contrast, laceration of the vascular anterior portion of the ciliary body by surgical mishap, penetrating wound, or contusion rupture will predictably cause massive bleeding. This ciliary body origin of hyphemas has been established by pathologic and gonioscopic studies and may be reconfirmed by adequate clinical study of injured eyes in any ophthalmic practice.

Continuing or recurrent bleeding must be caused by failure of fibrin clots to occlude the damaged vessels. The high fibrinolytic enzymatic activity of the uveal tract may contribute to the frequency of recurrent bleeding. The rapid disappearance of blood clots adherent to the iris has long been clinically recognized. This has sometimes been attributed (wrongly) to direct escape of the blood into the crypts of the iris or some such absorptive mechanism. The true explanation of the disappearance of these blood clots is provided by demonstration of the marked fibrinolytic activity associated with the iris vessels. If an 8 μ thick section of human iris is placed on a 0.06 mm thick layer of fibrin, the fibrin underlying the iris will be dissolved within an incubation time of 15 minutes (Fig. 36-1).[3] The fibrinolysis is a result of a plasminogen activator located in the vessels of the iris, ciliary body, scleral plexus, and endothelium of Schlemm's canal. Fibrinolytic activity is not possessed by the trabeculae, the ciliary processes, or the normal aqueous humor.

Interestingly, the first phase of blood coagulation and platelet adhesion is the antihemophilic factor A–von Willebrand. This factor is not present in the endothelium of Schlemm's canal or in the vessels of the ciliary processes but is characteristically found in all other blood vessel walls.[4]

Reasoning that inhibition of the fibrinolytic activity of the anterior chamber might reduce the frequency of secondary bleeding led to an evaluation of aqueous fibrinolytic activity in the presence of acetylsalicylic acid. This drug was chosen because it is known to inhibit many enzymes. Oral administration to rabbits of 35 mg/kg of acetylsalicylic acid every 6 hours for 48 hours resulted in a 90% increase in the time required for aspirated aqueous humor to lyse a standard fibrin clot. Of course, we do not know that fibrinolytic activity is the major cause of clot instability.[5] Also, the association of salicylates with delayed bleeding following tonsillectomy would concern the physician evaluating the clinical effect of aspirin on the course of a hyphema.

Defects of the normal clotting mechanism have not been incriminated as causative factors in the development of traumatic hyphema. Use of medications such as vitamin C, vitamin K, calcium, or rutin does not accelerate the functioning of an already normal clotting system and is irrational. Indeed, excessive amounts of vitamin K may cause a secondary hypoprothrombinemia.

Of course, a patient known to have a blood coagulation defect such as hemophilia will be unduly vulnerable to bleeding from trauma or surgery. Management or prevention of bleeding in hemophilia involves administration of factor VIII from cryoprecipitates of human donor blood.[6]

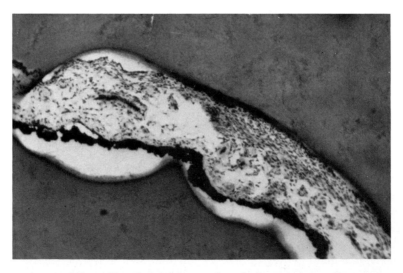

Fig. 36-1. Digestion of fibrin film (dark background) underlying section of human iris. Incubation time, 15 minutes. (From Pandolfi, M., and Kwaan, H. C.: Arch. Ophthalmol. 77:99, 1967.)

Because of the publicity received by conjugated estrogen hormonal treatment of hemorrhage, this subject deserves detailed consideration. The use of estrogenic substances (Premarin) in the control of bleeding does not have a known rationale. Proponents of this medication suggest that it increases the rate of clotting in some manner. The empirical use of Premarin in 22 patients with hyphema is reported to have prevented completely any secondary hemorrhage as compared to a 29% incidence in 41 control patients.[7] These patients received 20 mg intravenously, followed by 2.5 mg four times a day orally. Children under age 12 years were given half this dose. Unfortunately no mention of how patients were selected for treatment or to serve as controls is made. Although the fact that 20% of the control patients developed glaucoma and ultimate blindness is cited with the implication that this was the disastrous outcome of uncontrolled secondary bleeding, an equally tenable conclusion would be that a number of more severely injured patients existed in the control group. A truly controlled clinical study of the management of hyphema is most difficult because of the variable severity of injuries, their unpredictable course, differences in patient cooperation, and the relatively small numbers of available patients.

Estrogenic treatment (Premarin, 20 mg intravenously every day) was evaluated in 85 patients with traumatic hyphema in a well-standardized double-blind study.[8] This study concluded that estrogenic treatment of hyphema is of no value whatsoever. Bleeding time, clotting time, and prothrombin time were not altered by estrogenic treatment. Rebleeding, "eight-ball" hemorrhage, corneal bloodstaining, vitreous hemorrhage, retinal bleeding, and final outcome of the injured eye were not significantly different between the estrogen-treated and the placebo groups.

Intravenous injection of 20 mg of conjugated estrogens in 20 normal human subjects resulted in no demonstrable change in clotting mechanisms (prothrombin, factor V, and proconvertin levels) as measured during a 3-hour period after injection.[9] The authors concluded that conjugated estrogen therapy did not change plasma coagulation factors.

The use of estrogens to control nonuterine bleeding was not even mentioned in *New Drugs, Evaluated by the A.M.A. Council on Drugs,* 1966 edition,[10] nor has it been acknowledged since that time. Insofar as I can determine, the basis for the antihemorrhagic use of estrogens arises solely from the fact that the estrogen-stimulated endometrium bleeds on estrogen withdrawal. The portion of the medical literature that endorses estrogen treatment for nongenital bleeding appears to be uncritical and inadequately documented.

Whether bleeding can be arrested or recurrent bleeding prevented by minimizing movement of iris and ciliary body is not established. Theoretically, such movement could be arrested by either cycloplegic or miotic therapy. The literature (and everyday practice) supports the diverse approaches of cycloplegic therapy, miotic therapy, or neither. Parasympathomimetic drugs are known to increase the permeability of vessels, but no convincing data are available to indicate whether topical application of cycloplegics or miotics will increase, decrease, or leave unaltered the tendency to bleed from injured ciliary vessels.

For example, the use of topical epinephrine would seem to be a rational approach to the arrest of ciliary bleeding. All surgeons know of the effectiveness of this vasoconstrictor in stopping small vessel bleeding. Will topically applied epinephrine penetrate to the ciliary body? It is known to do so in the treatment of glaucoma, where up to a 40% decrease in the rate of aqueous secretion results from topically applied epinephrine. A friend of mine states that he has used epinephrine treatment of hyphema "successfully" for many years.[11] I know of no controlled data concerning this indication for epinephrine use.

Adrenochrome monosemicarbazone (an oxidation product of epinephrine) has been proposed for the control of capillary bleeding by systemic administration. Clinical studies supporting its effectiveness seem inadequately controlled. In a controlled study of 40 pairs of cataract extractions, adrenochrome monosemicarbazone has been shown to have no influence on the incidence of postoperative hyphema.[12]

Bed rest and binocular patching have been widely advocated as effective in reducing bleeding. For example, this limitation of activity was reported to prevent secondary hemorrhages in all but 20.5% of a series of patients, none of whom had visual acuity of 20/40 or less.[13] In contrast, 63.6% of ambulatory patients developed secondary hemorrhage, and 42.8% had visual acuity of 20/40 or less.

Advocates of limited activity indicate that rigid restriction of activity is important because of the disastrous consequences of a secondary hemorrhage.[13] (The presumption is made that activity, rather than spontaneous fibrinolysis, is responsible for the secondary hemorrhage.) While no one welcomes a secondary hemorrhage, our experience is that visual loss is caused by traumatic cataract and/or macular scarring from the original injury rather than by a complication of the secondary hemorrhage.[14]

Many ophthalmologists with wide practical experience have expressed reservations concerning rigid limitation of activity. Evanescent small hemorrhages are well known to affect various parts of the interior of the eye after many types of injury, including contusion, surgery, or even the normal birth process. Almost always such small hemorrhages (including hyphema) spontaneously cease and are more or less rapidly absorbed, depending on their location. Practical considerations such as availability and expense of hospital beds cannot be completely disregarded. When observing a frightened infant thrashing about in the confines of a net-covered hospital crib, I have often wondered if he would not be more quiet in the familiar surroundings of his own home. Use of that devil's own invention, the bedpan, is not completely devoid of stress. Finally, I have never understood why intraocular vascular pressure should be less when the patient is

recumbent than when he is erect—hydrodynamically, the reverse would be expected.

I advocate the compromise course of limiting the patient's activity after ocular contusion to home self-care, avoiding strenuous exertions for a period of a week. If the hyphema is sufficiently large to threaten glaucoma, daily observation is essential and hospitalization may be expedient.

Prevention of recurrent bleeding

Aspirin. Since many causes of hyphema are associated with pain, analgesics containing aspirin may commonly be ingested by the patient. Aspirin acetylation of the platelet impairs platelet aggregation induced by collagen. Defective platelet aggregation is demonstrable for a week after administration of only 150 mg aspirin. (The platelet life span is 9 to 11 days.) Inhibition of platelet aggregation begins as soon as 15 minutes after the first dose of aspirin.

A retrospective analysis[15] evaluated the frequency of rebleeding in hyphema with respect to aspirin therapy. Of 17 patients with mild hyphema receiving aspirin, seven had rebleeding. Of 71 patients with comparable hyphema but not receiving aspirin, only four had rebleeding. Avoidance of aspirin in patients with hyphema was recommended.

Alcohol. Ethanol inhibits collagen-induced platelet aggregation and also thrombin-induced aggregation. These platelet defects occur within several hours of intoxication and cause a prolonged bleeding time associated with normal platelet counts and normal prothrombin and thromboplastin times.

A spontaneous, nontraumatic hyphema occurred in a healthy 42-year-old woman taking three to five aspirin tablets weekly and drinking intermittently. The hyphema occurred 4 hours after consuming 15 ounces of ethanol. Her various clotting components were normal, but platelet aggregation was 85% decreased. Bleeding time was 9 minutes on admission (normal, less than 6) but dropped to 3 minutes after 2 weeks without aspirin or ethanol. She also had microscopic hematuria and ecchymoses of the extremities.[16]

Hyphema is rarely observed following cataract extraction performed by current surgical techniques. I have personally encountered three cases of serious postoperative hyphema associated with alcoholism, believe a causal relationship to exist, and advise against use of ethanol for 2 weeks prior to and subsequent to cataract surgery.

Aminocaproic acid. Aminocaproic acid inhibits the activating substance that converts plasminogen into the proteolytic enzyme plasmin. Another mode of action may be inhibition of fibrinolysis by plasmin. At any rate, oral administration of 1 g/hour of aminocaproic acid will inhibit systemic fibrinolysis. Inhibition of fibrinolysis in primary aqueous humor is achieved within 30 minutes of intravenous administration of aminocaproic acid. In treatment of hyphema, this drug may slow lysis of the original clot until repair of the damaged vessels occurs.

Of 59 patients with traumatic hyphema, 32 received aminocaproic acid (100 mg/kg every 4 hours orally, for 5 days). The other 27 (assignment determined by computerized randomization) received a placebo. The patients were hospitalized for prospective study. General treatment consisted of ambulation, 45 degree elevation of head of bed, with no eye drops of any kind. No patients received salicylates. The severity of the hyphemas in the two groups was considered to be the same. Rebleeding occurred in 33% of the placebo-treated patients and in only 3% of the aminocaproic acid group. The anterior chamber clots persisted for 2.8 days in the placebo group and 4.0 days in the treated group. There was no significant difference between the two groups in the other complications of the injury or in the final visual acuity.[17]

Aminocaproic acid has been used to decrease subarachnoid hemorrhage following ruptured intracranial aneurysms[18,19] and to help prevent bleeding in hemophiliac patients receiving factor VIII after surgery (4 g of aminocaproic acid every 6 hours for 2 weeks).[20]

Aminocaproic acid may be teratogenic and is contraindicated during early pregnancy. Cerebral arteriographic changes resembling intravascular thrombosis were noted in three patients with subarachnoid hemorrhages treated with aminocaproic acid.[21] Apparently no other significant thrombogenic complications have been noted.

Restricted activity. Physical strain on damaged vessels is popularly supposed to result in prolonged and increased amount of initial bleeding, as well as secondary bleeding. Such a conclusion seems obvious to a surgeon, who sees the operative field start to bleed anew when the patient bucks on the intratracheal tube. Still, this immediate bleeding may not be analogous to later bleeding. We do not, for instance, see renewed subconjunctival hemorrhage if the patient is active the next day.

A controlled, prospective study of 137 patients with hyphema[22] analyzed very carefully all the factors related to initial injury and the variations in clinical course. Only one variable was permitted in management; whether patients were confined to bed rest with binocular patching and sedation or whether they were up and moderately active. The duration of grossly visible hyphema averaged 5.6 days for the restricted group and 5.8 days for the active group. There was no significant difference in rebleeding, amount of hemorrhage, complications, or final visual acuity. In fact, there was only one significant difference: the duration of intraocular pressures above 24 mm Hg was 7.1 days in the restricted group, but only 5.0 days in the active group. This was clinically meaningless, however.

Insofar as I am aware, all recent controlled studies indicate that the outcome of hyphema is not significantly benefited by rigid, unpleasant, and expensive restrictions of activity.

Elimination of blood from anterior chamber

How does blood escape from the anterior chamber? Are the trabecular spaces large enough to permit the passage of a 7 μ red cell? Does iris phagocytosis account for the disappearance of a hyphema? What medications, if any, can accelerate clearing of a hyphema?

Anatomic descriptions of the microstructure and function of the anterior chamber angle differ considerably, depending on the techniques used. Injection into the anterior chamber of radiopaque particles of known size permits microradiography of the delicate passageways within the anterior segment of the eye.[23] Such microradiographs indicate that a system of ducts within the trabecular spaces empties into Schlemm's canal via small orifices measuring from 1.6 to 2.25 μ in diameter.

Intracameral injections of bacteria or of chromic phosphate particles of known size result in passage into Schlemm's canal of material up to 4 μ in size.[24] Tangential histologic sections demonstrate three layers of trabecular structure.[25] The uveal meshwork contains openings of 25 to 75 μ, the corneoscleral meshwork openings measure 10 to 30 μ, but the openings in the inner wall of Schlemm's canal are only 1 to 2 μ in size. Electron microscopy has demonstrated openings of 0.5 to 1.5 μ in size.[26]

Serial sections of human eyes demonstrate the presence of endothelial-lined canals passing from the trabecular spaces into the canal of Schlemm.[27,28] These canals (of Sondermann) are labyrinthine and require three-dimensional study for their recognition. Furthermore, only 20 to 25 such canals may exist in an eye; hence discovery of such an opening by the high magnification of electron microscopy would be most unlikely. Sondermann's canals are up to 12 μ in diameter. A number of excellent photographs demonstrating these canals in human eyes have been published. One such photograph actually shows red blood cells passing from the intratrabecular spaces via a Sondermann's canal into the canal of Schlemm.[28] Other studies[29] confirm the presence of 2 to 12 μ communications between the trabecular spaces and Schlemm's canal.

A form of glaucoma is caused by the entry of "ghost" degenerated red blood cells from the vitreous into the anterior chamber, where they clog the trabecular meshwork.[30] These dead skeletons are rigid, as are fixed red cells, do not readily escape from the an-

terior chamber, and are trapped within the trabecular meshwork. In contrast, under the same experimental conditions, living red cells easily escape via the trabecular meshwork, canal of Schlemm, and episcleral vessels of recently enucleated human eyes. Fresh red cells are extremely deformable and readily pass through a 5 μ Millipore filter.

Clinical evidence supports those anatomists who describe trabecular openings sufficiently large to permit the passage of a red cell. Retrograde passage of blood from the canal of Schlemm into the anterior chamber can be observed when external pressure causes the canal of Schlemm to fill with blood or when intraocular pressure is markedly reduced, as by paracentesis.[31] The characteristic very rapid (within several hours) rate of disappearance of small hyphemas is difficult to explain in any other way than by free outflow.

Escape of red cells from the anterior chamber of freshly enucleated human eyes can easily be demonstrated. To avoid confusion with the human red cells that might remain within the vessels of the eye, chicken red cells may be used. Chicken cells are nucleated and therefore are readily identified in histologic sections. They are elliptic, measuring 7 × 12 μ—slightly larger than a human red cell. Three eyes, obtained promptly after death from young patients (24 and 32 years old) with no known ocular disease, were perfused for 5 minutes with oxalated whole chicken blood at pressures of 10 to 15 mm Hg.[32] In all these eyes, the chicken red cells could be demonstrated on serial section to have penetrated from the anterior chamber into the trabecular meshwork, the canal of Schlemm, and the venous collector channels of the sclera.[32]

Electron microscopy of the monkey trabecular meshwork indicated the endothelium of Schlemm's canal to be a complete, nonfenestrated membrane. The trabecular meshwork was considered a dynamic biologic filter through which blood and particulate material do *not* pass freely from the anterior chamber into the systemic circulation.[33] These authors suggested that a previous study showing the escape of intact red cells from the anterior chamber represented artifactual rupture of the delicate endothelial lining of Schlemm's canal. As would be expected, the author of the previous study promptly presented a vigorous defense of his findings that radioactive chromium–labeled erythrocytes in the anterior chamber escape intact into the general circulation.[34]

Another route for the escape of blood from the anterior chamber—absorption by the iris—has been championed by many authors. Injection of particulate matter such as India ink or cinnabar into the anterior chamber results in deposition of some of this material within the stroma of the iris and ciliary body. Phagocytosis of foreign debris within the iris can be demonstrated histologically. The inflamed iris is well known to permit passage of the leukocytes that form a hypopyon. Absence of an endothelial lining on the iris surface supposedly would facilitate absorption of material from the anterior chamber. However, the concept of absorption of red cells by the iris should not be accepted uncritically. Modern theories of aqueous formation are based on the existence of a blood-aqueous barrier that is relatively impermeable to electrolytes. Red cells that are $7\,\mu$ will not be absorbed through the thick walls of an iris vessel that does not permit the passage of a sodium or chloride ion or of protein molecules. Using red cells tagged with radioactive phosphorus, it has been demonstrated[35] that blood injected into the anterior chamber reenters the circulation as whole cells, and that hemolysis is not the primary mechanism whereby the aqueous is cleared of blood.[35] Phagocytic absorption cannot account for the transfer of whole red cells from the aqueous via the iris into the circulating blood, since phagocytic ingestion requires at least partial destruction of the engulfed cells.

Histologic demonstration in injured eyes of blood adherent to the iris surface and within the iris crypts and stroma has erroneously been interpreted as indicating that the iris is the route of absorption. Published photomicrographs showing much blood in and on the iris but only a few red cells within the canal of Schlemm have been cited as evidence of iris absorption of hyphema.[36] Actually, such histologic findings prove exactly the opposite, for red cells will *not* accumulate in a channel from which they may readily escape, and they *will* remain in large numbers enmeshed in iris crypts from which there is no rapid absorption.

Further supporting the hypothesis that red blood cells escape from the anterior chamber by outflow is the demonstration that iridencleisis caused a 30% faster absorption of red cells. This was demonstrated in 43 rabbits with functioning iridencleisis by the injection of radioactive chromium–labeled cells.[37] A similar experiment in 48 rabbits with large iridectomies showed no significant difference in the rate of absorption of blood, indicating that red cells do not escape the anterior chamber via the iris.

An iris function in clearing blood from the anterior chamber is suggested by the more rapid disappearance of a blood clot overlying the iris than of the portions of the same clot overlying the pupil or iridectomy. Although this observation is accurate, its interpretation as signifying iris phagocytosis is not. The iris does contribute significantly to the absorption of a blood clot by providing fibrinolysin. Liberated from the fibrin clot, the red cells escape into the aqueous and are carried with it into the canal of Schlemm.

In conclusion, evaluation of all available data indicates that the escape of red cells from the anterior chamber occurs primarily via the canal of Schlemm. Iris absorption and phagocytosis may account for removal of only a small amount of hemolyzed debris. I have devoted so much attention to the consideration of the route of clearing of hyphema because of its obvious significance in determining medical therapy.

Medical therapy. Are there effective medical ways to eliminate blood from the anterior chamber? Can blood clots be caused to disintegrate, thereby hastening their absorption? Can the outflow channels of the eye be enlarged to enhance the escape of blood?

Fibrin clots within the anterior chamber enmesh red cells and prevent their escape from the eye. Experienced clinicians recognize that in serious anterior chamber hemorrhage (eight-ball), sufficient fibrin has accumulated to coagulate into a large clot. This clot blocks the trabecular meshwork, resulting in secondary glaucoma.

That clearing of a hyphema is slower when a fibrin clot exists within the anterior chamber seems clinically obvious and is experimentally demonstrable. Injection of a suspension of ^{51}Cr-labeled red cells into rabbit anterior chamber with and without thrombin injection (to form a clot) provided the data shown in Fig. 36-2.[38] The lower curve represents the rate of disappearance of radioactivity in nonclotted blood. Seventy-five percent

of the radioactivity of nonclotted blood had disappeared within 2½ days, whereas comparable clearing of the clotted blood required 9 days.

Anticoagulants. The clearing of experimental hyphema is more rapid when fibrin clotting in the anterior chamber is prevented by anticoagulants.[39] This finding is mainly of theoretical interest, indicating that the primary route by which blood escapes from the anterior chamber is mechanical outflow and that this route may be blocked by fibrin clots. Obviously, sodium warfarin (Coumadin) therapy of a bleeding eye would be contraindicated.

Proteolytic enzymes. The ability of proteo-

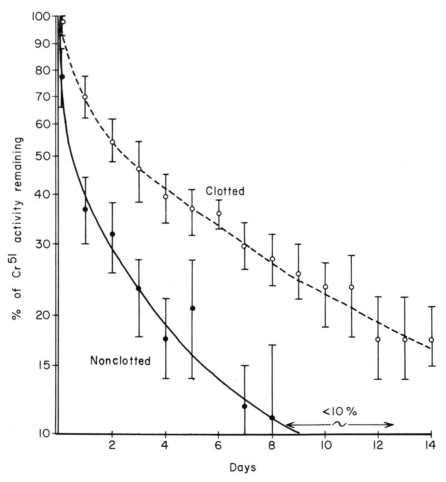

Fig. 36-2. Rate of disappearance of radioactivity from rabbit anterior chambers filled with clotted or unclotted ^{51}Cr-labeled red cells. (Modified from Schaeffer, E., and associates: Arch. Ophthalmol. **65:**699, 1961.)

lytic enzymes (streptokinase, streptodornase, trypsin, and chymotrypsin) to dissolve fibrin has suggested their use in the treatment of hyphema. Additionally, an anti-inflammatory effect has been attributed to such drugs by some clinicians, who advocate their use in the treatment of ocular contusions. Adequately controlled clinical evaluation of proteolytic enzyme treatment is difficult because of the varying severity of injuries. Most clinical reports describe a series of cases treated with "good results" with no attempt at devising a control series.

Carefully controlled animal experiments would be most likely to establish the effectiveness of proteolytic enzyme therapy of hyphema. The rate of clearing of experimental subconjunctival hemorrhage and anterior chamber hyphema was studied in 15 rabbits.[40] Five were treated with 10,000 units of streptokinase and 2500 units of streptodornase, injected parenterally daily for 10 days. Another group of five received 5000 units of trypsin injected daily for 10 days. The remaining five were controls. All eyes cleared in between 7 and 15 days, with no difference existing between the treated and the control groups. Although this study evaluated only a very small number of rabbits, the demonstrated failure of parenteral proteolytic enzyme therapy has been consistently confirmed by other authors.[40]

The subconjunctival injection of trypsin (4 mg) did not hasten the absorption of experimental hyphema in guinea pigs.[41]

Streptokinase, streptodornase, and fibrinolysin apparently penetrate into the anterior chamber after "subconjunctival" injection.[42] These enzymes were evaluated in the treatment of experimental hyphema (radioactive red blood cells in rabbits) because the absorption of red cells from the anterior chamber is impeded by fibrin. Subconjunctival injection of 1500 units of streptokinase-streptodornase (Varidase) increased the average rate of hyphema absorption over a 48-hour period by 41%. A 51% greater absorption resulted from subconjunctival injection of 3000 units, whereas 780 units caused no greater absorption than the controls. Between 1000 and 2000 units of Varidase was believed to be the optimal subconjunctival dosage, accelerating hyphema absorption and yet causing no toxic effect (other than mechanical trauma). Anterior chamber injection of 156 units of Varidase (0.05 ml) caused a 46% increase in hyphema absorption during 48 hours and was nontoxic. Retrobulbar injection of 12,500 units of Varidase did not increase the rate of hyphema absorption.

Subconjunctival fibrinolysin (plasmin, Actase), 15,000 units, caused a 55% increase in hyphema absorption during 48 hours (Fig. 36-3).[42]

Fibrinolysin irrigation. Irrigation of the anterior chamber with human fibrinolysin has been demonstrated to lyse fresh clots and aid in their surgical removal. The lysis of clots is greatly enhanced by the movement of the irrigating fluid. Stationary, incubated blood clots are lysed within 2 hours by 12,500 units of fibrinolysin/ml and do not dissolve at all in a concentration of 1500 units/ml. However, comparable clots may be broken up and removed from the anterior chamber within 15 to 90 minutes by gentle irrigation with fibrinolysin, 1250 units/ml. This latter concentration is nontoxic to the human anterior chamber structures.[43]

Fibrinolysin-induced clearing of experimental hyphema is most effective against fresh clots (1 to 2 days old). Organized 5-day-old clots are no more susceptible to removal by fibrinolysin than to the purely mechanical action of saline irrigation. This does not mean that fibrinolysin irrigation is contraindicated in the surgical treatment of a 5-day-old hyphema, since continued bleeding and fresh clot formation are common.

The complete and clean surgical removal of all clotted blood from the anterior chamber is not necessary, since scattered small remnants will spontaneously absorb. Fibrinolysin-aided surgical attack on a hyphema is not advisable except for the indication of medically uncontrollable glaucoma caused by complete obstruction of the angle by fibrin clots. Although paracentesis and irrigation seem to be relatively innocuous, corneal, iris, and lens injuries commonly complicate

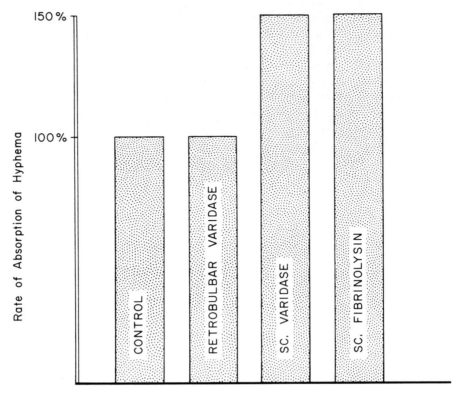

Fig. 36-3. Rate of absorption of experimental hyphema in control, after retrobulbar injection of 12,500 units of Varidase, after subconjunctival injection of 3000 units of Varidase, and after subconjunctival injection of 15,000 units of fibrinolysin. (Modified from Sinskey, R. M., and Krichesky, A. R.: Am. J. Ophthalmol. **54:**445, 1962.)

such surgery, which is actually highly dangerous.

Hemolysis. Theoretically, disintegration of the red cells would hasten absorption of a hyphema. Although hemolyzed red cells leave the anterior chamber of rabbit eyes much more rapidly than do whole red cells, this observation is not useful in the treatment of hyphema. Unfortunately chemicals (for example, benzalkonium chloride, cobra venom, and osmotic agents) that cause hemolysis are too toxic to intraocular tissues to permit clinical use.[44] Likewise, physical disruption of the red cells by ultrasound radiation damages ocular structure.

Corticosteroids. The rate of absorption of experimental hyphema (one half of rabbit anterior chamber filled with heparinized autologous blood) has been shown to be slowed by corticosteroid pretreatment.[45] Whereas con-

trol hyphemas disappeared in 2 days, 5 to 8 days were required in eyes pretreated with twice daily instillation of 0.17% betamethasone. Corticosteroid treatment *after* injection of the blood did not retard its disappearance. The mechanism of this corticosteroid effect is not clear. The coefficient of outflow of treated eyes was not different from that of the controls, nor was there any evidence of corticosteroid-induced glaucoma. Histologic study of the structure of the chamber angle showed no recognizable differences. Possibly pretreatment in some way changes the reaction of the eye to the trauma of injection. At any rate, this experiment cannot be interpreted to contraindicate (or indicate) corticosteroid treatment of clinical hyphema.

In another experiment, pretreatment of rabbit eyes with subconjunctival methylprednisolone doubled the rate of absorption of experimental hyphema. This was attributed to corticosteroid inhibition of clot formation within the anterior chamber. If given after clot formation had occurred, the methylprednisolone did not alter the rate of absorption of hyphema. The same author also reported that daily intravenous mannitol or urea tripled the rate of absorption of clotted blood from the rabbit anterior chamber.[46] The mechanism of this was unexplained; however, the possibility of secondary increase of aqueous outflow was postulated.

Spontaneous, nontraumatic hyphema during infancy may be caused by juvenile xanthogranuloma (nevoxanthoendothelioma). The diagnosis may be confirmed by biopsy of an iris tumor or of the typical yellowish or pink papular skin lesions (found in at least eight of 20 patients with eye lesions). Ideal treatment is not yet established, but a trial of topical corticosteroid therapy for several weeks has been suggested.[47] Whether this is effective therapy or simply permits time for spontaneous regression is not proved. Glaucoma secondary to xanthogranuloma may respond to x-ray therapy, not to exceed 500 rads given in divided doses of 200 rads or less.

Miotic therapy. The miotic-cycloplegic-nothing controversy in treatment of hyphema is one of the best-known subjects of therapeutic disagreement in ophthalmology. Theoretically, the escape of free red cells from the anterior chamber should be accelerated by miotics. (Obviously large fibrin clots cannot leave the anterior chamber while they are intact.) The increase in facility of outflow of aqueous caused by miosis is the accepted basis for the standard therapy of chronic simple glaucoma. Serial and tangential section of the trabecular meshwork establish that pilocarpine causes a stretching and spreading apart of the trabecular lamellae. As expected, atropine produces the opposite effect, of narrowing the trabecular openings. Early use of pilocarpine in the treatment of hyphema may encourage the escape of fibrin (and red cells) before it attains a concentration sufficient to form a clot within the anterior chamber.

Table 36-1. Percent of absorption of experimental hyphema as measured by disappearance of radioactivity (^{51}Cr-labeled red cells) from rabbit eyes treated by atropine or pilocarpine*

Hours	Cycloplegic (%)	Miotic (%)
20	0	35
23	28	54
27	44	66
28	30	51
	Loss of ^{51}Cr	

*From Bredemeyer, H.: Unpublished data, 1958; from New Orleans Academy of Ophthalmology: Symposium on ocular pharmacology and therapeutics, St. Louis, 1970, The C. V. Mosby Co.

With the aid of radioactive labeling, the absorption of heparinized blood cells from the rabbit anterior chamber has been studied under conditions of miosis and mydriasis. A total of 57 rabbits was used.[48] Sampling was done 1 to 7 hours after the injection of blood. Under these conditions the rate of escape of radioactivity from the anterior chamber was not affected by mydriatics or miotics.

In a comparable experiment of longer duration, miosis for 20 hours or longer resulted in a greatly accelerated escape of red cells from the anterior chamber.[49] One day after injection of the radioactive cells all the miotic eyes retained appreciably less radioactivity than the untreated eyes. The atropinized eyes retained more radioactivity than the untreated or miotic eyes. Differences in the amount of retained blood were grossly visible in most animals. Representative values are given in Table 36-1.

One of the most astute and experienced ophthalmologists of my acquaintance has used pilocarpine routinely in the management of hyphema during the past 20 years. He states that no single patient in whom pilocarpine was started early has required surgery for the complications of hyphema. (Surgery has been required for patients first seen late, however, when eight-ball hemorrhage and secondary glaucoma were already well established.) A commonly heard objection to pilocarpine therapy is that it could theoretically pull on the damaged vessel and cause rebleeding. Apparently this concern is unwarranted, since rebleeding has never been of sufficient severity to require surgery in this man's 20-year experience.[50]

My personal experience with pilocarpine treatment of hyphema, although far less extensive, has been equally encouraging. My present recommendation is that hyphema should be treated with sufficient pilocarpine to maintain good miosis (for example, 1% three times a day).

Just to confuse the issue, in another study the use of 1% atropine or 2% pilocarpine, assigned to alternate patients, was the variable under study.[51] The average clearing time for 1 mm hyphemas was 1.9 days for the cycloplegic eyes and 2.5 days for the miotic eyes. Although this was said to be "statistically significant," there were only 10 patients in each group, which seems rather small to me. The rationale of the cycloplegic is to relax the muscular pull exerted on the torn ciliary body, which is logical.

Control of secondary glaucoma

One of the most serious complications of hyphema is secondary glaucoma. This type of secondary glaucoma is caused by angle obstruction by blood clots. Whether angle obstruction occurs is determined by the amount and the rate of bleeding into the anterior chamber and by the rate of removal of fibrin and blood by outflow or by natural fibrinolysis.

Small hyphemas, filling less than one fourth of the anterior chamber, not infrequently follow contusions or intraocular surgery. Such small hyphemas almost invariably fail to cause secondary glaucoma. Presumably the ratio of fibrin entry to fibrin exit prevents accumulation of enough fibrin to form a clot large enough to block a critical portion of the trabecular drainage apparatus. The outflow potential of a healthy eye will maintain normal intraocular pressure even though more than half of the trabecular circumference is destroyed or temporarily occluded.

The eight-ball hemorrhage, a clot completely filling the anterior chamber and remaining there long enough for its hemoglobin to decompose to a black color, characteristically blocks the entire chamber angle with resultant glaucoma. Such increased intraocular pressure is not entirely disadvantageous, for it effectively arrests further bleeding and thereby may permit occlusion and healing of the bleeding site. Although glaucomatous optic atrophy is theoretically possible, glaucoma resulting from hyphema only rarely attains pressure heights or durations capable of recognizably damaging the optic nerve. The most distressing problem produced by the combination of glaucoma and hyphema is bloodstaining of the cornea. (If decomposing blood remains in the anterior chamber for long periods of time, corneal bloodstaining may occur without increased intraocular pressure.) The corneal opacity of bloodstaining is not permanent, but clearing of the cornea may require a year or more.

Pilocarpine. An obvious way to prevent clot formation in the anterior chamber would be to hasten the escape of fibrinogen and blood. That this can be accomplished by pilocarpine-induced miosis has previously been suggested. At the risk of repetition, let me spell out the distinction that pilocarpine treatment or prophylaxis of glaucoma secondary to hyphema is not designed primarily to enhance aqueous outflow. Its purpose is to hasten the elimination of fibrinogen and red blood cells.

Another mechanism whereby pilocarpine-induced miosis may accelerate the disappearance of a clotted hyphema is by enhanced fibrinolysis. Modern knowledge of iris physiology does not countenance the old theory that the increased surface of the miotic iris will phagocytose a clot more rapidly. However, the normal human iris can dissolve a 0.06 mm thick layer of fibrin within 15 minutes. Since this fibrinolytic activity is a function of surface contact, the larger area of a miotic iris will lyse more fibrin than will the smaller area of a cycloplegic iris. Unfortunately the trabecular meshwork does not have fibrinolytic capability.

Secretory inhibitors. Acetazolamide and

related drugs reduce intraocular pressure by decreasing aqueous secretion to as little as 40% of the normal rate. Such medications effectively reduce intraocular pressure if the trabecular outflow system is capable of handling 40% of the normal aqueous flow, but will be ineffective if the trabecular block is more complete. For example, a completely occluded narrow-angle acute glaucoma may respond poorly to acetazolamide. Similarly, glaucoma secondary to extensive fibrin occlusion of the angle may not be controlled by secretory inhibitors.

In theory, the reduced aqueous flow resulting from secretory inhibitors could be disadvantageous. One might speculate that fibrinogen and red cells would be washed out of the anterior chamber more rapidly by a greater volume of aqueous flow. Proof of such an untoward effect of acetazolamide would be almost impossible to establish clinically.

In practice, secretory inhibitors are commonly used to treat secondary glaucoma of all types. Whether such drugs benefit, hinder, or leave unaltered the spontaneous course of glaucoma secondary to hyphema is uncertain.

The rate of absorption of clotted blood from the rabbit anterior chamber was evaluated by a radioactive assay technique. Under the conditions of the experiment, half the blood was absorbed in 3 days. Treatment with 125 mg acetazolamide twice daily for 3 days reduced intraocular pressure by about 30% but neither accelerated nor retarded the absorption of the hyphema.[52]

Osmotic agents. Glaucoma secondary to traumatic hyphema may be treated successfully with intravenous mannitol or urea. Since the osmotic hypotensive effect is transitory, lasting only a few hours, one might logically expect the glaucoma to recur thereafter. Apparently such is not the case. Deepening of the anterior chamber through reduction of the vitreous volume may open the filtration angle, with subsequent permanent relief of the glaucoma. In a series of 14 eyes with hyphema and secondary glaucoma, intravenous urea controlled pressure in eight without subsequent need for surgery.[53] (The

other six eyes were irrigated with fibrinolysin.) These eyes regained 20/30 or better vision except in one eye that developed a detached retina. The same authors report useful vision in only one of 11 eyes treated by surgical evacuation of the clot. The other 10 eyes lost vision because of cataract, phthisis, or retinal detachment.

Unfortunately it is not uncommon to see eyes seriously damaged by poorly advised attempts at clot removal. Such a procedure is technically very difficult and should not be undertaken unless medical control is impossible. If pressure can be maintained at normal levels with the aid of mannitol (or other medications), surgical evacuation of the clot can safely be postponed and will often become unnecessary because of spontaneous reabsorption of the blood.[54]

Surgery. Routine extraction of a total black clot of the anterior chamber has been advocated, to be performed 4 days after hemorrhage. The reason for this timing is that recurrent bleeding may occur if the surgery is performed sooner, and adherence of the clot to intraocular structure occurs later.[55] Most ophthalmologists would not operate unless a painful increase in pressure persisted despite intravenous mannitol.

Prevention of corneal bloodstaining

Brownish gray opacification of the central corneal stroma occurs when sufficient amounts of hemosiderin accumulate in the anterior chamber, regardless of the intraocular pressure. Incubated in vitro at body temperature, fresh blood does not release significant amounts of hemosiderin for at least several days. If normal aqueous outflow is maintained, erythrocyte breakdown products cannot accumulate in sufficient concentration to cause corneal bloodstaining. Should blood clots block the escape of hemosiderin-filled aqueous from the anterior chamber there may simultaneously result a rising hemosiderin concentration and an elevation of intraocular pressure. Elevated intraocular pressure and corneal bloodstaining should be considered to result from a *common* cause, blocked aqueous outflow, rather than to have a cause and effect relationship.

The presence of old, black blood within the anterior chamber for several days should be considered to threaten development of corneal bloodstaining. Corneal bloodstaining may occur in a phthisical eye filled with old blood as well as in a glaucomatous eye.

Medical attempts to prevent corneal bloodstaining are based on the intent to enhance aqueous flow (and thereby remove hemosiderin concentrations from the anterior chamber). Obviously the appropriate medications are miotic drugs and osmotic agents. Pilocarpine may be administered any time after the hyphema is recognized, the sooner the better. Intravenous mannitol may be given whenever the anterior chamber is mostly filled with black blood clots; it is not necessary to wait for the onset of ocular hypertension.

An iron-chelating agent, desferrioxamine, has an iron-binding capacity greater than that of ferritin, hemosiderin, or other breakdown products of hemoglobin. Desferrioxamine will remove iron ions from these substances but not from hemoglobin or from other vital enzymes.

Experimental use of desferrioxamine has succeeded in removing corneal rust rings[56] and in extracting iron from intraocular fluids.[57] Unfortunately desferrioxamine has not been of practical clinical value in accelerating the disappearance of corneal bloodstaining.

Treatment of traumatic iritis

Fortunately, traumatic iritis is characteristically mild, is easily controlled, and shows little tendency to cause extensive formation of synechiae or inflammatory deposits (at least during short periods of time). Miotic treatment for several days does not cause this mild iritis to become significantly worse. Hence miotic treatment of a hyphema is possible without fear of causing damage from iritis.

Formation of posterior synechiae may be prevented by briefly dilating the pupil every few days with a short-acting drug (for example, tropicamide or cyclopentolate). Ideally, dilation of the pupil should be reserved for a time when the anterior chamber is free of blood.

Topical corticosteroids are well known to be effective in controlling anterior segment inflammation. Their effect in slowing absorption of hyphema is so minimal as to warrant disregard. Topical corticosteroid therapy of traumatic iritis is a recommended routine.

Late complications of contusion

The patient should be warned that an injured eye is predisposed to the late development of insidious and serious complications (such as chronic glaucoma or retinal detachment) and therefore requires periodic future examinations. Treatment of late traumatic glaucoma is comparable to that required by chronic simple glaucoma in both medical and surgical aspects.

Delayed detachments of the retina result from vitreous base disinsertion, consequent tearing of the peripheral retina (disinsertion), and traumatic liquefaction of the vitreous. The onset of both delayed detachments and late glaucoma is so insidious that it almost always goes unnoticed by the patient until irreparable damage has occurred. Some of our most tragic patients are children who have apparently recovered from a severe contusion with perfect sight. Years later, detected by routine school testing or by driver's license examination, the eye is found to have long-standing macular detachment. Presence of many demarcation lines testifies to the slow advance of the detachment, which could easily have been detected by routine rapid indirect ophthalmoscopy. But, alas, the parents must be told that macular function is forever gone, beyond the reach of successful detachment repair.

GENERAL EVALUATION OF THERAPY

A *prospective* study of 390 consecutive cases of traumatic hyphema evaluated the currently accepted methods of therapy as single variables. The format of this study is probably the most scientifically valid of any paper I have encountered on this subject. The conclusions are rather deflating—the spontaneous course of hyphema is totally unchanged by any form of medical management.

Final visual acuity and freedom from complications were better in ambulatory patients than those on bed rest; better if no eye pads were used than if one or both eyes were occluded (incidentally, the only logical reason for padding one eye is patient comfort); better if neither topical antibiotics nor corticosteroids were used; better if neither miotics nor mydriatics were used; better if trypsin, chymotrypsin, or papase enzyme therapy were not used; better if neither acetazolamide nor glycerol were used; and better if surgical evacuation of a three fourths to total hyphema was not performed.[58]

Are these results inexplicable, erroneous, illogical? They would seem entirely rational if we make the following assumptions, which I find plausible:

1. The severity of the initial injury determines the amount of ocular damage.
2. Rebleeding is correlated with spontaneous fibrinolytic clot dissolution rather than with external factors.
3. The natural course of healing of injured tissue is not accelerated by any known medical therapy.
4. Mechanical or chemical interference with normal physiologic functions is usually more detrimental than beneficial.

The usual excellent reviews of management of traumatic hyphema are at considerable variance with this nihilistic report.[59,60] Reconciliation of these differing points of view is difficult unless one dismisses all retrospective analyses as being uncontrolled and determined by artificial concentration of bad results in the casually managed group (casually managed successes not entering the statistics). This is rather a large assumption considering the consistency of most reports with respect to rest. On the other hand, the

arguments pro or con on a given medical regimen are certainly most impressive by their inconsistency. And it was not too long ago that newly delivered mothers and all recently operated general surgery (or eye) patients were supposed to spend days or weeks in bed.

Spontaneous hyphema

Infantile xanthogranuloma is a rare infiltrative iris lesion usually occurring before 1 year of age. Its main significance is that spontaneous anterior chamber hemorrhages occur, often of such severity as to cause glaucoma. The iris lesion responds to low doses of radiation. Corticosteroid therapy has been advised but is of doubtful benefit.[61]

A history of absence of injury is difficult to evaluate in an infant. Any parent knows that children are constantly bumping themselves. The possibility of the battered child syndrome must also be considered. Parents who mistreat their child are not apt to admit this.

In adults, spontaneous hyphema is usually a result of obvious ocular disease causing anterior segment neovascularization or vasodilation. A case has been reported of transient hemorrhage after routine ocular examination with the aid of phenylephrine followed by pilocarpine.[62] Presumably a fragile vessel spontaneously ruptured during the iris movements.

Rarely, faulty healing of the deep aspect of a cataract incision will predispose to recurrent bleeding from this same site on minor trauma. Gonioscopy may suffice to initiate such bleeding, which can be observed to confirm the diagnosis. Photographs of such a gonioscope-induced filiform hemorrhage have been published.[63] The condition is almost always benign, with spontaneous absorption of the blood, and does not require treatment. A single reported patient developed hemorrhagic glaucoma.

Of course, diabetic rubeosis iridis can be another cause of hyphema, especially following surgery. Unfortunately there is very little that can be done with medications to control the hemorrhages of diabetes.

REFERENCES

1. Benson, W. E., Wirostko, E., and Spalter, H. F.: The effects of inflammation on experimentally induced vitreous hemorrhage, Arch. Ophthalmol. **82:**822, 1969.
2. Dugmore, W. N., and Raichand, M.: Intravitreal urokinase in the treatment of vitreous hemorrhage, Am. J. Ophthalmol. **75:**779, 1973.
3. Pandolfi, M., and Kwaan, H. C.: Fibrinolysis in the anterior segment of the eye, Arch. Ophthalmol. **77:**99, 1967.
4. Pandolfi, M.: Coagulation factor VIII, localization in the aqueous outflow pathways, Arch. Ophthalmol. **94:**656, April 1976.
5. Smith, J. P., III, and Christensen, G. R.: The effect of salicylates on aqueous fibrinolysin, Invest. Ophthalmol. **10:**266, 1971.
6. Richards, R. D., and Spurling, C. L.: Elective ocular surgery in hemophilia, Arch. Ophthalmol. **89:**167, 1973.
7. Goldberg, J. L.: Conjugated estrogens in the prevention of secondary hyphema after ocular trauma, Arch. Ophthalmol. **63:**1001, 1960.
8. Spaeth, G. Link, and Levy, P. M.: Traumatic hyphema: its clinical characteristics and failure of estrogens to alter its course, Am. J. Ophthalmol. **62:**1098, 1966.
9. McGovern, J. J., Bunker, J. P., Goldstein, R., and Estes, J. W.: Effect of conjugated estrogens on the coagulation mechanism, J.A.M.A. **175:**1011, 1961.
10. New drugs, evaluated by A.M.A. Council on Drugs, Chicago, 1966, American Medical Association.
11. Magnuson, R. A.: Personal communication, 1968.
12. Swan, H. T., Nutt, A. B., Jowett, G. H., Wellwood-Ferguson, W. J., and Blackburn, E. K.: Monosemicarbazone of adrenochrome (Adrenoxyl) and cataract surgery, Br. J. Ophthalmol. **45:**415, 1961.
13. Smith, H. E.: Anterior chamber hemorrhages following nonperforating injuries, Trans. Pac. Coast Otoophthalmol. Soc. **38:**97, 1957.
14. Leone, C. R., Jr.: Traumatic hyphema in children, J. Pediatr. Ophthalmol. **3:**7, 1966.
15. Crawford, J. S., Lewandowski, R. L., and Chan, W.: The effect of aspirin on rebleeding in traumatic hyphema, Am. J. Ophthalmol. **80:**543, September 1975.
16. Kageler, W. V., Moake, J. L., and Garcia, C. A.: Spontaneous hyphema associated with ingestion of aspirin and ethanol, Am. J. Ophthalmol. **82:**631, October 1976.
17. Crouch, E. R., Jr., and Frenkel, M.: Aminocaproic acid in the treatment of traumatic hyphema, Am. J. Ophthalmol. **81:**355, March 1976.
18. Mullan, S., and Dawley, J.: Antifibrinolytic therapy for intracranial aneurysms, J. Neurosurg. **28:**21, 1968.
19. Levy, B. J., and Silver, D.: Treatment of subarachnoid hemorrhage: the ability of epsilon aminocaproic acid to cross the blood brain barrier and reduce the spinal fluid fibrinolytic activity, Surg. Forum **19:**413, 1968.
20. Cardamone, J. M., and Reese, E. P., Jr.: Ocular enucleation in a patient with severe classic hemophilia A, Am. J. Ophthalmol. **82:**767, November 1976.
21. Stein, V. K. H., and Stein, B. M.: Arteriopathic complications during treatment of subarachnoid hemorrhage with epsilon aminocaproic acid, J. Neurosurg. **40:**480, 1974.
22. Read, J., and Goldberg, M. F.: Comparison of medical treatment for traumatic hyphema, Trans. Am. Acad. Ophthalmol. Otolaryngol. **78:**OP-799, September-October 1974.
23. François, J., Neetens, A., and Collette, J. M.: Microradiographic study of the inner wall of Schlemm's canal, Am. J. Ophthalmol. **40:**491, 1955.
24. Huggert, A.: Pore size in the filtration angle of the eye, Acta Ophthalmol. **33:**271, 1955.
25. Flocks, M.: The anatomy of the trabecular meshwork as seen in tangential section, Arch. Ophthalmol. **56:**708, 1956.
26. Holmberg, A.: The fine structures of the inner wall of Schlemm's canal, Arch. Ophthalmol. **62:**956, 1959.
27. Theobald, G. D.: Further studies on the canal of Schlemm, Am. J. Ophthalmol. **39:**65, 1955.
28. Theobald, G. D.: The limbal area, with particular reference to the trabecular meshwork in health and disease, Am. J. Ophthalmol. **50:**543, 1960.
29. Ashton, N.: The exit pathway of the aqueous, Trans. Ophthalmol. Soc. U.K. **80:**397, 1960.
30. Campbell, D. G., Simmons, R. J., and Grant, W. M.: Ghost cells as a cause of glaucoma, Am. J. Ophthalmol. **81:**441, April 1976.
31. Kronfeld, P. C., McGarry, H. I., and Smith, H. E.: Gonioscopic studies of the canal of Schlemm, Am. J. Ophthalmol. **25:**1163, 1942.
32. Cahn, P. H., and Havener, W. H.: Factors of

importance in traumatic hyphema, Am. J. Ophthalmol. **55**:591, 1963.

33. Shabo, A. L., and Maxwell, D. S.: Observations on the fate of blood in the anterior chamber, Am. J. Ophthalmol. **73**:25, 1972.

34. Horven, I.: Erythrocyte passage into Schlemm's canal, Am. J. Ophthalmol. **74**:168, 1972.

35. Sinskey, R. M.: Experimental hyphema in rabbits, Am. J. Ophthalmol. **43**:292, 1957.

36. Philips, A. S.: Postcataract hyphema, Br. J. Ophthalmol. **24**:122, 1940.

37. Sinskey, R. M., and Krichesky, A. R.: Experimental hyphema in rabbits, Am. J. Ophthalmol. **52**:58, 1961.

38. Schaeffer, E., You, K., Bounds, G., and Heyssel, R. M.: Fibrinolysis in the anterior chamber of the rabbit eye, Arch. Ophthalmol. **65**:699, 1961.

39. Milthaler, C.: Anticoagulation and the resorption of hyphemas, Am. J. Ophthalmol. **60**:106, 1965.

40. Daily, L., and Tuttle, W. S.: Experimental use of enzymes for hyphemas and conjunctival hematomas, Arch. Ophthalmol. **65**:410, 1961.

41. Keeney, A. H.: The role of trypsin in experimentally induced hyphema, Am. J. Ophthalmol. **43**:275, 1957.

42. Sinskey, R. M., and Krichesky, A. R.: Experimental hyphema in rabbits, Am. J. Ophthalmol. **54**:445, 1962.

43. Podos, S. M., Liebman, S., and Pollen, A.: Treatment of experimental total hyphemas with intraocular fibrinolytic agents, Arch. Ophthalmol. **71**:537, 1964.

44. Sinskey, R. M., and Krichesky, A. R.: Experimental hyphema in rabbits, Am. J. Ophthalmol. **54**:1093, 1962.

45. Podos, S. M., Fingerman, L. H., and Becker, B.: The effect of corticosteroids on the resorption of partial hyphema in rabbit eyes, Invest. Ophthalmol. **4**:76, 1965.

46. Masket, S., Best, M., Fisher, L. V., Kronenberg, S. M., and Galin, M. A.: Therapy in experimental hyphema, Arch. Ophthalmol. **85**:329, 1971.

47. Gass, J. D. M.: Management of juvenile xanthogranuloma of the iris, Arch. Ophthalmol. **71**:344, 1964.

48. Sinskey, R. M.: Experimental hyphema in rabbits, Am. J. Ophthalmol. **48**:215, 1959.

49. Bredemeyer, H.: Unpublished data, 1958.

50. Magnuson, R. A.: Personal communication, 1968.

51. Bedrossian, R. H.: The management of traumatic hyphema, Ann. Ophthalmol. **6**:1016, October 1974.

52. Masket, S., and Best, M.: Therapy in experimental hyphema, Arch. Ophthalmol. **87**:222, 1972.

53. Cole, J. G., and Bryon, H. M.: Evaluation of 100 eyes with traumatic hyphema: intravenous urea, Arch. Ophthalmol. **71**:35, 1964.

54. Kwitko, M. L., and Costenbader, F. D.: Glaucoma due to secondary hyphema, Am. J. Ophthalmol. **53**:590, 1962.

55. Sears, M. L.: Surgical management of black ball hyphema, Trans. Am. Acad. Ophthalmol. Otolaryngol. **74**:820, 1970.

56. Galin, M. A.: Nonsurgical removal of corneal rust stains, Arch. Ophthalmol. **74**:674, 1965.

57. Wise, J. B.: Treatment of experimental siderosis bulbi, vitreous hemorrhage and corneal bloodstaining with deferoxamine, Arch. Ophthalmol. **75**:698, 1966.

58. Rakusin, W.: Traumatic hyphema, Am. J. Ophthalmol. **74**:284, 1972.

59. Edwards, W. C., and Layden, W. E.: Traumatic hyphema, Am. J. Ophthalmol. **75**:110, 1973.

60. Darr, J. L., and Passmore, J. W.: Management of traumatic hyphema, Am. J. Ophthalmol. **63**:134, 1967.

61. Sanders, T. E.: Infantile xanthogranuloma of the orbit, Am. J. Ophthalmol. **61**:1299, 1966.

62. Manor, R. S., and Sachs, W.: Spontaneous hyphema, Am. J. Ophthalmol. **74**:293, 1972.

63. Speakman, J. S.: Recurrent hyphema after surgery, Can. J. Ophthalmol. **10**:299, 1975.

37
LACRIMAL PROBLEMS

In general, the medical treatment of tear deficiency will consist of replacement solutions and that of lacrimal obstruction will be concerned with the use of appropriate antibiotics.

TEAR DEFICIENCY
Diagnosis

Schirmer test. Although the Schirmer test is the only objective criterion for the diagnosis of the "dry eye" syndrome, its limitations should be clearly recognized. In a series of 98 unselected clinic patients between 10 to 40 years of age, the average Schirmer measurement was 17 mm.[1] Five millimeters or less were wet in 17% of this group, and 3% produced no tears at all. Testing of 162 patients over 40 years old showed an average of 12 mm, with 39% (two fifths of this group) wetting 5 mm or less. Twelve percent produced no tears. Symptoms are not necessarily correlated with the Schirmer findings. Patients with no measurable tear production may be asymptomatic. Other individuals may show normal tear production and yet have complaints comparable to those of patients with "dry eyes," whose complaints are relieved by lubricant drops. In view of these findings, it was advised that lubricant therapy be prescribed on a symptomatic basis rather than because of the Schirmer test. Although it seems evident that the Schirmer test may lead to both false positive and false negative conclusions as to the existence of "dry eyes," I believe this diagnosis to be on a much

sounder basis if tear deficiency is measurable, and question whether a therapeutic response to lubricants used in a wet eye may not be simply a placebo effect.

The diagnosis of keratoconjunctivitis sicca on the basis of less than 5.5 mm of wetting of the Schirmer test strip gave false positive results in 17% of asymptomatic control patients and false negative results in 15% of patients diagnosed as having keratoconjunctivitis sicca on the basis of clinical characteristics and abnormally low lysozyme content of the tears (Fig. 37-1).[2] This figure suggests that it is reasonable to suspect a Schirmer test as being "abnormal" when wetting is less than 8 mm.

Vital staining. All of a series of 31 patients with keratoconjunctivitis sicca showed definite staining with 1% rose bengal.[3] In half of these patients, staining was distributed in discrete plaques located in the exposed portions of the cornea and conjunctiva. The other half showed staining of virtually the entire exposed cornea and conjunctiva. Fluorescein staining was a much less reliable indicator of epithelial abnormality in these patients.

Artifactual staining occurs in the portion of the conjunctiva irritated by the filter paper used in a Schirmer test. Tetracaine anesthesia also predisposes to exaggerated staining. However, rose bengal is quite irritating to patients with keratoconjunctivitis sicca, and anesthesia is desirable. Proparacaine is less toxic to the epithelium and may be less like-

720

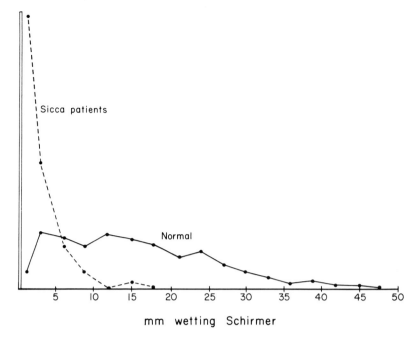

Fig. 37-1. Overlap of normal (550) and sicca (43) patients measured by Schirmer test. (Data from van Bijsterveld, O. P.: Arch. Ophthalmol. **82:**10, 1969.)

ly than tetracaine to cause artifactual staining.

Rose bengal staining was performed on 40 patients (ages 9 to 79 years) complaining only of errors of refraction. Unfortunately for the specificity of this test, 30% of these "normal" eyes retained considerable stain.

Apparently interpretation of rose bengal testing permits the following possibilities. Absence of staining excludes keratoconjunctivitis sicca. Presence of staining may indicate the diagnosis of keratoconjunctivitis sicca, may be an artifact of mechanical or anesthetic irritation, or may occur in as high as 30% of asymptomatic individuals.

Tear film breakup time. A more direct measure of the physiologic function of the tear film is the estimation of the tear film breakup time (BUT).[4] The BUT is defined as the interval between a complete blink and the appearance of the first *randomly* distributed dry spot. In normal eyes the BUT averages 25 to 30 seconds and is never less than 10 seconds.

The appearance of a dry spot is recognized by observation of the cornea with the biomicroscope using the cobalt blue filter and a broad beam. Fluorescein is applied by touching a *slightly* moistened fluorescein strip to the lower temporal conjunctival sac, following which the patient blinks several times. Artifactual defects in the tear film result if the patient does not distribute the fluorescein by blinking or if the fluorescein strip is excessively wet. The patient stares straight ahead without blinking during the measurement of the BUT time. Do *not* hold the lids open, for this disrupts the tear film meniscus and abnormally accelerates the BUT. Topical anesthesia greatly accelerates the BUT, presumably by damaging the corneal microvilli, which are necessary for proper mucin absorption.

Observation of the BUT is a simple and rapid clinical procedure that is indicated whenever the possibility of a surface corneal defect or a tear film deficiency is suspected. Repeat evaluations require simply a complete lid blink. A dry spot developing consistently in one area of the cornea indicates local disturbance of the surface and not a tear film deficiency.

Physiology of tear film. The tear film is not a homogeneous moist pool, as might be supposed, but rather consists of at least three layers.[5] The lipid, hydrophobic nature of the corneal epithelium is well known—such a surface cannot be wetted by water and would repel an aqueous tear. The deepest layer of the tear film is a thin sheet of mucus, probably derived from the conjunctival goblet cells. The function of the mucus is to increase the corneal surface tension sufficiently so that the aqueous lacrimal secretion will spontaneously spread on its surface. Note that this spreading occurs actively and is a function of the surface tension of the two interfaces. If the surface tension of the liquid is higher than that of the solid surface, the liquid will remain as circumscribed droplets on the solid (like water drops on a sheet of plastic). Conversely, the high surface tension of a mucous membrane surface results in great ease of wetting—water is literally pulled over the surface. Another feature of the mucus-covered surface is that the mucus clings tenaciously to the surface, does not spontaneously flow away, and is not easily wiped away.

The middle layer of the tear film is the aqueous secretion, coming primarily from the lacrimal gland. This aqueous layer is a rather passive component pulled across the cornea by surface tension forces and spread mechanically by blinking. Variations in the thickness of the tear film occur primarily in the aqueous layer, which is functional whether extremely thin or in excess. The physiologic surplus of lacrimal secretion remaining after evaporation is normally carried away by the tear ducts. By itself, a watery tear film is unstable and cannot protect the corneal surface from drying. So also, instillation of saline drops is not an effective treatment for a cornea deficient in mucus.

The oily surface layer of the tear film, the meibomian secretion, probably serves to stabilize the watery portion of the tear film. Having a relatively high surface tension, this oil tends to spread the aqueous middle layer, just as does the mucus on the other side.

The popular supposition that the oily layer retards evaporation is not supported by in vitro measurements, which indicate that the loss of water from experimental surfaces is identical whether or not they are covered by meibomian oils.[6] Two components of meibomian secretion exist. One is an oil with a hydrophilic end chain, a feature permitting spread as a monolayer over a watery surface. The bulk of the meibomian oil is nonpolar—this portion spreads on the surface of the hydrophilic monolayer. The total thickness of the oil layer can be measured by interference spectra and is about 0.2 μ deep. This corresponds to about 100 molecules.

Study of the hydrodynamics of blinking has confirmed the importance of the oily layer in spreading of the tear film.[7] As the upper lid lifts, its tear meniscus rises across the cornea, spreading a thin sheet of tear fluid. Additional thickening and stabilization of the tear film results from the surface tension effect of the oily layer, which pulls additional water upward in the middle layer of the tear film. This active pull resulting from surface tension forces helps to thicken the tear film only when a sufficient aqueous reservoir exists. When a film of water covering a relatively wettable surface decreases below a critical thickness, its own surface tension will cause it to retract to an equilibrium thickness. This phenomenon accounts for the sudden appearance of the holes in such a thin liquid film, as may be observed when studying the BUT.

Another surface tension phenomenon of significance to the tear film is meniscus-induced thinning.[8] A meniscus of fluid exists at any elevation from a surface. This meniscus may act as a source of fluid if it is drawn across the corneal surface by the moving eyelid. However, if the meniscus is not connected to a reservoir of fluid, it will have a detrimental effect on the tear film by pulling water from the surrounding film into the meniscus. Because of this negative pressure effect, a halo of thinner fluid will exist adjacent to any elevation or irregularity of the corneal surface. For example, a pterygium, an edematous conjunctival overhang following strabismus surgery, or the edge of a contact lens may cause such adjacent thinning of the aqueous layer of the tear film. (This is the mechanism of dellen formation after strabismus surgery.) Further thinning of the tear film by evaporation results in the initial retraction of the film from these thin spots.

Evaporation of water from the cornea and tear film is considerably more complex than being merely a function of the relative humidity of the environment. In vivo evaluation of the rate of surface evaporation indicates that the removal of the superficial lipid layer of the tear film results in a fourfold increase in the rate of evaporation, which returns to a normal rate after 5 minutes.[9] This somewhat puzzling result, in conflict with the previously mentioned failure of meibomian oils to retard evaporation in vitro, may have been an artifact caused by flushing the corneal surface with artificial tear solution. Removal of the epithelium resulted in a 20-fold increase in the evaporation rate from the exposed stroma. Another finding was that the tear film residue becomes more hypertonic with evaporation. This hypertonicity resists further evaporation and increases transcorneal fluid passage, thereby tending to maintain the tear film. The evaporation rate from the surface of the undisturbed rabbit cornea may amount to 2 to 4 μl/cm^2/hour. For comparison, the coefficient of aqueous outflow is about 3 μl/minute.

Etiology

Since every clinician is aware that dryness of the eyes becomes more frequent with increasing age, further comment on this factor is superfluous. Similarly, the close association between arthritis and keratoconjunctivitis sicca is well known.

The mechanisms whereby dry spots develop in such disorders can readily be inferred from the preceding discussion on the physiology of the tear film. Patients with clinical complaints from reduced tear flow (almost always less than 7 mm wetting of the Schirmer test strip) show dry spots in the tear film very quickly after blinking. Patients with unusually wide palpebral fissures (for example, thyrotrophic) or who do not close their lids completely with blinking will show dry spots in the exposed areas of the cornea. Trichiasis disrupts the surface tension of the tear film, resulting in local defects of the tear film. Surface irregularities of cornea and conjunctiva cause adjacent dry spots. Lid appositional faults (ectropion and marginal defects) cause corresponding dry areas. Whatever the cause of these dry spots, their persistence for only 2 or 3 seconds desiccates the underlying corneal epithelium, causing punctate staining. Decreased corneal sensation also contributes to the development of staining areas because it prevents the prompt blinking that is the normal response to the drying of the tear film.[10]

In 20 eyes of 25 patients with myotonic dystrophy the Schirmer test was positive (less than 10 mm in 5 minutes).[11] Four of these patients had clinically manifest keratoconjunctivitis sicca. Eight patients had chronic blepharitis. In the presence of major and unusual disorders we tend to overlook the possibility of treating coexistent minor and common problems. Often these minor problems are quite annoying to the patient, who will be grateful for their remedy. Obviously the patient with myotonic dystrophy should be evaluated as a possible condidate for lubricant therapy, just as we should also suspect arthritic, menopausal patients of having dry eyes.

Dryness of the eye is at least partially responsible for the damage resulting from neuroparalytic keratitis. The response of the lacrimal gland to systemically administered pilocarpine, 10 mg, and neostigmine, 1.5 mg, will indicate whether its innervation remains intact following neurosurgical procedures or disease. Damage to the great superficial petrosal nerve (the secretory nerve for the lacrimal gland) is common during operations on the gasserian ganglion. As measured by the Schirmer test, tear formation by a denervated lacrimal gland will be subnormal, will not increase in response to neostigmine, and will be greater than normal in response to pilocarpine. Neostigmine causes increased lacrimation if the lacrimal gland innervation is normal. The lacrimal response to pilocarpine or neostigmine may be measured 15 minutes after drug administration. Representative measurements are shown in Table 37-1.[12]

A very rare cause of the dry eye syndrome is familial dysautonomia (Riley-Day syndrome). These patients show denervation hypersensitivity to autonomic drugs. A unique and characteristic, easily observed physical finding is the absence of the fungiform papillae (the large round ones) of the tongue.[13]

Of course, destruction by disease of the lacrimal gland and the accessory secretory glands of the conjunctiva will cause a dry eye. Typical diseases capable of producing such damage include exfoliative dermatitis, Stevens-Johnson syndrome, trachoma, ocular pemphigoid, and vitamin A deficiency. Chronic herpetic keratoconjunctivitis includes a considerable component of dryness and trauma. Dellen of the cornea (erosions adjacent to elevated areas) are presumed to result from dehydration.

Severe keratitis sicca with a Schirmer test of only 1 mm was caused by sarcoidosis of the lacrimal gland.[14] Alternate day dosage of 60 mg of prednisone orally caused dramatic improval, with increase of Schirmer wetting to 18 mm in 5 minutes and disappearance of the dry eye symptoms. In another case of sarcoidosis with lacrimal glands so massive

that the tarsal plate was pushed away from the eye, the lacrimal glands returned to normal size after 2 months of alternate day dosage of 60 mg prednisone.

Management

Refer to the section on viscous medications for the properties of those fluids that may be used as artificial tears in replacement therapy.

Recent studies indicate the 24-hour volume of tear flow from one eye to be in the neighborhood of 14 to 28 ml.[15] Obviously, in severe deficiency of tear secretion, replacement therapy with 3 or 4 drops a day will not be adequate and symptoms will persist. Of even more serious import, deficiencies in the mucus and oil components of the tear film disrupt the surface tension mechanisms of fluid distribution. A few such patients present almost impossible therapeutic problems.

Fortunately the usual patient with keratoconjunctivitis sicca is considerably relieved by the occasional instillation of almost any type of artificial tear. Cold, moist compresses may also afford considerable symptomatic relief to patients with burning, dry eyes. Possibly humidification of the air might be of value in some cases. Recall that the relative humidity of an average northern home drops to 10% during the winter—roughly comparable to a desert atmosphere.

Unfortunately medical therapy is not effective in severe cases of tear film deficiency. In such instances the corneal surface may be protected by scleral contact lenses.[16] A variant of this method of management, the glued-on epikeratoprosthesis, was transiently advocated. "Bandage" soft contact lenses currently have replaced both types of hard lens in the management of difficult surface corneal problems.

Familial dysautonomia. Because of lacrimal deficiency and corneal anesthesia, patients with familial dysautonomia (Riley-Day syndrome) develop corneal scarring or even perforation. Medical treatment includes topical lubricants for protection and antibiotics prophylactically or certainly when-

Table 37-1. Schirmer test measurements in case of left lacrimal gland denervation, before and after neostigmine and pilocarpine*

Drug		OD	OS
Neostigmine, 1.5 mg	Initial	8	2
	16 min	25	3
Pilocarpine, 10 mg	Initial	20	2
	15 min	35	32

*Data from de Haas, E. B. H.: Arch. Ophthalmol. 67:439, 1962.

ever local infections develop in the eroded cornea. Tearing from the partially denervated but anatomically intact lacrimal gland may be induced by the use of methacholine eye drops or systemic neostigmine. Medical treatment is relatively ineffective, since significant corneal ulceration is reported in as high as 50% of cases. Hence the management of choice appears to be tarsorrhaphy performed with the patient under *local* anesthesia. Although these patients are seen in childhood and general anesthesia would seem appropriate, cardiac arrest occurred in eight of 27 operations on dysautonomic patients. This formidable anesthetic risk should be recognized by the surgeon before deciding on general anesthesia.[17]

Total xerophthalmia. Total xerophthalmia, as may result from the ocular complications of exfoliative dermatitis, cannot be controlled by artificial tears or lubricants for long periods of time. Parotid duct transplantation and conjunctivoantrorhinostomy represent the most successful current approach to management of the totally dry eye.[18]

Exposure keratopathy. Continuing corneal exposure almost always sooner or later results in corneal damage despite lubricants and patching. Appropriate surgical corrections by tarsorrhaphy are indicated. Particularly if corneal sensitivity is reduced or absent, exposure damage is nearly impossible to avoid by medical means.

The severity of ocular symptoms in 15 patients with Sjögren's syndrome was evaluated monthly for a year.[19] Each patient was treated for 6 months with 800 mg/day hydroxychloroquine and for 6 months with a placebo. An improvement in symptoms (burning, scratching, dryness, and photophobia) occurred in 12 patients during the period of hydroxychloroquine therapy and in six during placebo therapy. Hydroxychloroquine was selected for use because it is supposed to benefit rheumatoid arthritis and systemic lupus erythematosus, conditions possibly related to Sjögren's syndrome. (Six of the 15 patients had rheumatoid arthritis; four of these improved while on hydroxychloroquine.)

The only objective measurement that showed improvement was the erythrocyte sedimentation rate. There was no consistent improvement in the Schirmer test, the area of rose bengal stain, or the appearance of the precorneal tear film. The correlation between the physical measurements (rose bengal stain and Schirmer test) and the symptoms was very poor. This suggests that factors other than tear deficiency contribute to the symptoms of keratoconjunctivitis sicca. (One patient with a Schirmer test of 5 mm showed improvement to 15 mm with therapy; however, 3 weeks after the accidental death of a relative, her Schirmer test had dropped to 3 mm and her symptoms were worse.) Emotional factors seem to be related to the eye symptoms of Sjögren's syndrome.

Although twice as many patients improved while on hydroxychloroquine as during the placebo period, the improvement was incomplete, only two patients being able to stop using the lubricating drops. Furthermore, symptoms returned within several months after discontinuing therapy. Because of this limited response and the potential retinotoxic effect of hydroxychloroquine, I doubt this method of therapy will gain popularity. However, the demonstrated fact that half the patients with severe keratoconjunctivitis sicca improve spontaneously during a 6-month period is important to the future clinical evaluation of other methods of treatment.

EPIPHORA CAUSED BY LACRIMAL OBSTRUCTION

Although organisms recovered from an infected lacrimal sac may simply be secondary contaminants growing in an area of stasis, the primary cause of occlusion of canaliculi or the nasolacrimal duct may be infection. From the practical clinical standpoint, irrigation of the obviously infected lacrimal sac with antibiotic solution, followed by the topical instillation of antibiotics at home, will eliminate infections caused by common susceptible bacteria. Therapeutic failure will require the further expense of cultures and microscopic study.

The usual method of lacrimal irrigation,

with the patient's head positioned face up, washes away irrecoverably the sac contents, which may be of sufficient diagnostic value to guide the therapy of chronic conjunctival and lacrimal infection. A much more valuable method positions the patient face down, thereby permitting the irrigation fluid to run from the nose into a basin held by the patient.[20] If the basin is of dark color, identification of pus, mucus, fungus casts, or other debris is easier. Appropriate smear and culture study of material obtained by this simple technique is advised in the management of patients with chronic external infection that has failed to respond to the usual antibiotic therapy.

The rare but stubborn condition of actinomycosis of the lacrimal canaliculi ("Streptothrix" canaliculitis) may be diagnosed by the recognition of some or all of the following clinical features:

1. Persistent tearing
2. Chronic inflammation of the medial conjunctiva
3. Prominence and redness of the punctum
4. Mucopurulent or mucoid discharge
5. Swelling and tenderness of the canaliculi

Characteristically, concretions of fungus growth develop within the canaliculi and lacrimal sac or within diverticulae. These concretions are soft and readily crushed for diagnostic examination. The organism is pleomorphic and may exist in the form of branched mycelia, filaments, or beadlike structures closely resembling a string of gram-positive streptococci. Because of the variable appearance and because of the slow growth of this anaerobic organism, bacteriologic studies may be misleading.

Although this is a localized infection, topical instillation of antibiotic drops is not usually considered to be effective treatment. Mechanical removal of the concretions by curettage or surgical incision is ordinarily necessary to effect a cure. Whether postoperative irrigation with an antibiotic or with mild iodine solutions is additionally helpful is uncertain. The surgical approach to the

canaliculus should preserve the punctum and its capillary action.[21] The canaliculus may be opened by cutting down on the conjunctival side of a lacrimal probe within the canaliculus. Do not cut the punctum. Through this incision, the fungus deposits are readily and completely removed. Interrupted 6-0 sutures close the conjunctival wound. Dacryocystography may disclose the size and extent of the canalicular mass.[22]

Mycotic genital infections in the female may be a source of persistent or recurrent ocular infection. *Candida parakrusei* has been isolated from a cast of the left lacrimal sac and from vaginal culture.[23] The same patient had previously required a right dacryocystorhinostomy at which time a cast of unidentified fungus material was removed. Prior to the left dacryocystorhinostomy, the same fungus was cultured from fluid expressed from the sac. Only temporary relief from obstruction was achieved by preoperative irrigations. No antifungal medications were used in the treatment of this 24-year-old patient. Fungus cultures and local antifungal therapy (following positive cultures) would seem appropriate in the management of lacrimal drainage problems. Good personal hygiene and avoidance of spread from genital infection (self or marital partner) should be emphasized in such cases.

Canalicular infection by viruses such as herpes simplex or zoster may also cause lacrimal stenosis and epiphora.[24] These case reports suggest that IDU therapy of acute viral canaliculitis is ineffective in preventing subsequent stenosis.

Just as the pigmented oxidation products of epinephrine may be deposited in the conjunctiva, so also they may accumulate within the lacrimal sac and nasolacrimal duct to form large brownish black casts. Three of 27 patients (11%) receiving topical epinephrine for a year or longer were found to have epiphora resulting from lacrimal obstruction from such casts.[25] Irrigation of the lacrimal passages resulted in immediate or delayed expulsion of relatively huge casts (one measured 25 × 3 mm). Tearing was relieved by removal of the casts, but in one patient the same condition recurred several months later. From the clinical viewpoint, any patient who develops epiphora while using topical epinephrine should be irrigated with the intent of removal of such a melanin cast.

Stenosis or occlusion of the lacrimal puncta may result from severe allergy to cyclopentolate (Cyclogyl), may follow chemical burns or Stevens-Johnson disease, or can be congenital. Needle puncture through the punctum to the patent canaliculus followed by a one-snip procedure may solve the problem.[26]

Inasmuch as the evaluation and management of most patients with lacrimal obstruction are surgical procedures rather than medical problems, they are beyond the scope of this text. However, I do want to remind the reader that the diagnosis of the location and severity of the obstruction is fairly simple, requiring only the appropriate use of the primary and secondary dye tests and the fluorescein disappearance test.[27-30]

Instillation of a drop of 0.5% to 2% fluorescein (or its equivalent from a fluorescein paper strip) followed by intranasal insertion of a small tuft of cotton on a wire applicator (position in inferior meatus to contact the opening of the nasolacrimal duct) is called the "primary dye test." A positive primary

dye test results in visible staining of the cotton within 5 minutes and proves functional patency of the lacrimal excretory system.

The "secondary dye test" consists of irrigating the lacrimal sac with normal saline solution (*not* fluorescein) immediately after a negative primary dye test. During irrigation the patient's head is tipped forward to permit the irrigating fluid to run from the nose into a white basin or white tissue. A positive secondary dye test produces stained fluid. This indicates functioning canaliculi but nonfunctioning (yet patent) nasolacrimal duct. Nonstained nasal fluid from the secondary dye test indicates failure of the fluorescein used in the primary test to enter the lacrimal sac and therefore identifies the fault as existing in punctum, canaliculus, or lacrimal pump.

Immunologic mechanisms

The remarkable resistance of the delicate, moist ocular surface to infection is significantly related to immunologic capability within the tears. An anatomic basis for this was demonstrated by count of plasma cell populations. (The presence of plasma cells indicates immunologic activity.) Specimens from human autopsies showed the average lacrimal

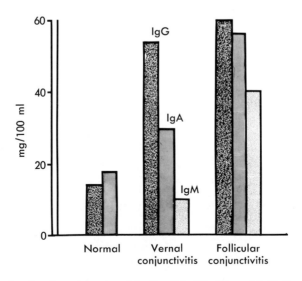

Fig. 37-2. Average levels of tear immunoglobulin. (Modified from McClellan, B. H., and associates: Am. J. Ophthalmol. **76:**89, July 1973.)

gland to contain over 3,000,000 plasma cells; the conjunctiva was found to contain over 2,000,000.[31] Comparative numbers of plasma cells in other tissues are not stated, but the report implies that this is a relatively high plasma cell concentration.

Immunoglobulin G is found in normal human tears, averaging 14.1 mg/100 ml. IgA averages 17.1 mg/100 ml.[32] These levels are only slightly increased in blepharoconjunctivitis or herpetic keratitis but are markedly elevated in vernal conjunctivitis and acute follicular conjunctivitis (Fig. 37-2).

Although the physician may be tempted to prescribe corticosteroids for chronic local allergic ocular problems, this choice is unwise because of the threat of glaucoma, increased susceptibility to infection, and possibly cataract. The local use of sympathomimetic drugs (for example, 0.12% phenylephrine) will provide relief from allergic symptoms actually more promptly than can be obtained by corticosteroid therapy and is far preferable.

REFERENCES

1. Wright, J. C., and Meger, G. E.: A review of the Schirmer test for tear production, Arch. Ophthalmol. **67**:564, 1962.
2. van Bijsterveld, O. P.: Diagnostic tests in the sicca syndrome, Arch. Ophthalmol. **82**:10, 1969.
3. Lansche, R. K.: Vital staining in normal eyes and in keratoconjunctivitis sicca, Am. J. Ophthalmol. **60**:520, 1965.
4. Lemp, M. A., and Jamill, J. R., Jr.: Factors affecting tear film breakup in normal eyes, Arch. Ophthalmol. **89**:103, 1973.
5. Lemp, M. A., Holly, F. J., Iwata, S., and Dohlman, C. H.: The precorneal tear film, Arch. Ophthalmol. **83**:89, 1970.
6. Brown, S. I., and Dervichian, D. G.: The oils of the meibomian glands, Arch. Ophthalmol. **82**:537, 1969.
7. Brown, S. I., and Dervichian, D. G.: Hydrodynamics of blinking, Arch. Ophthalmol. **82**:541, 1969.
8. McDonald, J. E., and Brubaker, S.: Meniscus-induced thinning of tear films, Am. J. Ophthalmol. **72**:139, 1971.
9. Iwata, S., Lemp, M. A., Holly, F. J., and Dohlman, C. H.: Evaporation rate of water from the precorneal tear film and cornea in the rabbit, Invest. Ophthalmol. **8**:613, 1969.
10. Brown, S. I.: Further studies on the pathophysiology of keratitis sicca of Rollet, Arch. Ophthalmol. **83**:542, 1970.
11. Burian, H. M., and Burns, C. A.: Ocular changes in myotonic dystrophy, Am. J. Ophthalmol. **63**:22, 1967.
12. de Haas, E. B. H.: Desiccation of cornea-conjunctiva, Arch. Ophthalmol. **67**:439, 1962.
13. Goldberg, M. F., Payne, J. W., and Brunt, P. W.: Ophthalmologic studies of familial dysautonomia, Arch. Ophthalmol. **80**:732, 1968.
14. Cook, J. R., Brubaker, R. F., Savell, J., and Sheagren, J.: Lacrimal sarcoidosis treated with corticosteroids, Arch. Ophthalmol. **88**:513, November 1972.
15. Norn, M. S.: The conjunctival fluid, its height, volume, density of cells, and flow, Acta Ophthalmol. **44**:212, 1966.
16. Gould, H. L.: The dry eye and scleral contact lenses, Am. J. Ophthalmol. **70**:37, 1970.
17. Howard, R. O.: Familial dysautonomia (Riley-Day syndrome), Am. J. Ophthalmol. **64**:392, 1967.
18. Bennett, J. E.: The management of total xerophthalmia, Arch. Ophthalmol. **81**:667, 1969.
19. Heaton, J. M.: The treatment of Sjögren's syndrome with hydroxychloroquine, Am. J. Ophthalmol. **55**:983, 1963.
20. Fasanella, R. M.: Complications of eye surgery, ed. 2, Philadelphia, 1965, W. B. Saunders Co.
21. Ellis, P. P., Bausor, S. C., and Fulmer, J.: Streptothrix canaliculitis, Am. J. Ophthalmol. **52**:36, 1961.
22. Richards, W. W.: Actinomycotic lacrimal canaliculitis, Am. J. Ophthalmol. **75**:155, 1973.
23. Buesseler, J. A., and Godwin, I. D.: Chronic dacryocystomycosis due to Candida parakrusei, Trans. Am. Acad. Ophthalmol. Otolaryngol. **67**:173, 1963.
24. Bouzas, A.: Canalicular inflammation, Am. J. Ophthalmol. **60**:713, 1965.
25. Spaeth, G. L.: Nasolacrimal duct obstruction caused by topical epinephrine, Arch. Ophthalmol. **77**:355, 1967.
26. Putterman, A. M.: Treatment of epiphora with absent lacrimal puncta, Arch. Ophthalmol. **89**:125, 1973.
27. Zappia, R. J., and Milder, B.: Lacrimal drainage function. I. The Jones fluorescein test, Am. J. Ophthalmol. **74**:154, 1972.
28. Zappia, R. J., and Milder, B.: Lacrimal drain-

age function. II. The fluorescein dye disappearance test, Am. J. Ophthalmol. **74:**160, 1972.

29. Jones, L. T., and Linn, M. L.: The diagnosis of the causes of epiphora, Am. J. Ophthalmol. **67:**751, 1969.
30. Putterman, A. M.: Evaluation of the lacrimal system, Eye Ear Nose Throat Mon. **51:**31, 1972.
31. Allansmith, M. R., Kajiyama, G., Abelson, M. B., and Simon, M. A.: Plasma cell content of main and accessory lacrimal glands and conjunctiva, Am. J. Ophthalmol. **82:**819, December 1976.
32. McClellan, B. H., Whitney, C. R., Newman, L. P., and Allansmith, M. R.: Immunoglobulins in tears, Am. J. Ophthalmol. **76:**89, July 1973.

38
UVEITIS

The frequency of occurrence of uveitis has been studied in Rochester, Minnesota.[1] The prevalence of uveitis in this community was 0.2% of the population. At this rate, 29,000 new cases of uveitis would be expected annually in the United States and the prevalence of uveitis would be one third of a million persons. Nine percent of the blindness in the United States is attributed to uveitis.

ETIOLOGY

Of 1559 referrals to the Ohio State University Uveitis Clinic, 899 were posterior uveitis, 263 were anterior uveitis, and 397 (25%) were macular degenerative changes, retinal detachments, or some other nonuveitic condition. Discussion of uveitis presupposes the ability to make an accurate diagnosis and to differentiate simulating conditions. Patients with acute glaucoma have been atropinized under the mistaken diagnosis of iritis. Such an elementary error is cited as an example of the potentially disastrous results of incorrect diagnosis. Recognition of the presence of uveitis and the clinical assessment of a likely etiology is dependent on capable use of ophthalmologic examining instruments rather than on consultation with medical specialists or laboratory reports. For instance, the presently popular diagnosis of toxoplasmic or histoplasmic posterior uveitis is largely based on ophthalmoscopic findings.

In Finland during 1964 to 1974, 653 patients with uveitis were reviewed. Diagnosed etiologies were rheumatoid (7%), tubercu-losis (3.7%), and toxoplasmosis (3.3%). Most cases (75%) were of undetermined etiology.[2]

Frustrated by the difficulty of the etiologic diagnosis of uveitis, the practicing ophthalmologist views with great interest such reports as that of the Academy Uveitis Survey.[3] It was claimed that this standard survey will identify the cause of approximately 80% of cases of granulomatous uveitis and 60% of nongranulomatous uveitis. The incidence of the various causes of 432 cases of granulomatous uveitis is given in Table 38-1. Nongranulomatous uveitis was attributed to bacterial sensitivity, primarily streptococcal. Interestingly, it has not been possible to differentiate granulomatous from nongranulomatous uveitis on the basis of any laboratory tests or examinations. This differentiation rests entirely on clinical criteria and probably has no etiologic significance.

Critical evaluation suggests the probability that the skin testing methods employed in diagnosis do not necessarily indicate a relationship between the uveitis and the existence of a previous or concurrent systemic infection. Attention should be called to the etiologic diagnoses made in the same institution in 1941 and 1953.[4] In 1941, tuberculosis accounted for 79% of cases of granulomatous uveitis and no cases were caused by toxoplasmosis. By 1953, tuberculosis accounted for only 23% of the cases and 26% were attributed to toxoplasmosis. This change is not one of disease frequency but rather of diagnostic criteria. Predictably, the future development of a skin

Table 38-1. Etiology of incidence in 432 cases of granulomatous uveitis*

Etiology	Percentage incidence
Toxoplasmosis	30.9
Tuberculosis	21.7
Questionable toxoplasmosis or tuberculosis	6.7
Syphilis	4.6
Sarcoidosis	4.4
Brucellosis	4.9
Histoplasmosis†	3.9
Miscellaneous (viral, sympathetic, etc.)	7.4
Undetermined (negative surveys)	15.5

*Data from Woods, A. C., and Abrahams, I. W.: Am. J. Ophthalmol. **51**:761, 1961.
†Tests for histoplasmosis in 186 patients only.

test diagnostic of some newly discovered common infection will again alter the incidence of etiologies diagnosed by such criteria.

Although an enormous amount has been written concerning the diagnostic techniques in uveitis, practicing physicians will find it difficult or impossible to establish the etiology of a given case of uveitis. Realizing this, they will usually undertake only medically justifiable studies, leaving the "complete diagnostic surveys" to the research institutes. Only rarely does information obtained from a diagnostic work-up significantly alter the final outcome.

Why, then, do any work-up at all, beyond the usual thorough eye examination? In a great many cases, particularly those which do not threaten eyesight and respond within a few weeks to corticosteroid and cycloplegic therapy, there is no necessity to do additional studies. Those patients whose sight is threatened or who suffer frequent recurrences are themselves realistically concerned and excite feelings of uncertainty and inadequacy within their physician. These compelling emotional reasons lead to the "work-up" of such patients. A *complete general physical examination* is certainly appropriate and will

often lead to the discovery of some condition, treatment of which is of benefit to the patient, although not to the uveitis. Examples of this include the medical care of hypertension or diabetes, dental treatment for bad teeth, and elimination of throat, sinus, or genitourinary infections.

Consultation with an otolaryngologist, dentist, urologist, gynecologist, or other specialist is indicated only if the history or the general examination has suggested the possibility of trouble in any of these areas.

Until sex ceases to be a popular pastime, routine *serology* should be part of all thorough examinations. A fluorescent antibody dark-field technique showed spirochetes to be present in the aqueous humor of six of 50 patients with active uveitis.[5] The authors pointed out the difficulty of identifying these organisms and suggested that probably this 12% frequency of syphilitic etiology was an underestimate of the true prevalence of this type of infection. Fifteen of the 50 patients had positive or borderline serologic tests. Of the six patients with spirochetes recoverable from their aqueous, only three had borderline positive serologic tests (FTA-ABS) and none gave any history of syphilis. Perhaps the ophthalmologists of the pasts were correct in their frequent diagnosis of luetic uveitis.

Not only is the *chest x-ray film* a desirable general screening test, but also it is valuable in detecting tuberculous lesions that require special attention during corticosteroid therapy. Remember that corticosteroid therapy of patients with old inactive tuberculosis may require them to take a year-long course of isoniazid! Urinalysis may detect diabetes, which is also of significance during corticosteroid administration. Skin tests for tuberculosis, toxoplasmosis, and histoplasmosis may help to support a presumptive diagnosis.[6]

The erythrocyte sedimentation rate is supposed to detect a wide variety of underlying chronic inflammatory or degenerative diseases. Sedimentation rates were performed on 169 adult patients with no known diseases. As shown in Fig. 38-1, the normal values for this test rise with age.[7] Knowledge of

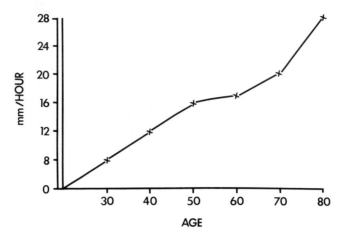

Fig. 38-1. The relationship of the erythrocyte sedimentation rate to age. (Modified from Hayes, G. S., and Stinson, I. N.: Arch. Ophthalmol. **94:**939, June 1976. Copyright 1976, American Medical Association.)

this rise in normal test values with age indicates that the sedimentation rate in an older patient must exceed 30 mm/hour before it can be considered to be abnormal. At any rate, the test is so nonspecific as to be of no value in diagnosis of uveitis. Its main use in ophthalmology is to enhance the suspicion of temporal arteritis.[7]

Nonspecific inflammatory response

The classification of inflammation as granulomatous or nongranulomatous is supposed to differentiate the presence or absence (respectively) of intraocular organisms. That such etiologic differentiation is unreliable is suggested by the fact that both nongranulomatous and granulomatous inflammation may be produced in rabbits of a series injected intravitreally with 0.1 ml horse serum.[8]

If a significant proportion of uveitis is on an allergic basis, a higher prevalence of other types of allergic disease might reasonably be expected in uveitis patients. Study of 420 uveitis patients and 209 controls revealed no significant difference in the frequency of recognized allergic disorders (for example, hay fever, allergic rhinitis, urticaria, etc.).[9] I seriously doubt that allergy is the cause of endogenous uveitis and prefer to believe in the actual presence of fungi, molds, viruses, protozoa, and the other microorganisms that have often been isolated from human eyes.

For example, the frequency of herpetic keratouveitis is well established. That herpes simplex could cause anterior iritis in the absence of corneal activity is easily imagined.[10]

An attractive explanation for recurrent uveitis proposes that increased uveal vascular permeability is induced by the primary inflammatory agent. This increased vascular permeability is thereafter reactive to many etiologically unrelated insults, which may be immunologic, the presence of living microorganisms, or purely mechanical. Experimental confirmation of this explanation has been termed the Auer reaction, in which vasodilation induced by xylene will result in a severe local reaction to any systemic antigenic challenge. Experimental nonspecific recurrent uveitis can easily be produced in accord with this hypothesis of localized vascular and tissue susceptibility.[11,12] Of course, such a mechanism would also explain the response of the disease to corticosteroid therapy.

SPECIFIC INFECTIOUS AGENTS

Proof that a *Candida albicans* infection of the retina was the cause of a retinochoroiditis was obtained at autopsy.[13] The ocular picture was that of a severe granulomatous uveitis. The organisms were confined to the retina and did not extend into choroid or sclera.

Bilateral posterior uveitis was present in a patient with *Candida* septicemia.[14]

A section of retina obtained from a healthy 10-year-old boy diagnosed as having Coats' disease showed branching fungi; the condition was tentatively identified as mucormycosis. (The eye was removed for painful glaucoma.) The condition originally presented as paramacular retinochoroiditis and ultimately caused total retinal detachment.[15]

Another fungus that has been demonstrated to grow within the retina is *Cryptococcus neoformans*.[16] Although this is usually recognized as part of cryptococcal meningitis, the infection may be localized to the eye.

A case of disseminated coccidioidomycosis with associated chorioretinitis responded to therapy with systemic amphotericin B; however, more than 2 years of treatment was required.[17]

Blastomycotic uveitis has been reported.[18]

A case of "toxoplasmic" retinochoroiditis in a healthy 42-year-old man progressively worsened despite corticosteroid, pyrimethamine, and sulfonamide therapy. On enucleation, the eye was found to contain *Sporotrichum schenkii*.[19]

Cytomegalovirus was recovered from the aqueous humor of a 25-year-old renal transplant patient on immunosuppressive therapy who was suffering from an extensive exudative retinochoroiditis. At autopsy, typical cytomegalic inclusion bodies were found in the retina. Over 90% of the population older than 50 years of age have antibodies to cytomegalovirus, indicating that it is an ubiquitous virus causing inapparent infection until host resistance is severely compromised.[20]

The classic congenital cytomegalovirus syndrome includes prematurity, microcephaly, intracranial calcifications, anemia, hepatosplenomegaly, chorioretinitis, and optic atrophy. The virus may be isolated from urine, saliva, or tears of infected children.[21] Treatment with idoxuridine and adenosine arabinoside did not benefit two patients with chorioretinitis.

Eleven days after exposure to the nasal secretions of cows infected with toxoplasmosis, a 33-year-old man developed acute juxtapapillary retinochoroiditis. During 9 days of prednisone treatment, the lesion steadily increased in size, involving the macula. Pyri-

methamine, sulfa, and prednisone therapy caused the lesion to localize after 16 days and thereafter to gradually resolve, leaving a large central scar. The patient had toxoplasma antibody titers rising from 1:2048 to 1:8192. Several days after exposure he had typical acute toxoplasmosis symptoms of rhinitis, sore throat, macular pains, fatigue, headache, lymphadenitis, and myocarditis (attack simulating angina pectoris). This case[22] illustrates the worsening of acute toxoplasmosis caused by corticosteroid therapy alone. Characteristically, corticosteroid therapy may cause temporary improvement, but progressively more severe relapses follow. Periocular corticosteroid depot injections are particularly apt to cause such an exacerbation.[23]

Granulomatous uveitis, with nodules on ciliary body and iris, is a helpful finding in sarcoid.[24]

Juvenile xanthogranuloma was diagnosed by paracentesis in a 9-year-old child with flare, cells, keratitic precipitates, and iris mass. Topical prednisolone 1% given every 2 hours resulted in rapid quiescence of the inflammation.[25]

The literature continues endlessly with such reports, which prove that active infection with microorganisms, as well as poorly understood inflammatory disorders, may cause uveitis.

Constitutional factors

Human leukocyte antigens have been found to be characteristically associated with certain diseases. For example, HLA-W27 antigen is found in 96% of patients with ankylosing spondylitis, but in only 9% of the general population. W27 antigen is also found in 74% of patients with Reiter's syndrome. The significance of this genetic immunologic response is not yet fully understood, although it is very clear that it is associated with the frequent occurrence of uveitis.[26-28]

Prostaglandin mechanism of inflammation

Prostaglandins may be found in many body tissues and are not unique to seminal vesicle secretions. They cause contraction of smooth muscle, antagonize catecholamines, result in vasodilation, break down the blood-eye barrier, increase intraocular blood flow, and elevate intraocular pressure.[29]

Topical application of prostaglandin E_2 (dinoprostone) (100 μl of 2 mg/ml solution) to the rabbit conjunctiva will cause massive swelling of the ciliary processes, resulting in marked protein leakage into the aqueous humor.[30] This response is already evident at 5 minutes and reaches a maximum within 15 minutes, causing the swollen ciliary processes to become confluent and press against the lens.

Doses of less than 200 μg of various prostaglandins injected into the vitreous caused minimal changes of the retinal vessels, although massive exudative reaction of the anterior chamber resulted.[31] Higher dosage caused fluorescein leakage from the retinal vessels, hemorrhage, vascular occlusion, and retinal detachment.

Prostaglandins may be opposed by drugs such as indomethacin and aspirin. Both indomethacin and aspirin inhibit the synthesis of prostaglandins. For example, following the trauma of cataract surgery, the protein content of the aqueous humor is elevated by an average of 53%. If the patient is pretreated with aspirin, 0.65 g orally every 4 hours for 12 hours just before surgery, the increase of aqueous protein is only 7%.[32] The clinical value of such pretreatment is not established, but might this be useful in operating a case of chronic uveitis?

The effect of daily subconjunctival injection of 15 mg of indomethacin in rabbits was evaluated by studying the response of the eye to intracorneal injection of BCG. Corneal scarring and vascularization, as well as iritis, were significantly reduced by the indomethacin.[33]

The inflammatory reaction subsequent to cryoapplication to the rabbit eye may be substantially reduced by pretreatment with aspirin (0.65 g suppository given to the 1.5 kg animal 1 hour before cryotherapy). The treated animals had obviously less ocular redness and edema. Furthermore, the average protein level in the aqueous humor 45 minutes after cryotherapy was 1.75 g/100 ml in the treated animals and 3.5 g/100 ml in the controls.[34] The practical intent of this work

was to determine whether there was an experimental basis for aspirin treatment of patients before clinical application of cryotherapy.

THERAPY
Anterior uveitis

For practical purposes, the therapy of anterior uveitis consists of cycloplegics and topical corticosteroids. Cycloplegics are useful whenever there is anterior segment inflammation. The most sensitive index of this is the presence of flare or cells as observed by the slit lamp. Redness of the eye, pain, or photophobia also indicate anterior inflammation that will benefit from cycloplegia. Cycloplegics are of no value in the treatment of chorioretinitis with no evidence of aqueous flare or cells. Secondary glaucoma does not prohibit the use of cycloplegics but calls for acetazolamide or, as a last resort, paracentesis. Glaucoma secondary to acute iridocyclitis is caused by angle block by inflammatory deposits, which clear best with cycloplegics. Miotics only make such a problem eye worse.

Severe iridocyclitis requires the use of a long-acting cycloplegic such as 1% atropine three times daily. Supplementary treatment with 10% phenylephrine or 1% cyclopentolate is helpful in breaking resistant synechiae. Initially, more intensive mydriatic instillation should be employed if fresh synechiae are present. Occasional constriction of the pupil may prevent posterior synechiae from forming in the dilated position.

During prolonged use of atropine for iridocyclitis, the possibility of glaucoma should be considered and excluded by periodic pressure estimations. The mechanism of such glaucoma may be the formation of peripheral anterior synechiae or the deposition of inflammatory debris on the relaxed trabecular spaces. In two cases of glaucoma appearing after several months of atropinization of iridocyclitis, the pressure abnormality was promptly controlled by echothiophate, 0.0625%, used once daily.[35] Possibly this complication could be avoided by intermittent use of atropine.

Epinephrine, 1:100, may be used topically in the therapy of glaucoma secondary to uveitis.[36] Presumably it acts by shrinking the volume of the angle structures, reducing further exudation, decreasing the rate of aqueous secretion, and dilating the pupil. Although effective, the use of epinephrine in uveitis has been largely replaced by other synthetic sympathomimetic drugs such as phenylephrine.

Although corticosteroid therapy does *not* cure uveitis, it causes a nonspecific reduction in the severity of inflammation and in the extent of final scarring. Probably the length of a given attack is not shortened by corticosteroids. Iritis and iridocyclitis usually respond well to topical corticosteroids, although severe cases are benefited by the addition of systemic corticosteroid. Frequency of instillation is more essential than the concentration or type of corticosteroid chosen, and hourly medication may be necessary initially. For practical purposes, corticosteroids should be used for both granulomatous and nongranulomatous anterior uveitis. Indeed, sympathetic ophthalmia and Boeck's sarcoid, which are classic examples of granulomatous uveitis, are well recognized to respond better to corticosteroids than to any other therapy. If a specific etiology is suspected, such as tuberculosis, specific drugs such as isoniazid or streptomycin may be employed—in addition to corticosteroids. Because of the recognized difficulty of making a specific diagnosis, it is almost certain that the benefit of the universal use of topical corticosteroids in therapy of anterior uveitis will outweigh the infrequent case that seems to be made worse. Very often an increase in dose will help a patient who seemed unresponsive to corticosteroids. It may be better to start with a high initial level of corticosteroid and taper down when response is obtained than to raise the dose slowly. Duration of therapy is judged by the appearance of the inflammation and should continue for at least several weeks of minimal dosage after all signs of activity have disappeared. Usually a month or more will be required to treat a severe iridocyclitis.

Shotgun antibiotic therapy does not help uveitis. After the discovery of penicillin, as would be expected, this antibiotic was used in the treatment of uveitis. It was soon evident that penicillin did not cure or improve uveitis. In a series of 56 patients having uveitis treated with penicillin the response "appeared to be no greater than would be expected with ordinary forms of treatment such as atropine, heat, and foreign protein."[37,38]

When uveitis is caused by the same organism causing a systemic infection, effective therapy of the general disease can reasonably be expected to cure the uveitis. For example, tetracycline therapy rapidly cured a case of Rocky Mountain spotted fever and its associated anterior uveitis.[39]

Although no medical treatment is necessary for heterochromic cyclitis, its recognition may spare the patient much diagnostic and therapeutic expense and trauma. For example, one such patient underwent extensive skin testing, was diagnosed as having tuberculosis, received streptomycin (a seriously toxic drug) and isoniazid, was desensitized to tuberculin, and suffered the inconvenience of prolonged atropinization.[40] Heterochromic eyes respond well to cataract surgery but are prone to develop destructive glaucoma that is unusually difficult to control.

As would be expected, ophthalmia nodosa, the toxic reaction to embedded caterpillar hairs, responds to appropriate topical corticosteroid and cycloplegic therapy. Prolonged treatment is necessary, often for several months. Relapses occur whenever additional hairs migrate to the interior of the eye.[41]

Behçet's disease (a form of hypopyon iritis associated with aphthous ulcers of mucous membranes and systemic vascular disorders) does not respond favorably to any known form of therapy.[42,43] Symptomatic therapy with topical corticosteroids and atropine is advocated.

Subconjunctival injection of 10 mg of methylprednisolone acetate (Depo-Medrol) did not decrease the severity of uveitis after experimental electric shock in rabbit eyes.[44]

Peripheral uveitis

Recognition of the site of focal activity of uveitis has been greatly aided by the indirect ophthalmoscope. The ability of this instrument to penetrate hazy media enables the ophthalmologist to make a more accurate differential diagnosis and to follow the course of the disease better. Combined with scleral depression, the indirect ophthalmoscope has led to the description of peripheral uveitis. Peripheral uveitis should be suspected in cases showing one or more of the following signs without obvious reason: flare or cells in aqueous or vitreous, peripheral anterior synechiae, vitreous opacities, posterior complicated cataract, macular edema, or retinal detachment without retinal breaks.[45] Confirmation of the diagnosis is by means of indirect ophthalmoscopy with scleral indentation and by contact lens mirror observation of the peripheral fundus.

The presumptive etiologic causes of peripheral uveitis are closely similar to those of posterior uveitis and include tuberculosis (14% of 100 patients), toxoplasmosis (8%), streptococcal infection (11%), assorted other infections, and unknown (61%).[46] Specific treatment of these patients with a presumptive etiologic diagnosis was not notably successful (two of eight "tuberculosis" patients improved; one of six "toxoplasmosis" patients improved). Fourteen of 19 patients with disease of minimal severity responded well to local corticosteroid treatment, and 15 of 32 severe cases were temporarily improved by systemic corticosteroids.

As is well known clinically, the presence of an aqueous flare in an intact inflamed eye suggests the diagnosis of iritis or iridocyclitis. A chorioretinitis without associated cyclitis does not cause aqueous flare unless the inflammation is exceptionally severe. The anatomic basis for this characteristic separation of posterior and anterior inflammations is the relative impermeability of the zonular region of the vitreous body. The dense zonular portion of the vitreous has been demonstrated to be an effective barrier to the passage of small protein molecules.[47] In contrast, even large protein molecules diffuse freely within the main vitreous structure. Peripheral uveitis is so situated as to cause both posterior and anterior inflammatory signs.

A series of 100 cases of peripheral uveitis indicated that this condition may persist for many years with spontaneous exacerbations and remissions and causes progressive damage to the lens, choroid, and retina.[48] Although corticosteroids may be useful during exacerbations to improve vision and minimize tissue damage, long-term corticosteroid therapy did not cure any of these 100 patients. Uveitis surveys proved no specific cause for uveitis in any of these patients.

Although systemic and topical corticosteroid therapy is traditionally advised for peripheral uveitis (pars planitis), even the most enthusiastic advocate of such treatment must admit the response of this disease is less than overwhelming. I doubt that chronic peripheral uveitis is a medical disease. Diathermy destruction of the involved periphery has been reported to give prolonged remissions.[49,50] The involved areas, including the vitreous base, must be completely encompassed by the freeze. Skill in scleral depression is mandatory for the surgeon performing this procedure.

The concept of cryotherapy for peripheral uveitis is deceptively simple. Actually, the precise, adequate, overlapping, complete cryotherapy of these lesions is technically difficult and much more time-consuming than would be expected. Failure to freeze the entire affected area permits persistence of the disease. As might be expected, the eye becomes appreciably more inflamed for some weeks after cryoapplication, but then clears remarkably as a quiet scar replaces the active lesion. Actually, "basal vitreopathy" would more accurately describe this lesion, which consists of a gelatinous deposit in the vitreous base, just internal to the peripheral retina and pars plana. Successful treatment requires that the cryotherapy include the involved areas of vitreous base.

Vigorous cryotherapy of 23 eyes with peripheral uveitis resulted in decreased inflammatory activity in all cases. One third of the treated eyes showed a complete remission during more than a year of followup.[51]

Photocoagulation is not useful in peripheral uveitis because of the technical problems of heating pale lesions in the far periphery, particularly when the vitreous is hazy. Equatorial chorioretinitis may respond to treatment by photocoagulation, diathermy, or cryotherapy. However, the value of such treatment has not been established by controlled studies and may well represent the spontaneous variable course of the disease.

Intravenous injection of *Candida albicans* will reproducibly cause focal disseminated exudative chorioretinitis in rabbits. Laser photocoagulation of such lesions destroyed the infection in small foci. Larger lesions with vitreous reaction could not be successfully treated by photocoagulation. Presumably this is because of the inability to heat such a large pale lesion sufficiently to kill the microorganisms.[52]

Coats' disease is an example of an exudative lesion, usually equatorial or somewhat peripheral, responsive to photocoagulation, diathermy, or cryotherapy.[53] Unfortunately this disease has a tendency to recur.

Posterior uveitis

The treatment of posterior uveitis could be summarized in one word—unsatisfactory.[54] Macular lesions presumably resulting from toxoplasmosis or histoplasmosis do not respond predictably to specific therapy—which is so toxic as to require hesitation before use. Surgical destruction of the lesion is apt to reduce vision abruptly. Systemic or retrobulbar corticosteroid therapy is often given in high dosage and may or may not be of help or hindrance to the patient. Often the macula is already totally destroyed when the patient is first seen. Should there be no hope of restoring central vision, the risk of poisoning the patient with pyrimethamine or corticosteroids is not really justified. Surprisingly often, a patient is treated until Cushing's syndrome develops even though there is no possibility of regaining useful acuity. A comparable regrettable error is prolonged corticosteroid therapy of senile macular degeneration.

Fortunately the inflammation in about 90% of patients with posterior uveitis will spontaneously quiet in about 3 months regardless of therapy.[55]

The possibility of enhancing host resistance by nonspecific stimulation with BCG was explored in rabbits.[56] Suprachoroidal injection of living *Toxoplasma* organisms in normal rabbits resulted in severe retinochoroiditis in two thirds of the animals, as compared with less than one third of the vaccinated animals. The onset of inflammation was within 2 days in the normal animals, but not until 6 days in the treated group.

Although it might be expected that the highly penicillin sensitive *Treponema pallidum* would cause a susceptible ocular inflammation, this is not always the case. More than half of patients with luetic uveitis had relapses after 10 days of therapy with ampicillin, 1.5 g, and probenecid, 0.5 g, every 6 hours orally for 10 days.[57]

Inasmuch as sensitivity to pine pollen has been suggested as a possible etiology of sarcoidosis, the effects of corticosteroid therapy on experimental pine pollen–induced uveitis may bear a relationship to the clinical treatment of sarcoidosis. Intravitreal injection of pine pollen produces granulomatous uveitis in guinea pigs previously sensitized by systemic injections of pine pollen.[58] This reaction is sufficiently severe to cause phthisis within 3 months. Prednisolone, 2 mg/kg/day, was given intramuscularly to these animals, beginning at various times in relationship to the pine pollen injections. When corticosteroid treatment was started before, with, or 3 days after pollen injection, the uveitis was much worse than in untreated animals and resulted in phthisis within 1 month. If prednisolone was not given until 1 or 2 weeks after the pollen, the ocular reaction was less severe than in controls. Increase of prednisolone to 8 mg/kg/day begun simultaneously with sensitization also caused worsening of the inflammation. Since about 90 guinea pigs were used in this study, the results seem reasonably substantiated. There is no obvious explanation of the variable effects of prednisolone. Unfortunately this study does not answer the question of corticosteroid treatment of sarcoid uveitis.

Homoimmune uveitis may be produced in the guinea pig by repeated intramuscular injection of uveal tissue and Freund's adjuvant.

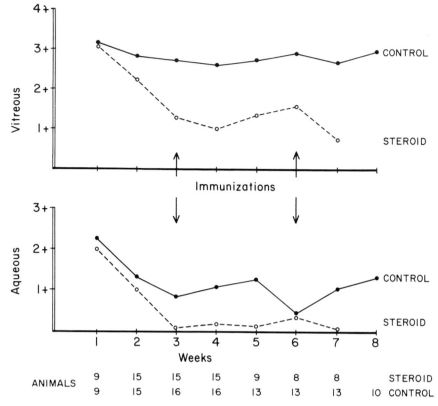

Fig. 38-2. Response of homoimmune uveitis to hydrocortisone. (Modified from Aronson, S. B., Hogan, M. J., and Zweigart, P.: Arch. Ophthalmol. **69:**379, 1963.)

This type of uveitis is greatly benefited by corticosteroid therapy. Fig. 38-2 compares the vitreous and aqueous inflammatory changes in control animals and in those treated with daily subcutaneous injection of 24 mg of hydrocortisone.[59]

It is not at all certain that the results of such an experiment can be cited in support of corticosteroid therapy of human endogenous uveitis, which I think is more likely to be caused by local infection than by autoallergy; however, this experimental model may resemble sympathetic uveitis.

Should the diagnosis of amebic chorioretinitis be considered sufficiently established to warrant specific therapy, systemic treatment is advised. Diiodohydroxyquin, 650 mg three times a day, is given for 20 days, together with chloroquine, 0.5 g at bedtime.

After a 1-week rest period, carbarsone, 250 mg three times a day, and chloroquine, 0.5 g at bedtime, are given for 10 days. If infection persists, the entire routine is repeated after a month's rest interval.

Such treatment was given to five patients diagnosed as having macular amebic chorioretinitis on the appearance of a large cystic macular lesion surrounded by many small hard exudates, increased eosinophil count, presence of *Entamoeba histolytica* in the purged stool, and positive serum hemaglutination test.[60] Within several months after therapy was started, three of the five patients regained considerable vision, improving to 20/30, 20/30, and 20/50. Systemic corticosteroids were given to three of these patients, following which their chorioretinitis became definitely worse. This is in agreement with previous observations that corticosteroid treatment was detrimental to amebic chorioretinitis.[61]

Unfortunately we cannot know with certainty that these cases were of amebic etiology or that their course was favorably altered by specific therapy.

Lens-induced uveitis

Lens-induced uveitis, at least in a mild form, is apparently not uncommon after extracapsular cataract extraction with retained cortex. Of 64 patients suffering such extracapsular extraction, 43% developed a postoperative inflammation considered to represent lens-induced uveitis.[62] Serologic study of these 28 patients with presumed lens-induced uveitis demonstrated specific antilens antibodies in 13, or approximately one half. These antibodies had *not* been present in the serum obtained at the time of operation; therefore they presumably were proved to result from the retained cortex. The large mutton-fat keratitic precipitates of severe lens-induced uveitis may be mistaken for sympathetic ophthalmia.

Medical therapy of lens-induced uveitis is fairly effective, whether this occurs after extracapsular extraction or as a spontaneous complication of a hypermature cataract. Topical corticosteroid therapy combined with adequate cycloplegia will control lens-induced uveitis while the cortical material is absorbed. Prolonged treatment (months) will be necessary if much lens tissue is retained (in which case the possibility of surgical evacuation should be evaluated). Such medical treatment of acute phacolytic glaucoma will permit temporary postponement of surgery until the eye is less inflamed and will allow scheduling of the surgery at a convenient time rather than as an emergency. Presumably, the mechanism of action of corticosteroid therapy includes suppression of the formation of the antilens antibodies.

A phacoanaphylactic reaction is commonly present in eyes lost from sympathetic ophthalmia.[63] In addition to the usual medical therapy for sympathetic ophthalmia, no doubt these eyes should be watched closely for the possible development of lens-induced inflammation and cataract extraction performed as indicated.

Sympathetic ophthalmia

The management of sympathetic ophthalmia is essentially identical to that of any other severe chronic uveitis.[64] Sympathetic ophthalmia characteristically tends to have recurrences when therapy is discontinued, and it is therefore necessary to follow such cases closely for at least a year. Systemic and topical corticosteroids and cycloplegics must be used in sufficient amount to suppress evidence of active inflammation and thereby prevent permanent intraocular scarring. Prescription of bifocals for use during this prolonged period of atropinization may permit the patient (often a relatively young, one-eyed individual) to read and to continue employment. Although some physicians forbid the use of the eyes during active uveitis, I have never believed that use of the properly treated eye causes any adverse effects or that restriction of physical activity is beneficial.

Ophthalmologists are generally aware that enucleation of a hopelessly injured eye within 2 weeks will prevent development of sympathetic ophthalmia. Another commonly recognized fact is that the loss of accommodation is an early manifestation of sympathetic disease. For this reason, measurement of the near point of accommodation is an important part of the routine evaluation at each visit following a penetrating eye injury. Careful biomicroscopy is also necessary, since the appearance of flare or cells can be recognized in the earliest stages of inflammation. To be most effective, therapy must be started early, before irreversible scarring occurs.

It is not generally realized that approximately half of the persons having sympathetic ophthalmia retain useful vision even without corticosteroid therapy. Although reported cases are not numerous, corticosteroid treatment seems to increase the prognosis to about 75% retention of useful vision. Another pertinent fact is that enucleation of the exciting eye once sympathetic ophthalmia has developed does *not* improve the prognosis for the sympathizing eye. Clearly, therefore, if the injured eye has any prospect of useful vision, it should *not* be enucleated when the diagnosis of sympathetic disease is made.

Antibiotics do not alter the course of sympathetic ophthalmia.

Immunosuppressive agents

Unusually severe uveitis possibly of immunogenic origin, such as sympathetic ophthalmia, will respond to immunosuppressive therapy. Since this is inherently dangerous treatment, it should be reserved for serious inflammations.

The severe allergic uveitis caused by injection of extract of retina and choroid emulsified in Freund's adjuvant can be completely blocked by methotrexate therapy in guinea pigs.[65] The potential toxicity of the drug is indicated by the death of three of 10 treated animals.

Behçet's uveitis typically causes blindness within 3 years, on the average. In 14 patients treated with chlorambucil for up to 2 years, visual acuity was maintained or improved in all cases.[66]

Chlorambucil was used to treat 31 patients with intractable, corticosteroid-resistant uveitis.[67] Sustained decrease of inflammatory activity followed therapy in four of five patients with Behçet's syndrome, in three of five patients with sympathetic ophthalmia, in two patients with chronic cyclitis, and in one patient with rheumatoid sclerouveitis. Ten of the 31 patients responded to chlorambucil. No improvement occurred in the other 21 patients, who suffered from chronic iridocyclitis, chorioretinitis, retinal vasculitis, and Eales' disease. The initial dose of chlorambucil was 2 mg/day, gradually increased each week by 2 mg, to a usual maximum of 12 mg/day. The dosage level was titrated to the clinical response, being raised or lowered as indicated by exacerbation or improvement of the disease. Weekly platelet count and white count were used to monitor toxicity.

REFERENCES

1. Darrell, R. W., Wagener, H. P., and Kurland, L. T.: Epidemiology of uveitis, Arch. Ophthalmol. **68:**502, 1962.
2. Saari, M., Miettinen, R., and Alanko, H.: Uveitis: report of a 10-year survey in northern Finland, Can. J. Ophthalmol. **10:**356, 1975.
3. Woods, A. C., and Abrahams, I. W.: Uveitis survey, Am. J. Ophthalmol. **51:**761, 1961.
4. Woods, A. C.: Endogenous uveitis, Baltimore, 1956, The Williams & Wilkins Co.
5. Whitfield, R., and Wirostko, E.: Uveitis and intraocular treponemes, Arch. Ophthalmol. **84:**12, 1970.
6. Schlaegel, T. F., Jr.: The value of routine testing in the etiologic diagnosis of uveitis, Am. J. Ophthalmol. **60:**648, 1965.
7. Hayes, G. S., and Stinson, I. N.: Erythrocyte sedimentation rate and age, Arch. Ophthalmol. **94:**939, June 1976.
8. Larsen, G.: Experimental uveitis, Acta Ophthalmol. **39:**231, 1961.
9. Leira, H.: Studies on causal relations in endogenous, nonpurulent, ocular inflammations, Acta Ophthalmol. **85**(suppl.):1, 1965.
10. Sugar, H. S.: Herpetic keratouveitis, Ann. Ophthalmol. **3:**355, 1971.
11. Gamble, C. N., Aronson, S. B., and Brescia, F. B.: Experimental uveitis. I. The production of recurrent immunologic (Auer) uveitis and its relationship to increased uveal vascular permeability, Arch. Ophthalmol. **84:**321, 1970.
12. Gamble, C. N., Aronson, S. B., and Brescia, F. B.: Experimental uveitis. II. The pathogenesis of recurrent immunologic (Auer) uveitis, Arch. Ophthalmol. **84:**331, 1970.
13. McLean, J. M.: Oculomycosis, Trans. Am. Acad. Ophthalmol. Otolaryngol. **67:**149, 1963.
14. Bonatti, W. D., Jaeger, E. A., and Frayer, W. C.: Endogenous fungal endophthalmitis, Arch. Ophthalmol. **70:**772, 1963.
15. Wadsworth, J. A. C.: Ocular mucormycosis, Am. J. Ophthalmol. **34:**405, 1951.
16. Okun, E., and Butler, W. T.: Ophthalmologic complications of cryptococcal meningitis, Arch. Ophthalmol. **71:**52, 1964.
17. Green, W. R., and Bennett, J. E.: Coccidioidomycosis—report of a case with clinical evidence of ocular involvement, Arch. Ophthalmol. **77:**337, 1967.
18. Cassady, J. V.: Uveal blastomycosis, Arch. Ophthalmol. **35:**84, 1946.

19. Font, R. L., and Jakobiec, F. A.: Granulomatous necrotizing retinochoroiditis, Arch. Ophthalmol. **94**:1513, September 1976.

20. Chumbley, L. C., Robertson, D. M., Smith, T. F., and Campbell, R. J.: Adult cytomegalovirus including retino-uveitis, Am. J. Ophthalmol. **80**:807, November 1975.

21. Cox, F., Meyer, D., and Hughes, W. T.: Cytomegalovirus in tears from patients with normal eyes and with acute cytomegalovirus chorioretinitis, Am. J. Ophthalmol. **80**:817, November 1975.

22. Saari, M., Vuorre, I., Neiminen, H., and Raisanen, S.: Acquired toxoplasmic chorioretinitis, Arch. Ophthalmol. **94**:1485, September 1976.

23. Nozik, R. A.: 'Steroids only' may not be best toxoplasmosis therapy, J.A.M.A. **236**:2378, November 22, 1976.

24. Mizuno, K., and Watanabe, T.: Sarcoid granulomatous cyclitis, Am. J. Ophthalmol. **81**:82, January 1976.

25. Schwartz, L. W., Rodrigues, M. M., and Hallett, J. W.: Juvenile xanthogranuloma diagnosed by paracentesis, Am. J. Ophthalmol. **77**:243, February 1974.

26. Mills, D. M., Arai, Y., and Gupta, R. C.: HL-A antigens and sacroiliitis, J.A.M.A. **231**:268, January 20, 1975.

27. Danilevicius, Z.: HL-A system and rheumatic diseases, J.A.M.A. **231**:283, January 20, 1975.

28. Henlry, W. L., and Leopold, I. H.: The importance of HL-A antigens in ophthalmology, Am. J. Ophthalmol. **80**:774, October 1975.

29. Ernest, J. T.: Prostaglandins—a missing link? Am. J. Ophthalmol. **74**:992, November 1972.

30. Laties, A. M., Neufeld, A. H., Vegge, T., and Sears, M. L.: Differential reactivity of rabbit iris and ciliary process to topically applied prostaglandin E$_2$ (dinoprostone), Arch. Ophthalmol. **94**:1966, November 1976.

31. Peyman, G. A., Bennett, T. O., and Vlchek, J.: Effects of intravitreal prostaglandins on retinal vasculature, Ann. Ophthalmol. **7**:279, February 1975.

32. Zimmerman, T. J., Gravenstein, N., Sugar, A., and Kaufman, H. E.: Aspirin stabilization of the blood-aqueous barrier in the human eye, Am. J. Ophthalmol. **79**:817, May 1975.

33. Belfort, R., Jr., Smolin, G., Hall, J. M., and Okumoto, M.: Indomethacin and the corneal immune response, Am. J. Ophthalmol. **81**:650, May 1976.

34. Chavis, R. M., Vygantas, C. M., and Vygantas, A.: Experimental inhibition of prostaglandin-like inflammatory response after cryotherapy, Am. J. Ophthalmol. **82**:310, August 1976.

35. Gorin, G.: Glaucoma induced by prolonged use of atropine, Am. J. Ophthalmol. **56**:639, 1963.

36. Barkan, O., and Maisler, S.: Adrenalin chloride 1:100 in ophthalmology, Am. J. Ophthalmol. **20**:504, 1937.

37. Irvine, S. R., Maury, F., Schultz, J., Thygeson, P., and Unsworth, A.: The treatment of nonspecific uveitis with penicillin, Am. J. Ophthalmol. **28**:852, 1945.

38. Yasuma, E. R.: Danger of penicillin therapy in active uveitis, Arch. Ophthalmol. **37**:598, 1947.

39. Cherubini, T. D., and Spaeth, G. L.: Anterior nongranulomatous uveitis associated with Rocky Mountain spotted fever, Arch. Ophthalmol. **81**:363, 1969.

40. Makley, T. A., Jr.: Heterochromic cyclitis in identical twins, Am. J. Ophthalmol. **41**:768, 1956.

41. Watson, P. G., and Sevel, D.: Ophthalmia nodosa, Br. J. Ophthalmol. **50**:209, 1966.

42. Winter, F. C., and Yokins, R. E.: The ocular pathology of Behçet's disease, Am. J. Ophthalmol. **62**:257, 1966.

43. Mamo, J. G., and Baghdassarian, A.: Behçet's disease, Arch. Ophthalmol. **71**:4, 1964.

44. Long, J. C.: Electric cataract, Am. J. Ophthalmol. **56**:108, 1963.

45. Brockhurst, R. J., Schepens, C. L., and Okamura, I. D.: Uveitis, Am. J. Ophthalmol. **49**:1257, 1960.

46. Brockhurst, R. J., Schepens, C. L., and Okamura, I. D.: Peripheral uveitis, Am. J. Ophthalmol. **51**:19, 1961.

47. Suran, A. A., and McEwen, W. K.: Diffusion studies with ox vitreous body, Am. J. Ophthalmol. **51**:814, 1961.

48. Hogan, M., and Kimura, S.: Cyclitis and peripheral chorioretinitis, Arch. Ophthalmol. **66**:667, 1961.

49. Gitter, K. A., Slusher, M., and Justice, J., Jr.: Traumatic hemorrhagic detachment of retinal pigment epithelium, Arch. Ophthalmol. **79**:729, 1968.

50. Gills, J. P., Jr.: Combined medical and surgical therapy for complicated cases of peripheral uveitis, Arch. Ophthalmol. **79**:723, 1968.

51. Aaberg, T. M., Cesarz, T. J., and Flickinger, R. R.: Treatment of peripheral uveoretinitis

by cryotherapy, Am. J. Ophthalmol. **75:**685, 1973.

52. Santos, R., de Buen, S., and Juarez, P.: Experimental Candida albicans chorioretinitis treated by laser, Am. J. Ophthalmol. **63:**440, 1967.

53. Morales, A. G.: Coats' disease, Am. J. Ophthalmol. **60:**855, 1965.

54. Leopold, I. H.: Drug therapy in uveitis, Am. J. Ophthalmol. **56:**709, 1963.

55. Kaufman, H.: Uveitis, Am. J. Ophthalmol. **55:**1073, 1963.

56. Tabbara, K. F., O'Connor, G. R., and Nozik, R. A.: Effect of immunization with attenuated *Mycobacterium bovis* on experimental toxoplasmic retinochoroiditis, Am. J. Ophthalmol. **79:**641, April 1975.

57. Goldman, J. N.: Clinical experience with ampicillin and probenecid in the management of treponeme-associated uveitis, Trans. Am. Acad. Ophthalmol. Otolaryngol. **74:**509, May 1970.

58. Coleman, S. L., and Canaan, S.: The effects of cortisone on pine pollen-induced uveitis in guinea pigs, Invest. Ophthalmol. **1:**751, 1962.

59. Aronson, S. B., Hogan, M. J., and Zweigart, P.: Homoimmune uveitis in the guinea pig, Arch. Ophthalmol. **69:**379, 1963.

60. King, R. E., Praeger, D. L., and Hallett, J. W.: Amebic choroidosis, Arch. Ophthalmol. **72:**16, 1964.

61. Braley, A. E., and Hamilton, H. E.: Central serous choroidosis associated with amebiasis, Arch. Ophthalmol. **58:**1, 1957.

62. Wirostko, E., and Spalter, H. F.: Lens-induced uveitis, Arch. Ophthalmol. **78:**1, 1967.

63. Allen, J. C.: Sympathetic uveitis and phacoanaphylaxis, Am. J. Ophthalmol. **63:**280, 1967.

64. Makley, T. A., and Leibold, J. E.: Modern therapy of sympathetic ophthalmia, Arch. Ophthalmol. **64:**809, 1960.

65. McMaster, P. R. B., Wong, V. G., Owens, J. D., and Kyriakos, M.: Prevention of experimental allergic uveitis, Arch. Ophthalmol. **93:**835, September 1975.

66. Mamo, J.: Treatment of Behçet's disease with chlorambucil, Arch. Ophthalmol. **94:**580, April 1976.

67. Godfrey, W. A., Epstein, W. V., O'Connor, G. R., Kimura, S. J., Hogan, M. J., and Nozik, R. A.: The use of chlorambucil in intractable idiopathic uveitis, Am. J. Ophthalmol. **78:**415, September 1974.

INDEX

Foreign body
fluorescein in detection of, 415
intraocular, use of corticosteroids for, 378
nonmagnetic, use of cyanoacrylate adhesives in extraction of, 44-45
Formyl tetrahydropteroylglutamic acid, 166
Fuchs' heterochromic cyclitis, 377
Fundus photography, fluorescein in, 419-420
Fungal infections; *see* Infections, fungal
Fungal endophthalmitis, 33
Fungizone; *see* Amphotericin B
Fungus endophthalmitis, treatment of, 551
Furacin; *see* Nitrofurazone
Furacin soluble dressing, 141
Furaltadone, 141
Furmethide; *see* Furtrethonium
Furtrethonium, 287
Fusarium
pimaricin treatment of, 653
thiabendazole treatment of, 656
Fusarium solanae as cause of fungal infections, 659, 660
Fusarium solani, pimaricin treatment of, 158
Fusidium terricola, amphotericin B treatment of, 125

G

Galactokinase deficiency, 529
Galactose cataract, prevention of, 528-529
Gamma globulin, 333-334
in treatment of herpes simplex, 679
Gas gangrene antitoxin, 339
Gas gangrene panophthalmitis, 339
Generic inequivalence of drugs, 7-8
Gentamicin, 137-138
Gentian violet, 426
Germicides, 214-215, 425-437
chemical, summary of characteristics of, 426
metallic, 432-435
rate of destruction of bacteria by, 425
surface-active, 427-431
ultraviolet light as, 435-436
Gibberella fujkuroi, amphotericin B treatment of, 125
Glaucoma
absolute, urea in treatment of, 448, 449
acetazolamide in long- and short-term control of, 483
acute
phenylephrine in, 240
and pilocarpine, 282-283
air pupillary block, 448
alpha-chymotrypsin–induced, 540
angle-closure, 628-629
and atropine, 249
and betamethasone, 393
and carbachol, 266
chronic simple, 280-282, 482, 551
closed-angle, and echothiophate, 305-306
congenital, 627-628
corticosteroid-induced, 387-394, 551
and demecarium, 313-314
dexamethasone, 388, 389-390, 391
effect of phenylephrine on, 607
and epinephrine, 226-231
with episcleritis, 626
following interstitial keratitis, 626-627
infantile, 627-628
and isoflurophate, 295-297

Glaucoma—cont'd
"low pressure," 618-619
malignant, 630-631
medications for, 575-576
narrow-angle, 619-622
open-angle, 598-635
diagnosis of, 601-608
and echothiophate, 303-305
general recommendations for, 611-613
gonioscopy and, 608
ophthalmoscopy and, 605-608
perimetry in, 604-605
relationship between, and retinal detachment, 392
therapy of, 608-618
tonography in, 603-604
tonometry in, 601-603
visual field and, 604, 605
phacolytic, 630
postcontusion, 623-624
postoperative, and cataract, 551-552
pralidoxime prophylaxis of, 316
primary acute, urea treatment of, 445-446
prognosis of, 615-617
requiring surgery, 628-631
response of, to ethanol intake, 409-410
response of, to hyaluronidase, 85
secondary, 622-627
to hyphema, urea treatment of, 446
to inflammation, urea treatment of, 446
to traumatic hyphema, 714-716
surgery for, epinephrine toxicity during, 232-233
transient open-angle deep chamber, 551
visual field in, 282
and zonulysis, 58-62
Glaucomatocyclitic crisis, 624-626
Glaucon, 226; *see also* Hydrochloride
Globulin
gamma, 333-334, 679
human immune, 333-335
human tetanus immune, 337
measles (rubella) immune, 334
vaccinia immune serum, 334-335
Glucocorticoids, 393
Glues, synthetic surgical, 39-45
Glutethimide, diplopia resulting from, 291
Glycerin; *see* Glycerol
Glycerol, 451, 453-459, 537
and lens dehydration, 459
in management of acute glaucoma, 621
mechanism of action of, 455-456
and sodium ascorbate, 459
toxicity of, 456-459
use of, in corneal clearing, 459
Glycosides, digitalis, 491-493
Gonioscopy and primary open-angle glaucoma, 608
Gonorrhea, 647
Gonorrheal ophthalmia, 434
Gonorrheal ophthalmia neonatorum, 648
Granulomatosis, Wegener's, 202, 578
Granulomatous conjunctivitis, subacute nodular, 125
Griffin lens, 26-27
Guanethidine, 242, 317

H

Haemophilus
chloramphenicol treatment of, 130
penicillin treatment of, 145

Phenylephrine—cont'd
  in test for sickle cell anemia, 241
  use of, for mydriasis, 236-240
Phenylephrine mydriasis, 237
Phenylephrine pack, 237
Phialophora verrucosa, thiabendazole treatment of, 193-194
pHisoHex, 9, 430-431
Phlyctenular keratoconjunctivitis, 650
Phoria, effect of, on AC/A ratio, 587
Pholine; *see* Echothiophate
Phosphorus, radioactive, 470-472
Photocoagulation in treatment of toxoplasmosis, 670-671
Photodynamic inactivation in treatment of herpes simplex, 679
Photography, fundus, fluorescein in, 419-420
Phthiriasis palpebrarum, 663
Physostigmine, 287-290
  adult dose of, 253
  as antidote for anticholinergic toxicity, 253, 289-290
  clinical use of, 298-290
  pharmacology of, 287-289
  toxicity of, 290
Physostigmine ointment, 289
Physostigmine salicylate, 289-290
Pigment, effect of pilocarpine on, 277
Pilocarpine, 267-287, 541
  and accommodation, 285-286
  accommodative spasm resulting from, 29
  and acute glaucoma, 282-283
  allergy to, 287
  and anterior chamber, 275
  and aqueous veins, 278-279
  and blood-aqueous barrier, 279-280
  after cataract extraction, 286
  and chronic simple glaucoma, 280-282
  and ciliary body, 273-275
  clinical use of, 280-286
  commercial preparations of, 280
  and conjunctival vessels, 278-279
  and contact lenses, 27
  to counteract mydriasis, 283-285
  in diagnosis of Adie's pupil, 286
  in differential diagnosis of dilated pupil, 286
  and eserine, 270, 271
  facility of outflow of, 275-276
  and hyphema, 286
  inactivation of, 272-273
  and intraocular muscles, 269-272
  and intraocular pressure, 276-277
  and iris, 273-275
  and isoflurophate, 270
  and lens, 275
  molecular weight of, 27
  ocular penetration of, 268-269
  ocular responses of, 273-280
  pharmacology of, 267-268
  and phenylephrine, 240
  pigment effect of, 277
  rate of release of, from Ocusert, 27, 28
  secretory inhibition of, 277-278
  stability of, 280
  toxicity of, 286-287
  and trabeculum, 273-275
  in treatment of glaucoma secondary to traumatic hyphema, 714
Pilocarpine miosis, 272

Pimaricin, 158-159
  clinical use of, 158
  experimental combined therapy of, 158-159
  in treatment of fungal infections, 653
Pityrosporum ovale, 557
Placebo effect, 9-13
Plasma-lyte 148, 538, 539
Poisoning; *see also* Toxicity
  by aniline dyes, fluorescein as antidote to, 420-421
  anticholinergic, physostigmine as antidote for, 253
  ethylene glycol, use of ethanol in, 409
  methanol, 406-409
  parasympatholytic, 249
  quinine, 469
  scopolamine, 253
Poly I:C; *see* Polyinosinic-polycytidilic acid
Polyinosinic-polycytidilic acid, 690
Polymer derivatives, 508
Polymerized cyanoacrylate, acetone as solvent for, 42-43
Polymyxin B, 159-160
  and colistin, 135
  ocular penetration of, 159
  ocular tolerance of, 159
  use of, in treatment of corneal ulcers, 159-160
Polyphloretin phosphate, 626
Polyvinyl alcohol, 507
Pontocaine; *see* Tetracaine
Postcontusion glaucoma, 623-624
Posterior uveitis, 737-739
Postoperative edema of posterior pole and cataract, 552
Postoperative glaucoma and cataract, 551-552
Postoperative hyphema, 542-544
Postoperative infection and cataract, 549-551
Postoperative miotic iritis and cataract, 548-549
Postoperative shallow chamber, 544-548
Post's solution #4, 431
Potassium iodide in treatment of fungal infections, 656
Potassium penicillin G, 144
Potassium phenethicillin, 145
Povidone, 417-418
Povidone-iodine, 431
Pralidoxime, 314-317
  administration of, 315
  as antidote for systemic anticholinesterase poisoning, 316
  clinical use of, 316-317
  for improved mydriasis, 316-317
  mechanism of action of, 314-315
  neutralization of ocular anticholinesterase effects by, 316
  pharmacology of, 314-315
  prophylaxis of, during glaucoma therapy, 316
  stability of, 316
  toxicity of, 317
Preanesthetic preparation, 92-98
Pred Mild Suspension, 364
Prednisolone, 349, 362-364
Prednisone, 349, 359
  intraocular penetration of, 362-364
  molecular weight of, 27
Premarin, 705
Premedications, 92-98
Preoperative sedation and cataract, 534-535
Presbyopia and echothiophate, 306
Prescriptions of drugs, 522-523
Preservative, 427-429, 431
Pressor amines, 96